Pathy's Principles and Practice of Geriatric Medicine

FIFTH EDITION

Volume 2

To my mother, Ivy, and father, Radovan, for giving me the opportunity.

–Alan J. Sinclair

To all my older friends and patients who have taught me geriatrics, to my wife Pat and my children Robert, Susan and Jacqueline who have supported me throughout my career, and to my grandchildren Amanda, Conor, Katelyn, Nicole, Paige and John who are my eternal joy and hope for my future of elder care.

–John E. Morley

To all the teams working at the Gérontopôle, to my father Professor Pierre Vellas who created the Universities of the Third Age, and to Professor J.L. Albarede, our mentor.

–Bruno Vellas

Pathy's Principles and Practice of Geriatric Medicine

Edited by

Alan J. Sinclair
Dean and Professor of Medicine
Bedfordshire & Hertfordshire Postgraduate Medical School
University of Bedfordshire, Luton, UK

John E. Morley
Dammert Professor of Gerontology
Director, Division of Geriatric Medicine and Director, Endocrinology
Saint Louis University Medical Center
St Louis, MO, USA

Bruno Vellas
Professor of Medicine
Clinic of Internal Medicine and Gerontology
Gérontopôle, Toulouse University Hospital
Toulouse, France

FIFTH EDITION

Volume 2

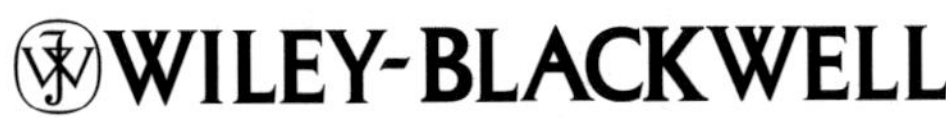

A John Wiley & Sons, Ltd., Publication

Wiley-Blackwell is an imprint of John Wiley & Sons, formed by the merger of Wiley's global Scientific, Technical and Medical business with Blackwell Publishing.

Registered office: John Wiley & Sons, Ltd, The Atrium, Southern Gate, Chichester, West Sussex, PO19 8SQ, UK

Editorial offices: 9600 Garsington Road, Oxford, OX4 2DQ, UK
The Atrium, Southern Gate, Chichester, West Sussex, PO19 8SQ, UK
111 River Street, Hoboken, NJ 07030-5774, USA

For details of our global editorial offices, for customer services and for information about how to apply for permission to reuse the copyright material in this book please see our website at www.wiley.com/wiley-blackwell

Library of Congress Cataloging-in-Publication Data
Pathy's principles and practice of geriatric medicine / edited by Alan J. Sinclair, John E. Morley, Bruno Vellas.–5th ed.
p. ; cm.
Principles and practice of geriatric medicine
Rev. ed. of: Principles and practice of geriatric medicine. 4th ed. c2006.
Includes bibliographical references and index.
ISBN 978-0-470-68393-4 (cloth)
I. Sinclair, Alan (Alan J.) II. Morley, John E. III. Vellas, B. J. (Bruno J.) IV. Pathy, M. S. J. V. Principles and practice of geriatric medicine. VI. Title: Principles and practice of geriatric medicine.
[DNLM: 1. Geriatrics–methods. WT 100]
LC classification not assigned
618.97–dc23

2011032652

A catalogue record for this book is available from the British Library.

Wiley also publishes its books in a variety of electronic formats. Some content that appears in print may not be available in electronic books.

Typeset in 9/12pt Palatino by Laserwords Private Limited, Chennai, India
Printed and bound in Singapore by Markono Print Media Pte Ltd

First Impression 2012

Cover design: image of coronal sections of brain at the level of the hippocampus, courtesy of Dr Jim Galvin

Contents of Volume 1

A colour plate section is to be found in Volume 2, between pages 1414 and 1415

Contents of Volume 2

A colour plate section is to be found in Volume 2, between pages 1414 and 1415

About the Editors

Alan Sinclair

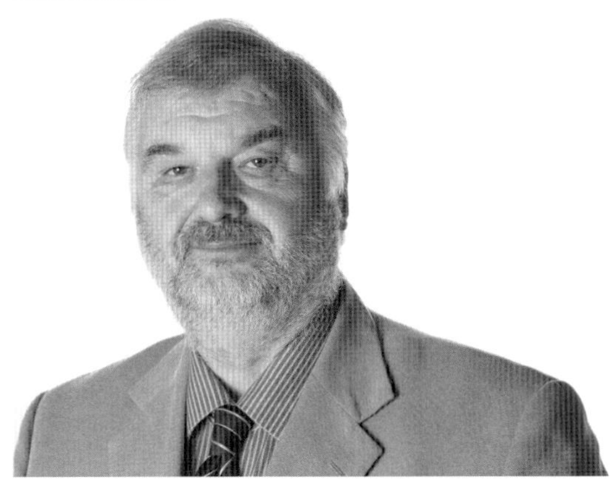

Alan Sinclair is Dean and Professor of Medicine at the Bedfordshire & Hertfordshire Postgraduate Medical School at the University of Bedfordshire, UK. He was a founding member and Academic Director of the European Union Geriatric Medicine Society (EUGMS) and previously Charles Hayward Professor of Geriatric Medicine at the University of Birmingham, UK. His principle research interests are in the areas of diabetes, older people, nutrition and frailty. He is the recipient of both national and international research awards. Alan recently established the Institute of Diabetes for Older People (IDOP), which is the first institute of its kind to be solely dedicated to the enhancement of quality diabetes care in older people.

John Morley

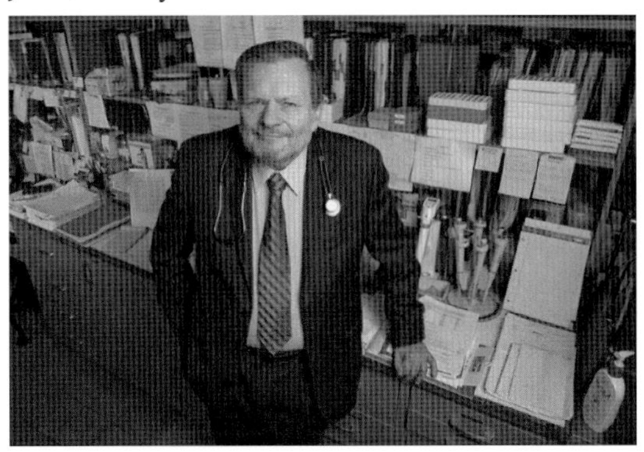

John Morley is the Dammert Professor of Gerontology, Director, Division of Geriatric Medicine and Director, Endocrinology at Saint Louis University Medical Center. Dr Morley is the Editor-in-Chief of the *Journal of the American Medical Directors Association.*

Bruno Vellas

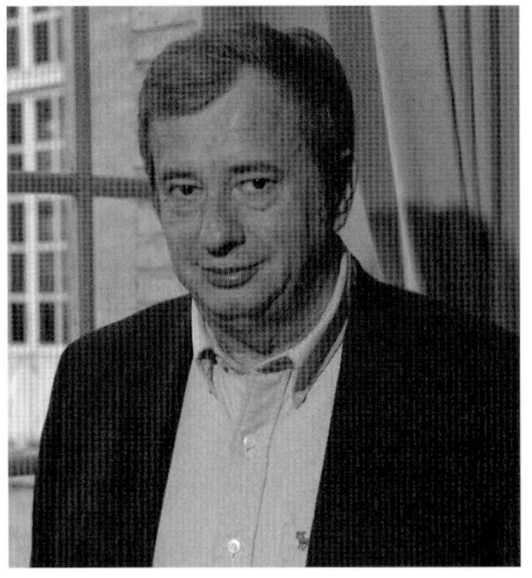

Bruno Vellas is Professor of Internal Medicine and Geriatrics, Chair of the Gérontopôle in Toulouse, France, including the Alzheimer's Disease Research and Clinical Centre. Professor Vellas is President of the IAGG (International Association of Gerontology and Geriatrics) and Editor-in-Chief of the *Journal of Nutrition, Health and Aging.*

List of Contributors

Ahmed H. Abdelhafiz
Rotherham General Hospital, Rotherham, Yorkshire, UK

Mohammed T. Abou-Saleh
St George's, University of London, London, UK

Charlotte Ågrup
University College of London Hospitals NHS Trust and University College London, London, UK

Avan Aihie Sayer
Southampton General Hospital, University of Southampton, Southampton, UK

Stewart G. Albert
Saint Louis University School of Medicine, St Louis, MO, USA

Suraj Alakkassery
Saint Louis University Medical Center, St Louis, MO, USA

Cristina Alonso Bouzón
Hospital Universitario de Getafe, Madrid, Spain

Sandrine Andrieu
University of Toulouse III, INSERM Unit 1027, Toulouse, France

Jean-Pierre Aquino
Clinique Médicale de la Porte Verte, Versailles, France

Hiroyuki Arai
Institute of Development, Aging and Cancer, Tohoku University, Sendai, Japan

H. James Armbrecht
St Louis Veterans' Affairs Medical Center and Saint Louis University School of Medicine, St Louis, MO, USA

Wilbert S. Aronow
New York Medical College, Valhalla, NY, USA

Jaffer Babaa
University of South Florida, pre-medical student, Tampa, FL, USA

Marco Baccini
University of Florence and Azienda Ospedaliero – Universitaria Careggi, Florence, Italy

Abhay Bajpai
St George's, University of London, London, UK

Laurent Balardy
Gérontopôle, CHU Toulouse, Toulouse, France

Mario Barbagallo
University of Palermo, Palermo, Italy

Karen F. Barney
Saint Louis University, St Louis, MO, USA

Bedanta P. Baruah
Cardiff University, Cardiff, Wales, UK

Nazem Bassil
Saint Louis University Medical Center, St Louis, MO, USA

Antony Bayer
Cardiff University, Cardiff and University Hospital Llandough, Penarth, UK

Joël Belmin
Groupe Hospitalier Pitié-Salpétrière-Charles Foix and Université Pierre et Marie Curie (Paris 6), Ivry-sur-Seine, France

Mario Belvedere
University of Palermo, Palermo, Italy

Susan Mary Benbow
Staffordshire University, Stafford, Staffordshire and Older Mind Matters Ltd, Manchester, UK

Rachelle E. Bernacki
Brigham and Women's Hospital, Boston, MA, USA

Chantal Bernard-Marty
Institut Claudius Regaud, Toulouse, France

Kimberly C. Berni
University of Missouri, Columbia, MO, USA

Peter McL. Black
Harvard Medical School, Boston, MA, USA

François Blanchard
Hôpital Maison Blanche, Reims, France

Michael Blank
Firelands Regional Medical Center, Sandusky, OH, USA

Dan G. Blazer
Duke University Medical Center, Durham, NC, USA

Martin M. Brown
Institute of Neurology, University College London, London, UK

Rhona Buckingham
Royal College of Physicians, London, UK

A. John Camm
St George's, University of London, London, UK

Elizabeth A. Capezuti
New York University, New York, NY, USA

Gideon A. Caplan
Prince of Wales Hospital, Sydney, Australia

David Carr
The Rehabilitation Institute of St Louis, St Louis, MO, USA

Marta Castro Rodríguez
Hospital Universitario de Getafe, Madrid, Spain

Pierre Celsis
INSERM Unit 825, Toulouse, France

Oscar A. Cepeda
Saint Louis University School of Medicine and St Louis Veterans' Affairs Medical Center, St Louis, MO, USA

Ian M. Chapman
University of Adelaide, Royal Adelaide Hospital, Adelaide, Australia

Richard Y.T. Chen
Changi General Hospital, Singapore

Antonio Cherubini
Perugia University Medical School, Perugia, Italy

Leung-Wing Chu
Sau Po Centre on Ageing, University of Hong Kong and Queen Mary Hospital, Hong Kong

Nicola Coley
University of Toulouse III, INSERM Unit 1027, Toulouse, France

Cynthia L. Comella
Rush University Medical Center, Chicago, IL, USA

Simon Conroy
University of Leicester, Leicester, UK

Claudia Cooper
University College London, London, UK

Cyrus Cooper
Southampton General Hospital, University of Southampton, Southampton, UK

Pamela M. Crawford
York Hospital, York, UK

Suzanne Crowe
Adelaide Meath and National Children's Hospital, Dublin, and University of Dublin, Dublin, Ireland

Alfonso J. Cruz-Jentoft
Hospital Universitario Ramón y Cajal, Madrid, Spain

Dulce M. Cruz-Oliver
Saint Louis University, St Louis, MO, USA

James M. Cummings
University of Missouri, Columbia, MO, USA

Lenise A. Cummings-Vaughn
Saint Louis University School of Medicine and St Louis Veterans' Affairs Medical Center, St Louis, MO, USA

Jean-François Dartigues
INSERM Unit 897, and Université Bordeaux Segalen, Bordeaux, France

Sam Dawkins
John Radcliffe Hospital, Oxford, UK

Lisette C.P.G.M. de Groot
Wageningen University, Wageningen, The Netherlands

Olivier Deguine
Hôpital Purpan and Université Toulouse III, CNRS, Toulouse, France

Julien Delrieu
Gérontopôle, Toulouse University Hospital and INSERM Unit 558, University of Toulouse III, Toulouse, France

Jean-François Démonet
Leenaards Memory Centre, CHUV, Lausanne, Switzerland

Michael J. Denham
Wellcome Trust Centre for the History of Medicine at UCL, London, UK

Abhilash K. Desai
Sheppard Pratt Hospital, and University of Maryland School of Medicine, Baltimore, MD, USA

David Doig
Institute of Neurology, University College London, London, UK

Ligia J. Dominguez
University of Palermo, Palermo, Italy

Richard L. Doty
Smell & Taste Center, University of Pennsylvania School of Medicine, Philadelphia, PA, USA

Nicolas Doumerc
Gérontopôle, CHU Toulouse, Toulouse, France

Christopher Dyer
Royal United Hospital, Bath, UK

Pamela M. Enderby
University of Sheffield, Sheffield, UK

Francesco Fattirolli
University of Florence and Azienda Ospedaliero – Universitaria Careggi, Florence, Italy

Maria A. Fiatarone Singh
University of Sydney, New South Wales, Australia; Hebrew Rehabilitation Center for Aged, Roslindale, MA, USA and Tufts University, Boston, MA, USA

Ilora G. Finlay
Cardiff University and Velindre Hospital, Cardiff, UK

Paul Finucane
Graduate-Entry Medical School, University of Limerick, Limerick, Ireland

Joseph H. Flaherty
Saint Louis University School of Medicine and St Louis Veterans' Affairs Medical Center, St Louis, MO, USA

Roger M. Francis
Institute for Ageing and Health, Newcastle University, Newcastle upon Tyne, UK

James E. Galvin
New York University Langone Medical Center, New York, NY, USA

Julie K. Gammack
Saint Louis University School of Medicine, and St Louis Veterans' Affairs Medical Center, Geriatric Research Education and Clinical Center, St Louis, MO, USA

Clement Gaudin
Gérontopôle, CHU Toulouse, Toulouse, France

Andrea R. Genazzani
University of Pisa, Pisa, Italy

Stephane Gerard
Gérontopôle, CHU Toulouse, Toulouse, France

George T. Griffing
Saint Louis University Medical Center, St Louis, MO, USA

George T. Grossberg
Saint Louis University School of Medicine, St Louis, MO, USA

Renato Maia Guimarães
Hospital Universitário de Brasília, Universidade de Brasília, Brasília, Brazil

Ramzi R. Hajjar
American University of Beirut Medical Center, Beirut, Lebanon and Saint Louis University School of Medicine, St Louis, MO, USA

Kingsley K. Hampton
Royal Hallamshire Hospital, Sheffield, UK

Arthur E. Helfand
Temple University, Philadelphia, Thomas Jefferson University Hospital, Philadelphia, and Philadelphia Corporation for Aging, Philadelphia, PA, USA

Robert D. Helme
Royal Melbourne Hospital, University of Melbourne, Melbourne, Victoria, Australia

David Hilton-Jones
John Radcliffe Hospital, Oxford; Milton Keynes Hospital Foundation Trust, Milton Keynes, Buckinghamshire; Muscular Dystrophy Campaign Muscle and Nerve Centre, Oxford, and Myasthenia Gravis Association Myasthenia Centre, Oxford, UK

Michael Horowitz
University of Adelaide, Royal Adelaide Hospital, Adelaide, Australia

Philippe Huber
University Hospital of Geneva, Geneva, Switzerland

Jonathan Ilowite
Winthrop University Hospital, Mineola, NY, USA

Radha Indusekhar
University Hospital of North Staffordshire, Stoke-on-Trent, UK

Donald F. Jessett
Formerly of University of Wales Institute, Cardiff, UK

David Jolley
Manchester University, Manchester, UK

Seema Joshi
Veterans Affairs Medical Center, Leavenworth, KS, USA

Lalit Kalra
King's College, London, UK

Anjali S. Kamat
Saint Louis University Health Sciences Center, St Louis, MO, USA

Benny Katz
St Vincent's Hospital and LaTrobe University, Melbourne, Victoria, Australia

Rafi T. Kevorkian
Saint Louis University School of Medicine and St Louis Veterans' Affairs Medical Center, St Louis, MO, USA

Joan Khoo
Changi General Hospital, Singapore

Heidi D. Klepin
Wake Forest University School of Medicine, Winston-Salem, NC, USA

Katie Kompoliti
Rush University Medical Center, Chicago, IL, USA

Christine Lafont
Toulouse University Hospital and Centre of Geriatric Medicine, Toulouse, France

James F. Lamb
Ohio State University College of Medicine and Public Health, Columbus, OH, USA

Andrew J. Larner
Walton Centre for Neurology and Neurosurgery, Liverpool, UK

Luc Letenneur
INSERM Unit 897, and Université Bordeaux Segalen, Bordeaux, France

Wee Shiong Lim
Tan Tock Seng Hospital, Singapore

Milta Oyola Little
Saint Louis University Medical Center, St Louis, MO, USA

Gill Livingston
University College London, London, UK

Susannah Long
Imperial College London, London, UK

Gordon D.O. Lowe
University of Glasgow, Glasgow, UK

Linda M. Luxon
University College of London Hospitals NHS Trust and University College London, London, UK

Gerald M. Mahon
Saint Louis University School of Medicine, St Louis, MO, USA

Suzanne M. Mahon
Saint Louis University, St Louis, MO, USA

Aneil Malhotra
John Radcliffe Hospital, Oxford, UK

Leocadio Rodríguez Mañas
Hospital Universitario de Getafe, Madrid, Spain

Robert E. Mansel
Cardiff University, Cardiff, Wales, UK

Kenneth G. Manton
Duke University, Durham, NC, USA

Niccolò Marchionni
University of Florence and Azienda Ospedaliero – Universitaria Careggi, Florence, Italy

Mathieu Marx
Hôpital Purpan and Université Toulouse III, CNRS, Toulouse, France

Giulio Masotti
University of Florence and Azienda Ospedaliero – Universitaria Careggi, Florence, Italy

Graydon S. Meneilly
University of British Columbia, Vancouver, BC, Canada

Jean-Pierre Michel
University Hospital of Geneva, Geneva, Switzerland

Paul Montgomery
University of Oxford, Oxford, UK

Kim J. Moon
Saint Louis University School of Medicine and St Louis Veterans' Affairs Medical Center, St Louis, MO, USA

Terry L. Moore
Saint Louis University Medical Center, St Louis, MO, USA

Jo Moriarty
King's College London, UK

John E. Morley
Saint Louis University School of Medicine and St Louis Veterans' Affairs Medical Center, St Louis, MO, USA

John S. Morris
Princess of Wales Hospital, Bridgend, UK

Loic Mourey
Institut Claudius Regaud, Toulouse, France

Emmanuel Moyse
Hôpital Purpan, Toulouse, France

Carlos G. Musso
Hospital Italiano de Buenos Aires, Buenos Aires, Argentina

Joseph M. Mylotte
University at Buffalo, Buffalo, NY, USA

Robert A. Norman
Dr Robert A. Norman & Associates, Tampa, FL, USA

Fatima Nourhashemi
Toulouse University Hospital, Toulouse, France

P.M. Shaughn O'Brien
University Hospital of North Staffordshire, Stoke-on-Trent, UK

Dennis S. Oh
Tufts University School of Medicine, Springfield, MA, USA

Takashi Ohrui
Institute of Development, Aging and Cancer, Tohoku University, Sendai, Japan

Fidelma O'Mahony
University Hospital of North Staffordshire, Stoke-on-Trent, UK

Desmond O'Neill
Trinity College Dublin, Dublin, Ireland

Dimitrios G. Oreopoulos
University Health Network, Toronto, ON, Canada

Francesco Orso
University of Florence and Azienda Ospedaliero – Universitaria Careggi, Florence, Italy

Roger Orpwood
University of Bath and Royal United Hospital, Bath, UK

Hardev S. Pall
University of Birmingham and University Hospital Birmingham Foundation Trust, Birmingham, UK

Miguel A. Paniagua
Saint Louis University School of Medicine, St Louis, MO, USA

Thomas T. Perls
Boston University School of Medicine, Boston, MA, USA

Horace M. Perry III
Saint Louis University School of Medicine and Geriatric Research, Education and Clinical Center, St Louis Veterans' Affairs Medical Center, St Louis, MO, USA

Ronald C. Petersen
Mayo Clinic, Rochester, MN, USA

Carolyn D. Philpot
Saint Louis University Medical Center, St Louis, MO, USA

Antoine Piau
Gérontopôle, Toulouse University Hospital, Toulouse, France

Nicola Pluchino
University of Pisa, Pisa, Italy

Jonathan Potter
Formerly Royal College of Physicians of London, London, UK

Bayard L. Powell
Wake Forest University School of Medicine, Winston-Salem, NC, USA

Charlene M. Prather
Saint Louis University, St Louis, MO, USA

Bernard D. Prendergast
John Radcliffe Hospital, Oxford, UK

Terence J. Quinn
Institute of Cardiovascular and Medical Sciences, University of Glasgow, Glasgow Royal Infirmary, Glasgow, Scotland, UK

Shobita Rajagopalan
Los Angeles County Department of Public Health, Los Angeles, CA, USA

Christopher K. Rayner
University of Adelaide, Royal Adelaide Hospital, Adelaide, Australia

Kathleen C. Reid
Women's College Hospital, Toronto, ON, Canada

Michael W. Rich
Washington University School of Medicine, St Louis, MO, USA

Lucio A. Rinaldi
University of Florence and Azienda Ospedaliero – Universitaria Careggi, Florence, Italy

Richard C. Roberts
University of Dundee, Dundee, Scotland, UK

Miriam B. Rodin
Saint Louis University Medical Center, St Louis, MO, USA

Yves Rolland
INSERM Unit 1027, F-31073; University of Toulouse III, Gérontopôle of Toulouse, France

David S. Rosenthal
Harvard Medical School, Boston, MA, USA

Philip A. Routledge
Cardiff University School of Medicine, Cardiff, Wales, UK

Geneviève Ruault
French Society of Geriatrics and Gerontology, Suresnes, France

Laurence Z. Rubenstein
University of Oklahoma College of Medicine, Oklahoma City, OK, USA

Natalie Sachs-Ericsson
Florida State University, Tallahassee, FL, USA

Abdi Sanati
Southwest London and St George's NHS Trust, Sutton Hospital, Sutton, UK

Sivakumar Sathasivam
Walton Centre for Neurology and Neurosurgery, Liverpool, UK

Eric Schmidt
Hôpital Purpan, Toulouse, France

Marie-Laure Seux
Assistance Public Hôpitaux de Paris, Hôpital Broca, Paris, France

Dennis J. Shale
Cardiff University, University Hospital of Wales, Cardiff, Wales, UK

Lindsay Dianne Shepard
University of Oxford, Oxford, UK

Hamsaraj G.M. Shetty
University Hospital of Wales, Cardiff, Wales, UK

Stephen D. Silberstein
Thomas Jefferson University, Philadelphia, PA, USA

Tomasso Simoncini
University of Pisa, Pisa, Italy

Alan J. Sinclair
Institute of Diabetes for Older People (IDOP), Luton, UK

Peter Spiegler
Winthrop University Hospital, Mineola, NY, USA

Richard M. Stone
Harvard Medical School, Boston, MA, USA

David J. Stott
Institute of Cardiovascular and Medical Sciences, University of Glasgow, Glasgow Royal Infirmary, Glasgow, UK

Elsa S. Strotmeyer
University of Pittsburgh, Pittsburgh, PA, USA

Andreas E. Stuck
Geriatrics Inselspital University Hospital, Bern, Switzerland

Adam Szafranek
University Hospital of Wales, Cardiff and Vale University Health Board, Cardiff, Wales, UK

Peggy A. Szwabo
Saint Louis University School of Medicine, St Louis, MO, USA

Eric G. Tangalos
Mayo Clinic, Rochester, MN, USA

Syed H. Tariq
Saint Louis University School of Medicine, St Louis, MO, USA

David R. Thomas
Saint Louis University Health Sciences Center, St Louis, MO, USA

Florian P. Thomas
St Louis Veterans' Affairs Medical Center and Saint Louis University School of Medicine, St Louis, MO, USA

Debbie T. Tolson
Glasgow Caledonian University, Glasgow, UK

Nina Tumosa
St Louis Veterans' Affairs Medical Center and Saint Louis University School of Medicine, St Louis, MO, USA

Allan R. Tunkel
Drexel University College of Medicine, Philadelphia, PA and Monmouth Medical Center, Long Branch, NJ, USA

Wija A. van Staveren
Wageningen University, Wageningen, The Netherlands

Bruno Vellas
Gérontopôle, Toulouse University Hospital and INSERM Unit 558, University of Toulouse III, Toulouse, France

Joe Verghese
Albert Einstein College of Medicine, Bronx, NY, USA

Adie Viljoen
Lister Hospital, Stevenage, Hertfordshire, and Bedfordshire and Hertfordshire Postgraduate Medical School, Luton, Hertfordshire, UK

Charles Vincent
Imperial College London, London, UK

Aaron I. Vinik
Eastern Virginia Medical School, Norfolk, VA, USA

Ladislav Volicer
University of South Florida, Tampa, FL, USA

Ulrich O. von Oppell
University Hospital of Wales, Cardiff and Vale University Health Board, and University of Cardiff, Wales, UK

Martha Wadleigh
Harvard Medical School, Boston, MA, USA

Adrian Wagg
University of Alberta, Edmonton, Alberta, Canada and Royal College of Physicians, London, UK

Laura M. Wagner
New York University, New York, NY, USA

Michael Watts
Graduate-Entry Medical School, University of Limerick, Limerick, Ireland

Ryan Westhoff
University of Kansas Medical Center, Kansas City, KS, USA

Victoria J. Wheatley
Aberdare General Hospital, Aberdare, UK

Anthony S. Wierzbicki
Guy's & St Thomas' Hospitals, London, UK

Tanya M. Wildes
Washington University School of Medicine, St Louis, MO, USA

Margaret-Mary G. Wilson
Formerly Saint Louis University Health Sciences Center and Veterans' Affairs Medical Center, St Louis, MO, USA

Gary A. Wittert
University of Adelaide, Adelaide, Australia

Thomas T. Yoshikawa
UCLA School of Medicine and VA Greater Los Angeles Healthcare System, Los Angeles, CA, USA

William B. Young
Thomas Jefferson University, Philadelphia, PA, USA

Preface to the Fourth Edition

"I offer no apology for the publication of this volume. The subject is one of the highest importance, and yet it has been strangely overlooked during the last half-century by the physicians of all countries."

–George Edward Day
(1815–1872)

George Day's introduction to his textbook *Disease of Advanced Life*, published in 1848, regrettably remains appropriate for textbooks published over 150 years later. Modern physicians can still fail to recognize the differences in disease presentation and management between middle-aged and older adults. It is our hope that this Fourth Edition of "Principles and Practice of Geriatric Medicine" will help increase the awareness of geriatric principles and improve the treatment of older individuals. John Pathy's original vision for the first edition was to provide, in a single volume, a comprehensive reference source for all those involved in the medicine of old age. We have endeavored to adhere to this vision, but inevitably the size of the textbook has grown. While in any text of this size some overlap with general texts of medicine will occur, the emphasis is on those assessments and disorders that are particularly of relevance to older persons.

Over the seven years since the last edition of this text was published, there have been dramatic advances in our understanding of the pathophysiology of disease as it interacts with the physiological processes of aging. There has been a continuing validation of assessment tools for older persons and the development of some new ones. Large-scale studies of the efficacy of various geriatric systems such as Acute Care for the Elderly Units, Geriatric Evaluation and Management Units, and Home Care Systems have been carried out. All of these have demonstrated the value and cost-effectiveness of the geriatric specialist approach to managing older people. In comparison, most studies assessing Coronary Care Units and Intensive Care Units have failed to come close to demonstrating the effectiveness that has been shown for geriatric units. Despite this, all major hospitals have highly expensive critical care units, while fewer have developed geriatric units. The last decade has also seen an increased awareness of the need to enhance the quality of long-term care. This increase in geriatric knowledge has been recognized by the addition of nearly 40 new chapters in this edition. In addition, many of the previous chapters have been totally rewritten to allow the recognition of the changes that have occurred in our understanding of the care of older persons.

Previous editions of this textbook were edited by a single person, John Pathy. With the rapid increase in geriatric knowledge and John's desire for the Fourth Edition to reflect the input of other academic minds, he has added two new editors to share the burden with him, namely, Alan Sinclair and John Morley. This has allowed a more even distribution of the editing tasks, though John Pathy has continued to carry the lion's share. In recognition of the globalization of the world, in general, and geriatrics, in particular, one of the new editors, John Morley, is from the United States, while Alan Sinclair draws on his European experiences. In addition, a major effort has been made at the end of the text to recognize the differences (as well as the similarities) of geriatrics as it is practiced around the world. The enormous good fortune the editors had in recruiting a stellar class of contributors from around the world has, we hope, allowed this text to be truly representative of a global view of geriatric medicine. From the beginning, John Pathy has made this a goal of his text, and the editors feel that this edition has truly achieved an international view of old-age medicine as originally developed by Marjorie Warren and her colleagues in the United Kingdom.

The general outline of the text still follows that of the first edition. The first sections provide a general perspective of old age, the processes of aging, and social and community perspectives. The chapter on preventive medicine now focuses on issues of particular importance to older persons. In Part III "Medicine in Old Age", the section "Eating Disorders and Nutritional Health" has been increased to recognize the increased importance and understanding of nutrition in old age. Chapters on frailty, sarcopenia, palliative care, and women's health have been added to recognize the increasing importance of these issues in older persons. The final part on ''Health Care Systems'' focuses first on the emergence of continuous quality improvement, geriatric systems and evidence-based medicine as the foundation of high-quality geriatric medicine. The development of novel education systems is discussed. Finally, unique aspects of geriatric care around the world are examined.

In an attempt to improve the readability of the text, we have asked the authors to make liberal use of tables and figures, and key points have been added at the end of each chapter. References have been limited, and at the beginning of the reference list, authors identify a few key references to allow for further reading. The new editors have tried to keep the easy reading style of the previous editions, but, as can be imagined, this has been a difficult task as we have increased the number of contributors from around the world.

Overall, we hope our readers enjoy and learn from this textbook; for the three of us, it has been a true labor of love. We particularly would like to thank our contributors for the excellent job they have done. We would also like to thank Layla Paggetti from John Wiley & Sons for her tireless efforts in making sure this book came to fruition. Finally, we would like to thank our families for their forbearance. This book is dedicated to all those who care for older persons.

M.S. John Pathy, Alan J. Sinclair, John E. Morley
December 2005

Preface to the Fifth Edition

The Fifth Edition of this widely known international textbook incorporates the latest evidence of research into the often complex management of common clinical problems in older people. We as Editors embarked on this edition with the knowledge that John Pathy would be there to guide us with all his wisdom and incredible grasp of the discipline of Geriatric Medicine. His untimely departure from this world left a major gap for us, but we have worked very closely as an editorial team, supported by Wiley-Blackwell, and hope that this edition fulfils all the expectations and objectives that were set when we originally sat down with John Pathy to discuss the textbook. We pay tribute to John Pathy as a tremendous role model for aspiring geriatricians all over the world and hope that his textbook will continue to educate all those who seek enlightenment in caring for older people.

We have used, wherever possible, an evidence-based approach to developing each chapter and asked all authors to think hard on what are the key messages. Chapters that have been revised and updated were edited closely to ensure that the clinical pathway is still highly relevant and that the references also reflected an in-depth revision process. A new layout of chapters will be apparent and is based on grouping chapters with similar clinical relevance and where similar pathophysiological mechanisms may be operating. In a majority of chapters, we have leading international authors who are experts in the field.

Wide clinical experience is the hallmark of a sound geriatrician or other healthcare specialist who claims expertise in managing older people who are hospitalized or who have clinically deteriorated in the community. This may take many years of training, although at an early stage of their careers, recognition of the varying nature of illness in old age and how both simple and focused interventions can lead to health gain are prerequisites for enhancing clinical care. This textbook should complement these activities irrespective of the status of the practitioner but, as always, reading a book and acquiring knowledge must be accompanied by a practical clinical care approach aligned with compassion and understanding of the critical issues affecting older people.

Professor Alan Sinclair would like to thank Caroline Sinclair, and Professor John Morley would like to thank Susan Brooks, for their tremendous assistance in helping them to complete their editorial tasks, and the Editors would like to express their appreciation of the incredible patience and support from Gill Whitley and Robyn Lyons at Wiley-Blackwell.

Alan J. Sinclair
John E. Morley
Bruno Vellas

Foreword

One of my earliest memories is of my father at work in his small study: he would be surrounded by what, to a child's eye, appeared to be a chaotic mass of books, journals, papers and slides. He never seemed to rest. The time not occupied by professional work was filled with hard labour in the garden or, with the constant support of his devoted wife Norma, in bringing up five children.

One of the results of the drive and determination in that time spent in his study was the first edition of *Principles and Practice of Geriatric Medicine* in 1985. I had become a medical student by that time, and remember the work involved in the production of that first edition. Twenty-five years on, I wonder at how my father managed to find the time, after completion of all his clinical and teaching tasks, even to contemplate such a *magnum opus* – however, many distinguished contributors may have been ready to assist.

The success of the first edition led to a request for a second, enlarged, edition, and then to a third edition. It was during the production of the third edition that my father himself required in-patient treatment. During this stay in hospital I called in to visit him, but found that he was not in bed but in the ward office on the telephone to a consultant at the hospital who was a contributor to the book, simply confirming that the contribution would be received by the deadline.

My father died before he could begin work himself on the fifth edition. Although by then he was no longer as physically fit as he would have wished, particularly for gardening, he remained mentally sharp, alert and energetic. Medicine remained his passion. He continued to be involved in research and remained abreast of the latest developments in professional literature. His private study, where he continued to beaver away energetically, remained as chaotic as ever.

Dr Damian Pathy FRCP

SECTION 7

Dementia and Cognitive Disorders

CHAPTER 71

Delirium

Joseph H. Flaherty

Saint Louis University School of Medicine and St Louis Veterans' Affairs Medical Center, St Louis, MO, USA

Overview

Delirium is a dangerous diagnosis. It is common; it is commonly missed; and it is associated with several adverse outcomes. Although most clinicians label patients with delirium as having an 'acute change in mental status', the formal diagnostic criteria according to the *Diagnostic and Statistical Manual of Mental Disorders* (DSM-IV-Text Revision) paints a more complete and descriptive picture of these patients if put into sentence form: 'A sudden onset of impaired attention, disorganized thinking or incoherent speech. The patient usually has a clouded consciousness, perceptual disturbances, sleep–wake cycle problems, psychomotor agitation or lethargy and is disoriented'.[1]

History and pathophysiology

Although the term 'delirium' was not used, references to patients with delirium date as far back as the time of Hippocrates. Delirium has only attracted attention as a syndrome or a diagnosis in the past three decades, with the first textbook dedicated solely to delirium being published in 1980.[2] The reasons for this long misunderstanding of what to call this constellation of symptoms are related to the various ways in which delirium can present (hypoactive, hyperactive or a combination of the two) and the complex pathophysiology that causes such a variety of presentations. Although research into the pathophysiology of delirium is in its infancy in clearly defining the contribution each neurotransmitter system and biochemical mechanism has on the clinical picture of delirium, one proposed pathoaetiological model of delirium (Figure 71.1) is important in helping clinicians understand the complexity of a patient with delirium.[3] By keeping the complex systems and mechanisms in mind when trying to diagnose or manage a patient with delirium, clinicians will better be able to understand the challenges in making an accurate diagnosis (especially in the face of dementia) and the significant limitations that medications have in the 'treatment' of delirium.

Prevalence and incidence for various sites and situations

Delirium is one of the most serious illnesses that patients can have or develop and one that clinicians should not miss at the reported rate of 32–66%.[4] Typical rates of delirium on admission to a medical unit are between 20 and 30%. In a thorough systematic review of 42 studies meeting selection criteria with a focus on medical inpatient settings, only eight performed delirium assessment within 24 h of admission. The prevalence of delirium on admission among these well-performed studies ranged from 10 to 31%, but the low 10% was thought to be an underestimate as this study had strict selection criteria. In the same systematic review, the incidence during hospitalization among 13 studies was 3–29%.[5]

In general, surgical patients have been found to have higher rates of delirium than medical patients. In a review of primary data-collection studies, Dyer *et al.* found that rates are highest postoperatively among coronary artery bypass graft patients, ranging from 17 to 74% (>50% in five of the 14 studies reviewed).[6] They also found that rates among orthopaedic surgical patients ranged from 28 to 53% (>40% in five of the six studies). Of the two urological studies reviewed, rates ranged from 4.5 to 6.8%. Past biases have blamed anaesthesia agents for most cases, which wrongly have kept alive the belief, like that in the case of the intensive care unit (ICU), that delirium is unpreventable. Several studies which have evaluated the association between routes of anaesthesia (general, epidural, spinal, regional) and the risk of postoperative delirium have found that the route of anaesthesia was not associated with the development of delirium.

Principles and Practice of Geriatric Medicine, Fifth Edition. Edited by Alan J. Sinclair, John E. Morley and Bruno Vellas.

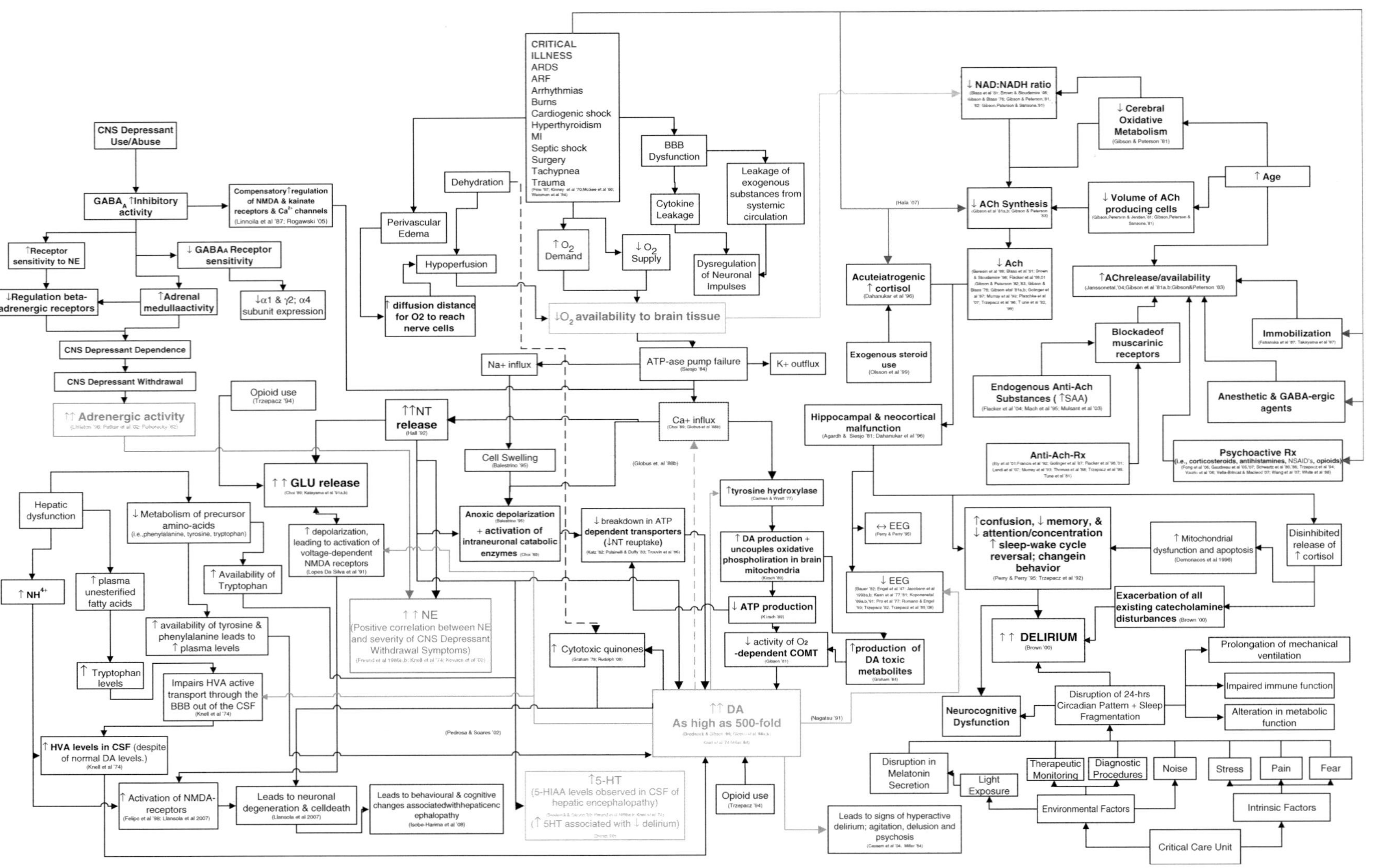

Figure 71.1 The pathoetiological model of delirium. Reprinted from Maldonado JR (2008).[3] Copyright (2008), with permission from Elsevier.

One of the sites with the highest rates of delirium, but perhaps the most controversial because of so many complicating factors, is the ICU. Rates as low as 19% and as high as 80% have been found.[7,8] For years, however, people have ignored these facts, have called it inevitable and unpreventable and have even labelled it 'ICU psychosis' so as to blame it on the ICU.

Discharge or 'transition' of patients out of the acute hospital setting has seen many changes over the past three decades. Data from post-acute care facilities (under such names as subacute-care facilities, skilled nursing facilities, rehabilitation centres and long-term care facilities) reveal two major issues: patients are discharged from acute hospitals with persistent delirium and delirium at these sites persists for an extended period of time. Kelly *et al.* found that 72% of 214 nursing home patients who were hospitalized for delirium still had delirium at the time of discharge back to the nursing home. The delirium persisted for 55% of the patients at 1 month and 25% at 3 months after discharge.[9] Marcantonio *et al.* found that 39% of 52 patients with hip fractures were discharged with delirium, which persisted for 32% of the patients at 1 month and 6% at 6 months after discharge.[10] In a large study of over 80 post-acute care facilities using the Minimum Data Set (MDS) to identify patients with any symptoms of delirium, Marcantonio *et al.* found a prevalence rate of 23% on admission. Among these patients, 52% still had the symptoms at 1 week follow-up.[11]

Two studies that looked at point of prevalence within nursing facilities discovered a similarly high rate of delirium. Mentes *et al.* evaluated 324 long-term nursing home residents using the MDS and found that 14% of patients had delirium.[12] Cacchione *et al.* prospectively evaluated 74 long-term nursing home patients and identified 24 (33%) with delirium.[13] While neither study could determine whether the delirium was a persistent one after a hospital stay or was an incident (new episode of) delirium, it is evident that delirium is common among nursing home residents.

Home care is an understudied site concerning delirium. However, two studies (detailed in the section 'Prevention and management interventions') showed lower rates of delirium among ill, older persons cared for at home compared with similarly ill, older persons cared for in the hospital. It is unclear whether something positive is being done in the home that prevents delirium or whether something negative is occurring in the hospital that contributes to the development of delirium.[14,15]

Associated adverse outcomes

Data about the adverse outcomes associated with delirium mainly come from studies of older patients in the hospital setting. Here, delirium has been found to be associated with hospital complications, loss of physical function, increased length of stay in the hospital, increased instances of discharge to a long-term care facilities and high mortality rates. Mortality rates for hospitalized delirious patients have been reported to be 25–33%, as high as the mortality rates for acute myocardial infarction and sepsis. There has been some question in the past about whether delirium was independently associated with these adverse outcomes or whether it was merely a marker of severe illness and physical frailty, since most studies identified older age, underlying cognitive impairment, severe, acute and chronic illness and functional impairment as the predisposing factors. However, when adjusting for these factors, delirium has been found to be independently associated with poor outcomes in most studies.

Associated adverse outcomes among delirious ICU patients have shown prolonged ICU stay, prolonged hospital stay and increased mortality compared with patients without delirium.[7,8] Data from post-acute facilities have also shown associated adverse outcomes, related to loss of physical function and mortality.[9,11,13]

The comprehensive approach to delirium

In order to improve the adverse outcomes associated with delirium, it is not enough just to improve our skills in diagnosing delirium and treating the underlying medical causes. The following are the necessary components of a comprehensive approach for those involved in the care of older persons and healthcare systems that interface with older persons:

1 *Awareness*: Be aware of how commonly delirium occurs and where it occurs and get others involved in the care of older persons to do the same.

2 *Diagnosis*: Know why it is important to differentiate and how to differentiate between delirium and dementia.

3 *Evaluation*: Identify and treat the underlying causes of delirium.

4 *Prevention*: Implement strategies or care systems that can prevent delirium.

5 *Management*: Manage patients who develop delirium.

Although there are no available studies to date that implement all five interventions, a multifaceted approach is warranted because of the nature of this multifactorial problem.

Awareness

Delirium should become part of the medical jargon for all who care for older persons. Furthermore, given the frequency with which delirium is seen and the seriousness of this diagnosis, a vital sign for mental status has been recommended,[16] and rates of incidence and outcomes associated with delirium could be considered as quality-of-care measures.

Diagnosis

Delirium is not dementia. There is no difference in the core features of delirium in the DSM-IV-TR version compared with the previous version, DSM-IV, except that the DSM-IV-TR version recognizes that delirium can arise during the course of dementia.[1] Although this appears to be a minor detail, the message that this gives to healthcare professionals is a critically important one: '*delirium is not dementia*'. Most types of dementia have a progressive downhill course. Delirium should be considered reversible. A mislabelling or lack of differentiation between these two diagnoses is thought to be the reason why delirium is missed by physicians and by nurses. Misdiagnosis or late diagnosis may also partly explain why delirium is associated with adverse outcomes. Table 71.1 details some of the differentiating characteristics between delirium and dementia, based on DSM criteria, keeping in mind that one of the criteria not in Table 71.1 is that delirium must occur in the context of a medical illness, metabolic derangement, drug toxicity or withdrawal.

Altered level of consciousness (LOC) is an excellent clue in differentiating delirium and dementia because it is not always possible to know the patient's baseline mental status. Without ever having seen the patient before, one can determine whether the patient's LOC lies towards the agitated or vigilant side of the spectrum of LOC or towards the lethargic, drowsy or stuporous side of the spectrum.

One can ask orientation questions, but since disorientation and problems with memory are present in both delirium and dementia, the key in determining delirium from dementia is *how* the patient answers. The delirious patient will often give disorganized answers, which can be described as rambling or even incoherent.

The classic identifiers of delirium are acute onset and fluctuating course, both of which are usually obtained by close caregivers (family or nurses). Although acute implies 24 h, the term subacute is used to emphasize that subtle mental status changes can be overlooked by caregivers. Over a period of many days, the patient may appear to be slowly declining mentally due to the underlying dementia. If left unchecked, the initial delirium may impair other necessary functions, leading to further medical problems, such as dehydration and malnutrition, further complicating the delirium. This snowball effect explains in part why the aetiology of delirium is typically multifactorial. Therefore, if it is unclear how long the change has been occurring, patients should be put in the category of delirium and an evaluation should be made.

Attention is also one of the classic identifiers of delirium, which may often be helpful if the patient's baseline mental status is not known. It can be tested by having a conversation. Patients may have difficulty maintaining or following the conversation, perseverate on the previous question or become easily distracted. Attention can also be tested with cognitive tasks such as days of the week backwards, spelling backwards or digit span.

Psychomotor agitation or lethargy, hallucinations, sleep–wake cycle abnormalities and slow or incoherent speech can all be seen in patients with delirium, but these features are not necessary for the diagnosis.

Table 71.1 Differentiating delirium from dementia.

	Delirium	Dementia
Consciousness	Decreased or hyper-alert 'Clouded'	Alert
Orientation	Disorganized	Disoriented
Course	Fluctuating	Steady, slow decline
Onset	Acute or subacute	Chronic
Attention	Impaired	Usually normal
Psychomotor	Agitated or lethargic	Usually normal
Hallucinations	Perceptual disturbances May have hallucinations	Usually not present
Sleep–wake cycle	Abnormal	Usually normal
Speech	Slow, incoherent	Aphasic, anomic, difficulty finding words

Evaluation

General guidelines for the medical evaluation of patients are to consider all possible causes, proceed cautiously with appropriate testing and keep in mind that delirium is usually caused by a combination of underlying causes.

After a physical check and ascertaining the history, which includes obtaining details from anyone considered a caregiver (e.g. family, nurse's aide) and a thorough medication list, the mnemonic D-E-L-I-R-I-U-M-S can be used as a checklist to cover most causes of delirium (Table 71.2). Drugs are notorious for causing delirium. According to most authors in this area, 'virtually any' and 'practically every' drug can be considered deliriogenic. Several drugs have been found *in vitro* to have varying amounts of anticholinergic properties. However, since the pathophysiological and neurotransmitter mechanisms of delirium go beyond anticholinergic mechanisms, a more practical approach is to remember certain categories of medications that have been reported to cause delirium, some more common than others. The mnemonic A-C-U-T-E C-H-A-N-G-E I-N M-S is long, as would be expected, but highlights why

Table 71.2 Causes of delirium.

D	Drugs
E	Eyes, ears
L	Low O_2 state (MI, stroke, PE)
I	Infection
R	Retention (of urine or stool)
I	Ictal
U	Underhydration/undernutrition
M	Metabolic
(S)	Subdural

Table 71.3 Medications that can cause (have been reported to cause) an A-C-U-T-E C-H-A-N-G-E I-N M-S (mental status).

A	Antiparkinson drugs
C	Corticosteroids
U	Urinary incontinence drugs
T	Theophylline
E	Emptying drugs (e.g. metoclopramide, compazine)
C	Cardiovascular drugs
H	H2 blockers
A	Antibiotics
N	NSAIDs
G	Geropsychiatry drugs
E	ENT drugs
I	Insomnia drugs
N	Narcotics
M	Muscle relaxants
S	Seizure drugs

drugs are such a common cause of delirium (Table 71.3). In order to be as inclusive as possible and because many older reports did not discuss strict delirium criteria or such criteria were not commonly used, the following paragraphs describe not just delirium as a side effect, but also psychiatric side effects that might indicate presence of delirium, such as hallucinosis, paranoia, delusions, psychosis, general confusion, aggressiveness, restlessness and drowsiness.[17]

Levodopa (an antiparkinson drug) has been reported to cause mental status changes at a rate of 10–60% and include hallucinosis on a background of a clear sensorium, delusional disorders and paranoia. Abnormal dreams and sleep disruption may precede the more frank delirium symptoms and may be an early clue to their onset. Selegiline has been reported to cause mental status changes described as psychosis, aggressiveness and even mania.

Corticosteroids have been reported to cause 'psychiatric complications' in up to 18% of patients with doses above 80 mg per day. The mental status changes seen have been described as depressive/manic, an organic affective disorder with associated paranoid-hallucinating features and general 'confusion'.

Although short-acting urinary incontinence drugs have a greater potential to cause delirium, newer sustained release agents have also been reported.

Theophylline 'madness' probably meets delirium criteria. One of the first case reports described a patient with a toxic blood level that correlated with hyperactive periods marked by flailing of limbs, intense emotional lability, incessant crying and ripping out of intravenous lines and nasogastric tubes.

'Emptying' drugs is a reminder that drugs such as metoclopramide and droperidol that are often used for nausea and vomiting have potential for mental status changes. Reported mental status side effects include restlessness, drowsiness, depression and confusion. The mechanism is likely because of their antidopaminergic properties.

Cardiovascular drugs rarely cause mental status problems, but because they are so commonly prescribed for older persons, it is worthwhile to remember that some are more likely to cause problems, and also a few that have been reported in case reports. One of the first reports of confusion due to digoxin toxicity was over 100 years ago. Since then, reports of confusion even at therapeutic levels have been published. Antihypertensive agents that may cause mental status changes have primarily been reported in the literature through case reports. However, since they are so commonly used, it is worthwhile being suspicious about a few of them. These include beta-blockers (including in the form of eye drops), angiotensin-converting enzyme inhibitors and calcium channel antagonists.

H2 blockers, because they are primarily renally excreted and may have some H1 activity (antihistamine receptor subtype-1), may cause delirium, especially if patients have underlying risk factors such as renal insufficiency and dementia.

Antimicrobials, like cardiovascular drugs, rarely cause mental status changes, but are very commonly used; some examples worth being aware of are penicillin, erythromycin, clarithromycin, gentamycin, tobramycin, streptomycin, trimethoprim-sulfamethoxazole, ciprofloxacin, some cephalosporins and the antiviral acyclovir, particularly at high doses. Most reports propose that the mechanisms by which antimicrobials cause mental status changes are related to impaired renal function, drug–drug interaction and occasionally idiosyncratic behaviour. Several types of non-steroidal anti-inflammatory drugs (NSAIDs) have been reported to cause delirium, even the selective cyclooxygenase-2 inhibitors.

'Geropsychiatric' medications are too large a category for an in-depth discussion, but a few comments are warranted to create some balance between reflexively blaming these drugs for the delirium just because 'any drug that works in the brain, can cause a problem in the brain' and understanding that although no centrally acting psychiatric medication is completely safe, certain ones may be safer than others and psychiatric illnesses, especially depression, need to be treated. Tricyclic antidepressants (TCAs) can cause delirium with an overall incidence ranging from 1.5 to 20%. The highest rates, of course, seem to be among older, previously cognitively impaired and medically ill patients. Serotonin selective reuptake inhibitor (SSRI) antidepressants have a much safer side effect profile than the TCAs as far as delirium is concerned. However, one of the main side effects of SSRIs, hyponatraemia, can present as delirium in older persons. This has been reported with fluoxetine, fluvoxamine, paroxetine and sertraline. Although frank delirium due to SSRIs is rare, most reported cases seem to point towards drug interactions as a plausible cause. However, to emphasize that no centrally acting drug is completely safe, in a study of 10 healthy volunteers, paroxetine increased ratings of confusion and fatigue. There are also case reports of confusion due to antidepressants such as mirtazapine and venlafaxine. SSRIs alone and combinations such as sertraline and tramadol (a mu-receptor pain medication), trazodone and buspirone, and trazodone and methylphenidate have been reported to cause symptoms similar to those described in the serotonin syndrome.

The use of benzodiazepines (BDZs) was associated with an increased relative risk of developing cognitive impairment in one study among hospitalized patients, even those with normal mini-mental status examination scores on admission. Postoperative use of BDZs has also been found to increase the risk of delirium. Short-acting BDZs, even in small doses, have been reported to cause problems and the clinician should be aware that withdrawal from BDZs in the elderly may also present as delirium, perhaps more so when discontinuing short-acting compared with long-acting BDZs. However, there are models of successfully withdrawing patients from BDZs and this should be attempted whenever possible.

Antipsychotics can cause delirium, even the low-potency antipsychotic agents. Whether the antipsychotic prescribed is considered a typical or an atypical antipsychotic, the clinician needs to keep in mind that none of these drugs have pure mono-neurotransmitter activity. Rather, they have varying degrees of activity, either agonist or antagonist to many of the neurotransmitters implicated in the pathophysiology of delirium, such as dopamine, acetylcholine, serotonin and histamine. Therefore, like other geriatric psychiatric medications, antipsychotic drugs can and should be considered as a potential cause of delirium. Patients with Lewy body dementia have an increased sensitivity to neuroleptics. The clinical challenge here is that sometimes it is difficult to differentiate between Alzheimer's dementia and Lewy body-type dementia.

The ENT drugs in the mnemonic are a reminder of the multiple drugs, in particular over-the-counter (OTC) medications, that are taken for respiratory or sinus illnesses. The most worrisome of these ENT medications are the combination formulas, which contain two and sometimes three or even four active ingredients. Antihistamines, particularly the drug diphenhydramine, can cause problems at high doses, at moderately high doses, after a first-time oral dose in compromised elderly patients and even with topical use. Mental status changes have been reported to occur at high doses, at low doses and even from overuse of nasal inhalation of common OTC decongestants such as pseudoephedrine, phenylpropanolamine and phenylephrine. Expectorants and antitussins are probably safe provided that they are only used by themselves. One of the most commonly used, if not overused, ENT medications is meclizine. It has the potential to cause mental status changes because of its central anticholinergic action at the chemoreceptor trigger zone. The anticholinergic properties were thought to be the cause of confusion and steady cognitive and functional decline in an older patient who had been on meclizine for 3 years. Within 1 month off the drug, the patient's function and mentation improved. When rechallenged, the patient had cognitive and functional decline within 1 week.

'I' is a reminder that medications used for insomnia because of their effect on sedation have the potential to cause varying degrees of delirium. Most OTC sleeping aids come under a multitude of brand names without specifying the potentially dangerous deliriogenic medications dyphenhydramine or scopolamine.

Narcotics can be used safely in older persons with little risk of developing delirium, but a few important details need to be remembered. Meperidine is particularly risky in older persons, likely due to the anticholinergic activity of its active metabolite normeperidine. The main problems associated with the use of narcotics are probably related to toxicity, overuse or overdosage in patients with impaired hepatic or renal function.

Muscle relaxant is a misnomer because these medications act centrally in the brain, not locally at the muscles. Some of the commonly used muscle relaxants include cyclobenzaprine, methocarbamol and carisoprodol and have been reported to cause delirium.

Seizure medications have been reported to cause various types of cognitive impairment, including drowsiness, agitation, depression, psychosis and delirium. The cognitive impairment is thought to be related to serum levels, but clinicians should keep in mind that most anticonvulsants are protein bound and if the patient's nutritional status is poor then there is potential that the amount of free drug will actually be higher than what is measured by the serum level.

In conclusion, although the list of medications that can cause delirium is long, the mnemonic A-C-U-T-E C-H-A-N-G-E I-N M-S can help clinicians recognize some of the more common and some of the rare offenders. For patients who present with delirium or for patients who are at risk for delirium, the following general guidelines concerning medication management can be used:

1 Use non-pharmacological interventions whenever possible instead of a medication.

2 Do not treat vague symptoms with a medication (for example, do not routinely give H2 antagonists for vague gastrointestinal complaints).

3 Include an assessment of OTC medications as potential offenders.

4 Evaluate all drugs for drug–drug and drug–disease interactions.

5 If a drug is started, decide on how long that drug will be used. The old rule of 'start low and go slow' needs to be expanded to 'start low, go slow and know when to stop'.

6 The justification for prescribing medications should be based on therapeutic reasons and not on preventive reasons and until the patient is no longer at risk for delirium or the delirium has resolved.

7 Do not treat adverse effects of drugs with another drug unless completely necessary (as may be the case with long-acting narcotics and laxatives).

The 'E' in the D-E-L-I-R-I-U-M mnemonic stands for emotions and reminds the clinician that depression can have psychotic features and as such may present similarly to patients with delirium. Although depression has classically been considered the masquerader of dementia, given some of the DSM-IV criteria for delirium such as disorganized thinking or psychomotor lethargy, depression should be considered a reversible cause of delirium.

Low O_2 (oxygen) states, 'L' in the mnemonic, should highlight to the clinician that older patients with acute cardiovascular or pulmonary illnesses can present with delirium. It could be said that 'delirium is as serious as a heart attack' because not only can the mortality rate of delirium be as high as that of myocardial infarction (MI) but also older delirious patients can have MIs that are commonly missed or present atypically. It is unclear whether patients, because of the delirium, cannot either describe or tell clinicians about chest pain or whether there exists a cardiocerebral syndrome in which the stress of the MI affects the adrenergic system causing a stress on the balance in the central nervous system, that is, in cognition. Not only are patients with stroke at risk of developing delirium as a complication of the stroke or the underlying comorbidities associated with the stroke but also delirium may be the presenting feature of some stroke patients.

Infections are one of the most common underlying causes of delirium among older people. The most common types of infections that cause delirium are urinary tract infections and respiratory infections. However, with the recent rise in antibiotic-associated diarrhoea due to *Clostridium difficile* bacteria, some clinicians have urged caution not to overdiagnose urinary tract infections that may be asymptomatic bacteriuria. Subtle infections such as cholecystitis and diverticulitis should be in the differential diagnosis. Although meningitis should also be considered, it is not clear whether or not cerebrospinal fluid analysis is warranted in the initial work-up of delirious patients without other symptoms that point towards a central nervous system infection.

Retention of urine and faeces can both cause delirium, although typically the presentations differ. Urinary retention causing delirium has been well reported in the literature under the term cystocerebral syndrome. The original report was of three cases, all involving older men who became acutely agitated and nearly mute. All three patients had large volumes of urine in their bladder and, in all three patients, the agitated delirium resolved within a short time after emptying the bladder. A proposed explanation is that the adrenergic tension related to the urinary retention might increase in the central nervous system and the consequent increase in catecholamines might produce delirium. Although this pathophysiological explanation has not been proven, clinicians should be very aware of this syndrome. One of the best ways to evaluate quickly for urinary retention is with a hand-held bladder ultrasound. Although the equipment has a fairly high initial cost, cost savings from the reduction in the use of straight catheterizations may help balance this issue.

Faecal retention as a cause of delirium has not been reported in the literature. However, since older patients, for multiple reasons, are at risk for faecal impactions, clinicians should be suspicious of this problem when the delirium is of the hypoactive type.

Ictal states are a rare cause of delirium and are not difficult to diagnose clinically for patients with tonic clonic seizures. However, patients who experience absence seizures may go unnoticed by caregivers and may only seem to have fluctuating mental status changes. Although an electroencephalogram (EEG) is not indicated in the initial medical evaluation of delirium, it should be considered when pertinent history is obtained.

Underhydration is used in the mnemonic, not only to emphasize the fact that dehydration can be one of the underlying causes of delirium but also to highlight the fact that those at risk for dehydration are at risk for delirium. Although there is much debate and consternation about which, if any, physical signs are pathomnemonic for dehydration among older persons, one quick method is to calculate the blood urea nitrogen (BUN) to creatinine ratio. Although there are several circumstances when the BUN/creatinine ratio may not be accurate, there are data to suggest that a ratio of greater than 17:1 puts the patient at risk for delirium.[18] Given this easy and commonly accessible parameter and given the data supporting the use of dehydration or difficulty with hydration as a target for

, as will be seen below, dehydration should d to be at the top of the list as a contributing ot only as a risk factor for delirium and should as aggressively as possible keeping in mind the s of each patient related to their cardiovascular

rnutrition or malnutrition is rather complex and it to understand as a cause of delirium, most likely se, unlike other causes of delirium, it is less likely to versed quickly. It is evident, however, that malnutri- among hospitalized patients is not only common but o is associated with longer hospital stays, postoperative mplications and even higher mortality. Clinicians and all iealthcare providers in the hospital should be aware that restricted diets are likely to exacerbate malnutrition. Malnutrition is most directly related to delirium probably through the issue of medications that are protein bound. Patients who are malnourished may have lower protein stores and therefore protein-bound drugs will have a higher free concentration that puts the patient at risk for delirium. Other proposed relationships between malnutrition and delirium, which have yet to be fully elucidated, include those mechanisms looking at cytokines. Metabolic abnormalities that cause delirium are not difficult to identify because of the availability of commonly used laboratory tests. A complete metabolic panel will usually identify hyponatraemia or hypernatraemia, hypocalcaemia or hypercalcaemia and abnormalities of liver function or renal function. Thyroid function tests and vitamin B_{12} are typically put in this category.

Although delirium is not spelled with an 's' at the end, using the mnemonic D-E-L-I-R-I-U-M-S emphasizes to the clinician that delirium usually has more than one cause. The 's' also reminds the clinician that a subdural haematoma can cause a mental status change. Although the mortality rate of subdural haematomas among younger people is fairly high, the prognosis for older people is quite good provided that the diagnosis is not missed. The other difference between older and younger patients with subdural haematomas is that older patients may develop the subdural haematoma over a period of a few hours or days. Although there could be some debate as to whether or not all older patients presenting to a hospital with delirium should have some sort of brain imaging, most would agree that because this is a very reversible problem and which would cease to be reversible if the diagnosis is delayed, imaging should be considered if there has been a history of head trauma or falls or any suspicion that there was an unwitnessed fall.

One of the other causes of delirium not represented in the mnemonic is pain. Recognition of pain is improving, now identified as the *fifth vital sign*, and should be considered as a readily treatable cause of delirium, especially associated with elective surgery.

Prevention and management interventions

Before identifying which interventions are effective and which are not, it is important to understand the goals of interventions concerning delirium. They are (1) to prevent the development of delirium, (2) to reduce the adverse outcomes associated with delirium in those patients for whom delirium is not prevented and (3) to provide healthcare professionals with alternatives to physical restraints and pharmacological methods in the management of delirium. It is also important to emphasize that delirium is a complex issue related to the challenge of identifying who is at risk of developing it, diagnosing it if it does develop and getting other healthcare professionals to do the same. Interventions that are successful will involve several components, many of which are not easily measured. These include education about the risk factors and diagnosis of delirium, a 'culture' change about how *not* to use what seems logical and protective (for example, physical restraints or pharmacological sedation) and a realization that multicomponent interventions are not simple but can be done.

The most consistent message about successful interventions is to use an interdisciplinary team approach and follow geriatric principles. One of the most rigorous studies to date because of the assessment methods used and the close follow-up of patients was a prospective study of a multicomponent intervention to prevent the development of delirium in hospitalized older patients.[19] The study identified patients at risk for delirium on the basis of a previously developed predictive model. The study used the following six out of seven risk factors for the development of delirium: baseline cognitive impairment, eye or visual problems, altered sleep–wake cycle, dehydration, restricted or decreased mobility or hearing impairment (Table 71.4). The seventh risk factor, addition of more than three medications, was not used in the study, but is included in Table 71.4 for completeness (B-E-W-A-R-E). The standardized intervention protocols that were used in the study included the first six targeted interventions as described in Table 71.4 (P-R-E-V-E-N-T). Delirium developed in 15% of 426 usual care patients compared with only 9.9% of 426 intervention group patients [odds ratio (OR), 0.60; 95% confidence interval (CI), 0.39–0.92). The total number of days of delirium and the total number of episodes of delirium were also significantly lower in the intervention group, but the severity of delirium and recurrence rates were not significantly different. The interdisciplinary team included a specialist geriatric nurse, two specially trained persons familiar with the standardized intervention protocols, a certified therapeutic recreation specialist, a physical therapy consultant, a geriatrician and trained volunteers. The importance of this study is twofold. This study probably underestimates the success of a multicomponent intervention such as this because of the likely contamination that occurred

Table 71.4 Risk factors for delirium (B-E A-W-A-R-E) and targeted interventions (P-R-E-V-E-N-T) based on an intervention trial to prevent delirium.

B	Baseline dementia?
E	Eye problems?
A	Altered sleep–wake cycle?
W	Water or dehydration problems?
A	Adding >3 medications, especially sedating and psychoactive ones?
R	Restricted mobility?
E	Ear problems?
P	Protocol for sleep (back massage, relaxation music, decreased noise, warm milk or caffeine-free herbal tea)
R	Replenish fluids and recognize volume depletion
E	Ear aids (amplifier or patient's own hearing aid)
V	Visual aids (patient's own glasses, magnifying lens)
E	Exercise or ambulation as soon as possible
N	Name person, place and time frequently for reorientation
T	Taper or discontinue unnecessary medications. Use alternative and less harmful medications

throughout the hospital through implementing some of the standardized protocols. Since the study was done within one hospital, it was unable to randomize patients to separate floors and, thus, some intervention patients were on floors that also included patients from the usual care group. This was evident based on the 15% rate of delirium in the usual care group, which is lower than in previous studies.

A pre–post-intervention trial that focused on education of emergency department staff and admission to an acute geriatric unit ($n = 374$) showed positive results. The incidence of delirium decreased from 41% in the pre-intervention group to 22.7% in the post-intervention group at 4 months and 19.1% at 9 months.[20]

A few studies have targeted a very high risk group for delirium: older patients with surgical repair of hip fractures. Two randomized trials have focused on the prevention and management of delirium. In one study, 126 patients who were 65 years or older and admitted for surgical repair of hip fracture were randomized to geriatric physician consultation or usual care. The geriatric consultation was 'proactive', which meant that the consultation began preoperatively (for 61% of the patients) or within 24 h of surgery and a geriatrician made daily visits for the duration of the hospitalization. Targeted recommendations were made on the basis of a structured protocol emphasizing geriatric principles as well as postoperative medical care. Recommendations covered areas such as treatment of severe pain, elimination of unnecessary medications, regulation of bowel/bladder function (including discontinuing bladder catheters by postoperative day 2), adequate nutritional intake and early mobilization. The overall adherence rate by the orthopaedics team to the recommendations was 77%. Delirium developed in 32% of the 62 consultation group patients compared with 50% of the 64 usual care group patients (OR, 0.64; 95% CI, 0.37–0.98). There was a greater reduction in severe delirium, occurring in 12% of the consultation group and 29% of the usual care group (OR, 0.40; 95% CI, 0.18–0.89). Median length of stay did not differ in the two groups (5 days).[10] In the other study ($n = 120$), the multicomponent interventions were education of nurses, systematic screening, consultation by a nurse specialist and scheduled pain protocol. Mortality rates were inconclusive and there was no change in hospital length of stay (LOS) or physical function. However, there was a decrease in delirium duration and severity, but not incidence.[21] One randomized trial with a focus on just the management of hip fractures patients with delirium used multiple strategies for recognition of delirium, staff education, cooperation between orthopaedics and geriatrics and management of delirium and complications ($n = 49$). The study showed improved function and decreased duration and incidence of delirium in the intervention group.[22]

Randomized trials for the management of medical inpatients who already have delirium have not been as successful. Two trials utilized the same multicomponent intervention of systematic detection of delirium, a geriatric physician consultation with a geriatric nurse specialist doing follow-up. The first trial ($n = 227$) showed no change in mortality, LOS, function, discharge location or delirium duration.[23] The second trial ($n = 88$) showed no change in mortality, LOS or function, but there was a minor change in delirium severity.[24] A third randomized trial ($n = 174$) performed comprehensive geriatric assessments in the intervention group compared with a control group. It also utilized individually tailored treatment directed at the management of delirium, which turned out to mean that a significantly higher percentage of patients in the intervention group compared with the control group received physiotherapy, nutritional supplements, hip protectors, acetylcholinesterase inhibitors for underlying dementia and atypical neuroleptics for the delirium (and lower percentage of typical neuroleptics). The study showed no change in mortality, LOS or rate of institutionalization. Delirium was 'alleviated' significantly faster in the intervention group.[25] Finally, a fourth trial ($n = 400$) that focused on both the management and prevention of delirium was successful. A multicomponent intervention targeted staff education, assessment, prevention and treatment of delirium with an additional intervention towards the caregiver. The study showed a decrease in mortality (two versus nine deaths, $p = 0.03$), decrease in LOS (10.8 versus 20.5 days) and a decrease in the percentage of patients with delirium at day 7 (30 versus 60%).[26]

Another approach in the management of delirium is the delirium room (DR). The DR is a specialized four-bed rovide 24 h nursing care and observation by ne nurse in the room and is completely free of restraints.[27] The hallmarks of the DR are the fol- The four-bed DR is an integral part of an acute or the elderly (ACE) unit. As such, the patients in DR receive not only 24 h close observation but also benefits of the geriatric principles for which the ACE t has been shown to be effective in preventing loss of nctional decline. Nursing inservices and protocols devel- ped by nurses on how to identify and manage delirious patients are necessary. The DR is not isolated from the rest of the floor, rather it is the closest room to the main nurses' station. Having a location on the floor called the *Delirium Room* (see Figure 71.1) raises the awareness among healthcare professionals that delirium is a serious diagnosis, with serious consequences. Putting delirious or potentially delirious patients together in a room does not increase agitation as previous literature might suggest. Although the report of the DR was descriptive, it showed that over a 12 month consecutive time frame, out of the 69 patients with a diagnosis (according to the *International Classification of Disease*, 9th edition) of delirium in the DR, negative associations found in other studies of delirious patients were minimized. No physical restraints were used and only 29% of the patients received new orders for medications considered to be pharmacological restraints (haloperidol, risperidone or lorazepam), all at total daily doses of less than 2.0 mg. Only 13% of the patients lost physical function and none of the 69 patients died during their stay in the hospital. Mean length of stay for these patients was not significantly different compared with the length of stay for all other patients over the age of 70 years during the same time frame.[27]

Two studies of 'home–hospital care' have shown lower rates of delirium among medical patients cared for in the home compared with similar patients cared for in the hospital.[14,15] In the study by Caplan *et al.*,[14] 100 patients with a mean age of 76 years (71% from home, 25% from nursing homes and 4% from hostels) with medical illnesses such as acute infections requiring intravenous antibiotics, deep venous thrombosis, minor cerebrovascular accidents or cardiac failure, were randomized within 24 h of diagnosis to either home or hospital. Although the researchers used the term 'confusion' instead of the formal diagnosis of delirium, they found a lower incidence of confusion (0 versus 20.4%; $p = 0.0005$) in the home group compared with the hospital group. Other geriatric complications were also found to be at a lower rate in the home group compared with the hospital group: urinary complications (incontinence or retention) (2.0 versus 16.3%; $p = 0.01$) and bowel complications (incontinence or constipation) (0 versus 22.5%; $p = 0.0003$).[14] The study by Leff *et al.*[15] identified older patients who required hospital-level care for pneumonia, congestive heart failure, chronic obstructive pulmonary disease and cellulitis. Of those who went home for treatments associated with hospital care, compared with patients who completed their treatments in the hospital (average length of stay 2.9 versus 4.9 days), the adjusted OR for incident delirium was 0.25 (adjusted 95% CI, 0.11 to 0.58).[15]

The take-home message for delirium is that although it is a difficult problem to prevent or manage when unpreventable, it can be done usually through a multicomponent intervention. No single simple intervention is likely to succeed and it is not possible to tease out which of the multiple components are having an effect and which are the detractors. Nonetheless, multicomponent interventions still need to be considered as the standard of care because delirium is such a complicated multifactorial problem.

Physical restraints

Physical restraints should not be used for patients who are at risk of developing delirium or who have already developed delirium (see Chapter 133, Restraints and immobility). The use of physical restraints is associated with developing delirium and is significantly related to severity of delirium. Furthermore, the proposed reason for the use of physical restraints among delirious patients, to prevent injury primarily related to falls, is misconceived. Of three studies of restraint reduction programmes in long-term care institutions, two showed no change in fall rate and one showed an increase in fall rate. However, all three studies showed a decrease in fall injury rates.[28–30] Of two studies in the hospital setting, restraint reduction was not associated with an increase in falls.[31,32] The rate of restraint use in the study by Powell *et al.*[31] went from 52 per 1000 patient-days to just 0.3 per 1000 patient-days. Although neither study reported injury rates before and after restraint reduction, Mion *et al.*[32] reported that injury rates after the restraint reduction programme were low. Importantly, they were modestly successful (≥20% reduction) in two of six ICUs in restraint reduction and reported that no deaths occurred as a result of a fall or disruption in therapy, including in the case of ICU patients on mechanical ventilators.[31,32] Furthermore, the fact that restraint-free environments can be achieved, as in some geriatric departments in European hospitals,[33] ACE units in United States hospitals[27] and some nursing facilities[34,35] adds to the evidence that restraint-free care should be the standard of care.

Pharmacological restraints

Currently, no antipsychotic or other pharmacological agent is approved by the US Food and Drug Administration (FDA) for the treatment of delirium. On the basis of the available data concerning medications used in the management of delirium and the commonly accepted reason to use them (for patients whose behaviour interrupts the necessary medical care or puts themselves or others at risk of physical harm), antipsychotics should be considered a form of restraint until further evidence shows otherwise. Delirium is not analogous to psychosis. In patients with schizophrenia, antipsychotics can improve behaviour and function, with sedation being a common side effect. In patients with delirium, antipsychotics have not been shown to do this. It is argued that they control behaviour, but it is unclear whether this is through the sedation effects of the drugs or their effect on the neurotransmitters thought to play a role in delirium. To complicate matters further for older persons, one of the main problems with antipsychotic drugs, whether atypical or typical, is that they are not pure in their mechanism of action. For example, although risperidone primarily affects serotonergic (5-HT2A) receptors, it also affects to some extent dopaminergic and alpha-1 receptors. Although olanzapine affects the 5-HT2A receptors, similarly to risperidone, its sedation properties are probably due to its effect on the histaminic receptors. Clozapine also affects histaminic and muscarinic receptors and quetiapine has varying effects on histaminic and alpha-1 receptors and also has a small affect on dopaminergic and 5-HT receptors.

The available data for the use of antipsychotics in the management of delirium are poor because of the populations studied, types of studies done or the presence of the common mistake of not including a placebo group in order to measure the natural course (duration) of delirium without pharmacological intervention. As can be seen in Table 71.5, although several studies have examined the effects of antipsychotics in delirium, none of them were placebo controlled. It is important to note in the table the number of days when improvement is seen. Without a placebo-controlled group, it is unclear from the current evidence whether improvement in these studies follows the natural course of delirium or if it is from the use of the antipsychotic. It is evident from the lack of evidence that randomized placebo-controlled trials are needed. It should be noted that in a randomized controlled trial of a non-pharmacological intervention to prevent delirium, Inouye *et al.* found that even in the control group patients who developed delirium, the average total number of days of delirium was ~2.5.[19] Although this study did not go into detail about the percentage of delirious patients who received antipsychotics or the dose, another study[27] found that only 29% of 69 delirious patients received any form of pharmacological restraint (antipsychotics, benzodiazepines, sedatives/hypnotics) and this group had an average length of stay in hospital <5 days.

The proper dosages of antipsychotics have also never been established. One recent text recommends that if severe agitation is present, haloperidol doses of 0.25–1.0 mg can be used as often as every 20–30 min with a maximum 24 h dose of 3–5 mg. This dose is recommended because D2-dopaminergic receptors are saturated at low doses and therefore, theoretically, doses above 5 mg over a 24 h period are likely only to increase adverse events without providing additional clinical benefit. The goal should be an awake patient who is manageable, not a sedated patient, and the drug should be tapered and discontinued as soon as possible.

On the basis of the currently available data, the following conclusions can be drawn:

1 There is not enough evidence for the routine use of antipsychotic or other pharmacological approaches in the management of delirium.

2 On the basis of general geriatric principles, non-pharmacological interventions that have no or less risk should be tried before any pharmacological approach.

3 If pharmacological agents are used, the lowest possible dose should be tried first, keeping in mind the goal that is intended (patient manageable and awake, not oversedated).

4 On the basis of the very limited data, the category of drug of choice *seems* to be antipsychotics, not benzodiazepines or sedative-hypnotics.

Key points

- Delirium is common among older persons in the hospital, especially in surgical patients and patients in the intensive care unit (ICU) and in post-acute care settings, but not so common among patients with acute illnesses cared for at home.
- Delirium is a dangerous diagnosis and has been found to be associated with hospital complications, loss of physical function, increased length of stay in the hospital and ICU, increased incidence of discharge from the hospital to a long-term care facility and even higher mortality.
- The comprehensive approach to delirium involves awareness, diagnosis, evaluation, prevention and management. The causes of delirium can be remembered using the two mnemonics D-E-L-I-R-I-U-M-S and A-C-U-T-E C-H-A-N-G-E I-N M-S.
- Successful prevention and management interventions include a multicomponent intervention with protocols targeting risk factors to prevent the development of delirium, a geriatric consultation service for patients with hip fracture and a specialized four-bed room to provide 24 h nursing care, called the *Delirium Room*.
- Physical restraints should not be used in patients with delirium and rarely should pharmacological restraints be used.

Table 71.5 Available clinical studies examining the use of antipsychotics in delirium[a].

Study (methods)	*N* Mean age ± SD (years) (Age range, years) Type of patients	Drugs	Placebo?	Outcome and time frame (if reported)
Breitbart, 1996[36] (prospective, blinded, randomized)	30 39 ± 9 (23–56) All patients had AIDS	Haloperidol Chlorpromazine Lorazepam	No	DRS: average scores decreased from 20 to 12 by day 2 for haloperidol and chlorpromazine. Lorazepam: 'all patients had treatment limiting adverse side effects'
Nakamura, 1997[37] (prospective, open-label, randomized)	66 68 ± 15 vs 64 ± 13 (40–92 vs 23–86) Post-surgical and medical patients	Haloperidol Mianserin	No	DRS: 70% in each group improved by day 3 (DRS scores decreased from 22 to 10 in both groups)
Sipahimalani, 1998[38] (retrospective)	22 64 ± 20 (19–89) Psychiatric consults	Haloperidol Olanzapine	No	DRS: >50% reduction in scores 5/11 haloperidol group 6/11 olanzapine group Peak response[b]: 6.8 days haloperidol; 7.2 days olanzapine
Schwartz, 2000[39] (retrospective)	22 54 vs 58 (21–74 vs 19–91) Psychiatric consults; various medical illnesses	Haloperidol Quetiapine	No	DRS: >50% reduction in scores 10/11 in both groups Peak response: 6.5 days haloperidol; 7.6 days quetiapine
Kim, 2001[40] (prospective, open-label)	20 46 ± 18 (19–74) 11/20 patients had leukaemia	Olanzapine	No	DRS: >50% decrease in scores = 14/20 Peak response: 3.8 ± 1.7 days
Breitbart, 2002[41] (prospective, open-label)	79 61 ± 17 (range 19–89) Cancer patients	Olanzapine	No	MDAS: 76% had 'resolution' by day 7 according to MDAS <10
Sasaki, 2003[42] (prospective, open-label)	12 67 ± 15 Post-surgical and medical patients	Quetiapine	No	DRS: Japanese version: 100% had resolution (DRS-J <12) Average 4.8 ± 3.5 days
Kim, 2003[43] (prospective, open-label)	12 74 ± 4 (64–88) Medical patients	Quetiapine	No	DRS: 'stable' (not clearly defined) by 5.9 ± 2 days
Parellada, 2004[44] (prospective, open-label)	64 67 ± 11 Medical patients	Risperidone	No	DRS: 90% had DRS <13 by day 3
Han, 2004[45] (prospective, blinded, randomized)	24 66 ± 8 vs 67 ± 16 Mostly medical; some fractures	Risperidone vs haloperidol	No	MDAS <13: 42% risperidone vs 75% haloperidol (no significant difference) Average time to MDAS <13 was 4 days
Liu, 2004[46] (retrospective)	77 68 ± 10 vs 50 ± 15 (40–85 vs 15–77) Psychiatric consults	Risperidone vs haloperidol	No	'Recovered' based on 10-point visual analogue scale and two psychiatrists: 7 ± 4 days risperidone 8 ± 5 days haloperidol

Table 71.5 (*continued*).

Study (methods)	*N* Mean age ± SD (years) (Age range, years) Type of patients	Drugs	Placebo?	Outcome and time frame (if reported)
Pae, 2004[47] (retrospective)	22 Mean 69 ± 10 (range 48–85) Neurosurgery, orthopaedic, oncology	Quetiapine	No	DRS: >50% decrease in scores: 19/22 Average scores from 22 to <15 in 7 ± 4 days
Lee, 2005[48] (prospective, open-label, randomized)	31 61 ± 18 vs 63 ± 15 Psychiatric consults	Amisulpride vs quetiapine	No	DRS-R-98: >50% decrease in scores 81% vs 80% 'Stabilization' based on DRS-R-98 in 6.3 vs 7.4 days
Straker, 2006[49] (prospective, open-label)	14 70 ± 11 (18–85) Medical patients	Aripiprazole	No	DRS: >50% decrease in scores 7/14 by day 5, 12/14 by day 7
Takeuchi, 2007[50] (prospective, open-label)	38 69 ± 10 Post-surgical and medical patients	Perisperone	No	DRS-R-98: >50% decrease in scores 27/38 Peak response: 5.1 ± 4.9 days

[a]Abbreviations: MDAS = Memorial Delirium Rating Scale. a 10-item scale integrating DSM-III criteria for delirium. Maximum score = 30. Scores of 10 or greater re consistent with delirium; DRS = Delirium Rating Scale, a 10-item scale integrating DSM-III criteria for delirium. Maximum score is 32. Scores of 13 or greater are consistent with delirium. DRS-R-98 = Delirium Rating Scale-Revised-98, a 16-item scale with a maximum score of 36. It is a revision of the original DRS by Trzepacz *et al.*[51]

[b]Peak response: number of days receiving an antipsychotic before achieving maximum response.

References

1. American Psychiatric Association. *Diagnostic and Statistical Manual of Mental Disorders: DSM-IV-TR*, 4th edn, American Psychiatric Association, Washington, DC, 2000.
2. Lipowski ZJ. *Delirium. Acute Brain Failure in Man*. Charles C. Thomas, Springfield, IL, 1980.
3. Maldonado JR. Pathoetiological model of delirium: a comprehensive understanding of the neurobiology of delirium and an evidence-based approach to prevention and treatment. *Crit Care Clin* 2008;**24**:789–856.
4. Inouye SK. Delirium in hospitalized older patients: recognition and risk factors. *J Geriatr Psychiatry Neurol* 1998;**11**:118–25.
5. Siddiqi N and House A. Delirium: an update on diagnosis, treatment and prevention. *Clin Med* 2006;6(6):540–3.
6. Dyer CB, Ashton CM and Teasdale TA. Postoperative delirium. A review of 80 primary data-collection studies. *Arch Intern Med* 1995;**155**:461–5.
7. Ely EW, Shintani A, Truman B *et al*. Delirium as a predictor of mortality in mechanically ventilated patients in the intensive care unit. *JAMA* 2004;**291**:1753–62.
8. Pisani MA. Considerations in caring for the critically ill older patient. *J Intensive Care Med* 2009;**24**:83–95.
9. Kelly KG, Zisselman M, Cutillo-Schmitter T *et al*. Severity and course of delirium in medically hospitalized nursing facility residents. *Am J Geriatr Psychiatry* 2001;**9**:72–7.
10. Marcantonio ER, Flacker JM, Wright RJ and Resnick NM. Reducing delirium after hip fracture: a randomized trial. *J Am Geriatr Soc* 2001;**49**:516–22.
11. Marcantonio ER, Simon SE, Bergmann MA *et al*. Delirium symptoms in post-acute care: prevalent, persistent and associated with poor functional recovery. *J Am Geriatr Soc* 2003;**51**:4–9.
12. Mentes J, Culp K, Maas M and Rantz M. Acute confusion indicators: risk factors and prevalence using MDS data. *Res Nurs Health* 1999;**22**:95–105.
13. Cacchione PZ, Culp K, Laing J and Tripp-Reimer T. Clinical profile of acute confusion in the long-term care setting. *Clin Nurs Res* 2003;**12**:145–58.
14. Caplan GA, Ward JA, Brennan NJ *et al*. Hospital in the home: a randomised controlled trial. *Med J Aust* 1999;**170**:156–60.
15. Leff B, Burton L, Guido S *et al*. Home hospital: a feasible and efficacious approach to care for acutely ill older persons. *J Am Geriatr Soc* 2004;**52**:S194.
16. Flaherty JH, Rudolph J, Shay K *et al*. Delirium is a serious and under-recognized problem: why assessment of mental status should be the 6th vital sign. *J Am Med Dir Assoc* 2007;**8**:273–5.
17. Flaherty JH. Psychotherapeutic agents in older adults. Commonly prescribed and over-the-counter remedies: causes of confusion. *Clin Geriatr Med* 1998;**14**:101–27.
18. Inouye SK, Viscoli CM, Horwitz RI *et al*. A predictive model for delirium in hospitalized elderly medical patients based on admission characteristics. *Ann Intern Med* 1993;**119**:474–81.

19. Inouye SK, Bogardus ST Jr, Charpentier PA *et al*. A multicomponent intervention to prevent delirium in hospitalized older patients. *N Engl J Med* 1999;**340**:669–76.
20. Naughton BJ, Saltzman S, Ramadan F *et al*. A multifactorial intervention to reduce prevalence of delirium and shorten hospital length of stay. *J Am Geriatr Soc* 2005;**53**:18–23.
21. Milisen K, Lemiengre J, Braes T and Foreman MD. Multicomponent intervention strategies for managing delirium in hospitalized older people. *J Adv Nurs* 2005;**52**:79–90.
22. Lundström M, Edlund A, Lundström G and Gustafson Y. Reorganization of nursing and medical care to reduce the incidence of postoperative delirium and improve rehabilitation outcome in elderly patients treated for femoral neck fractures. *Scand J Caring Sci* 1999;**13**:193–200.
23. Cole MG, McCusker J, Bellavance F *et al*. Systematic detection and multidisciplinary care of delirium in older medical inpatients: a randomized trial. *CMAJ* 2002;**167**:753–9.
24. Cole MG, Primeau FJ, Bailey RF *et al*. Systematic intervention for elderly inpatients with delirium: a randomized trial. *CMAJ* 1994;**151**:965–70.
25. Pitkälä KH, Laurila JV, Strandberg TE and Tilvis RS. Multicomponent geriatric intervention for elderly inpatients with delirium: a randomized, controlled trial. *J Gerontol A Biol Sci Med Sci* 2006;**61**:176–81.
26. Lundström M, Edlund A, Karlsson S *et al*. A multifactorial intervention program reduces the duration of delirium, length of hospitalization and mortality in delirious patients. *J Am Geriatr Soc* 2005;**53**:622–8.
27. Flaherty JH, Tariq SH, Raghavan S *et al*. A model for managing delirious older inpatients. *J Am Geriatr Soc* 2003;**51**: 1031–5.
28. Neufeld RR, Libow LS, Foley WJ *et al*. Restraint reduction reduces serious injuries among nursing home residents. *J Am Geriatr Soc* 1999;**47**:1202–7.
29. Capezuti E, Strumpf NE, Evans LK *et al*. The relationship between physical restraint removal and falls and injuries among nursing home residents. *J Gerontol Ser A Biol Sci Med Sci* 1998;**53**:M47–52.
30. Dunn KS. The effect of physical restraints on fall rates in older adults who are institutionalized. *J Gerontol Nurs* 2001;**27**:40–8.
31. Powell C, Mitchell-Pedersen L, Fingerote E and Edmund L. Freedom from restraint: consequences of reducing physical restraints in the management of the elderly. *CMAJ* 1989;**141**:561–4.
32. Mion LC, Fogel J, Sandhu S *et al*. Outcomes following physical restraint reduction programs in two acute care hospitals. *Jt Comm J Qual Improv* 2001;**27**:605–18.
33. De Vries OJ, Ligthart GJ and Nikolaus Th. European Academy of Medicine of Ageing-Course III. Differences in period prevalence of the use of physical restraints in elderly inpatients of European hospitals and nursing homes. *J Gerontol Ser A Biol Sci Med Sci* 2004;**59**:M922–3.
34. Gatz D. Moving to a restraint-free environment. *Balance* 2000;**4**:12–5.
35. Makowski TR, Maggard W and Morley JE. The Life Care Center of St. Louis experience with subacute care. *Clin Geriatr Med* 2000;**16**:701–24.
36. Breitbart W, Marotta R, Platt MM *et al*. A double-blind trial of haloperidol, chlorpromazine, and lorazepam in the treatment of delirium in hospitalized AIDS patients. *Am J Psychiatry* 1996;**153**:231–7.
37. Nakamura J, Uchimura N, Yamada S *et al*. Does plasma free-3-methoxy-4-hydroxyphenyl(ethylene)glycol increase in the delirious state? A comparison of the effects of mianserin and haloperidol on delirium. *Int Clin Psychopharmacol* 1997;**12**:147–52.
38. Sipahimalani A and Masand PS. Olanzapine in the treatment of delirium. *Psychosomatics* 1998;**39**:422–30.
39. Schwartz TL and Masand PS. Treatment of delirium with quetiapine. *Prim Care Companion J Clin Psychiatry* 2000; **2**:10–2.
40. Kim KS, Pae CU, Chae JH *et al*. An open pilot trial of olanzapine for delirium in the Korean population. *Psychiatry Clin Neurosci* 2001;**55**:515–9.
41. Breitbart W, Tremblay A and Gibson C. An open trial of olanzapine for the treatment of delirium in hospitalized cancer patients. *Psychosomatics* 2002;**43**:175–82.
42. Sasaki Y, Matsuyama T, Inoue S *et al*. A prospective, open-label, flexible-dose study of quetiapine in the treatment of delirium. *J Clin Psychiatry* 2003;**64**:1316–21.
43. Kim KY, Bader GM, Kotlyar V *et al*. Treatment of delirium in older adults with quetiapine. *J Geriatr Psychiatry Neurol* 2003;**16**:29–31.
44. Parellada E, Baeza I, de Pablo J *et al*. Risperidone in the treatment of patients with delirium. *J Clin Psychiatry* 2004; **65**:348–53.
45. Han CS and Kim YK. A double-blind trial of risperidone and haloperidol for the treatment of delirium. *Psychosomatics* 2004;**45**:297–301.
46. Liu CY, Juang YY, Liang HY *et al*. Efficacy of risperidone in treating the hyperactive symptoms of delirium. *Int Clin Psychopharmacol* 2004;**19**:165–8.
47. Pae CU, Lee SJ, Lee CU *et al*. A pilot trial of quetiapine for the treatment of patients with delirium. *Hum Psychopharmacol* 2004;**19**:125–7.
48. Lee KU, Won WY, Lee HK *et al*. Amisulpride versus quetiapine for the treatment of delirium: a randomized, open prospective study. *Int Clin Psychopharmacol* 2005;**20**: 311–4.
49. Straker DA, Shapiro PA, Muskin PR. Aripiprazole in the treatment of delirium. *Psychosomatics* 2006;**47**:385–91.
50. Takeuchi T, Furuta K, Hirasawa T. Perospirone in the treatment of patients with delirium. *Psychiatry Clin Neurosci* 2007;**61**:67–70.
51. Trzepacz PT, Mittal D, Torres R *et al*. Validation of the Delirium Rating Scale-revised-98: comparison with the delirium rating scale and the cognitive test for delirium. *J Neuropsychiatry Clin Neurosci* 2001;**13**:229–42.

CHAPTER 72

Memory clinics

Antony Bayer
Cardiff University, Cardiff and University Hospital Llandough, Penarth, UK

Introduction

Clinics specifically for the diagnosis and management of early dementia were first developed in the USA in the late 1970s. These were primarily research based, linked to developing Alzheimer's disease (AD) and ageing research centres and acted as a focus for expert assessment, investigation, treatment and advice.[1] Initially described as 'dementia clinics', the terminology soon changed to the more acceptable name of 'memory clinics' or 'memory assessment clinics'. Although the new titles are less stigmatizing, they run the risk of serving as a euphemism, avoiding an open and honest approach to the reality of dementia.

Predominantly service-oriented memory clinics were set up in the UK in the early 1980s,[2,3] offering multidisciplinary, outpatient-based assessment and diagnosis for mainly older people with memory and other cognitive problems, in an acceptable and accessible environment. At first, many of these clinics were funded from outside the National Health Service and were based mainly in university departments of geriatric medicine or old age psychiatry. Existing services tended to consider memory clinics to be a luxury, allowing academics to indulge their narrow clinical interests away from the reality of budgetary considerations and the priorities of practical dementia care. However, this reflected the concentration of service provision on dealing with the behavioural and psychological symptoms of advanced dementia and on crisis intervention and institutional-based management. The first memory clinics played an important role in raising awareness of the value of elective intervention and interdisciplinary care for people with early dementia and acted as a focus for the development of specialist knowledge and expertise in early diagnosis and management of people presenting with cognitive impairment.

Most of the early UK clinics were also very actively involved in research, especially recruitment into clinical trials of the emerging anti-dementia drugs. Largely thanks to the work of these centres, specific drug treatment for AD became available in the late 1990s and the focus of activity shifted towards the provision of an effective clinical service for patients presenting with memory disturbances and best use of medication, together with psychosocial interventions and patient and carer support and education.[4] The evolution of hospital-based memory clinics into more community-based memory teams was the natural consequence, working alongside or as an independent part of traditional mental health teams for older people.

Initially criticized for being too academic and isolated from mainstream practice, and ill-equipped to provide care after diagnosis, memory clinics have now become an integral part of quality dementia assessment and care services. The clinical guideline on the management of dementia published by the UK National Institute for Health and Clinical Excellence (NICE) and the Social Care Institute for Excellence (SCIE) in 2006 recommended the development of memory assessment services as the single point of referral for all people with a possible diagnosis of dementia.[5] They were seen as providing a responsive service to aid early identification, including a full range of assessment, diagnostic, therapeutic and rehabilitation services and an integrated approach to the care of people with dementia and the support of their carers, in partnership with local health, social care and voluntary organizations. The National Dementia Strategy in England, published in 2009,[6] suggested that memory clinics might form the core of new services for early diagnosis and identification of dementia in 'every town and city' in the country.

Although most memory clinics focus on the diagnosis of early dementia and mild cognitive impairment (MCI), some have a broader remit, whereas others target people with purely subjective memory loss or younger people with early-onset dementia or people with learning disabilities. Many concentrate on diagnosis and assessment with a view to best use of available medication and those in academic centres continue to conduct a lot of research, including clinical trials of newer drug treatments. The emphasis on assessment for drug treatment should not detract from

Principles and Practice of Geriatric Medicine, Fifth Edition. Edited by Alan J. Sinclair, John E. Morley and Bruno Vellas.

the importance of providing the holistic, multiprofessional and multiagency approach to dementia care that should be central to the activity of all clinics.

Referral may be open access (those willing to see all-comers) or restricted to secondary or tertiary referrals or to selected individuals who meet predetermined criteria. In general, patients referred by their general practitioners (GPs) seem more likely to have dementia than self-referrals, although the reassurance given to those without organic disease (the 'worried well') should not be underestimated.[7] Memory clinics should never be merely rebranded old age psychiatry outpatient clinics or community-based services solely monitoring anti-dementia drugs.

Developments around the world

Memory clinics are now a feature of health services for older people in centres around the world, but they vary in terms of case mix, types of activity undertaken, whether they are primarily based in neurology, psychiatry or geriatric settings and their interface with other relevant agencies. Nearly all involve multiprofessional assessment, often with everyone coming together to share results in a diagnostic consensus meeting. The subsequent input into long-term support and follow-up can be very different, with some clinics seeing diagnosis and immediate care as the limit of their responsibility and others taking on the role of planning optimal long-term management. Memory clinics are sometimes the centre of a broad model of care, with preliminary home visits by a nurse and/or psychologist before clinic attendance and further home visits afterwards to discuss assessment results and plan future management.

In some countries, sometimes with government support, networks of clinics have developed to coordinate clinical, research and educational activity related to dementia. For example, in The Netherlands, memory clinics are well established and have led to the development of quality markers to facilitate description and comparison of activities and quality standards.[8] Most Dutch clinics actively involve the general practitioner, routinely provide a home assessment visit and have a strong research emphasis. In France, the national Alzheimer Plan has supported a major effort to ensure that each health district has its own memory unit (Consultation Mémoire) for dementia diagnosis and follow-up, building upon the expert memory clinics developed in the 1990s. At a regional level there are specialist Centres Mémoire de Ressources et de Recherche (CMRR), providing diagnosis in the most complex cases and delivering research and training. Other initiatives have included use of standard assessment and follow-up documentation, common educational projects and multicentre clinical research projects.

In Switzerland there is a collaborative group of memory clinics, enabling an active programme of education and training for health professionals and clinical research. The primary care doctor plays an important role in initial assessment before comprehensive diagnosis and treatment recommendations are made in the memory clinic, including memory training and caregiver support activities. There is also close involvement with the national Alzheimer's Association. The limited number of memory clinics in Germany and Austria are mainly university based and research oriented and are not covered by statutory health insurance, so have yet to become a standard component of local dementia care. In rural and isolated areas in Europe, the structures necessary to provide services are often lacking and novel approaches are therefore needed. For example, in Lapland there is a memory clinic bus which tours around offering memory testing and counselling services.

In the southern hemisphere, memory clinics providing multidisciplinary assessment and management for community-living people with dementia are developing in every continent, although still mainly based within the private sector or university centres in the larger cities. In Australia, a government-funded regional network of Cognitive, Dementia and Memory Services (CDAMS) were established in the 1990s across the state of Victoria, although elsewhere in the country the development of memory clinics has been more sporadic. The multicultural nature of Australian society presents particular challenges to ensure equity of assessment, service provision and utilization and highlights the need for clinics to be sensitive to the needs of people from a range of cultural and linguistic backgrounds,[9] a challenge also being addressed in many clinics in North America and Southeast Asia.

Why the need?

The worldwide growth in memory clinics has largely developed because of increasing demand and expectations of patients and families, frustrated by the difficulties of obtaining informed diagnosis and advice from existing services. They are not a replacement or alternative to these, but rather a more focused service providing a consistent approach to assessment, more specific diagnosis and a single resource for expert information and support (Table 72.1). Demographic changes are rapidly leading to greater numbers of patients with age-related cognitive disorders and there is appropriate reluctance to attribute forgetfulness merely to age. The growing awareness that memory failure is not inevitable and that effective intervention is available has led to a desire for comprehensive assessment, diagnosis, advice and treatment to be provided by professionals with specific expertise.

In many areas, existing services for diagnosis and management of memory disorders have been inadequate, with no clear professional responsibility and a widespread lack of specialist expertise and experience. There is a growing

Table 72.1 Potential benefits of memory clinics.

Benefits for patients and families
Non-stigmatizing, specialist resource breaking down potential barriers to recognition/diagnosis
Increases choice and improves patient experience and engagement
Expert multidisciplinary assessment and diagnosis of cognitive disorders
Ensures treatable conditions are not overlooked
Early identification of dementia and intervention
Anti-dementia drugs are effectively targeted, monitored and stopped as appropriate
Education and practical support for patients and carers
Empowers people with dementia while they are still able to maintain control over their lives
Provides advice on memory aids and memory training
Opportunities for counselling and psychosocial management
Improves quality of life by promoting and maintaining independence for as long as possible
Continuing care in the community may reduce need for institutionalization
Access to research studies
Benefits for service provision
Addresses growing demand for specialist diagnosis and treatment
Encourages earlier referral and multidisciplinary management
Develops awareness of dementia in primary care
Cost-effective way of significantly increasing the number of people able to be seen
Provides standardized assessment and diagnosis
Gateway to services
Efficient targeting and monitoring of scarce resources (including medication and psychosocial interventions)
Expertise in legal and ethical issues
Facilitates audit, planning and evaluation of services
Elective decisions may help to avoid crises in care
May reduce hospitalizations and lengths of stay
Postponement of institutionalization may reduce costs
Focus for professional education and research activity

appreciation of the complexity of the needs of these patients and that optimal assessment and management requires a multidisciplinary rather than a monodisciplinary approach.

Even in expert hands, assessment and management of mild cognitive disturbance are not always straightforward, with a difficult differential diagnosis ranging from the trivial to the very serious and from the easily reversible to the irreversible. Not all forgetful old people have dementia and not all demented old people have AD (Table 72.2). Comprehensive assessment reduces the chances of inappropriate labelling. There is a multiplicity of available assessment tools and investigations and, without access to the definitive diagnostic test of histopathology, some informed selection needs to be made. Once a working diagnosis has been reached, there is also a wide spectrum of available medical,

Table 72.2 Diagnoses to be considered in people presenting to memory clinics.

Neurodegenerative dementias
Alzheimer's disease
Dementia with Lewy bodies
Parkinson's disease dementia
Fronto-temporal dementia
Frontal variant
Primary progressive aphasia
Semantic dementia
Parkinson's-plus syndromes
Progressive supranuclear palsy
Corticobasal degeneration
Multiple system atrophy
Huntington's disease
Mild cognitive impairment (MCI)
Amnestic single-domain MCI
Amnestic multi-domain MCI
Non-amnestic single-domain MCI
Non-amnestic multi-domain MCI
Vascular cognitive impairment
Single stroke
Strategic infarct
Multiple cortical infarction
Multiple subcortical lacunes
CADASIL
Cerebral amyloid angiopathy (CAA)
Haemodynamic dementia
Neurological
Tumour
Normal pressure hydrocephalus
Multiple sclerosis
Motor neurone disease
Paraneoplastic
Mitochondrial encephalopathies
Learning disability
Post-traumatic
Subdural haematoma
Post-head injury
Dementia pugilistica
Functional/psychiatric
Depression
Anxiety
Stress and overwork
Adjustment disorder
Delusional disorder
Alzheimer phobia
Drugs/toxins
Prescribed medication
Alcohol-related
Substance abuse

(continued overleaf)

Table 72.2 (*continued*).

Endocrine/metabolic
Hypo-/hyperthyroidism
Hypo-/hyperparathyroidism
Hypo-/hyperadrenalism
Hepatic failure
Renal failure
Vitamin B_{12} deficiency
Thiamine deficiency/Korsakoff syndrome
Inflammatory
Rheumatoid cerebrovasculitis
Lupus cerebrovasculitis
Neurosarcoidosis
Infection
Post-encephalitis
HIV/AIDS
Neurosyphilis
Prion dementia (CJD)

psychological and social interventions that require tailoring to the individual.

The availability of specific drug treatment for AD and some other dementias and the need to identify suitable patients and to monitor drug efficacy are the most obvious justifications for early diagnosis. However, the emphasis on a medical model of care and the perceived influence of the pharmaceutical industry in driving forward the expansion of memory clinics should not detract from the broader psychosocial benefits of early recognition and intervention.

Although reversible dementia is uncommon, nearly all patients will have problems that can be helped and appropriate intervention can be instigated at a stage when it is likely to be most effective. A positive diagnosis reduces the risk of inappropriate management and avoids wrong assumptions being made. It empowers people with dementia to become involved in decision-making while they are still able to do so. The opportunities for forward planning may improve the psychosocial health of carers and also help to lessen the risk of crises in care at a later stage. Certainly a proactive approach is likely to be more efficient and also more humane than one that is crisis driven.

Are they effective?

In common with most health service developments, the rapid growth in memory clinics has occurred despite lack of evidence of effectiveness from randomized controlled comparisons with usual care. However, lack of evidence does not mean that they are ineffective and, given growing societal pressures and the considerable evidence on the effectiveness of the individual elements of memory clinics, the odds are in favour of their benefit.[10] A recent model suggested that memory services need only achieve a modest increase in average quality of life of people with dementia, plus a 10% diversion of people with dementia from residential care, to be cost-effective.[11] There is certainly evidence that community-living older people with cognitive impairment have fewer hospitalizations and nights hospitalized if their problem is diagnosed, compared with those who have never received such a diagnosis.[12]

Two completed randomized controlled trials have looked at the benefits of diagnosis of dementia in a memory clinic. A cluster randomized trial in The Netherlands showed that in comparison with usual care, an integrated multidisciplinary approach to dementia diagnosis in a hospital-based memory clinic setting increased health-related quality of life of the dementia patients for at least 12 months.[13] An Australian trial looked at the quality of life for carers of community-dwelling patients with mild to moderate dementia, who were randomized to attend a memory clinic or act as a control group. Those carers attending the memory clinic were found to have significant improvement in psychosocial health-related quality of life, particularly in the domains of alertness behaviour and social interaction, which was maintained at 12 months. However, there was no significant improvement in carer burden or knowledge of dementia.[14] The ongoing AD-Euro trial is comparing the clinical and cost effectiveness of post-diagnostic dementia guidance and treatment by memory clinics to usual care.[15]

Luce *et al.*[16] compared consecutive referrals to the memory clinic in Newcastle upon Tyne with referrals to the traditional and well-established old age psychiatry service in the same city. Memory clinic patients were younger, had lower levels of cognitive impairment and a wider range of diagnoses, with those diagnosed as having dementia being at least 2 years earlier in the course of the disease than those seen in the standard service. The authors concluded that memory clinics target a distinct patient group compared with traditional old age psychiatry services, identifying cases of dementia much earlier and having the potential to make valuable contributions to patient care in terms of access to treatments, services and support networks and in terms of obtaining information and preparing for the future.

Another British study in the more rural area of Dorset[17] compared consecutive new referrals to a memory clinic with consecutive new domiciliary requests within the same old age psychiatry service over the same period of time. The clinic patients had fewer behavioural and psychological symptoms of dementia, but were otherwise similar in demographic and clinical characteristics. Subsequently they were less likely to have a psychotropic drug prescribed, but were more likely to have documented risk management, care planning and follow-up, with a trend towards fewer moves into residential care and psychiatric ward admissions.

Surveys of memory clinic users' opinions of their experiences are generally very positive. van Hout *et al.*[18] used questionnaires with patients, relatives and GPs to measure their perception of the quality of care of an outpatient memory clinic. Positive opinions were recorded on the way in which the results were communicated, the usefulness of the assessment and the attitude of the clinicians. In contrast to GPs and relatives, patients were less positive about the clarity of the diagnostic information received and both relatives and GPs were negative on information and advice given to relatives. A subsequent study by the same researchers highlighted the importance of providing information not only on issues considered relevant by clinicians, but also tailored to the individual needs of patients and carers.[19] An Australian study of GPs' satisfaction with services provided by memory clinics also found them to be positive about the completeness and utility of the assessment and diagnostic information provided, but relatively less satisfied with advice regarding the family's coping and community support services for the patient.[20] It was considered that the service enhanced the capacity of GPs to provide ongoing care to people with dementia, but that the establishment of firmer communication and collaborative protocols between the clinics and GPs would improve their usefulness.

The memory clinic team

In order to provide a comprehensive service, memory clinics are characteristically multidisciplinary in nature, with a number of different professionals, each offering a particular expertise. Involvement is often based less on possession of any specific sub-specialist qualification than on interest and knowledge. In some centres the medical input may be from a geriatrician, in others from a neurologist and in others from a psychiatrist. Ideally there should be all three specialties involved. The other constant member of the memory clinic team tends to be a psychologist, not just to carry out neuropsychological assessment to aid diagnosis and management, but also to advise on and to undertake psychosocial interventions with both patient and family. Another invaluable team member is a specialist nurse, who can help with both the medical and psychological assessment and management. This can be carried out beyond the physical confines of the clinic, facilitating and reinforcing the process in the patient's own environment. Finally, dedicated administrative help is essential, not only to ensure the efficient running of the clinic, but also to cope with the forgetful patients who phone repeatedly to check the time of their appointments.

Beyond these core team members, there needs to be easy access to other professionals, such as speech and language therapists, occupational therapists and social workers. Increasingly there is also a need for someone competent to provide genetic counselling and advice to worried relatives. Developments in drug therapy suggest an important potential role for the pharmacist and newer diagnostic techniques may require greater involvement of radiologists and neurophysiologists. Volunteers and support workers from the local Alzheimer's Society are becoming closely associated with some clinics, providing additional practical support and counselling to newly diagnosed patients and their families.

The optimum size of the team is likely to be between four and seven, united by a common feeling of direction and purpose. Although each member should be able to identify the specific and general contribution they can make, a flexible working style which crosses conventional professional boundaries will provide greatest job satisfaction and most effective care for patients.

As in other aspects of geriatric practice, getting the multidisciplinary team to work effectively is essential for the smooth running of the clinic. Good teamwork takes time to develop and whoever is the team leader (usually the senior physician or psychiatrist) needs to strike a balance between over-structuring clinic activities and allowing individuals to function totally independently. The team will not work effectively when one particular professional (or profession) considers the guarding of their perceived area of expertise as a priority, setting up artificial borders which others fear to cross. A belief in the importance of professional hierarchies, concerns over territory and differences in terminology will act as barriers to effective care delivery and can lead to wasteful duplication of effort and apparently contradictory management advice. Individual members should be encouraged to view the value of their contribution as depending on the functioning of the whole team.

What happens in a memory clinic?

There would seem to be general agreement that a memory clinic can provide in one setting all the essential components of comprehensive assessment leading to diagnosis for older people presenting with memory problems, followed by appropriate interventions (Table 72.3). The assessment will include full history and medical examination, detailed neuropsychological and neurobehavioural assessment and appropriate laboratory tests and neuroimaging. Some clinics have a totally standardized approach, where everyone gets everything, whereas others will tailor the assessments to what is specifically indicated and what has not been done before. Whereas some clinics will restrict themselves to a one-off evaluation, confirming a diagnosis and perhaps recommending an appropriate intervention, others will aim to provide ongoing support and more comprehensive management. Certainly diagnosis divorced from effective intervention is likely to be unsatisfactory for all.

Table 72.3 Stages in memory clinic evaluation and management.

History (from patient and reliable informant), including functional and social background
Cognitive assessment (and mood)
Relevant physical examination
Investigations (including neuroimaging)
Formulate diagnosis and discuss appropriately (with patient and family with consent)
Provide relevant written information and contact details of local contacts
Consider management options:

- Treat comorbid medical conditions appropriately
- Review existing medication and consider anti-dementia drugs
- Ensure good nutrition and hydration
- Psychotherapeutic interventions
- Memory aids and problem-solving skills
- Safety issues (including driving) and promotion of independence
- Legal and financial/estate planning and eligibility for benefits
- Social interventions (home care, social clubs, respite)
- Carer education and practical and emotional support

Arrange appropriate follow-up

Clinics should be held close to the community they serve. Holding them away from the stigmatising settings of geriatric or psychiatric hospitals will help to encourage referral and attendance. Remembering to keep appointments is an obvious problem for this client group and sending reminders a few days before and asking people to confirm that they will be coming will help to reduce non-attendance. Forewarning people about how long the assessment will take is advisable. In some clinics assessments take all day, moving from one professional to another, and many patients find this tiring and cannot cooperate fully. Some psychometric tests need to be repeated at a set interval, so initial assessment will require more than one visit. Certainly, given the gravity of the potential diagnoses, a case can be made for all patients to be tested on at least two occasions a few weeks apart. We have found that a maximum of 60–90 min per visit (of which 30 min may be taken up with cognitive testing) is optimum.

Patients should be asked to come with someone who knows them well and can provide corroborative background. The presence of a close relative or carer will also help to ensure that advice and information provided in the clinic are acted upon. Ideally there need to be two clinic rooms, allowing an opportunity for patient and informant to talk separately to different team members.

History and medical examination

The essential first step in clinic assessment must be to obtain a detailed and accurate history. Cognitive impairment in elderly patients is often unrecognized. A patient who superficially appears alert, pleasant and cooperative and denies any significant symptoms is too often assumed to have no problems and mild dementia is easily overlooked. Establishing the reason for referral is a good place to start.

The onset and duration of symptoms are crucial and claims that difficulties date from some seemingly relevant event such as an accident, bereavement or hospital admission must not be accepted unquestioningly. Often a sudden change in circumstances merely draws attention for the first time to pre-existing problems. Changes in role are often of significance and questions should be asked about loss of competence in everyday skills and activities (e.g. driving, travelling away from home, handling correspondence and finances, taking medication regularly). The nature and progress of any changes should be established.

It is essential to take a history from both the patient and from a carer or friend (a neighbour may be of more value than an uninvolved relative) and specific examples of practical difficulties should be elicited. Associated mood disturbances, personality change and behavioural difficulties must be sought. Specific questions should be asked about delusions and hallucinations. Present and past consumption of alcohol, use of prescribed and non-prescribed drugs and the patient's general medical condition need to be established. A family history may give pointers to the diagnosis and sometimes explains a patient's excessive concern or apprehension. Much useful information is often available in previous medical records.

The Cambridge Mental Disorder of the Elderly Examination (CAMDEX) attempts to standardise the clinical information gathered in the course of a diagnostic interview with history being obtained from both the patient and a relative. Some details are therefore duplicated, but it serves as a useful starting place for those less confident in eliciting all the relevant issues. Informant questionnaires, such as the Informant Questionnaire on Cognitive Decline in the Elderly (IQCODE) can be completed by relatives before clinic attendance as an aid to establishing their report of changes in everyday cognitive function compared with 10 years before. Numerous other assessment scales, for example of neuropsychiatric symptoms, depression, activities of daily living, quality of life and carer burden, are available[21] and can be incorporated into clinic practice. They are valuable as an objective basis for documenting change and as a source of data for audit and research.

A medical examination, with particular attention to the cardiovascular system, central nervous system and special senses (eyes and ears) is also required. This may help to elucidate the cause of the memory problems, may identify physical consequences of the condition (poor nutrition, neglected personal hygiene, signs of physical abuse) or may identify coexisting morbidities. Focal neurological signs will suggest vascular disease or a space-occupying lesion and extrapyramidal signs will raise the possibility of Parkinson's disease or dementia with Lewy bodies (DLB). Primitive reflexes (e.g. palmo-mental, grasp, pout, rooting) are common in most forms of dementia, although not always easy to elicit. Myoclonus may be seen in prion disease, Huntington's disease and early-onset AD and muscle fasciculation may suggest motor neurone disease associated with fronto-temporal dementia (FTD).

Cognitive assessment

Following the history, an objective assessment of cognitive functioning is required. This will aim to establish strengths and weaknesses of a variety of functions relative to a standardized, norm-referenced scoring system. In this way, the nature and extent of cognitive deficits can be determined, informing diagnosis and management and acting as a comparator for past and future assessments. Ideally an experienced psychologist should undertake testing, although much useful information can still be obtained by any suitably trained professional. The Addenbrooke's Cognitive Examination Revised (ACE-R)[22] is an easy to use and acceptable screening measure with good sensitivity and specificity in clinic settings and incorporates the Mini Mental State Examination (MMSE) and clock face drawing. A simple screen of executive function, such as verbal fluency, will help to identify subcortical deficits. When possible, assessment should be made of premorbid intellectual status, to assist in the satisfactory interpretation of other test scores. Tests must also be appropriately selected to take account of limitations imposed by deficits such as language impairment and dyspraxia. For example, recognition memory tests may reduce the demand on expressive language, normally required in recall memory tests. A standardized measure of mood is also desirable.

There is a very wide choice of psychometric tests suitable for use with memory clinic patients and choice will be governed by the main purpose of the examination and the time available, and also personal preference and experience. Computer-based assessment of cognitive function is becoming more available and has the advantage of being sensitive to small changes in performance and allowing detailed assessment of attention and motor responses. At present its use is still confined mainly to research settings. An outline of the assessments used routinely in the Cardiff memory clinics is shown in Table 72.4.

Whatever tests are chosen, they must be acceptable to the person being tested and with no content that belittles their adult status. Consent to the assessment procedure needs to be obtained and the tester should spend some time in explanation of the purpose of specific tests and be competent to answer queries regarding their usefulness and acceptability. Sensory and physical limitations should be accommodated as much as possible, by the provision of adequate lighting, additional specialist earphone amplifiers, suitable seating and minimum distractions. During testing, realistic reassurance should be provided, with feedback phrased positively to highlight strengths as much as weaknesses. At the end of testing, patients should be given an opportunity to make their own observations on their performance.

Table 72.4 Cognitive tests commonly used in the memory clinics in Cardiff.

Premorbid ability
National Adult Reading Test (NART)
Cognitive screen/test battery
Mini-Mental State Examination (MMSE)
Addenbrooke's Cognitive Examination Revised (ACE-R)
Repeatable Battery for the Assessment of Neuropsychological Status (RBANS)
Frontal Assessment Battery (FAB)
Specific cognitive abilities
Story recall (immediate and delayed)
Irving Names Learning Test (NLT)
Kendrick Cognitive Tests (object learning and digit copying)
Rey–Osterrieth Complex Figure Test (ROCF)
Clock drawing
Verbal fluency (controlled oral word association test and category)
Trail-making Test A and B
Graded Naming Test (GNT)
Mood
Geriatric Depression Scale (GDS-15)

Observations of the person's concentration, cooperation, anxiety and motivation during assessment should be carefully weighed against performance. The approach of the patient to each test and his or her satisfaction with the outcome is often as revealing as the particular score obtained. Results should be considered in the context of the patient's previous education and experience, their age and presence of sensory impairments and comorbidity and diagnostic cut-offs for each score treated as guides rather than absolutes. In particular, a 'normal' score does not exclude the possibility of significant problems, including dementia. In such cases, more detailed testing will often reveal minor detriments in a range of tests, which are inconsistent with the patient's expected level of functioning. It is nearly always desirable, and sometimes essential, for assessment to be repeated at a future date in order to detect any progressive deterioration. Longitudinal follow-up increases the accuracy of diagnosis, particularly in mild dementia.

Laboratory tests

A routine screening battery of laboratory tests will be indicated in most patients when first seen.[5] These should include a full blood count, urea and electrolytes, liver function tests, calcium and phosphate, random blood glucose, thyroid function and vitamin B_{12} and folate. A more extensive range of tests may be indicated in younger people with dementia and in those with atypical presentations or signs and evidence of systemic illness. These might include plasma viscosity or C-reactive protein and autoantibodies for inflammatory disease and tumour markers for malignancy and paraneoplastic syndromes. Syphilis serology is now not carried out as a routine, but still needs to be considered. Genetic testing, for example for apolipoprotein genotype, is not yet diagnostically useful, but may be rarely indicated to look for known APP and PS-1 and PS-2 mutations when familial dementia is suspected. It should only be undertaken after appropriate counselling, preferably in collaboration with a specialist genetics service.

An electrocardiogram is desirable in any patient with possible vascular disease and in patients with a bradycardia or history of dysrhythmia who are being considered for acetylcholinesterase inhibitor (AChEI) drug treatment. An electroencephalogram is rarely indicated, but may be useful in suspected encephalitis, metabolic encephalopathy, seizures or prion disease and in confirming the presence or absence of delirium, in which it is almost always abnormal. Examination of cerebrospinal fluid is indicated in patients with suspected infectious, inflammatory, autoimmune or demyelinating disease and is used in some centres to measure amyloid and tau levels to improve diagnosis of early AD and identify patients with MCI who are more likely to convert. In normal pressure hydrocephalus (NPH), lumbar puncture may help to predict suitability for surgery. Rarely, nerve conduction studies may help to diagnose FTD associated with motor neurone disease, muscle biopsy may be useful in mitochondrial disorders and even cerebral biopsy may be justified in suspected primary cerebral vasculitis.

Neuroimaging

The role of neuroimaging in the routine management of memory clinic patients is largely determined by its availability. Certainly neuroimaging no longer merely fulfils the negative role of excluding 'treatable' conditions that mimic or cause dementia, but contributes positively to differential diagnosis and provides useful prognostic information. Depending on availability, computed tomography (CT), magnetic resonance imaging (MRI) and single photon emission computed tomography (SPECT) might all contribute to clinical care. Various other techniques are available in research centres. Recent diagnostic guidelines suggest that at least one structural CT or MRI examination should be made over the course of a dementing illness to rule out space-occupying or vascular lesions and that SPECT (or PET) may be used in cases of significant diagnostic uncertainty.[5]

Imaging with CT is probably the radiological investigation most often used in memory clinic patients, owing to its wide availability. It can show good detail of the brain structure and is especially useful in identifying dementia due to space-occupying lesions, hydrocephalus or large cerebral infarcts. Smaller lacunar infarcts are less easily seen and absence of infarcts does not exclude the possibility of vascular disease. Cortical atrophy is a common finding in older patients, not necessarily associated with clinically abnormal brain function. Some patients with AD will have a normal scan, but the presence of medial temporal lobe atrophy is usual. The presence of localized atrophy will also lend support to diagnoses of FTDs and focal syndromes such as posterior cortical atrophy. Overall, CT may be expected to impact on diagnosis and treatment in about one in eight of dementia cases.

MRI is less widely available, less tolerated by patients and more expensive than CT. However, contrast sensitivity and spatial resolution are better, even without the use of contrast agents, and it does not suffer from bone artefacts. Evidence of generalized atrophy is no more diagnostically useful than with CT, but measurement of the size of the hippocampus and entorhinal cortex plays an important role not only in diagnosis of AD, but also in identifying patients with mild cognitive impairment who are at risk of progressing to dementia. Smaller infarcts can be seen more clearly than with CT and MRI has the potential to detect focal signal abnormalities that may assist the clinical differentiation between AD and vascular dementia (VaD). Severe temporal lobe atrophy and hyperintensities involving the hippocampal or insular cortex are more frequently noted in AD. Basal ganglionic/thalamic hyperintense foci, thromboembolic infarctions, confluent white matter and irregular periventricular hyperintensities (leukoencephalopathy) are more common in VaD. Leukoencephalopathy involving at least 25% of the total white matter must be present to diagnose small-vessel cerebrovascular disease.

Functional imaging using HMPAO-SPECT allows regional cerebral blood flow to be visualized and quantified. In established AD there is a reduction of flow in mainly temporo-parietal regions, although this finding is inconsistent in the early stage of the disease when diagnosis is most problematic. In FTD, SPECT shows diminished perfusion anteriorly. In VaD, multiple focal deficits may be seen. FP-CIT SPECT distinguishes DLB and Parkinson's syndromes from AD. PET scans are largely limited to research centres. FDG-PET shows characteristic alterations in cerebral glucose metabolism early in AD and FTD. PET imaging of amyloid binding (PIB-PET) appears to be highly sensitive and specific for AD, even at preclinical stages. This seems likely to play an important role in diagnosis and treatment decisions in future years.[23]

What interventions can be offered?

At the very least, patients assessed in memory clinics should receive an informed discussion of their diagnosis and prognosis, with arrangements made for ongoing review, support and management. In a few patients, there will be a reversible cause for their symptoms (e.g. medication side effects, hypothyroidism, vitamin B_{12} deficiency, cerebral vasculitis, Wernicke–Korsakoff syndrome) that will respond to specific treatment. The proportion of patients with reversible dementia is probably less than 4%, but concurrent medical conditions causing mild cognitive disturbances are much more common and are potentially treatable.[24] Although treatment of these conditions may not always lead to complete resolution of cognitive symptoms, it is important to identify any concomitant conditions to avoid unnecessary disability and misdiagnosis.

Depression, whether primary or secondary, is especially deserving of energetic treatment, generally using a selective serotonin reuptake inhibitor (SSRI), such as citalopram or sertraline, or the noradrenergic and specific serotonergic antidepressant (NaSSA) mirtazapine, that are free of significant cognitive side effects. Even in patients with established dementia, appropriate medical intervention may help cognition and slow progression of the disease. Control of vascular risk factors, especially hypertension, may favourably influence the clinical course of both degenerative and vascular cognitive impairment. Timely use of specific drug treatments for AD and probably VaD and DLB will give significant benefit to a majority of patients taking them.

Certainly all patients with cognitive difficulties and their carers will benefit from informed discussion about their problems and appropriate psychosocial interventions.[25] Advice can be given on the appropriate use of memory aids, memory training and specific psychological interventions for patients and families. Financial and legal advice will usually be appropriate and practical suggestions to help with problems of daily living and safety concerns, particularly the advisability of continued driving. Issues surrounding advanced directives are attracting growing attention. Meeting the needs of carers is also important, by providing information, individual counselling, access to support groups and respite care through contact with local Alzheimer's organizations and relevant community services.

Diagnostic disclosure and meeting information needs

Most advocates for people with dementia and their carers now believe that, in most cases, patients should be told what is wrong with them, what the implications are, what can be done for them and what treatment is likely to involve. Breaking the news in a timely and tactful manner is an important role for memory clinic staff. Reactions of AD patients to being told their diagnosis include relief (as the diagnosis provides an explanation for their difficulties), disbelief (as they may lack insight and do not feel ill), loss (grieving for failing intellectual abilities and limitations in the future) and fear of becoming a burden. All can be satisfactorily addressed.

Practice of diagnosis disclosure amongst specialists is changing. In the 1990s, less than one-third of old age psychiatrists and geriatricians 'usually told' people with mild dementia their diagnosis, whereas recent studies report that a majority of specialists now regularly disclose diagnosis.

Memory clinic patients should be given the opportunity to learn as much or as little as they want to know about their condition, with information provided in a sensitive and measured way[26] (Table 72.5). Patients and carers both have individual needs and each should be addressed separately. In addition to clearly describing diagnosis, specific attention should be given to comprehensible and practical information about coping strategies, care services, likely course of the disease and treatment, specific drug treatment and follow-up. Wald *et al.*[27] proposed the 'rule of threes' for information provision to carers of people with dementia. At diagnosis, they want information about what dementia is, what medications are available and explanation about behavioural and psychiatric symptoms of dementia. At an early follow-up appointment, they want information about services, the course of the illness and what to do in a crisis. At a later follow-up appointment, they want information about support groups, benefits and financial and legal issues. At a later stage, they want information about psychological therapies, the effects of the illness on carers and complementary therapies.

Information giving is not only a medical responsibility. All members of the multidisciplinary team should consider every therapeutic encounter to be an opportunity for education and information provision. Dedicated time should be put aside during every memory clinic consultation for information provision – it should never be merely an after-thought at the end of the assessment. Verbal information should be backed up by written information, with recommendations for further reading. Increasingly people are turning to the Internet for more detailed information and trustworthy websites should be recommended to those interested. Mention should be made of local support groups and meetings and contact details of local Alzheimer support organizations. A telephone contact number for information and advice is always appreciated and unlikely to be abused.

Memory aids

The most simple and effective methods of helping patients with cognitive difficulties are the establishment of regular

Table 72.5 Recommendations for telling a diagnosis of dementia to patients and family.

Communication of the diagnosis should ordinarily occur in a *joint meeting with patient and family*
Use *simple language*. Avoid technical jargon that may conceal the truth
Use a graded approach that is patient led and allows the information given to be matched to what the patient wants to know
Allow sufficient time to explain and to answer questions from the patient and family
Assess the patient's and the family 's *understanding* and arrange *follow-up* (to reinforce information provided, clarify misunderstandings and answer questions that are outstanding)
Use the term 'Alzheimer's disease' (or other appropriate medical diagnosis) rather than just dementia and ensure that they understand the sense of both terms
Mellow the bad news with the possibility of therapeutic approaches (not just drugs). Avoid conveying the feeling that 'nothing more can be done'
Make it clear that a reorganized family network can *alleviate burden and maintain quality of life*
Inform the patient about the possibility of taking decisions about his/her future.

Adapted from OPDAL Study Group.[26]

routines, the careful organization of daily activities and the use of environmental cues and external memory aids. None of these require the patient to learn new strategies of thinking or remembering and may therefore be potentially useful in those with even moderately severe dementia. Written aids such as diaries, checklists and carefully positioned notes as reminders are often of benefit and reusable sticky note pads are ideal for sticking in conspicuous places. Labelling or colour coding of switches and doors may sometimes be helpful. A timer or digital alarm watch may act as a reminder to take medication, to attend to cooking or other household tasks or to refer to an appointments diary for guidance as to planned activities. In the kitchen, use of a microwave cooker may avoid food being incinerated in a conventional oven, red warning lights on electrical appliances may help to remind when they are on and use of kettles that whistle may ensure that a planned cup of tea is made and prevent open pans boiling dry. More sophisticated electronic devices and programmable organizers are generally too unfamiliar to the present generation of older people to prove useful, but assistive technology that does not require the person to operate it is attracting much interest. Such telecare can be used to monitor people's activities and trigger an alarm if there is a potential risk, such as flooding from taps left running, gas left on or leaving the house unexpectedly. Sensors and tracking devices can follow people's movements, but raise ethical issues if informed consent cannot be obtained.

Memory training

The idea of cognitive training as a method of improving, retaining or regaining skills is attractive to those worried about memory loss and to relatives who hope that developing problems might be minimized. Recent evidence suggesting that education and continued intellectual activity may reduce the risk of developing AD has further increased interest in this area. Computer-aided brain-training programmes are widely promoted, but so far they seem to meet best the needs of healthy elderly (and not so elderly) people and the worried well.

Experience of formal training programmes designed to improve the cognitive skills of healthy elderly subjects and those with cognitive deficits is limited.[28] Those most likely to gain appear to be well motivated, healthy individuals wishing to conserve their mental faculties as a prophylactic measure. There is little evidence of sustained benefit or generalizability in those with established dementia and regular tests and 'exercises' for the memory can easily become counterproductive. Positive benefits to patients may even be at the cost of increased distress to carers.

Specific approaches have included relaxation techniques, organization of material (e.g. with the use of categorization, associative cues and mnemonics), regular and repeated practice sessions, using spaced retrieval to rehearse information, techniques for improving visual imagery (e.g. pegword methods, face–name association) and verbal strategies (rhymes, first letter cueing, alphabet searching, etc.). Reactivating therapy, including manual and creative activities, self-management skills and orientation tasks, has been claimed to improve cognitive performance and psychosocial functioning of people with mild dementia. Training in groups with other people with memory impairment or with family members and carers may provide opportunities to harness a wider range of training resources and facilitate expression of mutual support. Another approach is to involve family members in providing the cognitive training at home.

Drug treatments

Memory clinics are now central to the effective prescribing of specific anti-dementia drug treatments. Careful initial assessment and diagnosis are essential before any pharmacological intervention is considered and the impact of treatment and the indication for its continuing use must be kept under regular review. The size of any drug effect that can be considered worthwhile is open to debate. Statistically significant improvement on psychometric tests does not necessarily equate with meaningful change in quality of life and a noticeable improvement or stabilization is more important than change in test score. Patients and carers tend to be more positive than professionals when assessing apparently small benefits of treatment, with three-quarters believing that halting progression of symptoms of early dementia for about 6 months justifies intervention. Such modest effect would seem comparable to that achieved by the drugs now available

The AChEI drugs have become the mainstay of treatment for AD and may also have benefits in mixed dementia, Parkinson's disease dementia and DLB. They act by inhibiting the breakdown of acetylcholine within the synapse, increasing its availability to muscarinic and nicotinic receptors. In mild to moderate AD, the available AChEI (donepezil, rivastigmine and galantamine) have all been shown to be clinically effective and safe compared with placebo, with improvements in cognition, ADL and overall clinical global impression. There had been some disagreement about their cost-effectiveness but NICE guidance in the UK now supports their use in mild and moderate AD.[29] All AChEIs have qualitatively similar cholinergic adverse effects, including nausea, vomiting, diarrhoea, fatigue and dizziness. These are generally mild and short-lived, resolving despite continued therapy. Caution with the use of AChEIs should be observed in the presence of bradycardia and atrial or ventricular conduction disorders. Muscle cramps, insomnia and nightmares are more common with donepezil and can sometimes be reduced by administering the drug in the morning rather than at night. About 40–60% of AD patients respond to AChEIs. Although similarities appear to be greater than the differences between the available AChEIs, it may be reasonable to consider switching drugs if patients do not tolerate or respond to the first drug used.

Memantine is a non-competitive NMDA (glutamate) receptor antagonist that blocks pathologically elevated glutamate. Glutaminergic overstimulation and consequent calcium overload have been implicated in neurodegeneration and memantine offers neuroprotection, while still allowing physiological receptor activation. The drug is licensed for treatment of moderately severe to severe AD, with patients on memantine in clinical trials showing significantly less deterioration in functional, cognitive and global measures. The emergence of troublesome behavioural symptoms, especially agitation, may also be less, with reduced need for institutionalization and less demands on caregiver time. The addition of memantine to donepezil treatment may show benefit over donepezil alone.

There are many drugs for dementia undergoing research, not only for symptomatic relief but also for disease modification, for example, through interference with amyloid or tau processing in AD and amnestic MCI. Memory clinics continue to provide an ideal setting for patient recruitment and involvement in phase 2 and 3 clinical trials and opportunities for involvement in research should be encouraged.

Over-the-counter medications that have been used to treat mild cognitive impairment and dementia include *Gingko biloba*, vitamin E, folic acid and omega-3 fish oils, but there is no good evidence of efficacy. Often patients and carers will be interested in the effectiveness of complementary and alternative medicine. These non-conventional therapies include herbal medicine, aromatherapy and massage, acupuncture, dietary supplements and melatonin and bright light therapy. The evidence base supporting their use is poor, but there have been few rigorous studies of good scientific design, with adequate patient numbers and using robust outcome measures. Patients and families are attracted by the 'natural' image of these therapies and may feel they have nothing to lose given the inadequacy of conventional treatments. Some will find considerable benefit from them and staff in memory clinics should be able to provide informed information about their safety and local availability, while not necessarily promoting their use.

The memory clinic as part of local dementia services

The World Health Organization and World Psychiatric Association consensus statement[30] on care for elderly people with mental health problems highlighted specific principles that should underpin service development. Good-quality dementia care should be comprehensive, taking into account not just the medical aspects of the problem but also the psychological and social consequences. It should be accessible and user friendly, minimizing obstacles to effective assessment and intervention. It should be responsive, listening to and understanding the problems brought to its attention, and able to act promptly and appropriately. Finally, assessment and care should be individualized, tailored to the needs of the patient and their family.

The consensus document emphasizes that a team approach is essential, not just multidisciplinary but trans-disciplinary, going beyond traditional professional boundaries and providing responsive, coordinated and community-orientated intervention. An effective memory clinic team can be the foundation of a comprehensive dementia service, encouraging early recognition and specialist referral, providing thorough initial assessment and careful diagnosis and ensuring appropriate high-quality support and care which can be flexibly integrated with other local service providers.

Key points

- Memory clinics offer responsive assessment, diagnosis, treatment and advice for people with memory disorders and for their families. They also act as a focus for professional education and clinical research.
- Most clinics centre on diagnosis and management of mild cognitive impairment and dementia, emphasizing the benefits of early presentation, psychometric assessment, differential diagnosis, appropriate use of drug treatments and psychosocial interventions.
- They have a multidisciplinary approach, with medical, psychology and nursing input and close working relationships with other professionals and dementia services.
- Potential benefits include improved quality of life of patients, reduced carer burden, less hospitalization and possible postponement of need for institutional care.

References

1. Larrabee GJ, Pathy MSJ, Bayer AJ and Crook TH. Memory clinics: state of development and future prospects. In: M Bergener and SI Finkel (eds), *Clinical and Scientific Psychogeriatrics*, Vol. 1, Springer, New York, 1990, pp. 83–97.
2. Bayer AJ, Pathy MSJ and Twining C. The memory clinic: a new approach to the detection of early dementia. *Drugs* 1987;**22**(Suppl 2):84–9.
3. Van der Cammen TJ, Simpson JM, Fraser RM *et al.* The memory clinic. A new approach to the detection of dementia. *Br J Psychiatry* 1987;**150**:359–64.
4. Wilcock GK, Bucks RS and Rockwood K. *Diagnosis and Management of Dementia: a Manual for Memory Disorders Teams*, Oxford Medical Publications, Oxford, 1999.
5. National Institute for Health and Clinical Excellence. *Dementia: Supporting People with Dementia and Their Carers in Health and Social Care. NICE–SCIE Clinical Guideline 42*, National Institute for Health and Clinical Excellence, London, 2006.
6. Department of Health. *Living Well with Dementia: a National Dementia Strategy*, Department of Health, London, 2009.
7. Schmidtke K, Pohlmann S and Metternich B. The syndrome of functional memory disorder: definition, etiology and natural course. *Am J Geriatr Psychiatry* 2008;**16**:981–8.
8. Draskovic I, Vernooij-Dassen M, Verhey F *et al.* Development of quality markers for memory clinics. *Int J Geriatr Psychiatry* 2008;**23**:119–28.
9. LoGiudice D, Hassett A, Cook R *et al.* Equity of access to a memory clinic in Melbourne? *Int J Geriatr Psychiatry* 2001; **16**:327–34.
10. Melis RJF, Meeuwsen EJ, Parker SD and Olde Rikkert MGM. Are memory clinics effective? The odds are in favour of their benefit, but conclusive evidence is not yet available. *J Roy Socf Med* 2009;**102**:456–7.
11. Banerjee S and Wittenberg R. Clinical and cost effectiveness of services for early diagnosis and intervention in dementia. *Int J Geriatr Psychiatry* 2009;**24**:748–54.
12. Caspi E, Silverstein NM, Porell F and Kwan N. Physician outpatient contacts and hospitalizations among cognitively impaired elderly. *Alzheimers Demen* 2009;**5**:30–42.
13. Wolfs CAG, Kessels A, Dirksen CD *et al.* Integrated multidisciplinary diagnostic approach for dementia care: randomised controlled trial. *Br J Psychiatry* 2008;**192**:300–5.
14. LoGiudice D, Waltrowicz W, Brown K *et al.* Do memory clinics improve the quality of life of carers? A randomized pilot trial. *Int J Geriatr Psychiatry* 1999;**14**:626–32.
15. Meeuwsen EJ, Melis RJF, Adang EM *et al.* Cost-effectiveness of post-diagnosis treatment in dementia coordinated by multidisciplinary memory clinics in comparison to treatment coordinated by general practitioners: an example of a pragmatic trial. *J Nutr Health Aging* 2009;**13**:242–8.
16. Luce A, McKeith I, Swann A *et al.* How do memory clinics compare with traditional old age psychiatry services? *Int J Geriatr Psychiatry* 2001;**16**:837–45.
17. Simpson S, Beavis D, Dyer J and Ball S. Should old age psychiatry develop memory clinics? A comparison with domiciliary work. *Psychiatr Bull* 2004;**28**:78–82.
18. van Hout H, Vernooij-Dassen M, Hoefnagels W and Grol R. Measuring the opinions of memory clinic users: patients, relatives and general practitioners. *Int J Geriatr Psychiatry* 2001;**16**:846–51.
19. Verooij-Dassen MJ, van Hout HP, Hund KL *et al.* Information for dementia patients and their caregivers: what information does a memory clinic pass on and to whom? *Aging Mental Health* 2003;**7**:34–8.
20. Gardner IL, Foreman P and Davis S. Cognitive dementia and memory service clinics: opinions of general practitioners. *Am J Alzheimer's Dis Other Demen* 2004;**19**:105–10.
21. Burns A, Lawlor B and Craig S. *Assessment Scales in Old Age Psychiatry*, 2nd edn, Martin Dunitz, London, 2004.
22. Mioshi E, Dawson K, Mitchell J *et al.* The Addenbrooke's Cognitive Examination Revised (ACE-R): a brief cognitive test battery for dementia screening. *Int J Geriatr Psychiatry* 2006;**21**:1078–85.
23. Small GW, Bookheimer SY, Thompson PM *et al.* Current and future uses of neuroimaging for cognitively impaired patients. *Lancet Neurol* 2008;**7**:161–72.
24. Hejl A, Hogh P and Waldemar G. Potentially reversible conditions in 1000 consecutive memory clinic patients. *J Neurol Neurosurg Psychiatry* 2001;**72**:390–4.

25. Moniz-Cook E and Manthorpe J. *Early Psychosocial Interventions in Dementia: Evidence-Based Practice*, Jessica Kingsley, London, 2009.

26. OPDAL Study Group. *Optimisation of the Diagnosis of Alzheimer's Disease*, Alzheimer Europe, Luxembourg, 2003.

27. Wald C, Fahy M, Walker Z and Livingston G. What to tell dementia caregivers – the rule of threes. *Int J Geriatr Psychiatry* 2003;**18**:313–7.

28. Clare L and Woods RT. Cognitive rehabilitation and cognitive training for early-stage Alzheimer's disease and vascular dementia. *Cochrane Database Syst Rev* 2003;(4):CD003260.

29. National Institute for Health and Clinical Excellence. *Donepezil, Galantamine, Rivastigmine and Memantine for the Treatment of Alzheimer's Disease, Review of NICE Technology Appraisal Guidance 111*. National Institute for Health and Clinical Excellence, London, 2011.

30. World Health Organization and World Psychiatric Association. Organisation of care in psychiatry of the elderly – a technical consensus statement. *Ageing Mental Health* 1998;**2**:246–52.

CHAPTER 73

Alzheimer's disease

James E. Galvin
New York University Langone Medical Center, New York, NY, USA

Introduction

Alzheimer's disease (AD) is the most common form of dementia in older adults.[1] AD symptoms include a loss of memory, impaired judgment and decision-making capacity, a decline in the ability to perform activities of daily living (ADLs), changes in behaviour, mood and personality and increasing dependence on caregivers with expanding degrees of burden and stress.

Alois Alzheimer described the first case in 1906, characterizing a 51-year-old woman who presented with delusions of spousal infidelity, memory and language problems. After her death, using recently developed silver staining techniques, Alzheimer described numerous senile plaques and neurofibrillary tangles characteristic of the disease.[2] For the next 60 years, AD was thought to be an infrequent pre-senile cause of dementia until it was recognized that the clinical symptoms and course and neuropathological findings of disease in individuals younger than 65 years was identical with those found in older adults.

The Alzheimer Association estimates that there are over 5 million people in the USA with AD and that within a generation the number of AD patients will exceed 15 million people.[3] In the USA, AD is the fifth leading cause of death, after cardiovascular disease, cancer, cerebrovascular disease and bronchopulmonary diseases. AD is the third most expensive disease after cardiovascular disease and cancer in terms of total dollars with an annual total (direct and indirect) cost of approximately $172 billion. While the costs of AD increase across the stages of severity, AD patients currently fill nearly half of all nursing home beds. This economic impact will continue to grow as the US population continues to age and the number of AD patients increases. At the time of writing, the cumulative costs of care for people with AD from 2010 to 2050 in the USA will exceed $20 trillion.[3] At present, only symptomatic therapies are available that provide cognitive, functional and behavioural benefits but do not alter the disease course.

Neuropathology

Macroscopically, AD is characterized by cortical atrophy and ventricular dilatation (Figure 73.1a). Volume is most noticeable on coronal sections with shrinkage of medial temporal lobe structures including hippocampus. The characteristic pathological changes in the AD brain are the accumulation of amyloid β-protein in the form of senile plaques and of tau protein in the form of neurofibrillary tangles. Amyloid β-protein (Aβ) is a 39–43 amino acid peptide cleaved from a larger precursor protein [amyloid precursor protein (APP)] found on chromosome 21.[2] Aβ deposits extracellularly as senile plaques that can be visualized by haematoxylin and eosin staining (Figure 73.1b), with the fluorescent dye thioflavin S (Figure 73.1c), by immunohistochemistry using antibodies raised against Aβ epitopes (Figure 73.1d) or with silver impregnation (Figure 73.1e). Amyloid can appear either as loose, non-fibrillar diffuse plaques (Figure 73.1d) or a more compacted, fibrillar form (Figure 73.1b), often with dystrophic neurites coursing through the plaque (neuritic plaque, Figure 73.1e). Cerebral amyloid angiopathy (CAA) is due to the deposition of amyloid in the walls of arteries and arterioles and, less often, capillaries and veins of the central nervous system (Figure 73.1d). The walls of these vessels become very fragile and have a propensity to rupture, leading to superficial cortical haemorrhages. In addition to focal motor and sensory symptoms, repeated haemorrhages can lead to cognitive decline.

Tau protein is a microtubule-associated protein encoded on chromosome 17.[2] Its normal function is to stabilize microtubules and it has numerous sites available for phosphorylation. When hyperphosphorylated, tau forms insoluble filaments that deposit in the cell body of the neuron as a neurofibrillary tangle (NFT) and in the axons and dendrites as neurophil threads (NTs). NFTs in AD are composed primarily of paired helical filaments (two strands of 10 nm diameter filaments that twist around each other

Principles and Practice of Geriatric Medicine, Fifth Edition. Edited by Alan J. Sinclair, John E. Morley and Bruno Vellas.

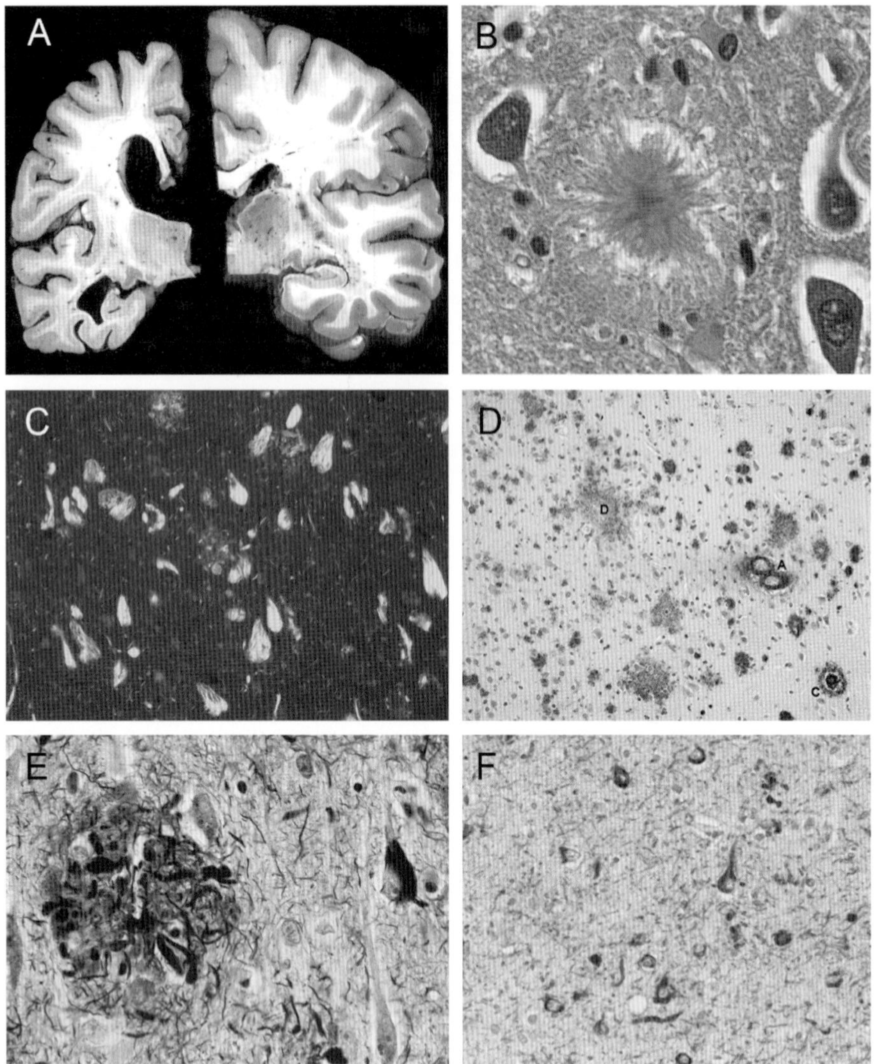

Figure 73.1 The neuropathology of AD. (a) Coronal sections of brain at the level of the hippocampus. On the left is a patient with AD, and on the right is an age-matched individual without cognitive impairment. Note the cortical atrophy and dilatation of the ventricles in the AD patient. (b) Extracellular Aβ senile plaques visualized with haematoxylin and eosin stain. (c) Thioflavin S fluorescent staining of amyloid plaques and neurofibrillary tangles. (d) Immunohistochemistry using Aβ antibodies demonstrating extracellular diffuse and fibrillar amyloid plaques and amyloid deposition in cerebral vessels. (e) Silver impregnation demonstrating fibrillar amyloid with dystrophic neurites and neurofibrillary tangles. (f) Immunohistochemistry using tau antibodies demonstrating neurofibrillary tangles and dystrophic neurites. See plate section for a colour version of these images.

like a helix). NFTs first appear in the hippocampus and entorhinal cortex in the AD brain (Figure 73.1f) and later involve the limbic and neocortex as the severity of dementia worsens. Hyperphosphorylated tau can be visualized by the same methods as amyloid since both proteins undergo transformations to a β-pleated sheet.

Epidemiology and genetics

A number of risk factors have been associated with AD (Table 73.1).[4] Age is clearly the most predictive risk factor. Although cases have been described as early as the third decade, the majority of cases occur after age 65 years. The prevalence of AD doubles each decade from 5% before age 65 years to nearly 50% at age 85 years. After age 85 years, studies are inconclusive as to whether the risk continues to increase; however, pathology characteristic of AD is frequently found in the brains of individuals over 90 years of age. In the oldest old, the course and progression of AD appear to be slower than for those individuals who develop the disease at younger ages. Family history of dementia in first-degree relatives appears to increase the risk of

Table 73.1 Alzheimer risk factors.

Age
Female gender
Family history
Low education
Head injury
Apolipoprotein E ε4 allele
Cardiovascular risk factors: hypertension, diabetes, hyperlipidaemia, homocysteine
Late-life depression
Trisomy 21 (Down syndrome)
Mutations in amyloid precursor protein (APP), presenilin 1 (PS1) or presenilin 2 (PS2)

developing AD. Up to 25% of patients are able to identify a family member with the disease. There is an association between female gender and AD that persists after correction for differences in life expectancy between men and women. The reason for this remains unknown. Earlier epidemiological studies supported a role of postmenopausal estrogen levels; however, the Women's Health Initiative found that estrogen replacement in later life increased rather than decreased the risk for AD.

Low educational attainment may also increase the risk of AD. There is increasing evidence supporting the hypothesis of cognitive reserve, that is, individuals with greater education are better able to stave off the effects of AD pathology in the early stages. Head injury associated with a loss of consciousness has been associated with increased risk of AD. Depression, particularly developing in late life, appears to be a prodromal symptom of AD. There is recent evidence to suggest that the same risk factors for cardiovascular disease may be important contributors to the risk of developing AD, including hypertension, high cholesterol, diabetes and homocysteine.[1,4] Epidemiological studies and chart-reviews have suggested that long-term use of non-steroidal anti-inflammatory drugs (NSAIDs) may reduce the risk of AD; however controlled clinical trials have failed to replicate these results and instead suggest that the use of NSAIDs may increase risks of gastrointestinal, cardiovascular and cerebrovascular disease.

There are also several genetic risk factors. The best characterized risk for late-onset disease is associated with epsilon 4 (ε4) allele of apolipoprotein E (ApoE).[5] ApoE is a cholesterol-carrying protein that may also play a role in handling of Aβ. Three isoforms of ApoE are present, ε2, ε3 and ε4. The ε3 allele is the most common, the ε2 is the least common and the ε4 allele is found in ~20% of the population. The ε4 allele is over-represented in AD, with ~60% of patients carrying at least one ε4 allele. Conversely, the presence of at least one ε2 allele appears to confer some protection. In Caucasians, compared with the ε3/ε3 genotype, individuals with one ε4 allele have a threefold increased risk whereas individuals with two ε4 alleles have a 15-fold increased risk of AD. This relationship holds true across most racial and ethnic groups.[5] The linkage between ApoE and senile plaques suggests that cholesterol homeostasis may play either a direct or indirect role in the pathogenesis. However, because the ApoE genotype is not causative, genetic testing is not recommended as it neither improve diagnostic certainty nor changes the management of the disease. Additional risk genes are being investigated and validated with genome-wide association studies.[6]

Autosomal dominant, early-onset cases of AD are associated with mutations in the amyloid precursor protein (chromosome 21), presenilin 1 (chromosome 14) and presenilin 2 (chromosome 1).[7] These three mutations appear to increase the production of the 42 amino acid long Aβ protein which has an increased propensity to aggregate. These mutations are rare, but can be suspected in a strong family history of AD with age of onset before 65 years. Even so, the mutations account for a small proportion of AD cases. The real value of the mutations has been in the creation of cell culture lines and transgenic animals that has greatly advanced research efforts. Associated with these genetic risk factors is the virtually certainty of AD developing in individuals with trisomy 21 (Down syndrome) with an additional copy of the region encoding the amyloid precursor protein. By the late 20s, Down syndrome patients begin to accumulate amyloid in their brains and nearly all patients are symptomatic by their mid-50s.[1]

Diagnostic criteria

Although AD can only be definitively diagnosed by autopsy, current clinical criteria permit experienced clinicians to make accurate diagnoses most of the time: 92% or more of the time, an expert clinician's diagnosis is confirmed by autopsy findings. The diagnosis of AD is one of inclusion using standardized clinical criteria: the *Diagnostic and Statistical Manual of Mental Disorders* (DSM-IV-TR)[8] and the National Institute on Ageing – Alzheimer's Association (NIA-AA).[9] The DSM criteria are broader in nature and capture more impaired individuals whereas the NIA-AA criteria apply more rigorous definitions that incorporate new findings regarding the use of biological markers of disease. In general, the current diagnostic criteria are characterized by a two-step procedure with (1) the identification of a dementia syndrome and (2) the exclusion of other aetiologies of a dementia syndrome, using biological and neuroimaging examinations.

The diagnosis can also be based on the criteria of the DSM-IV-TR[8] (Table 73.2). According to the DSM, the essential feature of dementia is impairment in short- and long-term memory, associated with impairment in abstract thinking, impaired judgment, other disturbances of

Table 73.2 DSM-IV criteria for dementia of the Alzheimer type.

The development of multiple cognitive deficits manifested by both
1 Memory impairment (impaired ability to learn new information or to recall previously learned information)
2 One or more of the following cognitive disturbances:
 a Aphasia (language disturbance)
 b Apraxia (impaired ability to carry our motor activities despite intact motor function)
 c Agnosia (failure to recognize or identify objects despite intact sensory function)
 d Disturbances in executive functioning (i.e. planning, organizing, sequencing, abstracting)

The cognitive decline causes significant impairment in social or occupational functioning and presents a decline from a previous level of functioning

The course is characterized by gradual onset and continuing cognitive decline

The cognitive deficits above are not caused by any of the following:
1 Other central nervous system conditions that cause progressive deficits in memory and cognition
2 Systemic conditions that are known to cause dementia
3 Substance abuse conditions

The deficits do not occur exclusively during the course of a delirium

The deficits are not better accounted for by another Axis I disorder (depression, schizophrenia)

Adapted from American Psychiatric Association, Task Force on DSM-IV. *Diagnostic and Statistical Manual of Mental Disorders: DSM-IV*, 4th edn, American Psychiatric Association, Washington, DC, 1994.

higher cortical function or personality change. Disturbances in these cognitive domains should be severe enough to interfere with social or occupational functioning or disrupt interpersonal relationships with others. An important caveat in the DSM criteria is that the diagnosis cannot be made in the presence of a delirium.[8] There are plans to update the DSM criteria but these are not available at the time of writing.

According to NIA-AA guidelines, the diagnosis is first established by determining the presence of dementia. Dementia is defined as cognitive or behavioural symptoms that (1) interfere with social or occupational functioning, (2) represent a decline from previous level of functioning and (3) are not explained by another disorder. Dementia is established by a combination of a detailed history from the patient and a knowledgeable informant and an objective assessment of cognitive ability. Changes in cognitive ability should involve at least two of the following domains: memory, reasoning and problem solving, visuospatial abilities, language and/or changes in personality, behaviour or social comportment. Once the dementia syndrome is established, the diagnosis of probable AD can be made when the patient has (1) dementia, (2) an insidious onset with gradual progression and (3) worsening of symptoms over time either by observation or report of patient and/or informant. The presentation of deficits can either by amnestic (memory impairment) or non-amnestic (language, visuospatial, executive dysfunction).[9] The diagnosis of AD should not be applied when there is clear evidence of cerebrovascular disease, Lewy body dementia, frontotemporal degeneration or another concurrent neurological, psychiatric or medical condition that can affect condition.[9] If the patient meets criteria for probable AD but has evidence of other disorders that can affect cognition, a mixed dementia syndrome is most likely present.

More importantly, the NIA-AA criteria take into consideration the role of biological markers of disease (biomarkers).[10] Recent advances in biomarker research such as magnetic resonance imaging (MRI), positron emission tomography (PET) scans and cerebrospinal fluid (CSF) biomarkers characterize the underlying pathophysiological processes associated with AD such as evidence of Aβ deposition measured by CSF Aβ levels or PET scans or markers of neuronal injury by CSF tau levels, glucose hypometabolism by PET or cortical atrophy by MRI.[9] Although the use of biomarkers is not advocated for routine clinical use, these tests may increase the diagnostic certainty of AD in difficult cases (Table 73.3).[9]

Evaluation of the AD patient

Clinical evaluation

Knowing that the risk of AD increases with age, older adults are a natural choice for screening for AD. At present, however, there are no formal recommendations for or against dementia screening. The US Preventive Services Task Force (http://www.ahrq.gov/clinic/3rduspstf/dementia/dementrr.pdf) concluded that the evidence is insufficient to recommend for or against routine screening for dementia in older adults. Many of the current brief screening measures such as the Mini-Mental State Examination (MMSE)[11] have good sensitivity but only fair specificity in detecting cognitive impairment and dementia.[12,13] The accuracy of the MMSE depends on a person's age and educational level: using an arbitrary cut-point (typically $\leq$23) may potentially lead to more false-positives among older people with lower educational levels and more false negatives among younger people with higher educational levels.[12]

On the other hand, the early recognition of dementia, in addition to helping make diagnostic and treatment decisions, allows clinicians to anticipate problems the patients may have in understanding and adhering to recommended therapy. Early diagnosis is also beneficial to the patient's caregiver(s) and family member(s) in helping to anticipate

Table 73.3 Probability of AD with biomarkers (NIA-AA criteria).[a]

Diagnostic category	Probability of AD based on biomarkers	Measurements of Aβ (CSF or PIB-PET)	Measurements of neuronal injury or degeneration (CSF tau, FDG-PET, MRI)
Probable AD			
Based on clinical criteria	Not helpful	–/?	–/?
With three levels of evidence based on AD pathology	Intermediate	–/?	++
	Intermediate	+	–/?
	High	+	+
Possible AD			
Based on clinical criteria	Not helpful	–/?	–/?
With evidence based on AD pathology	High (rule out secondary causes)	+	+
Unlikely to be AD	Low	–	–

[a]AD, Alzheimer's disease; Aβ, amyloid beta-protein; CSF, cerebrospinal fluid, PIB, Pittsburgh Compound B (Aβ ligand); PET, positron emission tomography; FDG, [^{18}F]fluorodeoxyglucose; MRI, magnetic resonance imaging;–/?, conflicting or indeterminate; +, positive.
Adapted from McKhann *et al.*[9]

and plan for future problems that may develop as a result of progression of cognitive impairment and for long-term care. Long-term care planning and advanced care decisions are important in all forms of chronic diseases, many of which are treated by neurologists and psychiatrists. Discussions covering these topics early in the course of chronic disease should probably be considered part of the norm, rather than the exception. Organizations such as the American Medical Association, American Geriatrics Society, American Academy of Neurology and American Academy of Family Physicians all recommend that clinicians remain diligent in the early identification of symptoms of AD in their patients.

So who should be evaluated for AD? The Alzheimer Association has published 10 warning signs of symptoms that are most commonly seen in AD (Table 73.4).[3] Although not every individual needs to be extensively worked up, developing a working list of reasons to consider AD as a possible diagnosis is reasonable (Table 73.5). Individuals with identified risk factors warrant further evaluation, as do individuals with memory complaints, with or without functional impairment. Additionally, even if an individual does not complain of memory or cognitive problems, informant complaints (spouses, adult children) should trigger further investigation. Evaluation should include a detailed history from the patient in addition to another source (spouse, caregiver, adult child) to gain insight into how the patient has changed from prior level of function. Historical points should highlight memory impairment (repetition; trouble remembering recent conversations, events, appointments; frequently misplacing items), executive function (deterioration of complex task performance; decreased ability to solve problems; difficulty with calculations; impaired driving), use of alcohol, prescription drugs and over-the-counter medications and the presence of focal neurological symptoms. A complete neurological examination will help to identify other causes of dementia (Table 73.6). Characteristic features of the four most common causes of dementia are given in Table 73.7 to help with differentiation.

Table 73.4 Ten warning signs.

Memory loss
Difficulty in performing familiar tasks
Problems with language
Disorientation with respect to time and place
Poor or decreased judgement
Problems with abstract thought
Misplacing things
Changes in mood or behaviour
Changes in personality
Loss of initiative

Source: Alzheimer's Association.

Cognitive evaluation

Performance-based tools

In terms of assessing cognitive function, the 30-item MMSE test, which takes around 10 min to complete, has frequently been used for initial assessment of AD, and its sensitivity increases if a decline of the score over time is taken into account.[11] The MMSE covers six areas: (1) orientation, (2) registration, (3) attention and calculation, (4) recall, (5) language and (6) ability to copy a figure. However, although the MMSE is quick and easy to administer and can track the

Table 73.5 Indications for evaluating for AD.

Physician observations
Difficulty in learning and retaining new information
Difficulty in performing complex tasks
Impaired reasoning
Problems with orientation and spatial abilities
Language difficulties, particularly word-finding
Behaviour or personality changes
Late-life depression, anxiety or apathy
Previous well-controlled medical conditions now more difficult to manage
Poor medication adherence/compliance
Patient complaints
Memory problems
Work difficulties
New-onset depression, anxiety or apathy
Sleep changes (insomnia, nocturnal movements, unusual dreaming)
Informant complaints
Changes in memory or cognitive abilities
Changes in functional abilities
Changes in mood, personality or behaviour

overall progression of cognitive decline, it is not considered to be a good test for definitive AD diagnosis,[14] particularly because of its greater emphasis on orientation (10 of 30 points), which is typically not impaired in the earliest stages of dementia. In addition, there are several issues associated with the MMSE, including bias according to age, race, education and socioeconomic status.[15]

Several diagnostic tests are now available for use in primary care as alternatives to the MMSE; these are continually being updated and simplified in order to provide brief, easy to administer and effective diagnostic tools.

The Mini Cognitive Assessment Instrument (Mini-Cog) combines an uncued three-item recall test with a clock-drawing test that serves as a recall distractor; it can be administered in about 3 min and requires no special equipment.[15] The Mini-Cog and the MMSE have similar sensitivity (76 versus 79%) and specificity (89 versus 88%) for dementia, comparable to those achieved using a conventional neuropsychological battery (75% sensitivity, 90% specificity). The Mini-Cog's brevity is a distinct advantage when the goal is to improve recognition of cognitive impairment in primary care, particularly in milder stages of impairment.[15] It has also been suggested that cognitive impairment assessed by the Mini-Cog is a more powerful predictor of impaired ADLs than disease burden in older adults. In addition, the Mini-Cog also has proven good performance in ethnically diverse populations of the USA in which widely used cognitive screens often fail, and is easier to administer to non-English speakers.[15] Furthermore, low educational status, which has been shown to impair

Table 73.6 Differential diagnosis of dementia.

Neurodegenerative disease
Alzheimer's disease
Dementia with Lewy bodies/Parkinson's disease dementia
Frontotemporal dementia
Huntington's disease
Progressive supranuclear palsy
Corticobasal degeneration
Multiple system atrophy
Wilson's disease
Haemochromatosis/haemosiderosis
Neuronal ceroid lipofuscinosis
Vascular disease
Vascular dementia
Cerebral amyloid angiopathy
CADASIL
Vasculitis
Prion disease
Creutzfeldt–Jacob disease
Gerstmann–Straussler–Scheinker disease
Kuru
Fatal familial insomnia
Hydrocephalus
Demyelinating disorders
Multiple sclerosis
Leukodystrophies
Traumatic brain injury
Metabolic disorders
Hepatic encephalopathy
Hypothyroidism
Storage disorders
Nutritional disorders
Vitamin B_{12} deficiency
Wernicke–Korsakoff syndrome (thiamine)
Mitochondrial disorders
Toxic disorders
Alcoholism
Drugs
Heavy metals
Neoplasia
Primary brain tumours (meningiomas, gliomas)
Metastatic disease
Paraneoplastic syndromes
Infection
HIV/progressive multifocal leukoencephalopathy
Neurosyphilis
Subacute sclerosing panencephalitis
Whipple's disease

Table 73.7 Characteristic features of the four leading causes of dementia.

Cause of dementia	Symptoms
Alzheimer's disease	Early failure of information storage and new memory creation. Disturbances in attention. May include early language or behavioural disturbances
Frontotemporal dementia	Early behavioural disturbances, particularly social misconduct and eating changes. Early language problems that may be fluent or non-fluent
Lewy body dementia	Early extrapyramidal signs (slowness, stiffness, tremor), visual hallucinations, visuospatial impairment, REM sleep behavioural disorders and fluctuations in attention and concentration
Vascular dementia	Early executive dysfunction usually associated with a focal neurological sign. Presence of vascular lesions in neuroimaging and temporal relationship between focal neurological signs and onset of cognitive symptoms

detection using the MMSE, does not affect the Mini-Cog, which is thus less biased by low educational status and literacy level.

Newer instruments, such as the Montreal Cognitive Assessment (MoCA), are gaining credibility owing to improvements in sensitivity, addressing frontal/executive functioning and decreasing susceptibility to cultural and educational biases.[16] The MoCA is a 10 min cognitive screening tool developed to assist first-line physicians in the detection of MCI. It has high sensitivity and specificity for detecting MCI in those patients who perform within the normal range of the MMSE. Compared with the MMSE, which had a sensitivity of 18% to detect MCI, the MoCA detected 90% of MCI subjects and, in patients with mild AD, the MMSE had a sensitivity of 78%, whereas the MoCA detected 100%.[16]

Informant-based tools

Another key test used in primary care is the AD8 screening interview, which is a brief, sensitive measure that reliably differentiates between individuals with and without dementia by querying memory, orientation, judgment and function.[12,13] The AD8 (Table 73.8) comprises eight Yes/No questions asked of an informant to rate change and takes ~2–3 min for the informant to complete. In the absence of an informant, the AD8 can be directly administered to the patient as a self-rating tool. The AD8 has a sensitivity of 74–80% and a specificity of 80–86%, with excellent ability to discriminate between non-demented older adults and those with mild dementia (92%), and is highly correlated with AD imaging and CSF biomarkers.[13] Use of the AD8 in conjunction with a brief assessment of the participant, such as a word list, could improve the detection of dementia in the primary setting to 97% for dementia and 91% for MCI.[12]

Laboratory Evaluation

In terms of laboratory evaluation for dementia, testing for comorbid medical illnesses that may cause or contribute to onset or progression of dementia is generally recommended.[17] Depression is a common, treatable comorbidity in patients with dementia and should be screened for in older adults. Vitamin B_{12} insufficiency is common in the elderly and vitamin B_{12} levels should be included in routine assessments of the elderly, but screening for other vitamin and nutritional deficiencies is not recommended unless historical information suggests these deficiencies as a clinical possibility. Because of its frequency, hypothyroidism should be screened for in elderly patients. Lastly, unless the patient has some specific risk factor or evidence of prior syphilitic infection or resides in one of the few areas in the USA with high numbers of syphilis cases, screening for the disorder in patients with dementia is generally not justified.[17] This includes collecting spousal history of exposure when applicable.

Genetic testing for patients with suspected dementia is not recommended unless there is clear, generational evidence of an autosomal dominant form of dementia. Even then, genetic counselling is recommended, prior to testing. The routine use of ApoE genotyping in patients with suspected AD is not recommended at present because of cost and because it adds little to the diagnostic accuracy.[17] In patients with clinical diagnoses of AD, the addition of ApoE testing increased the positive predictive value (using the prevalence of AD in this dementia autopsy series) of a diagnosis of AD by ~4% (from 90 to 94%) if an ApoE ε4 allele was present. In patients with a clinical diagnosis of non-AD, the absence of an ApoE ε4 allele increased the negative predictive value by 8% (from 64 to 72%).[18] No other serum or CSF biomarkers have established clinical validity at present and are therefore not recommended, although this is likely to change in the future.

Making the diagnosis

As shown in the algorithm in Figure 73.2, each of the above steps can help to identify the patient-at-risk, establish a likely diagnosis and further treatment recommendations. After establishment of a diagnosis of possible or probable

Table 73.8 The AD8 dementia screening test.

Remember, 'Yes, a change' indicates that there has been a change in the last several years caused by cognitive (thinking and memory) problems	**YES, a change**	**NO, no change**	**N/A, don't know**
1. Problems with judgment (e.g. problems making decisions, bad financial decisions, problems with thinking)			
2. Less interest in hobbies/activities			
3. Repeats the same things over and over (questions, stories or statements)			
4. Trouble learning how to use a tool, appliance or gadget (e.g. VCR, computer, microwave, remote control)			
5. Forgets correct month or year			
6. Trouble handling complicated financial affairs (e.g. balancing chequebook, income taxes, paying bills)			
7. Trouble remembering appointments			
8. Daily problems with thinking and/or memory			
TOTAL AD8 SCORE			

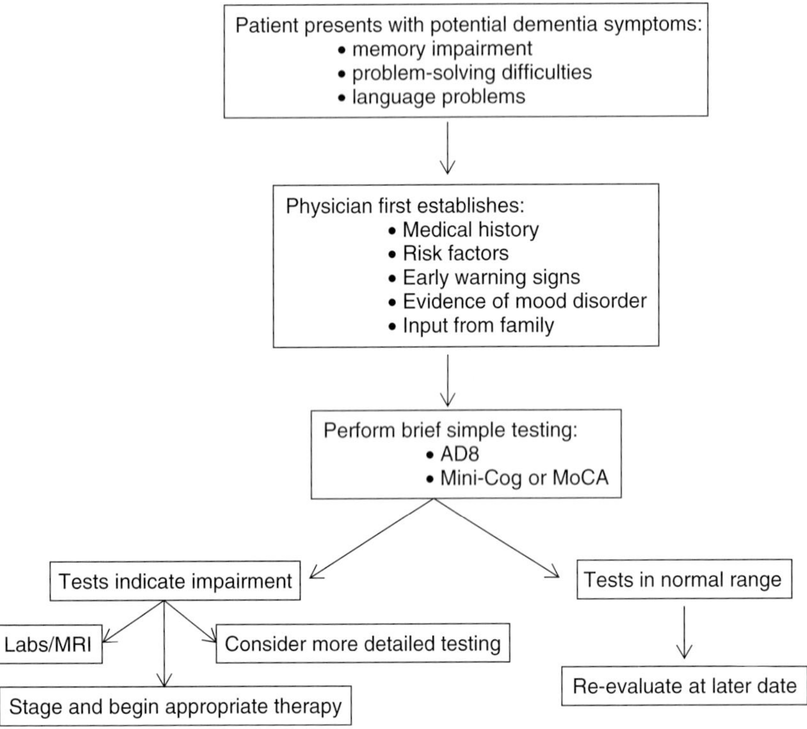

Figure 73.2 Algorithm for the diagnosis of AD in the office setting. This algorithm outlines steps for evaluating older adults for AD or other causes of cognitive impairment. Upon presentation of a patient with dementia-related symptoms elicited by from the patient or caregiver, the physician should first review the medical history to discover the onset, presentation and progression of symptoms, review potential risk factors and evaluate for confounding conditions such as depression. Simple office testing with a performance measure (Mini-Cog or MoCA) and an informant questionnaire (AD8) will enhance the clinician's ability to detect early impairment. If the patient performs in the normal range, periodic reassessment is warranted. If tests indicate cognitive impairment, the clinician should complete the work-up with routine laboratory tests to rule out reversible causes of dementia and neuroimaging. Additionally, the physician can refer to a specialist for more detailed neuropsychological testing. If AD is suspected, the patient should be staged and started on appropriate therapies and referral to community resources.

AD, the patient should be staged to assist in selection of appropriate pharmacotherapies, make referrals to community resources and assist in prognosis (Table 73.9).

There are barriers to the early detection of dementia for the clinician to consider. The first is misidentification of the early stages of dementia by patients and family members as the normal ageing process.[1] Forgetfulness is not a normal part of ageing but is often accepted as an inevitable consequence of growing old. If a patient or family member does not perceive the presence of a memory disorder, they are much less likely to come to medical attention until more advanced stages. A second issue is that social skills are often maintained in the early stages of AD. If a person lives alone, friends and acquaintances may not be able to detect cognitive decline due to lack of exposure. This and the fact of denial and lack of insight by the patient as to the extent of the cognitive problems may also lead physicians to miss early stages of dementia since the patient may not complain and cognitive screening is not part of a routine medical visit in most instances. Even if symptoms are identified by the patient and/or the family, there may be a reluctance to report them due to the social stigma of being diagnosed

Table 73.9 Simple staging scheme for AD.

Stage[a]	Characteristics	Example signs
Mild MMSE 19–27 CDR 0.5 or 1 GDS 3 or 4	• Symptoms are subtle • Self-care capacity, social skills and neurological function remain generally intact • Difficulty with complex tasks; if still working, a decline in job performance • Depression and apathy	• Repeating questions, statements or stories • Misplacing items • Forgetting recent events or conversations • Trouble operating household appliances • Less interest in hobbies
Moderate MMSE 10–18 CDR 2 GDS 5 or 6	• Ability to think, reason, communicate and function deteriorates dramatically • Beginning of behavioural symptoms	• Difficulty in using household appliances • Unable to travel alone • Difficulty in telling time • Restlessness, wandering, insomnia
Severe MMSE 0–9 CDR 3 GDS 7	• Individuals lose capacity for self-care and become completely dependent • Long-term care placement common	• Difficulty in eating, dressing • Incontinence • Cannot answer the telephone • Gait disturbances • Aggression, agitation, irritability

[a]MMSE, Mini-Mental State Examination; CDR, Clinical Dementia Rating; GDS, Global Deterioration Scale.

with AD. The diagnosis can also have consequences for obtaining insurance, employment and driving privileges. These factors can all contribute to delay in diagnosis and should be discussed with the patient and caregiver.

Biomarkers of AD

Cerebrospinal fluid biomarkers

According to the NINCDS–ADRDA guidelines, CSF examination is recommended as an exclusion procedure, largely undertaken to rule out other potentially correctable causes of cognitive decline, such as infection.[9] Since then, research has focused on the validity of AD-specific biomarkers that are reflective of the central pathogenic processes of β-amyloid aggregation and hyperphosphorylation of tau protein. These markers have included β-1–42-amyloid, total tau and phospho-tau: a decrease in the β-1–42-amyloid peptide and an increase in the tau and phospho-tau proteins may be the earliest signs of AD.[13,19] Indeed, both tests produce results with very good sensitivity and specificity. However, at present, these tests are probably not an option owing to patients' reluctance to undergo lumbar puncture and the costs associated with the assays.

Structural brain imaging

Structural brain imaging tests, which include non-contrast computed tomography (CT) or MRI, can evaluate changes consistent with AD and eliminate alternative causes of cognitive impairment.[17] Whenever possible, an MRI scan will provide a greater assessment of regional atrophy and periventricular vascular changes than can be gained from a CT scan. Quantitative MRI and PET amyloid imaging are recent techniques currently being developed to diagnose AD earlier in clinical practice. Within an AD diagnostic framework, the ideal role of structural brain imaging tests is to increase the specificity of clinical criteria.[17]

Functional brain imaging

PET scanning appears to have promise for use as an adjunct to clinical diagnosis, but further prospective studies with PET are needed to establish the value that it brings to diagnosis over and above a competent clinical diagnosis. One of the largest series of dementia cases that underwent PET scans and also had autopsy confirmation yielded a sensitivity of 93% and a specificity of 63%.[20] PET diagnostic accuracy increases with more advanced stages of dementia (87.2% for MMSE score >20 and 100% for MMSE score <20).[21] There are somewhat specific patterns of brain hypometabolism for each dementia subtype. In AD, hypometabolism is noted in the posterior temporoparietal cortices.[21] Fluorodeoxyglucose (FDG) PET may also be superior to MRI measures of hippocampal atrophy because changes in cerebral glucose metabolism antedate the onset of memory decline, whereas the MRI hippocampal changes may not reflect early disease.

Management

Disclosing the diagnosis

Disclosure of the diagnosis of AD to the patient and family may be difficult and consideration of the emotional responses should be taken into account. A family conference may be the most appropriate setting and the physician should be prepared to answer questions from the patient and family regarding the certainty of the diagnosis, the prognosis and implications for care. Recent research suggests that there is little long-term psychological effect of disclosing an AD diagnosis and both caregiver and patient self-ratings of depression and anxiety may be alleviated by having a frank, honest discussion about the disease.[22]

Setting treatment goals

Setting realistic treatment goals is critical to increasing patient and caregiver adherence. Because the currently available medications are symptomatic, it is important that the patient and family do not leave the physician's office under the impression that they will 'get better' by taking the medications. Although some patients do show improvement in different cognitive areas, the goal of current therapy for AD is to stabilize the patient for a period of time or to progress at a slower rate. As each patient has unique living and social situations, the clinician can work with the family to set expectations and discuss the limitations of current therapy.

Therefore, treatment goals should be discussed at the time of diagnosis. The first is to establish realistic expectations of treatment and review the course and complications of the disease. Goals should be set to (1) maintain quality of life, (2) maximize function and ADLs, (3) stabilize cognition, (4) treat mood and behavioural problems and (5) reduce caregiver burden.[1] Other discussion topics should include advanced directives, financial planning, referral to community resources, driving, durable power of attorney and discussion of long-term care planning. Addressing issues early in the diagnosis will empower the patient and caregiver to participate in the decision-making process.

Currently available management options for dementia

Although current pharmacological and behavioural interventions do not prevent eventual disease progression, they arguably lead to improvements in understanding, self-efficacy and quality of life for the patient and family. Recognizing dementia in its early phase may provide substantial benefits, including financial, medical and legal planning. It will also enable patients, their families and their caregivers to understand and deal better with the nature of the condition and subsequent changes in behaviour, allow caregivers to become familiar with appropriate support and social services and help maintain patients' functioning at the highest level possible.[23]

Managing mood disorders and behaviour problems

Traditionally, cognitive function has been the main focus of interest in treatment and research for people with dementia. It is becoming increasingly recognized, however, that non-cognitive symptoms are those that are most disturbing to families and caregivers and may seriously impact not only the patient's wellbeing, but also the family's, caregivers' and providers' approaches to managing the patient.[24] The most common symptoms are agitation, aggression, mood disorders/behavioural disturbance, apathy, depression, psychosis and hallucinations, with sexual disinhibition, elation/euphoria, appetite and eating disturbances and abnormal vocalizations occurring less frequently.[1,24] These have been grouped together under the umbrella term 'behavioural and psychological symptoms of dementia' by the International Psychogeriatric Association.[25] As the disease progresses, these symptoms become predominant problems and impose an enormous toll both emotionally and financially. They are also a common reason for institutionalization of people with dementia and they increase the burden and stress of caregivers.

Non-pharmacological interventions

Non-pharmacological interventions are recommended as the most appropriate initial strategy for managing inappropriate behaviours in dementia for the following reasons: (1) they address the psychosocial/environmental underlying reason for the behaviour and (2) they avoid the limitations of pharmacological interventions, namely adverse side effects, drug–drug interactions and limited efficacy.[24,26] Increased involvement of caregivers often has a secondary benefit of providing overburdened caregivers with an opportunity to receive support, information and skills. Further, environmental factors (e.g. confusing or noisy surroundings) or interpersonal factors (e.g. arguing with the patient) are often the primary triggers of behavioural problems. Attention to these factors through non-pharmacological approaches can be effective in alleviating or preventing behavioural problems in individuals with dementia. Unfortunately, in practice, pharmacological approaches involving psychotropic or sedative medications are often used as the first-line treatment, despite the modest evidence of efficacy from clinical trials where high placebo response rates are frequently seen, rather than first attempting a non-pharmacological approach.

An increasing number of non-pharmacological therapies are now available for people with dementia (Table 73.10). It should be noted that there are several areas of overlap between these therapies, hence each approach is rarely

Table 73.10 Non-pharmacological approaches and principles to behavioural therapies.

Standard therapies
Behavioural therapy
Reality orientation
Validation therapy
Reminiscence therapy
Alternative therapies
Art therapy
Music therapy
Activity therapy
Dance therapy
Aromatherapy
Bright-light therapy
Multisensory approaches
Brief psychotherapies
Cognitive behavioural therapies
Interpersonal therapy
Reducing behavioural symptoms
Provide the patient with a predictable routine (e.g. exercise, meals and bedtime should be routine and punctual)
Allow the patient to dress in his or her own clothing and keep possessions
Ask permission before touching patient or their belongings
Explain instructions to the patient in simple language
Simplify tasks; break up a complex task into steps and provide instruction for each step
Use distraction and redirection of activities to divert the patient's attention
Ensure that comorbid conditions are optimally treated
Provide a safe environment (e.g. no sharp-edged furniture, no throw rugs)
Equip doors and gates with safety locks
Install grab bars by the toilet and in the shower
Use calendars, clocks, labels and newspapers for orientation to time
Use colour-coded or graphic labels as cues for orientation in the home environment
Use lighting to reduce confusion and restlessness at night
Avoid glare from windows and mirrors, noise from a television and household clutter
Reduce excess stimulation and outings to crowded places
Consider using a day-care programme

used in isolation. It is therefore important for a clinician to have some knowledge of a number of these approaches, enabling a combination of treatments tailored to the individual requirements of the patient to be offered.[24] Therapy is now directed towards person-centred forms of care and, using this approach, greater attempts are made to understand the individual's experience of dementia and to employ strategies to improve quality of life.[26]

Pharmacological interventions

There are currently no means of reversing the pathological processes of AD. Therefore, the specific goals of therapy are to preserve cognitive and functional ability and to minimize behavioural disturbances and slow disease progression with maintenance of patients' and caregivers' quality of life. Early initiation of cholinesterase inhibitors (ChEIs) may temporarily stabilize or delay disease progression, which provides obvious desirable benefits for patients and caregivers. Studies have shown that both caregiver burden and overall cost are reduced by anticholinesterase therapy.[27] Beneficial response to a ChEI (i.e. stabilization or delayed deterioration of cognitive or behavioural problems) may be assessed from the physician's global assessment of the patient, the primary caregiver's report, a neuropsychological assessment or mental status questionnaire or evidence of behavioural or functional changes.

Five drugs have been approved for treating AD: four ChEIs approved for mild to moderate disease, one of which is also approved for severe AD, and a glutamate *N*-methyl-D-aspartate (NMDA) antagonist approved for moderate to severe disease (Table 73.11).

Mild to moderate disease

ChEIs have been the cornerstone of treatment for patients with mild to moderate AD for over a decade. Four ChEIs are currently available: tacrine (Cognex), donepezil (Aricept), rivastigmine (Exelon) and galantamine (Reminyl). These agents raise acetylcholine levels in the brain by inhibiting acetylcholinesterase, they tend to stabilize memory during the first year of treatment and they may slow the subsequent decline.

The systematic reviews and randomized controlled trials carried out to date, all of which involved at least 6 months of follow-up, found a significant difference that favoured the ChEI compared with placebo, ranging from 2.12 to 3.4 points on the ADAS-Cog scale. Donepezil 5 and 10 mg per day doses have been associated with significant improvements of–2.01 and–2.80 points, respectively, on the ADAS-Cog scale at 24 weeks, compared with placebo; donepezil 10 mg per day was also associated with a significant 1.84-point improvement over placebo on the MMSE at 52 weeks.[28] In addition to their effects on cognition, these agents have also demonstrated beneficial effects on measures of behaviour, ADLs and global patient function.

A meta-analysis which analyzed clinical results from 29 randomized, placebo-controlled trials of patients with mild to moderate AD found that ChEI therapy was associated with significant modest benefits in terms of neuropsychiatric and functional outcomes.[29] Current guidelines acknowledge that preventing or delaying further loss

Table 73.11 Pharmacological therapies for AD.

Drug	Approved indication	Suggested dosage	Side effects	Additional notes/caution
Cholinesterase inhibitors				
Tacrine (Cognex)	Mild to moderate AD	Four times daily dosing regimen	Poor tolerability and significant hepatotoxicity	Second-line agent owing to pharmacological characteristics and side effects Causes elevation of liver enzyme levels in 40% of patients; therefore, biweekly liver tests are necessary during dosage escalations and every 3 months thereafter
Donepezil (Aricept)	Mild to severe AD	Once daily, beginning with 5 mg per day, which can be increased to 10 mg per day (maximum dosage) after 4 weeks. Also available as an oral disintegrating tablet	Adverse effects are mild and include nausea, vomiting and diarrhoea	Gastrointestinal-related adverse effects can be reduced if the medication is taken with food Some patients exhibit an initial increase in agitation, which subsides after the first few weeks of therapy
Rivastigmine (Exelon)	Mild to moderate AD	*Oral* Twice daily, beginning with 1.5 mg twice daily. Also available as a 2 mg ml^{-1} oral solution *Transdermal patch* Once daily, 4.6 or 9.5 mg The target dose is 9.5 mg per 24 h patch (a 10 cm^2 patch) and requires a simple one-step dose titration to the therapeutic dose	Adverse effects include nausea, vomiting, diarrhoea, weight loss, headaches, abdominal pain, fatigue, anxiety and agitation. Gastrointestinal-related adverse effects less prominent with patch	Higher dosages are more efficacious than lower dosages No laboratory monitoring is required
Galantamine (Razadyne)	Mild to moderate AD	Twice daily, beginning with 4 mg twice daily After 4 weeks, the dosage is increased to 8 mg twice daily to a maximum of 12 mg twice daily Available in an extended-release formulation (8, 16 and 24 mg) that can be taken once daily. Also available as a 4 mg ml^{-1} oral solution	Most common side effects are nausea, vomiting and diarrhoea	Gastrointestinal-related adverse effects can be minimized by titrating the dosage gradually and taking the medication with meals
NMDA antagonists				
Memantine (Namenda)	Moderate to severe AD	Twice daily, beginning with 5 mg twice daily, increasing the dose to 10 mg twice daily over 3 weeks	Adverse effects include fatigue, pain, hypertension, headache, constipation, vomiting, back pain, somnolence	Moderate to severe AD may respond better with memantine–donepezil combination than with donepezil alone

of ADL function is an important goal of AD therapy and significant preservation of ADL function has been observed with donepezil, galantamine and rivastigmine compared with placebo. Patients treated with ChEIs and/or memantine may also experience behavioural benefits in terms of reduced severity of existing behavioural disturbances and fewer new behavioural symptoms, usually agitation/aggression and irritability, whereas depression, apathy and anxiety do not respond.[27] In an open-label study using the neuropsychiatric inventory (NPI), donepezil was shown to reduce significantly the severity of neuropsychiatric symptoms in patients with mild to moderate AD (mean total score: 25.4 versus 15.2 at baseline versus 12 weeks; $p<0.001$). With the exception of elation, all domains of the NPI were significantly improved from baseline. During the subsequent 12 week period, in which patients either continued with donepezil therapy or switched to placebo, these improvements were sustained with donepezil therapy, whereas patients receiving placebo experienced significant worsening in NPI scores.[30]

ChEIs have also been shown to reduce AD caregiver burden: in patients with moderate to severe AD, donepezil treatment for 24 weeks significantly reduced caregiver time spent assisting patients with basic and instrumental ADLs (−52 min per day; $p<0.005$). A small study has demonstrated that rivastigmine treatment reduces caregiver time spent assisting with ADLs (up to 690 h over 2 years).

Long-term treatment with ChEIs may also decrease the risk for nursing home placement.[31] A retrospective analysis of a large US medical claims database showed that over a 27 month follow-up period, more patients who were not treated with ChEIs were placed in nursing homes (11.0%) than those who received either rivastigmine (3.7%) or donepezil (4.4%).[32] These studies suggest that ChEIs enable patients to live longer in community settings, with associated personal, social and economic benefits.

Moderate-to-severe disease

Memantine is approved for the treatment of moderate to severe AD, based on a study in which patients with moderate to severe AD who received 20 mg memantine monotherapy showed less decline in cognition and function, while maintaining good tolerability, after 6 months than those who received placebo.[32] The ChEI donepezil has also recently been approved for use in severe AD. Donepezil has also been associated with reduced burden for caregivers of patients with moderate to severe AD. In one trial, the caregivers of patients receiving donepezil therapy reported spending almost 1 h less per day on assisting with ADLs than the caregivers of placebo-treated patients.[33]

There is also evidence that combination therapy with ChEIs plus memantine improves clinical and functional outcomes compared with placebo or ChEIs alone.[34]

Medical foods

Medical foods represent a new alternative to be considered for integration into a comprehensive therapeutic regimen for patients with AD. They comprise a US Food and Drug Administration (FDA)-regulated product defined by Congress as part of the Orphan Drug Act. Such products currently being marketed in the USA for the management of dementia include Axona (caprylic triglyceride) and CerefolinNAC. Other medical foods are also being developed, such as Souvenaid.

Axona has been developed for the clinical dietary management of the metabolic processes associated with mild to moderate AD. It is a formulation of caprylic triglyceride, a medium-chain triglyceride that is metabolized to ketone bodies, predominantly β-hydroxybutyrate (BHB). BHB is a common metabolic substrate that is normally produced by the body for neurons in starvation states where glucose is less available.[35] A double-blind crossover study conducted in patients with AD or MCI demonstrated that Axona therapy was associated with significant improvements in ADAS-Cog; however, the effect was only seen in patients who were ApoE ε4 non-carriers. Similar results were reported in a 90 day randomized, placebo-controlled study in patients with mild to moderate AD.[35] Gastrointestinal disturbances were the most commonly occurring adverse events in the clinical trials. In the 90 day study, one-quarter of patients taking Axona experienced diarrhoea compared with 14% in the placebo group. Gastrointestinal side effects are reportedly reduced by administration of Axona with a meal or mixing it with a drink.

CerefolinNAC, which contains L-methylfolate, methylcobalamin and *N*-acetylcysteine, is indicated for the distinct nutritional requirements of individuals under a physician's treatment for neurovascular oxidative stress and/or hyperhomocysteinaemia, including patients diagnosed with AD. The efficacy of its ingredients regarding cognitive performance has been assessed in various trials.[36]

Souvenaid combines omega-3 fatty acids, choline, uridine monophosphate and a mixture of antioxidants and B vitamins. In a randomized controlled trial involving more than 200 patients with very mild AD, Souvenaid was well tolerated and improved memory, compared with placebo.[37]

Behavioural management

Behavioural management with psychotropic agents

Pharmacological interventions are necessary when non-pharmacological strategies fail to reduce behavioural symptoms sufficiently. Although ChEIs and memantine may improve these symptoms, if behavioural disturbances persist despite their use then a psychotropic agent may be necessary.

If a psychotropic agent is needed, the rule 'start low and go slow, but go' (i.e. the agent should be initiated in a low dosage that should be increased slowly) should be followed and the patient should be closely monitored for side effects and adverse events. The dosage should be increased until an adequate response occurs or side effects emerge; potential drug interactions should also be considered. After behavioural disturbances have been controlled for 4–6 months, the dosage of psychotropic agent should be reduced periodically to determine whether continued pharmacotherapy is required. The choice of psychopharmacological agent is determined by specific target symptoms; some behaviours, such as wandering and pacing, are not amenable to drug therapy.

Atypical antipsychotics

Atypical antipsychotic drugs have been commonly used off-label in clinical practice for the treatment of serious dementia-associated agitation and aggression, although they have not been approved by the FDA for such use. The FDA analysis of the 17 registration trials across six antipsychotic drugs indicated a statistically significantly elevated risk of death in drug-treated patients (either heart-related or from infections) that was 1.6 times greater than in placebo-treated patients. These findings should be taken seriously by clinicians in assessing the potential risks and benefits of treatment in a generally frail population and in advising family members about treatment options. In general, psychotropic agents should be used only when non-pharmacological approaches have failed to control serious behavioural disruption adequately within 5–7 days.[38] A useful rule of thumb is that a behaviour needs to addressed pharmacologically when that behaviour interferes with patient care, patient safety or the safety of another individual. At all times, the prescriber in conjunction with the patient and caregiver should address the benefit–risk balance in this patient population. Other concerns regarding the use of antipsychotics involve a higher incidence of side effects in elderly patients, including sedation, falls and extrapyramidal signs, with recommendations that their use in this patient population should be carefully monitored.

Additional options for pharmacotherapy include trazodone, carbamazepine and valproate, although the data are inconclusive. Tricyclic antidepressants, antihistamines and benzodiazepines should be generally avoided in this population. Selective serotonin reuptake inhibitors appear to have efficacy for the treatment of agitation in patients with AD. Studies have demonstrated benefits for agitation with citalopram, compared with placebo, and similar efficacy, compared with risperidone.[39]

Future therapies

ChEIs and memantine are symptomatic therapies that help maintain neuronal function but do not have a significant impact on the underlying disease process. Their benefits are mild and treatments that modify the disease course are urgently needed. AD is currently thought to be a complex, multifactorial syndrome, unlikely to arise from a single causal factor; instead, a number of related biological alterations are thought to contribute to its pathogenesis. This may explain why the currently available drugs, developed according to the classic drug discovery paradigm of 'one molecule one target', have turned out to be palliative. In the light of this, drug combinations that can act at different levels of the neurotoxic cascade offer new avenues towards ameliorating the symptoms of AD.

Conclusion

The rising prevalence of AD suggests that all health providers will have an increasingly important role in the diagnosis and subsequent management of disease. A key factor in the optimal treatment and outcome of AD is the timely and accurate diagnosis of dementia, with diagnostic tools that can identify dementia early and precisely. There has been an unprecedented growth of scientific knowledge about AD. The distinctive and reliable biomarkers that are now available through structural brain imaging with MRI, PET and CSF analyses, along with a clearer definition of the clinical profile of amnestic disorders that occur early in the course of disease, have made it possible to identify AD with high accuracy, even in its early stages. New criteria for AD diagnosis are being proposed that may allow the detection of not only symptomatic disease but also prodromal states. Of the newly available diagnostic tools for use by primary care physicians, the Mini-Cog, MoCA and AD8 may be particularly useful as brief, easy to administer and effective diagnostic assessments that can be used in everyday clinical practice.

The treatment of AD consists of both pharmacological and non-pharmacological interventions. Non-pharmacological interventions are recommended as the most appropriate initial strategy for managing inappropriate behaviours in dementia. An increasing number of non-pharmacological therapies are now available. Given that there are currently no means of reversing the pathological processes of AD, the primary objectives of pharmacological interventions are to preserve cognitive and functional ability, minimize behavioural disturbances and slow disease progression. To date, five drugs have been approved for treating AD: four ChEIs, which have been the cornerstone of treatment for patients with mild to moderate AD for over a decade, and an NMDA antagonist. On occasions, it may be necessary to prescribe a psychotropic agent, with atypical antipsychotic agents commonly used off-label for serious dementia-associated agitation and aggression, and antidepressants, having been prescribed for patients with AD who also suffer from depression. Future therapies may include amyloid-modifying drugs, acetylcholine receptor agonists, mitochondrial inhibitors and tau-based and neuroprotective approaches.

> **Key points**
>
> - AD is the most common form of dementia.
> - Both pharmacological and behaviour therapies may improve the outcomes in AD.
> - Plaques are formed by amyloid β-protein.
> - Phosphorylated tau produces neurofibrillary tangles.

Acknowledgements

The author thanks Dr Nigel Cairns and the Neuropathology Core of the Alzheimer Disease Research Center at Washington University School of Medicine (funded by National Institutes of Health P50 AG05681) for the neuropathology images. This work was supported by grants from the National Institutes of Health (P30 AG008051 and R01 AG040211).

References

1. Galvin JE. Alzheimer disease: understanding the challenges, improving the outcome. *Appl Neurol* 2007;Suppl (Feb): 3–13.
2. Perl DP. Neuropathology of Alzheimer's disease. *Mt Sinai J Med* 2010;**77**:32–42.
3. Alzheimer's Association. *2010 Facts and Figures*, http://www.alz.org/documents_custom/report_alzfactsfigures 2010.pdf (last accessed 6 July 2010).
4. Bendlin BB, Carlsson CM, Gleason CE *et al*. Midlife predictors of Alzheimer's disease. *Maturitas* 2010;**65**:131–7.
5. Bertram L and Tanzi RE. Of replications and refutations: the status of Alzheimer's disease genetic research. *Curr Neurol Neurosci Rep* 2001;**1**:442–50.
6. Bertram L and Tanzi RE. Genome-wide association studies in Alzheimer's disease. *Hum Mol Genet* 2009;**18**(R2): R137–45.
7. Ryan NS and Rossor MN. Correlating familial Alzheimer's disease gene mutations with clinical phenotype. *Biomark Med* 2010;**4**:99–112.
8. American Psychiatric Association, Task Force on DSM-IV. *Diagnostic and Statistical Manual of Mental Disorders: DSM-IV*, 4th edn, American Psychiatric Association, Washington, DC, 1994.
9. McKhann G, Knopman DS, Chertkow H *et al*. The diagnosis of dementia due to Alzheimer's disease: recommendations from the National Institute on Aging–Alzheimer's Association workgroups on diagnostic guidelines for Alzheimer's disease. *Alzheimers Dement* 2011;**7**:263–9.
10. Dubois B, Feldman HH, Jacova C *et al*. Research criteria for the diagnosis of Alzheimer's disease: revising the NINCDS–ADRDA criteria. *Lancet Neurol* 2007;**6**:734–46.
11. Folstein MF, Folstein SE and McHugh PR. Mini-Mental State: a practical method for grading the cognitive status of patients for the clinicians. *J Psychiatr Res* 1975;**12**:189–98.
12. Galvin JE, Roe CM, Xiong C and Morris JC. The validity and reliability of the AD8 informant interview for dementia. *Neurology* 2006;**67**:1942–8.
13. Galvin JE, Fagan AM, Holtzman DM *et al*. Relationship of dementia screening tests with biomarkers of Alzheimer's disease. *Brain* 2010;**133**:3290–300.
14. deSouza L, Sarazin M, Goetz C and Dubois B. Clinical investigations in primary care. *Front Neurol Neurosci* 2009;**24**:1–11.
15. Borson S, Scanlan JM, Watanabe J *et al*. Simplifying detection of cognitive impairment: comparison of the Mini-Cog and Mini-Mental State Examination in a multiethnic sample. *J Am Geriatr Soc* 2005;**53**:871–4.
16. Nasreddine ZS, Phillips NA, Bedirian V *et al*. The Montreal Cognitive Assessment, MoCA: a brief screening tool for mild cognitive impairment. *J Am Geriatr Soc* 2005;**53**:695–9.
17. Knopman DS, DeKosky ST, Cummings JL *et al*. Practice parameter: diagnosis of dementia (an evidence-based review). Report of the Quality Standards Subcommittee of the American Academy of Neurology. *Neurology* 2001;**56**: 1143–53.
18. Devanand DP, Pelton GH, Zamora D *et al*. Predictive utility of apolipoprotein E genotype for Alzheimer disease in outpatients with mild cognitive impairment. *Arch Neurol* 2005; **62**:975–80.
19. Waldemar G, Dubois B, Emre M *et al*. Recommendations for the diagnosis and management of Alzheimer's disease and other disorders associated with dementia: EFNS guideline. *Eur J Neurol* 2007;**14**: e1–26.
20. Hoffman JM, Welsh-Bohmer KA, Hanson M *et al*. FDG PET imaging in patients with pathologically verified dementia. *J Nucl Med* 2000;**41**:1920–8.
21. Nordberg A, Rinne JO, Kadir A and Långström B. The use of PET in Alzheimer disease. *Nat Rev Neurol* 2010;**6**:78–87.
22. Carpenter BD, Xiong C, Porensky EK *et al*. Reaction to a dementia diagnosis in individuals with Alzheimer's disease and mild cognitive impairment. *J Am Geriatr Soc* 2008; **56**:405–12.
23. Fillit HM, Doody RS, Binaso K *et al*. Recommendations for best practices in the treatment of Alzheimer's disease in managed care. *Am J Geriatr Pharmacother* 2006;**4**(Suppl A): S9–24.
24. Douglas S, James I and Ballard C. Non-pharmacological interventions in dementia. *Adv Psychiatr Treat* 2004;**10**:171–9.
25. Finkel SI, Costa e Silva J, Cohen G *et al*. Behavioral and psychological signs and symptoms of dementia: a consensus statement on current knowledge and implications for research and treatment. *Int Psychogeriatr* 1996;**8**(Suppl 3): 497–500.
26. Cohen-Mansfield J. Nonpharmacologic interventions for inappropriate behaviors in dementia: a review, summary and critique. *Am J Geriatr Psychiatry* 2001;**9**:361–81.
27. Geldmacher DS. The cost benefit to health plans of pharmacotherapy for Alzheimer's disease. *Manag Care* 2005;**14**:44–46.

28. Birks J and Harvey R. Donepezil for dementia due to Alzheimer's disease. *Cochrane Database Syst Rev* 2006;(1): CD001190.
29. Trinh NH, Hoblyn J, Mohanty S and Yaffe K. Efficacy of cholinesterase inhibitors in the treatment of neuropsychiatric symptoms and functional impairment in Alzheimer disease: a meta-analysis. *JAMA* 2003;**289**:210–6.
30. Holmes C, Wilkinson D, Dean C *et al.* The efficacy of donepezil in the treatment of neuropsychiatric symptoms in Alzheimer disease. *Neurology* 2004;**63**:214–9.
31. Lopez OL, Becker JT, Saxton J *et al.* Alteration of a clinically meaningful outcome in the natural history of Alzheimer's disease by cholinesterase inhibition. *J Am Geriatr Soc* 2005; **53**:83–7.
32. Beusterien KM, Thomas SK, Gause D *et al.* Impact of rivastigmine use on the risk of nursing home placement in a US sample. *CNS Drugs* 2004;**18**:1143–8.
33. Atri A, Shaughnessy LW, Locascio JJ and Growdon JH. Long-term course and effectiveness of combination therapy in Alzheimer disease. *Alzheimer Dis Assoc Disord* 2008;**22**: 209–21.
34. Reisberg B, Doody R, Stoffler A *et al.* Memantine in moderate-to-severe Alzheimer's disease. *N Engl J Med* 2003;**348**: 1333–41.
35. Henderson ST, Vogel JL, Barr LJ *et al.* Study of the ketogenic agent AC-1202 in mild to moderate Alzheimer's disease: a randomized, double-blind, placebo-controlled, multicenter trial *Nutr Metab* 2009;**6**:31–56.
36. McCaddon A and Hudson PR. L-Methylfolate, methylcobalamin and *N*-acetylcysteine in the treatment of Alzheimer's disease-related cognitive decline. *CNS Spectr* 2010;**15** (1 Suppl 1):2–5.
37. Scheltens P, Verhey FRJ, Olde Rikkert MGM *et al.* The efficacy of a medical food (Souvenaid®) in Alzheimer's disease: results from the first trial and design of future trials *Alzheimer Dement* 2009;**5**:258–9.
38. Salzman C, Jeste DV, Meyer RE *et al.* Elderly patients with dementia-related symptoms of severe agitation and aggression: consensus statement on treatment options, clinical trials methodology and policy. *J Clin Psychiatry* 2008;**69**:889–98.
39. Pollock BG, Mulsant BH, Rosen J *et al.* A double-blind comparison of citalopram and risperidone for the treatment of behavioral and psychotic symptoms associated with dementia. *Am J Geriatr Psychiatry* 2007;**15**:942–52.

CHAPTER 74

Mild cognitive impairment

Eric G. Tangalos and Ronald C. Petersen
Mayo Clinic, Rochester, MN, USA

Introduction

The concept of mild cognitive impairment (MCI) as an intermediate state between normal cognition and dementia entered into the vernacular of geriatric medicine in the past 15–30 years. What this chapter may add to our understanding is that it is a relatively precise clinical diagnosis and a useful research tool. More often than not, the clinical diagnosis of MCI may have be applied to patients who are either normal or who have dementia. Although this misclassification may be a disservice to the diagnosis of MCI, the bigger disservice is to the patient. Geriatricians need to use the diagnosis appropriately for patient care, understand the treatment limitations, apply appropriate management strategies and embrace the research opportunities presented by this construct.

History

Mild cognitive impairment as a term was introduced into the literature in 1988 by Reisberg *et al.*,[1] but referred to a severity index of stage 3 as identified on the Global Deterioration Scale. Another instrument, the Clinical Dementia Rating Scale, sought to identify very early dementia given the possibility of identifying disease early and intervening as soon as possible.[2] By 1999, MCI had been proposed as a prodromal condition for Alzheimer's disease (AD) with the focus on memory as a chief clinical complaint for incipient disease.[3]

It was evident by the turn of the decade that not all forms of MCI evolved into AD. However, the general construct served most clinicians well enough. The difficulty was then, and still is today, that all too often MCI is used to soften a diagnosis of what should really be dementia. In 2004, Winblad *et al.*[4] sought to expand and revise the criteria.[5] From the symposium concerned, the criteria now used by the National Institute on Aging-Sponsored Alzheimer Disease Centers Program Uniform Data Set and the Alzheimer Disease Neuroimaging Initiative (ADNI)[6] have helped us design protocols to improve our understanding of the dementing process. The clinical phenotypes now include amnestic MCI (aMCI) and non-amnestic MCI (naMCI) with the subtypes of single- and multiple-domain classifications (Figure 74.1).

While specific changes in cognition are frequently observed in normal ageing, there is increasing evidence that some forms of cognitive impairment are recognizable as an early manifestation of dementia.[3] MCI is a heterogeneous state and there remains controversy over aspects of the construct. However, the utility of this paradigm is the recognition that dementia is not a dichotomous state and therefore refining our understanding of the layers of transition will improve the understanding of cognitive decline and ultimately benefit patients. Appropriate diagnosis lets us address our patients' needs with the best available therapies, be they drug or non-drug interventions.

In general, our shortcomings in approaching patients with cognitive decline have been to avoid a diagnosis and delay our interventions. The reasons are multiple, although taking the time to make a diagnosis means that much more time will be needed to explain the diagnosis and take action. Any assault on our independence with special concern regarding the loss of driving privileges plays poorly to the American mindset. We live in a land where our first right of passage is our driver's license and where all roads lead to the shopping mall. We do not live in walking communities and the last thing we give up is our driver's license. There have also been financial disincentives in the past when clinicians used a psychiatric code to define cognitive disease although MCI and the dementing syndromes can b now e classified with ICD-9 medical codes.

Although no symptomatic or disease-modifying drug therapies are available for MCI, there is much that can be done. The domains of cognition, function and behaviour define this population and where they reside in the spectrum of disease. Their preserved abilities can also

Principles and Practice of Geriatric Medicine, Fifth Edition. Edited by Alan J. Sinclair, John E. Morley and Bruno Vellas.

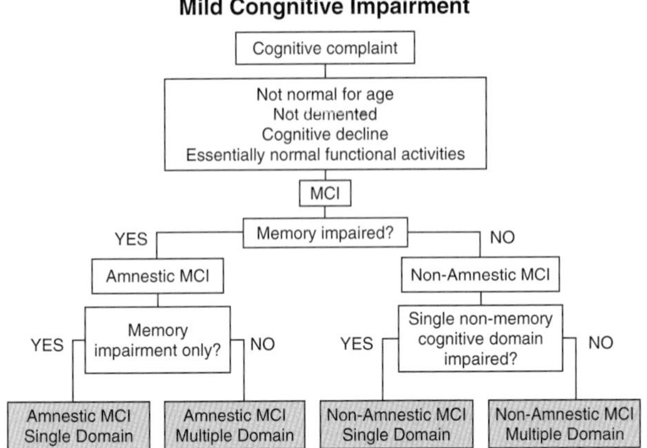

Figure 74.1 MCI flowchart. Reprinted from Petersen[5] with permission.

serve as markers for how the disease is progressing and how well they are living within a defined environment. Even without a drug treatment of MCI, understanding the environment that surrounds every one of these patients and how they function within their universe is most important. Overlearned behaviours and an environment that limit or prohibit excess disabilities should be stressed even for patients with MCI. Much can be done and running towards a diagnosis is better than running away from it.

Cognitive impairment, be it MCI or dementia, can still be defined by the capacities that are preserved and the capacities that are lost. This is where the issue of driving comes into play, but the concept applies to all kinds of tasks and opportunities. We counsel that a diagnosis is not an all-or-nothing phenomenon and many individuals with MCI or even early dementia sit on advisory boards to provide a patient voice in understanding better the needs of the patient. Unfortunately, explaining these concepts and what is both retained and what is lost takes time, especially for the primary care provider.

As our understanding of disease advances, the triad of cognition, function and behaviour not only defines the type of care that may be appropriate but also contributes to our understanding of where the best site of care might be. Our ability to address the environment early in the care of patients with MCI or other age-dependent deficiencies may improve the quality of life for our parents, avoid common pitfalls and provide for more cost-effective and successful management of the being, not just the disease they may have. A goal set by the Alzheimer's Association back in 1987 was to create an environment where a person can function with *minimal* failure and *maximal* use of retained abilities. There is even more opportunity today to create this success with earlier diagnosis and earlier intervention.

Our earliest work in the Mayo Alzheimer's Disease Research Center taught us that even normal individuals change as they get older. Not only does reaction time slow but on measures of Verbal IQ and measures of Performance IQ, the things we do day in and day out are better preserved.[7–9] In all of our attempts at providing care to the elderly, these are the principles that shaped us early and continue to play out in the advice we give out every day. Overlearned behaviours, repetitive tasks and rehearsed activities make it easy and comfortable for us to go about the routines of the day. The things we are confronted with that take an element of problem solving become all the more difficult as we age.

In addition, the concept of MCI plays extremely well as we design hypothesis-driven research; be it with regard to clinical markers, psychological assessment, neuroimaging, biomarkers or drug and non-drug interventions.[10] This is perhaps equally important as the clinical diagnosis and has generated research opportunities worldwide. The construct of MCI has been incorporated into research on ageing from multiple perspectives, including clinical research, epidemiology, neuroimaging, mechanisms of disease, clinical trials and caregiving.[10]

Definitions and terminology

Mild cognitive impairment (MCI) refers to cognitive impairment that does not meet the criteria for dementia. Various researchers have proposed several criteria for and subtypes of MCI.[3,11,12] These criteria and subtypes differ somewhat, although there is considerable overlap. The Mayo criteria are the ones most commonly applied in the literature:[13]

- memory complaint, preferably corroborated by an informant
- memory impairment documented according to appropriate reference values
- essentially normal performance in non-memory cognitive domains
- generally preserved activities of daily living
- not demented.

It is important to emphasize that these remain clinical criteria. Considerable judgment is involved in making the distinction between impairments that are normal for the elderly population and, at the other extreme, that do not represent dementia. However, it should be noted that this is the manner in which we apply criteria for dementia and AD also. Each follows a construct, has a literature base and serves the patient best when appropriately applied.

MCI is heterogeneous in terms of clinical presentation, aetiology, prognosis and prevalence.[12,14,15] In recognition of the narrower scope of the original Mayo criteria and others that relied heavily on memory problems, the concept was expanded. The intention of this was to broaden the scope and extend the emphasis of detection of other dementias in their prodromal stages.[5,13,16] A useful classification criteria separates MCI into amnestic and non-amnestic groups and further into single and multiple domains. The amnestic type of MCI is generally thought to represent prodromal AD.[17] Other subclasses may have different underlying mechanisms of cognitive impairment and may be associated with other non-AD disease processes [e.g. vascular dementia, frontotemporal dementia (FTD) or dementia with Lewy bodies (DLB)], but there is limited pathological evidence for this paradigm.[18]

The term MCI, without qualification, was traditionally and is still often used to refer to the amnestic type; however, using MCI without qualification is not the current state of affairs. This chapter includes the current breakdown into the various subtypes.

Single-domain amnestic MCI

Single-domain amnestic MCI (aMCI) refers to those individuals with significantly impaired memory who do not meet criteria for dementia. The criteria outlined above were initially developed to define MCI in general, but subsequently have been understood to identify only this type.[3,13]

Memory impairments that qualify for MCI are generally represented by defects that are 1.0–1.5 standard deviations (SDs) or more below age-corrected norms. Although this seems straightforward, different tests of memory likely have different sensitivity and specificity and norms are not available for all populations.[14]

Multiple-domain amnestic MCI

Many individuals with aMCI complain only of memory loss; however, they may have additional subtle impairments in other cognitive domains, for example, executive function, that are revealed with careful neuropsychological testing.[16,19–21] Some would interpret the latter finding as excluding patients from this subtype of MCI according to the criteria listed above.[14] This highlights the operational difficulties with the application of the criteria and was a primary reason for expanding the diagnostic categories to include single- and multiple-domain impairment.[5] Such persons may manifest subtle problems with activities of daily living, but they do not meet criteria for a formal diagnosis of dementia.[15] The multiple domains are, by definition, only slightly impaired (i.e. less than 0.5–1 SD below age- and education-matched normal subjects).

aMCI is often thought of as a precursor to AD.[17] Although memory performances are often similar in patients with aMCI and AD, the addition of impairments in multiple cognitive domains are also prominent in patients with AD.[3] Suffice it to say, the greater the extent of additional non-memory domains the smaller the distinction between MCI and AD becomes and the greater is the risk of conversion to dementia.

Often these individuals progress to meet criteria for AD or vascular dementia; in a minority of cases, the cognitive profile may simply reflect normal ageing.[15] The prognostic utility of the multiple-domain form of MCI remains unclear as some studies have identified this as the highest risk category for conversion to dementia whereas others have exposed instability, with some individuals returning to baseline level of function over time.[16,22,23] It may represent a progression of impairment from the memory domain alone to multiple domain involvement on the way to dementia.

Single-domain non-amnestic MCI

The concept of single-domain non-amnestic MCI (naMCI) is similar to that for aMCI, except that this form of MCI is characterized by a relatively isolated impairment in a single non-memory domain, such as executive functioning, language or visual spatial skills.[15] Depending upon the domain, individuals with this subtype of MCI may progress to other syndromes, such as FTD, including primary progressive aphasia, DLB, progressive supranuclear palsy (PSP) or even corticobasalganglionic syndrome (CBS). Individuals within this group appear to be at less of a risk for conversion to dementia, although supporting evidence is limited by the operationalization of MCI diagnosis.[18,24] Uncommonly, AD may present without a memory impairment initially, so naMCI can occasionally be a prodromal state of AD.

Multiple-domain non-amnestic MCI

As with aMCI, patients who meet this criterion are affected in multiple domains with a relative sparing of memory problems. The substrate of multiple-domain naMCI is felt to be that of degenerative disorders associated with tau, TAR DNA binding protein (TDP-43) and α-synuclein such as FTD and DLB.[25,26]

Although these criteria were developed as an ontological concept relating early changes in specific cognitive domains to those areas most commonly affected in the disorders, that is, memory problems and AD, there remains a significant amount of crossover between groups.[18] Additionally, in certain disorders, such as behavioural variant FTD, cognitive complaints are often preceded by significant alterations in behaviour and comportment. Hence some have proposed the concept of mild behavioural impairment as a similar paradigm to recognize an additional group with increased risk of dementia.[27]

Related terminology

There are a multitude of loosely related terms that have been used to describe constructs that are similar to or perhaps even the same as MCI, for example, incipient dementia, isolated memory impairment, dementia prodrome, minimal AD, predementia AD, prodromal AD and early AD.[3,12,13,15,28,29] In a glossary of these and other terms that describe cognitive impairment in elderly people without dementia, most of these definitions do not fully overlap with the definition of MCI.[30]

The concept of MCI perhaps reflects most closely the idea of 'cognitive impairment, no dementia' (CIND).[31] However, in contrast to the definition for the amnestic form of MCI, CIND relies less heavily on the presence of prominent memory deficits and includes in its definition the presence of a functional disability. It is a more inclusive definition than MCI and includes static encephalopathies, as is reflected by its higher prevalence.

'Age-associated memory impairment' (AAMI) and 'age-associated cognitive decline' (AACD) are also widely used and fairly well-known terms. However, these terms differ from MCI in that they were originally devised to define normal age-associated memory and cognitive changes in older adults as referenced to young normal adult individuals.[3,32,33] AACD was developed as a way of defining better the cognitive changes in elderly compared with age-adjusted norms. AACD has more recently been recognized as identifying a state of impairment similar to MCI.[34] In MCI, memory impairments are referenced to age-adjusted norms and require a decline from a previous level of functioning.

Studies of 'preclinical AD' should be distinguished from studies of MCI.[35] In MCI studies, patients meet cognitive criteria for diagnosis and are then followed prospectively to assess for conversion to AD. As we move forward with our understanding of disease, we expect presymptomatic cases to be described and defined by biomarker data.

Some investigators challenge the inclusion of intact activities of daily living as a criterion and have suggested further refining the concept of subjective cognitive complaint.[36–38] These and other judgments likely differ between assessors and account for some of the conflicting results in studies of this disorder. It is also important to note that an essential component of the diagnosis of MCI is based on the clinical history and should not rest on psychometric testing or a hesitancy to diagnose a dementia appropriately.

Case examples

The clinical presentation of a patient with MCI typically involves a cognitive complaint. Patients or family members commonly report difficulties with 'short-term memory' (by which they mean recent memory) but detailed history-taking should also ask about symptoms in other cognitive domains. Motor, neuropsychiatric, autonomic and sleep symptoms also may be present and should be elicited specifically during the initial evaluation. However, the field has expanded and the differential now includes a variety of subcategories including naMCI. Two examples may help in understand the current differentiations. Potential interventions as practiced by providers who wish to intervene early are included.

70-year-old man with amnestic MCI

This patient has a memory complaint and lacks other cognitive difficulties.

A 70-year-old right-handed male presents with a 2 year history of memory complaints. His wife mentions that he tends to misplace items, forget conversations and repeat himself. He maintains all activities of daily living and admits to having trouble with his memory. Although he finishes tasks with accuracy, he takes a slightly longer time to finish activities such as balancing the chequebook. He scores 34/38 on the Kokmen Short Test of Mental Status,[39] losing all four points on recall. His general neurological examination is within normal limits. Formal neuropsychological testing shows impairment only in the memory domain, with difficulties in delayed verbal recall. Performance on tests of attention-executive functioning, visuospatial skills and language is in the above-average range. Screening laboratory tests did not reveal a reversible cause for his cognitive difficulties. His brain magnetic resonance imaging (MRI) scan is significant for mild bilateral hippocampal atrophy.

Discussions were undertaken early on regarding the patient's cognitive complaints. He had preserved insight and was well aware that there was a problem. The discussion was 'hopeful' although his clinician was very clear that a diagnosis could already be established and that progression to a dementing syndrome still carried a strong likelihood. No drug therapy was offered and his type 2 diabetes had been well managed. An additional review of his medications revealed the use of oxybutynin for an overactive bladder and it was suggested that this drug be discontinued because of its anticholinergic burden. The family was most appreciative of this suggestion and had questioned whether the drug had provided any benefit in the first place. This discussion also provided the clinician with the opportunity to introduce the potential use of a cholinesterase inhibitor should the patient go on to manifest additional disease.

The opportunity also presented itself with regard to managing the environment of care. There had been some talk of moving to a warmer climate now that the patient was retired. They had vacationed in the previous two winters in a retirement community and enjoyed the experience. However, the patient had shown some reluctance in making a permanent move as he had misplaced the golf cart on more than one occasion. The conversation therefore turned to the most appropriate time to move and where to move. Patients with cognitive difficulties do best with stable and predictable environments. Learning becomes more difficult and the recommendation was either to move as soon as possible or not to move at all. In this way, the patient would have either the greatest opportunity to adjust to his new surroundings or benefit from the continuing, predictable and overlearned environment already surrounding him.

75-year-old woman with non-amnestic MCI

This patient's cognitive impairment is affecting attention-executive functioning and the visuospatial domain.

A 75-year-old right-handed female presents with a 2 year history of progressive cognitive difficulties. Her daughter reports that she does not multitask or make decisions as well as she did after her husband's death 10 years ago. She also takes longer to complete the laundry and finds it challenging to fix holiday meals. Otherwise, she maintains all activities of daily living independently and continues to drive to the grocery store. Both she and her daughter reported no problems with memory. On examination, she scores 33/38 on the Kokmen Short Test of Mental Status. Although she lost two points on learning, two points on calculation and one point on construction, she was able to state all four words on the delayed recall task. Her general neurological examination was significant for mild bradyphrenia, bradykinesia and hypomimia. Formal neurological testing showed impairment in attention-executive functioning and visuospatial skills, with above-average performance on measurements that tested the memory and language domains. Screening laboratory tests did not reveal a reversible cause for her cognitive difficulties. Her brain MRI scan also was unremarkable, without any evidence of cerebral or hippocampal atrophy.

The patient's daughter lives out-of-state and no close relatives or friends could be counted on for support. Power of attorney for healthcare had been established shortly after the husband's death and this was an opportunity to discuss additional advance directives. The patient had no plans for a living will but had talked extensively with the daughter about her husband's death. She did not want to go on a ventilator as he did after his heart attack and lived like a 'vegetable' after his subsequent stroke. They were both in agreement that it would be best if she moved closer to her daughter and with the clinician's support it was recommended that they do this sooner rather than later.

The daughter sought out local support and was a close friend of a social worker who worked at the neighbourhood hospital. As the mother was moving to a bigger city, there were many opportunities (none of which included living with the daughter). Both mother and daughter looked at a number of options together and, with advice provided by the social worker, chose a large campus that was essentially a continuing care retirement community. The rationale was that the mother would be able to live quite independently, although she planned to give up driving. Should her condition deteriorate, the campus had graduated programmes to attend to her needs. However, the entire campus maintained a unified philosophy, was easy to navigate and seemed to understand that patients should be left to function on their own whenever they had preserved abilities to do so. It was unlikely that the patient would ever leave the campus as a large, skilled nursing care facility was also part of the package.

Why does it matter?

If we wait for functional decline to define dementia, it may be too late to treat the underlying disease process.[40] Moreover, since functional decline is in the definition of dementia, it is best to work with a construct that would allow intervention sooner rather than later. With this theoretical framework, many studies have been conducted to investigate the utility and prognostic outcome of the diagnoses.[40]

Numerous investigations worldwide have used these criteria as an infrastructure for estimating the frequency of MCI and its subtypes.[14,18,20,41] Both prospective[18,42] and retrospective studies[36] have helped to define the subtleties of the diagnosis. A major factor in determining outcome depends on the source of the patient being studied. The closer one is to a community sample, the lower are the annual rates of progression (6–10%).[43] With referral-based studies, such as those that come from sampling a memory disorders clinic or AD centre, the progression rates rise to 10–15% per year, particularly for AD.[44] These differences reflect the probability of having an underlying disorder such as MCI when a participant or concerned family member seeks treatment at a referral clinic. The same phenomenon occurs at dementia 'screening' clinics that advertise their services and claim diagnostic rates approaching 50%. This is in the face of baseline incidence rates of dementia and AD of 1–2% per year.[3] Published rates of progression are summarized in Table 74.1.

Epidemiology

The Mayo Clinic Study of Aging was designed as a population-based study in Olmsted County, MN, USA, involving a random sample of nearly 3000 participants aged 70–89 years who were non-demented and cognitively normal or who had MCI at entry.[45,46] The prevalence of MCI from this study is estimated at ~15% of the non-demented population, with a 2:1 ratio of aMCI to naMCI. The most common putative cause is degenerative and this cause predominates to a greater extent for aMCI than for naMCI. There is evidence that these rates tend to hold up throughout the world at about 14–18% for individuals aged 70 years and older.[10] The overall progression rate for all MCI

Table 74.1 Rates of progression.

Source	Study location	No. of participants	Participant age range (years)	Reported rate of progression	Annual crude progression rate (%)[a]
Solfrizzi *et al.* (2004)[86]	Italy	1524	≥65	3.8/100 person-years	3.8
Busse *et al.* (2006)[18]	Leipzig, Germany	863	≥75	44% per 4.3 years	10.2
Tschanz *et al.* (2006)[87]	Cache County, UT, USA	3266	≥65	46% per 3 years	15.3
Fischer *et al.* (2007)[43]	Austria	476	75–76	33.9% per 30 months	13.6
Ravaglia *et al.* (2008)[88]	Italy	937	≥65	14% per 1 year	14
Farias *et al.* (2009)[89]	California	111	>60	3% per 1 year[b]	3.0
Petersen *et al.* (2010)[46]	Rochester, MN, USA	1969	70–89	7.5% per 1 year	7.5

[a]Annual crude progression rates (%) are reported in the data or estimated from the crude rates.
[b]In the Farias study, the rate of progression for the clinic cohort is reported as 13% per 1 year.

Table 74.2 Prevalence studies.

Source	Study location[a]	No. of participants	Participant age range (years)	Prevalence of MCI (%)
Unverzagt *et al.* (2001)[90]	Indianapolis, IN, USA	2212	≥65	23.4
Hanninen *et al.* (2002)[91]	Finland	806	60–76	5.3
Lopez *et al.* (2003)[42]	CHS	1690	≥75	22
Ganguli *et al.* (2004)[14]	MoVIES	1248	≥65	3.2
Busse *et al.* (2006)[18]	Leipzig, Germany	980	75–79	19.3
Das *et al.* (2007)[92]	India	745	≥50	14.9
Di Carlo *et al.* (2007)[93]	Italy	2830	65–84	16.1
Fischer *et al.* (2007)[43]	Austria	697	75	24.3
Manly *et al.* (2008)[94]	Manhattan, NY, USA	2364	≥65	21.8
Palmer *et al.* (2008)[95]	Kungsholmen, Stockholm, Sweden	379	75–95	11.1
Plassman *et al.* (2008)[96]	ADAMS	856	≥71	22.2
Roberts *et al.* (2008)[45]	Rochester, MN, USA	1969	70–89	14.8

[a]Abbreviations: ADAMS, Aging, Demographics and Memory Study; MoVIES, Monongahela Valley Independent Elders Survey; CHS, Cardiovascular Health Study.

by consensus is 8.5% and by concordance 9.4%. Published prevalence studies are summarized in Table 74.2.

Neuropathology

There are not many neuropathological studies to shed light on the clinical syndrome as patients survive much further into their disease course before succumbing to death and potential autopsy. The Religious Orders Study followed up a group of nuns and priests for many years and achieved high autopsy rates. The study reported that ~60% of the participants with MCI have neuropathological evidence of AD, but that vascular disease also accounts for significant pathology.[47] Other studies have implicated the importance and the findings of neurofibrillary tangle density to account for the symptoms of MCI.[48]

Two additional studies come from our own investigations. We evaluated participants who died while their clinical classification was MCI and found that most had a low probability of having the neuropathological features of AD at that point in time.[49] A second study observed participants who had been previously diagnosed with MCI and had progressed to dementia and characterized these participants as having diagnostic pathology. This study indicated that, while most of the participants with aMCI developed AD, another sizeable group (20–30%) developed another type of dementing disorder.[50] These studies remain in contrast to opinions that the discoverable pathology of MCI, albeit more advanced MCI, is only AD.[51,52]

Approaching the patient and their caregiver

The clinical history remains the mainstay in making a diagnosis of MCI. It is all about what insight the patient maintains in understanding their memory deficit. However, obtaining a history from both the patient and an informant may provide further support that a cognitive decline does exist.[53] Questions about cognition should address all major domains, including memory, attention-executive functioning, visuospatial skills and language. Common memory symptoms include the tendency for frequent repetition or forgetfulness of recent events.

Patients with attention-executive functioning impairment may have problems in making decisions, planning activities and multitasking. Visuospatial difficulties may be elicited by asking about a tendency to get lost while driving or an inability to track the lines on a page while reading. Word-finding difficulty, paraphasias, and/or anomia may indicate language dysfunction. The history taking should also focus on functional status, including the ability to drive, manage finances and maintain basic activities of daily living. Possible neuropsychiatric, motor and sleep issues should be addressed, as the presence of these symptoms may suggest a possible aetiology of an MCI subtype.

Language difficulties, disinhibition or socially inappropriate behaviour may be seen in those with FTD; REM sleep behaviour disorder (RBD), characterized by a tendency to act out dreams, has been associated with DLB. A past medical history may reveal cerebrovascular disease, seizures, head trauma, systemic cancer or infections that may be contributing to the cognitive impairment.

The time course of symptoms is also important. A gradual, insidious progression of symptoms may suggest a degenerative cause, whereas a more acute onset may indicate a vascular, inflammatory or infectious aetiology. Loss of concentration may be a presenting symptom, but it is more often associated with depression than with cognitive impairment. Good screening tests for depression are readily available and the PHQ-9 has found its way into many office practices.[29] The PHQ-9 is the nine-item depression scale of the Patient Health Questionnaire. It is a powerful tool for assisting primary care clinicians in diagnosing depression and also selecting and monitoring treatment.

The primary care clinician and/or office staff should discuss with the patient the reasons for completing the questionnaire and how to fill it out. It can be done by intact patients or used as a survey instrument and done by just about anyone. After the patient has completed the PHQ-9 questionnaire, it is simply scored. There are two components of the PHQ-9: (1) assessing symptoms and functional impairment to make a tentative depression diagnosis and (2) deriving a severity score to help select and monitor treatment. It also responds to treatment initiatives with clinically validated changes in the patient's response.

The PHQ-9 is based directly on the diagnostic criteria for major depressive disorder in the *Diagnostic and Statistical Manual of Mental Disorders*, 4th edition (DSM-IV). It is replacing the Geriatric Depression Scale in many situations and will soon become the depression scale on the nursing home Minimum Data Set 3.0. It offers better sensitivity than older tests and can be used across a greater age range. It is also used in many of the research protocols in evaluating mood in dementia states. No evaluation of a cognitive complaint is complete without an evaluation for depression.

After a history has been obtained that will also evaluate the impact of decline, a general neurological examination should be performed. Any practitioner with appropriate experience can do the examination. Although the examination may be normal, abnormalities could suggest a potential aetiology for the cognitive deficits. Parkinsonism may be seen with DLB and also other neurodegenerative disorders, motor neuron signs may be associated with FTD and focal deficit consistent with a specific vascular distribution may suggest a vascular cause for the cognitive impairment.

In addition to a general neurological examination, a screening mental status examination, such as the Mini-Mental State Examination (MMSE), 3MS, VA–St Louis University Mental Status Examination or Kokmen Short Test of Mental Status, should be administered.[39,54,55] Severity of symptoms may be determined using assessments such as the Clinical Dementia Rating scale (CDR).[2] A formal neuropsychological battery also can be performed and should include tests that sufficiently challenge a patient in each cognitive domain.

After adjusting for age and education, scores below 1.0–1.5 SDs below the mean typically indicate cognitive impairment on neuropsychological testing.[56,57] Learning and recall tasks may differentiate subjects with MCI from those experiencing normal ageing. On measures of general cognitive function such as the MMSE and full-scale IQ, the individual with MCI performs more similarly to a normal elderly subject, while memory function on delayed verbal recall (Logical Memory II) and non-verbal delayed recall (Visual Reproductions II) more closely resembles mild AD.[3]

Although the screening mental status examination and neuropsychological battery may be useful, it is important to remember that these tests may not be sensitive to cognitive impairment. Individuals may score within the 'normal' range, particularly those with high premorbid intellectual functioning. Despite normal scores, these patients may have MCI, if the clinician determines that there has been a change from baseline functioning. In these circumstances, it is usually best to follow these patients clinically, with repeat evaluations at regular intervals.

Laboratory tests used in the evaluation of dementia may identify medical issues that could affect cognitive function.[58] Basic laboratory tests that look for reversible causes of cognitive impairment include a complete blood count, basic metabolic panel, thyroid function tests, vitamin B_{12} levels and folate levels. Neuroimaging with MRI or computed tomography (CT) of the brain is also recommended to look for any structural abnormalities that may be contributing to symptoms.

Information from the history, screening mental status examination, neuropsychological testing and ancillary studies should be used to determine if cognitive function is changing, normal or impaired. Functional status can be obtained from the individual, the informant or both. If the patient has experienced cognitive decline but has maintained most daily activities, then that individual can be given an MCI diagnosis. Once an individual has been diagnosed as having MCI, the clinician can determine the MCI subtype based on which cognitive domains are impaired. From this determination, the MCI subtype can be made. If memory impairment is present, then the individual has an aMCI subtype. I f memory is preserved but evidence of decline is seen in other cognitive domains, then the subtype is naMCI.

After establishing the subtype as aMCI or naMCI, the next step is to determine if one or more cognitive domains are affected. If memory is the only domain affected, then the subtype would be single-domain aMCI; if at least one other cognitive domain is also affected, then the subtype would be an multiple-domain aMCI. If the impairment was isolated to one of the non-memory domains, then the subtype would be single-domain naMCI; if two or more non-memory domains were affected, then the subtype would be multiple-domain naMCI. Again, function must be essentially preserved to differentiate multiple-domain MCI from dementia.

The goal of such subtyping in clinical practice is to describe accurately the individual's clinical syndrome and to determine the possible aetiology of the patient's symptoms. Using the history, examination and ancillary data, the clinician can begin to deduce whether the cause of impairment is degenerative, vascular, psychiatric or secondary to concomitant medical disorders. Such deductions may assist in providing treatment options for each patient.

Natural progression of disease and outcomes

Since MCI is considered to be a transitional state between normal ageing and dementia, the aetiologies for dementia theoretically could be applied to MCI. While the construct has yet to be validated, aMCI due to a degenerative aetiology is thought to progress most likely to AD – an assertion that has been endorsed in a practice parameter from the American Academy of Neurology.[13]

Although a diagnosis of MCI places an individual at higher risk for developing dementia, it does not indicate that the patient necessarily will progress to a dementia state. Although the majority of the MCI subjects in one large prospective trial progressed to AD at a rate of 7–10% per year, a small percentage of these individuals improved to normal.[18] Others have been known to remain clinically stable for many years and may not develop dementia.[59] These potential outcomes should be discussed with patients and their families after a diagnosis of MCI has been made.

Genetic contributions

aMCI due to a degenerative cause most likely has similar features to clinically probable AD, with risk factors such as age, hypertension and diabetes.[60–62] Apolipoprotein ε4 (ApoE4) carrier status is a recognized genetic risk factor for the development of AD,[63] but its value for detecting progression to cognitive impairment is less clear. It has been a consistent predictor but has not found a useful way into clinical practice.

Some studies have suggested that ApoE4 carrier status may have assist in predicting those more likely to convert from MCI to AD,[64–66] and a synergistic effect with depression has been seen in cognitively normal individuals at risk for developing MCI. ApoE4 carrier status also may be associated both with hippocampal atrophy in MCI subjects and with higher rates of cognitive decline in cognitively normal adults.[67,68] However, others have shown that ApoE4 carrier status itself has not been demonstrated to predict cognitive decline or conversion to AD,[69] and its routine use is not recommended;[70] the diagnosis of MCI is made clinically.

Treatment

Early detection of cognitive decline theoretically may lead to the implementation of therapies that slow the progression of impairment. However, there currently is no FDA-approved treatment intervention for MCI. Since the aetiologies of MCI can be heterogeneous, medications targeting a neurodegenerative cause theoretically would be different from those targeting cognitive impairment due to vascular, psychiatric or other medical disorders. Clinical trials nevertheless have focused on the aMCI subtype, with the goal of slowing the progression to AD.

A number of studies have targeted medications used in the symptomatic treatment of clinically probable AD. These medications have included three of the cholinesterase inhibitors – donepezil, galantamine and rivastigmine.[71–73] Additionally, vitamin E and rofecoxib have been studied,[71,74] as both oxidative damage and inflammation have been implicated in the pathophysiology of AD.[75–78] Unfortunately, none of these interventions have shown a significant reduction in conversion rates of aMCI to AD, ranging from 6 to 17% in the medication arms versus from 4 to 21% with placebo. However, one study did find that donepezil reduced the progression risk for 12 months in those with aMCI – an effect that persisted up to 24 months in ApoE4 carriers.[71]

Despite the results of clinical trial data, these studies do support the construct of MCI as a transitional state between normal cognition and AD. The overall progression rates for MCI in these studies ranged from 5 to 16%, which are higher than the incidence rate for AD in the general population.[3,71] These rates suggest that patients who meet MCI criteria are at a higher risk for developing AD. Since not all of those with MCI develop AD pathology, more accurate identification of these subjects is essential. Incorporating potential predictive biomarkers in clinical trials may assist in testing compounds that target the underlying disease process of AD.[79]

A variety of non-drug interventions have also been tried on this population. Not surprisingly, cognitive training has been the most studied. The environment of care has been addressed and lifestyle management has been included. Interventions range from individualized therapy to group programmes that additionally address activity planning, self-assertiveness training, relaxation techniques, stress management, use of external memory aids and motor exercise. Multicomponent interventions seem to benefit activities of daily living, mood and memory performance. A standardized cognitive training manual has been proposed in addition to further studies utilizing larger sample sizes and more robust experimental designs.[80–82]

Advance care planning

Patients and families should be aware that those who have aMCI due to a degenerative cause may have a 10–15% chance of developing AD; however, it also should be noted that MCI is heterogeneous, with a number of potential outcomes.[59] Although some patients may not develop dementia, the label of 'mild cognitive impairment' nevertheless may lead to psychological consequences, such as a feeling of uncertainty or concerns of becoming burdensome to others.[83] Neuropsychiatric symptoms such as depression, anxiety, apathy and/or irritability may also be seen in those with MCI and may be associated with progression to AD.[84]

As identified in the two case examples above, encouraging patients and their families and caregivers to consider decisions about advance directives, future planning and finances is essential, especially if the cognitive impairment is thought to be due to a degenerative cause. Although definitive data are limited, patients should be encouraged to follow a heart-healthy diet and to remain active physically, intellectually and socially. Participation in a cognitive rehabilitation programme may also be useful in MCI subjects, with improvements in activities of daily living, mood and memory. Although these modifications may improve their overall quality of life, there has not been enough research to support a decreased progression from aMCI to AD.

Future directions

The MCI construct has become useful in the early detection of those at risk for developing dementia. Given the heterogeneity of the MCI subtypes and their potential aetiologies, identifying these individuals with more accuracy is essential. One area of future research is in developing a predictive profile for these patients. With aMCI, for example, a combination of ApoE4 genotypes, cerebrospinal fluid (CSF) biomarkers and neuroimaging findings on MRI, fluorodeoxyglucose positron emission tomography (FDG-PET) and Pittsburgh Compound B (PiB)-PET may identify those who are more likely to progress to AD, as opposed to some other pathology.

The Alzheimer's Disease Neuroimaging Initiative (ADNI), which began in October 2004, has gathered and analysed thousands of brain scans, genetic profiles and biomarkers in blood and CSF. Although the original goal was to define biomarkers for use in clinical trials to determine the best way to measure treatment effects of AD, it has been expanded to using biomarkers to identify AD at a predementia stage. There are over 800 participants comprised of 200 with AD, 400 with MCI (AD) and 200 with normal cognition. The next step is to scan and analyze the brains of people with early mild cognitive impairment (eMCI).

The scope of ongoing research has been expanded to enrol participants at an earlier stage of MCI, when symptoms are milder. Studies include PET, FDG-PET (which measures glucose metabolism in the brain), PET using a radioactive compound (PiB) that measures brain β-amyloid and structural MRI. Biomarkers in CSF are revealing other changes that could identify which patients with MCI will develop AD. Levels of β-amyloid and tau in CSF may also be predictive.

Longitudinal studies also need to be performed on the various MCI subtypes. Whereas there has been a plethora of research on aMCI and its association with AD, there is a lack of information on the outcomes of naMCI; some research has even suggested that both aMCI and naMCI subtypes may progress to AD.[43] Similarly to AD, other neurodegenerative disorders such as DLB and FTD may pass through an MCI state, although this presumption has not yet been validated. There is even ongoing work to help define stages of illness that precede MCI, such as subjective cognitive impairment (SCI).[85]

Finally, neuropsychological tests that are more sensitive in detecting cognitive impairment should be developed, as they may assist in identifying those with early MCI. In those with high intellectual premorbid functioning, scores on screening mental status examinations and formal neuropsychological batteries may be within normal limits. Nevertheless, these patients may still be diagnosed with MCI, especially if the clinician believes that there has been a decline from the individual's baseline cognition. More research is starting to be performed in this population of patients.

Being able to identify patients at risk for developing dementia is essential for clinical trials. Possible disease-modifying agents for AD currently are at various stages of investigation, including modulators of amyloid processing, active and passive immunization strategies and monoclonal antibodies. More accurate identification of MCI individuals may structure enrolment procedures and endpoints in future studies and hopefully will lead to better outcomes in subsequent treatment trials.

Conclusion

The MCI construct implies a intermediate state between normal cognition and dementia. Individuals with MCI have (a) a subjective cognitive complaint that is usually corroborated by an informant, (b) preserved general cognitive functioning, (c) impairment in one or more of the cognitive domains (memory, attention-executive function, visuospatial skills and/or language) and (d) essentially normal activities of daily living. Once the diagnosis of MCI has been made, the specific subtype can be determined, with aMCI referring to the presence of memory impairment and naMCI referring to the presence of impairment in one or more of the other domains with relative preservation of memory.

MCI remains a clinical diagnosis, aided by a thorough history, neurological examination, screening mental status examination and formal neuropsychological testing. Although an individual with high premorbid intellectual functioning may score within the normal range on bedside and formal testing, that patient may still be considered to have MCI based on the judgement of the clinician. Since there is subjectivity in the clinical diagnosis, creating an operational definition for clinical trials has been a challenge. In addition, a number of aetiologies can be associated with MCI, including degenerative and vascular processes, psychiatric causes and comorbid medical conditions.

The most researched subtype has been aMCI. Thought to be a risk factor for AD, the aMCI subtype has been associated with increased rates of progression to AD compared with the general population. A great deal of research has been performed to determine factors that may predict this progression, with more recent studies combining data on clinical, genetic, neuroimaging and surrogate biomarkers. While further studies clearly need to be performed in order to refine the MCI construct and its potential aetiologies, the ultimate goal is to use this construct as a tool in developing treatments that will potentially prevent or delay the progression of dementia. If a profile of neuroimaging and surrogate biomarkers can be used in conjunction with an MCI diagnosis and if that profile can indicate accurately which patients with MCI are most at risk for progressing to AD, then perhaps there is the potential for moving the AD diagnosis to an earlier stage and subsequently treating these patients even before they develop dementia.

Key points

- MCI is a relatively precise clinical diagnosis.
- Multiple-domain amnestic MCI has an increased likelihood of progressing to AD.
- Medications have failed to decrease conversion rates of MCI to dementia.
- Multicomponent interventions improve mood, memory performance and activities of daily living.

References

1. Reisberg B, Ferris S and de Leon MJ. Stage-specific behavioral, cognitive and *in vivo* changes in community residing subjects with age-associated memory impairment and primary degenerative dementia of the Alzheimer type. *Drug Dev Res* 1988;**15**:101–14.
2. Morris JC. The Clinical Dementia Rating (CDR): current version and scoring rules. *Neurology* 1993;**43**:2412–4.
3. Petersen RC, Smith GE, Waring SC *et al.* Mild cognitive impairment: clinical characterization and outcome. *Arch Neurol* 1999;**56**:303–8.
4. Winblad B, Palmer K, Kivipelto M *et al.* Mild cognitive impairment – beyond controversies, towards a consensus: Report of the International Working Group on Mild Cognitive Impairment. *J Intern Med* 2004;**256**:240–6.
5. Petersen RC. Mild cognitive impairment as a diagnostic entity. *J Intern Med* 2004;**256**:183–94.
6. Petersen R, Aisen P, Beckett L *et al.* Alzheimer's Disease Neuroimaging Initiative (ADNI): clinical characterization. *Neurology* 2010;**74**:201–9.
7. Ivnik RJ, Malec JF, Tangalos EG *et al.* The Auditory–Verbal Learning Test (AVLT): norms for ages 55 years and older. *Psychol Assess J Consult Clin Psychol* 1990;**2**:304–12.
8. Ivnik RJ, Smith GE, Tangalos EG *et al.* Wechsler Memory Scale (WMS): I.Q. dependent norms for persons ages 65–97 years. *Psychol Assess J Consult Clin Psychol* 1991;**3**:156–61.
9. Smith G, Ivnik RJ, Petersen RC *et al.* Age-associated memory impairment diagnoses: problems of reliability and concerns for terminology. *Psychol Aging* 1991;**6**(4):551–8.
10. Petersen R, Knopman D, Boeve B *et al.* Mild cognitive impairment: ten years later. *Arch Neurol* 2009;**66**:1447–55.
11. Apostolova LG, Thompson PM, Green AE *et al.* 3D comparison of low, intermediate and advanced hippocampal atrophy in MCI. *Hum Brain Mapp* 2010;**31**:786–97.
12. Bischkopf J, Busse A and Angermeyer MC. Mild cognitive impairment – a review of prevalence, incidence and outcome according to current approaches. *Acta Psychiatr Scand* 2002;**106**:403–14.

13. Petersen RC, Stevens JC, Ganguli M *et al.* Practice parameter: early detection of dementia: mild cognitive impairment (an evidence-based review). Report of the Quality Standards Subcommittee of the American Academy of Neurology. *Neurology* 2001;**56**:1133–42.

14. Ganguli M, Dodge HH, Shen C and DeKosky ST. Mild cognitive impairment, amnestic type: an epidemiologic study. *Neurology* 2004;**63**:115–21.

15. Petersen RC. Conceptual overview. In: Petersen RC (ed.), *Mild Cognitive Impairment: Aging to Alzheimer's Disease.* Oxford University Press, New York, 2003, pp. 1–14.

16. Salmon D and Hodges JR. Introduction: mild cognitive impairment – cognitive, behavioral and biological factors. *Neurocase* 2005;**11**:1–2.

17. Morris JC, Storandt M, Miller JP *et al.* Mild cognitive impairment represents early-stage Alzheimer's disease. *Arch Neurol* 2001;**58**:397–405.

18. Busse A, Hensel A, Guhne U *et al.* Mild cognitive impairment: long-term course of four clinical subtypes. *Neurology* 2006;**67**:2176–85.

19. Bozoki A, Giordani B, Heidebrink JL *et al.* Mild cognitive impairments predict dementia in nondemented elderly patients with memory loss. *Arch Neurol* 2001;**58**:411–6.

20. DeCarli C. Mild cognitive impairment: prevalence, prognosis, aetiology and treatment. *Lancet Neurol* 2003;**2**:15–21.

21. Nordlund A, Rolstad S, Hellstrom P *et al.* The Goteborg MCI study: mild cognitive impairment is a heterogeneous condition. *J Neurol Neurosurg Psychiatry* 2005;**76**:1485–90.

22. Rasquin SM, Lodder J, Visser PJ *et al.* Predictive accuracy of MCI subtypes for Alzheimer's disease and vascular dementia in subjects with mild cognitive impairment: a 2-year follow-up study. *Dement Geriatr Cogn Disord* 2005;**19**:113–9.

23. Alexopoulos P, Grimmer T, Perneczky R *et al.* Progression to dementia in clinical subtypes of mild cognitive impairment. *Dement Geriatr Cogn Disord* 2006;**22**:27–34.

24. Matthews FE, Stephan BC, McKeith IG *et al.* Two-year progression from mild cognitive impairment to dementia: to what extent do different definitions agree? *J Am Geriatr Soc* 2008;**56**:1424–33.

25. Kwong LK, Neumann M, Sampathu DM *et al.* TDP-43 proteinopathy: the neuropathology underlying major forms of sporadic and familial frontotemporal lobar degeneration and motor neuron disease. *Acta Neuropathol* 2007;**114**:63–70.

26. Molano J, Boeve B, Ferman T *et al.* Mild cognitive impairment associated with limbic and neocortical Lewy body disease: a clinicopathological study. *Brain* 2010;**133**(Pt 2):540–56.

27. Taragano FE, Allegri RF, Krupitzki H *et al.* Mild behavioral impairment and risk of dementia: a prospective cohort study of 358 patients. *J Clin Psychiatry* 2009;**70**:584–92.

28. Stokholm J, Jakobsen O, Czarna JM *et al.* Years of severe and isolated amnesia can precede the development of dementia in early-onset Alzheimer's disease. *Neurocase* 2005;**11**:48–55.

29. Nestor PJ, Scheltens P and Hodges JR. Advances in the early detection of Alzheimer's disease. *Nat Med* 2004;**10**(Suppl):S34–41.

30. Ritchie K and Touchon J. Mild cognitive impairment: conceptual basis and current nosological status. *Lancet* 2000; **355**:225–8.

31. Graham JE, Rockwood K, Beattie BL *et al.* Prevalence and severity of cognitive impairment with and without dementia in an elderly population. *Lancet* 1997;**349**:1793–6.

32. Crook T, Bartus RT, Ferris SH *et al.* Age-associated memory impairment: proposed diagnostic criteria and measures of clinical change – Report of a National Institute of Mental Health Work Group. *Dev Neuropsychol* 1986;**2**:261–76.

33. Levy R. Aging-associated cognitive decline. *Int Psychogeriatr* 1994;**6**:63–8.

34. Richards M, Touchon J, Ledesert B and Richie K. Cognitive decline in ageing: are AAMI and AACD distinct entities? *Int J Geriatr Psychiatry* 1999;**14**:534–40.

35. Small BJ, Mobly JL, Laukka EJ *et al.* Cognitive deficits in preclinical Alzheimer's disease. *Acta Neurol Scand Suppl* 2003;**179**:29–33.

36. Ritchie K, Artero S and Touchon J. Classification criteria for mild cognitive impairment: a population-based validation study. *Neurology* 2001;**56**:37–42.

37. Fisk JD, Merry HR and Rockwood K. Variations in case definition affect prevalence but not outcomes of mild cognitive impairment. *Neurology* 2003;**61**:1179–84.

38. Mitchell AJ. Is it time to separate subjective cognitive complaints from the diagnosis of mild cognitive impairment? *Age Ageing* 2008;**37**:497–9.

39. Kokmen E, Smith GE, Petersen RC *et al.* The short test of mental status: correlations with standardized psychometric testing. *Arch Neurol* 1991;**48**:725–8.

40. Gauthier S, Reisberg B, Zaudig M *et al.* Mild cognitive impairment. *Lancet* 2006;**367**:1262–70.

41. Larrieu S, Letenneur L, Orgogozo JM *et al.* Incidence and outcome of mild cognitive impairment in a population-based prospective cohort. *Neurology* 2002;**59**:1594–9.

42. Lopez OL, Jagust WJ, DeKosky ST *et al.* Prevalence and classification of mild cognitive impairment in the Cardiovascular Health Study Cognition Study. Part 1. *Arch Neurol* 2003;**60**:1385–9.

43. Fischer P, Jungwirth S, Zehetmayer S *et al.* Conversion from subtypes of mild cognitive impairment to Alzheimer dementia. *Neurology* 2007;**68**:288–91.

44. Ferris S, Mungas D, Reed BR *et al.* Progression of mild cognitive impairment to dementia in clinic vs community based cohorts. *Arch Neurol* 2009;**66**:1151–7.

45. Roberts RO, Geda YE, Knopman D *et al.* The Mayo Clinic Study of Aging: design and sampling, participation, baseline measures and sample characteristics. *Neuroepidemiology* 2008;**30**:58–69.

46. Petersen RC, Roberts RO, Knopman DS *et al.* Prevalence of mild cognitive impairment is higher in men: the Mayo Clinic Study of Aging. *Neurology* 2010;**75**:889–97.

47. Bennett DA, Schneider JA, Bienias JL *et al.* Mild cognitive impairment is related to Alzheimer disease pathology and cerebral infarctions. *Neurology* 2005;**64**:834–41.

48. Guillozet AL, Weintraub S, Mash DC and Mesulam MM. Neurofibrillary tangles, amyloid and memory in aging and mild cognitive impairment. *Arch Neurol* 2003;**60**:729–36.

49. Petersen RC, Parisi JE, Dickson DW *et al.* Neuropathology of amnestic mild cognitive impairment. *Arch Neurol* 2006; **63**:665–72.

50. Jicha GA, Parisi JE, Dickson DW *et al*. Neuropathological outcome of mild cognitive impairment following progression to clinical dementia. *Arch Neurol* 2006;**63**:674–81.
51. Morris JC. Mild cognitive impairment is early-stage Alzheimer disease: time to revise diagnostic criteria. *Arch Neurol* 2006;**63**:15–6.
52. Markesbery WR, Schmitt FA, Kryscio RJ *et al*. Neuropathologic substrate of mild cognitive impairment. *Arch Neurol* 2006;**63**:38–46.
53. Daly E, Zaitchik D, Copeland M *et al*. Predicting conversion to Alzheimer disease using standardized clinical information. *Arch Neurol* 2000;**57**:675–80.
54. Folstein MF, Folstein SE and McHugh PR. 'Mini-Mental State'. A practical method for grading the cognitive state of patients for the clinician. *J Psychiatr Res* 1975;**12**:189–98.
55. Teng E, Lu PH and Cummings JL. Neuropsychiatric symptoms are associated with progression from mild cognitive impairment to Alzheimer's disease. *Dement Geriatr Cogn Disord* 2007;**24**:253–9.
56. Ivnik RJ, Malec JF, Smith GE *et al*. Mayo's Older Americans Normative Studies: WAIS-R, WMS-R and AVLT norms for ages 56 through 97. *Clin Neuropsychol* 1992;**6**(Suppl):1–104.
57. Smith GE, Petersen RC, Parisi JE and Ivnik RJ. Definition, course and outcome of mild cognitive impairment. *Aging Neuropsychol Cogn* 1996;**3**:141–7.
58. Knopman DS, DeKosky ST, Cummings JL *et al*. Practice parameter: diagnosis of dementia (an evidence-based review): Report of the Quality Standards Subcommittee of the American Academy of Neurology. *Neurology* 2001; **56**:1143–53.
59. Panza F, D'Introno A, Colacicco AM *et al*. Current epidemiology of mild cognitive impairment and other predementia syndromes. *Am J Geriatr Psychiatry* 2005;**13**:633–44.
60. Reitz C, Tang MX, Manly J *et al*. Hypertension and the risk of mild cognitive impairment. *Arch Neurol* 2007;**64**:1734–40.
61. Luchsinger JA, Reitz C, Patel B *et al*. Relation of diabetes to mild cognitive impairment. *Arch Neurol* 2007;**64**:570–5.
62. Kryscio RJ, Schmitt FA, Salazar JC *et al*. Risk factors for transitions from normal to mild cognitive impairment and dementia. *Neurology* 2006;**66**:828–32.
63. Corder EH, Saunders AM, Strittmatter WJ *et al*. Gene dose of apolipoprotein E type 4 allele and the risk of Alzheimer's disease in late onset families. *Science* 1993;**261**:921–3.
64. Petersen RC, Smith GE, Ivnik RJ *et al*. Apolipoprotein E status as a predictor of the development of Alzheimer's disease in memory-impaired individuals. *JAMA* 1995;**273**:1274–8.
65. Tierney MC, Szalai JP, Snow WG *et al*. A prospective study of the clinical utility of ApoE genotype in the prediction of outcome in patients with memory impairment. *Neurology* 1996;**46**:149–54.
66. Aggarwal NT, Wilson RS, Bienias JL *et al*. The apolipoprotein E4 allele and incident Alzheimer's disease in persons with mild cognitive impairment. *Neurocase* 2005;**11**:3–7.
67. Jak AJ, Houston W, Nagel B *et al*. Differential cross-sectional and longitudinal impact of APOE genotype on hippocampal volumes in nondemented older adults. *Dement Geriatr Cogn Disord* 2007;**23**:282–9.
68. Caselli RJ, Reiman EM, Locke DE *et al*. Cognitive domain decline in healthy apolipoprotein E epsilon4 homozygotes before the diagnosis of mild cognitive impairment. *Arch Neurol* 2007;**64**:1306–11.
69. Devanand DP, Pelton GH, Zamora D *et al*. Predictive utility of apolipoprotein E genotype for Alzheimer disease in outpatients with mild cognitive impairment. *Arch Neurol* 2005;**62**:975–80.
70. Farrer LA, Cupples LA, Haines JL *et al*. Effects of age, sex and ethnicity on the association between apolipoprotein E genotype and Alzheimer disease. A meta-analysis. APOE and Alzheimer Disease Meta Analysis Consortium. *JAMA* 1997;**278**:1349–56.
71. Petersen RC, Thomas RG, Grundman M *et al*. Donepezil and vitamin E in the treatment of mild cognitive impairment. *N Engl J Med* 2005;**352**:2379–88.
72. Winblad B, Gauthier S, Scinto L *et al*. Safety and efficacy of galantamine in subjects with mild cognitive impairment. *Neurology* 2008;**70**:2024–35.
73. Feldman HH, Ferris S, Winblad B *et al*. Effect of rivastigmine on delay to diagnosis of Alzheimer's disease from mild cognitive impairment: the InDDEx study. *Lancet Neurol* 2007;**6**:501–12.
74. Thal LJ, Ferris SH, Kirby L *et al*. A randomized, double-blind, study of rofecoxib in patients with mild cognitive impairment. *Neuropsychopharmacology* 2005;**30**:1204–15.
75. Goodwin JS, Goodwin JM and Garry PJ. Association between nutritional status and cognitive functioning in a healthy elderly population. *JAMA* 1983;**249**:2917–21.
76. Gale CR, Martyn CN and Cooper C. Cognitive impairment and mortality in a cohort of elderly people. *BMJ* 1996;**312**:608–11.
77. La Rue A, Koehler KM, Wayne SJ *et al*. Nutritional status and cognitive functioning in a normally aging sample: a 6-y reassessment. *Am J Clin Nutr* 1997;**65**:20–9.
78. Morris MC, Beckett LA, Scherr PA *et al*. Vitamin E and vitamin C supplements use and risk of incident Alzheimer disease. *Alzheimer Dis Assoc Disord* 1998;**12**:121–6.
79. Cummings JL, Doody R and Clark C. Disease-modifying therapies for Alzheimer disease: challenges to early intervention. *Neurology* 2007;**69**:1622–34.
80. Belleville S. Cognitive training for persons with mild cognitive impairment. *Int Psychogeriatr* 2008;**20**:57–66.
81. Jean L, Bergeron ME, Thivierge S and Simard M. Cognitive intervention programs for individuals with mild cognitive impairment: systematic review of the literature. *Am J Geriatr Psychiatry* 2010;**18**:281–96.
82. Kurz A, Pohl C, Ramsenthaler M and Sorg C. Cognitive rehabilitation in patients with mild cognitive impairment. *Int J Geriatr Psychiatry* 2009;**24**:163–8.
83. Joosten-Weyn Banningh L, Vernooij-Dassen M, Rikkert MO and Teunisse JP. Mild cognitive impairment: coping with an uncertain label. *Int J Geriatr Psychiatry* 2008;**23**:148–54.
84. Lyketsos CG, Lopez O, Jones B *et al*. Prevalence of neuropsychiatric symptoms in dementia and mild cognitive impairment. *JAMA* 2002;**288**:1475–83.
85. Reisberg B and Gauthier S. Current evidence for subjective cognitive impairment (SCI) as the pre-mild cognitive impairment (MCI) stage of subsequently manifest Alzheimer's disease. *Int Psychogeriatr* 2008;**20**:1–16.

86. Solfrizzi V, Panza F, Colacicco AM *et al.* Vascular risk factors, incidence of MCI, and rates of progression to dementia. *Neurology* 2004;**63**:1882–91.

87. Tschanz JT, Welsh-Bohmer KA, Lyketsos CG *et al.* Conversion to dementia from mild cognitive disorder: the Cache County Study. *Neurology* 2006;**67**:229–34.

88. Ravaglia G, Forti P, Montesi F *et al.* Mild cognitive impairment: epidemiology and dementia risk in an elderly Italian population. *J Am Geriatr Soc* 2008;**56**:51–8.

89. Farias ST, Mungas D, Reed BR *et al.* Progression of mild cognitive impairment to dementia in clinic- vs community-based cohorts. *Arch Neurol* 2009;**66**:1151–57.

90. Unverzagt FW, Gao S, Baiyewu O *et al.* Prevalence of cognitive impairment: data from the Indianapolis Study of Health and Aging. *Neurology* 2001;**57**:1655–62.

91. Hänninen T, Hallikainen M, Tuomainen S *et al.* Prevalence of mild cognitive impairment: a population-based study in elderly subjects. *Acta Neurol Scand* 2002;**106**:148–54.

92. Das SK, Bose P, Biswas A *et al.* An epidemiologic study of mild cognitive impairment in Kolkata, India. *Neurology* 2007;**68**:2019–26.

93. Di Carlo A, Lamassa M, Baldereschi M *et al.* CIND and MCI in the Italian elderly: frequency, vascular risk factors, progression to dementia. *Neurology* 2007;**68**:1909–16.

94. Manly JJ, Tang MX, Schupf N *et al.* Frequency and course of mild cognitive impairment in a multiethnic community. *Ann Neurol* 2008;**63**:494–506.

95. Palmer K, Bäckman L, Winblad B and Fratiglioni L. Mild cognitive impairment in the general population: occurrence and progression to Alzheimer disease. *Am J Geriatr Psychiatry* 2008;**16**:603–11.

96. Plassman BL, Langa KM, Fisher GG *et al.* Prevalence of cognitive impairment without dementia in the United States. *Ann Intern Med* 2008;**148**:427–34.

CHAPTER 75

Vascular dementia

Marie-Laure Seux
Assistance Publique Hôpitaux de Paris, Hôpital Broca, Paris, France

Introduction

Considered in the past as the second most common cause of acquired dementia after neurodegenerative pathologies in the elderly, it is now recognized that cerebrovascular disease is associated with a heterogeneous group of cognitive impairment from mild cognitive impairment to dementia and/or mood disorders that share a presumed vascular cause and that extend well beyond the traditional concept of multi-infarct dementia (Figure 75.1).[1] There is also agreement that cerebrovascular disease contributes to cognitive impairment in neurodegenerative dementias, defining the so-called mixed dementia. The concept of vascular depression describing depression occurring in later life associated with vascular risk factors or white matter lesions is still debated.[2]

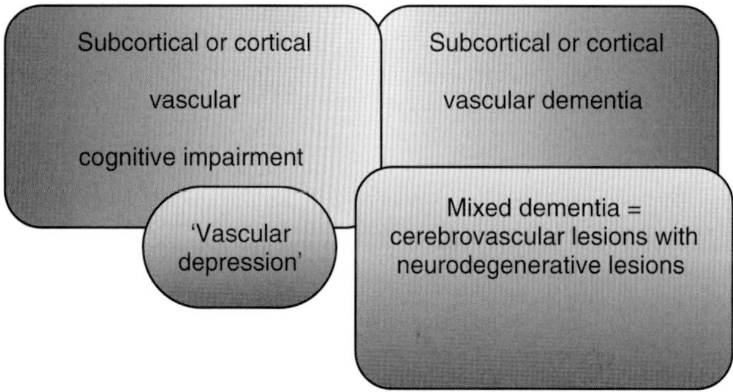

Figure 75.1 The broad spectrum of cognitive consequences of cerebrovascular disease.

Definition, physiopathology and classification

Vascular cognitive impairment (VCI), with or without dementia, is a multifactorial disorder related to a wide variety of lesions and causes. To take into account the heterogeneity of clinical, neuropsychological and radiological appearances related to the different vascular mechanisms and brain lesions, VCI could be defined as the loss of cognitive function resulting from ischaemic, hypoperfusive or haemorrhagic brain lesions due to cerebrovascular disease. Classification is based on the onset of cognitive impairment (acute or subacute), the location, type, number and size of brain lesions (cortical or subcortical, single or multiple stroke, lacuna), the mechanisms (ischaemic or haemorrhagic), the size of involved vessels (small or large vessels) and origin of vascular disease (atherosclerosis, arteriosclerosis, inflammation or genetic) (Table 75.1).[3]

The main cause of vascular dementia (VD) is related to vascular changes due to risk factors such as hypertension, diabetes and dyslipidaemia. Very rare causes due to inflammatory pathologies have been described, mainly in young people. Genetic forms of VD have been identified such as the cerebral autosomal dominant arteriopathy with subcortical infarcts and leukoencephalopathy (CADASIL) associated with a notch 3 family gene on chromosome 19.[4] Clinical manifestations include migraine with aura, recurrent ischaemic stroke, depression and progressive cognitive decline with early-onset VD. Other hereditary VDs are characterized by amyloid angiopathy leading to cerebral haemorrhages and dementia as in the amyloidosis-Dutch type, the BRI2 gene-related dementia (British and Danish type) and amyloidosis-Icelandic type due to variant cystatin C.[5] Sporadic cerebral amyloid angiopathy cases have also been described.[6]

A growing body of evidence suggests that cerebral white matter magnetic resonance imaging (MRI) grade abnormalities described as leukoaraiosis may also contribute to cognitive impairment. Periventricular and/or subcortical lesions are often seen with increasing age in demented and non-demented elderly people and seemed to be correlated with dysexecutive symptoms[7,8] and dementia.[9]

Principles and Practice of Geriatric Medicine, Fifth Edition. Edited by Alan J. Sinclair, John E. Morley and Bruno Vellas.

Table 75.1 Classification of vascular cognitive impairment aetiologies.

	Vessels involved	
	Large vessel disease	**Small vessel disease**
Location of lesions	Multiple cortical infarcts Single strategic stroke	Periventricular white matter lesions Thalamic infarct or lacuna in basal ganglia or in frontal white matter
Mechanisms and aetiologies	Ischaemia Extracerebral embolism: • Large artery atherosclerosis (carotid, ...) • Cardiac embolism, atrial fibrillation, ...	Ischaemia: • Arteriolosclerosis • Hypertensive arteriopathy • Inflammatory disease: primary vasculitis (giant cell arteritis, primary angiitis of CNS, periarteritis nodosa, ...) and vasculitis secondary to collagen vascular diseases, Behçet disease and other systemic conditions • CADASIL Haemorrhage: • Hypertension • Amyloid angiopathies, ...
Other haemorrhages	Traumatic subdural haematoma Subarachnoid haemorrhage	
Hypoperfusive	Diffuse anoxic encephalopathy (cardiac arrest)	

In CADASIL, cognitive decline and mood disturbances have been associated with extensive white matter hyperintensities on baseline MRI, clinically silent brain infarction, cerebral microhaemorrhages and changes in microstructure on diffusion imaging.[10] Cortical atrophy has also been implicated in cognitive impairment in VD.[11]

Numerous neuropathological studies have pointed out concomitant Alzheimer's lesions such as neurofibrillary tangles and neuritic plaques in VD or concomitant vascular lesions in Alzheimer's disease (AD), leading to the concept of mixed dementia. Both neurodegenerative and vascular brain injuries may have an additive effect or a synergistic effect to impair cognitive functioning.[12–16] However currently no precise knowledge exists regarding the extent to which the different vascular mechanisms and types of brain changes contribute to the cognitive loss.[17]

Diagnosis

Several criteria sets for VD have been defined according to the diagnostic procedure for AD.[18–21] The main differences in the four most common sets (Table 75.2) are the definition of cerebrovascular disease (clinical and/or neuroradiological), inclusion of white matter lesions in the criteria and precision of neuroimaging findings, description of the relationship between dementia and cerebrovascular disease and temporal relation or rater judgement. Their clinicopathological validation revealed great variations in the sensitivity and specificity of diagnosing probable VD, ranging from 20 to 50% and from 84 to 94%, respectively.[22]

Because of the lack of consensus regarding both the clinical and pathological definitions, diagnosis remains problematic in clinical practice.[23] The major difficulties are to document the vascular burden in case of diffuse white matter abnormalities and to determine the implications of documented cerebrovascular and neurodegenerative lesions in cognitively impaired subjects. Neuroimaging plays a fundamental role and MRI is the ideal imaging technique for cognitive disorders. MRI provides information about brain atrophy, ventricular size, medial temporal atrophy, white matter lesions and ischaemic changes or haemorrhagic lesions, including microbleeds. The radiological procedure should include the following sequences: 3D T1-weighted, T2-weighted, fluid attenuation inversion–recovery and gradient echo.[24] To assess the likelihood of concomitant AD, clinicians can also use anamnesis (progressive onset of memory impairment), neuropsychological profile demonstrating temporal dysfunction, brain metabolism investigations with positron emission tomography (PET) or single photon emission computed tomography (SPECT) imaging and biomarkers.

Epidemiology

In epidemiological surveys, prevalence and incidence vary according to the diagnosis criteria set and the included

Table 75.2 Comparison of clinical diagnosis sets for probable vascular dementia.

Probable VD	ICD-10	DSM-IV	ADDTC	NINDS–AIREN
Dementia	Decline in memory for at least 6 months, decline in general processing of information, judgement and thinking Significant impairment of social functioning Absence of clouding of consciousness	Memory impairment ≥1 disturbances: aphasia, apraxia, agnosia, executive functioning Significant impairment of social functioning Not occurring during the course of delirium	Decline in intellectual function not isolated to a single narrow intellectual performance Broad interference with patient's customary affairs of life Independent of level of consciousness	Cognitive decline Memory impairment ≥2 disturbances: orientation, attention, language, visuospatial or executive functions, motor control, praxis Interference with activities of daily living Exclusion of delirium, psychosis, . . .
Cerebrovascular disease: clinical evidence	Evidence from history, examination or tests: Focal signs Deterioration in emotional control, social behaviour, apathy	Focal neurological signs/symptoms OR Significant cerebrovascular diseases on imaging	Evidence of ≥2 infarcts: History, neurological examination History of multiple transient ischaemic attacks, vascular risk factors Elevated Hachinski scale AND/OR Cerebrovascular lesion on CT or MRI	Clinical examination: Focal signs or gait disturbance, falls, urinary symptoms, pseudobulbar palsy, mood changes, apathy, emotional inconsistency AND Relevant cerebrovascular lesion on CT or MRI
Cerebrovascular disease: brain imaging	Helpful but not required No precision	Multiple infarcts in the cortex and subcortical white matter	≥1 infarct in the cerebellum Multiple infarcts in brain regions known to affect cognition Further research for periventricular and deep white matter changes on T2-MRI	Multiple large-vessels infarcts Single strategic infarct Multiple basal ganglia and white matter lacunes or extensive periventricular lesions
Relationship	Reasonably judged to be aetiologically related to dementia Abrupt onset, stepwise deterioration	Judged to be aetiologically related to the disturbances	Clear temporal relationship required if a single stroke	Onset 3 months after stroke Abrupt deterioration or stepwise progression

cohort (population-based, individuals with vascular risks factors, stroke cohort).[25]

In a large survey, the Cardiovascular Health Study,[25] the different criteria sets identified 9% (NINDS–AIREN), 13% (DSM-IV) and 24% (ADDTC) incident cases of probable VD. The proportion of AD was 55%, probable VD 12% and mixed dementia 33% according to the ADDTC criteria combined with the NINCDS–ADRDA criteria for AD.[26]

The prevalence of dementia 3 months after an ischaemic cerebrovascular event in a stroke cohort varied from 6% (ICD-10) to 21.1% (NINDS–AIREN) and 25.5% (DSM-III).[27] In a population-based study, the risk of dementia in the year following stroke was nine times greater than expected with a persistent increased risk after the first year.[28] Retrospective evaluation using informant questionnaires showed that one-sixth of stroke patients had previous cognitive impairment before an acute cerebrovascular event, in favour of mixed dementia.[29] Episodes of stroke are known to worsen cognitive decline in patients with pre-existing AD and the risk of AD is also significantly increased after acute events such as stroke or transient ischaemic attack.[30] Stroke subtypes, volume of damaged brain tissue, functional tissue loss and location of the lesions in strategic areas were reported to be the major determinants of dementia, with inconsistent results in neuropathological and epidemiological studies.[31] White matter changes and associated Alzheimer pathology, cardiovascular risk factors, low educational level, female gender and apolipoprotein E4 may also contribute to cognitive impairment in stroke patients.[32]

Table 75.3 Risk factors associated with vascular cognitive impairment and vascular dementia.

Hypercholesterolaemia
Hypertension
Diabetes mellitus
Metabolic syndrome
Smoking
Atrial fibrillation
Hyperhomocysteinaemia
ApoE4 polymorphism
Systemic inflammation

VD and AD share common risk factors predisposing to cerebrovascular disease and stroke (Table 75.3), their correlation with cognitive deterioration was demonstrated in longitudinal studies, offering some promise for prevention of both pathologies.[33]

Since VCI without dementia was recently identified without any agreement on diagnosis, little is known about progression and risk of VD. In a population-based study, 42% of subjects with vascular mild cognitive impairment developed dementia within 5 years.[34]

Clinical and neuropsychological features

Clinical manifestations are related to the type of cerebrovascular disease (acute or subacute) and the brain areas involved.

Some clinical symptoms, such as gait disturbances, parkinsonism, dysarthria, dysphagia, urinary incontinence and pseudobulbar palsy were previously described in Binswanger disease or lacunar state and can be observed in association with periventricular white matter lesions.[35] In the case of a progressive, slow decline of cognitive function, evidence of those signs supports the diagnosis of subcortical VD rather than AD. By contrast, hemianopsia, reflex asymmetry, hemimotor or hemisensory dysfunction and aphasia are more often observed in the case of cortical cerebral infarct.[36]

The cognitive decline observed in patients with white matter lesions has been suggested to be due to disruption of subcortical–cortical pathways producing dysfunction of frontal lobe structures. That is why the major neuropsychological feature in VCI is executive dysfunction with decreased psychomotor speed, impairment of planning and switching from one task to another, deficit in working memory and reduced verbal fluency. Since memory tasks require concomitant executive functioning, impairment in episodic memory may also be observed even without dysfunction of the medial temporal lobe. Fluctuation of performances is another key feature of VCI.

Neuropsychological testing has to be adapted to this specific profile (verbal phonemic and semantic fluencies, trailmaking test, digit symbol, etc.) as proposed by the National Institute of Neurological Disorders and Stroke–Canadian Stroke Network.[24] For clinicians, management of patients with vascular risk factors, particularly hypertension, should include cognitive screening with the aim of detecting early signs of cognitive impairment and dementia.[37] For brief testing, the previous group suggested using the Montreal Cognitive Assessment, which is more sensitive than the Mini Mental State Examination to executive function (www.mocatest.org: free access to translations of tests and instructions for clinical and educational purposes).[38]

Finally, non-cognitive features such as apathy and depressed mood are very common in vascular cognitively impaired patients.

Preventive and curative therapies

Preventive approaches to VCI rely mainly on the identification and treatment of risk factors. Given the high proportion of dementia attributable to possibly reversible vascular causes, it has been suggested that vascular risk manipulation may result in up to a 50% reduction in the dementia prevalence rate in the elderly.[39]

Prevention strategies should focus on reduction of stroke and cerebrovascular disease, with attention to control of risk factors such as hypertension, diabetes mellitus, hypercholesterolaemia, atrial fibrillation and hyperhomocysteinaemia.

The benefit of antihypertensive drugs on dementia or cognitive decline prevention was demonstrated in three studies conducted in elderly hypertensives,[40] in high-risk subjects with previous ischaemic cerebral attack[41] and in patients with vascular disease or with diabetes associated with another vascular risk factor.[42] However, inclusion of patients with pathophysiologically heterogeneous types of vascular cognitive decline, prescription of active antihypertensive drugs in placebo groups and short duration of follow-up could explain the negative results in other studies.[43–47] Since dependency in VD is due to both cognitive impairment and stroke-related physical disability, the impact of such therapies on dependency is very positive.[48]

Studies concerning lipid-lowering agents on cognitive performance are rare. The PROSPER study did not show any effect of pravastatin on cognitive function as compared with placebo in 70–80-year-old subjects followed over 3 years.[49] Moreover, in patients with AD the LEADe study did not demonstrate any benefit regarding cognition of atorvastatin compared with placebo and anti-diabetes therapies in particular.[50]

Even though aspirin is widely prescribed in VD for stroke prevention, its effect on cognitive functioning or the impact on prognosis remain unclear.[51,52] Considering the risk of cerebral haemorrhage in patients with amyloid angiopathy, antithrombotic agents should be used with caution when lobar microbleeds are observed on brain MRI.[53]

Whether progression of white matter lesions could be a significant surrogate endpoint with regard to cognitive protection has to be elucidated, even though promising results were observed in a study conducted with blood pressure-lowering regimen in patients with previous cerebrovascular disease.[54,55]

Early detection is important to improve the observance of the action of drugs and will become increasingly important as preventive therapies become available. In a preventive trial. the benefit of lowering blood pressure on cognitive function was even higher in hypertensive patients with previous intellectual impairment, but not in another study conducted in patients with cerebrovascular lesions and decreased levels of cognitive functioning.[56,57]

A number of drugs have also been tested with the aim of improving or slowing cognitive decline in patients affected by various forms of cerebrovascular disease. Most of these trials, using nootropics (propentofylline,[58] pentoxifylline[59]) or other metabolically active compounds (nicergoline, Ginkgo biloba[60]) or calcium antagonists (nimodipine[61]), yielded unsatisfactory results.

Since cholinergic deficits are also encountered in VD, the response to cholinesterase inhibitors was investigated, with discrepancies in the results due to heterogeneous cerebrovascular disease or mixed dementia cases in the included subjects.[62,63] Furthermore, the primary endpoint has to be adapted to the specific neuropsychometric profile of VCI. However, in a double-blind, placebo-controlled trial avoiding all these biases, donepezil did not show any significant benefit in CADASIL.[64] So far, there has been no recommendation to prescribe cholinesterase inhibitors in the pure form for VD, but they should be used in mixed dementia with both AD and VD lesions.

Similarly, insufficient benefit of memantine in mild to moderate VD was observed to be able to recommend glutaminergic therapy.[65]

Concerning other strategies, such as cognitive training or physical activity, no definite conclusion can be drawn about their efficacy on cognitive functioning in patients suffering from VD.[66] Management of depression is often difficult, with a low efficacy of antidepressants.

Conclusion

Prevention had dramatically decreased mortality due to stroke in subjects with vascular risk factors by the end of the twentieth century. However, since the beginning of the present century, VCI, a more silent and progressive disorder, has become a major public health challenge, in association with other cognitive disorders such as AD. Clinicians must pay attention to the risk of cognitive impairment in patients with vascular risk factors in order to prevent dependency due to intellectual disability. Strategies that aim to reduce this risk have to be established, with special interest in blood pressure-lowering treatments.

Key points

- VCI, with or without dementia, is defined by the loss of cognitive function resulting from ischaemic and/or haemorrhagic brain lesions due to cerebrovascular disease.
- In subjects with cardiovascular risk factors, such as hypertension, focal ischaemic lesion (lacuna) or extensive subcortical or periventricular white matter, lesions are frequent.
- Brief cognitive testing oriented to executive and episodic memory evaluation is recommended in patients with vascular risk factors to detect potentially vascular and neurodegenerative symptomatic brain lesions.
- The impact of vascular risk factor management on cognitive impairment has to be evaluated.
- The benefit of blood pressure-lowering drugs on dementia has been demonstrated in elderly hypertensive patients and in subjects with a previous cerebrovascular event.

References

1. Moorhouse P and Rockwood K. Vascular cognitive impairment: current concepts and clinical developments. *Lancet Neurol* 2008;**7**:246–55.
2. Baldwin RC and O'Brien J. Vascular basis of late-onset depressive disorder. *Br J Psychiatry* 2002;**180**:157–60.
3. Roman GC, Erkinjunti T, Wallin A *et al.* Subcortical ischaemic vascular dementia. *Lancet Neurol* 2002;**1**:426–36.
4. Chabriat H, Joutel A, Dichgans M *et al.* CADASIL. *Lancet Neurol* 2009;**8**:643–53.
5. Revesz T, Holton JL, Lashley T *et al.* Genetics and molecular pathogenesis of sporadic and hereditary cerebral amyloid angiopathies. *Acta Neuropathol* 2009;**118**:115–30.
6. Iemolo F, Duro G, Rizzo C *et al.* Pathophysiology of vascular dementia. *Immun Ageing* 2009;**6**:13.
7. de Leeuw FE, de Groot JC, Achten E *et al.* Prevalence of cerebral white matter lesions in elderly people: a population-based magnetic resonance imaging study. The Rotterdam Scan Study. *J Neurol Neurosurg Psychiatry* 2001;**70**:9–14.
8. Prins ND, van Dijk EJ, den Heijet T *et al.* Cerebral white matter lesions and the risk of dementia. *Arch Neurol* 2004;**61**: 1531–4.
9. Söderlund H, Nilsson L-G, Berger K *et al.* Cerebral changes on MRI and cognitive function: the CASCADE study. *Neurobiol Aging* 2006;**27**:16–23.

10. Viswanathan A, Godin O, Jouvent E *et al.* Impact of MRI markers in subcortical vascular dementia: a multi-modal analysis in CADASIL. *Neurobiol Aging* 2010;**31**:1629–36.
11. Fein G, Di Sclafani V, Tanabe J *et al.* Hippocampal and cortical atrophy predict dementia in subcortical ischemic vascular disease. *Neurology* 2000;**55**:1626–35.
12. Snowdon DA, Greiner LH, Mortimer JA *et al.* Brain infarction and the clinical expression of Alzheimer disease. The Nun Study. *JAMA* 1997;**277**:813–7.
13. Neuropathology Group of the Medical Research Council Cognitive Fucntion and Ageing Study (MRC CFAS). Pathological correlates of late-onset dementia in a multicentre, community-based population in England and Wales. *Lancet* 2001;**357**:169–75.
14. Petrovitch H, Ross GW, Steinborn SC *et al.* AD lesions and infarcts in demented and non-demented Japanese-American men. *Ann Neurol* 2005;**57**:98–103.
15. Jellinger KA and Attems J. Prevalence and pathogenic role of cerebrovascular lesions in Alzheimer disease. *J Neurol Sci* 2005;**229–230**:37–41.
16. Giannakopoulos P, Gold G, Kövari E *et al.* Assessing the cognitive impact of Alzheimer disease pathology and vascular burden in the aging brain. *Acta Neuropathol* 2007;**113**:1–12.
17. Erkinjuntti T and Hachinski V. Rethinking vascular dementia. *Cerebrovasc Dis* 1993;**3**:3–23.
18. World Health Organization. *IC-10 Classification of Mental and Behavioral Disorders: Diagnostic Criteria for Research.* WHO, Geneva, 1993, pp. 36–40.
19. American Psychiatric Association. *Diagnostic and Statistical Manual of Mental Disorders*, 4th edn, American Psychiatric Association, Washington, DC, 1994, pp. 143–6.
20. Chui HC, Victoroff JI, Margolin D *et al.* Criteria for the diagnosis of ischemic vascular dementia proposed by the State of California Alzheimer's Disease Diagnostic and Treatment Centers. *Neurology* 1992;**42**:473–80.
21. Roman GC, Tatemichi TK, Erkinjuntti T *et al.* Vascular dementia: diagnostic criteria for research studies. Report of the NINDS–AIREN International Workshop. *Neurology* 1993;**43**:250–60.
22. Gold G, Bouras C, Canuto A *et al.* Clinicopathological validation of four sets of clinical criteria for vascular dementia. *Am J Psychiatry* 2002;**159**:82–7.
23. Chui HC. Vascular cognitive impairment: today and tomorrow. *Alzheimers Dement* 2006;**2**:185–94.
24. Hachinski V, Iadecola C, Petersen RC *et al.* National Institute of Neurological Disorders and Stroke–Canadian Stroke Network Vascular Cognitive impairment harmonization standards. *Stroke* 2006;**37**:2220–41.
25. Lopez OL, Kuller LH, Becker JT *et al.* Classification of vascular dementia in the Cardiovascular Health Study Cognition Study. *Neurology* 2005;**64**:1539–47.
26. McKhann G, Drachman DA, Folstein MF *et al.* Clinical diagnosis of Alzheimer's disease: report of the NINCDS–ADRDA Work Group under the auspices of the Department of Health and Human Services Task Force on Alzheimer's Disease. *Neurology* 1984;**34**:939–44.
27. Pohjasvaara T, Erkinjuntti T, Vataja R and Kaste M. Dementia three months after stroke. Baseline frequency and effect of different definitions of dementia in the Helsinki Stroke Aging Memory Study (SAM) Cohort. *Stroke* 1997;**28**:785–92.
28. Kokmen E, Whismant JP, O'Fallon WM *et al.* Dementia after ischemic stroke: a population-based study in Rochester, Minnesota (1960–1984). *Neurology* 1996;**46**:154–9.
29. Hénon H, Pasquier F, Durieu I *et al.* Preexisting dementia in stroke patients. Baseline frequency, associated factors and outcome. *Stroke* 1997;**28**:2429–36.
30. Kalaria RN. The role of cerebral ischemia in Alzheimer's disease. *Neurobiol Aging* 2000;**21**:321–30.
31. Zekry D, Duyckaerts C, Belmin J *et al.* The vascular lesions in vascular and mixed dementia: the weight of functional neuroanatomy. *Neurobiol Aging* 2003;**24**:213–9.
32. Pohjasvaara T, Mäntylä R, Salonen O *et al.* How complex interactions of ischemic brain infarcts, white matter lesions and atrophy relate to post-stroke dementia. *Arch Neurol* 2000;**57**:1295–300.
33. Casserly I and Topol E. Convergence of atherosclerosis and Alzheimer's disease: inflammation, cholesterol and misfolded proteins. *Lancet* 2004;**363**:1139–46.
34. Wentzel C, Rockwood K and MacKnight C. Progression of impairment in patients with vascular cognitive impairment without dementia. *Neurology* 2001;**57**:714–6.
35. Pohjasvaara TI, Mäntylä R, Ylikoski R *et al.* Clinical features of MRI-defined subcortical vascular disease. *Alzheimer Dis Assoc Disord* 2003;**17**:236–42.
36. Staekenborg SS, van der Flier WM, van Straaten EC *et al.* Neurological signs in relation to type of cerebrovascular disease in vascular dementia. *Stroke* 2008;**39**:317–22.
37. Rockwood K, Middleton LE, Moorhouse PK *et al.* The inclusion of cognition in vascular risk factor clinical practice guidelines. *Clin Interv Aging* 2009;**4**:425–33.
38. Nasreddine ZS, Phillips NA, Bédirian V *et al.* The Montreal Cognitive Assessment (MoCA): a brief screening tool for mild cognitive impairment. *J Am Geriatr Soc* 2005;**53**:695–9.
39. Stephan BCM, Matthews FE, Khaw K-T *et al.* Beyond mild cognitive impairment: vascular cognitive impairment, no dementia (VCIND). *Alzheimer's Res Ther* 2009;**1**:4.
40. Forette F, Seux M-L, Staessen JA *et al.* Prevention of dementia in randomised double-blind placebo-controlled Systolic Hypertension in Europe (Syst-Eur) trial. *Lancet* 1998; **352**:1347–51.
41. Tzourio C, Anderson C, Chapman N *et al.*; PROGRESS Collaborative Group. Effects of blood pressure lowering with perindopril and indapamide therapy on dementia and cognitive decline in patients with cerebrovascular disease. *Arch Intern Med* 2003;**163**:1069–75.
42. Bosch J, Yusuf S, Pogue J *et al.*; HOPE Investigators. Outcomes prevention evaluation. Use of ramipril in preventing stroke: double-blind randomised trial. *BMJ* 2002;**324**: 699–702.
43. Inzitari D, Erkinjuntti T, Wallin A *et al.* Subcortical vascular dementia as a specific target for clinical trials. *Ann N Y Acad Sci* 2000;**903**:510–21.
44. Lithell H, Hansson L, Skoog I *et al.* for the SCOPE Study Group. The Study on Cognition and Prognosis in the Elderly (SCOPE): principal results of a randomized double-blind intervention trial. *J Hypertens* 2003;**21**:875–86.

45. Peters R, Beckett N, Forette, F *et al.* for the HYVET Investigators. Incident dementia and blood pressure lowering in the Hypertension in the Very Elderly Trial Cognitive Function Assessment (HYVET-COG): a double-blind, placebo, controlled trial. *Lancet Neurol* 2008;**7**:683–9.
46. McGuinness B, Todd S, Passmore P and Bullock R. Blood pressure lowering in patients without prior cerebrovascular disease for prevention of cognitive impairment and dementia. *Cochrane Database Syst Rev* 2009;(4):CD004034.
47. Diener HC, Sacco RL, Yusuf S *et al.* Prevention Regimen for Effectively Avoiding Second Strokes (PRoFESS) Study Group. Effects of aspirin plus extended-release dipyridamole versus clopidogrel and telmisartan on disability and cognitive function after recurrent stroke in patients with ischaemic stroke in the Prevention Regimen for Effectively Avoiding Second Strokes (PRoFESS) trial: a double-blind, active and placebo-controlled study. *Lancet Neurol* 2008;**7**:875–84.
48. Perindopril Protection Against Recurrent Stroke Study (PROGRESS) Collaborative Group. Effects of a preindopril-based blood pressure-lowering regimen on disability and dependency in 6105 patients with cerebrovascular disease, a randomized controlled trial. *Stroke* 2003;**34**:2333–8.
49. Trompet S, van Vliet P, de Craen AJM *et al.* Pravastatin and cognitive function in the elderly. Results of the PROSPER study. *J Neurol* 2010;**257**:85–90.
50. Feldman HH, Doody RS, Kivipelto M *et al.* Randomized controlled trial of atorvastatin in mild to moderate Alzheimer disease: LEADe. *Neurology* 2010;**74**:956–64.
51. Williams PS, Rands G, Orrell M and Spector A. Aspirin for vascular dementia. *Cochrane Database Syst Rev* 2000;(4): CD001296.
52. Devine ME and Rands G. Does aspirin affect outcome in vascular dementia? A retrospective case-notes analysis. *Int J Geriatr Psychiatry* 2003;**18**:425–31.
53. Vernooij MW, Haag MD, van der Lugt A *et al.* Use of antithrombotic drugs and the presence of cerebral microbleeds: the Rotterdam Scan Study. *Neurology* 2001;**66**:714–6.
54. Schmidt R, Scheltens P, Erkinjuntti T *et al.* for the European Task Force on Age-Related White Matter Changes. White matter lesion progression, a surrogate endpoint for trials in cerebral small-vessel disease. *Neurology* 2004;**63**:139–44.
55. Dufouil C, Chalmers J, Coskun O *et al.*; PROGRESS MRI Substudy Investigators. Effects of blood pressure lowering on cerebral white matter hyperintensities in patients with stroke: the PROGRESS (Perindopril Protection Against Recurrent Stroke Study) Magnetic Resonance Imaging Substudy. *Circulation* 2005;**112**:1644–50.
56. Skoog I, Lithell H, Hansson L *et al.* for the SCOPE Study Group. Effect of baseline cognitive function and antihypertensive treatment on cognitive and cardiovascular outcomes: Study on Cognition and Prognosis in Elderly (SCOPE). *Am J Hypertens* 2005;**18**:1052–9.
57. Tzourio C, Anderson C, Chapman N *et al.*; PROGRESS Collaborative Group. Effects of blood pressure lowering with perindopril and indapamide therapy on dementia and cognitive decline in patients with cerebrovascular disease. *Arch Intern Med* 2003;**163**:1069–75.
58. Frampton M, Harvey RJ and Kirchner V. Propentofylline for dementia. *Cochrane Database Syst Rev* 2003;(2):CD002853.
59. Sha MC and Callahan CM. The efficacy of pentoxifylline in the treatment of vascular dementia: a systematic review. *Alzheimer Dis Assoc Disord* 2003;**17**:46–54.
60. Weinman S, Roll S, Scwarzbach C *et al.* Effects of Ginkgo biloba in dementia: systematic review and meta-analysis. *BMC Geriatr* 2010;**10**:14.
61. Lopez-Arrieta JM and Birks J. Nimodipine for primary degenerative, mixed and vascular dementia. *Cochrane Database Syst Rev* 2002;(3):CD000147.
62. Wilkinson D, Doody R, Helme R *et al.*; the Donepezil 308 Study Group. Donepezil in vascular dementia, a randomized, placebo-controlled study. *Neurology* 2003;**61**:479–86.
63. Craig D and Birks J. Galantamine for vascular cognitive impairment. *Cochrane Database Syst Rev* 2006;(1):CD004746.
64. Dichgans M, Markus HS, Salloway S *et al.* Donepezil in patients with subcortical vascular cognitive impairment: a randomised double-blind trial in CADASIL. *Lancet Neurol* 2008;**7**:310–8.
65. Orgogozo J-M, Rigaud A-S, Stöffler A *et al.* Efficacy and safety of memantine in patients with mild to moderate vascular dementia. A randomized, placebo-controlled trial (MMM 300). *Stroke* 2002;**33**:1834–9.
66. Clare L and Woods B. Cognitive rehabilitation and cognitive training for early-stage Alzheimer's disease and vascular dementia. *Cochrane Database Syst Rev* 2003;(4):CD003260.

CHAPTER 76

Mental stimulation and dementia

Joe Verghese
Albert Einstein College of Medicine, Bronx, NY, USA

Introduction

Owing to the rapid greying of populations worldwide, dementia has become a major global public health issue. Age-associated cognitive decline and primary dementia syndromes such as Alzheimer's disease are major sources of morbidity and mortality worldwide. They pose a significant burden not only on affected individuals, but also on their caregivers and society in general. In 2006, the worldwide prevalence of Alzheimer's disease was estimated to be 26 million.[1] It has been predicted that by 2050, the prevalence of Alzheimer's disease will quadruple, by which time one in 85 persons worldwide will be living with the disease.[1] The global burden and impact of dementia coupled with the paucity of effective pharmacological interventions lends a new urgency to discover new preventive strategies for dementia. It has been estimated that if interventions could be developed to delay both disease onset and progression by a modest 1 year, there would be nearly nine million fewer cases of Alzheimer's disease worldwide in 2050.[1]

Mentally stimulating activities in this chapter are defined as those activities that individuals engage in for enjoyment, mental health and wellbeing, which are independent of work, household chores or activities of daily living. These activities are popular, enjoyable, widely available and can be easily incorporated into lifestyles. Mentally stimulating activities run the gamut from board games such as chess to card games such as bridge, reading, playing musical instruments, listening to music, knitting, painting or doing crossword puzzles. There is growing interest among the scientific community and also the general public in understanding and defining the role of mentally stimulating activities as a preventive strategy for cognitive decline.

In this chapter, types of mental stimulation interventions, supporting evidence, possible mechanisms of action, targets of intervention and steps to consider in implementing mentally simulating activities for older adults in community or clinical settings are discussed.

Cognitive (mental) interventions

Clare and Woods categorized mental stimulation interventions into three types based on the mode of delivery and the goals of the intervention: cognitive stimulation, cognitive rehabilitation and cognitive training.[2]

Cognitive stimulation refers to the involvement in group activities that are designed to increase cognitive and social functioning in a non-specific manner. Examples of cognitive stimulation activities include participation in group discussions, supervised leisure activities, list memorization with no particular support and also more structured activities such as reminiscence therapy that involves the discussion of past activities, events and experiences.

Cognitive rehabilitation involves individually tailored programmes centred on specific activities of daily life. Examples include learning the name of a new caregiver, balancing a chequebook or improving conversational fluency.[2] Cognitive rehabilitation is a more individualized approach to helping people with cognitive impairments in which those affected and their families work together with healthcare professionals to identify personally relevant goals and devise strategies for addressing these. The emphasis of cognitive rehabilitation is not on enhancing performance in cognitive tasks as such, but on improving mental functioning of the patient in realistic situations.

Cognitive training involves teaching theoretically motivated strategies and skills in order to optimize cognition functioning. Cognitive training is most often provided individually or in small groups. Cognitive training typically involves guided practice on a set of standard tasks designed to reflect particular cognitive functions, such as memory, attention or problem solving. The underlying assumption is that practice has the potential to improve or at least maintain functioning in the given cognitive domain. The training is occasionally facilitated by family members with therapist support. Tasks may be presented in paper-and-pencil or computerized form or may involve analogues of activities

Principles and Practice of Geriatric Medicine, Fifth Edition. Edited by Alan J. Sinclair, John E. Morley and Bruno Vellas.

of daily living. Usually a range of difficulty levels is available within a standardized set of tasks to allow for selection of the level of difficulty that is most appropriate for a given individual. The Advanced Cognitive Training for Independent and Vital Elderly (ACTIVE) Study, which randomized 2832 non-demented elderly participants to a 6 week intervention, focused on memory, reasoning and speed of processing, is an example of this form of intervention.[3]

Supporting evidence

Support for the potential role of mentally stimulating activities in preventing or mitigating cognitive decline comes from animal studies and also observational studies in humans and, to a lesser extent, randomized clinical trials.

Animal studies

Exposure to environments enriched with various sensory stimuli and motor demands (*enriched environment*) is considered the animal equivalent of participation in mentally stimulating leisure activities by humans, although obvious species differences limit direct extrapolation of findings from rodents to humans.[4] In the 1960s, Rosenzweig and colleagues reported changes in brain neuroanatomy and neurochemistry in rats exposed to enriched environments, including increased cerebral cortex thickness.[5,6] In the 1970s, Greenough *et al.* reported finding greater synapse density, glial cell proliferation and structural changes in nerve cells, including increased dendritic branching in rats exposed to enriched environments compared with rats living in standard housing.[7] Recent studies have found increases in levels of acetylcholine, a neurotransmitter involved in cognition and in various neurotrophic factors, in rodents exposed to enriched environments.[4] Environmentally enriched conditions have been shown to reduce cognitive deficits in young and adult animals.[4] Neurogenesis has been demonstrated not only in the adult rodent hippocampus, olfactory bulb and cerebral cortex, but also in primates and humans.[4,8] These findings indicate a substantially important role of the external environment in inducing neurochemical, morphological and behavioural changes in the brain.[4,8]

Observational studies

There is increasing evidence for the role of lifestyle factors as moderators of differences in cognitive ageing and as protective agents for the development of Alzheimer's disease from observational studies in older adults. Lifestyle factors that have been extensively studied in the context of cognitive decline include education, occupational status and participation in leisure activities. Previous observational studies have found that high levels of participation in mentally stimulating leisure activities decreased the risk of dementia or cognitive decline. For instance, one study found leisure activities such as travelling, doing odd jobs, knitting and gardening to be associated with a reduced risk for dementia. In another study, frequency of participation in common cognitive leisure activities (e.g., reading books; playing games such as cards, checkers/draughts, crosswords or other puzzles; and going to museums) was assessed at baseline for 801 elderly Catholic nuns, priests and brothers without dementia.[9] During follow-up, a one-point increase in the cognitive activity score was associated with a 33% reduction in the risk for Alzheimer's disease. Additionally, engagement in cognitive leisure activities was also associated with slower rates of cognitive decline. In another prospective study, participation in a variety of leisure activities characterized as either intellectual (such as reading, playing games or going to classes) or social (such as visiting friends or relatives, going to movies or restaurants or doing community volunteer work) was assessed in a population study of 1772 non-demented elderly people living in New York city.[10] During follow-up, subjects who reported higher levels of participation in these activities at baseline had a 38% less risk of developing dementia.

Table 76.1 summarizes our own experience in assessing the association between participation in mentally stimulating activities and risk for various cognitive syndromes in a cohort of older adults participating in the Bronx Aging Study. The Bronx Aging study enrolled community residing subjects between 75 and 85 years of age.[11] Exclusion criteria included severe visual or hearing loss, idiopathic Parkinson's disease, liver disease, alcoholism or known terminal illness. Subjects were screened to rule out the presence of dementia. The inception cohort was middle-class, predominantly Caucasian (91%) and mostly women (64%). Self-reported frequency of participation in leisure activities was coded to generate a scale with one point corresponding to participation in one activity for one day per week.[12] For each activity, subjects received seven points for daily participation, four points for participating several days per week, one point for weekly participation, and zero points for participating occasionally or never. The number of activity days for each activity was summed to generate a Cognitive Activity Scale. Participants received detailed clinical, medical and cognitive assessments at baseline and at 18 -month follow-up visits. Over the study follow-up, a one-point increase in Cognitive Activity Scale scores was associated with reduced risk of developing not only various dementia syndromes[12] but also intermediate cognitive impairment states such as mild cognitive impairment (MCI) syndrome,[13,14] as presented in Table 76.1.

Table 76.1 Participation in mentally stimulating activities and risk of cognitive syndromes in the Bronx Aging Study[a].

Syndrome	Hazard ratio	95% CI
Any dementia[12]	0.93	0.89–0.96
Alzheimer's disease[12]	0.93	0.88–0.98
Vascular dementia[12]	0.92	0.86–0.99
Amnestic mild cognitive impairment syndrome[13]	0.95	0.91–0.99
Vascular cognitive impairment syndrome[14]	0.93	0.89–0.97

[a]Hazard ratios and 95% confidence intervals (CI) are reported for each one-point increase in the Cognitive Activity Scale score and were obtained from Cox proportional hazard models adjusted for several potential confounders such as age, gender, education and the presence or absence of medical illnesses.

Clinical trials

Numerous cognitive training interventions have been conducted in laboratory or small-scale clinical settings. In general, these studies showed that cognitive training helps normal elderly individuals to improve performance on the specific task for which they were trained as compared with untrained individuals. Near transfer of training effects refers to improvements in cognitive domains that are closely related to the cognitive processes trained. Far transfer refers to improvements in domains that are distal from the cognitive processes trained. Although some studies showed that near transfer effects can be retained for months,[15] no-one has conclusively proved that the improvement in any of the cognitive domains can be transferred to real-world situations.

The ACTIVE study reported beneficial effects on cognition in 2832 non-demented older adults following a 6 week cognitive training intervention, especially in the cognitive domains directly related to the intervention, and these effects were found to last up to 5 years. There were also modest effects on everyday functioning.[3,15] A randomized controlled study in 487 older adults that compared an 8 week computerized cognitive training programme with a general cognitive stimulation programme found that the intervention group improved on untrained measures of memory and attention.[16] In contrast, a 6 week study in which 11 430 participants self-trained three times each week for a minimum of 10 min per day on online cognitive tasks showed improvements in tasks trained, but no evidence was found for transfer effects to untrained tasks.[17] This study included participants with a wide age range (18–60 years), training sessions were not supervised and the duration of training (dose) was not standardized across participants, which may limit the generalizability of the results of this study to elderly populations.

The above clinical trials enrolled elderly individuals without dementia. Another clinical trial reported the effect of a programme of mental stimulation in nursing home residents with Alzheimer's disease. Following the intervention, the 115 Alzheimer's disease patients who received mental stimulation therapy showed improvements in global measures of cognition and also in quality of life compared with the 86 Alzheimer's disease patients in the usual care control group.[18] This trial indicates that engagement in mentally stimulating activities may have behavioural benefits beyond cognition.

Mechanisms

Given the wide range of mentally stimulating activities available to older adults, it is likely that multiple mechanisms are involved in the cognitive benefits reported in previous observational studies. The three main mechanisms that have often been invoked to explain cognitive benefits of mentally stimulating activities are improving or building cognitive reserve, improving vascular health or mitigating effects of vascular insults to the brain and via stress mechanisms.

Cognitive reserve

The concept of cognitive reserve has been proposed to account for the fact that there is no direct relationship between the degree of brain damage or pathology and its clinical manifestations. For example, a head injury of the same magnitude can result in different levels of cognitive impairment in different individuals. Several prospective studies of ageing have reported that up to 25% of older adults whose neuropsychological testing is unimpaired prior to death meet full pathological criteria for Alzheimer's disease,[19] suggesting that this degree of pathology does not invariably result in clinical dementia.

Cognitive reserve postulates that individual differences in the cognitive processes or neural networks underlying task performance allow some people to cope better than others with brain damage. Katzman proposed that highly educated individuals are more resistant to the effects of dementia as a result of having greater cognitive reserve and increased complexity of neuronal synapses.[20] When regional cerebral blood flow was compared in different groups of Alzheimer's disease patients with the same degree of cognitive deterioration but different levels of education, it was observed that the patients with a high level of education had a more severe deficit of parietotemporal perfusion, indicating that Alzheimer pathology was more advanced in these subjects.[21]

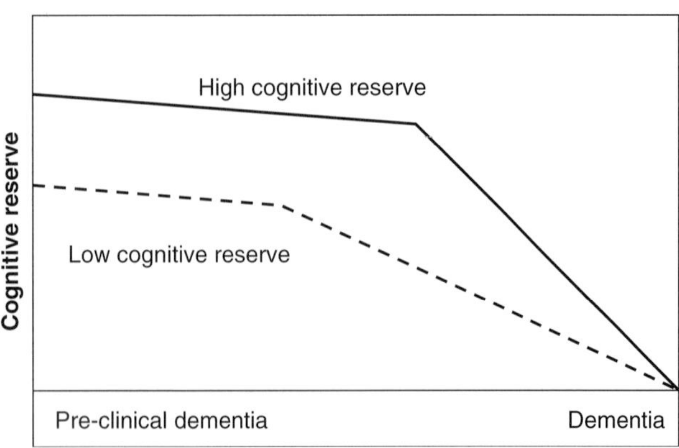

Figure 76.1 Cognitive reserve.

Figure 76.1 illustrates a hypothetical scenario comparing two older adults with high and low levels of cognitive reserve. The individual with higher cognitive reserve, who is able to resist the effects of dementia longer, develops cognitive decline later in life compared with the individual with low cognitive reserve. Since the duration of the dementia is assumed to be similar in both individuals, the patient with higher cognitive reserve will decline more rapidly than the patient with low cognitive reserve once that subject starts to manifest clinical symptoms.

Stern hypothesized that the neural implementation of cognitive reserve takes two forms, neural reserve and neural compensation.[22] In *neural reserve*, pre-existing brain networks that are more efficient or have greater capacity are less susceptible to disruption by age-related pathology such as Alzheimer's disease. Although healthy individuals may utilize these networks when coping with increased task demands, the networks could also help an individual cope with increasing brain pathology. In *neural compensation*, alternative brain networks compensate for pathology's disruption of pre-existing brain networks. Older adults show less specificity in many cognitive operations than young adults in brain regions that are recruited to carry out that task. This dedifferentiation has also been interpreted by some researchers as a compensatory function.

Accumulating evidence concerning brain plasticity in adults demonstrates the existence of several mechanisms that may augment cognitive reserve: angiogenesis, synaptogenesis and neurogenesis.[8] The widely held belief that the adult brain cannot develop new neurons is challenged by an increasing number of observations that at least some regions of the adult brain can respond to environmental stimuli by adding new neurons.[8]

Vascular

In the Bronx Aging Study, older adults who reported high levels of participation in cognitive leisure activities were at reduced risk of developing vascular cognitive impairment syndrome (cognitive impairment that is caused by or associated with vascular risk factors) with and without dementia.[14,23] Epidemiological studies have suggested that vascular disorders and vascular risk factors are involved in the pathogenesis and progression of Alzheimer's disease. Evidence from experimental, neuropathological and epidemiological studies supports both a direct or indirect effect of severe atherosclerosis on dementia and Alzheimer's disease in older adults.[23,24] As there is substantial clinical and neuropathological overlap between Alzheimer's disease and other dementias, the additive or synergistic interactions between vascular factors and Alzheimer pathology may be relevant in the clinical expression of dementia syndromes including Alzheimer's disease.[24,25] Mentally stimulating activities might be markers for healthy ageing; older adults who take part in mentally stimulating activities might also exercise more, have healthy diets or manage their comorbid medical illness better. Mentally stimulating activities may also promote vascular health by improving cognitive functions that are necessary to manage activities of daily living successfully. Interestingly, exposure to enriched environments was reported to improve functional outcomes after experimental brain infarctions in animal models.[4,26] This result suggests that mentally stimulating activities may help mitigate the effects of vascular insults to the brain, although this association has not been established in humans.

Stress

A high proneness to stress has been reported to be associated with increased risk of developing Alzheimer's disease.[27] The hippocampus is involved in stress response via glucocorticoids. Corticosterone hypersecretion due to stress downregulates hippocampal steroid receptors, which in turn can damp the feedback inhibition of the adrenocortical axis, leading to further hypersecretion, which finally can cause permanent loss of hippocampal neurons.[28] Associations between elevated cortisol levels, impaired cognitive function and hippocampal atrophy have been found in human studies involving dementia, depression, post-traumatic stress disorder and Cushing's disease.[28] Individuals who actively engage in mentally stimulating activities have more frequent contacts and have more opportunities to engage with others, leading to positive emotional states such as self-esteem, social competence and adequate mood, which lead to lower stress.

Targets of intervention

Disease prevention involves governments, professional organizations, public health professionals, healthcare

Table 76.2 Levels of prevention.

Level of prevention	Target population	Goals
Primary	Healthy seniors 'Worried well'	Prevent development of dementia Prevent age-associated cognitive decline
Secondary	Mild cognitive impairment (MCI) syndrome	Prevent conversion to dementia Prevent further cognitive decline
Tertiary	Dementia Alzheimer's disease	Prevent further cognitive decline Prevent behavioural disturbances Improve quality of life

professionals and individuals working at three levels to maintain and improve the health of individuals and communities. The first level, known as primary prevention, aims to prevent the development of disease before it occurs by eliminating or treating specific risk factors which may decrease or delay the development of disease, and usually targets healthy individuals. Secondary prevention refers to measures that target interventions at the preclinical stages of the disease, which is identified by clinical markers or biological tests. Tertiary prevention efforts focus on people already affected by disease and attempts to reduce resultant disability and restore functionality.

Table 76.2 lists target audiences and goals for each of these levels of prevention in the context of cognitive decline and dementia in older adults. Most drugs currently available for treating dementia patients have modest effects at best and do not substantially impact disease progression. Hence all forms of prevention for cognitive decline and dementia need to be explored more rigorously.

Implementing interventions

Exercise interventions are typically described in terms of dose ('how much?'), frequency ('how often?') and intensity ('how hard?'). There is limited evidence to recommend optimal dose, frequency and intensity for mentally stimulating activities to prevent cognitive decline. Although the optimal dose (how much?) of mental stimulation has not been established, findings from recent studies suggest that short duration of training or infrequent number of sessions may not be adequate to provide meaningful cognitive benefits.[2,16,17] In the Bronx Aging Study, participants whose cognitive activity levels were in the top third (greater than 11 points) of the group had a 63% reduced risk of dementia compared with those with activity levels in lowest third (fewer than 8 points).[12] Even participants with activity levels in the middle third (8–11 points) had a 52% reduced risk of dementia compared with those in the lowest third. These results indicate that the higher the frequency of participation, the better are the cognitive benefits of mentally stimulating activities.

Although engagement in mentally stimulating activities carries a very low risk of side effects, it is possible that some patients, who have not previously engaged in these types of activities, may be intimidated or stressed by starting these activities for the first time. Hence it is important to tailor mentally stimulating activities to the skill level and interests of the individual. The goal is to maximize participation and also the degree of mental stimulation. Depending on available resources or opportunities, patients could participate in these activities at home, local senior centres or in nursing home settings. The activities could be done either alone or with supervision. Formal cognitive rehabilitation programmes supervised by health professionals are also another option.

A discussion with the individual and/or family will be helpful in discovering current hobbies and interests or possible new areas or activities that might be of interest to the individual. It is important for the individual to choose mentally stimulating activities that are not only enjoyable, but also challenging. If a particular activity does not suit a patient, then they could be encouraged to try another mentally stimulating activity. Gradually increasing the duration and the level of difficulty of the activity will help prevent dropout. Involving the family and caregivers in the process is also important to ensure that the patient maintains participation. In the Bronx Aging Study, reading, playing board games such as chess or card games such as bridge and playing a musical instrument were the individual mentally stimulating activities that were associated with reduced risk of dementia.[12] However, other mentally stimulating leisure activities such as gardening, travelling, visiting museums or doing crossword puzzles have also been found to have beneficial effects on cognition in other epidemiological studies. Leisure activities that combine physical and mental effort, such as dancing, have also been reported to have cognitive benefits.[12] The use of computerized 'brain fitness' programmes have also become more popular in recent years.[16] A United States Census Bureau community survey in 2003 reported that 35% of adults over age 65 years and 63% of adults between ages 55 and 64 years had a computer at home, indicating a huge potential audience for computerized brain fitness programmes. It has been our experience that basic computing skills to play computerized brain games can be taught to older adults who are computer novices in one or two sessions. Hence the choice of mentally simulating activity may be less important than the dose, frequency and intensity of participation.

Conclusion

There is a paucity of high-quality clinical trials of mental stimulation in dementia. Large-scale population-based studies and controlled clinical trials are critically needed to investigate strategies to maintain cognitive function in individuals at risk for decline, to identify factors that may delay the onset of Alzheimer's disease among individuals at risk and to identify factors that may slow the progression of Alzheimer's disease among individuals already diagnosed with the disease.

Key points

- Observational studies support a link between increasing levels of participation in mentally stimulating activities and reduced risk of cognitive decline and dementia.
- Mentally stimulating activities may exert their protective effects on cognitive decline via improving cognitive reserve, promoting vascular health and reducing stress.
- Given the low risks associated with participation in mentally stimulating activities, clinicians should consider encouraging participation of older adults in such activities. The specific activities recommended should be tailored to the individual's interests, capacities and background. The duration and degree of difficulty of the activity should be gradually increased to provide increasing levels of challenge.
- However, it should be noted that there is a paucity of high-quality clinical trials of mental stimulation in dementia to support evidence-based recommendations at present.

Acknowledgement

The author is supported by grants from the National Institute on Aging, USA (grant numbers AG03949 and RO1 AG025119).

References

1. Brookmeyer R, Johnson E, Ziegler-Graham K and Arrighi HM. Forecasting the global burden of Alzheimer's disease. *Alzheimers Dement* 2007;**3**:186–91.
2. Clare L and Woods B. Cognitive rehabilitation and cognitive training for early-stage Alzheimer's disease and vascular dementia. *Cochrane Database Syst Rev* 2003;(4):CD003260.
3. Ball K, Berch DB, Helmers KF *et al*. Effects of cognitive training interventions with older adults: a randomized controlled trial. *JAMA* 2002;**288**:2271–81.
4. Petrosini L, De Bartolo P, Foti F *et al*. On whether the environmental enrichment may provide cognitive and brain reserves. *Brain Res Rev* 2009;**61**:221–39.
5. Diamond MC, Law F, Rhodes H *et al*. Increases in cortical depth and glia numbers in rats subjected to enriched environment. *J Comp Neurol* 1996;**128**:117–26.
6. Rosenzweig MR and Bennett EL. Psychobiology of plasticity: effects of training and experience on brain and behavior. *Behav Brain Res* 1996;**78**:57–65.
7. Greenough WT, Volkmar FR and Juraska JM. Effects of rearing complexity on dendritic branching in frontolateral and temporal cortex of the rat. *Exp Neurol* 1973;**41**:371–8.
8. Klempin F and Kempermann G. Adult hippocampal neurogenesis and aging. *Eur Arch Psychiatry Clin Neurosci* 2007;**257**:271–80.
9. Wilson RS, Mendes de Leon CF, Barnes LL *et al*. Participation in cognitively stimulating activities and risk of incident Alzheimer disease. *JAMA* 2002;**287**:742–8.
10. Scarmeas N, Levy G, Tang MX *et al*. Influence of leisure activity on the incidence of Alzheimer's disease. *Neurology* 2001; **57**:2236–42.
11. Katzman R, Aronson M, Fuld P *et al*. Development of dementing illnesses in an 80-year-old volunteer cohort. *Ann Neurol* 1989;**25**:317–24.
12. Verghese J, Lipton RB, Katz MJ *et al*. Leisure activities and the risk of dementia in the elderly. *N Engl J Med* 2003; **348**:2508–16.
13. Verghese J, LeValley A, Derby C *et al*. Leisure activities and the risk of amnestic mild cognitive impairment in the elderly. *Neurology* 2006;**66**:821–7.
14. Verghese J, Cuiling W, Katz MJ *et al*. Leisure activities and risk of vascular cognitive impairment in older adults. *J Geriatr Psychiatry Neurol* 2009;**22**:110–8.
15. Willis SL, Tennstedt SL, Marsiske M *et al*. Long-term effects of cognitive training on everyday functional outcomes in older adults. *JAMA* 2006;**296**:2805–14.
16. Smith GE, Housen P, Yaffe K *et al*. A cognitive training program based on principles of brain plasticity: results from the Improvement in Memory with Plasticity-based Adaptive Cognitive Training (IMPACT) study. *J Am Geriatr Soc* 2009;**57**:594–603.
17. Owen AM, Hampshire A, Grahn JA *et al*. Putting brain training to the test. *Nature* 2010;**465**:775–8.
18. Spector A, Thorgrimsen L, Woods B *et al*. Efficacy of an evidence-based cognitive stimulation therapy programme for people with dementia: randomised controlled trial. *Br J Psychiatry* 2003;**183**:248–54.
19. Ince P. Pathological correlates of late-onset dementia in a multicentre, community-based population in England and Wales. Neuropathology Group of the Medical Research Council Cognitive Function and Ageing Study (MRC CFAS). *Lancet* 2001;**357**:169–75.
20. Katzman R. Education and the prevalence of dementia and Alzheimer's disease. *Neurology* 1993;**43**:13–20.

21. Stern Y, Alexander GE, Prohovnik I and Mayeux R. Inverse relationship between education and parietotemporal perfusion deficit in Alzheimer's disease. *Ann Neurol* 1992; **32**:371–5.
22. Stern Y. Cognitive reserve. *Neuropsychologia* 2009;**47**: 2015–28.
23. Erkinjuntti T and Gauthier S. The concept of vascular cognitive impairment. *Front Neurol Neurosci* 2009;**24**:79–85.
24. Kalaria R. Similarities between Alzheimer's disease and vascular dementia. *J Neurol Sci* 2002;**203–204**:29–34.
25. Snowdon DA, Greiner LH, Mortimer JA *et al*. Brain infarction and the clinical expression of Alzheimer disease. The Nun Study. *JAMA* 1997;**277**:813–7.
26. Buchhold B, Mogoanta L, Suofu Y *et al*. Environmental enrichment improves functional and neuropathological indices following stroke in young and aged rats. *Restor Neurol Neurosci* 2007;**25**:467–84.
27. Wilson RS, Evans DA, Bienias JL *et al*. Proneness to psychological distress is associated with risk of Alzheimer's disease. *Neurology* 2003;**61**:1479–85.
28. Lupien SJ, McEwen BS, Gunnar MR and Heim C. Effects of stress throughout the lifespan on the brain, behaviour and cognition. *Nat Rev Neurosci* 2009;**10**:434–45.

CHAPTER 77

Exercise and dementia

Yves Rolland

Inserm U1027, F-31073; University of Toulouse III, Gérontopôle of Toulouse, France

Introduction

The incidence and prevalence of dementia are expected to increase dramatically in the coming decades. In the absence of curative treatment, risk factor modification remains the cornerstone for dementia prevention. Population studies and randomized controlled trials have recently indicated that people who are cognitively, socially and physically active have a reduced risk of cognitive impairment. Dementia is now considered as a long process resulting from accumulation of both risk and protective factors during lifespan (Figure 77.1).[1] Physical activity appears to be one of the main factors that contribute to the maintenance of a healthy ageing brain. Basic research trials also confirmed that an enriched environment and physical activity enhance the proliferation of new brain cells and promote brain repair in animal models.[2] Some of the most promising strategies for the prevention of dementia include vascular risk factor control, but also cognitive activity and physical activity.

Physical activity is already known as a cost-effective practice that has demonstrated during the past 30 years numerous physical benefits in the field of heart disease and cancer. The benefits of physical activity on brain functioning have been reported more recently.

Results from clinical and basic research facilitated by new technological approaches such as functional magnetic resonance imaging (fMRI) support the benefit of physical activity on cognitive decline in humans. However, none of the clinical research has clearly demonstrated that physical activity can prevent dementia. Nevertheless, growing evidence supports the view that physical activity may, at least, slow cognitive decline. Even a small delay of the onset of cognitive decline or a slowing of the disease progression would have a significant impact on this major public health priority.

Physical activity has also been shown to improve function even in frail nursing home residents[3] and Alzheimer's disease (AD) patients.[4] Physical activity yields an important and potent protective factor against functional decline and various frequent and devastating complications of the disease such as falls, fractures, malnutrition and behavioural disturbances, such as depression and anxiety. For demented patients, physical activity may also prevent key problems and have a major impact on the burden of the disease and quality of life.

Physical activity and the prevention of dementia in clinical research

Evidence that physical activity prevents cognitive decline is difficult to obtain. Results from epidemiological studies must be considered carefully as numerous biases may influence the relationship between exercise and the risk of dementia: the lifestyle of sedentary participants usually differs from that of exercisers in many ways. Many potential confounders between physical activity and the risk of dementia exist. Moreover, in most epidemiological studies, the assessment of physical activity is questionable. Involvement in physical activity varies substantially during a lifetime. The assessment of physical activity may not correspond to the mean long-term regular activity and even less to activity over the subject's past lifetime. Conclusions about the impact of different types, intensity and duration of the past physical activity are even more difficult to draw. An important limitation of most epidemiological studies is also that elderly subjects in the preclinical stage of dementia usually reduce their physical activity. Inactivity is a symptom frequently reported in the early phase of dementia rather than a risk factor. Behaviour disturbances such as depression or apathy usually precede the diagnosis of dementia and result in low physical activity. Finally, it is nearly impossible to discriminate between the effects of physical activity *per se* and the effects related to cognitive stimulation during physical activities that involve cognitive functions. It is therefore difficult to ascertain the specific effects of mobility and energy expenditure on brain functioning.

Principles and Practice of Geriatric Medicine, Fifth Edition. Edited by Alan J. Sinclair, John E. Morley and Bruno Vellas.

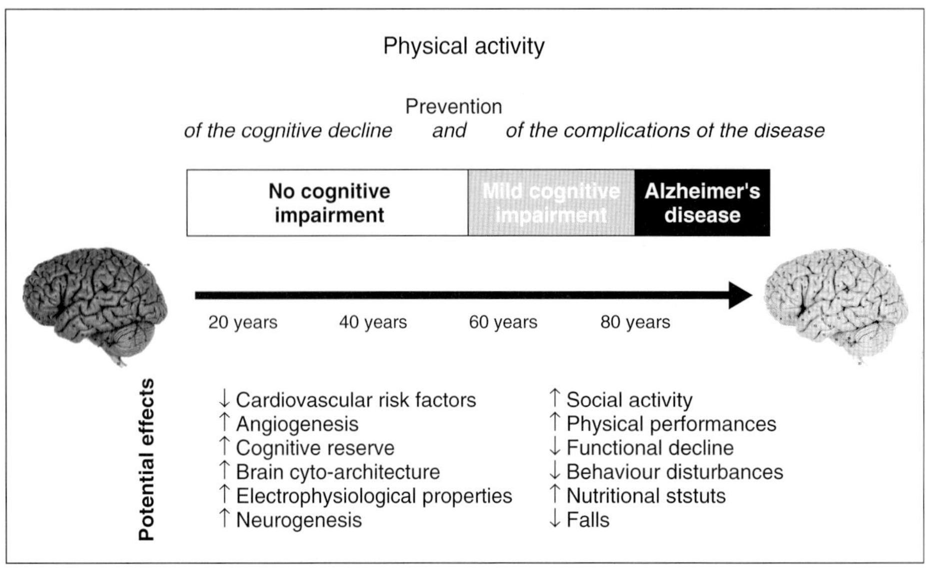

Figure 77.1 Alzheimer's disease and the potential roles of physical activity during lifespan.

Despite these limitations, many authors have examined the association between participation in physical activity and cognitive function in large groups of elderly people. Most of the time, the relationship between participation in physical activity and cognitive function is strong. Physically active aged individuals performed better in cognitive tests than their sedentary counterparts, especially in executive tests.[5] In several cross-sectional studies, cardiovascular fitness was associated with attention and executive function or visuospatial function. However, the cross-sectional design of these studies precludes inferences about causality in the relationship between physical activity and cognitive function. These cross-sectional studies are also subject to important methodological bias.

Table 77.1 reports most of the longitudinal epidemiological studies published during the past 10 years which have evaluated the association between physical activity and dementia or cognitive decline. Most of these epidemiological studies were controlled for potential confounders and suggest a protective effect of physical activity.

Currently, no randomized controlled trial (RCT) has ever concluded that physical activity prevents dementia or AD. Several randomized trials have reported a beneficial effect of a physical exercise programme on the cognitive performances of non-demented participants whereas other randomized trials have reported no cognitive improvement after a physical activity programme. None of these trials were designed to assess incidence of AD or dementia as the main outcome.

In 2003, Colcombe *et al.*,[24] in a meta-analysis of 18 interventional studies with a randomized design published between 1996 and 2001, Christie concluded that there is a significant effect of aerobic exercise training on cognitive function. In a Cochrane review published in 2008, Angevaren *et al.*[25] assessed the effectiveness of physical activity on cognitive function in people older than 55 years of age without known cognitive impairment. Eight out of 11 RCTs that compared aerobic physical activity programmes with any other intervention or no intervention reported an improvement in cognitive capacity that coincided with the increased cardiorespiratory fitness of the intervention group.

Since the above meta-analysis and systematic review, three large RCTs have reinforced these conclusions in non-demented elderly persons but also in patients with mild cognitive impairment (MCI). Patients with MCI are known to be at high risk for cognitive decline and AD and may be a target population for prevention programme.

Lautenschlager *et al.* reported that about 20 min per day of physical activity improved the cognitive function of 170 older adults with MCI.[26] The size of the effect of 6 and 18 months of a physical programme was modest but comparable to the benefit usually reported with the use of donepezil. Other authors have also reported that a high-intensity aerobic exercise programme (75–85% of heart rate reserve for 45–60 min per day, 4 days per week for 6 months) results in an improvement of executive control processes in older women with MCI.[27]

Finally, in the Lifestyle Interventions and Independence for Elders pilot (LIFE-P) study, 102 older adults at risk for mobility disability were randomized to a moderate-intensity physical activity intervention during 1 year. It was reported that the improvements in cognitive scores were associated with improvements in physical function.[28]

Table 77.1 Observational epidemiological studies on physical activity and risk of dementia or cognitive decline.

Study	Longitudinal non-demented population-based study	Summary of major findings (adjusted for confounders)
Physical activity as a significant preventive factor for dementia		
Hisayama Study (Yoshitake, 1995)[6]	828 individuals aged 65 years or over	Physical activity was associated with reduced risks of AD
Paquid study (Fabrigoule, 1995)[7]	2040 individuals aged 65 years or over	Physical activity was associated with reduced risks of dementia
Canadian Study of Health and Aging (Laurin, 2001)[8]	6434 individuals aged 65 years or over	High levels of physical activity were associated with reduced risks of cognitive impairment, AD and dementia of any type
Health Care Financing Administration Study (Scarmeas, 2001)[9]	1772 individuals aged 65 years or over	Leisure physical activities (walking for pleasure or going for an excursion) were associated with reduced risks of dementia
Bronx Aging Study (Yamada, 2003)[10]	469 individuals aged 75 years or over	Dancing was the only physical activity associated with a lower risk of dementia
Honolulu–Asia Aging Study (Abbott, 2004)[11]	2257 men aged 71–93 years	Walking more than 2 miles per day was associated with a lower risk of dementia
Cardiovascular Health Cognitive Study (Podewils, 2005)[12]	3375 individuals aged 65 years or over	Individuals engaged in more than four physical activities had lower risk of dementia
Cardiovascular risk factors, Aging and Incidence of Dementia (CAIDE) (Rovio, 2005)[13]	1449 individuals aged 65–79 years	Leisure-time physical activity, at least twice per week, was associated with a reduced risk of dementia and AD
The INVADE Study (Etgen, 2010)[14]	3903 individuals aged 55 years or over	Moderate or high physical activity was associated with a reduced incidence of cognitive impairment
Adult Change in Thought (Larson, 2006)[15]	1740 individuals aged 65 years or over	Physical activity at least three times per week was associated with a reduced risk of dementia
Physical activity as a non-significant preventive factor for dementia		
Sydney Older Persons Study (Broe, 1998)[16]	327 individuals aged 75 years or over	No statistically significant association between physical activity and dementia
Radiation Effect Research Foundation Adult Health Study (Yamada, 2003)[10]	1774 individuals	No statistically significant association between physical activity and dementia
Kungsholmen Project (Wang, 2002)[17]	776 individuals aged 75 years or over	Daily physical activity was associated with a no significant reduction risk of dementia
Physical activity as a significant preventive factor for cognitive decline		
MacArthur Study (Albert, 1995)[18]	1192 individuals aged 70 to 79 years	Strenuous physical activity was associated with a reduced risk of cognitive decline
Study of Osteoporotic Fractures (Yaffe, 2001)[19]	5925 individuals aged 65 years or over	Highest quartile of blocks walked per day was associated with a lower risk of cognitive decline
Brescia Study (Pignatti, 2002)[20]	364 individuals aged 70–85 years	Inactivity was associated with a higher risk of cognitive decline
Sonoma Study (Barnes, 2003)[21]	349 individuals aged 55 years or over	High peak oxygen consumption (VO_2) was associated with a lower risk of cognitive decline
Monongahela Valley Independent Elders Survey (MoVIES) (Lytle, 2004)[22]	1146 individuals aged 65 years or over	Exercising five times per week or more was associated with a lower risk of cognitive decline
Nurses' Health Study (Weuve, 2004)[23]	18 766 women aged 70–81 years	Walking at least 1.5 h per week at a pace of 21–30 min per mile was associated with a lower risk of cognitive decline
Physical activity as non-significant preventive factor for cognitive decline		
Sydney Older Persons Study (Broe, 1998)[16]	327 individuals aged 75 years or over	No statistically significant association between physical activity and cognitive decline

Physical activity and executive function

Most of the epidemiological studies and RCTs support the idea that the effects of physical activity were greatest for those tasks involving executive control processes.[24] Physical activity may influence structures and functions of the brain differently than other stimulation such as cognitive stimulation. In the MOBILIZE Boston Study, the neuropsychological executive tests were positively associated with participation in physical activity. In contrast, delayed recall of episodic memory was not associated with physical activity.[5] Other studies have reported that aerobic exercise intervention enhances executive function, whereas other cognitive functions seem to be less sensitive or insensitive to physical exercise. Using fMRI, it was recently demonstrated that physical activity enhances plasticity in prefrontal cortical regions that support executive function.[29] A physical activity programme also results in an increased grey matter volume mainly in prefrontal and cingulate regions and changes in brain-derived neurotrophic factor (BDNF) levels.[30] Colcombe *et al.*[24] reported that fitter older subjects had a greater grey matter volume in the prefrontal, parietal and temporal regions and a greater white matter volume in the genu of the corpus callosum than their less fit counterparts after controlling for potential confounders. These regions of the brain may retain more plasticity. These results support the notion of a specific biologically determined relationship between executive function and physical activity.

Further research is still required to increase our knowledge regarding the relationship between exercise and cognitive function in humans. However, clinical research and recent research on neuroimaging provide convincing support for the hypothesis that physical activity affects cognitive and neural plasticity in later life and prevents age-related cognitive decline.

Frailty, physical activity and cognitive reserve

Frailty is a clinical syndrome manifested by weight loss, weakness, fatigue, slow walking speed and low physical activity. These factors diminish the physiological reserves in elderly patients and put them at risk for adverse health outcomes such as disability, hospitalization and death when confronted by a stressor. Frailty has also been reported to be an independent predictor of cognitive decline[31] and dementia.[32] Low physical activity is one of the main factors for poor physical performances and frailty. Observation studies have reported that high physical performances are associated with lower rates of cognitive decline and dementia. A poor score on tests such as walking speed or poor results on the timed chair–stand test, standing balance or grip strength tests or other strength tests is associated with higher rates of cognitive decline and dementia. No study has reported that the prevention of frailty results in a reduced risk of dementia or cognitive decline. However, these studies support the hypothesis of a cross-talk between muscles and the central nervous system and that high functioning improves the cognitive reserve.

A higher cognitive reserve may help the subject engaged in regular physical activity to cope with the first cognitive symptoms of AD. This effect may delay the onset of the clinical manifestations of the disease, which may become apparent only later. Recent basic research has yielded convincing arguments that physical activity acts as a stimulus of neurogenesis, enhances the brain cytoarchitecture and electrophysiological properties and may influence neuropathological processes such as the formation of β-amyloid protein during AD.

Biological mechanisms of physical activity in preventing cognitive decline

Numerous hypotheses have been put forward to explain the relation between physical activity and brain function. Physical activity could protect against cognitive decline and dementia through a reduction of various cardiovascular risk factors such as hypertension, diabetes, hypercholesterolaemia and obesity. However, most epidemiological studies report a protective effect after adjustment for these cardiovascular risk factors, suggesting that physical activity has an independent preventive role. A review published in 2007 by Cotman *et al.*[33] examined the multiple underlying mechanisms promoted by physical activity to ensure brain health. Growing evidence from animal research suggests that physical activity directly modulates in the central nervous system, angiogenesis, neurogenesis and synaptogenesis. These responses to stress stimulated by physical activity may explain brain plasticity. Participation in physical activity may thus lower the risk of cognitive decline and dementia by improving cognitive reserve.

During a motor task and also for a brief period after a physical activity session, a transient increase in cerebral blood flow is observed in humans. In rats, aerobic training also enhances vascularization of the motor cortex but also of other regions of the brain. Angiogenesis may occur when the levels of neuronal activity of an area of the brain require an increased amount of oxygen that cannot be sufficiently delivered by the vessels. The lack of sufficient vascularization leads to the formation of new blood vessels and this occurs even in the elderly. During this process, the vascular endothelial growth factor (VEGF) seems to play an important role.[34]

In 1999, van Praag *et al.* reported that an exercise wheel enhances neurogenesis in mice.[2] Subsequent studies have confirmed that physical activity acts on proliferating precursor cells inducing neurogenesis.[34] Growing evidence suggests that this neurogenesis process integrates the neural networks which become functional. The neurogenesis seems to be mediated by many substances such as insulin-like growth factor 1 (IGF-1) and the brain-derived neurotrophic factor (BDNF). The neurotrophin BDNF is considered to be a crucial factor upregulated by physical activity.

The role of physical activity in synaptogenesis seems to be less important. Several studies have suggested that physical activity prevalently acts on neurogenesis whereas cognitive stimulation promotes synaptogenesis.[34]

Clinical practical applications: physical activity and prevention of AD

The basic recommendations from the American College of Sports Medicine (ACSM) and the American Heart Association (AHA) are to do moderately intense cardio training 30 min per day, 5 days per week *or* do vigorously intense cardio training 20 min per day, 3 days per week *and* do 8–10 strength training exercises per week, with 8–10 repetitions of each exercise. However, it remains actually unclear how much, what type and at what time of lifespan physical activity is optimally effective in preventing cognitive decline and dementia. No specific guidelines with a view to preventing cognitive decline, dementia or AD have been released.

Exercise programmes and assessment vary widely across experiments. Hence current epidemiological, interventional and animal studies can only suggest conditions under which physical activity (intensity, type, frequency and duration) may reduce the risk of dementia. The optimal exercise programme that would produce the maximal benefits is not known. This information may have important implications for the prevention of cognitive decline in the elderly. It also remains to be determined whether voluntary and forced exercise results in the same improvement.

Intensity and frequency

A relevant measure of intensity and duration or a standardized physical activity assessment scale is generally lacking in most longitudinal studies. They have not been designed to determine a threshold of physical activity that starts to protect against cognitive decline or AD.

Whether low-intensity physical activity, such as walking, cycling or swimming, or high-intensity activity, such as weight training, protects brain function is an important practical question. Some authors have reported that strenuous, but not moderate, physical activity was associated with less cognitive decline in a prospective study. However, organizing high-intensity activity may be challenging in frail elderly. Recommendations on physical activity have to be easily adopted by the population to be relevant.

Most epidemiological data suggest that the intensity threshold of physical activity required for a statistically significant impact on cognitive decline or dementia prevention is low. Physical activity such as playing golf, walking 1.6 km per day, playing tennis twice per week, walking at least 1.5 h per week at a pace of 21–30 min per mile, doing at least 15 min of activity at a time, three times per week, and per year amongst the physical activities walking, hiking, cycling, aerobics or calisthenics, swimming, water aerobics, weight training or stretching or other exercise was associated with a significantly lower risk of dementia in several epidemiological studies. In the LIFE pilot study, persistent engagement in physical activity was associated with beneficial effects on psychomotor processing speed and brain activation, even for moderate levels.[35]

Colcombe *et al.* also reported that a 1 h aerobic exercise training session [40–50% heart rate (HR) reserve increasing to 60–70% HR reserve over the course of the trial] three times per week over 6 months increased brain volume.[36] In this study, no dose-related response between physical activity and prevention of cognitive decline was found.

In the INVALIDE study, moderate activity (physical activity such as <3 times per week) and high activity (physical activity ≥ 3 times per week) was associated with a reduced incidence of cognitive impairment after 2 years in a large population-based cohort of elderly subjects.[14] Once again, no dose–response relationship between physical activity and incident cognitive impairment was found. In a recent interventional study, it was reported that physical activity conveys beneficial effects on memory function independently of its intensity, possibly mediated by local grey matter volume and neurotrophic factors.[30]

Other authors have reported significant trends for increased protection with greater intensity of physical activity. In the Canadian Study of Health and Aging, regular physical activity was associated with a lower risk of AD than no activity. In addition, an increased level of physical activity was associated with a decreased risk of cognitive impairment and dementia. In this cohort, risk of AD was reduced by half in subjects with higher levels of physical activity.

These results all suggest that the threshold of intensity that reduces the risk of cognitive decline and dementia is probably low. Previous studies have suggested that moderate activity could reduce dramatically the risk for other chronic diseases such as coronary heart disease. The same seems to be true for brain health. It should also be stated that, besides the benefit on brain health, exercise does not have to be performed at a specific intensity to confer a significant health benefit. However, the optimal intensity of physical activity required to maximize the slowing of cognitive decline and reduce the risk of dementia remains unclear.

Type of activity

The ACSM and the Centers for Disease Control (CDC) suggest that the benefit of physical activity is related to the amount of activity per day (energy expenditure), rather than to the type and modality of activity. Most epidemiological studies have investigated the role of physical activity on cognition using a composite score. None of these approaches make it possible to assess the influence of any specific activity on cognition.

Some specific physical activities may result in better brain functioning through social interaction and cognitive training. The psychological dimension of physical activity appears to be an important issue. In rodents, voluntary exercises have more benefit than forced exercises. Engagement in various physical activities, but not total energy expenditure, was significantly associated with the risk of dementia in the Cardiovascular Health Cognition Study (CHCS). Compared with participants engaged in one or no activity, the risk of dementia decreases by half in those engaged in four or more different activities, even after adjustment for energy expenditure. In the Bronx Aging study, dancing was the only physical activity that significantly reduced the risk of dementia.

Amongst the 13 different leisure activities of the Health Care Financing Administration (HCFA) study, walking for pleasure or going for an excursion was one of the activities the most strongly associated with a reduced risk of incident dementia. These results reinforce the hypothesis that physical activity may impact on cognition through its social interactions or cognitive training during the activity. However, other studies also suggest that simple tasks of a physical activity programme such as walking prevent cognitive decline.

Duration

Most of the studies that have investigated the association between mid-life physical activity and cognitive impairment have found that mid-life activity is associated with a lower incidence of both AD and all-cause dementia. A meta-analysis concluded that people who were not previously physically active can show improved cognitive functioning after exercising for as little as 4 months.[25]

Currently, we do not know at what period of life physical activity may have the most benefit against the risk for dementia. However, the pathophysiological process of AD begins long before cognitive decline is evident and the diagnosis established. It is probably necessary to begin being physically active early in life. According to the cognitive reserve hypothesis, physical activity performed across the whole lifespan may contribute to maintaining cognitive function in old age.

Physical activity in AD populations

Several studies have also confirmed the benefit of physical activity in older adults with dementia.[25,37] Older people with poor cognition had a steeper decline in physical performance than those with good cognition. Falls, malnutrition, behavioural disturbances or depression are frequent and severe consequences of the disease. These complications of the disease result in a high rate of functional decline. Their prevention may improve the course of dementia and the quality of life of the patients and reduce the burden on relatives. In this population, slowing the cognitive decline may not be the primary objective of physical activity.

On the other hand, depression, poor physical performance, malnutrition and behavioural disturbances are all linked to faster cognitive decline. In the REAL FR study, an abnormal one-leg balance predicts a higher rate of cognitive decline. Thus, in addition to the prevention and management of complications of the disease, physical activity may also be a realistic approach to delaying cognitive decline.[25,37] It seems reasonable to assume that physical activity in demented patients improves bowel movements and the appetite, some psychological factors (sleep, agitation and mood) and physical performance (balance, gait or strength). These effects may finally result in better cognitive functioning.

Large RCTs in AD patients are scarce, but most report significant improvements in psychological performances and mobility (Table 77.2). In a meta-analysis performed by Heyn *et al.*, it was shown that even in people with cognitive impairment or dementia, exercise training improves behavioural disturbances, physical function and cognitive function.[37] The mean time of most training programmes to achieve these results was less than 4 months. Even a programme including low-intensity physical activity may improve cognitive reserve in AD patients. It is very unlikely that physical activity reverses the pathophysiological process of dementia during this lapse of time. On the other hand, in this very sedentary population, especially in institutions, even a small amount of physical activity radically changes their way of life. In institutions, demented residents spent only 12 min a day in any constructive activity other than watching television.

Current RCTs on AD and physical activity have been short-duration trials with small samples of participants and left many questions unresolved. They need to be replicated in large future RCTs. Moreover, in most of these trials, physical activity was part of a combined intervention such as physical activity plus sensory environmental stimulation, behaviour management or social interaction. The impact of physical training on improved physical health, mood or functional mobility is then impossible to ascertain.

Table 77.2 Randomized controlled trials on physical activity in nursing-home demented residents.

First author	No. of residents	Mean MMSE	Intervention	Summary of major findings in the physical activity group
Molloy, 1988[38]	15	24/30	Light aerobic training 45 min once per week over 2 weeks	Modest improvement of word fluency
Friedman, 1991[39]	30	Moderate to severe	Walking 30 min 3 times per week over 10 weeks	Improvement of communication performances
Mulrow, 1994[40]	194	21/30	Strength, balance, transfer, mobility exercise 45 min 3 times per week over 16 weeks	Modest mobility benefits
Fiatarone, 1994[41]	100	22/30	Resistance training or nutritional supplementation or both, 45 min 3 times per week over 10 weeks	Improved physical performance and muscle mass
Tappen, 42[42]	42	6/30	Skill training 150 min 5 times per week over 20 weeks	Functional improvement
Alessi, 1995[43]	65	14/30	Sit-to-stand, walking and transferring exercise 120 min 5 times per week or rowing and walking 60 min 3 times per week over 9 weeks	Improved mobility, no improvement in sleep disruption
McMurdo, 1995[44]	55	15/30	Seated exercise 45 min twice per week over 6 months	Improved quadriceps strength, no change in cognitive function
Schnelle, 1995[45]	76	12/30	Functional incidental training (FIT) 30–55 min 5 times per week over 8 weeks	Reduced agitation, improved endurance and physical activity
MacRae, 1996[46]	37	20/30	Walking 30 min 5 times per week over 12 weeks	Improved endurance and walking distance
Lazowski, 1999[47]	68	–	Functional for Long Term Care (FFLTC) programme 45 min 3 times per week over 4 months	Improved mobility, balance, flexibility, lower extremities strength
Alessi, 1999[48]	29	13/30	Daytime aerobic exercise plus night-time intervention to decrease noise over 14 weeks	Improved sleep and decreased agitation
Tappen, 2000[49]	65	11/30	Walking or walking + conversation 30 min 3 times per week over 16 weeks	More compliance and less functional mobility decline in the walking + conversation group
Schnelle, 2002[50]	256	12/30	Incontinence care and exercise 60 min 5 times per week over 8 months	Improved continence and physical performance
Van de Winckel, 2004[51]	15	13/30	Physical activity + music 30 min per day over 3 months	Improved MMSE, no effect on behaviour
Stevens, 2006[52]	75	9–23/30	Physical activity 30 min 3 times per week over 12 weeks	Slower cognitive and disability decline
Williams, 2007[53]	90	10/30	Walking plus strength, balance, flexibility exercises 30 min 5 times per week over 16 weeks	Positive effect on mood
Rolland, 2007[4]	134	9/30	Collective exercise (walking, strength, balance and flexibility) 60 min twice per week over 12 months	Slower functional decline, increased gait speed
Dechamps, 2010[3]	160	16/30	Tai chi programme (4 times 30 min per week) or a cognition–action programme (30–45 min twice per week) over 6 months	Slowing of the decline in health-related quality of life based on activities of daily living and neuropsychiatric inventory

Table 77.3 Suggested rules for physical activity programme for demented patients in a nursing home.

Organize a physical activity committee

Identify leaders and organize a physical activity committee for exercise in the nursing home (occupational therapist, physiotherapist, nurse, nurse aids, geriatrician, nursing home director, caregiver, family, animation, volunteers, others)

Be aware that organizing an exercise programme takes effort and planning

Define the outcomes of the exercise programme and the role of each member

Organize a tracking system of the physical activity programme (adherence, side or adverse events, falls)

Organize education training for the staff about the benefits of physical activity in older people with dementia

Plan to buy few foam-rubber groundsheets, cones, easy to grasp soft balls and hoops

Schedule the nursing home physical activity programme

Adjust the sessions of physical activity to the schedule of the nursing home

Plan session of 1 h during the afternoon, twice per week, separated by at least 2 days (it is effective and realistic, but more frequent sessions would probably be better)

Define groups of residents

Inform the staff, the patients and their relatives

Define exercise groups according to their baseline physical performance scores, MMSE score and behaviour disturbances and the affinity between participants

Groups may be between 2 and 10 individuals

Improve adherence

Make the programme enjoyable and accessible

Begin at light intensity and gradually increase over the first month of the programme

Try the music during the sessions

Organize individualized exercises

Give favour to the participants' behavioural readiness for the proposed programme. Add a meaning to exercise in relation to everyday actions

Assess the physical performances of the residents before and regularly during the exercise programme (for example, gait speed, one-leg balance, short physical performance test)

Ritualize the session (same place, people, music, organization)

Finish the session by a snack time

Walking trail may pass the room of each exerciser to encourage joining the group

Inform (balance risks/benefits) and involve the family

Ensure that the intervention will be safe (comorbidities, architecture of the facility, shoes and behaviour disturbances between the residents)

Prescribe hip protectors if needed

Define an exercise programme

Define an inside (and/or an outside) circular walking trail in the nursing home (using the same trail to improve confidence) and an area dedicated to the exercise session

Define an organization to prepare (walking shoes) and group the participants

Duration of the session may be different between the participants

Start by a stretching warm-up

Subjects are encouraged to walk fast to reach moderate breathlessness but not exhaustion. Walking is required for at least half of the session

The walk can be interspersed with strength, flexibility and balance training (predetermined stations along the trail where guardrails in the corridor or foam rubber ground sheets can be used for safety)

Provide fun instructions that participants can enjoy

Encourage communication between the residents and staff during the session

Adapt strength training to the participant and focus on lower extremity strength (squatting at different levels or repeated standups from a chair, lateral elevation of the legs in a standing position and rising on the toes)

Flexibility (imitate simple flexibility exercises demonstrated by the therapist)

Balance training (adapted tai chi exercises, small step trial exercises using cones and hoops on the ground and one- or two-leg balance exercises on the ground or on foam-rubber groundsheets if possible)

Propose easy-to-remember movements that are repeated during training sessions and from one session to another

Adapt the programme as changes occur

Encourage the family to walk with the resident during their visit

Provide memory aides such as visual cues to remember to do the exercises

Physical activity training ranges from 150 min five times per week to 20 min three times per week. Population-based studies differ in terms of age, cognitive impairment severity or type of dementia and outcomes of the trial. Most studies have been organized in nursing home facilities and few in the community (Table 77.2). Only one clinical RCT of exercise for community-dwelling individuals with dementia has been reported.[54] This study involved 153 individuals and their family caregivers. Participants were assigned to an exercise and behaviour management treatment programme. The physical activity programme consisted in an individualized programme of walking, strength training, balance and flexibility exercises. Post-test, the exercisers had better physical functioning and fewer depressive symptoms than the control group. At 24 months, the exercisers were less likely to have been institutionalized.

Practical clinical applications: physical activity for demented patients

It is difficult to propose, on the basis of the literature, a specific kind of physical programme for AD patients. However, intensive exercise programmes may not be practical in some nursing-home settings in the long term. Simple programmes such as an aerobic exercise, twice per week, have been reported to slow the progression of the disease in nursing-home residents. Most RCTs suggest that aerobic exercise such as walking may promote cognitive and functional capacities in people with AD.

Compliance is another key issue for physical activity programmes. In this population, compliance seems to be a major limitation, more than cognitive status. The physical programme has to be enjoyable and accessible. Individualized exercises, based on the participant's behavioural readiness for the proposed training, and music during the session seem to increase compliance. Successful and safe interventions including strength, flexibility and balance training have been reported in this frail and cognitively impaired population. Compliance with the physical activity programme appeared better when the staff assigned to this task communicated with the resident at the same time.

Table 77.3 lists suggested rules for physical activity programme for demented patients in a nursing home.

Conclusion

In addition to its cardiovascular benefits, physical activity may also slow cognitive decline and the incidence of dementia. No RCTs have yet demonstrated that regular physical activity prevents dementia, but increasing evidence suggests that an easy to perform physical activity programme can result in a healthy ageing brain. This argument may convince sedentary individuals to change their lifestyle habits. During AD and dementia, physical activity can slow the rapid functional decline and improve the quality of life of the patient. This approach should be systematically proposed as a key non-pharmacological treatment for this population.

Key points

- Risk factor modification is an important part of dementia prevention.
- Sustained aerobic exercise in mid-life may have a role in preventing cognitive decline.
- Prevention of other risk factors for functional decline may also have benefits in reducing cognitive problems in later life.

References

1. Fratiglioni L and Wang HX. Brain reserve hypothesis in dementia. *J Alzheimers Dis* 2007;**12**:11–22.
2. van Praag H, Kempermann G and Gage F. Running increases cell proliferation and neurogenesis in the adult mouse dentate gyrus. *Nat Neurosci* 1999;**2**:266–70.
3. Dechamps A, Diolez P, Thiaudière E *et al.* Effects of exercise programs to prevent decline in health-related quality of life in highly deconditioned institutionalized elderly persons: a randomized controlled trial. *Arch Intern Med* 2010;**170**:162–9.
4. Rolland Y, Pillard F, Klapouszczak A *et al.* Exercise program for nursing home residents with Alzheimer's disease: a 1-year randomized, controlled trial. *J Am Geriatr Soc* 2007; **55**:158–65.
5. Eggermont LH, Milberg WP, Lipsitz LA *et al.* Physical activity and executive function in aging: the MOBILIZE Boston Study. *J Am Geriatr Soc* 2009;**57**:1750–6.
6. Yoshitake T, Kiyohara Y, Kato I, *et al.* Incidence and risk factors of vascular dementia and Alzheimer's disease in a defined elderly Japanese population: the Hisayama Study. *Neurology* 1995;**45**:1161–8.
7. Fabrigoule C, Letenneur L, Dartigues JF *et al.* Social and leisure activities and risk of dementia: a prospective longitudinal study. *J Am Geriatr Soc* 1995;**43**:485–90.
8. Laurin D, Verreault R, Lindsay J *et al.* Physical activity and risk of cognitive impairment and dementia in elderly persons. *Arch Neurol* 2001;**58**:498–504.
9. Scarmeas N, Levy G, Tang MX *et al.* Influence of leisure activity on the incidence of Alzheimer's disease. *Neurology* 2001;**57**:2236–42.
10. Yamada M, Kasagi F, Sasaki H *et al.* Association between dementia and midlife risk factors: the Radiation Effects Research Foundation Adult Health Study. *J Am Geriatr Soc* 2003;**51**:410–4.
11. Abbott RD, White LR, Ross GW *et al.* Walking and dementia in physically capable elderly men. *JAMA* 2004;**292**:1447–53.
12. Podewils LJ, Guallar E, Kuller LH, *et al.* Physical activity, APOE genotype, and dementia risk: findings from

the Cardiovascular Health Cognition Study. *Am J Epidemiol* 2005;**161**:639–51.

13. Rovio S, Kareholt I, Helkala EL, *et al.* Leisure-time physical activity at midlife and the risk of dementia and Alzheimer's disease. *Lancet Neurol* 2005;**4**:705–11.
14. Etgen T, Sander D, Huntgeburth U *et al.* Physical activity and incident cognitive impairment in elderly persons: the INVADE study. *Arch Intern Med* 2010;**170**:186–93.
15. Larson EB, Wang L, Bowen JD, *et al.* Exercise is associated with reduced risk for incident dementia among persons 65 years of age and older. *Ann Intern Med* 2006;**144**:73–81.
16. Broe GA, Creasey H, Jorm AF, *et al.* Health habits and risk of cognitive impairment and dementia in old age: a prospective study on the effects of exercise, smoking and alcohol consumption. *Aust N Z J Public Health* 1998;**22**:621–3.
17. Wang L, van Belle G, Kukull WB and Larson EB. Predictors of functional change: a longitudinal study of nondemented people aged 65 and older. *J Am Geriatr Soc* 2002;**50**:1525–34.
18. Albert MS, Jones K, Savage CR, *et al.* Predictors of cognitive change in older persons: MacArthur studies of successful aging. *Psychol Aging* 1995;**10**:578–89.
19. Yaffe K, Barnes D, Nevitt M *et al.* A prospective study of physical activity and cognitive decline in elderly women: women who walk. *Arch Intern Med* 2001;**161**:1703–8.
20. Pignatti F, Rozzini R and Trabucchi M. Physical activity and cognitive decline in elderly persons. *Arch Intern Med* 2002;**162**:361–2.
21. Barnes DE, Yaffe K, Satariano WA and Tager IB. A longitudinal study of cardiorespiratory fitness and cognitive function in healthy older adults. *J Am Geriatr Soc* 2003;**51**:459–65.
22. Lytle ME, Vander Bilt J, Pandav RS *et al.* Exercise level and cognitive decline: the MoVIES project. *Alzheimer Dis Assoc Disord* 2004;**18**:57–64.
23. Weuve J, Kang JH, Manson JE *et al.* Physical activity, including walking, and cognitive function in older women. *JAMA* 2004;**292**:1454–61.
24. Colcombe S and Kramer AF. Fitness effects on the cognitive function of older adults: a meta-analytic study. *Psychol Sci* 2003;**14**:125–30.
25. Angevaren M, Aufdemkampe G, Verhaar HJ *et al.* Physical activity and enhanced fitness to improve cognitive function in older people without known cognitive impairment *Cochrane Database Syst Rev* 2008;(2):CD005381.
26. Lautenschlager NT, Cox KL, Flicker L, *et al.* Effect of physical activity on cognitive function in older adults at risk for Alzheimer disease: a randomized trial. *JAMA* 2008; **300**:1027–37.
27. Baker LD, Frank LL, Foster-Schubert K *et al.* Effects of aerobic exercise on mild cognitive impairment: a controlled trial. *Arch Neurol* 2010;**67**:71–9.
28. Williamson JD, Espeland M, Kritchevsky SB *et al.*; LIFE Study Investigators. Changes in cognitive function in a randomized trial of physical activity: results of the lifestyle interventions and independence for elders pilot study. *J Gerontol A Biol Sci Med Sci* 2009;**64**:688–94.
29. Carlson MC, Erickson KI, Kramer AF *et al.* Evidence for neurocognitive plasticity in at-risk older adults: the Experience Corps Program. *J Gerontol A Biol Sci Med Sci* 2009;**64**:1275–82.
30. Ruscheweyh R, Willemer C, Krüger K *et al.* Physical activity and memory functions: an interventional study. *Neurobiol Aging* 2011;**32**:1304–19.
31. Samper-Ternent R, Al Snih S, Raji MA *et al.* Relationship between frailty and cognitive decline in older Mexican Americans. *J Am Geriatr Soc* 2008;**56**:1845–52.
32. Buchman AS, Boyle PA, Wilson RS *et al.* Frailty is associated with incident Alzheimer's disease and cognitive decline in the elderly. *Psychosom Med* 2007;**69**:483–9.
33. Cotman CW, Berchtold NC and Christie LA. Exercise builds brain health: key roles of growth factor cascades and inflammation. *Trends Neurosci* 2007;**30**:464–72.
34. Lista I and Sorrentino G. Biological mechanisms of physical activity in preventing cognitive decline. *Cell Mol Neurobiol* 2010;**30**:493–503.
35. Rosano C, Venkatraman VK, Guralnik J *et al.* Psychomotor speed and functional brain MRI 2 years after completing a physical activity treatment. *J Gerontol A Biol Sci Med Sci* 2010;**65**:639–47.
36. Colcombe SJ, Erickson KI, Scalf PE *et al.* Aerobic exercise training increases brain volume in aging humans. *J Gerontol A Biol Sci Med Sci* 2006;**61**:1166–70.
37. Heyn P, Abreu BC and Ottenbacher KJ. The effects of exercise training on elderly persons with cognitive impairment and dementia: a meta-analysis. *Arch Phys Med Rehabil* 2004;**85**:1694–704.
38. Molloy DW, Richardson LD and Crilly RG. The effects of a three-month exercise program on neuropsychological function in elderly institutionalized women: a randomized controlled trial. *Age Ageing* 1988;**17**:303–10.
39. Friedman R and Tappen RM. The effect of planned walking on communication in Alzheimer's disease. *J Am Geriatr Soc* 1991;**39**:650–4.
40. Mulrow CD, Gerety MB, Kanten D *et al.* A randomized trial of physical rehabilitation for very frail nursing home residents. *JAMA* 1994;**271**:519–24.
41. Fiatarone MA, O'Neill EF, Ryan ND *et al.* Exercise training and nutritional supplementation for physical frailty in very elderly people. *N Engl J Med* 1994;**330**:1769–75.
42. Tappen RM. The effect of skill training on functional abilities of nursing home residents with dementia. *Res Nurs Health* 1994;**17**:159–65.
43. Alessi CA, Schnelle JF, MacRae PG *et al.* Does physical activity improve sleep in impaired nursing home residents? *J Am Geriatr Soc* 1995;**43**:1098–102.
44. McMurdo ME and Johnstone R. A randomized controlled trial of a home exercise program for elderly people with poor mobility. *Age Ageing* 1995;**24**:425–8.
45. Schnelle JF, MacRae PG, Ouslander JG *et al.* Functional incidental training, mobility performance and incontinence care with nursing home residents. *J Am Geriatr Soc* 1995; **43**:1356–62.
46. MacRae PG, Asplund LA, Schnelle JF *et al.* A walking program for nursing home residents: effects on walk endurance, physical activity, mobility and quality of life. *J Am Geriatr Soc* 1996;**44**:175–80.
47. Lazowski DA, Ecclestone NA, Myers AM *et al.* A randomized outcome evaluation of group exercise programs in long-term care institutions. *J Gerontol A Biol Sci Med Sci* 1999;**54**:M621–8.

48. Alessi CA, Yoon EJ, Schnelle JF *et al*. A randomized trial of a combined physical activity and environmental intervention in nursing home residents: do sleep and agitation improve? *J Am Geriatr Soc* 1999;**47**:784–91.

49. Tappen RM, Roach KE, Applegate EB and Stowell P. Effect of a combined walking and conversation intervention on functional mobility of nursing home residents with Alzheimer disease. *Alzheimer Dis Assoc Disord* 2000;**14**:196–201.

50. Schnelle JF, Alessi CA, Simmons SF *et al*. Translating clinical research into practice: a randomized controlled trial of exercise and incontinence care with nursing home residents. *J Am Geriatr Soc* 2002;**50**:1476–83.

51. Van de Winckel A, Feys H, De Weerdt W and Dom R. Cognitive and behavioural effects of music-based exercises in patients with dementia. *Clin Rehabil* 2004;**18**:253–60.

52. Stevens J and Killeen M. A randomised controlled trial testing the impact of exercise on cognitive symptoms and disability of residents with dementia. *Contemp Nurse* 2006;**21**:32–40.

53. Williams CL and Tappen RM. Effect of exercise on mood in nursing home residents with Alzheimer's disease. *Am J Alzheimers Dis Other Demen* 2007;**22**:389–97.

54. Teri L, Gibbons LE, McCurry SM *et al*. Exercise plus behavioral management in patients with Alzheimer disease: a randomized controlled trial. *JAMA* 2003;**290**:2015–22.

CHAPTER 78

Drug development and Alzheimer's disease

Julien Delrieu[1,2], Antoine Piau[1] and Bruno Vellas[1,2]

[1]Alzheimer's Disease Clinical Research Centre, Gérontopôle, Toulouse University Hospital, Toulouse, France
[2]INSERM Unit 558, University of Toulouse III, Toulouse, France

Introduction

Alzheimer's disease (AD) mainly affects elderly individuals. Because of the ageing of populations worldwide, this disorder is reaching epidemic proportions, with a large human, social and economic burden. The progressive degeneration of neurons in AD causes abnormalities of the systems of neurotransmitters, and a combination of cholinergic and glutamatergic dysfunction appears to underlie the symptomatology of AD. Current drugs for AD target cholinergic and glutamatergic neurotransmission. Cholinesterase inhibitors (ChEIs) and/or butyrylcholinesterase are widely prescribed as symptomatic treatments for AD. Donepezil (Aricept), rivastigmine (Exelon) and galantamine (Reminyl) were approved by the US Food and Drug Administration (FDA) for the treatment of mild to moderately severe AD in 1996, 2000 and 2001, respectively. The use of donepezil for the treatment of severe AD has already been approved in the USA. Memantine [Ebixa and Axura (Europe) and Namenda (USA)] was approved in 2002 by the European Agency for the Evaluation of Medical Products (EMEA) for the treatment of moderately severe to severe AD and in 2003 by the FDA for the treatment of moderate to severe AD.

However, the effects of these treatments are limited or controversial as they do not modify disease progression.[1] Currently, much effort is directed towards identifying disease-modifying therapies. The use of biomarkers of plasma, cerebrospinal fluid (CSF) or neuroimaging [magnetic resonance imaging (MRI) and positron emission tomography (PET)] could play an important role in estimating their efficiency and their potential disease-modifying effect.

This chapter discusses general classes of potential disease-modifying drugs under investigation for the treatment of AD, and also the contribution of the non-pharmacological approach. Compounds and studies selected for this review were identified by systematic searches using PubMed. Only publications in English were reviewed. The ClinicalTrials.gov (http://www.clinicaltrials.gov) website was used for information on ongoing randomized controlled trials (RCTs).

Impact on cholinergic deficit

The mainstays of current pharmacotherapy for AD are compounds aimed at increasing the levels of acetylcholine (ACh) in the brain, thereby facilitating cholinergic neurotransmission through inhibition of the cholinesterases. Other drugs that can increase the ACh levels in brain include ACh precursors, muscarinic agonists and nicotinic agonists.

Recent reports suggest that AChEIs could affect the underlying disease processes[2,3] through neuroprotective and disease-modifying properties.[4] Huperzine A is a selective AChEI with potential properties that include modification of β-amyloid (Aβ) peptide processing, reduction of oxidative stress, neuroprotection and regulation of nerve growth factor (NGF) expression.[5,6] Clinical trials of its derivative, ZT-1, have demonstrated an improvement in cognitive function of AD patients.[7] Phenserine, a derivative of physostigmine, has a dual mode of action: AChEI and inhibitor of the formation of Aβ precursor protein (APP).[8,9] Phenserine is dose-limited in animals by its cholinergic actions. The (+)-phenserine enantiomer (Posiphen), which has weak activity as an AChEI and is potent on Aβ levels and amyloid processing, can be dosed much higher,[10,11] but clinical trials are required. Butyrylcholinesterase may play a role in attention, executive function, emotional memory and behaviour. Furthermore, butyrylcholinesterase activity progressively increases as the severity of dementia advances, whereas acetylcholinesterase activity declines. Therefore, inhibition of butyrylcholinesterase may provide additional benefits.[12] Structural analogues of phenserine,

Principles and Practice of Geriatric Medicine, Fifth Edition. Edited by Alan J. Sinclair, John E. Morley and Bruno Vellas.

cymserine and bisnorcymserine, proved to be potent inhibitors of human butyrylcholinesterase in comparison with phenserine.[13,14] *Salvia officinalis* (sage), which has cholinergic properties, is also under clinical investigation for AD.

Several M1 receptor agonists, such as Lu 25–109 (a compound that directly stimulates muscarinic cholinergic receptors), have been tested in clinical trials without much success.[15] Recent studies which suggest the role of muscarinic agonists in regulating the production of Aβ again raise the possibility that selective M1 agonists could be useful in AD.[16] The M1 muscarinic agonists are neurotrophic, elevate the nonamyloidogenic APP *in vitro*, decrease Aβ levels *in vitro* and *in vivo* and restore cognitive impairments in animal AD models.[17,18]

Nicotinic acetylcholine receptors (nAChRs), which are essential for learning and memory, are reduced in AD brains and research implicates a role for nAChRs in neuroprotection. Targeting nAChRs is an attractive therapeutic approach and several selective ligands for nAChRs have been developed, but a challenge has been the reduction of side effects.[19-22] ABT-089, a selective neuronal nicotinic receptor modulator which shows positive effects in rodent and primate cognitive models,[23] is a candidate for further evaluation as a treatment for AD.[24] GTS-21 (DMXBA) is a selective agonist of alpha7 nicotinic receptors which enhances a variety of cognitive behaviours in mice, monkeys, rats and rabbits. It also displays neuroprotective activity *in vitro* and has shown promising characteristics during phase 1 clinical tests.[25] Ispronicline (TC-1734, AZD-3480) is a selective neuronal nicotinic agonist that is neuroprotective *in vitro* and exhibits memory-enhancing properties *in vivo*. Ispronicline also had a beneficial effect on cognition in subjects with age-associated memory impairment in a phase 2 trial.[26] Other nicotinic agents under clinical evaluation are summarized in Table 78.1.

Anti-amyloid therapies

AD drug development is driven mainly by the amyloid hypothesis. In fact, currently available evidence strongly supports the position that the initiating event AD is related to abnormal processing of β-amyloid (Aβ) peptide, ultimately leading to the formation of Aβ plaques in the brain.[27] This process occurs while individuals are still cognitively normal. After a lag period, which varies from patient to patient, neuronal dysfunction and neurodegeneration become the dominant pathological processes. Anti-amyloid agents target production, accumulation, clearance or toxicity associated with Aβ peptide.

Drugs to promote Aβ clearance

Active and passive immunizations were developed to inhibit generation of toxic Aβ aggregates and to remove soluble and aggregated Aβ.

Active immunization

Active immunization of APP transgenic (Tg) mice before they had amyloid plaque deposits resulted in significantly reduced amyloid deposits and neuritic pathology, and Aβ immunization of older mice with pre-existing plaques also resulted in a reduction in plaque pathology. This suggests that this approach is able to slow the progression of amyloid deposition and even reverse it.[28] Subsequent studies have shown that Aβ immunization can also prevent or improve learning deficits in AD Tg mice.[29,30] A phase 1 human trial using an active immunization strategy against Aβ was promising but the phase 2a immunization trial with a synthetic Aβ peptide called AN-1792 was stopped after reports of meningoencephalitis in 6% of the treated patients.[31] The first analysis of efficacy in this trial, reported for a small subset of patients, was suggestive of a slowing cognitive decline, particularly in patients generating the highest antibody titres.[32] A more recent and complete analysis of all treated patients demonstrated no significant efficacy except in the small subset of subjects who had CSF examinations, CSF tau was decreased in antibody responders versus placebo subjects ($p < 0.001$).[33] Immunization strategies research in Tg mouse models has been refocused to establish safer therapeutic approaches.[34] A new generation of AD vaccines has been designed to try to prevent the induction of Aβ reactive T cells, which is thought to have been critical in AN-1792 failure.[35]

Passive immunization

It is also possible to bypass the immune response by direct administration of anti-Aβ antibodies with a passive immunization approach. This approach seems to be as effective as active immunization in Tg mice[36] and could potentially eliminate toxic T-cell-mediated responses to Aβ. In preclinical studies, passive immunization of APP Tg mice with pre-existing evidence of cerebral amyloid angiopathy resulted in an increased severity and incidence of microhaemorrhages, but the physiological implications of these findings remain unclear.[37,38] Antibodies against the β-secretase cleavage site of the APP are another way to limit APP processing. They inhibit Aβ formation *in vitro* and their long-term administration to Tg mice improved cognitive functions associated with a reduction in brain inflammation and incidence of microhaemorrhage.[39] Classical human immunoglobulin (Ig) preparation can also be investigated as a passive

Table 78.1 Ongoing clinical research on new drugs (based on ClinicalTrials.gov website)[a].

Agent/drug	Title	Outcome measures	Reference	Condition	Start date–completion date	Sponsor	Phase
Cholinergic agents							
Nicotinic modulator: MEM-3454	A Study of RO5313534 as Add-on to Donepezil Treatment in Patients with Mild to Moderate Alzheimer's Disease	ADAS-Cog, CANTAB tests, MMSE, ADCS CGIC, Behave-AD-FW, ADCS-ADL, Zarit Burden interview, AEs, laboratory parameters, suicidal risk, concomitant medications, physical and neurological examinations	NCT00884507	AD	May 2009–July 2011	Hoffmann-La Roche	2
EVP-6124	Safety and Cognitive Function Study of EVP-6124 in Patients with Mild to Moderate Alzheimer's Disease	ADAS-cog-13	NCT01073228	AD	April 2010–October 2010	EnVivo Pharma-ceuticals.	2
Antiamyloid agents							
Active immuniza-tion/V950	A Study of V950 in People with Alzheimer Disease	General safety and tolerability after each dose and throughout the study; immunogenicity after each dose and throughout the study	NCT00464334	AD	April 2007–February 2012	Merck	1
Active immuniza-tion/CAD106	Safety, Tolerability and Abeta-specific Antibody Response of Repeated i.m. Injections of Adjuvanted CAD106 in Mild Alzheimer Patients	Safety and tolerability assessments (physical/neurological examinations, ECG, vital signs, standard and special laboratory evaluations, MRIs, AE/SAE monitoring)	NCT01097096	AD	March 2010–?	Novartis	2
Active immunization/ ACC-001	A Long-Term Extension Study Evaluating ACC-001 with QS-21 in Subjects with Mild to Moderate Alzheimer's Disease	Incidence and severity of treatment-emergent adverse events; clinically important changes in safety assessment results including adverse events, vital signs, weight, clinical laboratory tests, ECGs, MRI scans and physical and neurological examinations.; Change from baseline levels of anti-A-beta IgG, anti-A-beta IgM and IgG subclass antibody levels at selected time points	NCT00960531	AD	July 2010–July 2014	Wyeth	2
Active immunization/ UB-311	Study to Evaluate Safety, Tolerability and Immunogenicity of Vaccine in Subjects with Alzheimer's Disease	To evaluate safety and tolerability of the vaccine	NCT00965588	AD	February 2009–December 2010	United Biomedical	1

(continued overleaf)

Table 78.1 *(continued)*.

Agent/drug	Title	Outcome measures	Reference	Condition	Start date–completion date	Sponsor	Phase
Active immunization/AFFITOPE AD02	Clinical- and Immunological Activity, Safety and Tolerability of Different Doses/Formulations of AFFITOPE AD02 in Early Alzheimer's Disease	Cognitive (ADAS-cog modified) and functional (ADCS-ADL modified)	NCT01117818	Early AD, (based on episodic memory deficit and hippocampal atrophy)	May 2010–April 2012	Affiris	2
Passive immunization/monoclonal antibody GSK933776A	A Clinical Study to Assess Single and Repeat Doses of a New Medication (GSK933776) in Patients with Alzheimer's Disease	AE. Changes suggesting potential adverse events detected in the physical and neurological examination, brain MRI, cognitive status, laboratory parameters, ECG and vital signs; Plasma pharmacokinetic parameters. Pharmacodynamic effects. CSF detectable levels. Effects on plasma and CSF biomarkers. Titre and neutralizing activity. Exploratory PET scan	NCT00459550	AD	March 2007–November 2010	GlaxoSmithKline	1
Passive immunization/monoclonal antibody PF-04360365	Multiple IV Dose Study of PF-04360365 in Patients with Mild to Moderate Alzheimer's Disease	Safety/tolerability in subjects with mild to moderate AD dosed for 18 months. (AE, physical/neurological examinations, vital signs, 12-lead ECG, clinical laboratories, brain MRI, cognitive assessments); pharmacokinetics following administration of multiple doses in subjects with mild to moderate AD. ADAS-cog, DAD, plasma/CSF Aβ, CSF tau and phosphotau, CSF protein, RBCs, WBCs and glucose, immunogenicity (anti-drug antibodies)	NCT00722046	AD	May 2010–August 2011	Pfizer	2
Passive immunization/monoclonal antibody PLY2062430 (solanezumab)	Effect of LY2062430 on the Progression of Alzheimer's Disease	ADAS-Cog, ADCS-ADL, CDR-SB, NPI, volumetric MRI, MMSE, RUD-Lite, EQ-5D Proxy, QoL-AD, change from baseline to end point in plasma LY2062430 to investigate a relationship between plasma LY2062430 and plasma Aβ levels, change from baseline to end point in plasma Aβ	NCT00904683	AD	May 2009–September 2012	Eli Lilly	2

Passive immunization/monoclonal antibody AAB-001 (bapineuzumab)	Study Evaluating the Efficacy and Safety of Bapineuzumab in Alzheimer Disease Patients	ADAS-Cog, DAD, Neuropsychological Test Battery, CDR	NCT00667810	AD	May 2008 – June 2014	Elan Pharmaceuticals	3
Passive immunization/monoclonal antibody MABT5102A	A Study of the Safety, Pharmacokinetics, Pharmacodynamics, and Immunogenicity of Anti-Abeta in Patients with Alzheimer's Disease	Safety and tolerability of single and multiple doses of MABT5102A	NCT00736775	Mild to moderate AD	August 2008–?	Genentech	1
Passive immunization/monoclonal antibody R1450 (gantenerumab)	A Multiple Ascending Dose Study of R1450in Patients with Alzheimer Disease	AEs, laboratory parameters, vital signs. Pharmacokinetic parameters of R1450 in plasma	NCT00531804	AD	December 2006–?	Hoffmann-La Roche	1
α-Secretase activator bryostatin-1	Safety, Efficacy, Pharmacokinetics, and Pharmacodynamics Study of Bryostatin 1 in Patients with Alzheimer's Disease	AEs, ADAS, CIBIC, CDR, ADCS-ADL, SIB, Hopkins Verbal Learning Test – Revised, temperature, respiratory rate, blood pressure, heart rate, ECG, physical examination, haematology, blood chemistry, urinalysis, pharmacokinetics, protein kinase C activity (pharmacodynamics)	NCT00606164	AD	April 2008–December 2008	Blanchette Rockefeller Neurosciences Institute	2
β-Secretase inhibitor thiazolidinedione, rosiglitazone	Rosiglitazone Effects on Cognition for Adults in Later Life	Cognitive measures: delayed list recall, Stroop Interference Test. Biological outcomes: plasma insulin, IDE, Aβ-40, Aβ-42, inflammatory cytokines and F2-isoprostanes. MRI outcome: whole brain and medial temporal lobe atrophy rate. Cognitive measures: ADAS-cog total score, story recall verbal fluency, paired associate learning, SOPT, rating scales	NCT00242593	MCI	June 2006–July 2010	GlaxoSmithKline	2
γ-Secretase inhibitor LY450139	Effects of LY450139, on the Progression of Alzheimer's Disease as Compared with Placebo	ADAS-Cog. ADCS-ADL, CDR, NPI, RUD-Lite, EQ-5D Proxy, Qol-AD, MMSE, a chemical marker of AD in the blood which may be lowered by LY450139, FDG-PET, vMRI, AV-45-PET, CSF tau, safety, to measure levels of LY450139 and their effect on safety, chemical markers and effectiveness	NCT00762411	AD	September 2008–March 2012	Eli Lilly	3

(*continued overleaf*)

Table 78.1 *(continued)*.

Agent/drug	Title	Outcome measures	Reference	Condition	Start date–completion date	Sponsor	Phase
γ-Secretase inhibitor BMS-708163	Study to Evaluate the Pharmacokinetics, Safety, and Tolerability of BMS-708163	Safety assessments will be based on adverse event reports and the results of vital sign measurements, ECGs, physical examinations and clinical laboratory tests	NCT01079819	AD	April 2010–July 2010	Bristol-Myers Squibb	1
γ-Secretase modulator CHF-5074	Safety, Pharmacokinetics and Pharmacodynamics Study of Treatment with CHF 5074 in Healthy Young Male Subjects	AEs	NCT00954252	Young healthy male volunteers	October 2009–December 2009	Chiesi Pharma-ceuticals	1
Anti-aggregation and anti-fibrillization agents ELND005 (AZD-103)	ELND005 Long-Term Follow-up Study in Subjects with Alzheimer's Disease	Safety and tolerability analyses will be based on the frequency and severity of AEs and on clinically important changes in laboratory assessment results	NCT00934050	AD	June 2009–April 2011	Elan Pharmaceu-ticals	2
Epigallocatechin-3-gallate (EGCg)	Sunphenon EGCg (in the Early Stage of Alzheimer's Disease) (SUN-AK)	ADAS-Cog	NCT00951834	Early stage of AD (Diagnosis DSM-IV and NINCDS/ADRDA, Dubois criteria 2007)	November 2009–April 2011	Charite University, Berlin	2
NIC5-15	Development of NICS-15 in the Treatment of Alzheimer's Disease	Pharmacokinetic analysis, safety assessments including vital signs, physical examination, symptom checklist, complete blood count, serum chemistries, urinalysis, ECG, ADAS-Cog	NCT00470418	AD	January 2007–March 2010	Department of Veterans' Affairs	2
Tau aggregation inhibitor							
Nicotinamide	Safety Study of Nicotinamide to Treat Alzheimer's Disease	ADAS-Cog	NCT00580931	AD	January 2008–January 2011	University of California	2
Neuroprotective agents							
Vitamin E and memantine (TEAM-AD)	A Randomized, Clinical Trial of Vitamin E and Memantine in Alzheimer's Disease	ADCS/ADL	NCT00235716	AD	August 2007–July 2012	Department of Veterans' Affairs	3
Docosahexaenoic acid (DHA)	Lipoic Acid and Omega-3 Fatty Acids for Alzheimer's Disease	ADL, ADAS-Cog	NCT01058941	AD	April 2010–April 2013	Oregon Health and Science University	1-2

EGB 761 (*Ginkgo biloba* extract)	Effect of EGb761® on Brain Glucose Metabolism in Three Groups of Elderly with Memory Complaint, Mild Alzheimer's Disease, and Cognitively Normal	18FDG-PET, change in brain atrophy; incidence of AEs	NCT00814346	Cognitive impair-ment, AD	October 2008–June 2012	Ipsen	2
T-817 MA (benzothiophene derivative)	Efficacy and Safety of T-817 MA in Patients with Mild to Moderate Alzheimer's Disease	ADAS-cog; secondary objectives are to evaluate the safety ADCS-ADL and ADCS-CGIC	NCT00663936	AD	April 2008–September 2011	Toyama Chemical	2
Resveratrol supplement	Randomized Trial of a Nutritional Supplement in Alzheimer's Disease	ADAScog, CGIC	NCT00678431	AD	January 2008–June 2011	Department of Veterans' Affairs	3
Curcumin	Efficacy and Safety of Curcumin Formulation in Alzheimer's Disease	To determine if curcumin formulation affects mental capacity in Alzheimer's patients based on mental examinations; to determine if curcumin formulation changes blood concentrations of Aβ	NCT01001637	AD	October 2009–November 2010	Jaslok Hospital and Research Centre	2
Neurorestorative factors							
Neurotrophic growth factor: CERE-110	Randomized, Controlled Study Evaluating CERE-110 in Subjects with Mild to Moderate Alzheimer's Disease	ADAS-Cog, Neuropsychological Test Battery, MMSE, NPI, ADCS-ADL	NCT00876863	AD	September 2009–July 2012	Ceregene	2
NsG0202	Encapsulated Cell Biodelivery of Nerve Growth Factor to Alzheimer's Disease Patients	AEs	NCT01163825	AD	January 2008–December 2011	NsGene	1
Other treatments							
Hormone therapy SERMs: raloxifene	Raloxifene for Women with Alzheimer's Disease	ADAS, CDR, ADCS-ADL, NPI, cognitive subscale of the Alzheimer's Disease Assessment Scale, other cognitive tests (East Boston Memory Test, digit ordering, category fluency, Trail Making Test, Boston Naming Test short version, MMSE, narrative writing, semantic binding), caregiver burden interview	NCT00368459	AD	August 2006–July 2010	National Institute on Aging	2

(*continued overleaf*)

Table 78.1 *(continued)*.

Agent/drug	Title	Outcome measures	Reference	Condition	Start date–completion date	Sponsor	Phase
Hormone therapy: testosterone (Androgel 1%)	Hormone and Information Processing Study	Behavioural and mood measure: Profile of Mood States (POMS), cognitive changes measured by neuropsychological tests: ADAS-Cog (MCI version), route test, paragraph recall, CSF, APOE genotyping	NCT00539305	MCI, AD	July 2009–June 2012	Solvay Pharmaceuticals	3
5-HT 6 receptor antagonist: SB-742457	A Study of SB-742457, Added to Donepezil for the Treatment of Mild-to-moderate Alzheimer's Disease	Change in cognition and function after 24 weeks, change in cognition and function after 12, 24, 36 and 48 weeks, safety and tolerability, pharmacokinetics and exploratory pharmacogenetics	NCT00710684	Mild-to-moderate AD	July 2008–December 2010	GlaxoSmithKline	2
5-HT 6 receptor antagonist: SAM-531	Study Comparing 3 Dosage Levels of SAM-531 in Outpatients with Mild to Moderate Alzheimer Disease	ADAS-Cog; they include the changes from baseline to week 24 in the DAD and in the NPI, ADCS-CGIC, CANTAB and the responder rate at week 24	NCT00895895	AD	April 2009–June 2011	Wyeth	2
Selective histamine H3 receptor antagonist: GSK239512	Study to Evaluate the Efficacy and Safety of GSK239512 in Alzheimer's Disease	Change from baseline in composite score of Cogstate battery; Change from baseline in ADAS-Cog total score at weeks 8 and 16; CIBIC+ score at weeks 8 and 16; safety measures: AEs, 12-lead ECG, vital signs (systolic and diastolic blood pressure, heart rate), clinical laboratory evaluations	NCT01009255	AD	November 2009–January 2011	GlaxoSmithKline	1
Anti-histamine agent: Dimebon	Safety and Efficacy Study Evaluating Dimebon in Patients with Mild to Moderate Alzheimer's Disease on Donepezil	ADCS-ADL, ADAS-Cog, CIBIC-plus, NPI, RUD-Lite, EQ-5D	NCT00829374	AD	March 2009–December 2011	Medivation	3
PF-04447943 in phase 2 (phosphodiesterase 9A inhibitors)	A Study of PF-04447943 Compared to Placeboin Subjects with Mild to Moderate Alzheimer's Disease	ADAS-Cog	NCT00930059	AD	September 2009–September 2010	Pfizer	2

RAGE inhibitor: TTP488 (PF 04494700)	A Phase 2 Study Evaluating the Efficacy and Safety Of PF 04494700 in Mild to Moderate Alzheimer's Disease	Evaluate the efficacy of PF 04494700 relative to placebo. Change from baseline in a standardized cognitive measure after 18 months of treatment. Examine the safety and tolerability of PF 04494700 relative to placebo. AEs, vital signs, physical examination, neurological examination, 12-lead ECG, laboratory tests (haematology, blood chemistry, urinalysis) and brain MRI. Evaluate the effects of PF 04494700 on potential biomarkers of RAGE inhibition and amyloid imaging (AV-45, F18 PET). Evaluate the potential dose response of PF 04494700. Evaluate the pharmacokinetics and characterize the pharmacokinetic/pharmacodynamic relationship of PF 04494700 to potential biomarkers and relevant efficacy and safety end points	NCT00566397	AD	December 2007–March 2011	Pfizer	2

[a]Magnetic resonance imaging (MRI); adverse event/serious adverse event (AE/SAE); Alzheimer's disease (AD); mild cognitive impairment (MCI); electrocardiogram (ECG); cerebrospinal fluid (CSF); positron emission tomography (PET); Alzheimer's Disease Assessment Scale-Cognitive Subscale (ADAS-cog); Disability Assessment for Dementia (DAD); Alzheimer's Disease Cooperative Study-Activities of Daily Living Inventory (ADCS-ADL); Clinical Dementia Rating-Sum of Boxes (CDR-SB); Neuropsychiatric Inventory (NPI); Mini Mental State Examination (MMSE); Resource Utilization in Dementia-Lite (RUD-Lite); EuroQol 5-Dimensional Health-related Quality of Life Scale Proxy version (EQ-5D Proxy); Quality of Life in Alzheimer's Disease (QoL-AD); Clinician's Interview Based Impression of Change (CIBIC); Severe Impairment Battery (SIB).

immunization therapy in AD, as a small percentage of antibodies are directed against Aβ peptide sequences. Intravenous infusion of Igs in five AD patients over a 6 month period prevented further cognitive decline,[40] suggesting that this approach could potentially act like a passive immunotherapy. Human trials of passively administered anti-Aβ antibodies are now being initiated. Other antibodies have recently reached clinical evaluation: GSK933776A, PF-04360365, PLY2062430 (solanezumab) and AAB-001 (bapineuzumab) (Table 78.1). In a recent RCT that enrolled patients with mild-to-moderate AD, treatment with bapineuzumab for 78 weeks reduced cortical 11C-PiB retention compared with both baseline and placebo.[41]

Drugs to reduce Aβ production

α-Secretase activators

APP processing by α-secretase is a non-amyloidogenic pathway, because the α-secretase cleavage site is within the Aβ sequence of APP. Enhanced cleavage at this site may represent a potential disease-modifying strategy. Bryostatin 1, a macrolide lactone, exhibits high affinity for protein kinase C and dramatically enhances the secretion of the α-secretase product in patients' fibroblasts[42] (Table 78.1). Etazolate (EHT-0202), a selective GABA receptor modulator, stimulates neuronal α-secretase and increases sAPPα production.[43] This drug, which is orally bioavailable, has recently been tested in a phase 2 RCT in patients with mild-to-moderate AD (NCT00880412, results not available). Talsaclidine, an M1 agonist that stimulates the non-amyloidogenic α-secretase processing *in vitro* and decreases CSF Aβ in AD patients following chronic treatment,[44,45] holds potential disease-modifying properties.

β-Secretase inhibitors

β-secretase has been shown to be a transmembrane aspartic protease, β-site Aβ cleaving enzyme 1 (BACE1). BACE-1 processing of Aβ precursor protein is the first step in the pathway leading to the production of Aβ. BACE-1 knockout mice develop normally and appear to have completely abolished Aβ production.[46] A selective BACE-1 inhibitor, GSK188909, reduced levels of secreted and intracellular Aβ40 and Aβ42 *in vitro* and also in APP transgenic mice brains.[47] Thiazolidinediones also act as β-secretase inhibitors by stimulating peroxisome proliferator-activated receptor-γ (PPARγ). PPARγ agonists, such as rosiglitazone, also have anti-inflammatory effects.[48,49] Thiazolidinediones are under evaluation in AD, but recent data have shown a potential higher risk of myocardial infarction with these compounds.[50] To compensate for the brain's reduced ability to use glucose in AD, administration of ketone bodies or their metabolic precursors such as medium-chain triglycerides (MCTs) might be another strategy. In a preliminary study with 20 subjects with AD or mild cognitive impairment (MCI), single doses of MCTs demonstrated pharmacological activity and significant efficacy in cognitive performance.[51] A phase 2b clinical trial in AD patients confirmed ketone bodies' safety and efficacy on cognition. A pivotal phase 3 clinical trial in AD patients is planned.[52]

γ-Secretase inhibitors and modulators

Inhibition of γ-secretase targets the generation of Aβ42, but other proteins are also substrates of this enzyme and particularly the transmembrane Notch receptor, involved in vital functions.[53–55] Abnormalities in the gastrointestinal tract, thymus and spleen in animal models result from inhibition of Notch cleavage.[56,57] Preclinical studies established that γ-secretase inhibitors can reduce brain Aβ and reverse Aβ-induced cognitive deficits in transgenic mice. LY450139 dihydrate, a γ-secretase inhibitor, inhibits Aβ formation *in vitro* and *in vivo*. In phase 1 volunteer studies, a dose-dependent reduction in plasma Aβ was demonstrated. However, Aβ concentrations were unchanged in CSF.[58,59] In an RCT of AD patients treated with LY450139 dihydrate, Aβ40 decreased significantly in plasma and decreased in a non-significant manner in CSF.[60] Single doses of GSI-953, a selective γ-secretase inhibitor, also produced dose-dependent reductions of plasma but not CSF Aβ peptides in humans.[61] Tarenflurbil is the pure *R*-enantiomer of flurbiprofen and is the first in a novel class of selective Aβ-42-lowering agents. It modulates γ-secretase and is highly specific for its effects on Aβ-42 and, unlike the γ-secretase inhibitors, does not interfere with the function of Notch. In a phase 2 study, tarenflurbil was well tolerated for up to 24 months of treatment in 210 AD patients, with evidence of a dose-related effect on measures of daily activities and global function in patients with mild AD,[62] but a phase 3 clinical trial was negative. Table 78.1 gives an overview of drugs that are currently in research and development in this field.

Anti-aggregation and anti-fibrillization agents

An alternative approach to secretase inhibition, which raises the problem of interfering with normal enzymatic reactions, is to inhibit Aβ aggregation into neurotoxic oligomers. Tramiprosate (NC-531 or 3APS) is a glycosaminoglycan mimetic that binds to Aβ and inhibits amyloid plaque formation.[63] Preclinical data have shown that tramiprosate reduces brain and plasma levels of Aβ and prevents fibril formation.[64] In a phase 2 trial, long-term administration of tramiprosate was safe, well tolerated and reduced CSF Aβ-42 levels in patients with AD. Tramiprosate has reached phase 3 clinical trials.[65] However, a phase 3 trial in the USA was negative and was stopped in Europe. Dysregulation of cerebral metal ions (Fe^{2+}, Cu^{2+} and Zn^{2+}) and their interactions with Aβ may contribute to AD by playing a role in the precipitation and cytotoxicity of Aβ.[66] Metal ions are required for Aβ protein oligomerization and recent studies showed that metal chelators could produce a significant reversal of Aβ deposition *in vitro* and *in vivo*.[67] XH1 and DP-109, both metal chelators, attenuated Aβ pathology in APP Tg mice.[68,69] Clioquinol (PBT-1) is a Cu/Zn chelator that promotes Aβ dissolution. In a pilot phase 2 clinical trial in AD patients, this fibrillization inhibitor shows a significant efficacy in the more severely affected group according to the authors[70] but this point is discussed.[71] Another chelator, desferioxamine, has shown some benefit in AD, but also severe adverse effects.[72] PBT-2, another metal protein-attenuating compound, was tested in a phase 2 trial in patients with early AD. PBT-2 affects the Cu^{2+}-mediated and Zn-mediated oligomerization of Aβ protein. The safety profile was favourable. Cognitive efficacy was restricted to two measures of executive functioning. The effect on putative biomarkers for AD in CSF but not in plasma was suggestive of a central effect of the drug on Aβ metabolism.[73] Another compound interfering with the aggregation and fibrillization of Aβ, ELND005 (AZD-103), is under evaluation in a clinical trial (Table 78.1).

Drugs to target tau protein

Microtubule-associated protein (MAP) tau is abnormally hyperphosphorylated in AD. Several kinases are reported to phosphorylate tau *in vitro*, including glycogen synthase kinase-3 (GSK-3), cyclin-dependent kinase-5 (CDK-5), mitogen-activated protein kinase family members (MAPK), casein kinase, calcium calmodulin-dependent kinase II, protein kinase A and others. Some of them, such as GSK-3, could be also involved in Aβ generation, promoting cell death, production of inflammatory molecules and cell migration.[74] Phosphoseryl/phosphothreonyl protein phosphatase-2A (PP-2A), which is co-localized with tau and microtubules in the brain, is apparently the most active enzyme in dephosphorylating the abnormal tau to a normal-like state.[75] Other phosphatases have also been implicated.[76] Reducing abnormal phosphorylation and restoring or stimulating phosphatase activity are promising therapeutic strategies. Lithium reduces tau phosphorylation *in vitro*, promotes microtubule assembly through inhibition of GSK-3[77] and has been shown to reduce tau phosphorylation in APP Tg mice.[78] In a preliminary clinical trial of lithium in AD patients, no effect of lithium on tau and Aβ-42 in the CSF was observed, which does not support the notion that lithium may lead to reduced hyperphosphorylated tau in AD after short-term treatment.[79] Methylthioninium chloride (Trx0014) has been shown *in vitro* to prevent aggregation of tau into tangles. It has demonstrated cognitive and behavioural benefits in animal models.[80]

Neuroprotective agents

Another alternative approach involves protection against cellular damage caused by oxidative, inflammatory or other toxic stressors.

Antioxidants

Genetic and lifestyle-related risk factors for AD could be associated with an increase in oxidative stress, suggesting that oxidative stress is involved in the early stage of the pathology.[81] Individuals with MCI or very mild AD show increased levels of lipid peroxidation and nucleic acid oxidation in postmortem brain and plasma.[82] Free radicals and oxidative injury to neurons could chronologically precede Aβ plaque deposition and tau phosphorylation.[83] Several antioxidants that have been investigated for their potential to reduce the risk of AD include vitamins A, C and E, coenzyme Q, selenium and polyunsaturated fatty acids. Vitamin E had been show to slow progression of the disease in patients with moderately severe AD.[84] However, recent meta-analysis and trial results suggest that vitamin E increases morbidity and mortality[85] and a Cochrane review does not support the use of vitamin E to treat AD.[86] The lack of consistent efficacy data for vitamin C and its questionable safety could also discourage its use.[87] Most of the published epidemiological studies are consistent with a positive association between high reported omega-3 polyunsaturated fatty acid consumption and a lower risk of developing cognitive decline or AD later in life.[88] Docosahexaenoic acid (DHA) is the most abundant omega-3 fatty acid in the brain. DHA acts in the brain via neurotrophic and anti-apoptotic pathways. In addition, DHA may act through anti-neuroinflammatory pathways, as DHA possesses anti-inflammatory properties in the periphery. The results from the first randomized, double-blind, placebo-controlled clinical trial evaluating the effects of dietary omega-3 fatty acid supplementation on cognitive functions in patients with mild to moderate AD showed no significant efficacy of daily intake of DHA and eicosapentaenoic acid. However, in a subgroup of patients with very mild cognitive dysfunction [Mini Mental State Examination (MMSE) >27 points], a significant reduction in MMSE decline rate was observed in the omega-3 fatty acid-treated group compared with the placebo group.[89] α-Lipoic acid (LA), an essential cofactor in mitochondrial dehydrogenase reactions, functions as an antioxidant and reduces oxidative stress.[90] LA seems to exert a cellular protective effect as evidenced by decreases in apoptotic markers in fibroblasts from AD patients.[91] Clinical preliminary data show that LA might be a successful therapy for AD.[92] EGb761, a *Ginkgo biloba* extract that has free radical scavenging properties, inhibits the formation of Aβ fibrils, attenuates mitochondrion-initiated apoptosis and decreases the activity of caspase-3, a key enzyme in the apoptosis cell signalling cascade.[93] Mitoquinol, an antioxidant that targets mitochondrial dysfunction, has demonstrated encouraging preclinical results. Mitoquinol mimics the role of the endogenous mitochondrial antioxidant coenzyme Q10 and augments its antioxidant capacity to supraphysiological levels.[94] Melatonin, an indolamine secreted by the pineal gland, may also protect neuronal cells from Aβ-mediated toxicity via antioxidant properties and could attenuate tau hyperphosphorylation.[95] Isoflavones are also under clinical evaluation for their antioxidant properties (Table 78.1). Other clinical trials with antioxidants are on the way (Table 78.1).

Anti-inflammatory drugs

Laboratory evidence shows that inflammatory mechanisms contribute to neuronal damage in AD. Epidemiological evidence[96] suggests that non-steroidal anti-inflammatory drugs (NSAIDs) may favourably influence the course of the disease. In a 1993 trial, indomethacin appeared to protect AD patients from cognitive decline, according to the authors,[97] but this point of view is not shared by Cochrane reviewers.[98] Another trial with indomethacin failed to show any efficacy in the progression of AD.[99] Ibuprofen, celexocib, rofecoxib and naproxen did not slow the progression of AD.[100–102] In a phase 2 AD clinical trial with (*R*)-flurbiprofen, a few subsets of patients who had high blood concentrations of this drug demonstrated a benefit in cognitive and behavioural performance.[103] However, Myriad Genetics has discontinued the development of (*R*)-flurbiprofen (Flurizan or MPC-7869). Cyclophosphamide is a potent anti-inflammatory and immunomodulatory drug acting primarily by inhibiting the proliferation of immune cells.[104] Excess tumour necrosis factor-alpha (TNF-α) has been shown to mediate the disruption in synaptic memory mechanisms caused by Aβ in addition to its proinflammatory functions.[105] Etanercept, an antagonist of TNF-α, delivered by perispinal administration in AD patients, showed great potential in a pilot study. Among traditional medicine products, resveratrol, a component of grapes, berries and other fruits, is a polyphenol that has been shown to mediate its effects through modulation of many different pathways. For instance, resveratrol has been shown to reduce the expression of inflammatory biomarkers and induce antioxidant enzymes.[106] Lastly, curcumin, a polyphenolic molecule safely used as a food colouring, proved to be immunomodulatory and has shown Aβ-40 aggregation inhibition properties *in vitro* and *in vivo*.[107]

Glutamate-mediated neurotoxicity

The glutamatergic system has long been recognized for its role in learning and memory and recent studies indicate the involvement of glutamate-mediated neurotoxicity in the pathogenesis of AD.[108,109] The neurotransmitter glutamate activates several classes of receptors and especially three major types of ionotropic receptors: α-amino-3-hydroxy-5-methyl-4-isoxazolepropionic acid (AMPA), kainate and *N*-methyl-D-aspartate (NMDA). Chronic activation of receptors, in particular of the NMDA type, ultimately leads to neuronal damage. Complete NMDA receptor blockade has also been shown to impair neuronal plasticity. Thus, both hypo- and hyperactivity of the glutamatergic system lead to dysfunction. Memantine is an uncompetitive NMDA receptor antagonist and has been approved for the symptomatic treatment of AD. Most other centrally acting NMDA antagonists have been discarded because of severe adverse psychomimetic and cardiovascular effects. A series of second-generation memantine derivatives are currently under development and may have greater neuroprotective properties than memantine. Neramexane is a new NMDA receptor antagonist that is currently under development. *In vivo*, neramexane enhances long-term spatial memory in adult rats.[110] Its clinical development seems to be completed. Another mode of action is the positive modulation of AMPA receptors.[111] LY404187, a selective positive modulator of AMPA receptors, improved the performance of cognitive function in animal models.[112] LY451395, an AMPA receptor potentiator, administered to AD patients did not show a statistically significant difference in effect versus placebo on cognitive functions in a clinical trial.[113] CX516 (Ampalex) enhances brain activity by positive modulation of AMPA receptors.

Neurorestorative approaches

NGF promotes survival and differentiation of neurons and neurotrophic factors have been suggested as contributors to AD pathophysiology. In rhesus monkeys, ageing is associated with a significant reduction in cortical cholinergic innervation, but this reduction is reversible by NGF delivery to cholinergic somata in the basal forebrain.[114] Phenotypic knockout of NGF activity in transgenic anti-NGF mice results in a progressive neurodegenerative AD-type phenotype and the neurodegeneration induced by the expression of anti-NGF antibodies can be largely reversed by NGF delivery.[115] A phase 1 trial evaluated NGF gene delivery in eight individuals with mild AD, by implanting autologous fibroblasts genetically modified to express human NGF into the forebrain. The results suggested improvement in the rate of cognitive decline after a mean follow-up of 22 months.[116] AIT-082 (Neotrofin) increases levels of NGF and stimulates nerve sprouting in the brain. A phase 1 study of AIT-082 was conducted in 36 mild AD patients with no significant side effects.[117] Growth factor modulators are also under clinical development for AD treatment (Table 78.1).

Animal studies show that human neural stem cells transplanted into animal brains differentiated into neural cells and significantly improved the cognitive functions. Neural stem cell grafts present a potential strategy of treatment. This raises the possibility of stimulating inherent precursor cells to replace lost neurons.[118,119]

Other potential therapeutic strategies

Hormonal therapy

RCTs suggest a very limited effect of estrogens on attention and verbal performance when administered to postmenopausal women with AD.[120] The efficacy of selective estrogen receptor modulator (SERMs) that exert tissue-specific estrogenic effects has also been investigated in AD RCTs (Table 78.1). It also appears that estrogens may work in conjunction with gonadotropins, such as luteinizing hormone (LH). LH, which can modulate cognitive behaviour, is present in the brain and has one of the highest receptor levels in the hippocampus.[121] It has been suggested that the increase in gonadotropin concentrations, following menopause, could be one of the causative factors for the development of AD.[122] The reduction in neurodegenerative disease among prostate cancer patients who are frequently treated with gonadotropin-releasing hormone (GnRH) agonist supports the role of LH and GnRH in AD.[122] Testosterone supplementation may also benefit cognitive function in men with AD.[123] In healthy older men, short-term testosterone administration enhances cognitive function.[124] Among other hormonal compounds, insulin-like growth factor-1 (IGF-1) is supposed to increase clearance of Aβ. Preliminary evidence shows that the growth hormone secretagogue MK-677 (ibutamoren mesylate), a potent inducer of IGF-1 secretion, could improve cognitive function in cognitively impaired patients.[125] However, MK-677 was ineffective at slowing the rate of progression of AD in a clinical trial.[126] Excessive levels of corticosteroid have been associated with impaired attention, concentration and memory and *in vivo* studies suggest that prolonged exposure to high circulating levels of glucocorticoid may be associated with a faster progression of AD.[127] Mifepristone is a glucocorticoid receptor antagonist and could improve cognition in AD. Pilot trials in patients with AD provide data on the safety and feasibility of this approach, but more extensive studies are needed.[128]

Drugs to target mitochondrial dysfunction

Attention and short-term memory-enhancing effects of H3 receptor antagonists are well described. Dimebon is a molecule previously approved in Russia as a non-selective antihistamine. The molecular mechanism by which Dimebon exerts its effects is not known, but the most potent pharmacological activities established *in vivo* is the stabilization of mitochondrial membrane depolarization in the setting of molecular stress and neurite outgrowth, which may be a consequence of its mitochondrial action. Dimebon has been shown to bind with high potency to serotonin (5-HT6 and 5HT-7) and α-adrenergic receptors (subtypes 1A, 1B, 1D, 2B), both implicated in cognitive pathways. Binding to histamine receptors is not believed to play a role in its therapeutic activity. Dimebon demonstrated cognition-enhancing properties *in vivo* and in a human pilot clinical trial in AD.[129] In a randomized, double-blind, placebo-controlled study,[130] patients showed significant improvements for five outcome measures, including assessment of cognition (ADAS-cog and MMSE), function (ADCS-ADL) and behaviour (NPI). It showed a significant drug–placebo difference in change from baseline on the ADAS-cog at week 26 which was not driven by worsening in the placebo group as patients given Dimebon were improved from their baseline values. The difference observed in the clinician- assessed global function scale (CIBIC-plus) supports the clinical relevance of this effect.

Statins

Epidemiological evidence suggests that statins may reduce the risk of developing AD. The mechanism of this putative protective effect is not completely understood, but may be related to the relationship between elevated cholesterol and amyloid deposition. Amyloidogenic APP processing may also occur preferentially in the cholesterol-rich regions of membranes known as lipid rafts. A placebo-controlled 1 year study of atorvastatin calcium showed a positive effect on decline on the ADAS-cog compared with placebo at 6 and 12 months follow-up in 63 patients with AD.[131] In *post hoc* analysis of a placebo-controlled study, simvastatin significantly decreased Aβ-40 levels in the CSF of patients with mild AD.[132] A major phase 3 study of atorvastatin[133] was negative.

Receptor for advanced glycation end product inhibitors

The receptor for advanced glycation end products (RAGE) is a cell-bound receptor of immunoglobulin which may be activated by a variety of pro-inflammatory ligands including advanced glycation end products leading to secretion of cytokines, which may link the amyloid pathway to the inflammatory pathway.[134] RAGE-mediated inflammation caused by glial cells and subsequent changes in neuronal glucose metabolism are likely to be important contributors to neurodegeneration in AD.[135] These pathways are considered interesting drug targets for the treatment of AD. RAGE inhibitor: TTP488 (PF04494700) is now under clinical development (Table 78.1).

Others

Recent studies have suggested modifications of serotonin cerebral metabolism in MCI and AD. Lecozotan (SRA-333), a selective serotonin 1a receptor antagonist, was developed for the treatment of AD after promising results in animal studies.[136] On the other hand, xaliproden (SR57746A), a 5-HT1a receptor agonist which appears either to mimic the effects of neurotrophins or to stimulate their synthesis, has reached phase 3, but its development is over. Both monoamine oxidase (MAO) A and MAO B have been implicated in AD pathogenesis and rasagiline, an MAO B inhibitor which exhibits neuroprotective and anti-apoptotic activity *in vitro* and *in vivo*,[137] is under clinical evaluation. Antihypertensive medications are associated with a lower incidence of AD and some of them as angiotensin-converting enzyme inhibitors or calcium channels blockers have become a source of interest. A phase 2 clinical trial in AD with MEM 1003, the (+)-enantiomer of a dihydropyridine, that has been optimized for central nervous system activity, is planned (Table 78.1). Blood levels of homocysteine may contribute to AD pathophysiology by vascular and direct neurotoxic mechanisms. Even in the absence of vitamin B deficiency, homocysteine levels can be reduced by administration of high-dose supplements of vitamin B. However, in a recently published RCT trial, high-dose B vitamin supplements failed to show any effect in cognitive decline in AD. Folate deficiency also induces an imbalance of sadenosyl-L-methionine (SAM) which could have an impact on cognitive functions. Dietary supplementation with SAM in the absence of folate attenuated these consequences *in vivo*.[138] Other agents are also under evaluation and Table 78.1 gives an overview of the drugs that are currently in research and development.

Non-pharmaceutical therapies

Several studies are ongoing to evaluate the impact of cognitive intervention (NCT00646269, NCT00319891) and physical activity (NCT00403507, NCT01061489, NCT01128361) on the memory and cognitive abilities of patients diagnosed with AD. The approach based on the transcranial or deep brain stimulation seems promising.

Repetitive transcranial magnetic stimulation (rTMS) to the prefrontal cortex could improve language performance in patients with AD.[139] Although the mechanisms of rTMS-induced naming facilitation in these patients are unknown, the procedure may be worth testing as a novel approach to the treatment of language dysfunction. This procedure seems to have persistent beneficial effects on sentence comprehension in AD patients. rTMS in conjunction with other therapeutic interventions (drug or cognitive brain training), may represent a novel approach to the treatment of cognitive dysfunction in AD patients (NCT01168245, NCT01179373). Several studies are ongoing to assess the ability of rTMS with H2 coil to prefrontal and parieto-temporal cortex (NCT00753662) to improve cognitive performance in patients with AD.

Fornix/hypothalamus deep brain stimulation (DBS) could modulate neurophysiological activity in these pathological circuits and possibly produce clinical benefits. In a phase 1 trial in six patients with mild AD, they received continuous DBS for 12 months.[140] DBS drove neural activity in the memory circuit, including the entorhinal and hippocampal areas, and activated the brain's default mode network. PET scans showed an early and striking reversal of the impaired glucose utilization in the temporal and parietal lobes that was maintained after 12 months of continuous stimulation. Cognitive evaluation (ADAS-Cog and MMSE) suggested possible improvements and/or slowing in the rate of cognitive decline at 6 and 12 months in some patients. Modulating pathological brain activity in AD with DBS merits further investigation. Several studies are ongoing to evaluate DBS with bilateral electrode implantation in the nucleus basalis Meynert (NCT01094145) and in the fornix/hypothalamus (NCT00888056).

Prevention and AD

Because no effective curative approaches are available, preventive approaches in the field of AD are needed. Indeed, because AD is a slowly progressing and age-dependent disease, delaying onset by as little as 5 years could halve the number of people afflicted with the illness.[141]

Epidemiological data suggest a preventive effect of EGb 761 in AD,[142] but RCT results evaluating EGb 761 for the treatment of AD are contradictory. The aim of the GuidAge Study is to evaluate the efficacy of 240 mg per day of EGb 761 in the prevention of AD.[143] Previous studies suggested that many factors may be involved in the occurrence of AD at late ages. Because of the probable multifactorial nature of AD, it seems logical to initiate multidomain interventions to examine their potential synergistic effects. The Multidomain Alzheimer Preventive Trial (MAPT) is an ongoing study which aims to evaluate the efficacy of a multidomain intervention (nutritional, physical and cognitive training) and omega-3 treatment in the prevention of cognitive decline in frail elderly persons aged 70 years or over.[144]

The PREADVISE study is trying to establish whether taking selenium and/or vitamin E supplements can help to prevent memory loss and dementia such as AD (NCT00040378). Other ongoing trials are assessing the effects of antihypertensives on individuals at risk for AD (NCT00980785) and simvastatin on CSF AD biomarkers in cognitively normal subjects (NCT01142336).

Conclusion

AD is an increasingly important issue in our societies. Many clinical studies are ongoing with numerous new compounds, but still no disease-modifying drug is available at present. To explain the disappointing results of several RCTs, researchers have highlighted different errors, both in drug choice and development programmes. Indeed, because of the complexity of AD, it is clear that multi-target therapies could be the future treatment approach. Multi-target therapies[145] can be designed in several ways. (1) The most conventional strategy is to prescribe several individual drugs. This approach is already used in AD, where ChEIs can be given together with NMDA receptor antagonists for better symptomatic effects. (2) Another strategy is to develop drugs that contain two or more active ingredients delivered in the same device. (3) The third strategy is to design a single compound with selective polypharmacology. Drugs such as memoquin (ChEI, β-secretase inhibitor, Aβ anti-aggregant, antioxidant properties and decreases tau hyperphosphorylation), talsaclidine (M1 agonist, α-secretase) and M-30 (monoamine oxidase inhibitor, antioxidant and iron-chelating properties and modulation of APP processing) are now in preclinical stages of testing.

A majority of the recent drugs under evaluation seem to act on multiple targets. The pharmacological field needs to be explored carefully, specifically with regard to new drug tolerability and security of use. Therefore, it needs to be shown that the benefits of such treatments outweigh the risk of side effects before they can be recommended for patients with AD. The publication of negative data is also an important issue and could enlighten researchers' ability to improve their knowledge about drug actions.

Key points

- Although a great deal of progress has been made with our understanding of the pathophysiological processes in involved in Alzheimer's Disease (AD), there has been little advancement in the use of effective disease-modifying agents.
- The mainstays of current pharmacotherapy for AD are compounds aimed at increasing the levels of acetylcholine (ACh) in the brain.
- It is clear that multi-target therapies could be the future for effective treatment approaches.

References

1. Mori E, Hashimoto M, Krishnan KR and Doraiswamy PM. What constitutes clinical evidence for neuroprotection in Alzheimer disease: support for the cholinesterase inhibitors? *Alzheimer Dis Assoc Disord* 2006;**20**(2 Suppl 1): S19–26.
2. Rees TM and Brimijoin S. The role of acetylcholinesterase in the pathogenesis of Alzheimer's disease. *Drugs Today (Barc)* 2003;**39**:75–83.
3. Ballard CG, Greig NH, Guillozet-Bongaarts AL *et al.* Cholinesterases: roles in the brain during health and disease. *Curr Alzheimer Res* 2005;**2**:307–18.
4. Mori E, Hashimoto M, Krishnan KR and Doraiswamy PM. What constitutes clinical evidence for neuroprotection in Alzheimer disease: support for the cholinesterase inhibitors? *Alzheimer Dis Assoc Disord* 2006;**20**(2 Suppl 1): S19–26.
5. Zhang HY and Tang XC. Neuroprotective effects of huperzine A: new therapeutic targets for neurodegenerative disease. *Trends Pharmacol Sci* 2006;**27**:619–25.
6. Li J, Wu HM, Zhou RL *et al.* Huperzine A for Alzheimer's disease. *Cochrane Database Syst Rev* 2008;(2): CD005592.
7. Wang R and Tang XC. Neuroprotective effects of huperzine A. A natural cholinesterase inhibitor for the treatment of Alzheimer's disease. *Neurosignals* 2005;**14**:71–82.
8. Greig NH, Sambamurti K, Yu QS *et al.* An overview of phenserine tartrate, a novel acetylcholinesterase inhibitor for the treatment of Alzheimer's disease. *Curr Alzheimer Res* 2005;**2**:281–90.
9. Kadir A, Andreasen N, Almkvist O *et al.* Effect of phenserine treatment on brain functional activity and amyloid in Alzheimer's disease. *Ann Neurol* 2008;**63**:621–31.
10. Lahiri DK, Chen D, Maloney B *et al.* The experimental Alzheimer's disease drug posiphen [(+)-phenserine] lowers amyloid-beta peptide levels in cell culture and mice. *J Pharmacol Exp Ther* 2007;**320**:386–96.
11. Klein J. Phenserine. *Expert Opin Investig Drugs* 2007;**16**: 1087–97.
12. Lane RM, Potkin SG and Enz A. Targeting acetylcholinesterase and butyrylcholinesterase in dementia. *Int J Neuropsychopharmacol* 2006;**9**:101–24.
13. Kamal MA, Al-Jafari AA, Yu QS *et al.* Kinetic analysis of the inhibition of human butyrylcholinesterase with cymserine. *Biochim Biophys Acta* 2006;**1760**:200–6.
14. Kamal MA, Klein P, Yu QS *et al.* Kinetics of human serum butyrylcholinesterase and its inhibition by a novel experimental Alzheimer therapeutic, bisnorcymserine. *J Alzheimers Dis* 2006;**10**:43–51.
15. Thal LJ, Forrest M, Loft H *et al.* Lu 25-109, a muscarinic agonist, fails to improve cognition in Alzheimer's disease. *Neurology* 2000;**54**:421–6.
16. Messer WS Jr. The utility of muscarinic agonists in the treatment of Alzheimer's disease. *J Mol Neurosci* 2002;**19**: 187–93.
17. Fisher A, Pittel Z, Haring R *et al.* M1 muscarinic agonists can modulate some of the hallmarks in Alzheimer's

disease: implications in future therapy. *J Mol Neurosci* 2003;**20**:349–56.

18. Caccamo A, Oddo S, Billings LM *et al.* M1 receptors play a central role in modulating AD-like pathology in transgenic mice. *Neuron* 2006;**49**:671–82.
19. Arneric SP, Sullivan JP, Decker MW *et al.* Potential treatment of Alzheimer disease using cholinergic channel activators (ChCAs) with cognitive enhancement, anxiolytic-like and cytoprotective properties. *Alzheimer Dis Assoc Disord* 1995;**9**:50–61.
20. Lippiello PM, Bencherif M, Gray JA *et al.* RJR-2403: a nicotinic agonist with CNS selectivity II. *In vivo* characterization. *J Pharmacol Exp Ther* 1996;**279**:1422–9.
21. Bencherif M, Bane AJ, Miller CH *et al.* TC-2559: a novel orally active ligand selective at neuronal acetylcholine receptors. *Eur J Pharmacol* 2000;**409**:45–55.
22. Lippiello P, Letchworth SR, Gatto GJ *et al.* Ispronicline: a novel alpha4beta2 nicotinic acetylcholine receptor-selective agonist with cognition-enhancing and neuroprotective properties. *J Mol Neurosci* 2006;**30**:19–20.
23. Lin NH, Gunn DE, Ryther KB *et al.* Structure–activity studies on 2-methyl-3-(2(*S*)-pyrrolidinylmethoxy)pyridine (ABT-089): an orally bioavailable 3-pyridyl ether nicotinic acetylcholine receptor ligand with cognition-enhancing properties. *J Med Chem* 1997;**40**:385–90.
24. Rueter LE, Anderson DJ, Briggs CA *et al.* ABT-089: pharmacological properties of a neuronal nicotinic acetylcholine receptor agonist for the potential treatment of cognitive disorders. *CNS Drug Rev* 2004;**10**:167–82.
25. Kem WR. The brain alpha7 nicotinic receptor may be an important therapeutic target for the treatment of Alzheimer's disease: studies with DMXBA (GTS-21). *Behav Brain Res* 2000;**113**:169–81.
26. Dunbar GC, Inglis F, Kuchibhatla R *et al.* Effect of ispronicline, a neuronal nicotinic acetylcholine receptor partial agonist, in subjects with age associated memory impairment (AAMI). *J Psychopharmacol* 2007;**21**:171–8.
27. Jack CR, Knopman DS, Jagust WJ *et al.* Hypothetical model of dynamic biomarkers of the Alzheimer's pathological cascade. *Lancet Neurol* 2010;**9**:119–28.
28. Schenk D, Barbour R, Dunn W *et al.* Immunization with amyloid-beta attenuates Alzheimer-disease-like pathology in the PDAPP mouse. *Nature* 1999;**400**:173–7.
29. Morgan D, Diamond DM, Gottschall PE *et al.* A beta peptide vaccination prevents memory loss in an animal model of Alzheimer's disease. *Nature* 2000;**408**:982–5.
30. Lavie V, Becker M, Cohen-Kupiec R *et al.* EFRH-phage immunization of Alzheimer's disease animal model improves behavioral performance in Morris water maze trials. *J Mol Neurosci* 2004;**24**:105–13.
31. Orgogozo JM, Gilman S, Dartigues JF *et al.* Subacute meningoencephalitis in a subset of patients with AD after ABeta42 immunization. *Neurology* 2003;**61**:46–54.
32. Hock C, Konietzko U, Streffer JR *et al.* Antibodies against beta-amyloid slow cognitive decline in Alzheimer's disease. *Neuron* 2003;**38**:547–54.
33. Gilman S, Koller M, Black RS *et al.* Clinical effects of ABeta immunization (AN1792) in patients with AD in an interrupted trial. *Neurology* 2005;**64**:1553–62.
34. Woodhouse A, Dickson TC and Vickers JC. Vaccination strategies for Alzheimer's disease: a new hope? *Drugs Aging* 2007;**24**:107–19.
35. Pride M, Seubert P, Grundman M *et al.* Progress in the active immunotherapeutic approach to Alzheimer's disease: clinical investigations into AN1792-associated meningoencephalitis. *Neurodegener Dis* 2008;**5**:194–6.
36. Bard F, Cannon C, Barbour R *et al.* Peripherally administered antibodies against amyloid beta-peptide enter the central nervous system and reduce pathology in a mouse model of Alzheimer disease. *Nat Med* 2000;**6**:916–9.
37. Goni F and Sigurdsson EM. New directions towards safer and effective vaccines for Alzheimer's disease. *Curr Opin Mol Ther* 2005;**7**:17–23.
38. Racke MM, Boone LI, Hepburn DL *et al.* Exacerbation of cerebral amyloid angiopathy associated microhemorrhage in amyloid precursor protein transgenic mice by immunotherapy is dependent on antibody recognition of deposited forms of amyloid beta. *J Neurosci* 2005;**25**:629–36.
39. Rakover I, Arbel M and Solomon B. Immunotherapy against APP beta-secretase cleavage site improves cognitive function and reduces neuroinflammation in Tg2576 mice without a significant effect on brain abeta levels. *Neurodegener Dis* 2007;**4**:392–402.
40. Dodel RC, Du Y, Depboylu C *et al.* Intravenous immunoglobulins containing antibodies against beta-amyloid for the treatment of Alzheimer's disease. *J Neurol Neurosurg Psychiatry* 2004;**75**:1472–4.
41. Rinne JO, Brooks DJ, Rossor MN *et al.* ^{11}C-PiB PET assessment of change in fibrillar amyloid-beta load in patients with Alzheimer's disease treated with bapineuzumab: a phase 2, double-blind, placebo-controlled, ascending-dose study. *Lancet Neurol* 2010;**9**:363–72.
42. Etcheberrigaray R, Tan M, Dewachter I *et al.* Therapeutic eff ects of PKC activators in Alzheimer's disease transgenic mice. *Proc Natl Acad Sci U S A* 2004;**101**:11141–6.
43. Marcade M, Bourdin J, Loiseau N *et al.* Etazolate, a neuroprotective drug linking GABA(A) receptor pharmacology to amyloid precursor protein processing. *J Neurochem* 2008;**106**:392–404.
44. Hock C, Maddalena A, Raschig A *et al.* Treatment with the selective muscarinic M1 agonist talsaclidine decreases cerebrospinal fluid levels of A beta 42 in patients with Alzheimer's disease. *Amyloid* 2003;**10**:1–6.
45. Wienrich M, Meier D, Ensinger HA *et al.* Pharmacodynamic profile of the M1 agonist talsaclidine in animals and man. *Life Sci* 2001;**68**:2593–600.
46. Luo Y, Bolon B, Kahn S *et al.* Mice deficient in BACE1, the Alzheimer's betasecretase, have normal phenotype and abolished beta-amyloid generation. *Nat Neurosci* 2001;**4**:231–2.
47. Hussain I, Hawkins J, Harrison D *et al.* Oral administration of a potent and selective non-peptidic BACE-1 inhibitor decreases beta-cleavage of amyloid precursor protein and amyloid-beta production *in vivo*. *J Neurochem* 2007;**100**:802–9.
48. Watson GS and Craft S. The role of insulin resistance in the pathogenesis of Alzheimer's disease: implications for treatment. *CNS Drugs* 2003;**17**:27–45.

49. Watson GS, Cholerton BA, Reger MA *et al.* Preserved cognition in patients with early Alzheimer disease and amnestic mild cognitive impairment during treatment with rosiglitazone: a preliminary study. *Am J Geriatr Psychiatry* 2005;**13**:950–8.

50. Nissen SE and Wolski K. Effect of rosiglitazone on the risk of myocardial infarction and death from cardiovascular causes. *N Engl J Med* 2007;**356**:2457–71.

51. Reger MA, Henderson ST, Hale C *et al.* Effects of beta-hydroxybutyrate on cognition in memory-impaired adults. *Neurobiol Aging* 2004;**25**:311–4.

52. ClinicalTrials.gov. http://www.clinicaltrials.gov (last accessed 8 July 2011).

53. Comery TA, Martone RL, Aschmies S *et al.* Acute gamma-secretase inhibition improves contextual fear conditioning in the Tg2576 mouse model of Alzheimer's disease. *J Neurosci* 2005;**25**:8898–902.

54. Dovey HF, John V, Anderson JP *et al.* Functional gamma-secretase inhibitors reduce beta-amyloid peptide levels in brain. *J Neurochem* 2001;**76**:173–81.

55. Hartmann D, Tournoy J, Saftig P *et al.* Implication of APP secretases in notch signaling. *J Mol Neurosci* 2001;**17**:171–81.

56. Barten DM, Meredith JE Jr, Zaczek R *et al.* Gamma-secretase inhibitors for Alzheimer's disease: balancing efficacy and toxicity. *Drugs R D* 2006;**7**:87–97.

57. Wong GT, Manfra D, Poulet FM *et al.* Chronic treatment with the gamma-secretase inhibitor LY-411,575 inhibits beta-amyloid peptide production and alters lymphopoiesis and intestinal cell differentiation. *J Biol Chem* 2004;**279**:12876–82.

58. Siemers E, Skinner M, Dean RA *et al.* Safety, tolerability and changes in amyloid beta concentrations after administration of a gamma-secretase inhibitor in volunteers. *Clin Neuropharmacol* 2005;**28**:126–32.

59. Siemers ER, Dean RA, Friedrich S *et al.* Safety, tolerability and effects on plasma and cerebrospinal fluid amyloid-beta after inhibition of gamma-secretase. *Clin Neuropharmacol* 2007;**30**:317–25.

60. Siemers ER, Quinn JF, Kaye J *et al.* Effects of a gamma-secretase inhibitor in a randomized study of patients with Alzheimer disease. *Neurology* 2006;**66**:602–4.

61. Frick G., Raje S., Wan H. *et al.* P4-366: GSI-953, a potent and selective gammasecretase inhibitor: modulation of beta-amyloid peptides and plasma and cerebrospinal fluid pharmacokinetic/pharmacodynamic relationships in humans. *Alzheimer's Dementia* 2008;**4**: T781.

62. Wilcock GK, Black SE, Hendrix SB *et al.* Efficacy and safety of tarenflurbil in mild to moderate Alzheimer's disease: a randomised phase II trial. *Lancet Neurol* 2008;**7**:483–93.

63. Aisen PS. The development of anti-amyloid therapy for Alzheimer's disease: from secretase modulators to polymerisation inhibitors. *CNS Drugs* 2005;**19**:989–96.

64. Gervais F, Paquette J, Morissette C *et al.* Targeting soluble Abeta peptide with tramiprosate for the treatment of brain amyloidosis. *Neurobiol Aging* 2007;**28**:537–47.

65. Wright TM. Tramiprosate. *Drugs Today (Barc)* 2006;**42**: 291–8.

66. Finefrock AE, Bush AI and Doraiswamy PM. Current status of metals as therapeutic targets in Alzheimer's disease. *J Am Geriatr Soc* 2003;**51**:1143–8.

67. Cuajungco MP, Frederickson CJ and Bush AI. Amyloid-beta metal interaction and metal chelation. *Subcell Biochem* 2005;**38**:235–54.

68. Dedeoglu A, Cormier K, Payton S *et al.* Preliminary studies of a novel bifunctional metal chelator targeting Alzheimer's amyloidogenesis. *Exp Gerontol* 2004;**39**:1641–9.

69. Lee JY, Friedman JE, Angel I *et al.* The lipophilic metal chelator DP-109 reduces amyloid pathology in brains of human beta-amyloid precursor protein transgenic mice. *Neurobiol Aging* 2004;**25**:1315–21.

70. Ritchie CW, Bush AI, Mackinnon A *et al.* Metal–protein attenuation with iodochlorhydroxyquin (clioquinol) targeting Abeta amyloid deposition and toxicity in Alzheimer disease: a pilot phase 2 clinical trial. *Arch Neurol* 2003;**60**:1685–91.

71. Sampson E, Jenagaratnam L and McShane R. Metal protein attenuating compounds for the treatment of Alzheimer's disease. *Cochrane Database Syst Rev* 2008;(1): CD005380.

72. Liu G, Garrett MR, Men P *et al.* Nanoparticle and other metal chelation therapeutics in Alzheimer disease. *Biochim Biophys Acta* 2005;**1741**:246–52.

73. Lannfelt L, Blennow K, Zetterberg H *et al.* Safety, efficacy and biomarker findings of PBT2 in targeting Abeta as a modifying therapy for Alzheimer's disease: a phase IIa, double-blind, randomised, placebo-controlled trial. *Lancet Neurol* 2008;**7**:779–86.

74. Phiel CJ, Wilson CA, Lee VM *et al.* GSK-3alpha regulates production of Alzheimer's disease amyloid-beta peptides. *Nature* 2003;**423**:435–9.

75. Zhao WQ, Feng C and Alkon DL. Impairment of phosphatase 2A contributes to the prolonged MAP kinase phosphorylation in Alzheimer's disease fibroblasts. *Neurobiol Dis* 2003;**14**:458–69.

76. Wei Q, Holzer M, Brueckner MK *et al.* Dephosphorylation of tau protein by calcineurin triturated into neural living cells. *Cell Mol Neurobiol* 2002;**22**:13–24.

77. Hong M, Chen DC, Klein PS *et al.* Lithium reduces tau phosphorylation by inhibition of glycogen synthase kinase-3. *J Biol Chem* 1997;**272**:25326–32.

78. Rockenstein E, Torrance M, Adame A *et al.* Neuroprotective effects of regulators of the glycogen synthase kinase-3beta signaling pathway in a transgenic model of Alzheimer's disease are associated with reduced amyloid precursor protein phosphorylation. *J Neurosci* 2007;**27**:1981–91.

79. Hampel H, Ewers M, Bürger K *et al.* Lithium trial in Alzheimer's disease: a randomized, single-blinded, placebo-controlled, parallel group multicentre 10-week study. *Alzheimer's Dementia* 2008;**4**: T782.

80. Deiana S, Harrington CR, Wischik CM *et al.* Methylthioninium chloride reverses cognitive deficits induced by scopolamine: comparison with rivastigmine. *Psychopharmacology (Berl)* 2009;**202**:53–65.

81. Nunomura A, Castellani RJ, Zhu X *et al.* Involvement of oxidative stress in Alzheimer disease. *J Neuropathol Exp Neurol* 2006;**65**:631–41.

82. Keller JN, Schmitt FA, Scheff SW *et al*. Evidence of increased oxidative damage in subjects with mild cognitive impairment. *Neurology* 2005;**64**:1152–6.
83. Nunomura A, Perry G, Aliev G *et al*. Oxidative damage is the earliest event in Alzheimer disease. *J Neuropathol Exp Neurol* 2001;**60**:759–67.
84. Sano M, Ernesto C, Thomas RG *et al*. A controlled trial of selegiline, alpha-tocopherol or both as treatment for Alzheimer's disease. *N Engl J Med* 1997;**336**:1216–22.
85. Miller ER III, Pastor-Barruiuso R, Dalal D *et al*. Meta analysis: high dosage vitamin E supplementation may increase all-cause mortality. *Ann Intern Med* 2005;**142**:37–46.
86. Isaac M, Quinn R and Tabet N. Vitamin E for Alzheimer's disease and mild cognitive impairment. *Cochrane Database Syst Rev* 2000;(4): CD002854.
87. Lee DH, Folsom AR, Harnack L *et al*. Does supplemental vitamin C increase cardiovascular disease risk in women with diabetes? *Am J Clin Nutr* 2004;**80**:1194–200.
88. Barberger-Gateau P, Raffaitin C, Letenneur L *et al*. Dietary patterns and risk of dementia: the Three-City cohort study. *Neurology* 2007;**69**:1921–30.
89. Freund-Levi Y, Eriksdotter-Jönhagen M, Cederholm T *et al*. Omega-3 fatty acid treatment in 174 patients with mild to moderate Alzheimer disease: OmegAD study: a randomized double-blind trial. *Arch Neurol* 2006;**63**:1402–8.
90. Holmquist L, Stuchbury G, Berbaum K *et al*. Lipoic acid as a novel treatment for Alzheimer's disease and related dementias. *Pharmacol Ther* 2007;**113**:154–64.
91. Moreira PI, Harris PL, Zhu X *et al*. Lipoic acid and *N*-acetylcysteine decrease mitochondrial-related oxidative stress in Alzheimer disease patient fibroblasts. *J Alzheimers Dis* 2007;**12**:195–206.
92. Hager K, Kenklies M, McAfoose J *et al*. Alpha-lipoic acid as a new treatment option for Alzheimer's disease – a 48 months follow-up analysis. *J Neural Transm Suppl* 2007;**72**:189–93.
93. Ramassamy C, Longpré F and Christen Y. Ginkgo biloba extract (EGb 761) in Alzheimer's disease: is there any evidence? *Curr Alzheimer Res* 2007;**4**:253–62.
94. Tauskela JS. MitoQ – a mitochondria-targeted antioxidant. *IDrugs* 2007;**10**:399–412.
95. Wang S, Zhu L, Shi H *et al*. Inhibition of melatonin biosynthesis induces neurofilament hyperphosphorylation with activation of cyclin-dependent kinase 5. *Neurochem Res* 2007;**32**:1329–35.
96. in't Veld BA, Ruitenberg A, Hofman A *et al*. Nonsteroidal antiinflammatory drugs and the risk of Alzheimer's disease. *N Engl J Med* 2001;**345**:1515–21.
97. Rogers J, Kirby LC, Hempelman SR *et al*. Clinical trial of indomethacin in Alzheimer's disease. *Neurology* 1993;**43**:1609–11.
98. Tabet N and Feldman H. Indomethacin for Alzheimer's disease. *Cochrane Database Syst Rev* 2002;(2): CD003673.
99. De Jong D, Jansen R, Hoefnagels W *et al*. No effect of one-year treatment with indomethacin on Alzheimer's disease progression: a randomized controlled trial. *PLoS ONE* 2008;**3**: e1475.
100. Reines SA, Block GA, Morris JC *et al*. Rofecoxib: no effect on Alzheimer's disease in a 1-year, randomized, blinded, controlled study. *Neurology* 2004;**62**:66–71.
101. Soininen H, West C, Robbins J *et al*. Long-term efficacy and safety of celecoxib in Alzheimer's disease. *Dement Geriatr Cogn Disord* 2007;**23**:8–21.
102. Aisen PS, Schafer KA, Grundman M *et al*. Effects of rofecoxib or naproxen vs placebo on Alzheimer disease progression: a randomized controlled trial. *JAMA* 2003;**289**: 2819–26.
103. Geerts H. Drug evaluation: (*R*)-flurbiprofen – an enantiomer of flurbiprofen for the treatment of Alzheimer's disease. *IDrugs* 2007;**10**:121–33.
104. Brode S and Cooke A. Immune-potentiating effects of the chemotherapeutic drug cyclophosphamide. *Crit Rev Immunol* 2008;**28**:109–26.
105. Tobinick EL and Gross H. Rapid cognitive improvement in Alzheimer's disease following perispinal etanercept administration. *J Neuroinflammation* 2008;**5**: 2.
106. Harikumar KB and Aggarwal BB. Resveratrol: a multitargeted agent for age-associated chronic diseases. *Cell Cycle* 2008;**7**:1020–35.
107. Yang F, Lim GP, Begum AN *et al*. Curcumin inhibits formation of amyloid beta oligomers and fibrils, binds plaques and reduces amyloid *in vivo*. *J Biol Chem* 2005;**280**:5892–901.
108. Greenamyre JT and Young AB. Excitatory amino acids and Alzheimer's disease. *Neurobiol Aging* 1989;**10**:593–602.
109. Chohan MO and Iqbal K. From tau to toxicity: emerging roles of NMDA receptor in Alzheimer's disease. *J Alzheimers Dis* 2006;**10**:81–7.
110. Zoladz PR, Campbell AM, Park CR *et al*. Enhancement of long-term spatial memory in adult rats by the noncompetitive NMDA receptor antagonists, memantine and neramexane. *Pharmacol Biochem Behav* 2006;**85**:298–306.
111. Dicou E, Rangon CM, Guimiot F *et al*. Positive allosteric modulators of AMPA receptors are neuroprotective against lesions induced by an NMDA agonist in neonatal mouse brain. *Brain Res* 2003;**970**:221–5.
112. Quirk JC and Nisenbaum ES. LY404187: a novel positive allosteric modulator of AMPA receptors. *CNS Drug Rev* 2002;**8**:255–82.
113. Chappell AS, Gonzales C, Williams J *et al*. AMPA potentiator treatment of cognitive deficits in Alzheimer disease. *Neurology* 2007;**68**:1008–12.
114. Conner JM, Darracq MA, Roberts J *et al*. Nontropic actions of neurotrophins: subcortical nerve growth factor gene delivery reverses age-related degeneration of primate cortical cholinergic innervation. *Proc Natl Acad Sci U S A* 2001;**98**:1941–6.
115. Capsoni S, Giannotta S and Cattaneo A. Nerve growth factor and galantamine ameliorate early signs of neurodegeneration in anti-nerve growth factor mice. *Proc Natl Acad Sci U S A* 2002;**99**:12432–7.
116. Tuszynski MH, Thal L, Pay M *et al*. A phase 1 clinical trial of nerve growth factor gene therapy for Alzheimer disease. *Nat Med* 2005;**11**:551–5.
117. Grundman M, Capparelli E, Kim HT *et al*. A multicenter, randomized, placebo controlled, multiple-dose, safety and pharmacokinetic study of AIT-082 (Neotrofin) in mild Alzheimer's disease patients. *Life Sci* 2003;**73**:539–53.

118. Elder GA, De Gasperi R and Gama Sosa MA. Research update: neurogenesis in adult brain and neuropsychiatric disorders. *Mt Sinai J Med* 2006;**73**:931–40.

119. Lovell MA, Geiger H, Van Zant GE *et al.* Isolation of neural precursor cells from Alzheimer's disease and aged control postmortem brain. *Neurobiol Aging* 2006;**27**:909–17.

120. Hogervorst E, Williams J, Budge M *et al.* The nature of the effect of female gonadal hormone replacement therapy on cognitive function in post-menopausal women: a meta-analysis. *Neuroscience* 2000;**101**:485–512.

121. Webber KM, Perry G, Smith MA *et al.* The contribution of luteinizing hormone to Alzheimer disease pathogenesis. *Clin Med Res* 2007;**5**:177–83.

122. Casadesus G, Garrett MR, Webber KM *et al.* The estrogen myth: potential use of gonadotropin-releasing hormone agonists for the treatment of Alzheimer's disease. *Drugs R D* 2006;**7**:187–93.

123. Cherrier MM, Matsumoto AM, Amory JK *et al.* Testosterone improves spatial memory in men with Alzheimer disease and mild cognitive impairment. *Neurology* 2005;**64**:2063–8.

124. Cherrier MM, Asthana S, Plymate S *et al.* Testosterone supplementation improves spatial and verbal memory in healthy older men. *Neurology* 2001;**57**:80–8.

125. Merriam GR, Schwartz RS and Vitiello MV. Growth hormone-releasing hormone and growth hormone secretagogues in normal aging. *Endocrine* 2003;**22**:41–8.

126. Sevigny JJ, Ryan JM, van Dyck CH *et al.* Growth hormone secretagogue MK-677: no clinical effect on AD progression in a randomized trial. *Neurology* 2008;**71**:1702–8.

127. Green KN, Billings LM, Roozendaal B *et al.* Glucocorticoids increase amyloid-beta and tau pathology in a mouse model of Alzheimer's disease. *J Neurosci* 2006;**26**:9047–56.

128. Pomara N, Doraiswamy PM, Tun H and Ferris S. Mifepristone (RU 486) for Alzheimer's disease. *Neurology* 2002;**58**: 1436.

129. Bachurin S, Bukatina E, Lermontova N *et al.* Antihistamine agent Dimebon as a novel neuroprotector and a cognition enhancer. *Ann N Y Acad Sci* 2001;**939**:425–35.

130. Doody RS, Gavrilova SI, Sano M *et al.* Effect of Dimebon on cognition, activities of daily living, behaviour and global function in patients with mild-to-moderate Alzheimer's disease: a randomised, double-blind, placebo-controlled study. *Lancet* 2008;**372**:207–15.

131. Sparks DL, Sabbagh MN, Connor DJ *et al.* Atorvastatin for the treatment of mild to moderate Alzheimer disease: preliminary results. *Arch Neurol* 2005;**62**:753–7.

132. Simons M, Schwärzler F, Lütjohann D *et al.* Treatment with simvastatin in normocholesterolemic patients with Alzheimer's disease: a 26-week randomized, placebo-controlled, double-blind trial. *Ann Neurol* 2002;**52**: 346–50.

133. Jones RW, Kivipelto M, Feldman H *et al.* The Atorvastatin/Donepezil in Alzheimer's Disease Study (LEADe): design and baseline characteristics. *Alzheimers Dement* 2008; **4**:145–53.

134. Stuchbury G and Münch G. Alzheimer's associated inflammation, potential drug targets and future therapies. *J Neural Transm* 2005;**112**:429–53.

135. Maczurek A, Shanmugam K and Münch G. Inflammation and the redox-sensitive AGERAGE pathway as a therapeutic target in Alzheimer's disease. *Ann N Y Acad Sci* 2008; **1126**:147–51.

136. Schechter LE, Smith DL, Rosenzweig-Lipson S *et al.* Lecozotan (SRA-333): a selective serotonin 1A receptor antagonist that enhances the stimulated release of glutamate and acetylcholine in the hippocampus and possesses cognitive-enhancing properties. *J Pharmacol Exp Ther* 2005;**314**:1274–89.

137. Youdim MB. The path from anti Parkinson drug selegiline and rasagiline to multifunctional neuroprotective anti Alzheimer drugs ladostigil and m30. *Curr Alzheimer Res* 2006;**3**:541–50.

138. Chan A and Shea TB. Folate deprivation increases presenilin expression, gammasecretase activity and Abeta levels in murine brain: potentiation by ApoE deficiency and alleviation by dietary *S*-adenosylmethionine. *J Neurochem* 2007;**102**:753–60.

139. Cotelli M, Manenti R, Cappa SF *et al.* Transcranial magnetic stimulation improves naming in Alzheimer disease patients at different stages of cognitive decline. *Eur J Neurol* 2008;**15**:1286–92.

140. Laxton AW, Tang-Wai DF, McAndrews MP http://www.ncbi.nlm.nih.gov/pubmed?term=%22Zumsteg%20D%22%5BAuthor%5D *et al.* A phase I trial of deep brain stimulation of memory circuits in Alzheimer's disease. *Ann Neurol.* 2010;**68**:521–34.

141. Brookmeyer R, Johnson E, Ziegler G *et al.* Forecasting the global burden of Alzheimer's disease. *Alzheimers Dement* 2007;**3**:186–91.

142. Andrieu S, Gillette S, Amouyal K *et al.* Association of Alzheimer's disease onset with ginkgo biloba and other symptomatic cognitive treatments in a population of women aged 75 years and older from the EPIDOS study. *J Gerontol A Biol Sci Med Sci* 2003;**58**:372–7.

143. Vellas B, Andrieu S, Ousset PJ *et al.* The GuidAge study: methodological issues. A 5-year double-blind randomized trial of the efficacy of EGb 761 for prevention of Alzheimer disease in patients over 70 with a memory complaint. *Neurology* 2006;**67**(9 Suppl 3): S6–11.

144. Gillette-Guyonnet S, Andrieu S, Dantoine T *et al.* Commentary on 'A roadmap for the prevention of dementia II. Leon Thal Symposium 2008. The Multidomain Alzheimer Preventive Trial (MAPT): a new approach to the prevention of Alzheimer's disease.' *Alzheimers Dement* 2009;**5**: 114–21.

145. Mangialasche F, Solomon A, Winblad B *et al.* Alzheimer's disease: clinical trials and drug development. *Lancet Neurol* 2010;**9**:702–16.

CHAPTER 79

Other dementias

Wee Shiong Lim
Tan Tock Seng Hospital, Singapore

Introduction

Dementia is an acquired syndrome in which there is impairment of cognitive abilities, severe enough to interfere with the individual's occupational, social and functional abilities. As conventionally used, the term dementia implies 'degenerative' and 'progressive', but it is also often used in the context of static conditions (such as post-stroke cognitive impairment) or reversible conditions (such as depression or medication-related cognitive impairment). Table 79.1 provides a list of the many causes of dementing illnesses that can occur in older individuals.

Because Alzheimer's disease (AD) is widely reported as the commonest cause of dementia worldwide, it may be tempting for clinicians to make this diagnosis routinely without systematically considering alternative or additional diagnoses. Such a practice, although probably fortuitously correct most of the time, would fail to detect reversible diseases that affect cognition (which often occur concomitantly with AD) and other non-AD aetiologies that may confer different prognosis and necessitate different treatment modalities from AD.

Population-based studies on Western and Asian cohorts indicate that vascular dementia (VaD) is often the commonest reported dementia aetiology after AD. When actively sought for with standard criteria, the prevalence of dementia with Lewy bodies (DLB) and frontotemporal dementia (FTD) may be higher than previously thought. For example, the Islington study of community-dwelling elderly revealed the following distribution of dementia subtypes: AD 31.3, VaD 21.9, DLB 10.9 and FTD 7.8%.[1] Specialized memory clinic-based estimates differ somewhat from population-based studies in having a relatively higher prevalence of non-AD aetiologies and concomitant potentially reversible conditions, especially depression and metabolic abnormalities. Generally, however, only a small percentage of these conditions have been found to be completely reversible, most notably hypothyroidism and vitamin B_{12} deficiency. The prevalence of aetiologies in demented patients presenting to private practitioners has not been estimated, but would likely reflect values intermediate between population- and specialized outpatient-based estimates.

This chapter discusses some conditions that are commonly encountered in clinical practice, notably vascular cognitive impairment and non-AD neurodegenerative dementias. We focus on conceptual advances and clinical gems that can help in the diagnosis and management of these conditions and conclude with a general approach to the evaluation of dementia with parkinsonism.

Vascular cognitive impairment/vascular dementia

Epidemiological studies in the West indicate that VaD is second in prevalence to AD, accounting for 12–20% of dementia cases. The incidence of VaD increases with age, but much less steeply than AD. Unlike AD, men are disproportionately more affected, especially at younger ages. Earlier international comparative studies revealed a higher frequency of VaD in Asian countries, notably Japan and China. The ratio of AD to VaD varied from 1.4 in Beijing, China, to 2.8 in Korea, compared with the ratio of 3.4 in Europe. However, a recent study from China reported a higher prevalence of AD than VaD (3.5 versus 1.1%) in the population older than 65 years.[2] Whether this portends an epidemiological shift towards Western trends or is due to methodological differences is unclear.

Despite being described by Alois Alzheimer more than a century ago, the role of cerebrovascular disease (CVD) in dementia has been dogged by misconception. For the greater part of the twentieth century, it was commonly held that the most frequent cause of late-onset dementia was arteriosclerosis. Seminal work in the late 1960s challenged this assumption, establishing that the main type of pathology underlying late-onset dementia was degenerative and of Alzheimer type rather than vascular. This led to

Principles and Practice of Geriatric Medicine, Fifth Edition. Edited by Alan J. Sinclair, John E. Morley and Bruno Vellas.

Table 79.1 Causes of dementia other than Alzheimer's disease.

1 Other degenerative dementias
  a Dementia with parkinsonism
    i Diffuse Lewy body disease
    ii Parkinson's disease dementia
    iii Progressive supranuclear palsy
    iv Corticobasal degeneration
    v Multiple system atrophy
  b Frontotemporal dementia
  c Huntington's disease
  d Hallervorden–Spatz disease
  e Kufs' disease
2 Vascular dementia
3 Other CNS causes
  a Normal-pressure hydrocephalus
  b Epilepsy
  c Traumatic dementia
    i Acute and chronic subdural haematoma
    ii Dementia pugilistica
    iii Craniocerebral injury
  d Tumours
    i Primary CNS tumours: gliomas, meningiomas
    ii Metastatic tumours, lymphoma, leukaemia
    iii Paraneoplastic limbic encephalitis
4 Psychiatric disorders
  a Depression
  b Others: schizophrenia, mania, other psychoses
5 Inflammatory
  a Cerebral vasculitis
    i Primary angiitis of the CNS
    ii Part of systemic involvement: disseminated lupus erythematosus, temporal arteritis, Behçet's disease, Wegener's granulomatosis, Churg–Strauss disease
  b Multiple sclerosis
6 Metabolic
  a Endocrinopathies
    i Hyper- and hypothyroidism
    ii Glucose disorders: hyper- and hypo- states
    iii Cushing's disease
    iv Addison's disease
  b Electrolyte abnormalities
    i Hypo- and hypernatraemia
    ii Hypercalcaemia
  c Inherited
    i Wilson's disease
    ii Mitochondrial disorders
    iii Adult lysosomal diseases (particularly metachromatic leukodystrophy)
    iv Peroxisomal disorders
7 Nutritional deficiency
  a Thiamine deficiency
  b Vitamin B_{12} deficiency
  c Folate deficiency
  d Vitamin B_6 deficiency (pellagra)

(*continued overleaf*)

Table 79.1 (*continued*).

8 Infective
  a Neurosyphilis
  b Human prion disease
  c HIV-associated dementia
  d Progressive multifocal leukoencephalopathy
  e Post-meningitic/post-encephalitic dementia
9 Drugs (remembered by the mnemonic ACUTE CHANGE IN MS[30])
  a **A**ntiparkinsonian drugs
  b **C**orticosteroids
  c **U**rinary incontinence drugs
  d **T**heophylline
  e **E**mptying (motility) drugs
  f **C**ardiovascular drugs
  g **H**2 blockers
  h **A**ntimicrobials
  i **N**SAIDs
  j **G**eropsychiatric drugs
  k **E**NT drugs
  l **I**nsomnia drugs
  m **N**arcotics
  n **M**uscle relaxants
  o **S**eizure drugs
10 Toxins
  a Alcohol
  b Heavy metals: lead, aluminium, mercury
  c Carbon monoxide poisoning
11 Others
  a Obstructive sleep apnea
  b Whipple's disease
  c Neurosarcoidosis

a redefinition of late-onset dementia as primarily the result of AD, with the result that the nosological status of vascular dementia became uncertain.

The field moved forward when the concept of *multi-infarct dementia* (MID) was described to reflect dementia due to multiple large and small strokes. The field further evolved with the recognition that MID was just one of many subtypes of VaD (Table 79.2).[3] VaD encompasses several clinicopathological subtypes, ranging from haemorrhagic (including hypertension, cerebral amyloidal angiopathy, subarachnoid haemorrhage, post-haemorrhagic obstructive hydrocephalus, subdural haematoma and haematological causes) to ischaemic and combinations of ischaemia and haemorrhage (such as cortical vein and sinus thromboses). Ischaemic forms of VaD can be further divided into large-vessel, small-vessel and strategic infarct subtypes (Table 79.2). Among the hereditary group, the most extensively studied condition is cerebral autosomal dominant arteriopathy with subcortical infarcts and leukoencephalopathy (CADASIL), a genetically transmitted small-vessel disorder that has

Table 79.2 Subtypes of vascular dementia (VaD).

Subtype	Description
Multi-infarct dementia (cortical VaD)	Predominantly resulting from large cortical infarcts
Small-vessel dementia (subcortical VaD)	Predominantly resulting from subcortical lacunes, white and/or deep grey matter lesions
Strategic infarct dementia	Resulting from a unilateral or bilateral infarct in a strategic area
Hypoperfusion dementia	Resulting from brain damage due to hypoperfusion
Haemorrhagic dementia	Resulting from intracerebral haemorrhage
AD with CVD	Presence (or presumption on the basis of clinical picture and brain imaging) of both significant Alzheimer and vascular pathology, both of which are thought to contribute to dementia
Hereditary dementia	Genetic causes of VaD, such as CADASIL due to mutation in the NOTCH 3 gene in chromosome 19

been mapped to chromosome 19q12 with mutations in the Notch 3 gene.

To make a diagnosis of VaD, three elements are necessary: presence of dementia, presence of cerebrovascular lesions and a temporal relationship between the two. Traditional diagnostic criteria for VaD can be broadly divided into two groups.[4] The *Diagnostic and Statistical Manual of Mental Disorders*, 4th edition (DSM-IV), and the *Classification of Mental and Behavioural Disorders*, 10th Revision, under the International Classification of Diseases (ICD-10), are general diagnostic tools that outline criteria without operationalizing them. The second set, such as the widely used National Institute of Neurological Disorders and Stroke and the Association Internationale pour la Recherche et l'Enseignement en Neurosciences (NINDS–AIREN) criteria (Table 79.3),[5] is a development of the first two and offers operational criteria. Autopsy studies have shown that although these criteria are generally able to exclude about 90% of AD, they have only modest sensitivity (50–70%) in diagnosing VaD. There is a tendency to misclassify mixed dementia (AD with CVD) as VaD (54% for ADDTC and 29% for NINDS–AIREN), especially in the 'possible VaD' category. Application of the NINDS imaging criteria also did not distinguish between demented and non-demented patients.

Advances in the past decade have consolidated our understanding of the contribution of CVD in cognition in three key areas.[6] First, *vascular cognitive impairment (VCI)* is a more comprehensive and appropriate concept than VaD. VCI is an umbrella term that includes VCI-no dementia,

Table 79.3 NINDS–AIREN criteria for probable and possible vascular dementia (VaD).[5]

Probable VaD

1 Dementia

2 Cerebrovascular disease
- Focal neurological signs consistent with stroke
- Neuroimaging evidence of clinically relevant vascular lesions

3 Temporal relationship between dementia and CVD, as evidenced by one or more of the following:
- Onset of dementia within 3 months of a recognized stroke
- Abrupt deterioration
- Fluctuating or stepwise progression

Clinical features consistent with diagnosis:
- Early presence of gait disturbance
- History of unsteadiness, frequent and unprovoked falls
- Early urinary frequency, urgency and other urinary symptoms not explained by urological disease
- Pseudobulbar palsy
- Personality and mood changes, abulia, depression, emotional incontinence and subcortical deficits, including psychomotor retardation and abnormal executive function

Criteria for relevant cerebrovascular disease on brain imaging
- Topography
  - a Large-vessel strokes
  - b Extensive white matter change
  - c Lacunes (frontal/basal ganglia)
  - d Bilateral thalamic lesions
- Severity
  - a Large-vessel lesion of dominant hemisphere
  - b Bilateral strokes
  - c White matter lesions affecting> 25% of white matter

Possible VaD

1 Dementia with focal neurological signs but without neuroimaging confirmation of definite CVD

2 Dementia with focal signs but without a clear temporal relationship between dementia and stroke

3 Dementia and focal signs but with subtle onset and variable course of cognitive deficits

Alzheimer's disease with cerebrovascular disease

1 Clinical criteria for possible AD

2 Clinical and imaging evidence of CVD

VaD and mixed dementia (Figure 79.1). About 5% of VCI people over the age of 65 are estimated to have VCI; in patients under 74, VCI may be the single most common cause of cognitive impairment.[7] The inclusion of VCI-no dementia, a subset with less severe cognitive impairment that do not meet formal criteria for dementia, is analogous to the concept of the pre-dementia stage of amnestic MCI in AD and serves to emphasize the preventable nature of VCI and the importance of early diagnosis. This concept can be taken further: while the progression of VCI is analogous

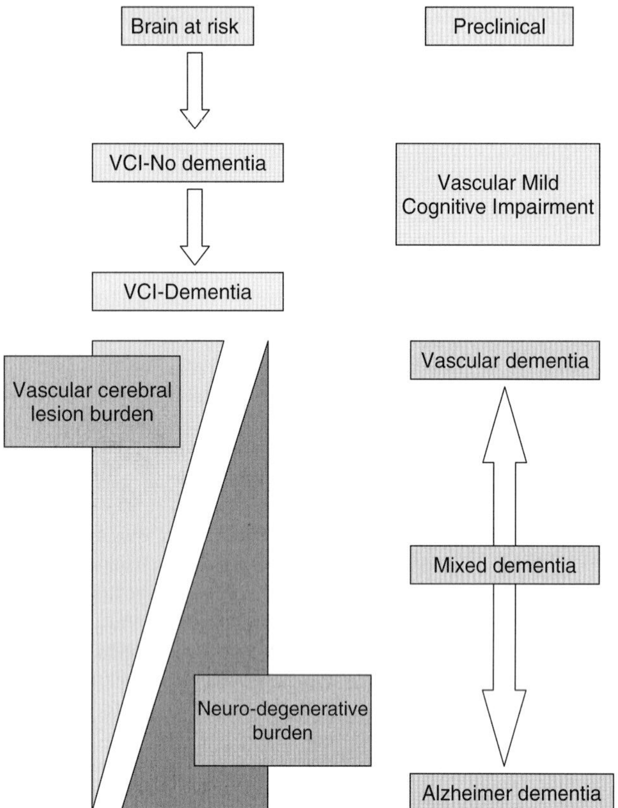

Figure 79.1 Schematic diagram depicting the spectrum of vascular cognitive impairment (VCI) and the overlap between vascular dementia (VaD) and neurodegenerative disease using Alzheimer's disease (AD) as an example. In this conceptual model, AD and VaD fall on a continuous spectrum of disease. The gradient of features, driven by the underlying burden of vascular (lacunes, white matter disease and cerebral microhaemorrhage) and neurodegenerative (amyloid plaques and neurofibrillary tangles) pathology, would then determine the phenotype and nosologic classification (VaD, mixed or AD).

to secondary prevention, primary prevention requires the recognition of the presence of risk factors in an asymptomatic susceptible host, termed 'brain-at-risk'.

Second, with increasing recognition of the overlap between AD and VCI in terms of predisposing factors and pathophysiology, these two disorders are currently conceptualized as a continuous spectrum rather than coexisting unrelated conditions (Figure 79.1).[8] Apart from the ends of the spectrum where pure AD or pure VaD lie, mixed dementia constitutes the majority of patients who cannot easily be classified as being in one group or the other. Limited data suggest that patients with mixed dementia outnumber those with pure AD.[6] Within the mixed group, vascular brain injury acts additively or synergistically with concomitant AD pathology to produce more severe cognitive dysfunction than either process alone. In support of this, clinicopathological data such as the Nun Study indicate that subjects with both vascular disease and AD pathology exhibit either more severe cognitive impairment during life than those with pure AD or require less pathology to produce the same amount of cognitive impairment. This suggests that in AD patients with concomitant CVD, both conditions require treatment, even if the vascular component may appear trivial.

Third, our understanding of the pathophysiology of VCI has evolved to distinguish VCI associated with large vessel disease from that associated with small vessel disease, including subcortical ischaemic vascular disease (SIVD) and non-infarct ischaemic changes such as leukoaraiosis. SIVD includes the lacunar state and Binswanger's disease, characterized, respectively, by multiple lacunes and periventricular leukoencephalopathy that typically spares the arcuate subcortical U fibres. Limited data from clinical samples indicate that SIVD is the most common subtype.[4] A recent study reported that 82.2% had small-vessel VaD whereas only 25.9% had large-vessel VaD.

Although there is some degree of overlap, large-vessel strokes tend to yield a clinical picture of cortical dementia, as opposed to the subcortical dementia of small-vessel forms (Figure 79.2). These can be reasonably differentiated by a combination of cognitive features, neurological features and clinical course (Table 79.4).[9] SIVD typically causes a slow, subacute-onset dementia that is characterized by executive dysfunction, impaired attention and impaired processing speed, with a comparatively milder memory deficit. There may be 'lower-half parkinsonism' producing characteristic gait changes of hesitation, *marche à petit pas* (walking with hurried small steps) and diminished step height. In fact, the triad of dementia, urinary incontinence and gait disturbance, is more often produced by small-vessel VaD than normal-pressure hydrocephalus (NPH). Neuropsychiatric disturbances such as depression, anxiety, agitation, disinhibition and apathy are not uncommon in VaD, especially the small-vessel subtype.

Dementia may occur in 25–33% of ischaemic stroke cases at ages 65 years and older. Predictors of the occurrence of dementia following stroke include older age, lower education level, non-White race, pre-existing cognitive decline, 'silent' infarcts on neuroimaging, ischaemic rather than haemorrhagic strokes, hemispheric rather than brainstem or cerebellar lesions, left rather than right hemispheric lesions, larger and recurrent strokes and more severe neurological deficit on admission. The number of vascular risk factors might be more important for predicting cognitive impairment than any individual factor. Apolipoprotein ε4 has been associated with increased risk for AD and mixed dementia, but not VaD. Leukoaraiosis may be an important predictor of cognitive decline in domains affected by cerebral small-vessel disease. There has been a continuing debate on whether periventricular or deep leukoaraiosis is more damaging to cognition. In the Rotterdam Study,

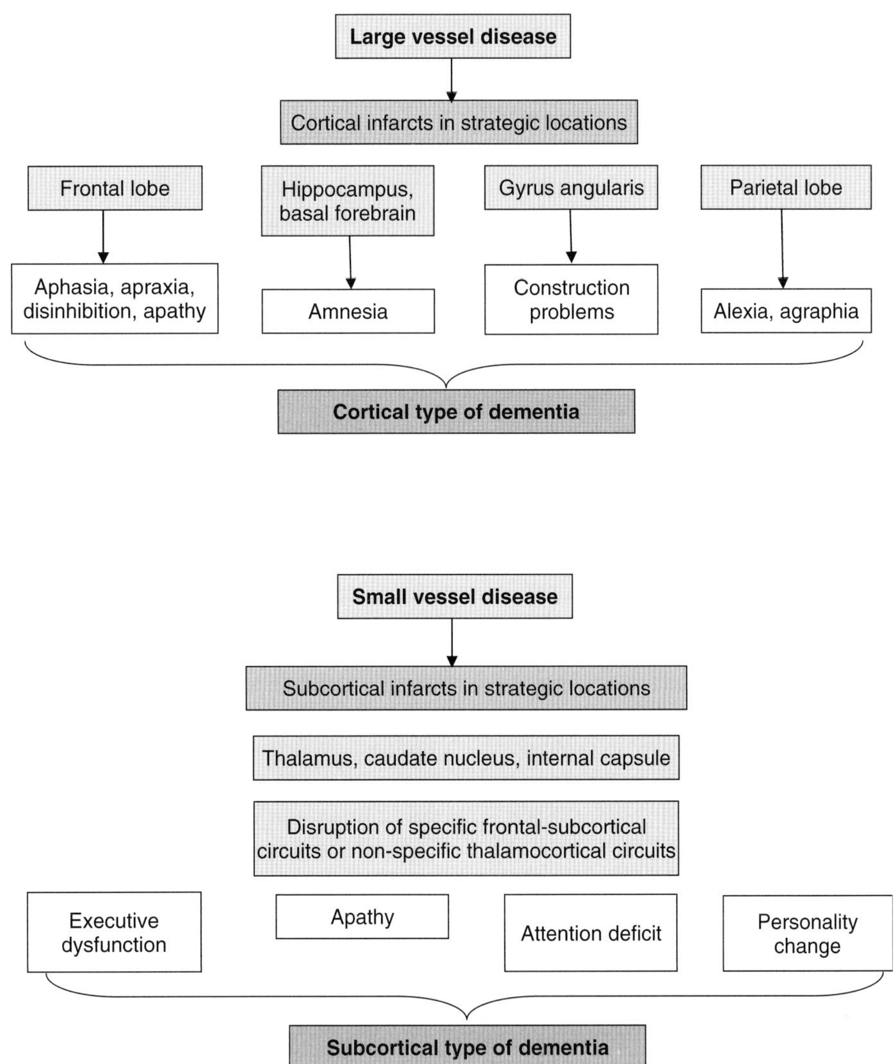

Figure 79.2 Differentiation of clinical features of vascular dementia by vessel size.

periventricular leukoaraiosis and infarcts but not subcortical white matter lesions were correlated with a decline in processing speed and general cognition.[10] The number of cerebral microbleeds as diagnosed by magnetic resonance imaging (MRI) study may be an independent predictor of cognitive impairment and severity of dementia. Patients undergoing coronary artery bypass grafting (CABG) may be at risk for both early (within 1 month) and late (beyond 5 or more years) cognitive decline. A recent observational study suggests that late cognitive decline after CABG is not specific to the use of cardiopulmonary bypass, because nonsurgical cardiac comparison patients also showed mild late cognitive decline.[10]

Management of VaD is multi-pronged and involves (1) symptomatic treatment for cognition, (2) management of neuropsychiatric disturbances, (3) stroke prevention strategies and (4) management of stroke-related disabilities such as spasticity, parkinsonism and incontinence. To date, three studies of donepezil in VaD and two of galantamine (one in VaD, the other in mixed dementia and VaD) have been completed.[7] A modest improvement in cognition analogous to 3 points on the ADAS-Cog has been found, but effects on other outcomes such as activities of daily living, behaviour and global assessment are inconsistent. Two studies in VaD of memantine, an NMDA antagonist that protects against glutamate-mediated excitotoxicity, show modest benefits in cognition, but no benefit on a global outcome measure. Depression is common in association with stroke and SIVD and is an eminently treatable condition; hence a course of antidepressant is justifiable if there is a suspicion of concomitant depression. Levodopa can be helpful in the treatment of apraxic gait in SIVD if the burden of vascular disease lies in the basal ganglia or substantia nigra.

Table 79.4 Characteristics of cortical and subcortical dementia.

Clinical feature	Cortical	Subcortical
Cognitive deficits	Memory impairment prominent	Executive dysfunction prominent
	Heteromodal cortical symptoms	Memory deficit milder
	Neuropsychological syndromes	Perseveration
	Executive dysfunction usually present	Mood changes (depression, emotional lability, apathy)
Neurological symptoms	Field cut	Imbalance/falls
	Lower facial weakness	Gait disturbance
	Upper motor neuron signs	Altered urine frequency
	Dominant/non-dominant lobe signs	Mild upper motor neurone signs
		Dysphagia
		Extrapyramidal signs
Clinical course	Abrupt onset	60%: slow, less abrupt onset
	Stepwise deterioration	80%: slow progression with or without stepwise decline
	Fluctuating course with plateaux	

Strategies for stroke prevention include anticoagulation in patients at risk of cardioembolism, antiplatelet agents, targeting modifiable risk factors (such as hypertension, diabetes, hyperlipidaemia and metabolic syndrome) and optimizing lifestyle factors (such as smoking cessation, physical activity, addressing mid-life obesity and fish consumption). Observational studies suggest a role for vitamin B_{12}, folic acid and homocysteine in VCI, although rigorous intervention studies are lacking.[10] Some studies suggest that treatment of hypertension may reduce the risk of incident dementia, although the recent HYVET-COG study of those aged $\geq$80 years treated with indapamide with option of perindopril or placebo found no effect on dementia. Despite the benefit of statins in reducing stroke by 30%, this did not translate into benefits in cognition in the PROSPER study.

In the later stages of disease, VaD is often associated with a greater degree of physical, behavioural and functional issues than in AD. The goal of treatment is then shifted to the alleviation of morbidity and caregiver burden and a multidisciplinary team input is often required.

Lewy body disease

There is growing appreciation that dementia with Lewy bodies (DLB) and Parkinson's disease dementia (PDD) are actually part of the spectrum of Lewy body disease (LBD).[11] Differences in early disease presentation in DLB and PDD gradually merge into a similar common pathway as the disease progresses, such that they share identical features in the end stage (Figure 79.3). The hallmark of both diseases is the presence of Lewy bodies, which are related to dysregulation of the synaptic protein, α-synuclein and suggest neurobiological links with other synucleinopathies such as multiple system atrophy (MSA). Recent evidence suggests that it is the presynaptic α-synuclein aggregates, rather than Lewy body pathology, that are synapto-toxic and cause neurodegeneration in LBD.

PDD should be used to describe dementia that develops in the context of established Parkinson's disease, whereas a diagnosis of DLB is appropriate when dementia precedes or coincides within 1 year of the development of motor symptoms.[12,13] Within these two 'extremes' of the DLB–PDD spectrum, considerable variation and overlap in disease presentation have been described, for instance, insidious onset of mild parkinsonism and forgetfulness or visual hallucinations early in the course of PD. The likelihood of clinically presenting as 'typical' DLB (Table 79.5) is directly related to the distribution of Lewy body pathology and inversely related to the severity of AD pathology.[12] Three patterns of Lewy body pathology have been described: (1) brainstem-predominant, corresponding to the clinical phenotype of PDD, (2) cerebral cortex-predominant, corresponding to the clinical phenotype of DLB, and (3) transitional pattern, with distribution of Lewy pathology and clinical phenotype intermediate between the other two subtypes. In addition, concomitant AD pathology is also present in 90% of LBD cases (more commonly β-amyloid plaques and, to a lesser extent, neurofibrillary tangles). Compared with those with mild or no neurofibrillary tangle pathology, DLB patients with marked concurrent tangle pathology often present with an insidious amnestic syndrome more suggestive of AD and there are also fewer cognitive fluctuations, fewer neuropsychiatric symptoms and less parkinsonism.[11]

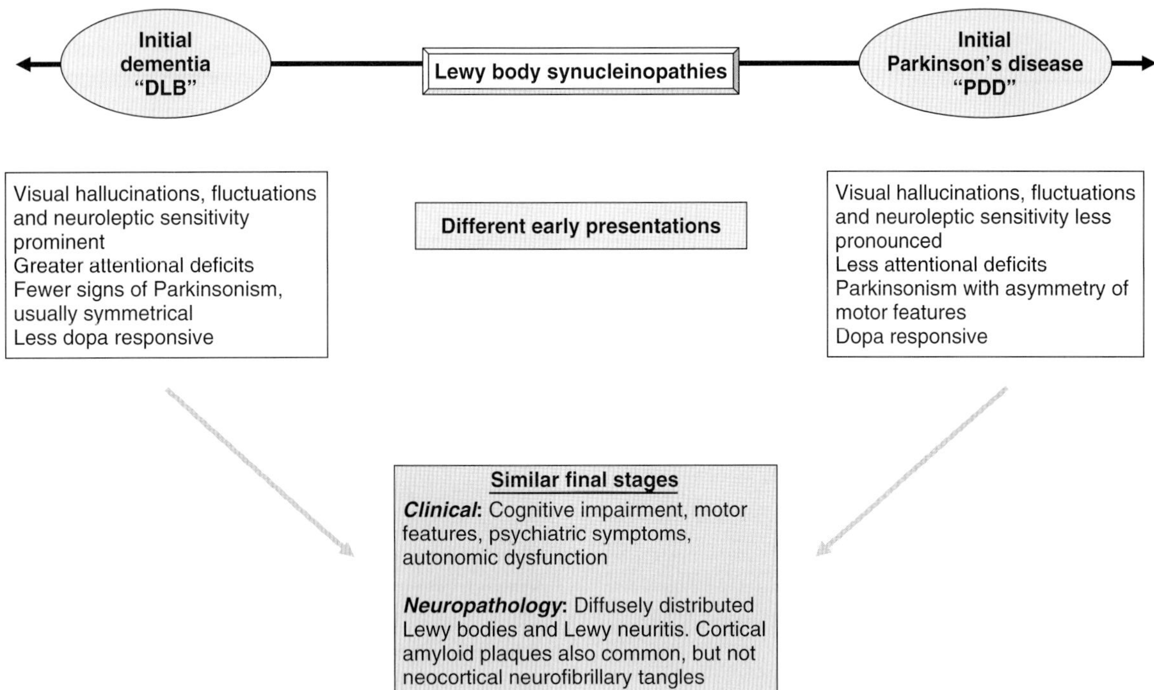

Figure 79.3 Schematic representation depicting how dementia with Lewy bodies (DLB) and Parkinson's disease with dementia (PDD) represent different points in the spectrum of Lewy body disease. Although the initial clinical manifestations of DLB and PDD differ, they are often indistinguishable in terms of clinical and neuropathological features by the end stage.

Dementia with Lewy bodies

DLB is now the preferred term for a series of diagnostic appellations that can be found in the older literature, including Lewy body variant of AD, Lewy body dementia, senile dementia of Lewy body type and cortical Lewy body disease. DLB represents the second most common cause of neurodegenerative dementia in older people after AD, accounting for ~15–20% in autopsy series. Onset of DLB is between 50 and 90 years of age and the duration of illness varies between 6 and 10 years.

Clinically, DLB is marked by a progressive dementia syndrome with fluctuating cognition and alertness, recurrent, well-formed visual hallucinations and parkinsonism (Table 79.5). Autopsy validation studies reported that previous criteria for DLB have high specificity (80–100%), but more limited sensitivity (35–80%). The latest consensus criteria were expanded to include suggestive features to address this limitation.[12]

The characteristic neuropsychological profile in early DLB is that of a 'dysexecutive' syndrome with prominent executive, attentional and visuospatial dysfunction. Amnesia may not be prominent or persistent in the early stages, but is usually evident with progression. Extrapyramidal motor symptoms in DLB are present in about 75% and consist primarily of bradykinesia, rigidity and postural instability. Compared with idiopathic Parkinson's disease, resting tremor is less common and, even if present, is never a prominent feature. Responsiveness to levodopa is also less pronounced.

Fluctuations in cognitive performance, attention and level of consciousness are the most characteristic feature of DLB. The marked amplitude between the best and worst performances distinguishes it from the minor day-to-day variations that commonly occur in dementia of any cause. Transient changes of consciousness in which patients are found mute and unresponsive for periods of several minutes may represent the extreme of fluctuation in arousal, but are often mistaken for transient ischaemic attacks despite a lack of focal neurological signs. One study reported that informant endorsement of at least three items out of four composite features of fluctuations (daytime drowsiness and lethargy, daytime sleep of $\geq$2 h, staring into space for long periods, episodes of disorganized speech) yielded a positive predictive value of 83% for DLB against the alternate diagnosis of AD.[14]

Prominent neuropsychiatric symptoms at time of presentation are among the defining features of DLB. Visual hallucinations are typically recurrent, well formed and detailed, and usually involve three-dimensional mute images of people and animals. Caregivers may under-report visual hallucinations, hence patient self-report can be useful. The presence of visual hallucinations is a marker of cortical LB pathology and greater cortical cholinergic deficits and

Table 79.5 Diagnostic criteria for dementia with Lewy bodies (DLB).

Central feature
Progressive cognitive decline with reduced social and occupational function
Core features
Fluctuating cognition with pronounced variations in attention and alertness
Recurrent vivid visual hallucinations
Spontaneous parkinsonism
Suggestive features
REM sleep disorder
Severe neuroleptic sensitivity
SPECT/PET imaging: low dopamine transporter uptake in basal ganglia
Probable DLB: 2 core OR at least 1 core plus 1 suggestive
Possible DLB: 1 core OR 1 suggestive
Supportive features
Repeated falls and syncope
Transient, unexplained loss of consciousness
Severe autonomic dysfunction, e.g. orthostatic hypotension, urinary incontinence
Systematized delusions
Hallucinations of other modalities
Depression
CT/MRI scan: relative preservation of medial temporal lobe structures
SPECT/PET perfusion scan: generalized low uptake with reduced occipital activity
EEG: prominent slow wave activity with temporal lobe transient sharp waves
Features less likely to be present
History of stroke
Any other physical illness or brain disorder sufficient to account for the clinical picture
If parkinsonism appears for first time only at severe stage of dementia

Modified from McKeith *et al.*[12]

predicts a good response to cholinergic therapy. Other common behavioural manifestations include hallucinations in other modalities, depression, misidentifications and systematized delusions. The most common form of delusions in DLB are misidentification delusions (i.e. delusions that someone is in the room, delusions that the home is not one's own or that television or movie personalities are actually present in the home), followed by persecutory/paranoid delusions, phantom boarder delusions (the belief that an unwanted person is living in the house) and abandonment delusions.

Rapid eye movement (REM) sleep behaviour disorder (RBD) is manifested by vivid and often frightening dreams during REM sleep. Because the usual limb atony in REM sleep is lost, patients are able to 'act out their dreams'. They may talk or shout in their sleep, strike out at their bed partner and even fall out of bed. As the patient may have little recall of these episodes, history is obtained from the bed partner. RBD is commonly a very early symptom that precedes the onset of dementia and parkinsonism by many years and, curiously, usually improves as the disease progresses. It is frequently associated with synucleinopathies (DLB, PD and MSA) and only rarely with other neurodegenerative disorders. Thus, a history of RBD, if present, is of great diagnostic utility because RBD can serve as a fairly specific antecedent biomarker of an underlying synucleinopathy.[15]

Approximately 50% of DLB patients do not react adversely to antipsychotic agents, hence a history of neuroleptic tolerance does not exclude a diagnosis of DLB. In contrast, a positive history of severe neuroleptic sensitivity is strongly suggestive. These range from sedation, increased confusion and worsening of parkinsonism, to more deleterious effects such as irreversible parkinsonism, impaired consciousness and marked autonomic disturbances. Autonomic dysfunction may occur early in DLB to produce orthostatic hypotension, urinary incontinence, constipation, impotence and swallowing difficulties. It can also contribute to repeated falls, syncope and transient loss of consciousness.

Differential diagnoses include other dementia syndromes such as AD and VaD, other causes of delirium, other neurological syndromes such as PD, progressive supranuclear palsy or Creutzfeld–Jakob disease and other psychiatric disorders such as late-onset delusional disorders, depressive psychosis and mania. Useful neuroimaging investigations in the diagnosis of DLB include (1) relative preservation of hippocampal and medial temporal lobe volume on MRI, (2) occipital hypoperfusion on SPECT imaging, compared with posterior parietotemporal hypoperfusion in AD, and (3) reduced dopamine transporter uptake in basal ganglia on SPECT/PET (single photon emission computed tomography/positive emission tomography) imaging. A multi-centre study reported the diagnostic utility of a ^{123}I-FP-CIT SPECT scan in the differential diagnosis of probable DLB and AD (sensitivity 78%, specificity 90%).[16] There is preliminary evidence that low α-synuclein levels in the cerebrospinal fluid may be a useful biomarker in the diagnosis of DLB.

Management of DLB involves the treatment of motor, cognitive, psychiatric and autonomic dysfunction. The clinician needs to be mindful of the tension between improving one symptom at the expense of worsening another – for example, aggravating hallucinations with levodopa. In the treatment of neuropsychiatric symptoms, conventional neuroleptic medications are best avoided, while atypical newer agents should be used judiciously. There is evidence that cholinesterase inhibitors (ChIs) are effective and relatively safe for the treatment of psychiatric and cognitive symptoms in DLB, with major side effects (mainly gastrointestinal) similar to those reported in AD. A recent case report highlighted that DLB patients may be more susceptible to bradyarrhythmic side effects from ChIs due to the associated autonomic dysfunction.[17] Memantine has recently been reported to produce cognitive and global benefits in DLB but without any significant improvement in psychiatric symptoms.[18] However, caution should be exercised as there are case reports of worsening of delusions and hallucinations with memantine use in DLB.

Parkinson's disease with dementia

It is now recognized that prevalence figures of 20–40% from earlier cross-sectional surveys of movement-disorder clinic populations underestimated the frequency of PDD. Subsequent long-term follow-up studies showed that 50–80% of PD patients will develop dementia, typically after 10–15 years of motor disability. Older age at PD onset, duration of motor symptoms, akinetic-rigid or postural instability gait disturbance phenotype (as opposed to the tremor-predominant subtype), reduced verbal fluency (naming the number of items belonging to a specific category, for example, animals, in 1 min), early hallucinations and mild cognitive impairment documented at first evaluation for PD increase the likelihood of PDD.[13]

Four salient issues related to the management of PDD are worth highlighting. First, from a diagnostic standpoint, clinical diagnostic criteria for PDD have been developed (Table 79.6).[19] Unlike AD, the initial impairment in PDD typically involves attention, executive function and visuospatial performance with only mild memory impairment in the initial stages. When evaluating cognitive function in PD, therefore, appropriate instruments that adequately evaluate the non-amnestic domains should be employed. In addition, tests that can be utilized by the clinician without the need for special expertise in neuropsychological testing have been proposed.[20] In the determination of dementia, it may also be difficult to judge the extent to which functional impairment is attributable to cognitive dysfunction rather than motor disability.

Second, the clinician should actively screen for and manage attendant neuropsychiatric and other non-motor issues that are common in PDD and can affect the quality of life of the patient and caregiver. The former include depression, anxiety, hallucinations, delusions and apathy. Among depressive mood disorders, dysphoria (40–58%) is more common than major depression (13%). Anxiety is common in PDD, especially in the 'off' period of treatment, and usually coexists with depression. The phenomenology of hallucinations is similar to DLB and comprises complex, formed visions of people or animals that are vivid in coloration. Delusions can be 'feeling of presence', phantom boarder, paranoid or grandiose type. Other non-motor complications in PDD include sleep disorders (such as restless leg syndrome, excessive daytime sleepiness and REM sleep disorders) and autonomic dysfunction.

Table 79.6 Diagnostic criteria for Parkinson's disease with dementia (PDD).

I Core features
1 Diagnosis of Parkinson's disease
2 Dementia syndrome developing within the context of established Parkinson's disease

II Associated clinical features

Cognitive features
- Impaired attention, executive function and visuospatial function
- Impaired retrieval failure-type memory (free recall that does not improve with cueing or in recognition tasks)

Behavioural features
- Apathy, depression, anxiety, delusions, hallucinations and excessive daytime sleepiness
- Presence of at least one behavioural symptom supports but is *not required* for the diagnosis of PDD

III Features that make the diagnosis uncertain but do not exclude PDD
1 Coexistence of another abnormality that may by itself cause cognitive impairment, e.g. presence of relevant vascular disease in imaging
2 Time interval between development of motor and cognitive symptoms not known

IV Features that are not compatible with diagnosis of PDD
1 Cognitive and behavioural symptoms appearing *solely* in the context of other exclusionary conditions, such as:
2 Drug intoxication
3 Acute delirium
4 Major depression
5 Probable vascular dementia by NINDS–AIREN criteria

Probable PD: criteria I–IV met
Possible PDD: criteria I and IV met, BUT II, III or both not met

Modified from Emre *et al.*[19]

Third, managing clinicians should be mindful of treatment-associated side effects that can occur with agents used for treatment of motor symptoms (such as levodopa, dopamine agonists and anticholinergic agents) and behavioural symptoms (such as antipsychotic agents). Severe neuroleptic sensitivity has been reported in up to 40% of exposed PDD patients. Among antipsychotic agents, clozapine and quetiapine have been reported to be better tolerated in PDD patients.

Fourth, there is evidence from randomized controlled trials of PDD patients that cholinesterase inhibitors can offer modest improvements in memory mirroring the degree seen in AD, and also attention and neuropsychiatric features (especially hallucinations). Tremors occurred more frequently with treatment, but the overall motor function did not decline. Although improved cognition has been reported in patients with mild Parkinson's disease following the administration of levodopa, mixed results have been found in moderately to severely affected PD patients. A small randomized controlled study of PDD or DLB patients reported that memantine produced cognitive and global benefits but not in psychiatric symptoms; preliminary subgroup analyses suggested a more pronounce global response in PDD than in DLB.[18]

Progressive supranuclear palsy

Progressive supranuclear palsy (PSP) is a tauopathy characterized neuropathologically by marked midbrain atrophy, neurofibrillary tangles or neuropil threads in the basal ganglia and brainstem and tau-positive astrocytes. Clinically, it is the degenerative disorder most commonly confused with PD. According to the National Institute of Neurological Diseases and Stroke–Society for Progressive Supranuclear Palsy (NINDS–SPSP) criteria, key clinical features for probable PSP are onset at age 40 years or later, a gradually progressive course, paralysis of vertical gaze and prominent postural instability with falls in the first year of disease onset.[21] Other pertinent features include dysphagia, dysarthria leading to unintelligible speech and a dysexecutive pattern of cognitive impairment. Unlike PD, which is associated with delusions, hallucinations and depression, PSP tends to exhibit more apathy, anxiety, obsessive–compulsive behaviour and disinhibition.

Two main clinical subtypes have been described: (1) Richardson's syndrome (54%), which features early appearance of falls, absence of tremor, symmetry of signs and poor response to levodopa; and (2) PSP-parkinsonism (32%), characterized by delayed onset of falls, presence of tremor, asymmetry and response to levodopa. The presenting symptoms of PSP are often non-specific and include falls (62%), personality change (22%), giddiness and gait disturbance. In the first 2 years of disease, characteristic signs of vertical gaze paresis, dysarthria and dysphagia are subtle or absent. About 40% of PSP cases do not exhibit falls in the first 2 years, especially in the PSP-parkinsonism subtype. It is therefore not surprising that the diagnosis of PSP is often delayed with a mean time of 3.9 years from symptom onset to a correct diagnosis.[22]

Several features may alert the astute clinician to the possibility of PSP. These include early instability and falls, especially in the first year of symptom onset, speech and swallowing difficulties early in the disease course, florid frontal lobe symptomatology such as apathy, impaired abstract thought, decreased verbal fluency or frontal release signs, and a predominantly axial pattern of parkinsonism that shows an absent, poor or waning response to levodopa. The hallmark of PSP is vertical supranuclear gaze palsy, which is characterized by disproportionate limitation of downward gaze (in contrast to the limitation of upward gaze that occurs in normal aging and PD) occurring in the presence of intact oculocephalic reflexes. Among the earliest signs of PSP is slowing of voluntary downward saccades, which appears long before the restriction in amplitude of vertical gaze range.[22] This is easily tested by asking the patient to shift gaze quickly from the primary position to the floor. MRI may show disproportionate atrophy of the dorsal midbrain ('hummingbird sign') or increased iron deposition in the lateral putamen ('eye of the tiger' sign). PET/SPECT imaging shows hypoactivity of the frontal lobes.

Treatment is supportive and centred on falls prevention, and also aggressive surveillance and management of dysphagia. Cholinesterase inhibitors have not been shown to be useful in PSP. Unfortunately, the prognosis in PSP is generally poor, with progression to a chairbound state in a median of 5 years after symptom onset. Death, occurring at a median of 7 years, is often due to the sequelae from falls or dysphagia.

Corticobasal degeneration

Corticobasal degeneration (CBD) is a tauopathy which has substantial overlap with FTD and PSP. The cardinal neuropathological features are asymmetric cortical degeneration involving primarily the frontal and parietal regions, severe neuronal loss in the substantia nigra, ballooned achromatic cells and also tau-positive astrocytic plaques, neurofibrillary tangles and neuropil threads in the cortex, subcortex and brainstem. Clinically, CBD presents in the sixth or seventh decade of life with the following classical features: (1) unilateral parkinsonism that is unresponsive to levodopa; (2) asymmetrical movement disorder such as rigidity, dystonia or focal myoclonus; (3) cortical features such as asymmetric apraxia, cortical sensory loss (for instance, impaired two-point discrimination, agraphesthaesia and astereognosis), visual or sensory hemineglect and alien limb phenomenon; and (4) late-onset cognitive impairment.[22] In addition, CBD can also mimic other clinical syndromes such as primary progressive aphasia, frontotemporal dementia, progressive orofacial apraxia and or posterior cortical atrophy. Given the heterogeneous clinical presentation of CBD, it is unsurprising that the sensitivity of diagnosis of CBD is disappointingly low (30%) and patients with CBD pathology are often misdiagnosed with other conditions, most commonly FTD and PSP. Conversely, the pathological heterogeneity of the corticobasal syndrome means that those receiving a clinical diagnosis of CBD commonly demonstrate alternative pathologies at autopsy such as AD, Pick's disease, PSP and prion disease.

The myoclonus of CBD is typically focal, confined to the limb (usually the arm) and most prominent during voluntary action. Apraxia is classically of the ideomotor type, referring to inability to perform movements on command that is not explained by motor or sensory abnormalities. The apraxia is most severe in the limb affected by dystonia or myoclonus and, rarely, can involve buccofacial structures. In the alien limb phenomenon, the affected limb performs actions that are not consciously intended by the patient. CBD has a unique cognitive profile of combined cortical and frontal-subcortical deficits that is marked by executive dysfunction, visuospatial disturbances, retrieval memory deficit and aphasia. Behaviourally, depression and apathy are frequent and often prominent. MRI may reveal asymmetric frontoparietal atrophy, while functional PET/SPECT neuroimaging shows asymmetric changes typically maximal in the frontoparietal cortex that are most severe on the side contralateral to the affected limb.

Treatment is largely supportive in nature. There is typically little or no levodopa response and disease duration is 7 years on average. Benzodiazepines, most notably clonazepam, may improve myoclonus. Botulinum toxin may be useful for the treatment of dystonia, eyelid movement disorders and drooling.

Multiple system atrophy

Multiple system atrophy is a synucleinopathy characterized by α-synuclein-positive glial cytoplasmic inclusions in glial cells with neurodegenerative changes in striatonigral or olivipontocerebellar structures. It is a sporadic, progressive, adult-onset disorder characterized by autonomic dysfunction that includes MSA with predominant parkinsonism (MSA-P) and MSA with predominant cerebellar ataxia (MSA-C).[23] Onset after age 75 years, hallucinations not induced by drugs and dementia make the diagnosis of MSA unlikely. Nonetheless, cognitive changes, particularly with executive function, have been reported in neuropsychological studies. Among subtypes, MSA-P tends to have more severe and more widespread cognitive dysfunction than MSA-C. MRI may demonstrate atrophy in the putamen, pontine and middle cerebellar peduncle and the hot cross bun sign on T2 images; marked cortical atrophy is unusual in MSA. SPECT/PET functional imaging shows striatal or brainstem hypometabolism. Progression is more rapid than idiopathic PD, with 40% of patients markedly disabled or wheelchair-bound within 5 years of onset. Treatment is mainly supportive. Fludrocortisone or midodrine may be used for treating symptomatic postural hypotension

Frontotemporal lobar degeneration

Frontotemporal lobar degeneration (FTLD) denotes a spectrum of neurodegenerative disorders that are characterized by a progressive dementia syndrome with prominent behavioural and/or language dysfunction early in the course of the disease arising from relatively circumscribed frontal and temporal atrophy. Clinically, the relatively younger age of onset, the typical presentation of syndromes and focal asymmetric frontotemporal atrophy hint at the diagnosis of FTLD. FTLD is superior to 'dementia' as a generic term for this group of disorders, since patients may have progressive neurological dysfunction for substantial periods of time before meeting criteria for a dementia syndrome.

FTLD is a neuropathologically, genetically and clinically heterogeneous group of disorders. Histopathologically, both familial and sporadic FTLD can be broadly divided into FTLD-tauopathy and FTLD-U/TDP-43 types on the basis of immunohistochemical analysis.[24] Historically, FTLD has been subdivided into either a tau-positive or tau-negative disorder on the premise of two pathologically distinct substrates: (1) tau-positive pathology with or without Pick's bodies and (2) dementia lacking distinctive histopathology (DLDH) in the absence of any defining inclusions. Recent advances in immunohistochemistry techniques have elucidated that in the majority of FTLD cases erstwhile subtyped as DLDH, ubiquitin-positive/tau-negative intra-neuronal inclusions are actually present; some of these cases have clinical or pathological evidence of motor neurone disease (FTLD-MND) whereas others do not (FTLD-U). The field moved further forward with the discovery of TAR DNA-binding protein 43 (TDP-43), which is the major pathogenic protein underlying sporadic and familial FTLD-U and FTLD-MND, and also in amyotrophic lateral sclerosis. More than 95% of FTLD cases are TDP-43 proteinopathies (50–60%) or tauopathies (35–45%), with DLDH and TDP-43 negative ubiquitinated inclusions comprising the remaining 5%.

A family history of dementia is present in about 40% of first-degree relatives. About 10% of the familial cases and 0–3% of sporadic cases have been linked to specific mutations. Many of these mutations occur in the microtubule-associated protein tau (*MAPT*) gene on chromosome 17 and have been collectively referred to as FTD with parkinsonism linked to chromosome 17 (FTDP-17) in familial cases with evidence of parkinsonism. Mutations that have been linked to TDP-43 proteinopathies include the progranulin (PRGN) gene on chromosome 17 and the valosin-containing (VCP) gene, which cause the rare autosomal dominant disorder of inclusion body myopathy associated with Paget's disease of bone and FTD (IBMPFD).

It is estimated that 3–20% of all cases of dementia may be FTLD. FTLD is the second most common form of dementia in those who are younger than 65 years (after AD) and widely regarded as the third most common cause of neurodegenerative dementia overall (after AD and LBD).[25] Onset occurs most commonly between ages 45 and 65 years, although FTLD can present before the age of 30 years and also in the elderly. An epidemiological study in the USA reported FTLD incidence rates of 2.2 in the 40–49 age class, 3.3 in the 50–59 age class and 8.9 in the 60–69 age class. There

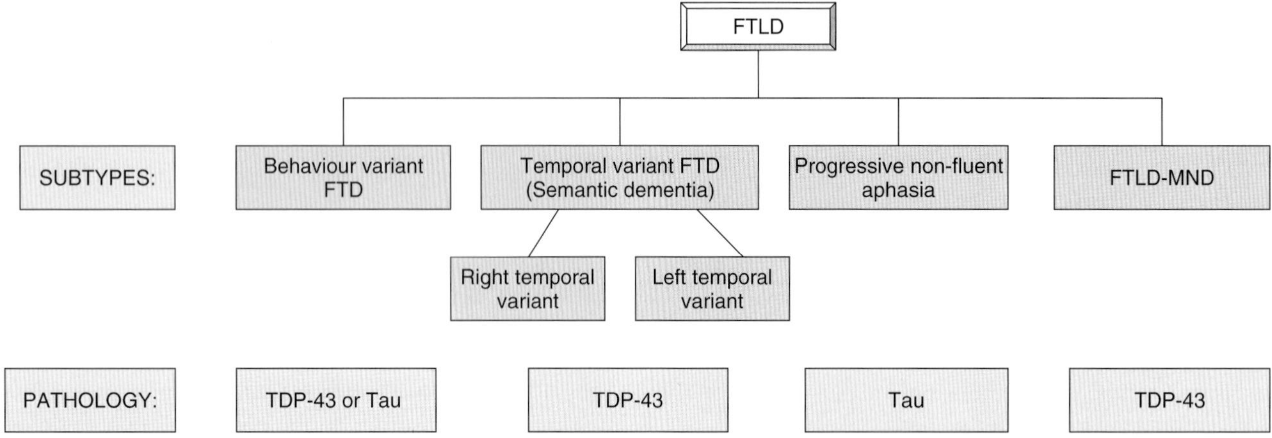

Figure 79.4 Clinicopathological correlation of the clinical subtypes of frontotemporal lobar degeneration (FTLD).

is an equal gender distribution. The duration of disease is in about 9 years in the FTLD-U and tau-positive groups, but significantly shorter at less than 3 years in FTLD-MND. Studies of age and education-adjusted autopsy-confirmed cases suggest that FTLD is associated with shorter survival and faster rates of cognitive and functional decline than AD.

There are three distinct clinical syndromes in FTLD, depending on the pre-eminent symptoms and the pattern of brain atrophy (Figure 79.4).[26] The commonest (at least 70%) is frontotemporal dementia (FTD), followed by semantic dementia (SD) (about 15%) and progressive non-fluent aphasia (PNFA) (about 10%). The right temporal variant of FTLD is a rare subtype characterized by asymmetric focal right temporal atrophy and can be considered to be the right hemispheric variant of SD. There can be substantial overlap between the three syndromes, and also with other clinical disorders, notably CBD and PSP. Motor neurone disease has been seen in combination with all three subtypes, but is most common with FTD and PNFA. All eventually worsen and produce a dementia syndrome. The clinical syndrome does not predict histological type, so that clinical distinctiveness itself does not imply aetiological difference.

Although there is too much overlap for reliable clinicopathological correlation, the clinical presentation may suggest which pathology is more likely (Figure 79.4).[27] Most patients with SD and FTLD-MND have TDP-43 proteinopathies, whereas PNFA (and CBD/PSP) is nearly always FTLD-tauopathy. The pathological correlate for bvFTD is evenly split between FTLD-tauopathy and FTLD-U/TDP-43. This concept of a TDP-43–tau pathological dichotomy has also been invoked in developing strategies for disease-modifying therapy that targets the underlying pathology in FTLD.

Frontotemporal dementia

Frontally predominant FTD, also known as behaviour variant FTD (bvFTD), is associated with atrophy of the frontal and/or anterior temporal cortex and subsequent involvement of the basal ganglia. Clinically, the salient characteristic is an early and profound alteration in personality and social conduct, occurring in the context of relative preservation of memory, spatial skills and praxis. Typical behaviours include disinhibition, apathy, social withdrawal, loss of empathy, hyperorality and dietary changes, diminished insight, neglect of personal hygiene, mental rigidity, perseveration, stereotypic behaviour and repetitive motor behaviours. Although repetitive and compulsive behaviours (such as tapping each wall twice upon entering a room, rereading the same book, walking to the same location repeatedly and clock-watching) can be present, bvFTD patients do not typically experience the feelings of anxiety and release from anxiety characteristic of obsessive–compulsive disorder. Dietary changes typically take the form of overeating, food fads and a preference for sweet foods. Utilization behaviours are common in the later stages; they refer to stimulus-bound behaviour in which patients grasp and use an object in their visual field despite its contextual inappropriateness (e.g. drinking from an empty cup). Also common are verbal stereotypies, involving the repeated use of a word, phrase or complete theme. When delusions occur, they are often bizarre and grandiose, but rarely persecutory. Progressive language loss or aphasia is often superimposed or appears simultaneously. Although there may be memory complaints, cognitive changes reflect frontal lobe dysfunction (inattention, poor abstraction, difficulty shifting mental set and perseverative tendencies) rather than a true amnestic syndrome. Table 79.7 summarizes the distinguishing features from AD.

Table 79.7 Distinguishing features between frontotemporal dementia and Alzheimer disease.

Clinical feature	Frontotemporal dementia	Alzheimer's disease
Cognitive		
Amnesia	Delayed until later in the course	Occurs early, *sine qua non* feature
Executive dysfunction	Early, progressive	Less prominent in early stages
Language	Reduction of speech output	Anomia with fluent aphasia; speech output preserved
Visuospatial skills	Relatively preserved	Involved early
Calculation	Relatively preserved	Involved early
Behavioural		
Disinhibition	Common	Occurs, but is less severe
Euphoria	Common	Rare
Stereotyped behaviour	Common and marked	Less common
Apathy	Common and severe with marked emotional blunting	Common, less severe
Dietary changes	Hyperorality and food fads (carbohydrate craving) common	Anorexia more common then overeating
Self-neglect	Common	Rare until late
Psychosis	Occurs, but is less common	Delusions and hallucinations more common
Imaging		
Structural MRI	Focal atrophy in frontal and/or anterior temporal lobes	Medial temporal lobe atrophy
	Usually asymmetric	Symmetrical
Functional. e.g. FDG-PET	Frontal and/or anterior temporal hypometabolism	Parietal and temporal hypometabolism

On physical examination, primitive reflexes such as grasping, pouting and sucking reflexes, occur earlier in the course then AD. Parkinsonian signs of akinesia, rigidity and tremor develop with disease progression. A minority of bvFTD patients develop fasiculations, wasting and weakness typical of motor neurone disease. Structural imaging with MRI is more sensitive than computed tomography (CT) in showing atrophy of the frontal and/or anterior temporal lobes, which is often asymmetric. Functional imaging such as PET or SPECT has high negative predictive value and a positive scan has high specificity for 'ruling in' FTD even in the absence of discernible atrophy on structural imaging. A longitudinal study of [^{18}F]fluorodeoxyglucose (FDG) PET imaging found that anterior hypometabolism progresses to include parietal and temporal regions over time, which may be mistaken for the parietal and temporal hypometabolism seen in AD. Functional imaging should therefore be performed early in the course of suspected FTD, when it is more likely to assist in differentiating FTD from AD.[25]

Semantic dementia

SD, also known as temporal variant FTD (tvFTD), begins with atrophy of the anterior temporal lobes with later involvement of the orbitofrontal cortex and basal ganglia. Clinically, patients with more significant *left* temporal atrophy present with progressive loss of ability to understand the meaning of words, although fluency is retained. Because of the loss of semantic knowledge, patients typically question the meaning of words they hear in conversation (for instance, 'What is spaghetti?'), giving the impression of impaired comprehension and repetition. Semantic paraphasic errors are common with word substitutions (such as 'food' for 'carrots') and later, fluent semantic jargon, often totally irrelevant to the questions asked or the topics discussed. They have difficulty reading irregular words due to the inability to move from orthograph to meaning (for example, 'gnat' is read as 'gunat'), although articulation, syntax and phonology remain intact. An unusual number of SD patients have an emergence of artistic talent in their dementia syndrome, reflecting the integrity and, possibly, disinhibition of right hemispheric activity. Clinical presentation in the *right* temporal variant includes prosopagnosia (impaired recognition of identity of familiar faces), topographic disorientation in familiar places, associative agnosia (impaired recognition of object identity) and, less commonly, complex visual hallucination. Typical behavioural changes in SD include irritability, impulsivity, bizarre alterations in dressing, mental rigidity and goal-directed compulsive collecting. Additionally, SD patients develop behavioural features that overlap considerably with bvFTD. The main differential diagnosis is AD, which can also manifest as a progressive fluent aphasic disorder. However, AD patients exhibit a greater degree of amnesia and concomitant visuospatial and calculation dysfunction. In addition, although both groups exhibit medial temporal lobe atrophy, there is asymmetric hippocampal atrophy and greater atrophy of the anterior temporal region in SD patients compared with AD.

Progressive non-fluent aphasia

PNFA is associated with atrophy of the left inferior frontal lobe, anterior insula and basal ganglia. The dominant feature is disorder of expressive language, presenting as progressively worsening non-fluent spontaneous speech with shortened phrase length, agrammatism (omission or incorrect use of grammatical terms including articles and prepositions), phonological paraphasia with sound-based errors and anomia. There is often accompanying stuttering, speech apraxia, impaired repetition with paraphasic intrusions, alexia and agraphia. In the early stages, comprehension is preserved for word meaning, but impaired for syntactic relationships. Often, executive function and working memory are impaired. Behaviourally, these patients may be impulsive, apathetic or depressed, but are generally appropriate and many have retained insight. Many patients with PNFA ultimately develop a clinical syndrome suggestive of either CBGD or PSP that is confirmed by neuropathology.

Treatment

As with other dementias, the management of FTLD is multifaceted. Caregiver education and support, and also optimization of non-pharmacological measures are paramount. Pharmacological treatment is currently aimed at symptomatic treatment with a focus on management of difficult behaviours and cognitive impairment. A host of disease-modifying strategies targeting the underlying pathology in FTLD are under investigation and tau-based therapies are already under way in the preclinical stage of investigation for FTLD.

Consistent with the selective vulnerability of serotonergic neurons in FTLD, a systematic review of selective serotonin reuptake inhibitors (SSRIs) and trazadone suggests that these medications offer modest benefits for improving the behavioural symptoms of bvFTD. The use of trazadone may be limited owing to its sedating side effects. Behaviours that may respond to SSRI treatment include impulsivity, disinhibition, repetitive stereotyped behaviours and obsessive–compulsive behaviour. Whereas depression is rare in bvFTD, it is more common in SD and PNFA patients and amenable to SSRI treatment. In general, apathy is recalcitrant to pharmacotherapy and can be a welcome relief for caregivers in the severely behaviourally disturbed patient. In some cases, bupropion (which has additional dopaminergic agonist properties) can be considered in FTLD patients with apathy and parkinsonism.[27] Atypical antipsychotic agents may be considered to treat delusions, severe agitation and aggression, but should be used sparingly in patients with FTLD owing to enhanced sensitivity to extrapyramidal side effects, somnolence, weight gain and exacerbation of apathy.

Less success has been reported in treating the cognitive symptoms of bvFTD. Unlike AD, there is no demonstrable cholinergic deficit in FTLD. Studies using cholinesterase inhibitors (ChIs) have produced mixed results. Although some open-label studies have reported a possible benefit, experience from a number of FTD-specialty clinics suggests that ChIs frequently worsen behavioural symptoms in bvFTD patients. Three open-label studies of memantine in bvFTD have been reported, all suggesting that memantine is well tolerated although no clear evidence of efficacy could be identified. A recent open-label study of memantine treatment in the three subtypes of FTLD demonstrated only a transient benefit in behaviour in bvFTD, but there was no other benefit in cognition, behaviour or motor symptoms in bvFTD and the other two subtypes.[28]

Motor impairments, including atypical parkinsonism or weakness from motor neuron involvement, are commonly observed with more advanced disease. When parkinsonism occurs early in the course of the disease, a trial of dopamine agonist therapy should be considered. Generally, axial instability and dysphagia are recalcitrant to such treatment, but patients may experience more fluidity of movements. Patients with FTLD should be evaluated thoroughly for signs of motor neuron disease and, when appropriate, referred to a neuromuscular specialist. Patients with FTD-MND can be started on riluzole, which is generally well tolerated and has low drug–drug interactions with antidepressants and memantine.[27]

Depression

Depression is common among the elderly. The term *pseudodementia* was coined to reflect impairment in thinking and memory that frequently accompanies depression. The cognitive domains affected in depression include slowed mental processing and deficits in attention and executive function. Individuals with late-onset depression tend to exhibit more significant cognitive impairment.

Making a diagnosis of depression in a patient presenting with cognitive impairment can be difficult, since the patient may not complain of classical mood changes or have comorbid medical conditions that confound interpretation of 'physical' symptoms of sleep, appetite/weight, psychomotor change and energy disturbance. Although certain clinical features can be helpful in the differential diagnosis of dementia and depression, none are diagnostic and frequent exceptions and overlaps exist. It is helpful to keep in mind three possible relationships that can exist between depression and dementia.

First, the two conditions often coexist. Epidemiological data indicate prevalence rates of 30–50% for depressive symptoms among AD patients, especially in the earlier stages of dementia where insight is often retained. Depression does not generally have a profound impact on cognitive performance in early-stage AD. Hence it is often the experience that while antidepressant treatment of concomitant depression in dementia can result in impressive improvement in mood and quality of life, the cognitive impairment remains relatively unchanged.

Second, there is a growing body of evidence that baseline depression is a risk factor for incident dementia and cognitive decline.[29] Therefore, dementia needs to be entertained as a differential diagnosis in cases of long-standing depression where there is lack of cognitive improvement, despite adequate treatment of the underlying affective disorder.

Third, owing to the considerable overlap in symptoms, some individuals with dementia may be erroneously diagnosed as having depression instead. Features of depression such as loss of interest, decreased energy, psychomotor changes and decreased concentration lose diagnostic specificity in the presence of dementia. Affective symptoms such as guilt, expressions of worthlessness and suicidal thoughts, if present, are more useful in distinguishing depression from dementia. It is also important to give appropriate consideration to the proxy informant's subjective reports of symptoms of depression in a demented patient, as the latter tends to minimize or under-report depressive symptoms, particularly when there is lack of insight into the underlying cognitive deficits.

Since depression in the elderly is not always easily diagnosed, particularly in the context of dementia, an empirical trial of antidepressant therapy in cases of diagnostic uncertainty is a reasonable strategy. A 6–8 week treatment trial of an appropriate antidepressant without significant anticholinergic properties, such as the SSRIs, is relatively safe and can sometimes provide considerable improvement.

Medications

Strictly, medications cause a state of cognitive impairment secondary to chronic confusion or delirium rather than an actual dementia. As with depression, cognitive impairment due to medications is often superimposed on other dementing disorders. Virtually any medication, including many over-the-counter drugs, has been implicated. The commonest culprits are drugs that affect the cholinergic, dopaminergic, serotonergic and noradrenergic systems and can be remembered by the mnemonic ACUTE CHANGE IN MS (mental status) (Table 79.1).[30] Medications are potentially reversible causes of cognitive impairment, hence a high index of suspicion is required, especially if there is a clear temporal relationship between the onset of symptoms and change in type or dosage of medications. Removing or reducing unnecessary medications may improve cognition, even in patients with underlying neurodegenerative diseases such as AD.

Dementia with parkinsonism

General approach

The principal causes of cognitive impairment with parkinsonism in the elderly are listed in Table 79.8. When confronted with this diagnostic conundrum, a systematic approach would be to (1) exclude easily identifiable secondary causes and then (2) determine if the clinical picture supports a diagnosis of Parkinson's plus syndrome as opposed to idiopathic PD. Useful discriminating features in favour of Parkinson's plus syndrome are symmetrical onset of parkinsonism, absence of resting tremors and the presence of concomitant atypical features (history of poor response to levodopa, predominantly axial involvement, early severe dementia, early marked autonomic disturbance, gaze palsies and upper motor

Table 79.8 Causes of parkinsonism with cognitive impairment in the elderly.

Parkinson's disease
- Idiopathic
- Familial

Parkinsonism in other neurodegenerative diseases

Dementia with Lewy bodies
- Progressive supranuclear palsy
- Frontotemporal dementia with parkinsonism
- Multiple system atrophy (MSA)
  - MSA with predominant parkinsonism (MSA-P)
  - MSA with predominant cerebellar ataxia (MSA-C)
- Corticobasal degeneration
- Hallervorden–Spatz disease

Vascular dementia with parkinsonism

Post-encephalitic parkinsonism
- Encephalitis lethargica
- Other encephalitides, e.g. syphilis

Secondary parkinsonism
- Pharmacological: antipsychotic agents, especially the high-potency conventional agents and other dopamine blocking drugs
- Toxins: carbon monoxide intoxication, cyanide poisoning, methanol, ethanol
- Post-anoxic parkinsonism
- Dementia pugilistica
- Normal-pressure hydrocephalus
- Space-occupying lesions: tumours, blood clot, abscess
- Metabolic (e.g. Wilson's disease)

neuron findings). In a clinicopathological study that examined patients who exhibited two out of the three classic signs of parkinsonism (tremors, rigidity and bradykinesia), the strongest additional bedside predictor for idiopathic PD is the combination of (1) asymmetric onset, (2) no atypical features and (3) no alternative diagnosis.

In the clinical history, it is important to ascertain the onset, duration and progression of the illness. A younger age of onset would alert the clinician to familial syndromes, hereditary illnesses (e.g. Wilson's disease) and certain neurodegenerative causes such as FTLD and MSA. Cognitive decline without significant progression over time is not, in general, likely to be secondary to neurodegenerative causes since once symptomatic, these tend to be progressive. Chronology of presenting symptoms, in particular the temporal relationship between the onset of parkinsonism and dementia, can yield useful information. For instance, dementia onset more than 12 months after the initial motor symptoms of parkinsonism favours the diagnosis of PDD rather than DLB. Marked fluctuations in cognition, attention and alertness are pathognomonic of DLB and PDD, although it is prudent to exclude delirium and its myriad causes if the duration is short. A history of frequent falls early in the course of disease suggests PSP, although this can also be seen in PD, DLB, MSA and NPH. Early dysphagia or dysarthria is characteristic of PSP. Compared with AD, the degree of memory impairment in the group of dementias with parkinsonism is comparatively milder by disease stage and there are usually more neuropsychiatric features at the time of presentation. FTD patients are more likely to manifest euphoria and disinhibition, whereas visual hallucinations, delusions and misidentifications are more common in DLB and PDD. A detailed family history and medication review cannot be overemphasized. Other relevant history includes occupational history (e.g. dementia pugilistica results from recurrent significant head trauma and classically occurs in boxers), ethanol ingestion and significant illnesses (e.g. strokes, encephalitis).

Pertinent pointers during physical examination include examination of the eyes (impairment of vertical gaze with intact oculocephalic reflex in PSP), cerebellar signs (MSA-C), pattern of extrapyramidal involvement (PSP is characterized by predominantly axial as opposed to appendicular rigidity), postural blood pressure (orthostatic hypotension from autonomic dysfunction is a feature of MSA, but can also occur in DLB and PD; it can also be secondary to drug treatment with levodopa and dopamine agonists), higher cortical function (asymmetric limb apraxia and cortical sensory loss in corticobasal degeneration) and gait (apraxic gait typically in NPH, but also seen in Binswanger's disease and SIVD). Structural neuroimaging with CT or MRI can yield useful information about the differential diagnosis: hydrocephalus, space-occupying lesions, evidence of cerebrovascular disease such as lacunar infarcts, white matter hyperintensities or cerebral microbleeds, midbrain atrophy which is typical of PSP, pontine and cerebellar atrophy and the hot cross bun sign evident in MSA. Hypointensity of the striatum on MRI is generally against the diagnosis of idiopathic PD.

Conclusion

Non-Alzheimer dementias constitute a significant proportion of dementia aetiologies in epidemiological studies. It is important to diagnose non-Alzheimer's dementias accurately, as they often carry different prognoses and entail different treatment considerations from AD. Atypical features that arouse a suspicion of non-Alzheimer's dementia are most salient early in the course of disease and include prominent executive dysfunction, marked speech disturbance, marked behavioural changes (such as disinhibition, euphoria, stereotyped behaviour, apathy and self-neglect), frequent falls, vivid visual hallucinations, focal neurological deficit, extrapyramidal signs, vertical gaze limitation and asymmetric apraxia/dystonia. The major degenerative subtypes are vascular dementia (VaD), dementia with Lewy bodies (DLB), Parkinson's disease dementia (PDD) and frontotemporal dementia (FTD). These conditions have distinct clinical features and can often be reliably distinguished clinically from AD through the use of standard criteria and ancillary structural and functional neuroimaging modalities. With data from recently completed studies, and also recent advances in histopathological and diagnostic techniques, there is now a broader evidence base that the clinician can draw upon to guide the evaluation and management of non-Alzheimer's dementia.

Key points

- Vascular dementia is the most common dementia other than Alzheimer's disease.
- Lewy body dementia is associated with abnormal behaviours.
- Frontotemporal dementia is associated with apathy.
- Atypical features of dementia should arouse the suspicion that it is not due to Alzheimer's disease.

References

1. Stevens T, Livingston G, Kitchen G *et al.* Islington study of dementia subtypes in the community. *Br J Psychiatry* 2002; **180**:270–6.
2. Zhang ZX, Zahner GE, Roman GC *et al.* Dementia subtypes in China: prevalence in Beijing, Xian, Shanghai and Chengdu. *Arch Neurol* 2005;**62**:447–53.

3. Kalaria RN, Kenny RA, Ballard CG *et al*. Towards defining the neuropathological substrates of vascular dementia. *J Neurol Sci* 2004;**226**:75–80.
4. O'Brien JT. Vascular cognitive impairment. *Am J Psychiatry* 2006;**14**:724–33.
5. Roman GC, Tatemichi TK, Erkinjuntti T *et al*. Vascular dementia: diagnostic criteria for research studies. Report of the NINDS–AIREN international workshop. *Neurology* 1993;**43**:250–60.
6. Bowler JV. Vascular cognitive impairment. *J Neurol Neurosurg Psychiatry* 2005;**76**(Suppl):v35–44.
7. Moorhouse P and Rockwood K. Vascular cognitive impairment: current concepts and clinical developments. *Lancet Neurol* 2008;**7**:246–55.
8. Viswanathan A, Rocca WA and Tzourio C. Vascular risk fact ors and dementia: how to move forward? *Neurology* 2009;**72**:368–74.
9. Roman GV. Vascular dementia: distinguishing characteristics, treatment and prevention. *J Am Geriatr Soc* 2003;**51**: S296–304.
10. Gorelick PB and Bowler JV. Advances in vascular cognitive impairment. *Stroke* 2010;**41**:e93–8.
11. McKeith I. Dementia with Lewy bodies and Parkinson's disease with dementia: where two worlds collide. *Pract Neurol* 2007;**7**:374–82.
12. McKeith I, Dickson D, Emre M *et al*. Diagnosis and management of dementia with Lewy bodies: Third Report of the DLB Consortium. *Neurology* 2005;**65**:1863–72.
13. Goetz CG, Emre M and Dubois B. Parkinson's disease dementia: definitions, guidelines and research perspectives in diagnosis. *Ann Neurol* 2008;**64**(Suppl): S81–92.
14. Ferman TJ, Smith GE, Boeve BF *et al*. DLB fluctuations: specific features that reliably differentiate DLB from AD and normal aging. *Neurology* 2004;**62**:181–7.
15. Boeve BF and Saper CB. REM sleep behavior disorder. A possible early marker for synucleinopathies. *Neurology* 2006;**66**:796–7.
16. McKeith I, O'Brien J, Walker Z *et al*. Sensitivity and specificity of dopamine transporter imaging with ^{123}I-FP-CIT SPECT in dementia with Lewy bodies: a phase III, multicentre study. *Lancet Neurol* 2007;**6**:305–13.
17. Rosenbloom MH, Finley R, Scheinman MM *et al*. Donepezil-associated bradyarrhythmia in a patient with dementia with Lewy bodies. *Alzheimer Dis Assoc Disord* 2010;**24**:209–11.
18. Aarsland D, Ballard C, Walker Z *et al*. Memantine in patients with Parkinson's disease dementia or dementia with Lewy bodies: a double-blind, placebo-controlled, multicentre trial. *Lancet Neurol* 2009;**8**:613–8.
19. Emre M, Aarsland D, Brown R *et al*. Clinical diagnostic criteria for dementia associated with Parkinson's disease. *Mov Disord* 2007;**22**:1689–707.
20. Litvan I, Agid Y, Calne D *et al*. Clinical research criteria for the diagnosis of progressive supranuclear palsy (Steele–Richardson–Olszewski syndrome): report of the NINDS–SPSP International Workshop. *Neurology* 1996;**47**: 1–9.
21. Golbe LI. Early diagnosis of progressive supranuclear palsy. Bucking the odds. *Neurology* 2008;**71**:1754–55.
22. Riley DE and Lang AE. Clinical diagnostic criteria. In: I Litvan, CG Goetz and AE Lang (eds), *Corticobasal Degeneration and Related Disorders*, Lippincott Williams & Williams, Philadelphia, 2000, pp. 29–34.
23. Gilman S, Wenning GK, Low PA *et al*. Second consensus statement on the diagnosis of multiple system atrophy. *Neurology* 2008;**71**:670–6.
24. Cairns NJ, Bigio EH, Mackenzie IR *et al*. Neuropathologic diagnostic and nosologic criteria for frontotemporal lobar degeneration: consensus of the Consortium for Frontotemporal Lobar Degeneration. *Acta Neuropathol* 2007;**114**:5–22.
25. Arvanitakis Z. Update on frontotemporal dementia. *Neurologist* 2010;**16**:16–22.
26. Neary D, Snowden JS, Gustafson L *et al*. Frontotemporal lobar degeneration: a consensus on clinical diagnostic criteria. *Neurology* 1998;**51**:1546–54.
27. Vossel KA and Miller BL. New approaches to the treatment of frontotemporal lobar degeneration. *Curr Opin Neurol* 2008;**21**:708–16.
28. Boxer AL, Lipton AM, Womack K *et al*. An open label study of memantine in three sub-types of frontotemporal lobar degeneration. *Alzheimer Dis Assoc Disord* 2009;**23**:211–7.
29. Saczynski JS, Beiser A, Seshadri S *et al*. Depressive symptoms and risk of dementia. The Framingham Heart Study. *Neurology* 2010;**75**:35–41.
30. Flaherty JH. Psychotherapeutic agents in older adults. Commonly prescribed and over-the-counter medications: causes of confusion. *Clin Geriatr Med* 1998;**14**:101–27.

CHAPTER 80

Treatment of behavioural disorders

Ladislav Volicer
University of South Florida, Tampa, FL, USA

Introduction

Behavioural disorders in elderly individuals are most commonly caused by a dementing process. Individuals who suffered from lifelong psychiatric diseases, such as schizophrenia, might continue to exhibit symptoms of these diseases even in old age, but management of these symptoms follows general psychiatric practice. Therefore, this chapter concentrates on behavioural disorders caused by a progressive degenerative dementia.

Problem behaviour is a serious aspect of progressive dementias and is the most common reason for institutionalization.[1] The most common progressive dementias are Alzheimer's disease, vascular dementia, dementia with Lewy bodies and frontotemporal dementia. A behavioural disorder may also be caused by a delirium that is induced by an acute medical or surgical condition (e.g. infections, dehydration, metabolic disorder) or by adverse effects of medications (e.g. drugs that have anticholinergic effect such as diphenhydramine, thioridazine and benztropine, cardiac medications such as digoxin and antihypertensive agents and drugs used to treat peptic ulcers such as cimetidine). Individuals with dementia are more sensitive to development of delirium and occurrence of delirium in cognitively intact individuals is an indication that the individual is at high risk of developing dementia.

Delirium is characterized by an acute onset of mental status change, fluctuating course, decreased ability to focus, sustain and shift attention and either disorganized thinking or an altered level of consciousness that resolves if the precipitating causes are removed (see Chapter 71, Delirium). However, diagnosis of delirium is not easy because some of these diagnostic criteria are not unique to delirium. Acute onset of mental status change may be caused also by a vascular dementia and fluctuating course of cognitive impairment is an important clinical diagnostic feature of dementia with Lewy bodies. Delirium is also not always a transient cognitive impairment because cognitive impairment resolves within 3 months in only 20% of patients with diagnosis of delirium. The specific symptoms of reversible dysfunction include plucking at bedclothes, poor attention, incoherent speech, abnormal associations and slow, vague thoughts. Delirium superimposed on dementia ranges from 22 to 89% of hospitalized and community populations aged 65 years and older with dementia and has several adverse consequences including accelerated decline, need for institutionalization and increased mortality. Therefore, the possibility that delirium is responsible for the onset of new behavioural symptoms should always be considered.

The diagnostic criteria for Alzheimer's disease include multiple cognitive deficits manifested by both memory impairment and at least one other cognitive disturbance (aphasia, apraxia, agnosia or disturbance of executive functioning). These cognitive deficits have to be severe enough to cause significant impairment in social or occupational functioning and have to represent a significant decline from a previous level of functioning. The course of Alzheimer's disease is characterized by a gradual onset and continuing cognitive decline. The cognitive impairment cannot be due to other brain disease, to systemic disturbances that can cause dementia or to drug-induced effects. Clinical diagnosis of the Alzheimer's disease is tentative and needs to be supported by neuropathological examination of the brain after the patient dies. Hence the most definite clinical diagnosis of Alzheimer's disease is 'probable Alzheimer's disease', which is made when there are no other possible aetiological factors and 'Possible Alzheimer's disease' when other possible aetiological factors are also present.

There are several diagnostic sets of criteria for vascular dementia and they differ from each other (see Chapter 75, Vascular dementia). Vascular changes are often present together with Alzheimer changes during brain autopsy. Hence it is difficult to exclude the possibility that a patient has Alzheimer's disease even when several criteria for vascular dementia are met.

Dementia with Lewy bodies (also sometimes called *diffuse Lewy body disease*) is characterized by a fluctuating course of cognitive impairment that includes episodic confusion with

Principles and Practice of Geriatric Medicine, Fifth Edition. Edited by Alan J. Sinclair, John E. Morley and Bruno Vellas.

lucid intervals similar to delirium (see Chapter 79, Other Dementias). The diagnosis of frontotemporal dementia is based on personality changes and the presence of atrophy of the frontal brain areas in neuroimaging studies [computed tomography (CT) or magnetic resonance imaging (MRI) scan].

Physical causes of behavioural symptoms

Before any behavioural symptoms are ascribed to underlying dementia, possible physical causes have to be eliminated. Behavioural symptoms may be induced by an acute illness or by an exacerbation of a chronic condition. These conditions include cardiovascular disease, brain tumours, sensory deprivation (see Chapter 85, Disorders of the eye; Chapter 86, Auditory system), metabolic disorders, chronic obstructive pulmonary disease and anaemia. Acute illness can be an infection, acute abdominal conditions or an injury. Unrecognized pain is a common cause of behavioural symptoms and treatment of behavioural symptoms with acetaminophen may decrease the inappropriate use of psychoactive medications (see Chapter 69, Control of chronic pain). The pain could result from faecal impaction, urinary retention or unrecognized fracture, but the most common cause of chronic pain in nursing home residents is arthritis, followed by old fractures, neuropathy and malignancy. Detection of pain is difficult in individuals with dementia who cannot describe the pain and its location. A comprehensive evaluation of pain in non-communicative individual relies on the observation of facial expression, vocalization and body movements and tension and may use one of recently developed scales.[2]

Conceptual framework of behavioural symptoms of dementia

Although progressive degenerative dementias differ in their early presentation, the behavioural disorders that they cause in later stages of dementia are very similar. Several conceptual frameworks were developed to classify and describe behavioural symptoms of dementia on the basis of nursing, psychological or psychiatric concepts. A model integrating all these approaches postulates a hierarchy of causes of behavioural symptoms (Figure 80.1). At the core of these symptoms is the dementing process itself, which may be modified by the underlying personality of the individual. Primary consequences of dementia are functional impairment, mood disorders and delusions/hallucinations. These primary consequences, alone or in combination, lead to secondary consequences, namely inability to initiate meaningful activities, dependence in activities of daily living (ADLs), spatial disorientation and anxiety. Primary and secondary consequences of dementia cause peripheral symptoms: agitation, apathy, insomnia, interference with other residents, rejection of care, food refusal and elopement.

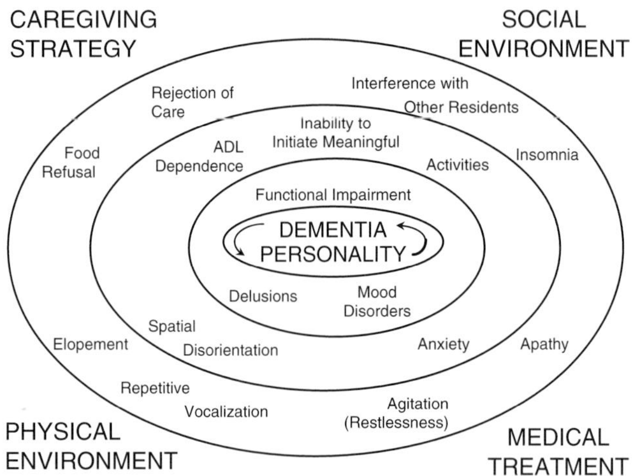

Figure 80.1 Comprehensive model of psychiatric symptoms of progressive degenerative dementias. Modified from Mahoney EK, Volicer L and Hurley AC. *Management of Challenging Behaviours in Dementia*, Health Professions Press, Baltimore, 2000, p. 2.

Peripheral symptoms may be caused by more than one of the primary and secondary consequences and each primary and secondary consequence can generate several peripheral symptoms. For instance, functional impairment may lead to an inability to initiate meaningful activities, dependence in ADLs and anxiety and agitation if stressful demands are made or agitation/apathy and repetitive vocalization if meaningful activities are not provided. Similarly, depression may lead to anxiety, worsening of the ability to initiate meaningful activities and to engage in ADLs, food refusal, agitation, insomnia and increased likelihood of rejection of care. Therefore, it is important to analyze the cause(s) of peripheral behavioural symptoms of dementia and treat effectively the primary or secondary consequences that are causing these symptoms instead of treating each peripheral symptom in isolation. Behavioural symptoms of dementia are influenced by four environmental factors: caregiving approaches, social environment, physical environment and medical interventions. The rest of this chapter describes in more detail elements of this model and therapeutic strategies that can be used.

Dementia and personality

Dementia is at the core of behavioural disorders. There is some evidence that premorbid personality traits are related to subsequent psychiatric symptoms. Patients who were more neurotic and less assertive before developing dementia are more likely to become depressed, whereas patients who were more hostile before developing dementia are more likely to have paranoid delusions. Patients who were neurotic and extroverted before developing dementia are more likely to engage in aggressive behaviour whereas previous agreeableness decreases the probability of aggression. Unfortunately, there is no treatment currently available that would stop or reverse the course of progressive degenerative dementias. However, there are currently two classes of medications approved for the treatment of Alzheimer's disease (Table 80.1). There is some evidence that cholinesterase inhibitors may also be useful for treatment of vascular dementia and dementia with Lewy bodies. Although the primary effect of cholinesterase inhibitors is the improvement of cognitive function, their administration also leads to some improvement in behavioural symptoms of dementia. Meta-analysis of published reports regarding the efficacy of cholinesterase inhibitors showed that the behaviour of patients treated with cholinesterase inhibitors improved significantly and there was no difference in efficacy among cholinesterase inhibitors.[3] Memantine treatment was associated with a reduced severity or emergence of specific symptoms, particularly agitation and aggression.[4]

Cholinesterase inhibitors may not be effective enough to control all behavioural symptoms of dementia, but they may be useful as a first-line treatment. Caregivers of individuals with dementia treated with donepezil report lower levels of behavioural disturbances than caregivers of individuals not receiving this treatment. Donepezil patients were described as significantly less likely to be threatening, to destroy property and to talk loudly. Cholinesterase inhibitors are usually well tolerated, with diarrhoea and nausea being the most common adverse effects.

Functional impairment

The presence of functional impairment that interferes with daily activities is necessary for the diagnosis of dementia. Functional impairment is a result of several deficits affecting both cognitive and physical functions. Memory impairment causes inability to remember appointments and prevents the individual from participating in social games, for example, bridge. Speech impairment interferes with social contact and may result in an inability to understand spoken or written language. Apraxia leads to the inability to use tools and to continue engagement in previous hobbies. Spatial disorientation leads to the inability to take independent walks. Executive dysfunction leads to deficits in problem solving and judgement and prevents the individual from planning and executing an activity.

Functional impairment may cause three secondary consequences of dementia: dependence in ADLs, inability to initiate meaningful activities and anxiety if a person with dementia recognizes his/her limitations or if a caregiver has unrealistic expectations about the abilities of the care recipient. These secondary consequences may cause several peripheral symptoms: rejection of care, agitation, repetitive vocalization, apathy and insomnia. Functional impairment may involve both cognitive and physical components.

Treatment of the cognitive component of functional impairment involves both behavioural and pharmacological approaches. Because of the progressive nature of dementia, the deficits cannot be reversed. However, they can be minimized and the function maintained for as long as possible by creating an environment in which the individual with dementia can experience positive emotions and by preventing excess disability that may be induced either by expecting too much or by expecting too little from the individual (see Chapter 141, Occupational therapy: achieving quality in daily living). In the mild to moderate stage of dementia, memory aids may be helpful. Verbal instructions, presented automatically through simple technology, were helping persons with mild to moderate Alzheimer's disease recapture independence in morning bathroom routine, dressing and table-setting.[5] Practice may also help maintain cognitive skills. Patients who performed exercises that included word fluency, immediate and long-term verbal and non-verbal recall and recognition and problem solving improved their cognitive function and had fewer

Table 80.1 Drugs for treatment of dementia.

Generic name	Trade name	Mechanism of action[a]	Daily doses (mg)	Maintenance dose[f]
Donepezil	Aricept	Inhibition of AChE	5, 10[b], 23[c]	10 or 23 mg QD
Galantamine	Razadyne	Inhibition of AChE, nicotinic	8, 16, 24[d]	8–12 mg BID
	Razadyne ER	receptor modulation		8–24 mg QAM with food
Rivastigmine	Exelon	Inhibition of AchE, inhibition of	3, 6, 9, 12[e]	4.5–6 mg BID
	Exelon patch	BChE	4.6–9.5[d]	9.5 mg QAM
Memantine	Namenda	Modulation of NMDA receptors	5, 10, 15, 20[d]	10 mg BID
	Namenda XR		7, 14, 21, 28[d]	28 mg QD

[a] AChE, acetylcholinesterase; BChE, butyrylcholinesterase; NMDA, *N*-methyl-D-aspartate.
[b] The dose should be increased after 4–6 weeks.
[c] The dose should be increased after 3 months of treatment with 10 mg dose.
[d] The dose should be increased if a lower dose is tolerated for 4 weeks.
[e] The dose should be increased every week.
[f] QD, once per day; BID, twice per day; TID, three times per day; QAM, every morning.

behavioural problems whereas the control group continued to decline. These results indicate that procedural learning can occur in individuals with dementia and that the rate of decline can be slowed by the prevention of excess disability. Individuals may also maintain ability to perform an activity (e.g. playing dominoes) even after they lose the ability to explain the rules.

Pharmacological management of cognitive component of functional impairment involves drugs used for treatment of dementia described above. There is good evidence that both cholinesterase inhibitors and memantine improve functional abilities temporarily or slow the rate of their loss. Multifactorial approaches to maintenance of cognitive function were also developed. In a study involving administration of *Ginkgo biloba*, vitamin C, vitamin E and low-fat diet and including meditation, mind-body exercises, physical exercises, stress reduction techniques and cognitive rehabilitation exercises, the experimental group improved in verbal fluency, controlled oral word association test and paired association.[6]

The physical component of functional impairment includes decreased ability to ambulate and eat. Individuals with dementia become unable to ambulate independently because they cannot recognize objects in their path and because neurological impairment leads to unsteady or narrow-based gait (see Chapter 91, Gait, balance and falls). Both of these consequences lead to an increased risk for falls. If the risk for falls is managed by restraints, the individuals deteriorate further because of deconditioning and forgetting how to walk. It is important to maintain ambulatory ability for as long as possible because walking represents meaningful activity and because inability to walk increases the risk of intercurrent infections and pressure ulcers. Ability to walk can be promoted by a regular walking programme and by assistive devices, such as a Merry Walker.

Mood disorders

Mood disorders that can occur in individuals with dementia include depressive disorders and bipolar disorder. Depressive disorders are major depression with or without psychosis, dysthymic disorder and minor depressive disorder (see Chapter 83, Depression in later life: aetiology, diagnosis and treatment). Depression is very common in community-dwelling individuals with dementia and should be considered even in individuals with advanced dementia. Depression can cause or aggravate the inability to initiate meaningful activity and dependence in ADLs and often has an anxiety component. These secondary consequences may lead to several peripheral symptoms, such as apathy, agitation, food refusal and repetitive vocalization. Depression may also increase the likelihood of rejection of care because depressed individuals ignore ADLs. Depression also increases the propensity for escalation of rejection of care into verbal or physical behaviours directed towards the caregivers because even cognitively intact depressed individuals are angry and do not tolerate others. Depression is one of the main risk factors for development of verbally and physically abusive behaviour.[7] Depressive symptomatology may be improved by providing sufficient meaningful activities, but often requires treatment with antidepressants.

The first-line drugs to use for treatment of depression in individuals with dementia are selective serotonin reuptake inhibitors (SSRIs) (Table 80.2). These medications are usually well tolerated, with the most common adverse effect

Table 80.2 Selected antidepressants for treatment of depression in individuals with dementia.

Drug class[a]	Name (trade name)	Dose range (mg per day)	Frequency[b]	Elimination half-life (h)
Tricyclics	Desipramine (Norpramin)	25–100	TID	14–25
	Nortryptyline (Pamelor)	25–50	BID–QID	15–39
SSRIs	Citalopram (Celexa)	20–60	QAM/QHS	33–37
	Escitalopram (Lexapro)	10–20	QAM/QHS	27–32
	Fluoxetine (Prozac)	10–40	QAM	4–6 days
	Fluvoxamine (Luvox)	50–300	QHS	15
	Paroxetine (Paxil)	20–50	QHS	15–22
	Sertraline (Zoloft)	50–200	QAM	22–32
SNRIs	Venlafaxine (Effexor)	25–75	BID/TID	3–7
	Duloxetine (Cymbalta)	30–90	AD-BID	11–16
Others	Bupropion (Wellbutrin)	150–300	QHS	12–30
	Mirtazepine (Remeron)	15–45	TID, QHS	25–40
	Trazodone (Desyrel)	50–300	BID-TID	8

[a]SSRIs, selective serotonin reuptake inhibitors; SNRIs, selective serotonin/norepinephrine reuptake inhibitors.

[b]QD, once per day; BID, twice per day; TID, three times per day; QID, four times per day; QAM, every morning; QHS, every evening.

being diarrhoea. Since many individuals with dementia suffer from constipation, this usually is not a problem. SSRIs have some differences in their effects. Fluoxetine is the most stimulating of them and may result in increased agitation while paroxetine is sedating. Both fluoxetine and paroxetine and to a lesser extent sertraline affect cytochrome P450 isoenzymes and interfere with the metabolism of several drugs. Escitalopram may be an improvement over the first-generation SSRIs because it is faster acting than citalopram.

In individuals who do not tolerate SSRIs, venlafaxine or bupropion may be used. Another option is mirtazepine, which may promote food intake in individuals with decreased appetite. Tricyclic antidepressants are used infrequently because they cause significant adverse effects that are partly mediated by an anticholinergic activity. Because of this activity, they are contraindicated in individuals treated with cholinesterase inhibitors. Trazodone is a relatively weak antidepressant but is useful for treatment of insomnia, as will be discussed below. Electroshock therapy is effective in the treatment of depression in elderly individuals but may increase memory loss caused by dementia. Treatment of psychotic depression requires the addition of antipsychotics to the antidepressant therapy. However, addition of an antipsychotic may be also effective in the treatment of resistant depression without psychotic features.

The prevalence of manic episodes in individuals with Alzheimer's disease and other dementias is relatively low and most of the individuals who exhibit them have a history of mania before the onset of Alzheimer's disease. Manic episodes are more common in people with cerebrovascular disease, especially when it involves the right hemisphere and orbitofrontal cortex. Manic symptomatology can be a significant cause of agitation and may also lead to interference with other residents, for example, unwelcome sexual advances.

Manic symptomatology is best treated with mood stabilizers (Table 80.3). Lithium is a drug of choice for the treatment of bipolar disorder in young individuals, but its use in older individuals is questionable because the elderly may have age-related decreased kidney function or diseases and drug treatments that affect lithium excretion. Valproate may have effects as good as or better than those with lithium in acute mania and carbamazepine is also effective. However, gabapentin, lamotrigine and topiramate were not found to be effective in the treatment of acute mania. Anticonvulsants are sometimes used to treat behavioural symptoms of dementia even when there is no evidence that mania is present. Topiramate was recently shown to be as effective as risperidone in the treatment of behavioural symptoms of dementia.

Carbamazepine is effective in the treatment of agitation in nursing home residents with dementia, but it has significant adverse effects that include rash, sedation, ataxia, agranulocytosis, hepatic dysfunction and electrolyte disturbance. Valproate may not be effective and high doses are associated with unacceptable rates of adverse effects, mainly sedation. Other potential adverse effects of valproic acid include weight gain, hair loss, thrombocytopenia and hepatic dysfunction. Gabapentin was reported to be effective in the management of behavioural problems in individuals with dementia in case reports and case series, but there is no randomized control study. Lamotrigine is also sometimes used for the treatment of behavioural symptoms of dementia but there are only limited data about its effectiveness and its use risks the development of life-threatening rash.

Delusions and hallucinations

Delusion is a false belief, based on incorrect inference about an external reality that is firmly sustained despite evidence to the contrary. Delusions are often combined with hallucinations, which are sensory perceptions occurring without the appropriate stimulation of the corresponding sensory organ. Delusions occur in about half of individuals with Alzheimer's disease. Most of them have only delusions, some have both delusions and hallucinations, while

Table 80.3 Selected mood stabilizers used in dementia.

Name (trade name)	Dose range (mg)	Frequency[a]	Elimination half-life (h)	Therapeutic level
Lithium (Eskalith, Lithobid, etc.)	100–300	BID–QID	22	0.6–1.2 mequiv. l^{-1}
Valproic acid (Depakene); divalproex sodium (Depakote)	100–300	BID–QID	9–16	50–125 $\mu g\, ml^{-1}$
Carbamazepine (Tegretol)	100–200	BID	25–65 (12–17)[b]	4–12 $\mu g\, ml^{-1}$
Gabapentin (Neurontin)	300–900	TID[c]	5–7	Not measured
Topiramate (Topamax)	100–400	BID	19–23	Not measured
Lamotrigine (Lamictal)	25–100	QD	24–34	Not measured

[a] BID, twice per day; TID, three times per day; QID, four times per day.
[b] After chronic administration.
[c] After titration phase (during titration, 300 mg once or twice per day).

isolated hallucinations are rare. Isolated hallucinations are more common in dementia with Lewy bodies. Delusions and hallucinations could be caused by other conditions. The most common one is delirium, which was described above.

Delusions may be divided into two types: simple persecutory delusions and complex, bizarre or multiple delusions (see Chapter 81, Geriatric psychiatry). Simple persecutory delusions include delusions of theft or suspicion. Suspicions involve beliefs such as being watched or having an unfaithful spouse. Complex delusions may include a conviction about a family member or a pet being injured, about plots against individuals of certain religious faith and about wild parties happening on a non-existing floor of the nursing home. An example of complex delusion is Capgras syndrome, which consists of a false belief that significant people have been replaced by identical-appearing impostors. Complex delusions may also present as grandiose delusions often connected with euphoria and hypomanic mood.

The most common delusions in Alzheimer patients are paranoid delusions and the most common of those are delusions of theft, which occurred in 28% of patients. The cause of these delusions may be a memory problem of the patient, who forgets where he or she has put personal belongings. Delusions of suspicion were seen in 9% of the patients and more complex delusions in 3.6%. A common delusion of suspicion is that other patients in a long-term care facility are criticizing the patient behind his or her back. A stimulus for this delusion may be an innocent conversation in the hallway that is not heard very well by the patient and is misinterpreted. A very common delusion is the belief that the patient is much younger than his or her actual age. This delusion may be connected with misidentification, for example, of the patient's wife as his mother.

Onset of hallucinations in Alzheimer's disease is usually later in the disease progression, more than 5 years after the onset of dementia or more than 1 year after diagnosis. In approximately half of the patients the hallucinations are temporary, whereas in other patients hallucinations persist until death. Therefore, it is important to re-evaluate frequently the need for pharmacological treatment in demented individuals. Hallucinations and delusions are associated with greater functional impairment and are more common in individuals who have extrapyramidal signs, such as muscle rigidity, and in individuals who have myoclonus. Delusions and hallucinations may cause several secondary and peripheral behavioural symptoms of dementia. They may induce anxiety and spatial disorientation and they may also interfere with ADLs because the individual does not believe that the activity is needed. This results in rejection of care that may result in physical or verbal behavioural symptoms directed towards the caregivers.[7] Delusions and hallucinations may also lead to food refusal if the individual believes that the food is poisoned and to attempts to leave a home or facility if the individual believes that they have to go to work or go 'home'. Misidentification of other residents and staff may lead to interference with other residents or inappropriate behaviour towards the staff.

Treatment of delusions and hallucinations should consider their relationship to other behavioural symptoms of dementia. Some individuals with dementia have many delusions or hallucinations but are not bothered by them and they do not affect them behaviourally. In that case, no treatment is necessary. Otherwise, it is important to attempt non-pharmacological management of delusions and hallucinations before initiating treatment with antipsychotic medications. Non-pharmacological management should include attention to sensory perceptions, environmental modifications and behavioural strategies. Improvement of vision or hearing may decrease auditory delusions or visual hallucinations. Increased lighting, decreased noise, safe space for ambulation and social environment of a dementia special care unit will decrease the need to treat delusions and hallucinations, which cause behaviours that may be distressing to other cognitively intact residents. Behavioural strategies should recognize that reasoning cannot change behaviour because the individual with dementia does not understand reasoning and does not remember what he or she was told; therefore, caregivers have to change their behaviour. Caregivers should avoid the word 'no' and instead of arguing distract the individual from undesirable activity. It is better to accept the individual's reality than to try to orient them to our reality. Also, the person with dementia should always be made comfortable by smiling, by a positive tone of voice and by answering in a positive way even if the individual's speech does not make sense.

Pharmacological treatment of delusions and hallucinations utilizes administration of antipsychotics (Table 80.4). Older antipsychotics, represented by haloperidol, were potent antagonists of dopamine receptors. This led to a high incidence of extrapyramidal side effects and akathisia. These drugs are mostly replaced by newer (atypical) antipsychotics that have a more beneficial adverse effect profile. This improvement is due to their effect on other than dopamine receptors. The most significant is blockade of the serotonin 2A receptors that prevents extrapyramidal side effects and may also lead to improvement in apathy. This activity is present in risperidone and olanzapine. However, activity at other receptors may lead to some adverse effects. Olanzapine and quetiapine block histamine 1 receptors, resulting in sedation and weight gain. The weight gain is especially troublesome in olanzapine, because it could lead to the development of diabetes. Blockade of noradrenergic alpha-1 receptors, that is present in quetiapine and risperidone, may lead to orthostatic

Table 80.4 Selected antipsychotics used for treatment in dementia.

Name (trade name)	Dose range (mg)	Frequency[a]	Elimination half-life (h)	Most common adverse effects
Aripiprazole (Abilify)	10–15	QD	75 (94)[b]	Insomnia, somnolence
Haloperidol (Haldol)	0.5–1	QD–TID	18	EPS[c], tardive dyskinesia
Olanzapine (Zyprexa)	2.5–10	QD	30	Weight gain, anticholinergic, sedation
Quetiapine (Seroquel)	25–100	BID–TID	6	Sedation, hypotension
Risperidone (Risperdal)	0.25–1	QD–BID	3–20 (21–30)[b]	EPS, hypotension
Ziprasidone (Geodon)	20–40	BID	4–10	QTc prolongation, hypotension, rash

[a]QD, once per day; BID, twice per day; TID, three times per day.
[b]Active metabolite.
[c]EPS, extrapyramidal side effects.

hypotension. Aripiprazole has a novel mechanism of action because it is a partial agonist on dopamine receptors. This effect prevents excessive dopamine activity while preserving normal dopamine function.

Antipsychotics are frequently used not only for the treatment of delusions and hallucinations but also for behavioural symptoms that may not be related to them, despite several meta-analysis studies indicating a moderate effect of only a few antipsychotics, namely olanzepine, aripiprazole and risperidone.[8] A nationwide study found that 32% of antipsychotic drug users had no identified clinical indication for this therapy and that prevalence of antipsychotic use differed significantly in different facilities. This prevalent use of antipsychotics mostly continues, despite recent warning about their serious side effects. Antipsychotics increase the risk of stroke and sudden cardiac death,[9] increase threefold the incidence of serious events in community-dwelling individuals and twice the incidence in nursing home residents, and increase the incidence of hip fractures and overall mortality rate. Therefore, it is important to avoid the use of antipsychotics if possible and to use the lowest effective dose when they are being used. Alternative medications that may be used instead of antipsychotics are described below in the section on rejection of care.

Dependence in activities of daily living (ADLs)

ADLs are the activities that are needed for self-care and independent living. They include instrumental activities of daily living (IADLs) and physical activities of daily living (PADLs) sometimes called *basic ADLs*. Dependence in ADLs is the result of functional impairment induced by dementia, but depression or delusions may aggravate the dependence, resulting in excess disability. Therefore, it is important to determine carefully the reasons for dependence. If the individual is dependent in PADLs, physical care has to be provided. The individual with dementia might not recognize the reason for this care and might reject it. This rejection may escalate into combative behaviour, as will be described below. Thus, ADL dependence may lead to significant behavioural changes.

IADLs include shopping, preparing meals, travelling, doing housework and laundry, using the telephone, taking medications and managing money. Continued participation in ADLs is important for the self-esteem of the individual with dementia, but safety and stress induced by these activities have to be considered. IADLs should be simplified because the individual with dementia may still be able to participate in some steps but not in the entire activity (Table 80.5). Supportive services, such as a homemaker or meals-on-wheels, may allow an individual with dementia to continue living in their own home. Assistance may come in many forms: encouragement, verbal cues, visual cues (gestures) and physical guidance.

PADLs include bathing, dressing, grooming, toileting, walking and eating. PADL functional abilities decline in a predictable temporal order according to the complexity of the ADL – bathing, dressing, grooming, toileting, walking and eating. Bathing is an activity that most often results

Table 80.5 Examples of IADL adaptations for individuals with dementia.

IADL	Suggested adaptations
Shopping	Plan and go shopping with others Continue to help choosing purchases
Meal preparation	Prepare one dish, with steps presented one at a time
Using telephone	Help person list things to talk about before making a call Help person call relatives and friends Put pictures of people on preprogrammed telephone buttons
Money management	Simplify bill-paying routine Carry small amount of money Make small purchases with assistance on shopping trips

in rejection of care. Strategies for bathing dependence are described below. A significant improvement in dressing performance can be achieved by implementing strategies that allow the person to dress themselves independently with as little help as possible. Strategies for toileting difficulties include behavioural interventions (prompted voiding), establishing a routine, clothing modifications, making going to the bathroom easier, becoming familiar with and watching for cues indicating that the individual needs to use the bathroom, preserving dignity and physical assistance to reach a bathroom. Independent eating is promoted by encouraging independence while providing supervision and assistance, by creating a social mealtime environment and by simplifying the eating process. Walking ability can be maintained for as long as possible by the use of assistive devices, such as a Merry Walker.

Inability to initiate meaningful activities

This inability is caused by functional impairment involving loss of executive function due to damage of the prefrontal cortex, but may also be aggravated by depression. Lack of meaningful activities may result in apathy or agitation, repetitive vocalization and insomnia, if the individual with dementia sleeps during the day. Involvement in meaningful activities is important for maintenance of functional abilities, social involvement, feeling of success and accomplishment, improvement in mood and reduction of disruptive behaviour.

Management goals for people with the inability to initiate meaningful activity are prevention of excess disability, improvement of their interaction with the environment and their quality of life. Excess disability may be caused by impaired hearing or sight and by depression. Therefore, it is important to correct sensory impairment and treat depression even in individuals with advanced dementia. Individuals with dementia who are unable to initiate meaningful activities may be unoccupied and appear bored or not engaged with the environment, sitting motionless or wandering around aimlessly with increased risk for falls. They spend more time in a state of inner retreat and this withdrawn behaviour may manifest itself as lack of behaviour, somnolence, perseveration or non-directed agitation.

The goal of management of the inability to initiate meaningful activities is to create an environment with optimal stimulation and a steady flow of meaningful activities that are adapted to the functional capacity of the individual with dementia. There is a need for three different programmes to meet the needs of individuals with different severities of dementia. Individuals with mild cognitive impairment and mild dementia may be unable to participate in regular activity programming that is targeted to cognitively intact residents. They may benefit from a memory enhancement programme that provides separate activities promoting cognitive functioning and a social environment providing contact with similarly impaired non-judgemental residents.[10]

As the dementia progresses, it becomes increasingly difficult to keep the individual engaged during activities because of their short attention span. An activity programme that provides continuous programming throughout the majority of residents' waking hours is not only an effective way to reduce psychotropic medication, reduce falls and social isolation,[11] but also helps individuals with dementia to live with some purpose and meaning in spite of the disease. General guidelines for planning activities for individuals with dementia are listed in Table 80.6. In an institution, the programming should take into consideration the routine that the individual had before admission for long-term care. The continuous programming for moderate dementia should begin with a morning routine that may include the Pledge of Allegiance (in the USA), a patriotic song, newspaper or weather report discussion. Exercise programmes, food and beverages served in a social atmosphere, word games and spelling bees should follow. All these programmes should be 'no fail' opportunities to have fun. An individualized programme that was found to decrease agitation and improve mood is Simulated Presence Therapy.[12] At the end of the day, active participants are tired and ready for a video or a movie, a snack and a peaceful sleep.

As dementia progresses into the severe stage, it becomes even more challenging to engage individuals in meaningful activities. They tend to sleep during programmes

Table 80.6 Guidelines for planning activities for people with dementia.

Principle	Rationale
Focus on enjoyment, not achievement	The goals of therapeutic programme are to prevent excess disability and help the person 'feel good'
Create a 'failure-free' environment	Helps person maintain self-esteem
Design therapeutic activities to stimulate multiple senses	The ability to experience a range of human responses (emotions, behaviour) continues across mild, moderate and severe stages of dementia
Make activities part of daily routine	Maintain home-like routines Make all activities (including ADLs) meaningful Not an extra burden for the caregiver
Plan structured activities that employ previously learned motor patterns	These tasks require no new learning, yet can make the person feel useful and productive

and may have difficulty communicating. Another level of programming, one that has more individual attention and has less physical activities, helps meet their needs at this stage. This programming may be provided by nursing staff in a special room reserved for residents who do not benefit from other activities. Namaste Care is a programme that provides continuous activity without the need for additional staff.[13] The staff provide more touch, respect when the resident needs to take short 'naps' and use more visual cues. Other activities useful in that stage include pet therapy, massage and Snoezelen.[14] Meaningful activities should be provided even for individuals in the terminal stage of dementia because Alzheimer's disease rarely, if ever, progresses to the persistent vegetative state.[15]

Anxiety

Anxiety is defined as a vague, uneasy feeling, the source of which is often non-specific or unknown to the individual who is experiencing it. Anxiety is a feeling of distress, subjectively experienced as fear or worry and objectively expressed through autonomic and central nervous system responses. Anxiety can be a symptom of depression or be caused by disturbing delusions and hallucinations. It also can be caused by a primary anxiety disorder such as generalized anxiety disorder, phobia, post-traumatic stress disorder and obsessive–compulsive disorder. However, new-onset primary anxiety disorders are unusual in older adults. In most instances, older people with primary anxiety disorders have a history of them and it is therefore important to obtain complete personal and family psychiatric history.

Anxiety may also be a symptom of physical illness or be caused by medications. It may be induced by decreased delivery of oxygen to the brain caused by cardiac or pulmonary disease and by endocrine disorders such as hyperthyroidism and hypoglycaemia. Medications that may cause anxiety as an adverse effect include anticholinergic drugs, caffeine, steroids, decongestants, bronchodilators, alcohol, narcotics, sedative–hypnotics and other psychotropic medications. Anxiety also may be a withdrawal symptom in individuals dependent on alcohol, benzodiazepines or sedatives/hypnotics.

Anxiety is very common in Alzheimer's disease, occurring in 52% of patients in mid and late stages of the disease. The prevalence of anxiety increases with the progression of the disease,[16] but it is present together with suspiciousness even in individuals with mild cognitive impairment. Anxiety is even more common in individuals with vascular dementia and frontotemporal dementia than in individuals with Alzheimer's disease.[16]

Presence of anxiety is associated with reduced functional status in performing ADLs and with sleep disturbances. Over half of individuals with Alzheimer's disease who were experiencing anxiety woke up their caregivers at least once at night during the past week. The awakenings are associated with higher levels of patient anxiety and impairment in ADLs. Anxiety may also lead to agitation and repetitive vocalization.

Non-pharmacological management of anxiety is based on decreasing the stress level to which the individual with dementia is exposed. This may be accomplished by rest periods that prevent fatigue, positive communication strategies, prevention of overstimulation by providing a low-stimulation environment and avoiding unfamiliar situations. Pharmacological management should first consider treatment of the primary consequences of dementia that may cause anxiety: mood disorders and delusions/hallucinations. Only if this approach is not effective or there is strong evidence that the anxiety is caused by a primary anxiety disorder should anxiolytic medications be used. These medications include administration of benzodiazepines and buspirone (Table 80.7). Only short-acting benzodiazepines should be used and they may be useful also for short-term treatment of an anxiety-induced catastrophic reaction that usually causes extreme agitation.

Table 80.7 Selected medication for treatment of anxiety.

Drug class	Name (trade name)	Dose range and frequency[a]	Elimination half-life (h)	Side effects
Benzodiazepines	Alprazolam (Xanax) Lorazepam (Ativan) Oxazepam (Serax)	0.25–0.5 mg TID 0.5–1 mg BID or TID 10–20 mg TID or QID	12 15 8	Sedation, impaired motor coordination, risk of falls, memory loss, respiratory depression, dependence, paradoxical reaction
Azapirones	Buspirone (Buspar)	5–20 mg TID	Onset of action 3–6 weeks	Headache, nausea, drowsiness, lightheadedness
Antidepressants	See Table 80.2			
Antipsychotics	See Table 80.4			

[a]QD, once per day; BID, twice per day; TID, three times per day.

Trazodone is another medication that may be useful on an as-needed basis because of its antidepressant and sedative effects.

Spatial disorientation

Spatial disorientation is the misperception of immediate surroundings; not being aware of one's setting or not knowing where one is in relation to the environment. Spatial disorientation may cause misunderstanding of the environment and lead to development of fear, anxiety, suspicions, delusions and safety problems such as getting lost. Getting lost may also lead to the occurrence of interference with other residents if an individual with dementia invades their space and the inability to find a bathroom contributes to ADL deficit. In the early stages of dementia, the individual may become confused when they are in an unfamiliar place. In the later stages, the individual becomes confused even in previously familiar places.

Spatial disorientation may be related to damage of a specific brain area, the posterior cingulate gyrus, because hypofunction of this area measured by positron emission tomography (PET) was associated with disorientation for place. Another brain area that is necessary for place navigation and is damaged severely in Alzheimer's disease is the hippocampus. A healthy hippocampus uses two mechanisms for spatial orientation: cognitive mapping and cue navigation. Cognitive mapping requires cognitive processing to identify and store mental images of the most frequently encountered elements in a particular environment and the ability to make the connections among those elements. Cue navigation works by selection of a single landmark that directs an individual towards a specific location in the environment. Individuals retain these cues longer when they are familiar and are strongly associated with an environmental landmark. Another factor that participates in spatial disorientation in Alzheimer's disease is impaired depth perception. Because of this impairment, a change in colour of a carpet or tile may be perceived as a step or obstacle.

Management of spatial disorientation utilizes information from these studies by using pop-up cues and environmental landmarks. The pop-up cues strategy attempts to simplify the detection of the cue by providing one salient feature and colour contrasts. If the cue is complex, it requires more cognitive processing than a simple cue. Individuals with dementia, who have impaired attention span and cognitive processing, may not recognize complex cues. Colour contrast improves detection of the cue. Thus, a white toilet in a red bathroom is easier to find than a white toilet in a white bathroom. Environmental landmark strategy utilizes long-term memory by either keeping the environment unchanged or by using familiar objects as landmarks in a new environment. Personal or emotionally charged objects should be used as orientation devices. It is also important to simplify the environment by removing clutter and scatter rugs. Spatial orientation is promoted by signs on doors of common rooms, personal pictures or items by the door of individual rooms, adequate lighting that does not cast shadows that may be misinterpreted and by establishing a walking area with colour-contrasting borders.

Rejection of care

'Reject evaluation or care' is a new terminology used in the Minimum Data Set (MDS) 3.0 instead of 'resist care' used in MDS 2.0. Therefore, rejection of care will be used in this chapter instead of resistiveness to care, but both of these terms describe the same behaviour. These behaviours occur primarily during hands-on care that includes bathing, dressing, toileting, eating and administering medication. They can also occur when the caregiver attempts to redirect the individual with dementia.

Rejection of care is caused by either misperception of the need for care activity or by misperception of the caregiver's intent (see Chapter 59, Communication disorders and dysphagia). Thus, an individual who does not recognize that they have soiled clothing will reject a caregiver's attempt to change their clothes. Communication difficulties may prevent the individual with dementia from recognizing what the caregiver's intent is. In both cases, the individual with dementia does not cooperate with the caregiver and actively resists the caregiver's approach. If the caregiver insists on providing care, the individual with dementia may defend themselves from this unwanted attention, becomes combative and even strikes out. Such an individual may be labelled 'aggressive'. However, the patient perceives the caregiver as the aggressor and just defends themselves. Most individuals with dementia are not aggressive unless provoked and most 'aggressive' behaviours reported in the literature occur in the context of personal care.

Several factors increase the probability of rejection of care. Delusions and hallucinations may prevent recognition of the need for care or lead to misidentification of a staff person. Depression increases rejection of care because depressed individuals are angry and do not tolerate others.[7] Spatial disorientation may result in increased need for toileting because the individual cannot find a bathroom. Management of these factors may decrease rejection of care but the most important factor for its management is the caregiver approach. Therefore, caregiver behaviour should always be evaluated when rejection of care occurs before initiation of any pharmacological therapy.

The goal of care is to prevent the escalation of rejecting behaviour into combative behaviour. The approach used by the caregiver is crucial. Relaxed and smiling caregiver behaviour is related to calm and functional behaviour of the individual with dementia. It is important to avoid making demands that create stress or are beyond the ability of the individual with dementia, avoid rushing through ADLs, avoid touching without warning, avoid painful procedures, avoid overstimulating the individual and express respect for the individual with dementia by allowing them to maintain some control. Distraction may be also used to direct the individual's attention away from the stressful stimulus. Engaging an individual in conversation on a favourite topic or reminiscing about happy memories that are retained takes the focus away from the task and places it on the person. This person-centred approach is effective even with individuals who have significant cognitive and language impairment. In an institutional setting, distraction may be accomplished by using two caregivers. While one caregiver engages the individual's attention by talking or singing, a second caregiver performs the ADL care.

Another important factor is the environment in which the care is provided. This is especially important for bathing. The bathroom should feel private and personal, it should be warm, have relaxing music, soft lighting, a low noise level, home-like furnishings, aromas to evoke memories and set mood and make the bathing experience pleasant, and the bathing equipment should be comfortable and functional. A very effective strategy for decreasing rejection of care is the modification of care procedures. Some individuals prefer to bathe in the morning and some in the afternoon or evening. It is also possible to make a shower more personal or to replace it with a bed bath that is much less stressful for an individual with dementia.

Pharmacological management should take into account the possible causes of rejection of care. A possibility that resistiveness is induced by pain that the individual experiences during care procedures should be considered and if pain is present premedication with analgesics before a care episode should be instituted. If symptoms of depression are present, antidepressant treatment often decreases the resistive behaviour. A double-blind randomized study indicated that citalopram is as effective as risperidone in the treatment of agitation and psychotic symptoms in patients with dementia. However, this effect requires effective antidepressant doses and duration of therapy as indicated by the DIADS study, where NPI score was improved only in those patients who obtained an antidepressant effect after treatment with sertraline.[17] Enhancement of antidepressant effect by addition of small doses of antipsychotics may be sometimes required.

There is also some evidence that inhibitors of cholinesterase have small beneficial effects on behavioural symptoms of dementia,[18] and one double-blind randomized study found that behavioural symptoms of dementia were improved by administration of prazosin.[19] Delusions are a common cause of resistive behaviour and, if the behaviour cannot be managed by behavioural strategies, antipsychotic therapy may be useful. In addition, treatment with mood stabilizers may also be effective since topiramide was recently shown to be as effective as risperidone in the treatment of behavioural symptoms of dementia.

Food refusal

One important goal of dementia care is to provide adequate nutrition by promoting eating and preventing food refusal. Food refusal may have several causes (see Chapter 16, The anorexia of ageing; Chapter 17, Weight loss; Chapter 59, Communication disorders and dysphagia). An individual with dementia may dislike institutional food, especially if they are of different ethnic background and were used to eating different food. Food refusal may also be caused by physical reasons, such as fatigue, overstimulation, constipation, medication-induced nausea, dehydration, toothache or ill-fitting dentures. Food refusal is an important symptom of depression and may also be caused by delusions about food being poisoned. In advanced dementia, when individuals develop swallowing difficulties, food refusal may be a consequence of choking on food and liquids. Finally, in the terminal stage of dementia, some individuals are unable to open the mouth and swallow.

Food refusal may lead to weight loss and malnutrition, although very often it is only occasional and the individual with dementia makes up for decreased food intake one day by eating more the next day. Management of food refusal should first consider personal and behavioural factors that may contribute to food refusal. It is important to obtain information about foods that the individual with dementia likes or dislikes, although sometimes food preferences change significantly as dementia progresses. Environmental factors that may cause food refusal are a chaotic or noisy dining area, inadequate staff time or staff knowledge of how to promote eating, unappealing food presentation and improper utensils. As dementia progresses, individuals become unable to use utensils and their failure to eat may not indicate food refusal. Serving finger food may allow them to eat independently for much longer.

If the behavioural and environmental interventions are ineffective, pharmacological management may be initiated. The most important is to eliminate depression and delusion as causes of food refusal by appropriate treatment with antidepressants or antipsychotics. If that approach is not appropriate or effective, food intake may be enhanced by administration of megestrol acetate or dronabinol. Megestrol acetate is a progesterone derivative with androgenic properties. It is used for the treatment of anorexia and cachexia in cancer and AIDS. Megestrol acetate improved appetite and wellbeing in nursing home patients.[20] Dronabinol is a cannabinoid derivative that is used for the treatment of anorexia in AIDS and the prevention of vomiting after chemotherapy for cancer. Dronabinol increased body weight of institutionalized individuals with Alzheimer's disease[21] and may also improve their problem behaviours.

Tube feeding is not an appropriate strategy for the management of food refusal in individuals with advanced dementia. Tube feeding does not have any benefits for these individuals.[22] Tube feeding does not prevent malnutrition or infections and it does not increase survival in individuals with progressive degenerative dementia (see Chapter 48, Aspiration pneumonia). Nasogastric tubes may cause infections of the sinuses and middle ear and gastrostomy tubes may cause cellulitis, abscesses and even necrotizing fasciitis and myositis. Contaminated feeding solution may cause gastrointestinal symptoms and bacteriuria. Insertion of a tube may actually cause death from arrhythmia during insertion of a nasogastric tube and from perioperative mortality in percutaneous endoscopic gastrostomy tube placement. The occurrence of pressure ulcers is not decreased by tube feeding and it may actually be increased because of the use of restraints and increased production of urine and stool (see Chapter 133, Restraints and immobility). There is also no evidence that tube feeding promotes healing of pressure ulcers or improves the functional status of individuals with advanced dementia.

Insomnia

Sleep disturbances are common in elderly and probably even more common in individuals with dementia (see Chapter 54, Sleep apnoea and sleep disorders). A survey of individuals aged 65 years or older who were living at home showed that 28% had difficulty in falling asleep and 42% had difficulty both in falling asleep and staying asleep. Ageing affects sleep structure, resulting in less time spent in deep sleep and slightly more time spent in lighter stages of sleep. The elderly experience frequent night-time awakenings and fragmentation of sleep. They also sleep less efficiently, with their actual time asleep being only 70–80% of the total time spent in bed.[23]

Insomnia could be a primary condition but it may also be caused by other factors, including medical and psychiatric illness, medication use, specific sleep disorders, psychosocial factors and circadian rhythm changes. Insomnia is associated with respiratory symptoms, physical disabilities, use of non-prescription medications, depressive symptoms and poor self-perception of health.[23] Many medications that are used for the treatment of chronic conditions may affect sleep. These medications include decongestants, antiasthmatics, corticosteroids, antihypertensives, alcohol, caffeine, nicotine and thyroid preparations. Sleep disorders include sleep apnoea and periodic limb movement in sleep. Both of these conditions are very common in the elderly. Psychosocial factors include loneliness, bereavement and the lack of physical activity. Circadian rhythm changes differently in normal ageing and in Alzheimer's disease. In normal ageing, there is an advance of the sleep phase with early evening sleepiness and early morning awakenings. Even if elderly persons go to bed later, they may wake up early in the morning and be unable to go back to sleep.

In Alzheimer's disease, there is a delay in circadian rhythm resulting in an inability to go to sleep in the evening. This rhythm shift may be so pronounced that it results in complete reversal of day and night activities, with the individual with dementia sleeping during the day and staying up during the night. The delay in circadian rhythm may also participate in increased behavioural disturbances in the afternoon and evening that are often called *sundowning*. In contrast, individuals with frontotemporal dementia have no change in circadian rhythm of body temperature but an advanced rhythm of motor activity. Institutionalized individuals with dementia have extremely fragmented sleep, barely sleeping for a full hour and barely staying awake for a full hour throughout the day and night.

Management of insomnia should first utilize behavioural modifications. This includes avoiding caffeine, heavy meals and excessive amounts of alcohol before going to sleep, avoiding nocturia by decreased fluid intake in the evening, reviewing medications and limiting day naps to 30 min.[24] If behavioural modifications are not effective in reducing insomnia, the use of hypnotic medications may be considered (Table 80.8). Antihistamines should not be used because they have strong anticholinergic effects that can aggravate memory problems and can also cause other adverse effects. Most common agents used in the management of insomnia are benzodiazepines. Only short-acting benzodiazepines should be used to avoid daytime sedation and increased risk for falls. The shortest acting agent, zaleplon, is especially useful in individuals who have difficulty falling asleep. Trazodone is a non-tricyclic sedative antidepressant. Although there are few data to support the use of trazodone in non-depressed individuals, trazodone is useful in the treatment of insomnia associated with administration of stimulating antidepressants. Melatonin was not found to be an effective sleep agent in individuals with Alzheimer's disease.

Table 80.8 Drugs for treatment of insomnia.

Name (trade name)	Dose range (mg)	Elimination half-life (h)
Trazodone	50–300	4–9
Triazolam (Halcion)	0.125–0.25	2–3
Zaleplon (Sonata)	5–10	1
Zolpidem (Ambien)	5–10	1.5–3.5
Eszopiclone (Lunesta)	1–3	5.8

Apathy and agitation

Agitation is sometimes used as a term to label all behavioural symptoms of dementia. However, such a use of this term does not take into consideration the context in which a behaviour happens and does not differentiate between behavioural symptoms induced by caregiving activity (rejection of care) and symptoms that occur without provocation or environmental triggers. Therefore, it is more useful to limit the term 'agitation' to behaviours that communicate to others that the individual with dementia is experiencing an unpleasant state of excitement and that are observable without subjective interpretation, are not strictly behaviours that are invoked by caregiving activities, are unrelated to known physical needs of the patient that can be remedied and are without known motivational intent.[25]

Apathy is also a very common behavioural symptom of dementia and it is present in 27% of individuals with dementia living in the community and up to 92% of patients with advanced dementia. It is less common in individuals with dementia who lived with their spouses than in individuals who lived with others.[26] Unfortunately, apathy is very often not diagnosed and treated because apathetic patients do not cause a disturbance that would attract the attention of the caregivers. Apathetic individuals appear passive, demonstrate inattention to the external environment (e.g. fixed staring or immobility) and are uninterested in what is happening around them. Apathy and depression are not synonymous and there is no significant correlation between them. Apathy and depression also result in a different pattern of brain blood flow changes.

Both agitation and apathy denote a lack of psychological wellbeing. The most common cause of agitation and apathy is functional impairment, resulting in inability to initiate meaningful activities. If these activities are not provided, the individuals with dementia experience boredom and become apathetic. Alternatively, the individuals attempt to stimulate themselves and that may result in repetitive behaviours or repetitive vocalization. Therefore, the most important intervention for both apathy and agitation is the availability of meaningful activities. An enhanced continuous activity programme decreased agitation and social isolation significantly.[11] Because lack of meaningful activities may induce both apathy and agitation, both of these symptoms are often present in the same individuals. Treatment of agitation with sedating medications results in an even more apathetic individual.

However, agitation may persist even in the presence of these activities and may actually interfere with participation in activities. In that case, the agitation may be a symptom of depression or a consequence of anxiety that may be induced by delusions or hallucinations. Therefore, careful analysis of the likely causes of agitation and treatment of the underlying cause are necessary. Agitation may also be induced by changes in circadian rhythms. Delay in circadian rhythm is related to agitation in the afternoon and evening, sundowning. Resetting of the circadian rhythm by bright light exposure may improve sundowning, although the effect is not very strong.

Elopement and interference with others

Unsupervised wandering away from a home or institution may have severe consequences for the individual with dementia. Elopement exposes the individual to a risk of injury if they walk into traffic, to hypothermia in cold climates and hyperthermia with dehydration in warm climates. Wandering into rooms of other residents leads to conflict between residents, especially if the other resident is cognitively intact and resents the intrusion.

Wandering commonly describes the ambulating behaviour of a person with dementia when that person walks away from one area or walks into an area 'without permission'. Wandering may be caused by spatial disorientation or by delusions and hallucinations. An individual may be searching for something, attempting to fulfil unmet needs, escaping a threatening situation, reacting to reminders of departure near an exit or carrying out a predementia lifestyle function.

Longitudinal studies indicate that wandering behaviour starts on average 10 months after diagnosis of dementia in 40% of individuals but eventually occurs in 80% of all patients with dementia. Cross-sectional studies find prevalence of wandering between 15 and 28% with wandering characteristics similar in nursing homes and assisted-living facilities.[27]

Some individuals with dementia walk back and forth as if following a rhythm or pattern. In that case, their activity is called *pacing*. Pacing often occurs with speed and a sense of urgency and may seem to represent hyperactivity or restlessness. Pacing may pose a problem for the individual with dementia if it occupies so much walking time that the individual becomes overtired. Pacing may also interfere with sitting down to eat and may result in weight loss. Pacing actually consumes a considerable amount of energy and it was estimated that up to an additional 1600 calories are required to maintain adequate nutrition in individuals who pace. Another adverse effect of pacing may be foot problems, such as blisters.

Both wandering and pacing should not be a problem if they occur in a safe environment and may actually provide beneficial physical exercise. Interference with other residents may be avoided by providing care for individuals with dementia in a dementia special care unit, where residents may not mind the intrusion because they themselves have spatial orientation difficulties. Hence the most important intervention for these behaviours is environmental modification. These modifications should provide a safe walking path away from exits and secure exits by disguising them or by a touch padlocking device. Wandering and pacing may also be a consequence of a lack of meaningful activities. Engaging an individual in activity might distract them from seeking an exit from a home or institution. Because an individual with dementia living in a community may wander away from a caregiver in public places and because the individual may elope from a home despite safety measures, it is important (in the USA) to register the individual with both the Alzheimer's Association Safe Return Program and the Medic Alert Program.

Environmental factors

Four environmental factors influence behavioural symptoms of dementia: caregiving approaches, social environment, physical environment and medical interventions. Each of them can be modified to prevent or improve behavioural symptoms. Caregiving approaches are most important for the rejection of care that may lead to verbal or physical behaviours directed towards the caregivers. The appropriate modification of caregiving approaches was described in the section Rejection of care.

Optimal social environment for care of individuals with dementia is a special care dementia unit (SCU). It eliminates problems related to interaction with cognitively intact nursing home residents who do not tolerate intrusion in their rooms and other people rummaging in their belongings. Research on the advantages of the SCU is not uniformly positive probably because of quality of care differences. When residents with dementia living on and off an SCU were compared, there was no difference in the use of physical restraints, but SCU residents were less likely to have had bed rails and to have been tube fed. SCU residents were more likely to be on toileting plans and less likely to use pads or briefs in the absence of a toileting plan. SCU residents were more likely to have received psychotropic medications, primarily antipsychotics.[28] Establishing an SCU increases occupancy rate and private pay census and decreases behavioural symptoms of dementia. The presence of an SCU also allows for the establishment of an activity programme specifically designed for individuals with moderate and severe dementia.[11]

The physical environment should prevent elopement and provide for safe ambulation and wandering. This environment is more easily created on an SCU. Using the Physical Environmental Assessment Protocol (PEAP), it was found that the SCUs were more supportive on six dimensions: maximizing awareness and orientation, maximizing safety and security, regulation of stimulation, quality of stimulation, opportunities for personal control and continuity of the self.[29] The environment should also help in the orientation of residents with dementia and provide stimulation by the presence of objects that may be handled safely by the residents.

Medical interventions may aggravate behavioural symptoms because demented individuals do not understand the need for these interventions and do not cooperate with diagnostic and therapeutic procedures. It is important to realize that even a routine intervention, such as measurement of blood pressure, causes some discomfort that may not be tolerated by individuals with dementia. Therefore, before any medical intervention is performed, its burden and benefits should be considered and compared with the goals of care for the individual patient. Some interventions may not be appropriate for a patient with advance dementia, for example, cardiopulmonary resuscitation.[30] Transfer to an acute care setting and use of antibiotics for treatment of generalized infections should be also considered carefully and not done as a default strategy. Tube feeding may not be indicated, as explained in the section on food refusal.

Key points

- Physical causes of problem behaviours need to be eliminated prior to attributing the causes to dementia.
- Demented persons may have concomitant depression or bipolar disorders.
- Caregiver behaviour may be responsible for rejection of care.
- The most important intervention for both apathy and agitation is the availability of meaningful activities.

References

1. Phillips VL and Diwan S. The incremental effect of dementia-related problem behaviors on the time to nursing home placement in poor, frail, demented older people. *J Am Geriatr Soc* 2003;**51**:188–93.
2. Volicer L. Do we need another dementia pain scale? *J Am Med Dir Assoc* 2009;**10**:450–2.
3. Birks J. Cholinesterase inhibitors for Alzheimer's disease. *Cochrane Database Syst Rev* 2006;(1):CD005593.
4. Grossberg GT, Pejovic V, Miller ML and Graham SM. Memantine therapy of behavioral symptoms in community-dwelling patients with moderate to severe Alzheimer's disease. *Dement Geriatr Cogn Disord* 2009;**27**:164–72.
5. Lancioni GE, Pinto K, LaMartire ML *et al.* Helping persons with mild or moderate Alzheimer's disease recapture basic daily activities through the use of an instruction strategy. *Disabil Rehabil* 2009;**31**:2119.

6. Bender RL, Moore R, Russell D *et al*. Multifaceted approach to cognitive decline. *Brain Aging* 2002;**2**:44–7.
7. Volicer L, Van der Steen JT and Frijters D. Modifiable factors related to abusive behaviors in nursing home residents with dementia. *J Am Med Dir Assoc* 2009;**10**:617–22.
8. Schneider LS, Dagerman K and Insel PS. Efficacy and adverse effects of atypical antipsychotics for dementia: meta-analysis of randomized, placebo-controlled trials. *Am J Geriatr Psychiatry* 2010;**14**:191–210.
9. Ray WA, Chung CP, Murray KT *et al*. Atypical antipsychotic drugs and the risk of sudden cardiac death. *N Engl J Med* 2009;**360**:225–35.
10. Simard J. The Memory Enhancement Program: a new approach to increasing the quality of life for people with mild memory loss. In: SM Albert (ed.), *Assessing Quality of Life in Alzheimer's Disease*, Springer, New York, 2000, pp. 153–62.
11. Volicer L, Simard J, Pupa JH *et al*. Effects of continuous activity programming on behavioral symptoms of dementia. *J Am Med Dir Assoc* 2006;**7**:426–31.
12. Camberg L, Woods P, Ooi WL *et al*. Evaluation of Simulated Presence: a personalized approach to enhance well-being in persons with Alzheimer's disease. *J Am Geriatr Soc* 1999;**47**:446–52.
13. Simard J. *The End-of-Life Namaste Care Program for People with Dementia*. Health Professions Press, Baltimore, 2007.
14. Staal JA, Sacks A, Matheis R *et al*. The effects of Snoezelen (multi-sensory behavior therapy) and psychiatric care on agitation, apathy and activities of daily living in dementia patients on a short term geriatric psychiatric inpatient unit. *Int J Psychiatry Med* 2007;**37**:357–70.
15. Volicer L, Berman SA, Cipolloni PB and Mandell A. Persistent vegetative state in Alzheimer disease – does it exist? *Arch Neurol* 1997;**54**:1382–4.
16. Porter VR, Buxton WG, Fairbanks LA *et al*. Frequency and characteristics of anxiety among patients with Alzheimer's disease and related dementias. *J Neuropsychiatry Clin Neurosci* 2003;**15**:180–6.
17. Lyketsos CG, DelCampo L, Steinberg M *et al*. Treating depression in Alzheimer disease – efficacy and safety of sertraline therapy and the benefits of depression reduction: the DIADS. *Arch Gen Psychiatry* 2003;**60**:737–46.
18. Sink KM, Holden KF and Yaffe K. Pharmacological treatment of neuropsychiatric symptoms of dementia: a review of the evidence. *JAMA* 2005;**293**:596–608.
19. Wang LY, Shofer JB, Rohde K *et al*. Prazosin for the treatment of behavioral symptoms in patients with Alzheimer disease with agitation and aggression. *Am J Geriatr Psychiatry* 2009;**17**:744–51.
20. Yeh SS, Lowitt S and Schuster MW. Usage of megestrol acetate in the treatment of anorexia–cachexia syndrome in the elderly. *J Nutr Health Aging* 2009;**13**:448–54.
21. Wilson MM, Philpot C and Morley JE. Anorexia of aging in long term care: is dronabinol an effective appetite stimulant? – a pilot study. *J Nutr Health Aging* 2007;**11**:195–8.
22. Candy B, Sampson EL and Jones L. Enteral tube feeding in older people with advanced dementia: findings from a Cochrane systematic review. *Int J Palliat Nurs* 2009;**15**: 396–404.
23. Dauvilliers Y. Insomnia in patients with neurodegenerative conditions. *Sleep Med* 2007;(Suppl 4):S27–34.
24. Deschenes CL and McCurry SM. Current treatments for sleep disturbances in individuals with dementia. *Curr Psychiatry Rep* 2009;**11**:20–6.
25. Hurley AC, Volicer L, Camberg L *et al*. Measurement of observed agitation in patients with Alzheimer's disease. *J Mental Health Aging* 1999;**5**:117–33.
26. Clarke DE, van Reekum R, Simard M *et al*. Apathy in dementia: clinical and sociodelmographic correlates. *J Neuropsychiatry Clin Neurosci* 2008;**20**:337–47.
27. Volicer L. Epidemiology of wandering. In: AL Nelson and DL Algase (eds), *Evidence-based Protocols for Managing Wandering Behaviors*, Springer, New York, 2007, pp. 53–64.
28. Gruneir A, Lapane KL, Miller SC and Mor V. Is dementia special care really special? A new look at an old question. *J Am Geriatr Soc* 2008;**56**:199–205.
29. Morgan DG, Stewart NJ, D'arcy KC and Werezak LJ. Evaluating rural nursing home environments: dementia special care units versus integrated facilities. *Aging Mental Health* 2004;**8**:256–65.
30. Volicer L. End-of-life care for people with dementia in long-term care settings. *Alzheimer's Care Today* 2008;**9**:84–102.

CHAPTER 81

Geriatric psychiatry

Abhilash K. Desai[1] and George T. Grossberg[2]

[1]Sheppard Pratt Hospital, and University of Maryland School of Medicine, Baltimore, MD, USA
[2]Saint Louis University School of Medicine, St Louis, MO, USA

Introduction

Care of older patients with mental health problems is immensely satisfying and rewarding. The most common mental health problems in older adults in the community include cognitive problems (e.g. dementia), depression and anxiety, alcohol and benzodiazepine misuse/abuse. In long-term care (LTC) settings, management of behavioural and psychological symptoms associated with dementia account for the majority of mental health problems. In acute care settings, delirium, depression and agitation in persons with dementia account for the majority of mental health problems in older adults. Abuse and neglect and severe mental illness (SMI), although less common in all settings, cause immense suffering and are associated with high health care utilization. Table 81.1 lists the most common mental health disorders in older adults. Thoughtful, individualized care of older adults with mental health problems takes time and can be facilitated by restructuring current practices (e.g. routine interdisciplinary assessment and management) and building new models of care (e.g. patient-centred medical home). Although old age may increase the likelihood of exposure to risk factors for the development of psychiatric disorders such as reduced social support, physical impairment and cognitive decline, it is important for primary care providers, patients and their families to realize that dementia and depression are not a normal part of ageing and that adequate treatment of these conditions can significantly enhance future health and wellbeing. Certain mental disorders are covered in greater detail in other chapters, although they are important disorders seen by geriatric psychiatry. These include depression, dementia and delirium.

Epidemiology

One in four older adults (aged 65 years and older) has at least one significant mental health problem/disorder.[1] The prevalence of mental health problems in the oldest old (aged 85 years and older) approaches 50%. The prevalence of mental health problems in the LTC population ranges from 65 to 100%. Older adults account for 14% of the population but almost 20% of all suicides. The prevalence of psychiatric disorders in older adults is expected to double over the next 30 years, making them a priority for healthcare and social care services.[2] The actual burden of mental disorders in older adults is probably underestimated because the stigma associated with mental disorders results in under-reporting of symptoms by older adults, under-diagnosis by healthcare providers (HCPs), clinical significance of sub-threshold symptoms and under-representation in epidemiological studies of high-risk older adults (e.g. medically ill, LTC residents).[3]

Challenges in geriatric psychiatry

There are a number of ways in which older adults uniquely express mental health disorders including under-reporting of symptoms, manifesting subclinical disorders and differential expression of symptoms based on age of onset. Clinically significant, subthreshold syndromes increase with age. Psychophysiological changes accompanying normal ageing, including alterations in sleep, appetite and psychomotor functioning, may make it difficult to diagnose clinically significant psychopathology. Cognitive impairment may further cloud the presentation of mood and psychotic symptoms. Late-life mental disorders often vary in their expression (e.g. less endorsement of affective symptoms in mood disorders) and treatment responsiveness (e.g. reduced response to antidepressants). In addition, the co-occurrence of general medical disorders with older age makes attributing functional limitations to mental health diagnoses more difficult. Common mental health problems (e.g. depression) often present atypically (e.g. with memory loss) in older individuals and loss of physical abilities, financial resources and family and friends can challenge even the most resilient amongst older persons. Many mental health problems (e.g. complicated grief) in older adults do not fit the conventional paradigm of disease. Older adults are

Principles and Practice of Geriatric Medicine, Fifth Edition. Edited by Alan J. Sinclair, John E. Morley and Bruno Vellas.

Table 81.1 Common mental health disorders in older adults.

Depressive disorders
- Complicated grief
- Major depression
- Depression secondary to a physical health condition (e.g. stroke, Parkinson's disease, chronic pain)
- Dysthymic disorder

Anxiety disorders
- Generalized anxiety disorder
- Phobias (including fear of falls)
- Panic disorder
- Post-traumatic stress disorder

Cognitive disorders
- Delirium
- Alzheimer's disease
- Vascular cognitive impairment
- Dementia with Lewy bodies
- Parkinson's disease dementia
- Frontotemporal dementia
- Mixed dementia
- Mild cognitive impairment

Behavioural and psychological symptoms associated with dementias
- Apathy/indifference
- Depressive symptoms
- Psychotic symptoms
- Anxiety symptoms
- Sleep disorders (e.g. insomnia, excessive daytime sleepiness, REM sleep behaviour disorder)
- Agitation (e.g. wandering, hoarding)
- Aggressive behaviours (e.g. verbal aggression, physical aggression)
- Sexually inappropriate behaviours
- Eating disorders (e.g. anorexia, hyperphagia, pica)

Severe mental illness
- Schizophrenia
- Schizoaffective disorder
- Bipolar disorder

Other disorders
- Prescription-drug and substance abuse and dependence
- Drug-induced psychiatric disorders
- Personality disorders
- Adjustment disorders
- Delusional disorder

also more susceptible to the adverse effects of psychotropic drugs. Psychotherapy may need to be modified to accommodate cognitive and sensory deficits. All HCPs working with older adults should be prepared for these challenges.

The psychiatric interview of an older adult

The foundation of the diagnostic work-up of the older adult experiencing a psychiatric disorder is the diagnostic interview. Input from a reliable informant who is familiar with the patient is often crucial for accurate diagnosis. To supplement the clinical interview, the use of standardized rating scales is recommended. Table 81.2 gives a list of scales recommended for use in primary care, and Table 81.3 presents the CAGE questionnaire. All complaints, whether on the part of the patient or the family, must be taken seriously as they may signal treatable mental and physical health conditions. A simple screening question asking about the patient's mood and memory state is often informative. Coexisting sensory deficits (e.g. hearing, vision) and comorbid medical conditions (e.g. heart failure, chronic kidney disease, sleep apnoea, nutritional deficiencies) can all negatively affect mental health and their identification should therefore be part of any comprehensive assessment. The interview should routinely assess both risk and protective factors for late-life mental disorders. Involving

Table 81.2 Common standardized scales recommended in primary care.

Cognition (delirium)
- Confusion assessment method[4]

Cognition (dementia)
- Screening tools:
  - AD8[5]
  - Mini-Cog[6]
- Assessment tools:
  - Saint Louis University Mental Status (SLUMS) Examination[7]
  - MMSE[8]
  - MoCA[9]

Depression
- Screening tools:
  - Patient Health Questionnaire - 2 (PHQ-2)[10]
- Assessment tools:
  - Patient Health Questionnaire - 9 (PHQ-9)[11]
  - Geriatric Depression Scale 15-item and 30-item versions (GDS-15 and GDS-30)[12]
  - Cornell Scale for Depression in Dementia (CSDD)[13]

Harmful alcohol use and alcohol abuse
- Screening tools:
  - CAGE questionnaire[14]
- Assessment tools:
  - Short Michigan Alcohol Screening Test – Geriatric Version (SMAST-G)[15]

Agitation in patients with dementia
- Cohen-Mansfield Agitation Scale – Short Form[16]

Table 81.3 CAGE questionnaire.

C	Have you ever felt you ought to CUT DOWN on your drinking?
A	Have people ANNOYED you by criticizing your drinking?
G	Have you ever felt bad or GUILTY about your drinking?
E	Have you ever had a drink first thing in the morning (EYE OPENER) to steady your nerves or get rid of a hangover?

HCPs from other disciplines in comprehensive assessment is strongly recommended because the majority of older adults with mental health problems have multiple physical, interpersonal, social and financial problems that need to be addressed simultaneously.

Work-up

Laboratory testing, neuropsychological testing and neuroimaging can further assist in accurate diagnosis and identification of prognostic and protective factors in older adults with mental health problems. A comprehensive metabolic panel (CMP), thyroid-stimulating hormone (TSH) and vitamin levels (B_{12}, folate, D) to assess the aetiology of new-onset or resistant mental health problems are recommended. Certain clinical situations may dictate ordering urine tests (analysis, culture and sensitivity) and other laboratory tests (e.g. free testosterone levels in older adults with depression and other symptoms of testosterone deficiency). Before initiating antipsychotics, a baseline electrocardiogram (ECG) is recommended due to recent reports of sudden cardiac death associated with antipsychotic use. For residents in a hospice and for residents in the terminal stages of dementia, these baseline blood tests may not be ordered. Subtle seizure disorder should also be considered in the differential diagnosis of new-onset or atypical mental health syndromes and may require an electroencephalogram (EEG) and a referral to a neurologist. In some situations, a polysomnogram or nocturnal pulse oximetry may need to be ordered to rule out sleep disorders such as obstructive sleep apnoea. Neuropsychological testing is often crucial for accurate early diagnosis of dementing disorders [especially Alzheimer's disease (AD) and vascular cognitive impairment (VCI)] and differentiating it from depression and mild cognitive impairment (MCI). As part of comprehensive diagnostic work-up, neuroimaging such as computed tomography (CT) or magnetic resonance imaging (MRI) scans is recommended for all older adults with significant cognitive deficits, new onset mood or psychotic symptoms.

Interdisciplinary approach and individualized care plan

Most behavioural and psychological symptoms are best treated by an interdisciplinary team. Table 81.4 delineates the members who may constitute an ideal interdisciplinary team. Although the role of most of the team members listed in Table 81.4 is recognized by primary care providers, it is important to recognize the role of some key team members who are particularly important in LTC psychiatry. Recreational therapists use a whole host of tools and interventions (e.g. air mat therapy, sensory stimulation box) to address behavioural problems in LTC residents after a comprehensive assessment to identify background factors (e.g. cognitive ability) and proximal factors (e.g. psychosocial need states). Music therapists may lead group music activities as a part of a daily continuous activity schedule and also provide one-to-one music therapy for specific LTC residents who have depression and/or agitation. Art therapists use a variety of media, including paints, ceramics, natural materials and fabrics, to guide residents through everything from one-to-one painting sessions to group quilting projects.

Table 81.4 Members of an ideal interdisciplinary team.

Members
Patient
Patient advocate, usually a family member/friend/caregiver
Geriatric psychiatrists/psychiatrists (Team Leader)
Nurse practitioners and physician assistants with geriatric mental health expertise
Primary care physician/geriatrician and physician extenders working with them
Pharmacists
Nurses
Certified nursing assistants
Social workers
Psychologists
Neuropsychologists
Registered dieticians
Chaplains and members of the clergy
Geriatric care manager
Physical therapist
Occupational therapist
Speech therapist
Music therapist
Recreational/activities therapist
Art therapist
Aromatherapist

The HCP should work with patient, their family members and other team members to develop and implement an individualized care plan for mental health problems and also for general medical and social problems. Determining which interventions are realistic and monitoring (and documenting) the response to the interventions are recommended. Trying to anticipate adverse events (such as constipation with pain medication) and planning interventions for the adverse event during care planning are also recommended.

Depression

Late-life depression is a heterogeneous group of disorders. Late-life depression is prevalent and eminently treatable. Late-onset depression may be a prodrome of late-life dementia and may also promote neuropathogenic processes that eventually cause dementia. Depression has been associated with increased rates of cardiovascular illness and mortality after myocardial infarction. Depression and anxiety typically co-occur. Electroconvulsive therapy (ECT) remains the most effective treatment for depression in older adults. Antidepressants (especially for severe and or chronic depression) combined with psychotherapy is recommended for cognitively intact older adults with depression. Newer brain stimulation therapies (e.g. repetitive transcranial magnetic stimulation, vagal nerve stimulation, magnetic seizure therapy and deep brain stimulation) have not been well studied in older adults with depression and hence their use is not recommended except in academic/research settings.

Bereavement

Bereavement is associated with declines in health, increased utilization of healthcare resources and increased risk of death. Complicated bereavement may be distinct from major depression and formal criteria have been proposed. Complicated bereavement includes symptoms such as extreme levels of 'traumatic distress', numbness, feeling that part of oneself has died, assuming symptoms of the deceased, disbelief or bitterness, and symptoms endure for 6 months. Brief dynamic psychotherapy, traumatic grief therapy, crisis intervention and use of support groups can significantly reduce grief symptoms. Antidepressants may also be considered to treat complicated bereavement.

Severe mental illness

About 1% of the US population above the age of 55 years have severe mental illness (SMI). Mental health disorders considered as SMI include bipolar disorder, schizophrenia and schizoaffective disorder. Cognitive deficits, poor physical health and movement disorders are also experienced by a majority of older adults with SMI and they worsen adaptive functioning. Although suicide remains an important cause of mortality for this population, cardiovascular disease is the leading cause of death. Cardiovascular death among those with SMI is 2–3 times that of the general population. This is in part due to poor access to and use of quality healthcare services and high rates of obesity, diabetes and hyperlipidaemia (often exacerbated by antipsychotics). Older adults with SMI have difficulty complying with care regimens for chronic medical conditions such as diabetes and hypertension and have poor dietary habits. Older adults with SMI commonly face, in addition to persistent symptoms, increasing medical morbidity, limited financial resources and social impoverishment. Among homeless older adults, there is a high prevalence of SMI and cognitive impairment. Poor adherence to medication treatment for both mental and physical health conditions is common in older adults with SMI and has devastating consequences. Adherence problems are complex, determined by multiple factors and thus require a high index of suspicion and customized interventions that are focused on the underlying causes.

Bipolar affective disorder and late-onset mania

When an older adult presents with manic symptoms in later life and has no past history of bipolar disorder, a thorough work-up is recommended to identify general medical conditions that could cause manic symptoms (e.g. right hemisphere stroke, frontotemporal dementia) or drug-induced mania (e.g. corticosteroids or stimulants). Most older adults with bipolar disorder have had the disorder from their young adulthood, although onset as late as in the ninth and tenth decades has been reported. Late-onset bipolar disorder (onset after age 50 years) is commonly associated with comorbidities such as hypertension, diabetes or coronary artery disease and neurological disorders. There is high prevalence of cognitive dysfunction (especially executive dysfunction), frequent abnormalities on structural neuroimaging (e.g. cerebral white matter hyperintensities) and association with stroke. It is less likely to be associated with a family history of mood disorders. Older manic patients seldom display racing thoughts or euphoric/elated mood characteristic of younger adults and are more likely to be irritable, argumentative, angry, paranoid and disorganized. Mixed states are more common than in the younger population and psychotic symptoms are less common. Older adults often have more frequent episodes of mania and depression, with a shorter (e.g. rapid cycling) duration of symptoms than younger patients. Pharmacological interventions (e.g. atypical antipsychotics, valproate) combined with psychosocial interventions (e.g. psychotherapy, family and patient education) are needed for successful outcomes. ECT should not be considered only as a last treatment option, but should be considered in all older adults with bipolar disorder (including those with mild to moderate symptom severity), especially in those with a history of previous good response to ECT.

Schizophrenia

Schizophrenia is less prevalent than dementias and depression in older adults. However, the total health expenditures for older adults with schizophrenia exceed those of older adults with dementia and depression. Onset of illness is typically in early adulthood, with a small but distinct subgroup developing disease after the age of 45 years. Late-onset schizophrenia has a higher prevalence of the paranoid type, less severe negative symptoms, over-representation of women and requires lower doses of antipsychotic medications compared with early-onset schizophrenia. Most of the older adults with schizophrenia have been active smokers for many years. Older adults with schizophrenia have a high prevalence of vascular risk factors (e.g. obesity, hypertension, diabetes, high cholesterol) and vascular disease (e.g. coronary artery disease). Therefore, treatment interventions should include efforts to control these risk factors optimally. Most older adults with schizophrenia live in the community, are stable, but remain symptomatic and functionally impaired. Sustained remissions, although uncommon, can occur even in older adults with chronic schizophrenia. Pharmacological interventions (primarily atypical antipsychotics) combined with interventions for psychosocial rehabilitation (such as social skills training, cognitive remediation, supported employment, residential alternatives) is often necessary for optimal outcomes. Assertive community treatment and case management greatly increase the success of these interventions.

Late-life psychosis

There is an increased incidence of psychotic symptoms (delusions and hallucinations) in older adults in contrast to younger adults. Older adults presenting with psychotic symptoms for the first time need a thorough evaluation to identify underlying causes such as dementia, delirium, depression, general medical conditions (e.g. cancer) or drug-induced psychoses. If the work-up is negative, a diagnosis of late-onset schizophrenia or delusional disorder may be entertained.

Cognitive disorders

These primarily include dementing disorders, delirium, cognitive impairment no dementia (CIND), mild cognitive impairment (MCI) and vascular cognitive impairment (VCI).

Dementing disorders

It is important to evaluate formally and diagnose specifically the type(s) of dementia. Comorbid physical and mental health conditions (e.g. nutritional deficiencies, depression) that may accelerate cognitive and functional decline should be looked for and promptly treated. There exists a minimal set of care principles for patients with AD and their caregivers that all clinicians are recommended to follow.[17] The goals of care are (1) to delay disease progression, (2) delay functional decline, (3) improve quality of life, (4) support dignity, (5) control symptoms and (6) provide comfort at all stages of dementia. Older adults with dementia-related symptoms of agitation and aggression should first be managed with psychosocial/environmental interventions. Pharmacological interventions (including antipsychotics) should be used only when psychosocial and environmental interventions have failed to control behavioural disruption adequately.[18] The findings related to antipsychotic drug safety (e.g. increased risk of mortality and stroke) should be taken seriously by clinicians in assessing the potential risks and benefits of treatment and in advising families about treatment. Better matching of the available psychosocial/environmental interventions to the patient's strengths and interests may not only reduce agitation but also prevent agitation and depression in persons with dementia.

Delirium

Although there are many potential causes of delirium, a 'final common pathway' involving a concomitant decrease in cholinergic tone and increase in dopaminergic tone in relevant brain regions has been hypothesized. Management of behavioural disturbances associated with delirium is primarily through psychosocial environmental interventions (e.g. improved sleep hygiene, range-of-motion exercises, ambulation, reorientation and cognitive stimulation).[19] Low doses of antipsychotics such as parenteral haloperidol may be needed for acute control of severe agitation.

Mild cognitive impairment (MCI) and cognitive impairment no dementia (CIND)

Many conditions may cause cognitive impairment, which may not meet current diagnostic criteria for dementia. Within this heterogeneous group CIND, there are disorders associated with an increased risk of progression to dementia. MCI represents several clinical subtypes, in which symptoms may relate directly to a transition to a more serious neurodegenerative disease. A substantial minority of MCI cases revert to 'normal' cognition over 1–2 years.

Vascular cognitive impairment (VCI)

Cerebrovascular disease is the second most common cause of acquired cognitive impairment and dementia (first being AD) and contributes to cognitive decline in the neurodegenerative dementias. The term vascular cognitive impairment (VCI), which is characterized by a specific cognitive profile involving preserved memory with impairments in attentional and executive functioning, has been proposed. Important non-cognitive features of VCI include depression and apathy.

Substance abuse

The need for substance abuse treatment among Americans over age 50 years is projected to double by 2020, according to a report by the Substance Abuse and Mental Health Services Administration (SAMHSA). Alcohol abuse is the most common form of substance abuse in older adults. The 1 -year prevalence rate for alcohol abuse and dependence in the community is 2.75% for elderly men and 0.51% for elderly women. The prevalence rates are higher in primary care settings, where at-risk drinking has been estimated to be 5–15%. The prevalence of substance abuse may be underestimated because of the limited applicability of *Diagnostic and Statistical Manual of Mental Disorders*, 4th edition text revised (DSM-IV TR) criteria to the older adult population. Primary care physicians (PCPs) and emergency care providers can play a crucial role in early identification and initial management of addiction problems in older persons. Among older adults with chronic physical and mental health disorders, even modest alcohol consumption can lead to excessive disability and poorer perceived health. PCPs rarely ask about when and how much their older patients drink or what effect alcohol may have on their lives. In addition, older adults and their relatives are often in denial about the extent and effects of their drinking habits because the same amount of alcohol now causing difficulties had no untoward social or physical effects in middle age. PCPs are often not aware of recommended upper limits of healthy intake of alcohol and are in denial regarding the harmful effects of even 'social drinking' that typically exceeds recommended upper limits of alcohol intake. Older adults with alcohol abuse also face greater risk for suicide. Older adults with alcohol abuse are more likely to present with physical symptoms and to be admitted to medical or surgical units than younger patients with alcohol abuse. A non-judgemental and tactful approach is recommended in asking about and attempting to treat alcohol abuse, especially in ageing women. There is insufficient evidence to endorse pharmacological interventions (e.g. disulfiram, naltrexone, acamprosate) for alcohol abuse in older adults. Brief interventions (5 min for five brief sessions) targeting a specific health behaviour (at-risk drinking) by primary care providers are often fairly effective. Specific advice about the dangers of combining alcohol with prescription and over-the-counter (OTC) medications, especially psychoactive agents, should be given and regularly reinforced.

As 'baby boomers' age, illicit drug use among the over-50 population is also rising. Illicit drugs include marijuana, cocaine and the non-medical use of prescription drugs. An estimated 4.3 million adults aged 50 years or older used an illicit drug in the past year, according to SAMHSA. Age-related physiological and social changes make older adults more vulnerable to the harmful effect of illicit drug use. All older adults with illicit drug use (current or past) should be screened for hepatitis C and HIV infections.

Misuse and inappropriate use of prescription medications (especially benzodiazepines but also opiates) are a substantial issue in this population. The presence of a psychiatric disorder is a risk factor for prescription drug dependence in older adults. Benzodiazepine use increases with age and older adults tend to be on higher doses. Depression in older adults often presents with features of anxiety disorder and may be inappropriately treated with benzodiazepines rather than an antidepressant and/or psychotherapy. Signs of prescription drug abuse in older people include loss of motivation, memory loss, family or marital discord, new difficulty with activities of daily living, trouble with sleeping, drug-seeking behaviour and doctor shopping. Most misuse can be treated outside specialized substance abuse treatment programmes through education of patients, families and providers. Self-help groups (e.g. Narcotics Anonymous) is unlikely to benefit an older adult with prescription opioid abuse. In older adults, safe withdrawal may take weeks to months compared with days to weeks in younger adults. Implementation of non-drug interventions to treat chronic pain and insomnia play an important role in treatment of benzodiazepine and opiate misuse.

Anxiety disorders

Anxiety disorders are the most prevalent but under-treated psychiatric disorders in older adults. Common themes of anxiety in older adults include worries about physical illness and its impact on quality of life, including pain, disability and the possibility of death. These feelings can often be exacerbated by feelings of isolation and dependence in the LTC or hospital setting. Substantial comorbidity of medical and anxiety disorders with the possibility that physiological symptoms of anxiety can be a manifestation of a medical condition or adverse effects of a drug frequently confound and complicate proper detection of anxiety disorders in older adults.

Generalized anxiety disorder (GAD) is the most common anxiety disorder in older adults. Half of older adults with GAD have had symptoms for most of their lives, whereas the remaining half report developing GAD within the last 5 years. Many older patients with onset of panic attacks in early life continue experiencing symptoms in later life. New onset of panic attacks in older persons requires a thorough evaluation to detect underlying general medical condition(s) as its cause. Phobias are prevalent, chronic and persist into old age. Fear of falling is a typical phobia seen in older adults (especially those with history of fall and fracture) but is rare in younger adults. Post-traumatic stress disorder symptoms may recur later in life and recent losses or dementia may trigger a recurrence or emergence of symptoms for the first time in older adults at risk (e.g. war veterans/survivors, victims of abuse).

Incapacitating anxiety symptoms are common in patients with certain general medical disorders (e.g. chronic obstructive pulmonary disease, patients with pacemakers, Parkinson's disease). Anxiety symptoms occasionally may be due to an underlying physical health condition (e.g. hyperthyroidism) or be drug induced (e.g. secondary to OTC sympathomimetics) or drug-withdrawal states (e.g. alcohol withdrawal).

Treatment of anxiety symptoms and disorders in older adults has typically involved the use of benzodiazepines, which are often effective but problematic because they are associated with a high risk of cognitive impairment, falls and fractures. Safer and equally effective (in the long term) alternatives to benzodiazepines include buspirone, antidepressants [e.g. selective serotonin reuptake inhibitors (SSRIs)], relaxation training and cognitive behaviour therapy. The therapeutic effects of antidepressants and buspirone may take up to 6 weeks to become noticeable. Judicious short-term use of short-acting benzodiazepines (e.g. lorazepam) may be necessary if symptoms are incapacitating until the other interventions become effective.

Geriatric psychiatry emergencies

Suicide

Some 20–50% of older adults who commit suicide have seen their PCPs within the week preceding their suicide. Older adults in general give fewer warnings, use deadlier methods (71% using firearms) and have lower attempts to completion ratios (4:1 versus 200:1 in adolescents), making it more difficult to identify older adults at risk of suicide. Clinicians are less apt to decide that suicidal thinking in an older adult is a serious condition which may respond to treatment. Depression is the strongest risk factor for suicide in older adults and for suicide's precursor, suicidal ideation. Other risk factors include, but are not limited to, alcohol abuse, loneliness, recent loss, previous suicide attempt, unrelenting pain and physical disability. Protective factors include strong ties to social and religious support networks. A thorough suicide risk assessment involves not only stated suicidal wishes but also behaviours indicating hopelessness and intention to end one's life. Collaborative assessment that involves other team members (e.g. family members, nurse, social worker) and prompt treatment of depression may reduce the risk of suicide.[20] Novel interventions (e.g. depression care managers, education of primary care providers on assessment and management of suicide and incorporation of such education into clinical practice) in community-based primary care offices can reduce suicidal risk regardless of depression severity.

Elder abuse

Older men and women of all socioeconomic and ethnic backgrounds are vulnerable to abuse and neglect and most often it goes undetected. Physical abuse is most recognizable, yet neglect is most common. Psychological and financial abuse may be more easily missed. Abused older adults are more likely to be physically dependent, cognitively impaired and have mental health problems than their non-abused counterparts. Although one in four vulnerable older persons is abused, only a small proportion of this abuse is currently reported. Most HCPs underestimate the prevalence of elder abuse. Asking older adults and their caregivers about abuse is probably the single most effective detection strategy. High index of suspicion combined with awareness of risk factors (e.g. cognitive impairment) and clinical manifestations (e.g. bruises) allows clinicians to provide early detection and intervention for abuse and neglect. Interventions that teach HCPs about the management of abuse by face-to face training rather than giving written information is recommended in order to increase the knowledge about elder abuse among HCPs.[21] Interdisciplinary collaboration between physicians, social workers and mental health professionals is crucial to detect and manage elder abuse.

Other common mental health problems in older adults

Psychological, behavioural and cognitive adverse effects of commonly prescribed medications and OTC drugs in older adults are prevalent and, in most instances, predictable and preventable. Drugs with significant anticholinergic properties (e.g. diphenhydramine), benzodiazepines and opiates are the usual suspects. Insomnia is prevalent in older adults. However, few mention their sleep problems to their primary care providers and most self-medicate with OTC medications. Many OTC sleep aids (such as diphenhydramine) have considerable psychiatric adverse effects (e.g. delirium). Sleep complaints in all older adults should be taken seriously and thoroughly evaluated to identify serious but eminently treatable conditions such as sleep apnoea and restless leg syndrome. Non-pharmacological interventions are first line in the treatment of chronic insomnia. These include improved sleep hygiene, cognitive behavioural interventions, bright light therapy, regular exercise and dietary changes (e.g. avoiding caffeine). Pharmacotherapy should be limited to short-term use of agents least likely to cause daytime sedation such as zolpidem, zaleplon and eszopiclone. Some older adults with chronic insomnia may benefit from these agents and also ramelteon. Personality traits that have been found frequently to affect the prevalence, course and prognosis of mental health disorders include neuroticism (tendency to experience negative emotions and emotional instability), extroversion (disposition toward sociability, positive emotions, dominance, high activity level), openness to experience (interest in new things, ideas and courses of action), agreeableness (deference, acquiescence, amiability, trust) and conscientiousness (diligence, reliability, organization, goal striving). Evaluation of these traits may help tailor treatment interventions to patients' strengths and weaknesses and thereby improve outcomes. For example, higher neuroticism and low conscientiousness confer a higher risk of depression higher extroversion may enhance the odds of accessing specialty mental health services, higher openness may raise the likelihood of acceptance of innovative interventions such as meditation, higher agreeableness may improve odds of smoother transition to LTC facilities and higher conscientiousness may reduce the risk of dementia through better management of cardiovascular risk factors.[22]

Special populations in geriatric psychiatry

LTC residents

Mental health disorders account for at least half of the morbidity among the LTC population and are the prime reason for admission to LTC facilities. Behavioural and psychological symptoms of dementia (BPSDs) are the most common psychiatric problems in nursing homes. Education and training of all healthcare providers working in LTC facilities in assessment of psychiatric symptoms and their management with evidence-based psychosocial environmental and when necessary pharmacological interventions are key to improving the quality of life of LTC residents.

Ageing ethnic minority groups

It is estimated that by 2060, a majority of Americans will be 'ethnic minorities', and this increase will be most pronounced for Latinos and African Americans. At present, these groups have higher than average mental healthcare needs compared with others and this seems to result from income disparities and certain behaviours and attitudes that may be culturally related. Regarding healthcare services and, in particular, mental health services, many of these groups may be better served by providers who understand the culture and by systems that are closely aligned with community needs. Unfortunately, disparities in the provision of care to racial and ethnic minorities remain. These inequalities translate into inferior outcomes in these populations, especially in the ageing ethnic minority groups.

Older adults visiting the Emergency Department (ED)

The prevalence of mental health problems (especially alcohol abuse, depression and delirium) in older adults visiting EDs is high. Thus, screening for depression, alcohol abuse and delirium for all elderly persons visiting the ED is recommended. Brief interventions to address these disorders in the ED, such as notification of the PCP and home health providers, and referrals as needed may improve outcomes (e.g. reduced risk of functional decline).

Older prisoners

Older prisoners are the fastest growing segment of the population in US federal and state prisons. It is increasingly recognized that older prisoners have a higher burden of mental health, physical health and social problems, in addition to different mental health needs than the mainly adult male population within prisons. Up to 20% of inmates older than 55 years have a significant mental illness.[23] Depression, guilt, worry and psychological stress are common. Older inmates also express stress of being away from their families, the stigma associated with their crime and depression related to the possibility of dying in prison as some of the largest factors in their problems with emotional wellbeing. Ethnic minorities are over-represented in prison populations. Involving clinical faculty and staff from academic medical centres to provide healthcare (including mental healthcare) to the ageing prison population can produce significant improvements in access to care and health outcomes. Thousands of older and medically frail prisoners are being released early from prisons following a court-ordered inmate reduction programme. Many of these older inmates will need immediate care at hospitals, dialysis units and mental health units and their first stop in freedom may be the ED.

Caregivers

Many older adults find themselves in the role of caring for their spouse or partner with dementia or older children with disability (e.g. mental retardation). Caregiving can take a toll on the mental health of caregivers and has been associated with an increased risk of depression and functional decline. Caregiving involves learning to 'bend without breaking'. Transition to institutional care is particularly difficult for spouses, almost half of whom visit the disabled spouse daily and continue to provide help with physical and emotional care during their visits. Symptoms of depression and anxiety often do not diminish after institutional placement, use of anxiolytic medications by caregivers increases and nearly half of the caregivers are at risk for clinical depression following placement of their loved one in LTC facilities. Clinical interventions that prepare the caregiver for a placement transition and treat their depression and anxiety following placement are recommended. Healthcare providers must help families work towards effectively coping with the disease in their family member, decreasing the harmful effects on the family and keeping family conflicts to a minimum. Interventions such as counselling, support groups, psychoeducational groups, training in contingency planning, respite services, skills training and family-directed treatments can alleviate caregiver stress, prevent caregiver depression and improve coping skills.

Oldest old

Oldest old refers to the 85 years and over age group, which is the fastest growing age group in the USA. This group has not been well studied and therefore is poorly understood by psychiatrists.[24] Although function varies widely among the oldest old, many quickly develop a serious decline in their cognitive and physical health, which in turn causes emotional suffering. This group also experiences loss of spouse and friends due to death and disability and therefore are at risk for bereavement- and depression-related morbidity and mortality. The boundaries between psychiatry and medicine become inextricably blurred at the most advanced ages. Once older people experience a serious general medical and/or psychiatric illness, physical, mental and social impairments coalesce and cascade, resulting in disability and premature death unless multimodal interventions are put in place. Oldest old patients receiving collaborative depression care were found to have a lower rate of long-term treatment response and complete remission in the long run compared with younger old.[25] Centenarians are proportionally the most rapidly growing segment of the oldest old. The majority of centenarians are in remarkably good emotional and cognitive health until the last few years of their life.

Palliative and end-of-life care

Conversations with patients and family about end-of-life care, the evaluation and treatment of suffering, including pain, depression, suicidality, anxiety and delirium, providing individual and family therapy to address conflicts, capacity determination, advance care planning, withholding life-sustaining treatments, palliative/hospice care and management of terminal agitation are some of the key areas where geriatric psychiatrists and other health professionals can contribute to a dignified and peaceful final phase of life for older adults.

Geriatric psychopharmacology

Older adults are substantial users of psychopharmacological agents. About 12–15% of older adults living in the community and up to 75% of LTC residents receive psychotropic medications at some point in their lives. All psychotropic agents should be prescribed judiciously and only for severe and/or chronic mental health symptoms because of the potential for serious adverse effects and even death associated with many psychotropic agents. Therefore, PCPs caring for older adults need to have a comprehensive knowledge of the risks and benefits of commonly prescribed psychotropic drugs (e.g. SSRIs, benzodiazepines, atypical antipsychotics). Table 81.5 summarizes the principles of psychopharmacotherapy in older adults. Benzodiazepines, commonly used for the treatment of anxiety and insomnia, are the most frequently prescribed psychotropic agents in older adults. Because of their potential to cause cognitive impairment and problems with balance which may increase the risk of falls and fractures, their use should be restricted to short-term treatment of incapacitating anxiety symptoms and/or insomnia.

Table 81.5 Principles of psychopharmacotherapy in older adults.

1. Perform a thorough evaluation prior to prescription of psychotropic agents
2. Optimize conditions for successful psychopharmacological outcomes:
   a. Reduce anticholinergic burden
   b. Discontinue unnecessary drugs
   c. Check liver and kidney functions prior to initiation of psychopharmacological therapy
3. Identify goals of psychopharmacological therapy and discuss them with the patient prior to initiation
4. Provide education regarding the importance of compliance and adverse effects to look for
5. Select a psychotropic agent based on evidence to date, patients' physical health conditions, risk of drug–drug interactions and response to previous agents that may have been tried
6. Start low and go slow
7. Give an adequate dose for an adequate duration
8. Combine psychopharmacological therapy with psychotherapy and or other psychosocial interventions
9. Monitor for adverse effects and drug–drug interactions
10. Measure response to treatment
11. Discontinue psychotropic agents if there is no response
12. Introduce/change one psychotropic agent at a time

Electroconvulsive therapy

Older adults constitute more than one-half of patients who receive ECT for the treatment of depression. ECT is an underutilized treatment options despite its relative safety and high effectiveness for relieving depression in older adults. Although ECT is often considered only when depression is life threatening (e.g. the patient is suicidal, not eating), it should be considered a first-line option in all patients with severe depressive symptoms, especially in the presence of psychotic symptoms. The efficacy of ECT does not diminish with advancing age but the seizure threshold increases.

Psychotherapy and other psychosocial interventions

Later life is increasingly seen as a time of vitality during which individuals can expect to explore and develop their potential. Psychotherapy can foster this. Society has made available social services and living options that did not exist a few decades ago. Although emotions are vital ingredients of all the therapies, focus is best directed at functional outcomes. Psychotherapeutic approaches in older adults need to be dynamic and sensitive to the existential issues of loss, dependency and change of status, yet fully aware of opportunities for growth and vigour. Psychotherapy can play a vital role in the relief of suffering for older adults, their families and palliative care staff. Existential anxiety of facing death in old age can also be addressed during psychotherapy. The use of psychotherapy in combination with medication can improve long-term outcomes and decrease disability in elderly depressed patients. The task in later life is the acceptance of life as a finite and almost completed product and, therefore, an acceptance of mortality. Usually, this is accomplished without help being needed from psychiatrists or psychotherapists. The burden of caring for older patients near death or actually dying requires an acute awareness and unusual flexibility on the part of the therapist. When the focus is changed to quality of life and decreasing suffering, even for just a few days, all mental health interventions in end of life become meaningful. Regardless of disability or age, hope and dignity can be maintained to the end. Cognitive behaviour therapy, interpersonal therapy, problem-solving therapy and family therapy appear well suited to addressing many physical, interpersonal, social and financial problems among older adults with depression and anxiety. Families are such important components of older adults' lives that they offer a powerful locus for intervention, in addition to powerful support for individual interventions. Clinicians need to 'think family' as they provide mental and physical health services to older adults, as older adults are highly likely to be intensively embedded in a family support and care structure.

Spirituality and geriatric psychiatry

A growing literature links religious participation and spirituality with better mental health among older adults. Religiosity/spirituality may (a) provide a sense of meaning or purpose that buffers stress and assists with coping; and (b) provide a network of like-minded persons who can serve as social resources and promote the development of psychological resources, including self-esteem and a sense of personal growth. Clinicians have a moral obligation to address patients' spiritual concerns. In considering the spiritual dimension of the patient, the clinician is sending an important message that he or she is concerned with the whole person. This enhances the patient–physician relationship and is likely to increase the therapeutic impact of interventions. Referring older adults suffering from depression, pain or other serious symptoms to chaplains or to their own personal clergy should be routinely considered.

Prevention in geriatric psychiatry

With the rapidly growing number of elderly individuals at risk for depression, delirium and dementia, finding ways to prevent these syndromes is a public health priority.[26] Older adults with multiple risk factors (e.g. chronic pain, stroke, dementia, hearing and vision deficits, residing in an LTC facility) may be considered a target population for prevention programmes. As we continue to understand risk factors better, it may be possible to personalize depression, suicide and dementia prevention. Other targets for prevention include premature institutionalization and alcohol or medication misuse. Table 81.6 highlights some of the evidence-based prevention interventions.

Best practice models for geriatric psychiatry services

Service needs of older adults with psychiatric disorders are complex. Older adults with psychiatric disorders commonly face, in addition to persistent symptoms, increasing medical morbidity, dwindling financial resources and social impoverishment. In addition, older adults are victims of a culture that has stigmatized both mental illness and advanced age. Older adults with psychiatric disorders are more susceptible to stigmatization than younger adults and therefore less likely to seek help. Older adults are less likely than younger persons to self-identify mental health problems or seek specialty mental health services. This problem is further compounded by family members and professional providers who share the misperception that mental disorders such as depression and dementia are a 'normal part of ageing'. Without addressing stigma, systemic reforms designed to improve access are unlikely to be successful. The use of community-based, multidisciplinary, geriatric mental health treatment teams is one of the ideal models of psychiatry service delivery in the community.[34] Hospital-based geriatric psychiatry consultation–liaison services are also recommended to meet the complex mental health needs of hospitalized older adults. Geriatric psychiatry subspecialty care for older adults needing treatment in an inpatient psychiatric unit appears to be associated with distinct clinically relevant assessment and treatment advantages (such as complete medical work-ups, structured cognitive assessment, ageing sensitive aftercare referral and monitoring of psychopharmacological side effects and blood levels) over general

Table 81.6 Examples of evidence-based prevention in geriatric psychiatry.

Interventions	Potential outcomes
Non-pharmacological multicomponent interventions[19]	Prevention of delirium
Telemedicine[27]	Prevention of psychiatric admissions from LTC facility
Family intervention[28]	Delay in institutionalization of patients with dementia
Exercise plus behavioural management[29]	Reduced disability in patients with dementia
Caregiver counselling and support[30]	Prevention of caregiver depression
Depression care managers in primary care[20]	Prevention of suicide
Comprehensive nutritional treatment[31]	Prevention of weight loss in patients with dementia
Exercise[32]	Prevention of depression
Adult day programme[33]	Reduced risk of accelerated cognitive decline associated with nursing home placement

psychiatry care. Best practice models for mental healthcare in LTC facilities include routine presence of qualified mental health clinicians in the nursing home, interdisciplinary and multidimensional approaches using innovative techniques in training and education and consultation and feedback on clinical practices. Model services to meet the growing needs of all older adults with psychiatric disorders will require a multidisciplinary approach to treatment, encompassing both the traditional models of psychiatric treatment and treatments that focus on medical, cognitive and social arenas.

Although there is considerable underutilization of mental health services by older adults in all settings (primary care, hospital, long-term care, home health, rehabilitation), older adults who receive treatment report benefiting from services at least as much as their younger counterparts. The President's New Freedom Commission on Mental Health urged the adoption of evidence-based practices (EBPs) across the lifespan and its Subcommittee on Older Adults identified the dissemination and implementation of EBPs as one of the most important initiatives for improving quality of care for older persons with mental disorders.[1]

Long-term care homes

Visionary and determined people are reinventing LTC facilities. These individuals believe that each of us, no matter how old, sick, frail, disabled or forgetful, deserves to have a loving home – not a facility. These individuals have pioneered long-term care homes (LTCHs) to replace long-term care facilities (LTCFs). Such LTCHs make the quality of life of their residents life affirming, create a culture that rekindles the human spirit and mend the frayed social fabric of our current society. Such transformational change is needed not only in LTCFs but also in the entire culture of ageing. There are several remarkable LTCHs led by people with vision and determination and staffed by compassionate, creative and competent individuals. Residents and staff members of such LTCHs have more friends than restrictions and rules to follow. Such LTCHs know that the single most important thing residents and caregivers (family and professional) value – more than good food, good medical care or clean facilities – is the warmth of a caring relationship. Such LTCHs sustain their high-quality care through relentless adherence to person-centred care (PCC). We need to give homes that have adopted PCC credit and create incentives and training for every home to begin its own journey towards PCC. An ideal LTCH not only becomes a home of choice in the community, but also reduces staff turnover and the cost of healthcare (e.g. reduced hospitalizations at the end of life).

Geriatric psychiatry in primary care offices

Approximately one-third of older primary care patients have significant mental health problems. There is high comorbidity of mental health disorders in older adults with medically unexplained symptoms. Utilization of herbal and nutritional compounds is very high (up to 30%) in older adults with mood disorders. Therefore, HCPs in primary care need to assess f routinely or their use, particularly with respect to potential drug–drug interactions. Many older adults prefer to receive mental health services in community-based settings (especially in their PCP offices) and home-based settings (e.g. home visits including psychotherapy for frail older adults). Care management models that integrate mental health providers (e.g. trained social workers) into the primary care setting to provide same-day mental health services show promise in enhancing access to high-quality mental healthcare.

Academic detailing, which consists of brief one-to-one educational sessions coupled with provider-specific feedback on treatment practices, is effective in influencing the practice behaviour of PCPs and can be used to improve the management of psychiatric disorders in primary care.

Successful ageing

Emotional and cognitive health as it pertains to the older adult should be defined not just as the absence of disease, but also as the development and preservation of the multidimensional emotional and cognitive structures that allow the older adult to maintain social connectedness, an ongoing sense of purpose and the abilities to function independently, to recover functionally from illness or injury; and to cope with residual functional deficits.[35] In daily life, the domains of emotional and cognitive health are inseparably linked. Therefore, promoting emotional wellbeing should be conceptualized hand in hand with promoting cognitive wellbeing. The ageing human brain has a surprising capacity to maintain plasticity. Although usually under-emphasized, positive personality changes, such as better tolerance, regulation of affect and ability to appreciate different points of view, occur with ageing and can contribute to successful adjustment and high quality of life. Older adults as a whole do not have more psychiatric disorders than younger adults, they do not see themselves as sick even when they take three to eight different medications, their fear of death declines and their spirituality and serenity increase. Improving levels of education may have a positive impact on late-life emotional and cognitive wellbeing. Researchers to date have identified many predictors of successful ageing (such as absence of alcohol abuse and of cigarette smoking before the age of 50 years) that are to a large extent under the individual's own control. Stable marriage and adaptive defences are also predictive of successful ageing, subjective satisfaction and objective mental health. Among factors outside the individual's control, only depression before the age of 50 years was a significant predictor of mortality, medical morbidity and sadness during late life. Older adults with strong feelings of personal control and self-efficacy (that is, the personal conviction that one can successfully execute behaviours required in novel or stressful situations) are more likely to cope successfully with late-life challenges and, consequently, more likely to maintain a high level of emotional wellbeing. The presence of a spiritual belief system has also been correlated with decreased depression, faster recovery from illness and increased longevity in later life. SECA may involve optimal balance between functions of phylogenetically more primitive brain regions (limbic system) and newer ones (prefrontal cortex).

An extract from a poem by the Indian poet Rabindranath Tagore reflects the attitude that many older adults who age successfully have toward life, death and disease. It is time geriatric psychiatry pays as much attention to health promotion as to disease.

On fear of death

Let me not pray to be sheltered from dangers but to be fearless in facing them.

Let me not beg for the stilling of my pain but for the heart to conquer it.

Let me not look for allies in life's battlefield but to my own strength.

Let me not crave in anxious fear to be saved but hope for the patience to win my freedom.

Grant me that I may not be a coward, feeling your mercy in my success alone; but let me find the grasp of your hand in my failure.

Rabindranath Tagore (in *Fruit Gathering*).

Future research

The DSM-IV TR has significant limitations relative to its utility in older adults with mental health problems. Future research needs to overcome these limitations. The most prevalent activity throughout our lives is work. Future studies need to clarify whether retirement has detrimental effects on emotional and cognitive wellbeing, especially for individuals who do not have resources to maintain a high level of activity and social participation. Only in the last few years has attention been paid to studying preserved emotional and cognitive health as an outcome in older adults. Future research needs to identify validated instruments to measure these outcomes. There is also an emerging realization that whenever emotional disorders (e.g. depression) and cognitive disorders (e.g. dementia) occur together, they worsen each other. More research is needed to clarify these complex interactions and identify interventions that prevent accelerated decline in function and premature death.

Key points

- Psychiatric disorders in older adults are prevalent and eminently treatable.
- Comprehensive assessment, an interdisciplinary approach and holistic multimodal interventions are the hallmarks of geriatric psychiatry.
- Evidence base is most developed for interventions addressing depression and dementia in older adults, although effective treatments and service models have been identified for a variety of psychiatric disorders in older adults.
- Overcoming barriers such as stigma, inadequate reimbursement for psychiatric services, lack of geriatric expertise, fragmented care and lack of integration of primary care and mental health services is crucial to preventing the upcoming crisis in geriatric psychiatry services.

References

1. Bartels SJ. Improving the system of care for older adults with mental illness in the United States. Findings and recommendations for the President's New Freedom Commission on Mental Health. *Am J Geriatr Psychiatry* 2003;**11**:486–97.

2. Jeste DV, Alexopoulos GS, Bartels SJ *et al.* Consensus statement on the upcoming crisis in geriatric mental health: research agenda for the next two decades. *Arch Gen Psychiatry* 1999;**56**:848–53.
3. Gum AM, Cheavens JS. Psychiatric comorbidity and depression in older adults. *Current Psychiatry Reports* 2008;**10**(1):23–29.
4. Inouye SK. Clarifying confusion: the confusion assessment method: a new method for detection of delirium. *Ann Intern Med* 1990;**113**:941–50.
5. Galvin JE, Roe CM, Powlishta KK *et al.* The AD8: a brief informant interview to detect dementia. *Neurology* 2005; **65**:559–64.
6. Borson S, Scanlan JM, Chen P *et al.* The Mini-Cog as a screen for dementia: validation in a population-based sample. *J Am Geriatr Soc* 2003;**51**:1451–4.
7. Tariq SH, Tumosa N, Chibnall JT *et al.* The Saint Louis University Mental Status (SLUMS) Examination for detecting mild cognitive impairment and dementia is more sensitive than the Mini-Mental Status Examination (MMSE) – a pilot study. *Am J Geriatr Psychiatry* 2006;**14**:900–10.
8. Folstein M, Folstein SE and McHugh PR. 'Mini-Mental State': a practical method for grading the cognitive state of patients for the clinician. *J Psychiatr Res* 1975;**12**;189–98.
9. Nasreddine ZS, Phillips NA, Bedirian V *et al.* The Montreal Cognitive Assessment (MoCA): a brief screening tool for mild cognitive impairment. *J Am Geriatr Soc* 2005;**53**:695–9.
10. Kroenke K, Spitzer RL and Williams JB. The PHQ-2. Validity of a two-item depression screener. *Med Care* 2003;**41**:1284–94.
11. Kroenke K and Spitzer R. The PHQ 9: A new depression diagnostic and severity measure. *Psychiatr Ann* 2002;**32**:1–7.
12. Yesavage JA, Brink TL, Rose TL *et al.* Development and validation of a geriatric depression screening scale: a preliminary report. *J Psychiatr Res* 1983;**17**:37–49.
13. Alexopolous G, Abrams R, Young R, and Shamoian C. Cornell scale for depression in dementia. *Biol Psychiatry* 1988;**23**:271–84.
14. Ewing JA. Detecting alcoholism: the CAGE Questionnaire. *JAMA* 1984;**252**:1905–7.
15. Blow FC, Gillespie BW, Barry KL *et al.* Brief screening for alcohol problems in elderly populations using the Short Michigan Alcohol Screening Test – Geriatric Version (SMAST-G). *Alcoholism Clin Experimental Res* 1998;**22**:31A.
16. Cohen-Mansfield J and Libin A. Assessment of agitation in elderly patients with dementia: correlations between informant rating and direct observation. *Int J Geriatr Psychiatry* 2004;**19**:881–91.
17. Lyketsos CG, Colenda CC, Beck C *et al.* Position statement of the American Association for Geriatric Psychiatry regarding principles of care for patients with dementia resulting from Alzheimer's disease. *Am J Geriatr Psychiatry* 2006;**14**:561–72.
18. Ballard C, Corbett A, Chitramohan R and Aarsland D. Management of agitation and aggression associated with Alzheimer's disease: controversies and possible solutions *Curr Opin Psychiatry* 2009;**22**:532–40.
19. Inouye SK, Bogardus ST Jr, Williams CS *et al.* The role of adherence on the effectiveness of nonpharmacologic interventions: evidence from the delirium prevention trial. *Arch Intern Med* 2003;**163**:958–64.
20. Alexopoulos GS, Reynolds CF III, Bruce ML *et al.* Reducing suicidal ideation and depression in older primary care patients: 24-month outcomes of the PROSPECT study. *Am J Psychiatry* 2009;**166**:882–90.
21. Cooper C, Selwood A, Livingston G. The prevalence of elder abuse and neglect: a systematic review. *Age Ageing* 2008;**37**(2):151–160.
22. Weiss A, Sutin AR, Duberstein PR *et al.* The personality domains and styles of the five-factor model are related to incident depression in medicare recipients aged 65 to 100. *Am J Geriatr Psychiatry* 2009;**17**:591–601.
23. Mitka M. Aging prisoners stressing health care system. *JAMA* 2004;**292**:423–4.
24. Blazer DG. Psychiatry and the oldest old. *Am J Psychiatry* 2000;**157**:1915–24.
25. Van Leeuwen Williams E, Unutzer E, Lee S and Noel P. Collaborative depression care for the old-old: findings from the IMPACT trial. *Am J Geriatr Psychiatry* 2009;**17**:1040–9.
26. Desai AK, Grossberg GT and Chibnall JT. Healthy brain aging: a road map. *Clin Geriatr Med* 2010;**26**:1–16.
27. Lyketsos CG, Roques C, Hovanec L and Jones BN III. Telemedicine use and the reduction of psychiatric admissions from a long-term care facility. *J Geriatr Psychiatry Neurol* 2001;**14**:1626–8.
28. Mittleman MS, Ferris SH, Shulman E *et al.* A family intervention to delay nursing home placement of patients with Alzheimer disease. A randomized controlled trial. *JAMA* 1996;**276**:1725–31.
29. Terri L, Gibbons LE, McCurry SM *et al.* Exercise plus behavioral management in patients with Alzheimer's disease: a randomized controlled trial. *JAMA* 2003;**290**:2015–22.
30. Mittelman MS, Roth DL, Coon DW and Haley WE. Sustained benefit of supportive intervention for depressive symptoms in caregivers of patients with Alzheimer's disease. *Am J Psychiatry* 2004;**161**:850–6.
31. Keller HH, Gibbs AJ, Boudreau LD *et al.* Prevention of weight loss in dementia with comprehensive nutritional treatment. *J Am Geriatr Soc* 2003;**51**:945–52.
32. Christmas C and Andersen RA. Exercise and older patients: guidelines for the clinician. *J Am Geriatr Soc* 2000;**48**:318–24.
33. Wilson RS, McCann JJ, Li Y *et al.* Nursing home placement, day care use and cognitive decline in Alzheimer's disease. *Am J Psychiatry* 2007;**164**:910–15.
34. Bartels SJ, Dums AR, Oxman TE *et al.* Evidence-based practices in geriatric mental health care. *Psychiatr Serv* 2002; **53**:1419–31.
35. Hendrie HC, Albert MS, Butters MA *et al.* The NIH Cognitive and Emotional Health Project: Report of the Critical Evaluation Study Committee. *Alzheimer's Dementia* 2006;**2**:12–32.

CHAPTER 82

Organization of services in geriatric psychiatry

Susan Mary Benbow[1] and David Jolley[2]

[1]Staffordshire University, Stafford, Staffordshire and Older Mind Matters Ltd, Manchester, Cheshire, UK

[2]Manchester University, Manchester, UK

Introduction

Old age psychiatry is a relatively young specialty of psychiatry: the first pioneers of 'psychogeriatrics' began to develop specialist services for older people in the UK in the 1960s and 1970s. Early service principles included:

- a comprehensive age-related catchment area service
- assessment at home before admission by a senior member of the team
- diagnosis followed by active treatment
- team working
- close liaison with GPs, geriatricians and social services.

In 1989, old-age psychiatry was recognized as a specialty by the UK Department of Health and by the millennium the Royal College of Psychiatrists recognized over 350 specialists in the psychiatry of old age. In 2004, the number of old age psychiatrists was given as 444[1] and in September 2007 there were 543 old age psychiatrists (representing 510 full-time equivalents) in England alone (see http://www.cfwi.org.uk/).

It is useful to revisit the reasons why old-age psychiatry first developed. Within an all-age adult psychiatry service, older adults were not receiving the dedicated care and attention they deserved, as they were in competition with younger adults for attention and resources. Younger psychiatric patients present high-profile risks and work with young people carries higher kudos, perhaps because they are economically active and conform to accepted ideals of attractiveness. This ignores the enormous contribution which older adults make to society: most voluntary organizations would disappear without the input they provide, many continue to work long after retirement age, many take up or continue roles as carers (to younger people, people with learning disabilities, to other elders). Others continue to make their wisdom and talents available to the rest of society.

Looking beyond these ageist and attitudinal obstacles, mental illness in late life offers additional challenges as it is often complicated by comorbid physical illnesses, the physical and psychological changes associated with ageing, and/or by the coexistence of cognitive impairment. These attributes demand special skills and organization of the mental health professionals who aim to provide a service orientated to the practical needs of many elders.

The National Service Framework for Older People (NSF-OP: www.dh.gov.uk/en/Publicationsandstatistics/Publications/PublicationsPolicyAndGuidance/DH_4003066) set out a service model for a comprehensive mental health service for older people. Components of the model service were to include:

- mental health promotion
- early detection and diagnosis
- assessment and treatment
- support for carers
- specialist mental health services, to include acute admission and rehabilitation beds, day hospitals and memory clinics, domiciliary and outreach care and outpatient/community clinics.

The NSF-OP was warmly received by many old age psychiatrists as it embedded mental health as integral to the health of older people and its core principles ('rooting out age discrimination' and 'person-centred care') are potentially powerful influences for positive change in older people's mental health.

The National Service Framework for Mental Health (http://www.dh.gov.uk/en/Publicationsandstatistics/Publications/PublicationsPolicyAndGuidance/DH-4009598) had been less warmly received as it excluded older adults and focused on services to working aged adults. Monies and developments associated with the NSF-MH therefore excluded older adult services and led to expansion of working-aged adult mental health services at the expense of services to older adults. The NSF-OP stated that older people with severe mental illness would require the packages of care set out in the NSF-MH, but this requirement went largely unnoticed at the time.

Principles and Practice of Geriatric Medicine, Fifth Edition. Edited by Alan J. Sinclair, John E. Morley and Bruno Vellas.

Developments in the UK 2005–2010

Over the 5 years between 2005 and 2010 much has happened. Policy never stands still. Securing better mental health for older adults (www.dh.gov.uk/en/Publicationsandstatistics/Publications/PublicationsPolicyAndGuidance/DH_4114989) and Everybody's Business (http://www.nmhdu.org.uk/silo/files/six-key-messages.pdf) set out useful details about the structure and aims of OPMH services. Our Health, Our Care, Our Say (http://www.behfuture.nhs.uk/archive/docs/appendix_2.pdf) highlighted the need to improve the health and care of people with complex long-term conditions and to provide good local community facilities. It recognized the need for a national framework for NHS continuing and nursing care and clarity regarding what the NHS will provide for those with the most complex long-term care needs – this includes those people who need long-term care for mental health problems in late life. The NSF-OP was followed by the dignity in care campaign (see www.dhcarenetworks.org.uk/dignityincare/DignityCareCampaign/), which straddles mental and physical healthcare services.

Alongside these developments sit professional initiatives. Useful professional documents produced by the Royal College of Psychiatrists include the Faculty of Old Age Psychiatry report Raising the Standard (www.rcpsych.ac.uk/PDF/RaisingtheStandardOAPwebsite.pdf), the report on older adult liaison services called Who Cares Wins (www.bgs.org.uk/PDF%20Downloads/WhoCaresWins.pdf), a report produced jointly with the Alzheimer's Society on services for younger people with dementia (www.rcpsych.ac.uk/publications/collegereports/cr/cr135.aspx), a report on transitions between general psychiatry services and older people's mental health services (www.rcpsych.ac.uk/files/pdfversion/CR153.pdf) and an updated report on services to ethnic elders (www.rcpsych.ac.uk/files/pdfversion/CR156.pdf).

The Mental Capacity Act of 2005 (www.opsi.gov.uk/acts/acts2005/ukpga_20050009_en_1) had far-reaching implications in England and Wales for the care of people who may be incapable of making decisions. It changed the legal context: there is an obligation to take 'all practicable steps' to help the person make their own decision and to consider whether the outcome could be achieved in a less restrictive way when doing something to someone or making a decision on their behalf. The Act was modified in 2007 to introduce safeguards for very vulnerable people at risk of being deprived of their liberty.

Meanwhile, social care has developed a new emphasis on personalization, which is sometimes seen purely in financial terms as putting people in charge of how money is spent on their care, but, in fact, potentially embraces a much wider move towards giving individuals more control and choice in respect of their support services. New Horizons (http://www.dh.gov.uk/en/Publicationsandstatistics/Publications/PublicationsPolicyAndGuidance/DH_109705) brings together a life course approach, which sees older people's mental health brought together with mental health at other stages of life and personalization.

With regard to dementia services, this period has seen the controversial 2009 updating of NICE's Technology Assessment of the anti-dementia drugs (http://guidance.nice.org.uk/TA111), which accepted that the anti-Alzheimer's drugs are clinically effective but restricted their use (on the grounds of dubious cost-effectiveness) to people with moderate dementia, resulting in a storm of protest in the media. The protests were muted somewhat by the commonsense approach of the dementia guideline (www.nice.org.uk/nicemedia/pdf/CG42Dementiafinal.pdf). Since then, an ambitious National Dementia Strategy (www.dh.gov.uk/en/Publicationsandstatistics/Publications/PublicationsPolicyAndGuidance/DH_094058) has been introduced, but in the prevailing economic climate it will be surprising if the strategy achieves its aspirations. Dementia 2010 (www.dementia2010.org/reports/Dementia2010Full.pdf) has recently highlighted how important it is for the country, financially and in human terms, to face the challenges posed by the dementias, which are costing the UK economy more than cancer and heart disease combined.

Changes in practice have occurred alongside these initiatives. Some services have subdivided into inpatient and community services or sponsored specialist teams for liaison mental health, home treatment[2,3] or even forensic problems.[4] There are some enthusiasts for specialist 'dementia-only services', a notion supported by some charities and managers. We would counsel the preservation and enrichment of services which are catholic in their acceptance criteria and comprehensive in their coverage.

The ageism saga continues

The exclusion of older people from the NSF-MH in 1999 was regarded by some as ageist and the New Horizons initiative (www.dh.gov.uk/en/Healthcare/Mentalhealth/DH_209) has since recognized that old-age psychiatry is firmly part of the family of psychiatry. However, there are hazards ahead: it is equally ageist to deny that older adults have special needs to which services should be sensitive and in dealing with which service organization and response must be competent. What is right for adults of working-age will not always be right for older people. Older people need services which are designed to meet their particular and often complex needs. These are not confined to dementia, so services should encompass the whole range of mental disorders of late life for a number of reasons:

• The distinction between depressive disorders and the dementias is not a clearly defined boundary. Many people present to services with a mixture of symptoms raising the classical old-age psychiatry conundrum – is this depression or is this dementia? (it may of course be both).
• Older adults with other mental health problems and without a dementia have special needs in service terms and should receive appropriate specialist help.
• Other mental illnesses also overlap with the dementias, for example, anxiety disorders, paranoid states.

Hence the issue of age discrimination in mental health is a challenge for services, which must be tailored to need and not to rigid age cutoffs or politically correct prejudices. This is an important principle in service planning and delivery.

Services

Community old-age psychiatry

Community treatment

One of the early principles of old-age psychiatry was assessment at home by a senior member of the old-age psychiatry team.[5] This led on to the concept of a community clinic[6] and many services carry out the majority of their assessment, treatment and follow-up by seeing people in their homes, coordinating the activity of different disciplines using IT support and close liaison between team members. Community treatment for older people involves close working with social services (particularly with day centres for older adults and domiciliary services) and voluntary organizations and close links between the CMHT-OP and places where older adults are resident, including sheltered and extra-care housing and the residential and care home sector.

Early detection and diagnosis: interface with primary care

The majority of people with mental health problems in late life are never seen by a specialist service. Many will remain unrecognized even when they have contact with primary and social care services (for more details, see www.nao.org.uk/publications/0910/improving_dementia_services.aspx).

Family doctors are, however, well placed to identify cognitive problems and mood disorders early, to provide people with information and to introduce them, where necessary, to further investigations, treatment and support. Those working in primary care see many elders with physical problems regularly and this gives the opportunity to assess and monitor the person's mental health in a familiar setting. An established relationship with their family doctor or practice nurse may also help an individual to accept the need for referral to specialist services for assessment, treatment or support or to social services or voluntary organizations. The family doctor is an essential and central person in care coordination. A useful opportunity for early detection presents when people are being seen in primary care for other reasons. For example, people at high risk for arteriosclerosis are also at high risk for developing a vascular dementia, and family doctors screen people routinely for cardiovascular disease. Those who are identified as at high risk are examined regularly and have renal function and lipid levels checked. Some family doctors add a cognitive test to the cardiovascular assessment and use this opportunity to detect cognitive problems. This practice is now rewarded within the QOF system (see www.qof.ic.nhs.uk).

One of the milestones set out in the Older People's NSF was that Primary Care Trusts (PCTs) were required by April 2004 to ensure that every general practice was using a protocol agreed with local specialist services for the diagnosis, treatment and care of older adults with depression or dementia. Protocols for the treatment of people with Alzheimer's disease aimed to set out physical investigations and cognitive testing which could be carried out in primary care, in order to facilitate early detection and rapid access to anti-dementia drug treatment if appropriate. Tucker *et al.*[7] found that fewer than 50% of their responding consultant old-age psychiatrists reported that GPs were using protocols for the care of people with depression or with dementia. Where are the protocols now?

A great deal of research is currently being directed towards improving the performance of primary care in identifying and caring for people with dementia.[8] Some specialist services have developed formal links with primary care.[9]

Community mental health teams for older people (CMHT-OP)

The NSF-OP set out who should be core members of the CMHT-OP: this included community mental health nurses, consultant old-age psychiatrists, clinical psychologists, social workers and occupational therapists. A range of other disciplines were listed as needing to have agreed working and referral arrangements with the team but not working as full members of it. One of the big issues for a CMHT-OP is that of 'integration'. In this context, integration usually refers to the integration of health and social care (for more information, see http://its-services.org.uk/silo/files/integrating-opmh-services.pdf). The Durham mapping project pilot in older people's mental health services used four main criteria for an integrated CMHT-OP:

• The team should include interagency multidisciplinary staff involving health and social services.
• It should provide integrated assessment, care planning and care coordination.
• It should use shared recording systems and IT, supporting both the Care Programme Approach (CPA) and the Single Assessment Process (SAP).

• There should be a single point of entry to specialist mental health assessment.

Integration remains an issue today, although, along with protocols, it has become less fashionable. A 'single point of access' has become a must-have for many managers who are rushing to introduce it despite feedback from a number of localities that it introduces a new raft of service problems.

How teams work in relation to team members' responsibility is another continuing question. This became increasingly important because of high consultant psychiatrist vacancy levels in the UK (running at around 12–14%) with associated problems of recruitment and retention, coupled with evidence that consultants were overburdened and stressed.[10] An initiative called New Ways of Working (see http://www.newwaysofworking.org.uk/component/option,com_docman/task,cat_view/gid,214/Itemid,412/) claimed to modernise mental health services by placing greater responsibilities on nurses and other non-medical staff. The aim has been to reduce pressure on consultant psychiatrists and to enable them to focus on more complex cases. Insensitive top-down insistence on imposing this model nationally and on including services for older people has not been appreciated.[11]

Specialist community teams

Some services for older people have claimed that there is an advantage in establishing specialist teams: examples include specialist home treatment teams,[2,3] crisis resolution and home treatment teams extended to cover older adults[12] and Care Homes Support teams (www.rcpsych.ac.uk/files/pdfversion/CR153.pdf). These initiatives are usually the product of opportunistic local service redesign and require rigorous objective evaluation. Most are conceived in the belief that they will enable more people to be treated in their own homes, thus avoiding hospital admissions and costing less.

Hospital

Hospital-based facilities

Acute inpatient beds

Community-orientated services need access to inpatient beds for the assessment and treatment of older people with a range of diagnoses who cannot be managed in the community. A small proportion will be detained under mental health legislation. The main distinction is between people who have an organic brain disorder and those with so-called functional disorders, the most common of which is depressive illness. Current thinking is said to support separate inpatient provision for people with organic brain disorders and those with other mental health problems in later life (www.audit-commission.gov.uk/health/nationalstudies/socialcare/pages/forgetmenot_copy.aspx). The distinction between the two is often neither clear nor absolute in practice, and flexibility and tolerance are needed when accommodating the changeable and complex needs of very ill/disturbed older people. It is not usually appropriate to care for older adults with complex needs on wards for younger adults. This would place them at risk and deprive them of the specialist nursing, medical and other care which they require.

Day hospitals

Day hospitals for older people are widely available across the UK, but the literature supporting their role is remarkably sparse. The Faculty of Old Age Psychiatry carried out a survey of old-age psychiatry day hospitals and published a report in June 2001 (see www.rcpsych.ac.uk/pdf/surveydayhospitals.pdf). Three-quarters of day hospitals operated a mixed service to people with organic and functional illnesses in late life. The study found that people attend day hospitals for a great many different reasons and for varying periods of time: over one-third of people attend for over 1 year. Carer support is a common feature of a day hospital service and some units aim to provide a respite service for people with dementia in association with particularly challenging behaviours which restrict their access to alternative sources of respite. Aims for an old-age psychiatry day hospital include the following:

• reduction of inpatient bed use by functionally ill older people
• prevention of admission: by supporting CMHTs in maintaining ill people in the community during crisis
• prevention of readmission through relapse prevention
• prevention of readmission through prevention of recurrence
• reduction of duration of an episode of inpatient treatment.

Outpatient clinics

For many services, the majority of activity takes place in the community using a community clinic model. Some older adults may prefer to be seen in a traditional hospital-based outpatient clinic. The hospital may also support specialist clinics, for example, clinics carried out jointly with geriatric physicians or neurologists, memory clinics or family therapy clinics.[13] Some outpatient clinics may be carried out in settings other than the hospital, for example, GP surgeries, day centres, nursing homes or residential homes.

Memory clinics

Memory clinics are imported from a North American tradition. Initially they were configured to attract people with mild memory problems who might become subjects of research, but they have spread in popularity and are seen to offer high-quality assessments, information, education and support to patients and carers.[14] Although memory clinics are closely associated with anti-dementia drug treatments, they are also linked with psychosocial interventions. The National Dementia Strategy (www.dh.gov.uk/en/Publicationsandstatistics/Publications/PublicationsPolicyAndGuidance/DH_094058) positions them as the preferred access point for assessment and specialist care, that is, preferable to the traditional community contacts of old-age psychiatry service.

Services to the general hospital

Older people are frequently admitted to hospital because of inter-current illness. Some will have pre-existing psychiatric problems; others may develop new mental health problems in association with their acute physical illness. All will require attention to the full range of their needs. Unhappily, the environment of large general hospitals is often less than helpful to frightened, confused old people (see http://alzheimers.org.uk/countingthecost). The pressure to move from assessment ward to treatment ward and out of hospital may compound their difficulties. Formal liaison psychiatry services did not, traditionally, take a major interest in older people and old-age psychiatry services often gave greater priority to patients in the community, thus leaving older people with mental problems on hospital wards to fall between the two services. This failing is being addressed by the development of old-age psychiatry liaison teams (see www.bgs.org.uk/PDF%20Downloads/WhoCaresWins.pdf)[15] and by broader initiatives within the organization of general hospitals encouraged by the National Dementia Strategy.

Intermediate care for older people with mental health problems

Intermediate care was conceived originally in response to the increasing demand for acute hospital services and aimed to promote faster recovery from illness, prevent unnecessary acute hospital admissions, support timely discharge and maximize independent living. After a decade of mixed experiences,[16] refined guidance (see www.dh.gov.uk/prod_consum_dh/groups/dh_digitalassets/@dh/@en/@pg/documents/digitalasset/dh_103154.pdf) confirms its place within the spectrum of healthcare and emphasizes that people with dementia or other mental disorders should be able to access this service and its benefits.

Special groups

Elders with learning disability

People with a learning disability are much more likely to survive into their sixties and beyond now than was the case in the past.[17] People with learning disability may develop problems characteristic of late life earlier than the general population; those with Down syndrome are particularly at risk of Alzheimer's disease,[18] which requires skilful care in its terminal phases. Thus, older people with learning disability may have complex needs which cross the interface between old-age psychiatry, geriatric medicine and learning disability services. Good practice will often require that services work together to meet an individual's needs best.[19] Flexibility and trust are vital. Users and their families need to be clear about care plans, about who is taking responsibility for what and how they might be contacted. Commissioners need to ensure that this group is not neglected in service planning.

Early-onset dementia

The Alzheimer's Society[20] provided a charter for younger people with dementia and their carers in 1996. This supports early diagnosis, assessment and referral and access to specialist services. In 2000, the Royal College of Psychiatrists published a Council Report which recommended that each district should have a named consultant responsible for the service for younger people with dementia and that old-age psychiatrists should take the lead. A postal survey demonstrated that awareness of the report was comparatively high, but no area met all the report's recommendations. There was evidence of improvement in service provision and many respondents outlined plans for future development. Progress since then has been patchy and disappointing. The Council Report has been revised and updated (see www.rcpsych.ac.uk/publications/collegereports/cr/cr135.aspx). It recommends that commissioners should have:

- a named individual who takes responsibility for commissioning services for younger adults with dementia
- specific contractual arrangements for a specialized service for younger people with Alzheimer's disease and other dementias, including programmed time from a named consultant (usually an old-age psychiatrist).

People with enduring or relapsing mental illness

Those individuals who lived out their lives with chronic schizophrenia, manic-depressive psychosis, brain damage or personality disorders in large mental hospitals were often overlooked by the psychogeriatric services of the 1970s and 1980s. Closure of the large mental hospitals and changing expectations have meant that new generations of 'graduates' with a psychosis live within the community, often in hostels or nursing homes. They may have remained in touch with mental health services or drifted out of touch. They are at risk of neglect or misunderstanding or of falling into a gap between different services.[21] Their plight has been recognized and existing guidance encourages all authorities to recognize them, discover their needs and agree the best arrangements for their care within the range of available local resources (see www.rcpsych.ac.uk/files/pdfversion/CR153.pdf).

People in residential and nursing care

Despite the emphasis on supporting people in their own homes and providing alternative and innovative housing solutions for older, frailer people, large numbers spend their last months or years in residential homes or nursing homes. In many residential homes, 40% or more of the residents have dementia and up to 20% are depressed or demonstrate other psychiatric morbidity.[22] Roughly half of the population with a diagnosis of dementia in the UK are in care at any one time. For most this is terminal care. The transfer of care from large, ill-sited, ill-equipped and poorly staffed mental hospitals to community-based residential homes nearer their families represents progress for many people, but there are continuing concerns over the quality of care available to residents and their quality of life. Scandals relating to hospital care in the past led to service improvement, yet scandals continue to be reported in a variety of institutional settings[23,24] (also http://www.elderabuse.org.uk/AEA%20Services/Useful%20downloads/Misc/CHI%20Rowan%20Ward.pdf). Recent concerns have focused on the excessive use of tranquillizing medication and the lack of alternative treatment strategies, particularly in nursing homes specialising in the care of people with dementia (www.dh.gov.uk/en/Publicationsandstatistics/Publications/PublicationsPolicyAndGuidance/DH_108303). It is essential that specialist services, both medical and mental health, take responsibility for the care of older people in the time of their greatest need, be this in residential or nursing homes or in the much diminished NHS continuing care sector.

Black and minority ethnic (BME) elders

The Royal College of Psychiatrists published a report on psychiatric services for BME elders in 2001 (see www.rcpsych.ac.uk/files/pdfversion/cr103.pdf). It was updated in 2009 (www.rcpsych.ac.uk/files/pdfversion/CR156.pdf) and made five main recommendations:

- Assessment and treatment should remain within mainstream psychiatric services.
- Continuing care services should be targeted at particular user groups.
- Services should endeavour to recruit a mix of staff reflecting the ethic mix of the local population.
- Good practice should be established and shared, perhaps using a website.
- staff should be trained in culturally sensitive issues.

There are already examples of good practice developing around the UK. In Wolverhampton alone there are several initiatives:

- Social services and health staff have jointly undertaken a course in basic Punjabi.
- Staff at a local day centre for Asian elders undertake exchanges with staff at the Resource Centre for older adults with mental health problems.
- A specialist CPN is employed to work with Asian elders presenting to old-age psychiatry.
- A support group for Asian carers of older adults with mental health problems has been established.

This experience must be multiplied many times around the country, as services increasingly address the needs of ethnic elders within their localities.

Patients' views and involvement

People with dementia and/or other mental health problems retain their individuality and views. The assumption that they are to be viewed as passive recipients of care (or neglect) has been strongly challenged recently. It is very clear that, until affected by the most severe stages of dementia, people want to (and should be able to) have a say in the life they are to lead. People are less afraid now to admit that they have a dementia and the emphasis on early diagnosis is likely to increase their demands. A number of publications have reported on subjective experiences of dementia, for example, Morgan.[25] Increasingly, services are encouraged to include patients within their planning and monitoring structures and the relevant charities sponsor and support patient action groups. Amongst these the Scottish Dementia Working Group is particularly impressive (see www.sdwg.org.uk/).

Carers

Carers in the UK have the right to an independent assessment of their needs (but not a right to services) under the Carers (Recognition and Services) Act of 1995 (see www.legislation.hmso.gov.uk/acts/acts1995/Ukpga_19950012_en_1.htm).

These rights have been further consolidated in England with the publication of the National Carers' Strategy (www.dh.gov.uk/en/Publicationsandstatistics/Publications/PublicationsPolicyAndGuidance/DH_085345). Many people who care for elders are themselves older adults (often spouses) and they may be stressed or have mental health problems. The National Institute for Social Work[26] identified 10 key requirements for carers (Table 82.1).

Thus carer support is a fundamental component of all aspects of service provision and carers are increasingly included in planning and monitoring services. The Alzheimer's Society (http://alzheimers.org.uk/) and Dementia UK: (www.dementiauk.org/) are charities strongly associated with supporting carers of people with dementia in England. They help individual carers, advise

Table 82.1 Key requirements for carers.

- Early identification
- Comprehensive assessment (including medical and social assessment)
- Medical treatment of treatable problems
- Prompt referral to other sources of help
- Information, advice and counselling
- Continuing support and review, preferably from a person known to and trusted by the carer
- Regular help with domestic tasks and personal care
- Regular breaks from caring (respite)
  Respite is seen as essential in sustaining informal carers of people with dementia and its impact and costs have been reviewed by colleagues at the University of York (see www.sdo.nihr.ac.uk/files/project/48-final-report.pdf)
- Financial support
- Access to permanent residential care when needed

and influence professionals and have the ear of government. There are equivalent international organizations. It is less easy to identify organizations specifically reaching out to families of people with other mental health problems in later life, but the general mental health charities and elder care charities do have special interest sections.

Additional responsibilities for geriatric psychiatry services

Health promotion

Mental health promotion is defined as 'any action to enhance the mental wellbeing of individuals, families, organizations and communities and a set of principles which recognize that: 'how people feel . . . (has) a significant influence on health'.[27] To promote mental health, rather than just treat mental illness, is a daunting challenge, yet aspects of mental health promotion are already incorporated into good service planning and operation. An approach which aims to promote health carries the potential for improving services and for improving the quality of life for people using those services. Mentality's briefing paper on evidence-based mental health promotion[28] set out a range of possibilities: opportunities for social and physical activities, access to information and practical help, volunteering and discussion and self-help groups are all linked with an evidence base showing a positive effect on mental wellbeing. The links between physical and mental health are also highly relevant to older adults who have factors known to predispose to vascular disorders; these are recognized to be associated with an increased incidence of dementia and mood disorders.[29]

Mental health professionals often encourage people to modify their lifestyle following an episode of mental ill-health, in order to improve their resilience. The challenge is to incorporate routine use of mental health promotion techniques into the design of clinical services and to promote health in those people who have an established dementia or an ongoing or recurrent functional mental health problem.

Training, education and continuing professional development (CPD)

Old-age psychiatry is one of the six specialties of psychiatry recognized within the UK National Health Service (General Adult, Old Age, Forensic, Child and Adolescent, Learning Disabilities and Psychotherapy). Specialist training in old-age psychiatry currently lasts 6 years: 3 years for core or generic training (as a Core trainee CT1-3) and 3 years for advanced training (as a Specialty Registrar ST4-6). Core training provides a range of experience across the whole of psychiatry and during this time a trainee prepares to take the examination for membership of the Royal College of Psychiatrists, which consists of three parts. The Clinical Assessment of Skills and Competencies (CASC) examination is taken after 30 months' experience in psychiatry and is required for entry into an advanced training programme. By the end of 3 years of training in approved and supervised placements and having passed the membership examination of the Royal College of Psychiatrists, a trainee who wishes to specialize in old-age psychiatry competes to enter a specialty training programme and then moves into advanced training, rotating through a series of approved and supervised placements, which will prepare them for independent practice as an old-age psychiatrist. After successfully completing their advanced training, trainees receive a Certificate of Completion of Training (CCT), which enables them to enter the General Medical Council's Specialist Register, a mandatory requirement for NHS consultants. Throughout their training, trainees undertake workplace-based assessments and are expected to develop research and audit skills and other special interests.

Once they start practice as independent specialists, learning does not stop; indeed, some might say that is when it really starts. Consultant old-age psychiatrists plan their CPD prospectively and in line with defined objectives throughout their careers. Many consultant old-age psychiatrists will take part in formal and informal education and teaching, of undergraduates studying medicine, of postgraduate doctors in psychiatry and perhaps related fields such as geriatric medicine and of a range of other professionals working in mental health and related fields. These activities will be included in their job plans and they may undertake additional training themselves in order to develop their skills as educators.

Research and audit

Research and audit are included in the training of old-age psychiatrists. Consultants will therefore have trained in the principles of research and audit and will be able to appraise scientific literature critically and use evidence-based treatments. Many will themselves engage in audit projects and clinical or scientific research while continuing to work as clinicians. In this they may be encouraged by involvement in a research network (www.dendron.org.uk).

Unfortunately, academic old-age psychiatry is under-developed and under-resourced. Perhaps this reflects the lack of priority given to older people's mental health in research funding generally: a recent report found that government and charitable spending on dementia research is 12 times lower than that spent on cancer research, despite the considerable cost of dementia to the country and the projected rising cost with projected population changes (see www.dementia2010.org/reports/Dementia2010Full.pdf).

Other issues

Legal framework

The legal framework within which services operate in England and Wales has changed with the introduction of the Mental Capacity Act (www.opsi.gov.uk/acts/acts2005/ukpga_20050009_en_1). This is particularly important to old-age mental health services since many older adult service users may be incapable of taking some decisions by virtue of a dementia or other severe mental illness. Services need to ensure that people are given the appropriate information to enable them to take out a Lasting Power of Attorney should they so wish and/or to make additional provisions through an Advanced Directive (www.direct.gov.uk/en/Governmentcitizensandrights/Death/Preparation/DG_10029683). After much discussion, the Mental Act of 1983 has been revised rather than replaced (www.opsi.gov.uk/acts/acts2007/ukpga_20070012_en_1).

Access to psychological therapies

The NSF-OP stated that a full range of psychological treatments should be available for older people with mental health problems; some years later, it appears that this aim has still not been achieved, although many memory clinics are reported to have links with psychological therapies. Evans[30] found that provision varied widely across the UK and was of unknown quality. Hepple[31] reviewed psychological therapies for older adults and stated that their slow development is due to ageism. Evans and Reynolds[32] found limited or no access to psychological therapies via older people's mental health services in some areas of Wales. Hilton[33] commented on government funding made available for the treatment of anxiety and depression which was targeted at adults of working age; she argued that the Human Rights Act has been largely ignored in the provision of older people's mental health services. It is likely that future cohorts of older adults will expect access to psychological therapies and that this aspect of service provision will need to respond to their demands. It will be interesting to see how recent moves towards age equality in health and social care (http://www.dh.gov.uk/prod_consum_dh/groups/dh_digitalassets/documents/digitalasset/dh_107398.pdf) impact on this and other areas of care provision.

Spirituality

Spirituality (and the need for services to address spiritual needs) has been increasingly recognized as an issue for services recently. There is research evidence that active involvement with faith organizations links to better health outcomes. Health and social care professionals now increasingly recognize that they should identify the spiritual needs of their patients/users and their family carers and work with colleagues who have expertise in faith and spirituality.

End of life Care

Mental disorders are associated with reduced life expectation. Dementia in particular can be conceived of as a slow-burn terminal illness.[34] The presence of psychological symptoms during the time that death is approaching is difficult for the individual and for their family and professionals caring for them. Death has begun to emerge from its status of taboo subject. An end of life strategy encourages a positive approach to death and dying, including death with dementia or other mental disorder (http://www.dh.gov.uk/en/Publicationsandstatistics/Publications/PublicationsPolicyAndGuidance/DH_086277). The loss of continuing care beds from the NHS Mental Health Services has meant that even difficult deaths are dispersed between home, care homes and general hospitals. Collaboration between old-age psychiatry and local hospices may provide a more appropriate model of care within this framework.[35]

An international perspective

Specialist mental health services for older people had their origins in the UK and have developed there as a model to which other countries can aspire. This account of services is based on the British scene as it has evolved from its roots in the late 1960s[36]. The UK model has been adopted in differing degrees in countries influenced by Tom Arie's British Council courses or lectures and publications from pioneers of the 1970s. There is, however, no international consensus on how best to provide services for older people with mental illness. The International Psychogeriatic Association (see www.ipa-online.org/) brings together professionals interested in improving geriatric psychiatry knowledge and services worldwide and enables people to learn from the different experiences in countries with widely differing healthcare contexts. Although we tend to think of dementia as being a problem for developed countries, improved life expectancy means that providing for the physical and mental health of older people is a global priority, growing in significance each year. In reality, most people with dementia live in developing countries[37] and older people's mental health is becoming increasingly important politically across the world as people recognize the potential future cost implications of providing services for older adults with dementia and other mental disorders. The 10/66 Dementia Research Group (see www.alz.co.uk/1066/) is part of Alzheimer's Disease International and is actively researching into ageing and dementia in low- and middle-income countries.

Conclusion

Old-age psychiatry has developed rapidly over the past 30 years in the UK and is a respected specialty with a distinctive community-orientated approach, a penchant for seizing opportunities and a tradition of attracting practitioners who are passionate advocates for older people with mental illness. Since its inception, there have been tensions in its relationships with general psychiatry and geriatric medicine and a lack of clarity about where it belongs – in services for older adults or with the rest of mental health? These tensions reflect the need for the specialty to cross boundaries and ensure that its staff and services are made available to older people with mental health problems wherever they might be. Another area of tension is the perceived split between the dementias and functional mental illness, but this highlights the need for an older people's mental health service to be inclusive in providing services across the range of mental illness in later life rather than expecting its users to fall neatly into one diagnostic category. Recently, some areas of psychiatry have suffered from a fashion for fragmentation and rigid access criteria. It is important to recognize that the strength of the specialty has been its inclusive, person-centred, collaborative and specialist approach, which must be valued and maintained within rapidly changing (and challenging) service contexts.

Key points

- Community services may now include various specialist teams.
- Hospital services operate with minimum beds and the assumption that a split between 'organic' and 'functional' beds is possible and useful.
- Memory clinics are regarded as a preferred first point of contact for those with cognitive problems and are likely to evolve further following the introduction of a National Dementia Strategy in England.
- General hospital care of older adults with a mental illness is an area of increasing focus. Alongside these developments, special groups in need of extra attention have been attracting interest.

References

1. Department of Health. *Better Health in Old Age. Report from Professor Ian Philp, National Director for Older People's Health to Secretary of State for Health*, Department of Health, London, 2004.
2. Fraser K, Clark, M, Benbow SM *et al.* Research Letter: Old Age Psychiatry Home Treatment Team – preliminary audit of a service improvement project. *Int J Geriatr Psychiatry* 2009; **24**:648–9.
3. Warner J and Lowery K. A successful older adult home treatment team. *Old Age Psychiatrist* 2008;(Spring): 10–11.
4. Yorston GA and Taylor PJ. Commentary: older offenders – no place to go ? *J Am Acad Psychiatry Law* 2006;**34**:333–7.
5. Arie T. The first year of the Goodmayes psychiatric service for old people. *Lancet* 1970;**ii**:1175–8.
6. Benbow SM. The community clinic – its advantages and disadvantages. *Int J Geriatr Psychiatry* 1990;**2**:119–21.
7. Tucker S, Baldwin R, Hughes J *et al.* Old age mental health services in England: Implementing the National Service Framework for Older People. *Int J Geriatr Psychiatry* 2007; **22**:211–7.
8. Downs M, Turner S, Bryans M *et al.* Effectiveness of educational interventions in improving detections and management of dementia in primary care. *BMJ* 2006;**332**:692–6.
9. Greening L, Greaves I, Greaves N and Jolley D. Positive thinking on dementia in primary care: Gnosall Memory Clinic. *Community Pract* 2009;**82**(5): 20–3.
10. Benbow SM and Jolley D. Old age psychiatrists: what do they find stressful ? *Int J Geriatr Psychiatry* 1997;**12**:879–82.
11. Hilton C. New ways not working and the consultoid. *Psychiatr Bull* 2009;**33**:356.
12. Dibben C, Saeed H, Konstantinos S *et al.* Crisis resolution and home treatment teams for older people with mental illness. *Psychiatr Bull.* 2008;**32**:268–70.
13. Benbow SM and Marriott A. Family therapy with elderly people. *Adv Psychiatr Treat* 1997;**3**:138–45.
14. Jolley D, Benbow SM and Grizzell M. Memory clinics. *Postgrad Med J* 2006;**82**:199–206.

15. Holmes J, Bentley K and Cameron T. A UK survey of psychiatric services for older people in general hospitals. *Int J Geriatr Psychiatry* 2002;**18**:716–21.
16. Young J. The development of intermediate care services in England. *Arch Gerontol Geriatr* 2009;**49**(Suppl 2):S21–7.
17. Collacott R. Psychiatric problems in elderly people with learning disability. In: O Russell (ed.), *Seminars in the Psychiatry of Learning Disabilities*, Royal College of Psychiatrists, London, 1997, pp. 136–47.
18. Holland AJ and Oliver C. Down's syndrome and the links with Alzheimer's Disease. *J Neurol Neurosurg Psychiatry* 1995;**59**:111–4.
19. Department of Health. *Valuing People: a New Strategy for Learning Disability*, HMSO, London, 2001.
20. Alzheimer's Society. *Younger People with Dementia: a Review and Strategy*, Alzheimer's Society, London, 1996.
21. Jolley D, Kosky N and Holloway F. Older people with long-standing mental illness: the graduates. *Adv Psychiatr Treat* 2004;**10**:27–36.
22. Mann A. Epidemiology. In: R Jacoby and C Oppenheimer (eds), *Psychiatry in the Elderly*. Oxford Medical Publications, Oxford, 1991, pp. 89–112.
23. Arie T and Isaacs A. The development of psychiatric service for the elderly in Britain. In: A Isaacs and F Post (eds), *Studies in Geriatric Psychiatry*, John Wiley and Sons, Ltd, Chichester, 1978, pp. 241–62.
24. Benbow SM. Failures in the system: our inability to learn from inquiries *J Adult Protect* 2008;**10**(3): 5–13.
25. Morgan K. Risks of living with Alzheimer's disease: a personal view. *J Adult Protect* 2009;**11**(3): 26–9.
26. Levin E. *Carers: Problems, Strains and Services*, Oxford University Press, Oxford, 1997.
27. Friedl L. Mental health promotion: rethinking the evidence base. *Ment Health Rev* 2000;**5**:15–8.
28. Mentality. *Making It Effective: a Guide to Evidence Based Mental Health Promotion. Radical Mentalities Briefing Paper 1*, Mentality, London, 2003.
29. Mentality. *Not All in the Mind: the Physical Health of Mental Health Service Users. Radical Mentalities Briefing Paper 2*, Mentality, London, 2003.
30. Evans S. A survey of the provision of psychological treatments to older adults in the NHS. *Psychiatr Bull* 2004;**28**: 411–4.
31. Hepple J. Psychotherapies with older people: an overview. *Adv Psychiatr Treat* 2004;**10**:371–7.
32. Evans C and Reynolds P. Survey of the provision of psychological therapies for older people. *Psychiatr Bull* 2006;**30**:10–3.
33. Hilton C. Psychological therapies, older people and human rights. *Psychiatr Bull* 2009;**33**:184–6.
34. Hughes J, Lloyd-Williams M and Sachs G (eds), *Supportive Care for the Person with Dementia*, Oxford University Press, Oxford, 2010.
35. Scott S and Pace V. The first 50 patients: a brief report on the initial findings from the Palliative Care in Dementia Project. *Dementia* 2009;**8**:435.
36. Pitt B, Arie T, Benbow SM and Garner J. The history of old-age psychiatry in the UK. *IPA Bull* 2006;**23**(2): 8–10.
37. Ferri CP, Prince M, Brayne C *et al.* Global prevalence of dementia: a Delphi consensus study. *Lancet* 2005;**366**:2112–7.

CHAPTER 83

Depression in later life: aetiology, epidemiology, assessment, diagnosis and treatment

Natalie Sachs-Ericsson[1] and Dan G. Blazer[2]
[1]Florida State University, Tallahassee, FL, USA
[2]Duke University Medical Center, Durham, NC, USA

Introduction

Depression, the most frequent cause of emotional suffering in later life, is associated with significant losses in health-related quality of life.[1] Depression adversely influences the outcome of comorbid health disorders.[2–4] Depression is related to an increased risk of mortality.[5] Among older adults, there is also a high comorbidity with cognitive decline and depression.[6] Depression in the medically ill elder also has negative consequences to their caregivers, who are typically family members. A diagnosis of major depression in older medical inpatients is associated with poor mental health in their informal caregivers, who also are typically comprised of family members.[7]

Varieties of late-life depression

Formal diagnostic criteria for depression are derived from the symptom criteria in the *Diagnostic and Statistical Manual*, 4th edition (DSM-IV).[8] *Major depression*, the most common mood disorder, is diagnosed when the individual exhibits, for at least 2 weeks, one or both of two core symptoms (depressed mood and lack of interest in most activities) along with four or more of the following symptoms: feelings of worthlessness or guilt; diminished ability to concentrate or make decisions; fatigue; psychomotor agitation or retardation; insomnia or hypersomnia; significant decrease or increase in weight or appetite; and recurrent thoughts of death or suicidal ideation.[8] For the most part, depression is similarly experienced by older adults if there are no comorbid conditions;[9] however, subtle differences with ageing may emerge. For example, depression with melancholia (symptoms of anhedonia, non-interactiveness and psychomotor retardation or agitation) appears to have a later age of onset than non-melancholic depression in clinical populations.[10,11] Older adults often experience depressive symptoms associated with bereavement after the loss of a loved one, symptoms consistent with those of a major depressive episode. Major depression may be diagnosed if the depressive symptoms are present at least 2 months or longer after the loss.

Minor, sub-syndromal or sub-threshold depression is diagnosed according to the Appendix of DSM-IV in the instance that one of the core symptoms is present (sad mood or loss of interest in most activities) along with one to three additional symptoms.[1,8] Other operational definitions of these less severe variants of depression include a score of 16 or more on the Center for Epidemiologic Studies Depression Scale (CES-D) but not meeting criteria for major depression,[12,13] a primarily biogenic depression not meeting criteria for major depression yet responding to antidepressant medication[14] or a score of 11–15 on the CES-D.[15]

Dysthymic disorder is a long-lasting chronic disturbance of mood, less severe than major depression that lasts for 2 years or longer.[8] It rarely begins in late life but may persist from mid life into late life.[1,16,17] To be diagnosed with dysthymic disorder, the older adult must experience a depressed mood for at least 2 years along with two of the following symptoms: eating disturbance, sleep disturbance, low energy or fatigue, low self-esteem, poor concentration or difficulty in making decisions and feelings of hopelessness. Finally, other investigators have suggested a syndrome of *depression without sadness*, thought to be more common in older adults,[18,19] or a depletion syndrome manifested by withdrawal, apathy and lack of vigour.[1,20–22]

Depression among individuals with dementia is fairly common, so much so that recently a group of investigators proposed a *depression of Alzheimer's disease (AD)*. In persons who meet criteria for dementia of the Alzheimer's type, three of a series of symptoms that include depressed mood, anhedonia, social isolation, poor appetite, poor sleep, psychomotor changes, irritability, fatigue or loss of energy, feelings of worthlessness and suicidal thoughts must be present for the diagnosis to be made.[1,23]

Principles and Practice of Geriatric Medicine, Fifth Edition. Edited by Alan J. Sinclair, John E. Morley and Bruno Vellas.

Depression in late life is frequently comorbid with physical conditions. When the depression derives from the physiological consequence of the medical condition, the disorder is diagnosed as *mood disorder due to general medical condition*.[8]

Depressive symptoms may also temporarily meet criteria for major depression in the midst of bereavement and acute adjustment disorders. The context of the depression therefore helps the clinician to determine whether a diagnosis of major depression should be made and treatment instituted or whether the symptoms will be expected to remit on their own when an appropriate time has elapsed. The clinician must remember, however, that what initially appears to be a case of bereavement or an adjustment disorder may evolve into major depression with time.

Epidemiology of late-life depression

Depressive symptoms are no more or less frequent in late life than in mid life.[1,24–26] Several large epidemiological studies have been conducted to assess the prevalence of affective disorders in older populations. Generally, among the elderly, the prevalence of major depression is ~1–3%[1,27,28] and reports of clinically significant depressive symptoms in community-dwelling elderly have been ~8–16%.[1,26,29–31] Further, among individuals aged 85 years or older, the incidence of major depression appears to increase among the oldest of old,[32] reaching ~13%.[33] However, this increased rate is explained by factors associated with ageing, including a higher proportion of women, more physical disability, more cognitive impairment and lower socioeconomic status.[34,35]

Higher rates of depression and depressive symptoms have been consistently found for women compared with men in the general population and for the elderly.[36,37] Whereas some studies of the elderly have found few racial differences in the frequency of depressive symptoms[29,38,39] or in the frequency of depressive diagnoses,[31,37,40] others have found African American elders to have a higher frequency of depressive symptoms than Caucasians.[41–44] Depressive symptoms may be greater in African Americans than Caucasians solely due to differences in socioeconomic status (SES).[45,46] Nevertheless, African Americans are generally thought by psychiatrists to have fewer depressive symptoms and are much less likely to be treated with antidepressant medications.[47,48] Some have also raised the issue of misclassification of African Americans as depressed.[49]

Comorbidity of depression with medical illness

Depression late in life often occurs within the context of physical impairment,[50] especially in the oldest individuals.[1,34] For example, in a study of patients hospitalized with acute myocardial infarction, investigators examined the degree of association between clinical depression and medical comorbidity and found that the adjusted odds ratios for having major depression increased linearly with medical comorbidity.[51] Depression also adversely influences the outcome of comorbid health disorders in the elderly.[1,2,52,53]

In a recent meta-analysis, chronic health problems were found to be a risk factor for depression among older adults.[54] The quantitative meta-analysis showed that, compared with the elderly without chronic disease, those with chronic disease were at higher risk for depression [relative risk (RR), 1.53; 95% confidence interval (CI), 1.20–1.97]. Compared with the elderly with good self-rated health, those with poor self-rated health were at higher risk for depression [RR, 2.40; 95% CI, 1.94–2.97).

We have found the perception that one's basic needs are not being met predicted future depressive symptoms in a highly controlled analysis. These results suggest that perception of inadequate basic needs, even when income and other known correlates of depression are controlled, is a strong predictor of future depressive symptoms.[55]

Depression and cognitive impairment

Depression is associated with both mild cognitive impairment[56] and dementia.[57] The prevalence of depression among the cognitively impaired has been found to range between 20 and 50%.[23,58,59] Depression among individuals with dementia may be more frequent in those with vascular diseases compared with those with AD.[60–62] Elevated rates of depression have also been found among individuals with dementia secondary to Parkinson's disease.[63a,64], Depression may signal the onset of AD and may represent prodromal signs of dementia.[65–67] Research suggests that depression initiated a glucocorticoid cascade that leads to damage of the hippocampus, a brain structure integral to memory, leading to subsequent cognitive decline.[68]

Major depression among those with dementia is associated with greater impairment of activities of daily living (ADLs), worse behavioural disturbance and more frequent wandering, even after adjusting for severity of dementia or comorbid health problems. Minor depression was also associated with non-mood behavioural disturbance and wandering.[69]

Course of late-life depression

Depression is a chronic and recurring illness.[70–75] In a meta-analysis[76] of the prognosis of elderly medical inpatients with depression, researchers found that at 3 months 18% of patients were well, 43% were depressed and 22%

were deceased. At 12 months or more, 19% were well, 29% were depressed and 53% were deceased. Factors associated with worse outcomes included more severe depression and more serious physical illness. Among those older depressed adults without significant comorbid medical illness or dementia and who are treated optimally, the outcome is more optimistic, with over 80% recovering and remaining well throughout follow-up.[75]

Medical comorbidity, functional impairment and comorbid dementing disorders all adversely influence the outcome of depression.[1] Depression also adversely affects the outcome of the comorbid problems such as cardiovascular disease[5] in which depressive disorder is associated with an increase in mortality,[77] particularly for women and less so for men.[78,79] Problems in meeting one's basic needs affects depression among older adults.[55]

Non-suicide mortality

Psychiatric disorders in general and severe depressive disorders increase the risk of non-suicide-related mortality.[1,5,80] For example, in a review of 61 reports of this relationship from 1997 to 2001, 72% demonstrated a positive association between depression and mortality in elderly people.[81a] Both the severity and duration of depressive symptoms predict mortality in the elderly population in these studies.[1,82] Other studies, however, have suggested that the association between depression and mortality is related to the high correlation between depression and other medical problems. In one study, depression at baseline predicted earlier (3 and 5 year) mortality but not later (10 year) mortality. The interaction between self-rated health and depression independently and strongly predicted mortality at all endpoints,[83] that is, depression impacts non-suicide mortality through intermediate risk factors.

In a recent study,[84] both moderate [multivariate hazard ratio (MHR), 1.29; 95% CI, 1.03–1.61] and severe depression (MHR, 1.34; 95% CI, 1.07–1.68) predicted 10 year mortality after multivariate adjustment. Chronic depression was associated with a 41% higher mortality risk in a 6 year follow-up compared with subjects without depression.

Suicide

The association of depression and suicide across the life cycle has been well established.[85–91] Older adults are at a higher risk for suicide than any other age group. While older Americans comprise ~13% of the US population, they account for 18% of all suicide deaths.[92] Increased risk for suicide attempts in late life is associated with being widow(er)s, living alone, perception of poor health status, poor sleep quality, lack of a confidant and experience of stressful life events, such as financial discord and interpersonal discord.[86,91]

The most common means of committing suicide in the elderly are use of a firearm[88] and drug ingestion.[1] Women attempt suicide more than men; however, men completed suicide more often than women.[93] Although completed suicides increase with age, suicidal behaviours do not increase.[94] This is consistent with the contention that older adults are more intent in their efforts to commit suicide.[95]

There are many risk factors for suicide, with depression being central.[96] Perhaps the best studied factor is pervasive feelings of hopelessness.[97,98] Other psychological constructs include emotional pain,[99] feelings of being a burden and social isolation.[100a] The lack of social networks and their disruption are significantly associated with risk for suicide in later life.[95] Joiner *et al.* have identified key risk factors for individuals at high risk for suicide,[101] and they (as others) have identified 'mattering to others' as an important protective factor.

Physical illness is strongly associated with suicide in the elderly. In one large epidemiological study the following medical illnesses were found to be associated with suicide:[102] congestive heart failure [odds ratio (OR), 1.73; 95% CI, 1.33–2.24], chronic obstructive lung disease (OR, 1.62; 95% CI, 1.37–1.92), seizure disorder (OR, 2.95; 95% CI, 1.89–4.61), urinary incontinence (OR, 2.02; 95% CI, 1.29–3.17), anxiety disorders (OR, 4.65; 95% CI, 4.07–5.32), depression (OR, 6.44; 95% CI, 5.45–7.61), psychotic disorders (OR, 5.09; 95% CI, 3.94–6.59), bipolar disorder (OR, 9.20, 95% CI, 4.38–19.33), moderate pain (OR, 1.91; 95% CI, 1.66–2.20) and severe pain (OR, 7.52; 95% CI, 4.93–11.46). Treatment for multiple illnesses was strongly related to a higher risk and these patients often saw a primary care physician in preceding months before suicidal behaviour, underscoring the physician's potential role in suicide. Indeed, almost half of the patients who committed suicide had visited a physician in the preceding week.

Older persons with mental disorders rarely seek help from mental health professionals, preferring to visit their primary care physician instead.[103] The majority of older adults who die by suicide have been seen recently by a healthcare provider. Suicide prevention strategies rely on the identification of specific, observable risk factors. Depression, hopelessness and self-harming behaviours (such as food refusal) are possible indicators of suicide risk.[95,104] Living alone, feeling like one is a burden to others and having few social ties are each a risk factor for suicide. Individuals with a previous history of suicide are more likely to attempt suicide again.[88] Increased risk is also associated with resolved plans, a sense of courage and/or competence regarding suicide and access to means of suicide (e.g. pills or gun).[105] Other variables that increase suicide risk include substance abuse,[106] marked impulsivity and personality disorder.[107]

Aetiology

Biological

As noted above, increased rates of depression are associated with many medical conditions, including dementing disorders,[57] cardiovascular disease,[81b] hip fractures[108] and Parkinson's disease.[109] Depression has been associated with pain in institutionalized elderly people[110] and is also common among home-bound elders with urinary incontinence.[111] In one study, initial medical burden, self-rated health and subjective social support were significant independent predictors of depression outcome.[112] Therefore, any exploration of the aetiology of late-life depression must begin with the possibility that the depression is caused in part, and perhaps wholly, by physical illness.

The role of heredity, that is, genetic susceptibility, has been of great interest in exploring the origins of depression across the life cycle.[113] Among elderly twins, genetic influences accounted for 16% of the variance in total depression scores on the CES-D and 19% of psychosomatic and somatic complaints. In contrast, genetics contributed minimally to the variance of depressed mood and psychological wellbeing.[114] Attention has been directed to specific genetic markers for late-life depression. For example, a number of studies have focused on the susceptibility gene APOE (the e4 allele) for AD. No association was found in a community sample between APOE e4 allele and depression;[115] however, the APOE e4 allele contributes to AD, which in turn is associated with increased rates of depression. In another study, hyperintensities in deep white matter but not in the periventricular white matter were associated with depressive symptoms, especially in elders carrying the e4 allele.[116]

Much attention has been directed to vascular risk for late-life depression, dating back at least 40 years, although the advent of magnetic resonance imaging (MRI) increased interest considerably.[73,117–120] Vascular lesions in some regions of the brain may contribute to a unique variety of late-life depression. MRI of depressed patients has revealed structural abnormalities in areas related to the cortical–striatal–pallidal–thalamus–cortical pathway,[121] including the frontal lobes,[122] caudate[123] and putamen.[124] These circuits are known to be associated with the development of spontaneous performance strategies demanded by executive tasks. Recent serotonin activity, specifically 5-HT2A receptor binding, decreases dramatically in a variety of brain regions from adolescence through mid life, but the declines slowly from mid life to late life. Receptor loss occurred across widely scattered regions of the brain (anterior cingulated, occipital cortex and hippocampus). Serotonin depletion can also be studied indirectly by the study of radioisotope-labelled or imipramine-binding (TIB) sites. There is a significant decrease in the number of platelet-TIB sites in elderly depressed patients compared with elderly controls and individuals.

In one study, healthy subjects showed a marked increase in cortisol levels 2–3 h into the procedure regardless of drink composition whereas recovered depressed subjects did not. In elderly patients who had recovered from depression, there was no evidence of greater vulnerability of hypothalamic 5-HT pathways to 5-HT depletion. However, they demonstrated reduced reactivity of the HPA axis compared with healthy subjects.[125]

Late-life depression is also associated with endocrine changes. Although the dexamethasone suppression test was long ago ruled out as a diagnostic test for depression, non-suppression of cortisol is associated with late-life depression compared with age-matched controls.[126] Depression is also associated with an increase in corticotrophin-releasing factor (CRF), which mediates sleep and appetite disturbances, reduced libido and psychomotor changes.[127] Ageing is linked to a heightened responsiveness of adrenocorticotropic hormone (ACTH), cortisol and dehydroepiandrosterone sulfate (DHEA-S) to CRF.[128] Low levels of DHEA have been associated with higher rates of depression and a greater number of depressive symptoms in community-dwelling older women.[129] Total testosterone levels have been found to be lower in elderly men with dysthymic disorder than in men without depressive symptoms.[130] However, the efficacy of testosterone in treating depression has not been established.[131]

In addition, Tsai's research suggests that decreased brain-derived neurotrophic factor (BDNF) is related to both AD and major depression.[132] The author suggests that BDNF could be a bridge between AD and depression, explaining both the depressive symptoms in AD and cognitive impairment in depression.

Dementia and depression

The prevalence of depression in dementia is estimated to range between 30 and 50%.[58] Symptoms of depression are common among individuals with dementia, complicating both the diagnosis and treatment, and are often associated with a more severe clinical course, higher cost of treatment, poorer quality of life and worse outcomes. Further, psychiatric symptoms that occur in individuals with dementia are often the primary cause of family burden and distress. Depression in dementia often goes unrecognized, resulting in less effective therapeutic interventions.[133] However, the identification and effective treatment of depressive disorder in individuals with dementia may substantially augment treatment outcome and improve the quality of life for the patient and family.

Depression among individuals with dementia may be more frequent in those with vascular diseases than in those with AD. Patients with vascular dementia have more frequent and more severe symptoms of depression, and also anxiety, than those with AD (after controlling for levels of cognitive impairment). Ballard *et al.* found that among patients with dementia, 25% had major depression and 27.4% had minor depression.[60] Major depression occurred significantly more often and was significantly more severe in patients with vascular dementia than in patients with AD.

Psychological and social

A variety of different psychological origins have been theorized for depression in later life, including behavioural, cognitive, developmental and psychodynamic theories. Among the behavioural explanations, learned helplessness[134] was originally used to describe the increasingly passive behaviour of dogs who were exposed to inescapable shock. The theory has been expanded, suggesting that one cause of depression is learning that initiating action in an environment that cannot be changed is futile.[134–136] As individuals face new challenges associated with ageing, coping strategies that were once useful may become less effective. Within this context, behavioural interventions (described below) encourage the individual to find new ways to cope successfully with environmental stress.

The most dominant current psychological model of depression is that of cognitive distortions.[137] Several researchers have found consistent differences in the cognitive styles of depressed individuals compared with non-depressed individuals. Beck and co-workers have described the cognitive schema of depressed persons as having logical errors that promote depression.[137–139] Cognitions may be distorted such that the elder has expectations that are not realistic, over-generalizes or over-acts to adverse events and personalizes events. Thus, in reaction to a negative life event (loss of a loved one, move into a nursing home, etc.), an individual's cognitive style may increase the likelihood of a depressive episode.

A developmental theory of ageing, the *disengagement theory* of ageing,[140] contends that there is a mutual social and affective withdrawal between the older adult and their social environment. Similarly, *gerotranscendence*[141] is a concept in which the older individuals are thought to narrow their personal social world and to have a decreased investment in activities that were once important in younger years. Others have conceptualized this withdrawal as a subtype of geriatric depression that has been termed *depletion*.[142] Some have attempted to couple the theory of social disengagement with ageing (much debated in the literature) with depression, suggesting that some symptoms of depression, such as lack of social interest and greater self-involvement, mirror attributes of older adults according to *disengagement theory*.[143,144] Other factors being equal, it is probable that elders who are less socially engaged are more depressed. For example, elders who stopped driving had a greater risk of worsening depressive symptoms.[145] A more recent yet controversial theory complements the depletion theory, suggesting that successful ageing is associated with *'selective optimization with compensation'*.[146] This model is based on the recognition by the elder of the realities of ageing, especially the losses. Such recognition leads to the selection of realistic activities, optimization of those activities and compensation for lost activities, which in turn leads to a reduced and transformed life. More recently, *socioemotional selectivity theory*[147,148] posits that decreasing rates of social contact reflect a greater selectivity in social partners.

Social engagement is a key concept related to depression and the association between late-life depression and impaired social support has been established for many years. Poor social support is strongly associated with depression in the elderly.[149,150] The quality of social support networks has been identified as an important factor in predicting relapse in depressive episodes and future levels of depressive symptoms.[151,152] Further, among the elderly, social support may serve as a buffer against disability,[153] while social disengagement may be a risk factor for cognitive impairment.[154]

Perceived negative interpersonal events are associated with depression among individuals in general and also among elders, particularly in those who demonstrate a high need for approval and reassurance in the context of interpersonal relationships. While social support has been found to be critical in buffering an individual against depression, ironically the interpersonal behaviours of individuals who become depressed are often associated with the withdrawal of social support from friends and family.[155]

Diagnosis

The diagnostic workup of late-life depression derives predominantly from what we know about symptom presentation and aetiology. The diagnosis is made on the basis of a history augmented with a physical examination and supplemented with laboratory studies. Importantly, there is no biological marker or test that creates the diagnosis of depression. However, for some subtypes of depression, such as vascular depression, the presence of subcortical white matter hyperintensities on MRI scanning are critical to confirming the diagnosis.[135,156]

There are several standardized screening measures for depression that are often used by primary care physicians.[157] Examples of such instruments include the Geriatric Depression Scale (GDS) and the Center for Epidemiologic Studies Depression Scale (CES-D).[13,158,159] Screening in primary care is critical. Not only is the frequency of depression high, but also suicidal ideation can be detected by screening.

Despite the centrality of the clinical interview, other diagnostic tools must be employed to assess the depressed elder. Cognitive status should be assessed with the Mini Mental State Examination (MMSE) or a similar instrument, given the high likelihood of comorbid depression and cognitive dysfunction.[57] Height, weight, history of recent weight loss, laboratory tests for hypoalbuminaemia and cholesterol are markers of nutritional status and are critical given the risk for frailty and failure to thrive in depressed elders, especially the oldest of old.[34,160] General health perceptions and also functional status (ADLs) should be assessed for all depressed elderly patients.[161,162] Assessment of social functioning,[163] medications (many prescribed drugs can precipitate symptoms of depression), mobility and balance, sitting and standing blood pressure, blood screen, urinalysis, chemical screen (e.g. electrolytes, which may signal dehydration) and an electrocardiogram if cardiac disease is present (especially if antidepressant medications are indicated) round out the diagnostic workup.

Differential diagnosis of depression and dementia

Dementia and depression have considerable symptom overlap.[63b] Hence distinguishing between late-life depression and depressive disorders in the elderly is one of the more challenging problems facing healthcare professionals.[164] There are a cluster of cognitive deficits that are common to both dementia and depression. Memory impairment is the most frequent shared symptom.[135,165] In addition, apathy is a common symptom among individuals with dementia, including those with and without comorbid depression, and also among non-demented elderly individuals with depression.[166]

As described elsewhere (Ref, 135, pp. 230–2), clinicians often have difficulty in their attempt to distinguish a primary mood disorder from other problems associated with depressed mood, in particular with what some have referred to as 'pseudodementia' (Ref. 135, pp. 349–72). Pseudodementia is a syndrome in which dementia is mimicked, but the underlying cause is a psychiatric disorder which is typically, but not always, depression.[167]

Memory problems accompanying depression in older age may be present and similar in form to symptoms of dementia. However, depressed elderly patients (without dementia) tend to focus on their memory problems. In contrast, patients with dementia are typically unaware of the extent and severity of their cognitive dysfunction and use strategies to conceal their cognitive dysfunction from others. Wells[167] compared the clinical features of patients with pseudodementia with those with true dementia and found that among the patients who present with depression and cognitive impairment, those who were eventually diagnosed with dementia were more likely to exhibit motivation-related symptoms, such as disinterest, low energy and concentration difficulties.

Treatment

Biological

Evidence-based guidelines for the prevention of new episodes of depression are available, as are care-delivery systems that increase the likelihood of diagnosis and improve the treatment of late-life depression. However, in North America, public insurance covers these services inadequately.[168]

There is clear and mounting evidence for the efficacy of antidepressant medications (both alone and in combination with psychotherapy) in the treatment of older adults with major depression and also for the treatment of dysthymia.[3] Antidepressant medications have become the foundation for the treatment of moderate to severe depression in older adults.[1] Although antidepressant medications are equally effective for treating serious major depression across the life cycle,[169–171] differences in side effects make some antidepressants more desirable. For example, although studies that compare tricyclic antidepressants (TCAs) and selective serotonin reuptake inhibitors (SSRIs) usually find equal efficacy, there are fewer side effects with SSRIs,[172] which make them the first choice for treatment of older adults.[173,174] The antidepressants even appear to be efficacious in subjects with AD and vascular depression.[175,176]

In a recent review of the literature on the effects of antidepressant medications in depressed older adults,[177] it was concluded that the available data, although limited, suggest that the dual-action agents [TCAs and serotonin norepinephrine reuptake inhibitors (SNRIs)] do not appear to confer any additional benefits in efficacy over single-action agents (SSRIs) in the treatment of depression in the elderly.

Interestingly, antidepressants appear less efficacious in treating less severe depression in older adults;[178] similar findings have recently been demonstrated in the general population. The overall evidence suggests that antidepressants and counselling have relatively small benefit in these less severe conditions.[179] However, in a study conducted in a primary care setting, paroxetine (compared with problem-solving therapy) was found to have moderate benefits for depressive symptoms in elderly patients with dysthymia and more severely impaired elderly patients with minor depression.[180] Most of the currently available SSRIs have been demonstrated to be efficacious in elderly people, including fluoxetine (10–20 mg daily),[181] sertraline (50–100 mg daily),[182] paroxetine (10–20 mg daily),[172,183] citalopram (10–20 mg daily)[184] and escitalipram (10–20 mg daily), whereas duloxetine has not been shown to be specifically efficacious in the elderly population, but studies are ongoing. Other newer-generation antidepressants that have been shown to be efficacious include venlafaxine,[185] mirtazapine[186,187] and buproprion.[188,189]

In a recent consensus of practising geriatric psychiatrists, the SSRIs along with psychotherapy were identified as the treatments of choice for late-life depression, along with venlafaxine. Buproprion and mirtazapine are alternatives [as was electroconvulsive therapy (ECT) in severe depression]. Medication (SSRI plus an antipsychotic, with risperidone and olanzapine being the antipsychotics most commonly recommended) and ECT are the suggested first-line treatments for major depression with psychotic features (yet these patients often must also receive ECT). Psychotherapy in combination with medication is recommended for dysthymic disorder. Education and watchful waiting, in contrast, are recommended for minor depression that lasts for less than 2 weeks (antidepressant medication plus psychotherapy are recommended for minor depression if symptoms persist).

In one consensus report, the preferred antidepressant for treating both major and minor depression is citalopram (20–30 mg) followed by sertraline (50–100 mg) and paroxetine (20–30 mg), with fluoxetine (20 mg) as an alternative. Escitalopram was not on the market when this survey was conducted.[100b]

Nortriptyline (40–100 mg) is the preferred tricyclic agent, with desipramine (50–100 mg) as the alternative. The consensus group recommended continuing the antidepressant for 3–6 weeks before a change in medications is made if the first-choice medication is not effective. If little or no response is observed, the consensus is to switch to venlafaxine (75–200 mg).[1] For a first episode of depression with recovery following antidepressant therapy, 1 year of continual therapy is recommended. For two episodes, 2 years of continual therapy and for three or more episodes, 3 years of continual therapy are recommended.[100b]

The new-generation antidepressants inhibit a number of the cytochrome P450 enzymes that metabolize most medications, such as CYP3A, CYP2D6, DYP2C, CYP1A2 and CYP2E1. The CYP3A enzymes metabolize 60% of the medications used today. Fluoxetine is a moderate inhibitor of CYP3A4. Approximately 8–10% of adults lack the CYP2dD6 enzyme and paroxetine is a potent inhibitor of this enzyme (which may explain, among some patients treated with paroxetine, the lack of efficacy of analgesics such as codeine that are metabolized by this enzyme). Citalopram and venlafaxine are the 'cleanest' of the medications in terms of inhibition of the cytochrome P450 enzymes.[190,191]

Hyponatraemia (39% in one study) poses a clear risk for the elderly on SSRIs or venlafaxine. Frail older adults and those with medical illness should have sodium levels checked before and after commencement of antidepressant medications.[192] The safest practice is to monitor all elders for sodium levels who are on these medications. This hyponatraemia is due to the syndrome of inappropriate secretion of antidiuretic hormone (SIADH). Other serious side effects reported with the SSRIs include the risk of falls (no less risk than with the tricyclics in one study),[193] the serotonin syndrome (lethargy, restlessness, hypertonicity, rhabdomyolysis, renal failure and possible death)[194] and gastrointestinal bleeding.[195] Less serious side effects include weight loss, sexual dysfunction, anticholinergic effects (most pronounced with paroxetine), agitation and difficulty in sleeping.

Psychotic depression in late life responds poorly to antidepressants but well to ECT.[196–199] In one study using bilateral ECT versus pharmacotherapy, the older age group had a better response to ECT than younger age groups.[200] Memory problems remain the major adverse effect from ECT that affects quality of life, but are usually transient and clear within weeks following treatment.

A repetitive transcranial magnetic stimulation (rTMS) could replace ECT in some situations.[201] TMS does not require anaesthesia and seizure induction is avoided. Although not studied specifically in elderly people, in one outcome study patients treated with rTMS compared with ECT responded equally well and their clinical gains lasted at least as long as those with ECT.[202] In another study, executive function improved in both middle-aged and elderly depressed subjects with rTMS compared with sham treatments.[203]

A variety of adjunct physical therapies may alleviate depression. In a community-based study, among subjects who were not depressed at baseline, those who reported a low activity level were at significantly greater risk for depression at follow-up.[204] An aerobic exercise training programme may be considered as an alternative to antidepressants for the treatment of depression in older persons with mild to moderate symptoms.[205] However, the advantages of exercise are not limited to aerobic activities. Unsupervised weight lifting has been found to decrease depressive symptoms up to 20 weeks after induction.[206] Light therapy may also be beneficial, especially if the depression follows a seasonal pattern. Exposure to bright light for 30 min per day improved depression among institutionalized elders in one controlled study.[207]

Psychological

The Prevention of Suicide in Primary Care Elderly Collaborative Trial[208] evaluated the impact of a care management intervention on suicidal ideation and depression in a large sample of older primary care patients. Participants were patients 60 years of age or older with depression identified after screening. The intervention consisted of services of 15 trained care managers, who offered algorithm-based recommendations to physicians and helped patients with treatment adherence over 24 months. Compared with patients receiving usual care, those receiving the intervention had a higher likelihood of receiving antidepressants and/or psychotherapy (84.9–89% versus 49–62%) and had a 2.2 times greater decline in suicidal ideation over 24 months. Among patients with major depression, a greater number achieved remission in the intervention group than in the usual-care group. Outcomes for those with minor depression were the same regardless of treatment.

Cognitive behavioural therapy (CBT) and interpersonal therapy (IPT) have been shown to be efficacious in the treatment of depression in the elderly, especially in combination with medications. Given that these therapies are short term (12–20 sessions), they are attractive to third-party payers. In addition, the educational (as opposed to a reflective) posture of the therapist employing such therapies is attractive to elders.[1]

CBTs focus on the patient's cognitions surrounding a given negative life event and assist the person to restructure their thought processes cognitively in a more realistic manner. The evidence is clear that treatments aimed at changing cognitive distortions can be fairly effective in decreasing depressive symptoms and even in preventing future relapse. Treatments that focus on problem solving and behavioural activation have also been found to be effective in the treatment of depression. For example, in a study to determine the effectiveness of a home-based programme for treating minor depression or dysthymia among older adults, patients were randomly assigned to an in-home based treatment (Program to Encourage Active, Rewarding Lives for Seniors, PEARLS) or usual care.[5] The PEARLS intervention consisted of problem-solving treatment, social and physical activation and recommendations to patients' physicians regarding antidepressant medications. The intervention was found to reduce depressive symptoms significantly and improve health status in chronically medically ill older adults with minor depression and dysthymia.

Another frequently used treatment for depression is IPT,[209,210] which has been adapted for older adults.[209,211] IPT focuses on four components hypothesized to lead to or maintain depression: grief (e.g. death of a loved one); interpersonal disputes (e.g. conflict with adult children); role transitions (e.g. retirement); and interpersonal deficits (e.g. lack of assertiveness skills). In a study of IPT and elderly depressed patients, clinicians determined that the most common problem areas in therapy were role transition (41%), interpersonal disputes (34.5%) and grief (23%).[212] Miller *et al.* found that IPT was an effective treatment not only with elderly patients with depression but also including those with moderate cognitive impairment.[213]

It is important to note that most studies of depression have found that a combination of psychotherapy and pharmacotherapy has a better outcome than either treatment alone.[214,215]

In a systematic review including 14 randomized controlled trials that assessed the efficacy of psychotherapy for treating depression in elderly people (55 years of age or older),[216] the results of the meta-analysis showed that, compared with a placebo, psychotherapy was more effective in reducing depression (standardized mean difference, – 0.92; 95% CI, – 1.21 to – 0.36). Subgroup analysis showed that cognitive behavioural therapy, reminiscence and general psychotherapy were all more effective than placebo; in contrast to other findings, psychotherapy as an adjunct to antidepressant medication did not increase effectiveness. However, a higher drop-out rate was observed in studies that did not include psychotherapy versus those that did.

The treatment of the elderly depressed has been shown to be cost-effective. In a randomized controlled trial, researchers recruited participants from 18 primary care clinics from eight healthcare organizations in five US States. A total of 1801 patients 60 years of age or older with major depression (17%), dysthymic disorder (30%) or both (53) were randomly assigned to the depression intervention ($n = 906$) or to usual primary care ($n = 895$). Intervention patients were provided access to a depression care manager supervised by a psychiatrist and primary care physician. Depression care managers offered education, support of antidepressant medications prescribed in primary care and problem-solving treatment in primary care (a brief psychotherapy). Relative to usual care, intervention patients experienced 107 (95% CI, 86 to 128) more depression-free days over 24 months. Total outpatient costs were $295 (95% CI, – $525 to $1115) higher during this period. The incremental outpatient cost per depression-free day was $2.76 (95% CI, – $4.95 to $10.47) and incremental outpatient costs per quality-adjusted life-year ranged from $2519 (95% CI, – $4517 to $9554) to $5037 (95% CI, – $9034 to $19 108). The authors concluded that the depression intervention is a high-value investment for older adults; it is associated with high clinical benefits at a low increment in healthcare costs.[217]

Conclusion

Depression has a profound negative impact on older adults, significantly decreasing their quality of life and functioning and increasing both medical morbidity and mortality.[1–5] Although rates of depressive disorders are no greater among the elderly than in the general population, significant rates of depressive symptoms have been identified in elderly populations. Older persons with mental disorders rarely seek help from mental health professionals, preferring to visit their primary care physician instead.[103] Nonetheless, depression among the elderly often goes unrecognized and untreated. However, when identified and addressed, depression, regardless of age, is a highly treatable illness. There are several psychotherapies that have been specifically developed for the treatment of depression, the most effective being cognitive behavioural therapy and interpersonal therapy. There are antidepressant medications that are efficacious in treating the depressed elderly patient; moreover, a combination of medication and psychotherapy has been shown to produce the most positive outcomes.

Key points

- Depression, the most frequent cause of emotional suffering in later life, is associated with significant losses in health-related quality of life.
- Depression is often comorbid with other disorders, including dementia and medical problems.
- Aetiological determinants of depression include psychological, biological and developmental life-span theories
- There is an association of suicide with depression.
- Depression often goes undetected and untreated; however, when identified it is a highly treatable illness.

References

1. Blazer DG. Depression in late life: Review and commentary. *J Gerontol A Biol Sci Med Sci* 2003;**58**:M249–65.
2. Cole MG and Dendukuri N. Risk factors for depression among elderly community subjects: a systematic review and meta-analysis. *Am J Psychiatry* 2003;**160**:1147–56.
3. Unützer J, Katon W, Callahan CM *et al*. Depression treatment in a sample of 1,801 depressed older adults in primary care. *J Am Geriatr Soc* 2003;**51**:505–14.
4. Unützer J, Patrick DL, Diehr P *et al*. Quality adjusted life years in older adults with depressive symptoms and chronic medical disorders. *Int Psychogeriatr* 2000;**12**:15–33.
5. Frasure-Smith N, Lesperance F and Talajic M. Depression following myocardial infarction. Impact on 6-month survival. *JAMA* 1993;**270**:1819–25.
6. Sachs-Ericsson N, Joiner T, Plant EA and Blazer D. The association of depression to cognitive decline in a community sample of elderly adults. *Am J Geriatr Psychiatry* 2005;**13**:402–8.
7. McCusker J, Latimer E, Cole M *et al*. Major depression among medically ill elders contributes to sustained poor mental health in their informal caregivers. *Age Ageing* 2007;**36**:400–6.
8. APA. *DSM-IV: Diagnostic and Statistical Manual of Mental Disorders*, 4th edn, American Psychiatric Association, Washington, DC, 1994.
9. Blazer D, Bachar J and Hughes D. Major depression with melancholia: a comparison of middle-aged and elderly adults. *J Am Geriatr Soc* 1987;**35**:927–32.
10. Parker G. Classifying depression: should paradigms lost be regained? *Am J Psychiatry* 2000;**157**:1195–203.
11. Parker G, Roy K, Hadzi-Pavlovic D *et al*. The differential impact of age on the phenomenology of melancholia. *Psychol Med* 2001;**31**:1231–6.
12. Beekman A, Deeg D, van Tilberg T *et al*. Major and minor depression in later life: a study of prevalence and risk factors. *J Affect Disord* **3** 1995;**6**:65–75.
13. Radloff L. The ces-d scale: A self-report depression scale for research in the general population. *Appl Psychol Meas* 1977;**1**:385–401.
14. Snaith R. The concepts of mild depression. *Br J Psychiatry* 1987;**150**:387–93.
15. Hybels C, Blazer D and Pieper C. Toward a threshold for subthreshold depression: an analysis of correlates of depression by severity of symptoms using data from an elderly community survey. *Gerontologist* 2001;**41**:357–65.
16. Blazer D. Dysthymia in community and clinical samples of older adults. *Am J Psychiatry* 1994;**151**:1567–9.
17. Devenand D, Noble M, Singer T *et al*. Is dysthymia a different disorder in the elderly? *Am J Psychiatry* 1994;**151**:1592–9.
18. Gallo J, Rabins P and Anthony J. Sadness in older persons: 13-year follow-up of a community sample in Baltimore, Maryland. *Psychol Med* 1999;**29**:341–50.
19. Gallo J, Rabins P and Lyketsos C. Depression without sadness: functional outcomes of nondysphoric depression in later life. *J Am Geriatr Soc* 1997;**45**:570–8.
20. Adams KB. Depressive symptoms, depletion or developmental change? Withdrawal, apathy and lack of vigor in the geriatric depression scale. *Gerontologist* 2001;**41**:768–77.
21. Newman J. Aging and depression. *Psychol Aging* 1989;**4**: 150–65.
22. Newman J, Engel R and Jensen J. Age differences in depressive symptom experiences. *J Gerontol* 1991;**46**:224–35.
23. Olin J, Schneider L, Katz I *et al*. Provisional diagnostic criteria for depression of Alzheimer disease. *Am J Geriatr Psychiatry* 2002;**10**:125–8.
24. Blazer D, Burchett B, Service C and George L. The association of age and depression among the elderly: an epidemiologic exploration. *J Gerontol Med Sci* 1991;**46**:M210–5.
25. Charles S, Reynolds C and Gatz M. Age-related differences and changes in positive and negative affect over 23 years. *J Personality Social Psychol* 2001;**80**:136–51.
26. Murrell S, Himmelfarb S and Wright K. Prevalence of depression and its correlates in older adults. *Am J Epidemiol* 1983;**117**:173–85.
27. Cole MG and Yaffe K. Pathway to psychiatric care of the elderly with depression. *Int J Geriatr Psychiatry* 1996; **11**:157–61.
28. NIMH. Diagnosis and treatment of depression of late life. *JAMA* 1992;**268**:1018–29.
29. Berkman L, Berkman C, Kasl S *et al*. Depressive symptoms in relation to physical health and functioning in the elderly. *Am J Epidemiol* 1986;**124**:372–88.
30. Blazer D, Swartz M, Woodbury M *et al*. Depressive symptoms and depressive diagnoses in a community population. *Arch Gen Psychiatry* 1988;**45**:1078–84.

31. Blazer D and Williams CD. Epidemiology of dysphoria and depression in an elderly population. *Am J Psychiatry* 1980;**137**:439–44.
32. Palsson S, Ostling S and Skoog I. The incidence of first-onset depression in a population followed from the age of 70 to 85. *Psychol Med* 2001;**31**:1159–68.
33. Meller I, Fichter M and Schroppel H. Incidence of depression in octo- and nonagenerarians: results of an epidemiological follow-up community study. *Eur Arch Psychiatry Clin Neurosci* 1996;**246**:93–9.
34. Blazer D. Psychiatry and the oldest old. *Am J Psychiatry* 2000;**157**:1915–24.
35. White L, Blazer D and Fillenbaum G. Related health problems. In: J. Cornoni-Huntley, D. Blazer, M. Lafferty *et al.* (eds), *Established Populations for Epidemiologic Studies of the Elderly*, National Institute on Aging, Bethesda, MD, 1990, pp. 70–85.
36. Steffens DC, Skook I, Norton MC *et al.* Prevalence of depression and its treatment in an elderly population: the Cache County Study. *Arch Gen Psychiatry* 2000;**57**:601–7.
37. Weissman M, Bruce M, Leaf P *et al.* Affective disorders. In: DA Regier and LN Robins (eds), *Psychiatric Disorders in America*, The Free Press, New York, 1991, pp. 53–80.
38. Blazer D, Landerman L, Hays J *et al.* Symptoms of depression among community-dwelling elderly African American and white older adults. *Psychol Med* 1998;**28**:1311–20.
39. Cummings SM, Neff JA and Husaini BA. Functional impairment as a predictor of depressive symptomatology: the role of race, religiosity and social support. *Health Soc Work* 2003;**28**:23–32.
40. Gallo J, Cooper-Patrick L and Lesikar S. Depressive symptoms of whites and African Americans aged 60 years and older. *J Gerontol B Psychol Sci Soc Sci* 1998;**53**:P277–86.
41. Baker FM, Parker DA, Wiley C *et al.* Depressive symptoms in African American medical patients. *Int J Geriatr Psychiatry* 1995;**10**:9–14.
42. Cochran D, Brown DR and McGregor KC. Racial differences in the multiple social roles of older women: implications for depressive symptoms. *Gerontologist* 1999;**39**:465–72.
43. Fabrega H, Mulsant BM, Rifai AH *et al.* Ethnicity and psychopathology in an aging hospital-based population: a comparison of African American and Anglo European patients. *J Nerv Ment Dis* 1994;**182**:136–44.
44. Kennedy GJ, Kelman HR and Thomas C. The emergence of depressive symptoms in late life: the importance of declining health and increasing disability. *J Community Health* 1990;**15**:93–104.
45. Plant EA and Sachs-Ericsson N. Racial and ethnic differences in depression: the roles of social support and meeting basic needs. *J Consult Clin Psychol* 2004;**72**:41–52.
46. Sachs-Ericsson N, Plant EA and Blazer DG. Racial differences in the frequency of depressive symptoms among community dwelling elders: the role of social economic factors. *Aging Ment Health* 2005;**9**:201–9.
47. Blazer D, Hybels C, Simonsick E and Hanlon J. Marked differences in antidepressant use by race in an elderly community sample: 1986–1996. *Am J Psychiatry* 2000;**157**:1089–94.
48. Teresi J, Abrams R, Holmes D *et al.* Influence of cognitive impairment, illness, gender and African American status on psychiatric ratings and staff recognition of depression. *Am J Geriatr Psychiatry* 2002;**10**:506–14.
49. Baker FM. Diagnosing depression in African Americans. *Community Ment Health J* 2001;**37**:31–8.
50. Hays J, Saunders W, Flint E and Blazer D. Social support and depression as risk factors for loss of physical function in late life. *Aging Ment Health* 1997;**1**:209–20.
51. Watkins L, Schneiderman N, Blumenthal J *et al.* Cognitive and somatic symptoms of depression are associated with medical comorbidity in patients after acute myocardial infarction. *Am Heart J* 2003;**146**:48–54.
52. Alexopoulos GS. Clinical and biological interactions in affective and cognitive geriatric syndromes. *Am J Psychiatry* 2003;**160**:811–4.
53. Finkel SI, Costa e Silva J, Cohen GD *et al.* Behavioral and psychological symptoms of dementia: a consensus statement on current knowledge and implications for research and treatment. *Am J Geriatr Psychiatry* 1998;**6**:97–100.
54. Huang C-Q, Zhang X-M, Dong B-R *et al.* Health status and risk for depression among the elderly: a meta-analysis of published literature. *Age Ageing* 2010;**39**:23–30.
55. Blazer D, Sachs-Ericsson N and Hybels C. Perception of unmet basic needs as a predictor of depressive symptoms among community-dwelling older adults. *J Gerontol Med Sci* 2007;**62**:191–5.
56. Lopez OL, Jagust WJ, Dulberg C *et al.* Risk factors for mild cognitive impairment in the Cardiovascular Health Study Cognition Study: Part 2. *Arch Neurol* 2003;**60**:1394–9.
57. Sachs-Ericsson N and Blazer DG. Depression and anxiety associated with dementia. In: G Maletta (ed.), *Geriatric Psychiatry: Evaluation and Management*, Lippincott Williams & Wilkins, Baltimore, 2006, pp. 591–603.
58. Olin J, Katz I, Meyers B *et al.* Provisional diagnostic criteria for depression of Alzheimer disease: rationale and background. *Am J Geriatr Psychiatry* 2002;**10**:129–41.
59. Zubenko GS, Zubenko WN, McPherson S *et al.* A collaborative study of the emergence and clinical features of the major depressive syndrome of Alzheimer's disease. *Am J Psychiatry* **1** 2003;**60**:857–66.
60. Ballard C, Bannister C, Solis M *et al.* The prevalence, associations and symptoms of depression amongst dementia sufferers. *J Affect Disord* 1996;**36**:135–44.
61. Cummings JL, Miller B, Hill MA and Neshkes R. Neuropsychiatric aspects of multi-infarct dementia and dementia of the Alzheimer type. *Arch Neurol* 1987;**44**:389–93.
62. Kim J, Lyons D, Shin I and Yoon J. Differences in the behavioral and psychological symptoms between Alzheimer's disease and vascular dementia: are the different pharmacologic treatment strategies justifiable? *Hum Psychopharmacol* 2003;**18**:215–20.
63. (a) Aarsland D, Tandberg E, Larsen JP and Cummings JL. Frequency of dementia in Parkinson disease. *Arch Neurol* 1996;**53**:538–42. (b) Aarsland D, Larsen JP, Lim N *et al.* Range of neuropsychiatric disturbances in patients with Parkinson's disease. *J Neurol Neurosurg Psychiatry* 1999;**67**:492–6.
64. Blazer D. *Depression in Late Life*, Mosby, St Louis, 1994.

65. Devanand D, Sano M, Tang M-X *et al*. Depressed mood and the incidence of Alzheimer's disease in the elderly living in the community. *Arch Gen Psychiatry* 1996;**53**:175–82.

66. Geerlings M, Schoevers R, Beekman A *et al*. Depression and the risk of cognitive decline and Alzheimer's disease: results of two prospective community-based studies in The Netherlands. *Br J Psychiatry* 2000;**176**:568–75.

67. Ritchie K, Gilham C, Ledesert B *et al*. Depressive illness, depressive symptomology and regional cerebral blood flow in elderly people with sub-clinical cognitive impairment. *Age Ageing* 1999;**28**:385–91.

68. Sachs-Ericsson N, Joiner T, Plant EA and Blazer DG. The influence of depression on cognitive decline in community-dwelling elderly persons. *Am. J. Geriatr. Psychiatry* 2005;**13**:402–8.

69. Lyketsos CG, Steele C, Baker L *et al*. Major and minor depression in Alzheimer's disease: prevalence and impact. *J Neuropsychiatry Clin Neurosci* 1997;**9**:556–61.

70. Alexopoulos G, Meyers B, Young R *et al*. Recovery in geriatric depression. *Arch Gen Psychiatry* 1996;**53**:305–12.

71. Baldwin R and Jolley D. The prognosis of depression in old age. *Br J Psychiatry* 1986;**149**:574–83.

72. Blazer D, Hughes D and George L. Age and impaired subjective support: predictors of depressive symptoms at one-year follow-up. *J Nerv Ment Dis* 1992;**180**:172–8.

73. Post F. *The Significance of Affective Symptoms at Old Age*, Oxford University Press, London, 1962.

74. Murphy E. The prognosis of depression in old age. *Br J Psychiatry* 1983;**142**:111–9.

75. Reynolds CF III, Frank E, Perel JM *et al*. Combined pharmacotherapy and psychotherapy in the acute and continuation treatment of elderly patients with recurrent major depression: a preliminary report. *Am J Psychiatry* 1992;**149**:1687–92.

76. Cole MG and Bellavance F. Depression in elderly medical inpatients: a meta-analysis of outcomes. *CMAJ* 1997;**157**:1055–60.

77. Romanelli J, Fauerbach J, Buch D and Ziegelstein R. The significance of depression in older patients after myocardial infarction. *J Am Geriatr Soc* 2002;**50**:817–22.

78. McGuire L, Kiecolt-Glaser J and Glaser R. Depressive symptoms and lymphocyte proliferation in older adults. *J Abnorm Psychol* 2002;**111**:192–7.

79. Williams S, Kasl S, Heiat A *et al*. Depression and risk of heart failure among the elderly: A prospective community-based study. *Psychosomc Med* 2002;**64**:6–12.

80. Bruce ML, Leaf P and Rozal G. Psychiatry status and 9-year mortality data in the New Haven epidemiologic catchment area study. *Am J Psychiatry* 1994;**51**:716–21.

81. (a) Schulz R, Drayer R and Rollman B. Depression as a risk factor for non-suicide mortality in the elderly. *Biol Psychiatry* 2002;**52**:205–25. (b) Schulz R, Beach S and Ives D. Association between depression and mortality in older adults: the Cardiovascular Health Study. *Arch Intern Med* 2000;**160**:1761–8.

82. Geerlings S, Beekman A, Beeg D *et al*. Duration and severity of depression predict mortality in older adults in the community. *Psychol Med* 2002;**32**:609–18.

83. Ganguli M, Dodge HH and Mulsant BH. Rates and predictors of mortality in an aging, rural, community-based cohort: the role of depression. *Arch Gen Psychiatry* 2002;**59**:1046–52.

84. Schoevers RA, Geerlings MI, Deeg DJ *et al*. Depression and excess mortality: evidence for a dose response relation in community living elderly. *Int J Geriatr Psychiatry* 2009;**24**:169–76.

85. Blazer D, Bachar J and Manton K. Suicide in late life: review and commentary. *J Am Geriatr Soc* 1986;**34**:519–26.

86. Conwell Y, Duberstein PR and Caine ED. Risk factors for suicide in later life. *Biol Psychiatry* 2002;**52**:193–204.

87. Conwell Y, Lyness J, Duberstein P *et al*. Completed suicide among older patients in primary care practices: a controlled study. *J Am Geriatr Soc* 2000;**48**:23–9.

88. Goldstein RB, Black DW, Nasrallah A and Winokur G. The prediction of suicide. Sensitivity, specificity and predictive value of a multivariate model applied to suicide among 1906 patients with affective disorders. *Arch Gen Psychiatry* 1991;**48**:418–22.

89. Murphy GE and Wetzel RD. Suicide risk by birth cohort in the united states, 1949 to 1974. *Arch Gen Psychiatry* 1980;**37**:519–23.

90. Raern M, Reneson B, Allebeck P *et al*. Mental disorder in elderly suicides: a case–control study. *Am J Psychiatry* 2002;**159**:450–5.

91. Turvey C, Conwell Y, Jones M *et al*. Risk factors for late-life suicide: a prospective, community-based study. *Am J Geriatr Psychiatry* 2002;**10**:398–406.

92. Arias E, Anderson RN, Kung HC *et al*. *Deaths: Final Data for 2001*, DHHS Publication (DHS), National Center for Health Statistics, Hyattsville, MD, 2001.

93. Sachs-Ericsson N. *Gender, Social Roles and Suicidal Ideation and Attempts in a General Population Sample*, Kluwer, Norwell, MA, 2000.

94. De Leo D, Padoani W, Scocco P *et al*. Attempted and completed suicide in older subjects: results from the WHO/Euro Multicentre Study of Suicidal Behaviour. *Int J Geriatr Psychiatry* 2001;**16**:300–10.

95. Conwell Y, Duberstein PR, Cox C *et al*. Age differences in behaviors leading to completed suicide. *Am J Geriatr Psychiatry* 1998;**6**:122–6.

96. Bruce ML, Ten Have TR, Reynolds CF III *et al*. Reducing suicidal ideation and depressive symptoms in depressed older primary care patients: a randomized controlled trial. *JAMA* 2004;**291**:1081–91.

97. Beck AT, Brown G, Berchick RJ *et al*. Relationship between hopelessness and ultimate suicide: a replication with psychiatric outpatients. *Am J Psychiatry* 1990;**147**:190–5.

98. Rifai AH, George CJ, Stack JA *et al*. Hopelessness in suicide attempters after acute treatment of major depression in late-life. *Am J Psychiatry* 1994;**151**:1687–90.

99. Shneidman E. What do suicides have in common? A summary of the psychological approach. In: B. Bongar (ed.), *Suicide: Guidelines for Assessment Management and Treatment*, Oxford University Press, New York, 1992, Chapter 1.

100. (a) Alexopoulos GS, Bruce ML, Hull J *et al*. Clinical determinants of suicidal ideation and behavior in geriatric depression. *Arch Gen Psychiatry* 1999;**56**:1048–53. (b) Alexopoulos

G, Katz I, Reynolds C *et al*. The Expert Consensus Guideline Series: Pharmacotherapy of Depressive Disorders in Older Patients. *Postgrad Med* 2001;(Special Issue, October):1–86.

101. Joiner T, Kalafat J, Draper J *et al*. Establishing standards for the assessment of suicide risk among callers to the national suicide prevention lifeline. *Suicide Life Threat Behav* 2007;**37**:353–65.

102. Juurlink DN, Herrmann N, Szalai JP *et al*. Medical illness and the risk of suicide in the elderly. *Arch Intern Med* 2004;**164**:1179–84.

103. Goldstrom ID, Burns BJ, Kessler LG *et al*. Mental health services use by elderly adults in a primary care setting. *J Gerontol* 1987;**42**:147–53.

104. Pearson JL and Brown GK. Suicide prevention in late life: directions for science and practice. *Clin Psychol Rev* 2000;**20**:685–705.

105. Joiner T, Walker R, Rudd MD and Jobes D. Scientizing and routinizing the outpatient assessment of suicidality. *Prof Psychol Res Pract* 1999;**30**:447–53.

106. Conwell Y and Brent D. Suicide and aging. I. Patterns of psychiatric diagnosis. *Int Psychogeriatr* 1995;**7**:149–64.

107. Duberstein PR. Openness to experience and completed suicide across the second half of life. *Int Psychogeriatr* 1995;**7**:183–98.

108. Whooley MA, Kip KE, Cauley JA *et al*. Study of Osteoporotic Fractures Research Group. Depression, falls and risk of fracture in older women. *Arch Intern Med* 1999;**159**:484–90.

109. Starkstein S, Preziosi T, Bolduck P and Robinson R. Depression in Parkinson's disease. *J Nerv Ment Disord* 1990;**178**:27–31.

110. Parmelee P, Katz I and Lawton M. The relation of pain to depression among institutionalized aged. *J Gerontol* 1991;**46**:15–21.

111. Endberg S, Sereika S, Weber E *et al*. Prevalence and recognition of depressive symptoms among homebound older adults with urinary incontinence. *J Geriatr Psychiatry Neurol* 2001;**14**:130–9.

112. Lyness JM, Heo M, Datto CJ *et al*. Outcomes of minor and subsyndromal depression among elderly patients in primary care settings. *Ann Intern Med* 2006;**144**:496–504.

113. Barondes S. *Mood Genes: Hunting for Origins of Mania and Depression*, Freeman, New York, 1998.

114. Gatz M, Pedersen N, Plomin R *et al*. Importance of shared genes and shared environments for symptoms of depression in older adults. *J Abnorm Psychol* 1992;**101**:701–8.

115. Blazer D, Burchette B and Fillenbaum G. APOE e4 and low cholesterol as risks for depression in a biracial elderly community sample. *Am J Geriatr Psychiatry* 2002;**10**:515–20.

116. Nebes R, Vora I, Melzer C *et al*. Relationship of deep white matter hyperintensities and apolipoprotein e genotype to depressive symptoms in older adults without clinical depression. *Am J Psychiatry* 2001;**158**:878–84.

117. Coffey C, Figiel G and Djang W. Subcortical hyperintensity on magnetic resonance imaging: a comparison of normal and depressed elderly subjects. *Am J Psychiatry* 1990;**147**:187–9.

118. Krishnan K, Goli V, Ellinwood E *et al*. Leukoencephalopathy in patients diagnosed as major depressive. *Biol Psychiatry* 1988;**23**:519–22.

119. Kumar A, Mintz J, Bilker W and Gottlieb G. Autonomous neurobiological pathways to late-life depressive disorders: clinical and pathophysiological implications. *Neuropsychopharmacology* 2002;**26**:229–36.

120. Kumar A, Thomas A, Lavretsky H *et al*. Frontal white matter biochemical abnormalities in late-life major depression detected with proton magnetic resonance spectroscopy. *Am J Psychiatry* 2002;**159**:630–6.

121. George M, Ketter T and Post R. Prefrontal cortex dysfunction in clinical depression. *Depression* 1994;**2**:59–72.

122. Krishnan K, McDonald W, Doraiswamy P *et al*. Neuroanatomical substrates of depression in the elderly. *Eur Arch Psychiatry Clin Neurosci* 1993;**243**:41–6.

123. Krishnan K, McDonald W, Escalona P *et al*. Magnetic imaging of the caudate nuclei in depression: preliminary observation. *Arch Gen Psychiatry* 1992;**49**:553–7.

124. Husain M, McDonald W, Doraiswamy P *et al*. A magnetic resonance imaging study of putamen nuclei in major depression. *Psychiatry Res* 1991;**40**:95–9.

125. Porter RJ, Gallagher P and O'Brien JT. Effects of rapid tryptophan depletion on salivary cortisol in older people recovered from depression and the healthy elderly. *J Psychopharmacol* 2007;**21**:71–5.

126. Davis K, David B, Mathe A *et al*. Age and the dexamethasone supression test in depression. *Am J Psychiatry* 1984;**141**:872–4.

127. Arborelius L, Owens M, Plotsky P and Nemeroff C. The role of corticotropin-releasing factor in depression and anxiety disorders. *J Endocrinol* 1999;**160**:1–12.

128. Luisi S, Tonetti A, Bernardi F *et al*. Effect of acute corticotropin releasing factor on pituitary-adrenocortical responsiveness in elderly women and men. *J Endocrinol Invest* 1998;**21**:449–53.

129. Yaffe K, Ettinger B and Pressman A. Neuropsychiatric function and dehydroepiandrosterone sulfate in elderly women: a prospective study. *Biol Psychiatry* 1998;**43**:694–700.

130. Seidman S, Araujo A, Roose S *et al*. Low testosterone levels in elderly men with dysthymic disorder. *Am J Psychiatry* 2002;**159**:456–9.

131. Seidman S, Spatz E, Rizzo C and Roose S. Testosterone replacement therapy for hypogonadal men with major depressive disorder: a randomized, placebo-controlled clinical trial. *J Clin Psychiatry* 2001;**62**:406–12.

132. Tsai S. Brain-derived neurotrophic factor: a bridge between major depression and Alzheimer's disease? *Med Hypotheses* 2003;**61**:110–3.

133. Evers MM, Purohit D, Perl D *et al*. Palliative and aggressive end-of-life care for patients with dementia. *Psychiatr Serv* 2002;**53**:609–13.

134. Seligman M and Maier S. Failure to escape traumatic shock. *J Exp Psychol* 1967;**74**:1–15.

135. Blazer D. *Depression in Late Life*, 3rd edn, Springer, New York, 2002.

136. Seligman MEP. Learned helplessness. *Annu Rev Med* 1972;**23**:407.

137. Beck AT. Cognitive model of depression. *J Cogn Psychother* 1987;**1**:2–27.

138. Beck AT. Thinking and depression. I. Idiosyncratic content and cognitive distortions. *Arch Gen Psychiatry* 1963;**9**:324–33.

139. Kovacs M and Beck AT. Maladaptive cognitive structures in depression. *Am J Psychiatry* 1978;**135**:525–33.

140. Adams K. Depressive symptoms, depletion or developmental change? Withdrawal, apathy or lack of vigor in the geriatric depression scale. *Gerontologist* 2001;**41**:768–77.

141. Tornstam L. Gero-transcendence: a reformulation of disengagement theory. *Aging* 1989;**1**:55–63.

142. Johnson CL and Barer BM. Patterns of engagement and disengagement among the oldest old. *J Aging Stud* 1992;**6**:351–64.

143. Cumming E and Henry W. *Growing Old: The Process of Disengagement*, Basic Books, New York, 1961.

144. Lewinsohn P, Rohde P, Seeley J and Fischer S. Age and depression: unique and shared effects. *Psychol Aging* 1989;**6**:247–60.

145. Fonda S, Wallace R and Herzog A. Changes in driving patterns and worsening depressive symptoms among older adults. *J Gerontol Psychol Soc Sci* 2001;**56**:S343–51.

146. Baltes P and Baltes M (eds), *Successful Aging: Perspectives from the Behavioral Sciences*, Cambridge University Press, Cambridge, 1990.

147. Carstensen L. Motivation for social contact across the life span: a theory of socioemotional selectivity. *Nebr Symp Motiv* 1992;**40**:209–54.

148. Frederickson BL and Carstensen LL. Choosing social partners: how old age and anticipated endings make people more selective. *Psychol Aging* 1990;**5**:335–47.

149. DuPertuis LL, Aldwin CM and Bosse R. Does the source of support matter for different health outcomes? Findings from the normative aging study. *J Aging Health* 2001;**13**:495–510.

150. Goldberg EL, Van Natta P and Comstock GW. Depressive symptoms, social networks and social support of elderly women. *Am J Epidemiol* 1985;**121**:448–56.

151. Holahan CJ, Moos RH, Holahan CK and Cronkite RC. Resource loss, resource gain and depressive symptoms: a 10-year model. *J Pers Soc Psychol* 1999;**77**:6209.

152. Joiner T and Coyne JC. *The Interaction Nature of Depression: Advances in Interpersonal Approaches*, American Psychological Association, Washington, DC, 1999.

153. Mendes de Leon CF, Glass TA and Berkman LF. Social engagement and disability in a community population of older adults: The New Haven EPESE. *Am J Epidemiol* 2003;**157**:633–42.

154. Bassuk SS, Glass TA and Berkman LF. Social disengagement and incident cognitive decline in community-dwelling elderly persons. *Ann Inter Med* 1999;**3**:165–73.

155. Joiner T and Metalsky GA. prospective test of an integrative interpersonal theory of depression: a naturalistic study of college roommates. *J Pers Soc Psychol* 1995;**69**:778–88.

156. Kraaij V and de Wilde E. Negative life events and depressive symptoms in the elderly: a life span perspective. *Aging Ment Health* 2001;**5**:84–91.

157. Williams JW Jr, Noel PH, Cordes JA *et al*. Is this patient clinically depressed? *JAMA* 2002;**287**:1160–70.

158. Koenig H, Cohen H, Blazer D *et al*. Cognitive symptoms of depression and religious coping in elderly medical patients. *Psychosomatics* 1995;**36**:369–75.

159. Yesavage J, Brink T and Rose T. Development and validation of a geriatric depression screening scale: a preliminary report. *J Psychiatr Res* 1983;**17**:37–49.

160. Fried L. Frailty. In: W. Hazzard, E. Bierman, J. Blass *et al*. (eds), *Principles of Geriatric Medicine and Gerontology*, 3rd edn, McGraw Hill, New York, 1994, pp. 1149–56.

161. Branch L and Meyers A. Assessing physical function in the elderly. *Clin Geriatr Med* 1987;**3**:29–51.

162. Fillenbaum G. *Multidimensional Functional Assessment of Older Adults: the Duke Older Americans Resources and Services Procedures*. Erlbaum, Hillsdale, NJ, 1988.

163. Blazer D. Social support and mortality in an elderly community population. *Am J Epidemiol* 1982;**115**:684–94.

164. Karlawish J and Clark C. Diagnostic evaluation of elderly patients with mild memory problems. *Ann Intern Med* 2003;**138**:411–9.

165. Knott P and Fleminger J. Presenile dementia: the difficulties of early diagnosis. *Acta Psychiatr Scand* 1975;**51**:210–7.

166. Starkstein SE, Petracca G, Chemerinski E and Merello M. Prevalence and correlates of parkinsonism in patients with primary depression. *Neurology* 2001;**57**:553–5.

167. Wells C. Pseudodementia. *Am J Psychiatry* 1979;**136**:895–900.

168. Alexopoulos GS. Depression in the elderly. *Lancet* 2005;**365**:1961–70.

169. Forlenza O, Junior A, Hirala E and Ferreira R. Antidepressant efficacy of sertraline and imipramine for the treatment of major depression in elderly outpatients. *Sao Paulo Med J* 2000;**118**:99–104.

170. Kyle C, Petersen H and Overo K. Comparison of the tolerability and efficacy of citalopram and amitriptyline in elderly depressed patients treated in general practice. *Depress Anxiety* 1998;**8**:147–53.

171. Salzman C, Wong E and Wright B. Drug and ECT treatment of depression in the elderly, 1996–2001: a literature review. *Biol Psychiatry* 2002;**52**:265–84.

172. Mulsant B, Pollock B, Nebes R *et al*. A twelve-week, double-blind, randomized comparison of nortriptyline and paroxetine in older depressed inpatients and outpatients. *Am J Geriatr Psychiatry* 2001;**9**:406–14.

173. Callahan C, Hendrie H, Nienaber N and Tierney W. Suicidal ideation among older primary care patients. *J Am Geriatr Soc* 1996;**44**:1205–9.

174. Koenig H, Cohen H, Blazer D *et al*. Religious coping and depression in elderly hospitalized medically ill men. *Am J Psychiatry* 1992;**149**:1693–700.

175. Lyketsos C, Sheppard J, Steele C *et al*. A randomized placebo-controlled, double-blind, clinical trial of sertraline in the treatment of depression complicating Alzheimer disease: initial results from the Depression in Alzheimer Disease Study (DIADS). *Am J Psychiatry* 2000;**157**:1686–9.

176. Reifler B, Teri L, Raskind M *et al*. Double-blind trial of imipramine in Alzheimer's disease patients with and without depression. *Am J Psychiatry* 1989;**146**:45–9.

177. Mukai Y and Tampi RR. Treatment of depression in the elderly: a review of the recent literature on the efficacy of single- versus dual-action antidepressants. *Clin Ther* 2009;**31**:945–61.
178. Ackerman D, Greenland S, Bystritsky A and Small G. Side effects and time course of response in a placebo-controlled trial of fluoxetine for the treatment of geriatric depression. *J Clinic Psychopharmacol* 2000;**20**:658–65.
179. Oxman T and Sungupta A. Treatment of minor depression. *Am J Geriatr Psychiatry* 2002;**10**:256–64.
180. Williams J, Barrett J, Oxman T *et al*. Treatment of dysthymia and minor depression in primary care: a randomized controlled trial in older adults. *JAMA* 2000;**284**:1519–26.
181. Feighner J and Cohn J. Double-blind comparative trials of fluoxetine and doxepin in geriatric patients with major depression. *J Clin Psychiatry* 1985;**46**:20–5.
182. Cohn C, Shrivastava R and Mendels J. Double-blind multicenter comparison of sertraline and amitriptyline in elderly depressed patients. *J Clin Psychiatry* 1990;**51**:28–33.
183. Katona C, Hunder B and Bray JA. double-blind comparison of paroxetine and imipramine in the treatment of depression with dementia. *Int J Geriatr Psychiatry* 1998;**13**:100–80.
184. Nyth A, Gottfried C and Lyby K. A controlled multicenter clinical study of citalipram and placebo in elderly depressed patients with and without concomitant dementia. *Acta Psychiatr Scand* 1992;**86**:138–145.
185. Mahapatra S and Hackett D. A randomized, double-blind, paralled-group comparison of venlafaxine and dothiepin in geriatric patients with major depression. *Int J Clin Pract* 1997;**51**:209–13.
186. Hoyberg O, Maragakis B, Mullin J *et al*. A double-blind multicentre comparison of mirtazapine and amitriptyline in elderly depressed patients. *Acta Psychiatr Scand* 1996; **93**:184–90.
187. Schatzberg A, Kremer C, Rodrigues H and Murphy G. Double-blind, randomized comparison of mirtazapine and paroxetine in elderly depressed patients. *Am J Geriatr Psychiatry* 2002;**10**:541–50.
188. Branconnier R, Cole J, Ghazviain S *et al*. Clinical pharmacology of buproprion and imipramine in elderly depressives. *J Clin Psychiatry* 1983;**44**:130–3.
189. Weihs K, Settle E, Batey S *et al*. Buproprion sustained release versus paroxetine for the treatment of depression in the elderly. *J Clin Psychiatry* 2001;**61**:196–202.
190. Greenblatt D, van Moltke L, Harmatz J and Shader R. Drug interactions with newer antidepressants: role of human cytochromes p450. *J Clin Psychiatry* 1998;**59**(Suppl 15):19–27.
191. Pollock B. Geriatric psychiatry: psychopharmacology: general principles. In B. Sadock and V. Sadock (eds), *Kaplan and Sadock's Comprehensive Textbook of Psychiatry/VII*. Williams & Wilkins, Baltimore, MD, 2000, pp. 3086–3090.
192. Kirby D, Harigan S and Ames D. Hyponatraemia in elderly psychiatric patients treated with selective serotonin reuptake inhibitors and venlafaxine: a retrospective controlled study in an inpatient unit. *Int J Geriatr Psychiatry* 2002;**17**:231–7.
193. Thapa P, Gideon P, Cost T *et al*. Antidepressants and the risk of falls among nursing home residents. *N Engl J Med* 1998;**339**:918–20.
194. Gillman P. The serotonin syndrome and its treatment. *J Psychopharmacol* 1999;**13**:100–9.
195. de Abajo F, Rodriguez L and Montero D. Association between selective serotonin reuptake inhibitors and upper gastrointestinal bleeding: population based case–control study. *BMJ* 1999;**319**:1106–9.
196. Benbow S. The use of electroconvulsive therapy in old-age psychiatry. *Int J Geriatr Psychiatry* 1987;**2**:25–30.
197. Flint A and Rifat S. The treatment of psychotic depression in later life: a comparison of pharmacotherapy and ECT. *J Geriatr Psychiatry* 1998;**13**:23–8.
198. Fraser R and Glass I. Unilateral and bilateral ECT in elderly patients. *Acta Psychiatr Scand* 1980;**62**:13–31.
199. Godber C, Rosenvinge H, Wilkinson D and Smithes J. Depression in old age: prognosis after ECT. *Int J Geriatr Psychiatry* 1987;**2**:19–24.
200. O'Conner M, Knapp R, Husain M *et al*. The influence of age on the response of major depression to electroconvulsive therapy: a C.O.R.E. Report. *Am J Geriatr Psychiatry* 2001;**9**:382–90.
201. McNamara B, Ray J, Arthurs O and Boniface S. Transcranial magnetic stimulation for depression and other psychiatric disorders. *Psychol Med* 2001;**31**:1141–6.
202. Dannon P, Dolberg O, Schreiber S and Grunhaus L. Three- and six-month outcome following courses of either ECT or RTMS in a population of severely depressed individuals – preliminary report. *Biol Psychiatry* 2002; **51**:687–90.
203. Moser D, Jorge R, Manes F *et al*. Improved exective functioning following repetitive transcranial magnetic stimulation. *Neurology* 2002;**58**:1288–90.
204. Camacho T, Roberts R, Lazarus N *et al*. Physical activity and depression: evidence from the Alameda County Study. *Am J Epidemiol* 1991;**134**:220–31.
205. Blumenthal J, Babyak M, Moore K *et al*. Effects of exercise training on older patients with major depression. *Arch Intern Med* 1999;**159**:2349–56.
206. Singh N, Clements K and Kingh M. The efficacy of exercise as a long-term antidepressant in elderly subjects: a randomized controlled trial. *J Gerontol Med Sci* 2001;**56**:M497–504.
207. Sumaya I, Rienzi B, Beegan J and Moss D. Bright light treatment decreases depression in institutionalized older adults: a placebo-controlled crossover study. *J Gerontol Med Sci* 2001;**56**:M356–60.
208. Alexopoulos GS, Reynolds CF III, Bruce ML *et al*. Reducing suicidal ideation and depression in older primary care patients: 24-month outcomes of the prospect study. *Am J Psychiatry* 2009;**166**:882–90.
209. Frank E, Frank N and Cornes C. Interpersonal psychotherapy in the treatment of late life depression. In: G Klerman and M Weissman (eds), *New Applications of Interpersonal Psychotherapy*, American Psychiatric Press, Washington, DC, 1993.
210. Klerman GL, Weissman MM, Rounsaville BJ and Chevron ES. *Interpersonal Psychotherapy of Depression*, Basic Books, New York, 1984.

211. Frank E and Spanier C. Interpersonal psychotherapy for depression: overview, clinical efficacy and future directions. *Clin Psychol Sci Pract* 1995;**2**:349–65.
212. Miller MD, Wolfson L, Frank E *et al.* Using interpersonal psychotherapy (IPT) in a combined psychotherapy/medication research protocol with depressed elders: a descriptive report with case vignettes. *J Psychother Pract Res* 1998;**7**:47–55.
213. Miller MD, Cornes C, Frank E *et al.* Interpersonal psychotherapy for late-life depression: past, present and future. *J Psychother Pract Res* 2001;**10**:231–8.
214. Reynolds CF III, Frank E, Perel JM *et al.* Nortriptyline and interpersonal psychotherapy as maintenance therapies for recurrent major depression: a randomized controlled trial in patients older than 59 years. *JAMA* 1999;**281**:39–45.
215. Thompson L, Coon D and Gallagher-Thompson D. Comparison of desipramine and cognitive/behavioral therapy in the treatment of elderly outpatients with mild-to-moderate depression. *Am J Geriatr Psychiatry* 2001;**9**: 225–40.
216. Peng XD, Huang CQ, Chen LJ and Lu ZC. Cognitive behavioural therapy and reminiscence techniques for the treatment of depression in the elderly: a systematic review. *J Int Med Res* 2009;**37**:975–82.
217. Katon WJ, Schoenbaum M, Fan M-Y *et al.* Cost-effectiveness of improving primary care treatment of late-life depression. *Arch Gen Psychiatry* 2005;**62**:1313–20.

CHAPTER 84

The older patient with Down syndrome

John E. Morley

Saint Louis University School of Medicine and Saint Louis Veterans' Affairs Medical Center, St Louis, MO, USA

Introduction

The association between trisomy 21 and Down syndrome was first recognized in 1959 by Lejeune, Gautier and Tarpin. In recent times, the number of fetuses conceived with Down syndrome has increased, but prenatal screening has resulted in a decline in the number of children conceived with this condition. Thus, the occurrence of Down syndrome has decreased from 1 in 700 to 1 in 1000 live births. In addition to the true trisomy, 3–4% of Down patients have translocation of a portion of chromosome 21 and 1% have mosaicism with some cells having 46 and other 47 chromosomes.

From 1983 to 1997, the median age of death of persons with Down syndrome increased from 25 to 49 years.[1] More recently, it was suggested that the average life expectancy for Down syndrome is 60 years.[2] The oldest reported person with Down syndrome lived until 83 years of age. Three factors make persons with Down syndrome of interest to the geriatrician: (1) the increasing life span; (2) the fact that these persons tend to develop early frailty and functional decline in their 40s; and (3) the early onset of Alzheimer's disease.

Genes and Down syndrome

There are 329 genes predicted to be on chromosome 21. Sixteen of these genes play a role in mitochondrial energy metabolism or the generation of free radicals. Abnormalities in these genes are thought to lead to increased free radical production, leading to premature ageing.

At least 10 genes on chromosome 21 play a role in brain development and neuronal loss. Two of these are associated with Alzheimer's disease, namely the amyloid precursor protein and the S100 calcium-binding protein. Overproduction of amyloid precursor protein and, thus, β-amyloid, is thought to play a key role in the early onset of Alzheimer's disease in persons with Down syndrome. In addition, excess production of β-amyloid has been shown to lead to problems with learning and memory, which may contribute to the cognitive problems seen in persons with Down syndrome.

There are six genes that are involved in folate and methyl group metabolism on chromosome 21. Elevated levels of homocysteine, which are seen in folate deficiency, are associated with Alzheimer's disease. In our clinical experience, elevated homocysteine levels are not rare in younger adults with Down syndrome.

The physician, and the patient with Down syndrome

Older persons with Down syndrome are usually easily recognized when they present to the physician, because of the classical facial features (brachycephaly, epicanthal folds and flat nasal bridge) and short stature. These persons also often have broad hands, lax ligaments and a wide gap between the first and second toes, brachydactyly and mental retardation. The majority of persons with Down syndrome live in the community. They may live in group housing and work in sheltered workshops. Physicians need to identify the person who accompanies the individual with Down to the office. This person often provides supervisory care for the individual with Down syndrome and can provide useful historical information on behavioural and other changes that may be occurring. We recommend office visits every 6 months for healthy persons with Down syndrome and every 3–4 months when functional or mental decline is present. This allows the patient to become comfortable with the healthcare provider. Many patients enjoy hugging and this can further increase trust in the physician. However, the physician must remember to ask the patient first if they wish to hug. The physician should always discuss the patient's work and how it is progressing. Also, note should be made of their recreational activities and how they are interacting with other persons within a group home. The quality of life of all patients should be assessed by probing multiple

Principles and Practice of Geriatric Medicine, Fifth Edition. Edited by Alan J. Sinclair, John E. Morley and Bruno Vellas.

areas such as 'things you do, your family and friends, your self-image, your leisure time, your employment and help you need' before exploring the person's health issues.

Always address the person with Down syndrome directly, before hearing the caregiver's story. This gains their confidence and allows observation of their language ability. Finally, never assume that changes in persons with Down syndrome are due to the condition itself before excluding other common medical causes. Problems with spatial memory are classical of Down syndrome and so should not be used in the diagnosis of Alzheimer's disease.[3] Aerobic exercise programmes may help improve both psychosocial and physical health.[4]

For some medical examinations, such as pap smears, and special tests, such as MRI or CT scan, or procedures such as dental care, persons with Down syndrome may require sedation. We have found that 0.5–1 mg of lorazepam orally is usually sufficient for this purpose and produces no adverse effects. Low-dose intravenous lorazepam can also be used in more difficult situations. Others have recommended oral ketamine and midazolam, given under the supervision of an anaesthetist.[5] Before undergoing a procedure requiring sedation, a risk–benefit evaluation should always be undertaken. Informed consent needs to be obtained from the patient or, where applicable, the court-appointed guardian.

Preventive measures for Down syndrome patients should be similar to those for the general adult population. This includes screening for hypertension and heart disease. Because obesity is a common problem in this population, regular counselling on the need for exercise is mandatory. Although, in our experience, most Down syndrome patients do not smoke or drink alcohol, this should be confirmed both from the patient and the caregiver.

Down syndrome adults tend to complain of pain, even when present, less often than other persons. Therefore, it is important to utilize facial expressions during the examination to obtain input concerning presence of pain. Also, such patients may stop using a limb when it is painful. Rocking and 'head banging' behaviours occur as visceral pain proxies. As is the case with older adults, middle-aged adults with Down syndrome often manifest medical problems as a delirium or other behavioural problem.

Persons with Down are a vulnerable population and therefore, like children and older people, are at increased risk for abuse. When adults with Down syndrome become withdrawn, this may suggest abuse or an unrecognized pain syndrome or depression. The presence of unexplained bruises, skin tears or fractures must increase the physician's suspicion of abuse. New-onset falls can suggest delirium, functional deterioration or abuse.

Health counselling includes decisions on advanced directives and guardianship. Financial support questions need to be addressed and relatives need to be aware of local resources. Estate planning, for example trusts, need to be created where appropriate, as Down syndrome persons are now regularly outliving their parents and other close relatives. Parent (caregiver) support groups can be invaluable as caregiver stress is common, particularly as the parent ages. Local and national societies for Down syndrome or for persons with developmental disabilities are an important resource. The physician needs to look for excess stress and/or depression in caregivers and advise treatment where appropriate.

Functional ability using at least basic activities of daily living (ADLs) and instrumental activities of daily living (IADLs) should be assessed yearly. Where possible, mental status screening using the Mini Mental Status Examination (MMSE) or the Saint Louis University Mental Status Examination and the Geriatric Depression Scale or the Cornell Depression Inventory should be done yearly.

There are a number of disease conditions that occur more commonly in adults with Down syndrome than in the general population (Table 84.1). 'Health-Care Guidelines for Individuals with Down Syndrome' were developed by a consensus panel of the Down Syndrome Medical Interest Group.[5] There is a lack of evidence in this area and so physician-substituted judgement is important in deciding

Table 84.1 Conditions that occur commonly in adults with Down syndrome.

Obesity
Periodontal disease
Hearing loss
Visual problems including early cataracts
Aortic valvular disease
– Mitral valve prolapse
– Aortic regurgitation
Arthritis
Hypogonadism (male)
Hypothyroidism
Hyperthyroidism
Diabetes mellitus
Early menopause
Osteoporosis
Coeliac disease
Sleep apnoea
Atlantoaxial subluxation
Testicular cancer
Seizures
Dermatological abnormalities
Depression
Alzheimer's disease
Delirium
Agitated behaviour
Foot problems

which healthcare screening approaches are most efficacious in this population.

Disorders associated with Down syndrome

Endocrinological

Congenital hypothyroidism occurs in one in 141 neonates with Down syndrome and the prevalence increases with age. In adults with Down syndrome, between 15 and 40% have hypothyroidism.[6] Its presentation is often insidious and many of the early signs and symptoms are difficult to detect in patients with Down syndrome. All patients with a recent decline in mental function need to be screened for hypothyroidism. Because of the frequency of hypothyroidism in this population, it is recommended that adult patients are screened by having a thyroid-stimulating hormone (TSH) blood test every year. All patients with a TSH $>10\,\mathrm{mU\,l^{-1}}$ should be treated, regardless of whether or not the thyroxine level is normal. Goitre and thyroiditis also commonly occur in this population. No studies have determined the utility of examining thyroid antibodies to determine which patients will progress to hypothyroidism. Thyroid cancer is extremely rare in this population.

Type 1 diabetes mellitus occurs in over 1% of young persons with Down syndrome. No studies have examined the prevalence of type 2 diabetes mellitus in adults with Down syndrome. However, in view of the high prevalence of obesity, it is generally believed that there is a higher prevalence. Similarly, the metabolic syndrome (insulin resistance, hypertension, hypertriglyceridaemia and hyperuricaemia) is not rare in this group of patients. Uric acid levels are increased in the serum of most patients with Down syndrome.

Male hypogonadism occurs fairly commonly in males in their 40s with Down syndrome. It is predominantly of the secondary hypogonadism type, with low lueinizing hormone and also low testosterone and bioavailable testosterone. Treatment with testosterone can stabilize mood and prevent loss of muscle and bone. Males with trisomy 21 have reduced fertility. Females have a premature menopause of 47.1 years compared with 51 years for the woman without developmental disabilities. At present, based on the findings of the Women's Health Initiative, we are not utilizing estrogen replacement in postmenopausal women with Down syndrome.

Persons with Down syndrome have lower peak bone mass and, therefore, are more likely to develop osteopenia and osteoporosis.[7] This is aggravated by the high use of anticonvulsant medicines in this age-group. Bone mineral density should be measured in all patients with Down syndrome at the age of 50 years. Calcium and vitamin D administration should be initiated at age 40 years for women. All Down syndrome patients should receive 1000 IU of vitamin D daily. The use of hip pads should be considered in Down patients who have frequent falls.

Otolaryngolical conditions

Hearing loss occurs in up to two-thirds of persons with Down syndrome.[8] This can worsen with ageing. In addition, many middle-aged patients have further hearing deterioration because of common impaction. Hearing loss can aggravate speech problems and make the person appear more cognitively impaired than they are or to appear unresponsive to simple requests.

As many as half of the adults with Down syndrome can have sleep apnoea.[9] This is related, in part, to mid-facial hypoplasia and also to their short neck and obesity. While in patients it is of the obstructive type, central sleep apnoea can also occur. Sleep apnoea presents with daytime fatigue and somnolence and night-time snoring with apnoeic periods. Behavioural changes such as irritability or withdrawal can result from sleep apnoea. Diagnosis is made with a sleep study. Some patients will tolerate continuous positive airways pressure, but this is often rejected.

Surgical approaches can help, but the failure rate is relatively high.

Joint problems

Children with Down syndrome can develop a condition similar to juvenile rheumatoid arthritis, associated with subluxation of joints. The diagnosis is often delayed. Similarly, arthritis is often only diagnosed late in adults with Down syndrome.

Atlantoaxial instability occurs in Down syndrome where there is excessive movement of the first cervical vertebra (atlas) on the second one (axis).[10] The diagnosis is made when there is increased space between the posterior segment of the anterior arch of C1 and the anterior segment of the odontoid process. This occurs in 15% of patients with Down syndrome. About 1–2% will have subluxation with neurological signs and symptoms consistent with spinal cord compression (Table 84.2). When this occurs, it is a neurosurgical emergency. However, outcomes of surgery are often poor.

Severe cervical and lumbar-sacral osteoarthritis are fairly common. This is associated with pain, gait disturbance, sometimes hand clumsiness, difficulty in moving and associated behavioural disturbances.

Coeliac disease

Coeliac disease is a malabsorption syndrome that occurs in response to the ingestion of gluten products. It occurs in as many as 7% of Down syndrome patients.[11] It is screened

Table 84.2 Presentation of spinal cord compression in persons with Down syndrome who have atlantoaxial subluxation.

Neck pain
Gait disturbance
Clumsiness of hands
Torticollis
Incontinence
Hyperreflexia
Clonus
Quadriplegia/paresis
Positive Hoffman's and Babinski reflexes

for at 24 months of age. Symptoms include diarrhoea and weight loss. Diagnosis is made by serum antibodies and intestinal biopsy. Coeliac disease can present for the first time later in life and should be considered as the diagnosis in any Down syndrome patients with unexplained weight loss or diarrhoea.

Dermatological conditions

Vitiligo and alopecia are seen in adults with Down syndrome. Dry skin is extremely common and often associated with pruritus. Fungal infections are common and often difficult to eradicate. Seborrheic and atopic dermatitis also occur frequently. A fissured or geographic tongue is present in almost one-third of patients with Down syndrome.

Cardiovascular disorders

Congenital heart disease occurs in about half of the children born with Down syndrome.[12] Some of these, such as isolated secundum atrial septal defects, may have been missed in childhood and present for the first time in adults. Mitral valve prolapse occurs in about half of patients and aortic regurgitation in 17%. In the presence of signs or symptoms, an echocardiogram should be carried out. Alterations in cardiac conduction are not rare and should be considered in those with new onset falls with or without syncope. In those with valvular defects, antibiotic prophylaxis needs to be given before dental care or other instrumentation.

The coronary artery disease death rate is low, possibly because of increased activity of the cystathionine-β-synthase gene, which accelerates the conversion of homocysteine to cysteine, thus reducing homocysteine levels.[13] Persons with Down syndrome are less likely to have hypertension due to a reduction in the expression of the type 1 angiotensin receptor gene.

Dental problems

Gingivitis and periodontal disease are common and lead to tooth loss. Orthodontic problems are common and may not have been able to be corrected during childhood. Bruxism is not rare.

Cancer

In children, both acute lymphoblastic and myeloid leukaemia occur with increased frequency.[14] Whereas most cancers occur with a decreased frequency in persons with Down syndrome,[15] testicular cancers appear to be more common.

Foot problems

These include hallux valgus, hammer toe deformities, plantar fasciitis and early onset of foot arthritis. All of these can result in unstable gait and increased falls. Feet should be examined regularly and the services of a podiatrist utilized when necessary.

Gynaecological problems

Where possible, as in any other adult, Papanicolaou smear and pelvic examination should be carried out. This is often extremely difficult and may need to be deferred. Similarly, mammography should be carried out when feasible. Breast examinations should be done yearly. Early age at menopause is associated with an increase in dementia and earlier mortality in Down patients.[16]

Eye disorders

Refractive errors are present in 40% of adults. Cataracts occur in 3% of patients and keratoconus is present in 15% of patients.

Alzheimer's disease

Alzheimer's disease occurs commonly in Down syndrome patients, starting at the age of 30 years (Table 84.3).[17] Over three-quarters of patients, by the time they reach 70 years of age, may have some symptoms of Alzheimer's disease, although a fairly recent study has suggested that this may be an overestimate.[18] While much of the blame for this has been placed on the trisomy of amyloid precursor protein, recent evidence has suggested that trisomy of DYRK1A leads to hyperphosphorylation of tau protein.[19] The diagnosis of Alzheimer's disease is very difficult to make in persons with Down syndrome. Common early changes are memory loss, loss of conversational skills, withdrawal and functional decline. Decline in executive function is a common early sign of Alzheimer's disease.[20] The diagnosis requires the careful exclusion of other causes of dementia, such as drugs, depression, hypothyroidism, vitamin B_{12} deficiency, visual and auditory problems, space-occupying lesions, for

Table 84.3 Approximate prevalence of Alzheimer's disease in persons with Down syndrome.

Age (years)	Alzheimer's disease (%)
41–50	8.9
51–54	17.7
55–59	32.1
≥60	25.6

example, bilatent subdural haematomas following a fall, or infections. Late presentations associated with Alzheimer's disease include seizures, apathy, focal neurological signs and personality changes.

Epilepsy

Seizures occur in about 8%, with half occurring with the first year of life and half in the third decade or later.[21] We are particularly impressed with the ease of use of keppra, compared with dilantin, in these patients.

Behaviour disorders

Depression occurs commonly. Loss of a parent or caregiver can precipitate depression, as can change in a familiar environment. Problems within the social environment of a group house can also precipitate depression. Most of those who are depressed are treated with selective serotonin reuptake inhibitors. These agents can cause hyponatraemia, leading to delirium.

Aggressive behaviour occurs in about 6% of adults with Down syndrome. Management is difficult. Valproic acid, trazadone, lorazepam and antipsychotics have all been tried but with limited success. Oversedation is often a complication of these treatments.

Delusions of things being stolen from them are common, with a prevalence of 14%. Visual hallucinations tend to be present in the late states of Down syndrome with Alzheimer's disease.[22]

Conclusion

Middle-aged persons with Down syndrome often present with all the special needs of frail older adults. For this reason, geriatricians are the ideal physicians for this group. In addition, some of the special needs of this population make it preferable for them to utilize a physician who cares for a number of patients with Down syndrome. The physician needs to work closely with the interdisciplinary team that provides day-to-day care for these individuals.

Key points

- Down syndrome (trisomy 21) is associated with early onset of frailty and Alzheimer's disease.
- Sleep apnoea occurs commonly in Down syndrome.
- Hypothyroidism, diabetes mellitus, osteoporosis and coeliac disease occur more commonly in Down syndrome patients.
- Subluxation of the cervical spine can lead to spinal cord damage in Down syndrome and is a neurosurgical emergency.

References

1. Yang Q, Rasmussen SA and Friedman JM. Mortality associated with Down's syndrome in the USA from 1983 to 1997: a population-based study. *Lancet* 2002;**359**:1019–25.
2. Bittles AH, Bower C, Hussain R *et al.* The four ages of Down's syndrome. *Eur J Public Health* 2007;**17**:221–5.
3. Edgin JO, Pennington BR and Mervis CB. Neuropsychological components of intellectual disability: the contributions of immediate, working and associative memory. *J Intellect Disabil Res* 2010;**54**:406–17.
4. Andriolo RB, El Dib RP, Ramos L *et al.* Aerobic exercise training programmes for improving physical and psychosocial health in adults with Down syndrome. *Cochrane Database Syst Rev* 2010;(5):CD005176.
5. Smith DS. Health care management of adults with Down syndrome. *Am Fam Physician* 2001;**64**:1031–8.
6. Karlsson B, Gustafsson J, Hedov G *et al.* Thyroid dysfunction in Downs syndrome – relation to age and thyroid autoimmunity. *Arch Dis Child* 1998;**49**:242–5.
7. Schrager S. Epidemiology of osteoporosis in women with cognitive impairment. *Ment Retard* 2006;**44**:203–11.
8. Venail F, Gardiner Q and Mondain M. ENT and speech disorders in children with Down's syndrome: an overview of pathophysiology, clinical features, treatments and current management. *Clin Pediatr* 2004;**43**:783–91.
9. Dahlqvist A, Rask E, Rosenqvist CJ *et al.* Sleep apnea and Down's syndrome. *Acta Otolaryngol* 2003;**123**:1094–7.
10. Ferguson RL, Putney ME and Allen BL Jr. Comparison of neurologic deficits with atlanto-dens intervals in patients with Down syndrome. *J Spinal Disord* 1997;**10**:246–52.
11. Carnicer J, Farre C, Varea V *et al.* Prevalence of celiac disease in Down's syndrome. *Eur J Gastroenterol Hepatol* 2001;**13**:263–7.
12. Howells G. Down's syndrome and the general practitioner. *J R Coll Gen Pract* 1989;**39**:470–5.
13. Vis JC, Duffels MGJ, Winter MM *et al.* Down syndrome: a cardiovascular perspective. *J Intellect Disabil Res* 2009;**53**:419–25.
14. Roizen NJ and Patterson D. Down's syndrome. *Lancet* 2003;**361**:1281–9.
15. Roberge D, Souhami L and Laplante M. Testicular seminoma and Down's syndrome. *Can J Urol* 2001;**8**:1203–6.

16. Coppus AM, Evenhuis HM, Verberne GJ *et al.* Early age at menopause is associated with increased risk of dementia and mortality in women with Down's syndrome. *J Alzheimers Dis* 2010;**19**:545–50.
17. Lott IT and Head E. Down syndrome and Alzheimer's disease: a link between development and aging. *Ment Retard Dev Disabil Res Rev* 2001;**7**:172–8.
18. Coppus AM, Evenhuis HM, Verberne GJ *et al.* Dementia and mortality in persons with Down's syndrome. *J Intellect Disabil Res* 2006;**50**:768–77.
19. Wiseman FK, Alford KA, Tybulewicz VLJ *et al.* Down syndrome – recent progress and future prospects. *Hum Mol Genet* 2009;**18**:R75–83.
20. Adams D and Oliver C. The relationship between acquired impairments of executive function and behavior change in adults with Down syndrome. *J Intellect Disabil Res* 2010; **54**:393–405.
21. Stafstrom CE. Epilepsy in Down syndrome: clinical aspects and possible mechanisms. *Am J Ment Retard* 1993;**98**(Suppl 1):12–26.
22. Urv TK, Zigman WB and Silverman W. Psychiatric symptoms in adults with Down syndrome and Alzheimer's disease. *Am J Intellect Dev Disabil* 2010;**115**:265–76.

SECTION 8

Special Senses

CHAPTER 85

Disorders of the eye

Nina Tumosa

Saint Louis Veterans' Affairs Medical Center and Saint Louis University School of Medicine, St Louis, MO, USA

Introduction

The positive association between visual impairment and mortality has been well documented in several longitudinal eye studies[1–7] although the mechanisms for this association are not as well understood.[8,9] Because visual impairment can predict mortality, a better understanding of the common types of visual impairment and their treatments and risk factors should assist practitioners in providing life prolonging medical care.

Five major disorders cause the greatest visual disability: cataracts, diabetic retinopathy, refractive error, macular degeneration and glaucoma. Increasing age is a major risk factor for all five of these disorders. The overall prevalence of refractive error resulting from these five causes of visual impairment is remarkably consistent around the world. Figure 85.1 shows average values for the prevalence of these disorders in people aged 75 and over in the American population gleaned from multiple sources of reviewed literature[10–13] (http://one.aao.org/CE/PracticeGuidelines/PPP.aspx). These numbers were determined from epidemiological studies done in the 1980s. It is reasonable to expect that these percentages may have decreased somewhat with improved treatment options, especially for diabetes mellitus. However, with the increase in persons now over age 75, the number of persons suffering from these visual impairments is still rising.

Visual impairment is often described as a person's most feared disability, and with good reason. In older persons, visual impairment is particularly devastating because it has been associated with dramatic reduction in QOL.[14] As vision declines, people are forced to curtail driving. Those who can no longer see clearly report having a reduction in mobility, and having difficulty walking and leaving their homes to participate in social and religious activities. They report a loss of ability to perform activities of daily living (ADL) such as dressing, shopping and getting in and out of bed safely. Poor vision interferes with the ability to take medications properly. It is also a leading risk factor for falls and fractures which, in turn, are risk factors for placement in both non-institutional and institutional extended care and for loss of independence. In addition, other conditions appear to be strongly comorbid with low vision. These include dementia, depression and delirium and other sensory losses, such as hearing and balance deficits. Thus, vision impairment has profound effects on the older person and it is incumbent upon healthcare providers to identify people at risk for leading causes of visual impairment, and to initiate treatments in a timely manner.

Definitions, treatments, and risk factors

Refractive errors

Refractive error can be described as visual acuity with best lens prescription worse than 20/40. It is the most frequent eye problem and is usually corrected with prescription eyewear. The percentage of people whose visual acuity cannot be improved beyond 20/40 increases dramatically with age: 0.8% for those between 43 and 54 years old, 0.9% for those between 55 and 64, 5% for those between 65 and 74, and 21.1% for those 75 and older. This increasing degree of uncorrected refractive error is due to a number of variables. For example, there is normally an increase in the against-the-rule astigmatism with age and it is often exacerbated during surgery that breaches the conjunctiva such as cataract and glaucoma[15] surgeries. The long-term effects of refractive surgeries such as laser-assisted *in situ* keratomileusis (LASIK) and epi-LASEK that many people are now undergoing for the correction of myopia, hyperopia and presbyopia is being studied.[16] Differences in sample sizes, age and sex distributions, length of follow-up and preoperative spherical equivalents have made it difficult to compare results. More follow-up studies are still needed to distinguish the effect of ethnicity on postoperative visual

Principles and Practice of Geriatric Medicine, Fifth Edition. Edited by Alan J. Sinclair, John E. Morley and Bruno Vellas.

Incidence rate of eye disorders in persons age 75 and older

- Cataracts (52%)
- Age-related macular degeneration (30%)
- Refractive error (21%)
- Glaucoma (3%)
- Diabetic retinopathy (1%)

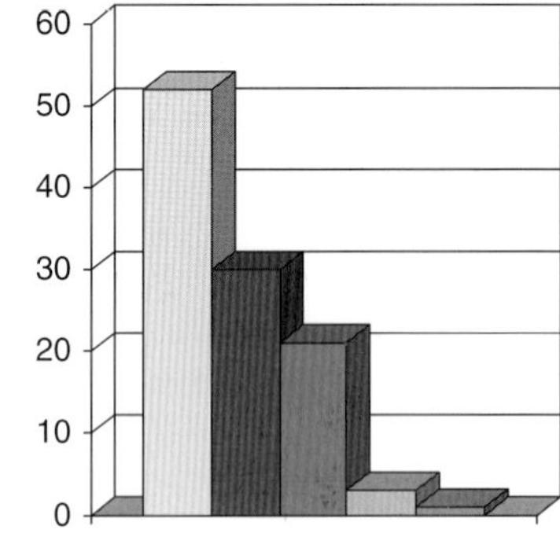

Figure 85.1 Over 50% of Americans aged 75 and older will suffer from visual impairment due to cataracts, 30% will lose central vision from age-related macular degeneration, 21% will have uncorrected refractive errors, 3% will report visual field loss due to optic nerve damage from glaucoma, and 1% will suffer vision loss due to diabetic retinopathy

Table 85.1 Medical risk factors for refractive errors.

- Dry eye
- Cataracts
- Increased glare
- Yellowing of lenses
- Reduction in dark adaptation
- Decreased pupil size (miosis)
- Decreased contrast sensitivity
- Normal hyperopic shift with age
- Increasing against-the-rule astigmatism with age

Table 85.2 Social risk factors for refractive errors.

- Cost of care
- Lack of access to care
- Living in institutional extended care settings
- Lower expectations of patients and providers with age
- Lack of ability to access transportation to receive care

outcomes and standards for reporting surgical outcomes must be set in order to be able to compare efficacy, stability and safety of the different procedures.

The most common refractive error is myopia, or nearsightedness. With this disorder a person has difficulty seeing distant objects clearly. Severe myopia carries with it a large risk of blindness because it is associated with ocular comorbidities such as retinal detachment, macular choroidal degeneration, premature cataract and glaucoma.[17] Genetic studies of myopia have identified several loci that are linked to myopia and a key environmental inverse determinant of myopia is total time spent outdoors.[18] Clearly there is great value in the next decade to performing research on assessing the role of early-age near work versus outdoor activity on genotypes for myopia. This research would provide valuable insight on how to reduce this worldwide epidemic of myopia and its associated high levels of blindness.

There is also a normal hyperopic shift in older adults that may be altered by cataract surgery.[19] Contrast sensitivity decreases with age, in part due to the increased prevalence of dry eye with age, and in part due to the smaller pupil size found in the older person. Dark adaptation also decreases with age and with diseases such as diabetic retinopathy and cancer. Finally, cataracts, yellow lenses and aberrations of the cornea, all of which increase with age, produce glare caused by excess light scattered within the eye. This glare can be debilitating. It can cause difficulty with driving and other tasks conducted in bright light. It can also cause headaches. As people who have been faithful contact lens wearers for decades enter their 70s and 80s, it will be interesting to determine whether the rate of corneal aberrations rises.

There are many risk factors for refractive errors in the older person. Many of the medical and social risk factors are listed in Tables 85.1 and 85.2. Most of these risk factors can be handled with annual dilated fundus eye exams and instructions to seek medical treatment at the first sign of worsening vision. For many persons, that translates into instructions to seek vision care when they notice that they are having more difficulty with their every-day activities due to vision changes.

Age-related macular degeneration

Age-related macular degeneration (AMD) is a disorder of the macula characterized by the presence of drusen, hypo- or hyper-pigmentation of the retinal pigment epithelium (RPE), local atrophy of the RPE and choriocapillaris, neovascularization of the macula, and a reduction or loss of central vision.[12] AMD is the leading cause of severe, irreversible vision impairment in developed countries. Ninety percent of the AMD cases are of the non-exudative (dry or atrophic) type. Ten percent are of the exudative (or wet) type. Non-exudative AMD is characterized by the presence of drusen and loss of RPE and photoreceptors. Sight in the central visual field is lost gradually. Exudative AMD is characterized by a much more rapid loss of central vision due to neovascularization of the choroid and its accompanying haemorrhages that lead to retinal and RPE detachments and scarring. Although non-exudative AMD is more prevalent, most of the people with severe vision loss have exudative AMD.

The National Eye Institute (2010) lists the risk factors for developing AMD as age over 60, obesity, Caucasian race, smoking, family history, being female[20] (although estrogen has not been implicated in increased AMD risk)[21] and exposure to sunlight.[22] Currently, there are no pharmaceutical treatments for AMD. However, patients with dry AMD should receive regular dilated fundus eye exams and should be encouraged to increase their consumption of antioxidants. They should be educated about how to use an Amsler grid to screen for the progression of dry AMD into wet AMD and encouraged to seek medical attention at the first sign of new symptoms. Dietary consumption of fresh fruits and vegetables is encouraged because they contain antioxidants such as Vitamin C, Vitamin E, carotenoids, selenium and zinc, which are thought to neutralize damage caused by free radicals. Those who have unilateral AMD should be encouraged to take supplements in order to reduce their chances of developing AMD in the other eye. Results from the National Eye Institute Age-related Eye Disease Study (AREDS) showed that supplements containing high levels of antioxidants and zinc significantly reduce the risk of advanced AMD and its associated vision loss.[23] (As an aside, it should be noted that the same nutrients had no significant effect on the development or progression of cataract.) If the patient requests it, advice on developing a diet to help maintain a healthy weight and increase consumption of antioxidants should be provided in written form.

Routine examinations for patients with wet AMD should include optical coherence tomography (OCT) in order to monitor changes in retinal thickness due to both the presence of drusen in the retinal pigment epithelium and blood caused by retinal bleeding. OCT allows the structural integrity of the retina to be followed during therapy. In an effort to preserve residual vision, retinal bleeding is currently controlled by laser photocoagulation but this is not a curative therapy.

There are several ongoing research studies on surgical treatments for wet AMD that is no longer responsive to diet and supplements. Wet, or neovascular, AMD is a complex disease. Several studies have looked at the role of angiogenic agents that probably contribute to choroidal neovascularization.[24–27] To date, no clear treatment guidelines have been developed for the anti-angiogenic therapies.

Although there are several environmental risk factors for AMD, the future of some treatments may indeed be rooted in the genome. To that end, researchers are looking at genotypic variation for AMD. Although AMD is a complex disease, about 40% of the genetic variance can be explained by variations in five common single-nucleotide polymorphisms (SNPs).[28] Other SNPs have been associated with risks for common treatments such as photodynamic therapy or bevacizumab treatment.[29] Recent advances in these inexpensive genetic technologies may allow medicine to produce personalized diagnosis and treatment plans for AMD.[30]

Finally, persons with advanced AMD may be classified as legally blind and often require assistance with ADLs even if the AMD is monocular because contrast sensitivity is affected, thereby reducing visual acuity in the unaffected eye. They are also at significant risk for depression. Vision can often be enhanced by the use of low vision aids such as magnifiers and bright lights. Motivated patients can be taught to read with the peripheral retina. Because functional status and QOL are related, every effort should be made to encourage patients to seek rehabilitation.

Risk factors for, and other factors associated with, AMD are listed in Tables 85.3 and 85.4.

Diabetic retinopathy

Diabetic retinopathy (DR) is a leading cause of blindness in the industrialized world in people between the ages of 25 and 74,[31] and the fourth leading cause of blindness in people of all ages in developing countries.[32] Annually, between 12 000 and 24 000 diabetic patients in the United States become legally blind as a result of complications of diabetic retinopathy.[33] Every diabetic patient is at risk for several changes to vision that occur as a result of uncontrolled systemic diabetes mellitus (DM) of long duration, including numerous ocular and periocular changes that characterize diabetic retinopathy. DR is a disorder of the retinal vasculature. Resulting changes are characterized by waxy exudates, micro-aneurysms, punctate haemorrhages and, less frequently, neovascularization, all of which lead to a decrease in visual acuity and, perhaps, to blindness. Indeed, the elderly diabetic patient is 1.5 times more likely to develop vision loss and blindness than is an age-matched non-diabetic person.[34]

DR can occur with both type 1 (insulin deficient) and type 2 (non-insulin dependent) diabetes mellitus. Despite

Table 85.3 Confirmed risk factors for AMD.

- Smoking
- Female sex
- Advanced age
- Caucasian race
- Low levels of antioxidants
- Exposure to sunlight in early adulthood

Table 85.4 Factors associated with AMD.

- High-fat diet
- Alcohol use
- Hormonal status
- Family history of AMD
- High levels of C-reactive protein
- High intake of saturated fats and cholesterol

the fact that type 1 diabetics develop the disease at an earlier age, a greater number of type 2 diabetics will develop DR because more than 90% of diabetics have type 2 diabetes. DR progresses from its mild, non-proliferative stage with increased vascular permeability, to severe, non-proliferative DR which is characterized by vascular closure, to proliferative DR with neovascularization in the retina and on the vitreous humour which tends to produce vitreal haemorrhages and resultant vision loss, retinal detachment and possibly, glaucoma. Vision loss can result in several ways: (1) central vision can be lost due to macular oedema or capillary loss; (2) neovascularization can lead to retinal detachment; (3) pre-retinal or vitreal haemorrhages can obstruct vision; (4) glaucoma can result in response to the damage caused by DR.

The retinal damage caused by DR cannot be cured. However, DR does respond favourably to early detection and treatment of diabetes and to case management of the disease.[35] Annual dilated fundus examinations are recommended for early detection and management of DR. Laser photocoagulation significantly reduces vision loss.[36] Finally, for those who have experienced vision loss, low-vision care and rehabilitation is recommended. These recommendations on how to minimize vision loss associated with DR are particularly significant in light of the research that shows that vision loss contributes significantly to poorer health, more disability and increased frequency of falls in diabetics[37] as well as restrictions in reading, mobility, work and leisure activities.[38]

Diabetics are at greater risk for comorbid conditions. The presence of diabetes mellitus increases the risk for the development of cataracts. In turn, the presence of cataracts complicates both the patient's and the provider's abilities to monitor vision changes due to DR. In addition, diabetics are at greater risks for complications during cataract surgery. Finally, comorbid conditions such as hypertension and hyperglycaemia can worsen DR and should be treated.[39] Risk factors of and other factors associated with diabetic retinopathy are listed in Tables 85.5 and 85.6.

Management and treatment of DR is multifold. It should include dietician-monitored diets that are individualized to the patient's diagnosis and treatment goals, taking into account eating habits and other lifestyle factors. A supervised exercise programme helps with glycaemic and blood pressure control which, in turn, delays both the onset and progression of DR. Currently, laser photocoagulation and vitrectomy remain the conventional management protocols for DR.[13] Many new studies on the treatment of DR have been initiated based on the observations that microvascular damage to patients with chronic hyperglycaemia is mediated by interrelated pathways involving aldose reductase, advanced glycation end products, protein kinase C (PKC) and vascular endothelial growth factor (VEGF). Many new pharmacological agents are currently being tested for their abilities to slow or reverse the progression of DR. However, the recent publication of results from a randomized, controlled study that compared the efficacy of photocoagulation versus intravitreal injection of triamcinolone acetonide indicates that although the triamcinolone acetonide appears to reduce the risk of progression of DR, it also causes adverse events such as cataract formation and glaucoma.[40] Preliminary data on the role of human erythropoietin (EPO), a primary regulator of erythropoiesis, in the pathophysiology of DR[41] indicates that researchers are continuing to search for pharmaceutical solutions to the progression of DR.

Table 85.5 Risk factors for diabetic retinopathy.

- Duration of diabetes
- Late diagnosis of diabetes
- No perception of vision problems
- Lack of frequent evaluation of vision
- Uncontrolled or poorly controlled blood sugar level (HbA1c)
- Presence of other systemic diseases such as hypertension and hyperglycaemia

Table 85.6 Factors associated with diabetic retinopathy.

- Age
- Race
- Obesity
- Smoking
- Clotting factors
- Renal disease
- Use of angiotensin-converting enzyme inhibitors

Glaucoma

Glaucoma is a general term that refers to a number of disorders of the optic nerve that are often accompanied by increased intra-ocular pressure (IOP) (ocular hypertension) and that results in a gradual and progressive visual field loss when the optic nerve is damaged. Glaucoma is the second leading cause of legal blindness in the United States and the leading cause of legal blindness in African-Americans.[42] The destruction of the optic nerve that occurs as glaucoma progresses causes gradual loss of peripheral vision. As the disease progresses, the field of vision gradually narrows and blindness can result. Glaucoma has no early symptoms so about half of the people who are affected are unaware they have the disease. By the time people experience problems with their vision, they usually have a significant amount of optic nerve damage.

Early detection of glaucoma is critical. If glaucoma can be controlled, serious vision loss can be prevented. Comprehensive dilated eye examinations are recommended at least once every two years for African-Americans over age 40 and all people over age 60. Primary open-angle glaucoma (POAG) is the most common form of glaucoma and one of the nation's leading causes of vision loss. POAG has a characteristic loss of retinal ganglion cells and atrophy of the optic nerve that occurs in the presence of an open and normal looking angle. The visual field loss may be monocular but if it is binocular, it may well be asymmetric[13] (http://www.aao.org/aao/CE/PracticeGuidelines/PPP.aspx).

Currently, there are no primary prevention strategies for glaucoma. Therefore, it is important to optimize early detection by understanding the risk factors for glaucoma.[42,43] These factors are listed in Table 85.7. The only modifiable risk factor is elevated baseline IOP. Perhaps in the next edition of this book more research will have been done on the effects of modifiable socioeconomic characteristics such as nutrition, exercise, smoking, sleep apnoea and body mass index (BMI).

Treatment to control IOP is helpful in reducing the visual field losses associated with glaucoma, regardless of whether the patient has elevated or normal (low-tension) glaucoma.[14] Drug therapy, in the form of eye drops, is normally initiated to reduce the production and/or increase drainage of aqueous humour. These drops may be beta-blockers, alpha-agonists, carbonic anhydrase inhibitors (CAIs), prostaglandin-like compounds, cholinergic agents, or epinephrine compounds. If these eye drops fail, CAI pills may be prescribed. This large choice of treatment agents hints at the variability found in the types of glaucoma. Research studies are just beginning to show us the genetic variability of glaucoma.[44–46] The efficacy of a drug has been shown to be affected by the genetic make-up of the recipient.[47,48] This concept that generic variation contributes to a person's response to therapy is both a boon and a bane. Personalized medicine is fast becoming the Holy Grail of effective medicine but the cost of that success will include the need for practitioners to become savvy about health legislation, discrimination, employment issues, insurance regulations and ethics, as well as medicine.[49] Surgery is recommended once a patient becomes intolerant of the drugs, is not compliant with the drug schedule, or is unresponsive to the drug. Trabeculoplasty is a form of laser surgery that opens clogged trabecular meshwork, thereby allowing aqueous humour to drain out of the anterior chamber more rapidly.

Table 85.7 Risk factors for glaucoma.

- Age greater than 60
- Central corneal thickness
- Elevated intraocular pressure
- African descent over age of 40
- Family history (parent or sibling)

Trabeculoplasty does not always give a permanent solution so eye drops are often continued or reinstated over time. When both the eye drops and the trabeculoplasty are no longer effective, a filtering procedure called trabeculectomy is done. This procedure cauterizes a part of the trabecular meshwork. For patients with secondary glaucoma or for children with glaucoma drainage implants are used to drain aqueous humour.

The efficacy of surgical interventions, the number of times each of the surgeries needs to be repeated, and the order in which the surgery types are offered in combination, differ for black and white patients.[50] Further study will undoubtedly fine-tune future surgical interventions.

Before determining whether the disease will be treated with eyedrops or surgery, an effort must be made to determine the patient's health status and life expectancy, how difficult daily treatment of eyedrops will be, how expensive the drug costs are, and what the possible side effects will be.

The use of marijuana as a complementary therapy for POAG glaucoma is not recommended. NEI studies have demonstrated that some derivatives of marijuana do result in lowering IOP for 3 to 4 hours when administered orally, intravenously, or by smoking. However, potentially serious side effects included increased heart rate, a decrease in blood pressure, impaired memory of recent events and impaired motor coordination.

Efforts to better understand the pathogenesis of glaucoma have led to attempts to locate gene anomalies associated with glaucoma. Defects in the *myocilin* gene (MYOC) have been associated with POAG and defects in PITX2, FOXC1 and CYP1B 1 are associated with anterior segment development.[51] The risk factors for and other factors associated with glaucoma are summarized in Tables 85.7 and 85.8.

Cataracts

Cataracts are a leading cause of blindness worldwide.[11] They are opacities of the lens or the lens capsule. Cataracts are *named* by the location of the opacity; the opacity may occur in the nucleus (nuclear cataract), in the lens cortex (cortical cataract), or in the lens periphery (coronary

Table 85.8 Other factors associated with glaucoma.

- Late onset menarche
- Migraine headaches
- Peripheral vasospasm
- Low diastolic perfusion pressure
- Presence of AMD, hypertension or diabetes
- High ratio of n-3 to n-6 polyunsaturated fat
- Suspicious optic nerve appearance (cup-to-disc ratio greater than 0.5)

cataract), or posterior (posterior subcapsular, posterior cortical and posterior polar cataracts).

Cataracts are caused by the hardening of the lens that occurs as a part of normal ageing. They also may occur as a result of blunt trauma, but the history of this type of cataract is a rapid onset and a rapid rate of progression. Normal cataracts progress slowly and may be present for years before they are noticed.

Cataracts are not normally life-threatening. No effective medical treatment for cataract exists, but a diet rich in lutein and zeaxanthin, carotene and Vitamin A, and long-term Vitamin C supplementation are thought to slow the progression of cataracts.

Once the patient reports a decreased QOL or impaired function, elective surgery can correct the visual impairment. For patients with glaucoma, AMD, or diabetes, where visualization of the fundus is necessary for continuing management and treatment, surgery may be indicated before the patient reports a decline in functional status.[12,13,52]

When vision becomes cloudy enough to bother the patient, surgery can remove the clouded lens and replace it with an IOL implant. Surgery is normally an outpatient procedure using local anaesthetic. Phacoemulsification (ultrasonic cataract removal) is used to emulsify the lens for easy removal (although promising research on the use of lasers to break up the lens is ongoing).[53] An IOL is then implanted within the empty lens capsule to serve as the new lens. Normally the incision is self-sealing. The surgical procedure is so safe that it has changed little in the past 10 years although lens implants of differing powers can reduce dependence upon glasses for either reading or distance work.

Many risk factors have been associated with cataracts although the studies have been largely observational. General risk factors for cataracts are listed in Table 85.9 and specific risk factors for cortical, nuclear and posterior subcapsular cataracts are listed in Tables 85.10–85.12.

Table 85.9 General risk factors for all cataracts.

- Age
- Diabetes
- Cost of treatment
- Low socioeconomic status
- Diet low in lutein and zeaxanthin
- Lack of education about cataracts

Table 85.10 Risk factors specific for cortical cataracts.

- Iris colour
- Hypertension
- Hyperglycaemia
- Family history
- Abdominal obesity
- Low body mass index
- Exposure to UV-B radiation

Table 85.11 Risk factors specific for nuclear cataracts.

- Smoking
- Iris colour
- Family history
- Low education level
- Non-professional occupation
- Occupational sun exposure in third decade of life

Table 85.12 Risk factors specific for posterior subcapsular cataracts.

- Smoking
- Hyperglycaemia
- Inhaled corticosteroid use
- Systemic corticosteroid use
- Alcohol consumption
- Exposure to UV-B radiation

Summary

Each type of eye disorder discussed above has unique risk factors, ranging from diet to environment. Increased age is associated with all of the eye disorders, that is, the frequency of the disorder in the population increases with age. In addition, some of the risk factors are shared by two of the eye disorders. Excessive exposure to sunlight is a risk factor for both cataracts and macular degeneration. Additionally, a particular symptom may have more than one cause. For example, glare may be caused by corneal aberrations or by the development of cataracts. A decrease in contrast sensitivity may be the result of decreased illumination to the retina because of a decreased pupil size, but it may also be caused by AMD, glaucoma, or diabetic retinopathy. A decrease in dark adaptation may be caused by a miotic pupil or it may also be caused by cataracts. Thus, treatment of a specific visual deficit may require more than one approach because due consideration must be given to how different disorders contribute to the resulting morbidity.

In addition to having shared risk factors, there is some degree of comorbidity between the eye disorders. Either cataracts or glaucoma may often co-occur with DR, and AMD often co-occurs with glaucoma. Interactions between diseases may complicate the treatments needed to prevent visual impairment and blindness. Finally, although there is little research about how comorbid eye disorders affect an already decreased level of function and QOL, the QOL of patients is dependent upon better understanding of the interactions between diseases and between their treatments.

For people who become blind from an eye disorder, there is some hope. Research on artificial vision techniques is ongoing. Artificial vision through the use of cortical implants is a promise of the future,[54] although it is designed to promote mobility, not reading. These cortical implants are contraindicated for people with severe chronic infections and for those blinded by stroke or cortical trauma. However, cortical models for patients without viable optic nerves (e.g. glaucoma patients) and retinal prostheses for those without viable photoreceptors (e.g. AMD patients) are under development. Research such as this should considerably brighten the future of visually impaired people.

Key points

- Increasing age is a risk factor for loss of vision due to the following eye disorders: cataract, age-related macular degeneration, refractive error, glaucoma and diabetic retinopathy.
- Poor vision due to refractive error and cataracts is often reversible.
- Loss of vision due to diabetic retinopathy, glaucoma and age-related macular degeneration is not recoverable.
- Vision impairment caused by these eye disorders has a negative impact on functional status, mobility, independence and cognitive status of elders.
- Education and visual rehabilitation play important roles in improving the quality of life of persons with visual impairments.

References

1. Clemons TE, Kurinji N, Sperduto RD. AREDS Research Group. Associations of mortality with ocular disorders and an intervention of high-dose antioxidants and zinc in the Age-Related Eye Disease Study. *Arch Ophthalmol* 2004;**122**:716–26.
2. Cugati S, Cumming RG, Smith W *et al.* Visual impairment, age-related macular degeneration, cataract, and long-term mortality: the Blue Mountains Eye Study. *Arch Ophthalmol* 2007;**125**:917–24.
3. Freeman EE, Egleston BL, Wet SK *et al.* Visual acuity change and mortality in older adults. *Invest Ophthalmol Vis Sci* 2005;**46**:4040–5.
4. Klein R, Klein BE. Moss SE. Age-related eye disease and survival: the Beaver Dam Eye Study. *Arch Ophthalmol* 1995;**113**:333–9.
5. Knudston MD, Klein BE, Klein R. Age-related eye disease, visual impairment, and survival: the Beaver Dam Eye Study. *Arch Ophthalmol* 2006;**124**:243–9.
6. McCarthy CA, Nanjan MB, Taylor HR. Vision impairment predicts five year mortality. *Arch Ophthalmol* 1995;**85**:322–6.
7. Wang JJ, Mitchell P, Simpson JM, Cumming RG, Smith W. Visual impairment, age-related cataract, and mortality. *Arch Ophthalmol* 2001;**119**:1186–90.
8. Christ SL, Lee DJ, Lam B *et al.* Assessment of the effect of visual impairment on mortality through multiple health pathways: structural equation modeling. *Invest Ophthalmol Vis Sci* 2008;**49**:3318–23.
9. Karpa MJ, Mitchell P, Beath K *et al.* Direct and indirect effects of visual impairment on mortality risk in older persons. *Arch Ophthalmol* 2009;**127**:1347–53.
10. AAO PPP (American Academy of Ophthalmology Preferred Practice Patterns). *Primary Open Angle Glaucoma*, 2005, http://one.aao.org/CE/PracticeGuidelines/PPP.aspx (accessed November 23, 2009).
11. AAO PPP (American Academy of Ophthalmology Preferred Practice Patterns). *Cataract in the Adult Eye*, 2006, http://one.aao.org/CE/PracticeGuidelines/PPP.aspx (last accessed 22 November 2011).
12. AAO PPP (American Academy of Ophthalmology Preferred Practice Patterns). *Age-related Macular Degeneration*, 2008, http://one.aao. org/CE/PracticeGuidelines/PPP.aspx (last accessed 22 November 2011.
13. AAO PPP (American Academy of Ophthalmology Preferred Practice Patterns). *Diabetic Retinopathy* 2008, http://one.aao.org/CE/PracticeGuidelines/PPP.aspx (last accessed 22 November 2011).
14. Lee AG, Coleman AL. Geriatric ophthalmology. In: DH Solomon, J LoCicero 3rd and RA Rosenthal (eds) *New Frontiers in Geriatric Research: An Agenda for Surgical and Related Medical Specialties*, American Geriatrics Society, New York, 2004, pp. 177–202.
15. Egrilmez S, Ates H, Nalcaci S, Andac K, Yagci A. Surgically induced corneal refractive change following glaucoma surgery: nonpenetrating trabecular surgeries versus trabeculectomy. *J Cataract Refract Surg* 2004;**30**:1232–39.
16. Ang EK, Couper T, Dirani M *et al.* Outcomes of laser refractive surgery for myopia. *J Cataract Refract Surg* 2009;**35**:921–33.
17. Kempen J, Mitchell P, Lee K *et al.* The prevalence of refractive error among adults in the United States, western Europe and Australia. *Arch Ophthalmol* 2004;**122**:495–505.
18. Hornbeak DM, Young TL. Myopia genetics: a review of current research and emerging trends. *Curr Opin Ophthalmol* 2009;**20**:356–62.
19. Guzowski M, Wang JJ, Rochtchina E *et al.* Five-year refractive changes in an older population: the Blue Mountains Eye Study. *Ophthalmology* 2003;**110**:1364–70.
20. National Eye Institute Facts about Age-related Macular Degeneration, 2010, http://www.nei.nih.gov/health/maculardegen/armd_facts.asp (last accessed 22 November 2011).
21. Abramov Y, Borik S, Yahalom C *et al.* The effect of hormone therapy on the risk for age-related maculopathy in postmenopausal women. *Menopause* 2004;**11**:62–8.
22. Tomany SC, Cruickshanks KJ, Klein R, Klein BE, Knudtson MD. Sunlight and the 10-year incidence of age-related

maculopathy: the Beaver Dam Eye Study. *Arch Ophthalmol* 2004;**122**:750–7.

23. Higginbotham EJ, Gordon MO, Beiser JA *et al*. for the Ocular Hypertension Treatment Study Group. The Ocular Hypertension Treatment Study. Topical medication delays or prevents primary open-angle glaucoma in African American individuals. *Arch Ophthalmol* 2004;**122**:813–20.
24. Bressler NM. Antiangiogenic approaches to age-related macular degeneration today. *Ophthalmology* 2009;**116**: S15–S23.
25. Do DV. Antiangiogenic approaches to age-related macular degeneration in the future. *Ophthalmology* 2009;**116**: S24–S26.
26. Lai TY, Liu DT, Chan KP *et al*. Visual outcomes and growth factor changes if two dosages of intravitreal bevacizumab for neovascular age-related macular degeneration. *Retina* 2009;**29**:1218–26.
27. Mohan KC, Shukla D, Namperumalsamy P, Kim R. Management of age-related macular degeneration. *J Indian Med Assoc* 2003;**101**:471–6.
28. Sobrin L, Maller JB, Neale BM *et al*. Genetic profile for five common variants associated with age-related macular degeneration in densely affected families: a novel analytic approach. *Eur J Hum Genet* 2010;**148**:869–74. [Epub 2009 Oct 1.doi:10.1038/ejhg.2009.15.]
29. Andreoli MT, Morrison MA, Kim BJ *et al*. Comprehensive analysis of complement Factor H and *LOC387715/ARMS2/HTRA1* variants with respect to phenotype in advanced age-related macular degeneration. *Am J Ophthalmol* 2009;**148**: 869–74.
30. Baird PN, Hageman GS, Guymer RH. New era for personalized medicine: the diagnosis and management of age-related macular degeneration. *Clin Experiment Ophthalmol* 2009; **37**:814–21.
31. National Institute of Health (NIH), 2010, www.nei.nih.gov/eyedata (last accessed 22 November 2011).
32. World Health Organization (WHO), http://www.who.int/mediacentre/factsheets/fs282/en/ (last accessed 22 November 2011).
33. Wild S, Roglic G, Green A *et al*. Global prevalence of diabetes: Estimates for the year 2000 and projections for 2030. *Diabetes Care* 2004;**27**:1047–53.
34. Sinclair AJ, Bayer AJ, Girling AJ, Woodhouse KW. Older adults, diabetes mellitus and visual acuity: a community-based case-control study. *Age Ageing* 2000;**29**:335–9.
35. Norris SL, Nichols PJ, Caspersen CJ *et al*. Task Force on Community Preventive Services. The effectiveness of disease and case management for people with diabetes. *Am J Prev Med* 2002;**22**(Suppl 1):15–38.
36. ETDRS (Early Treatment Diabetic Retinopathy Study Research Group). Early photocoagulation for diabetic retinopathy. ETDRS Report Number 9. *Ophthalmology* 1991; **98**:766–85.
37. Miller DK, Lui LY, Perry HM 3rd *et al*. Reported and measured physical functioning in older inner-city diabetic African Americans. *J Geront A Bio Sci Med Sci* 1999;**54**: M230–39.
38. Lamoureux EL, Hassell JB, Keeffe JE. The impact of diabetic retinopathy on participation in daily living. *Arch Ophthalmol* 2004;**122**:84–8.
39. Fong DS, Aiello L, Gardner TW *et al*. Diabetic retinopathy. *Diabetes Care* 2003;**26**: S99–S102.
40. Bressler NM, Edwards AR, Beck RW *et al*. Exploratory analysis of diabetic retinopathy progression through 3 years of a randomized clinical trial that compares intravitreal triamcinolone acetonide with focal/grid photocoagulation. *Arch Ophthalmol* 2009;**127**:1566–71.
41. Shah SS, Tsang SH, Mahajan VB. Erythropoetin receptor expression in the human diabetic retina. *BMC Res Notes* 2009;**2**:234–40.
42. Coleman AL, Miglior S. Risk factors for glaucoma onset and progression. *Surv Ophthalmol* 2008;**53**(Suppl 1): S3–S10.
43. Coleman AL, Kodjebacheva G. Risk factors for glaucoma needing more attention. *Open Ophthalmol J* 2009;**3**:38–42.
44. Baird PN, Foote SJ, Mackay DA *et al*. Evidence for a novel glaucoma locus on chromosome 3p21-22. *Hum Genet* 2005; **117**:249–57.
45. Craig JE, Baird PN, Healet DL *et al*. Evidence for genetic heterogeneity within eight glaucoma families, with the *GLC1A* Gln368STOP mutation being an important phenotypic modifier. *Ophthalmology* 2001;**108**:1607–20.
46. Jiao X, Yang Z, Yang X. Common variants on chromosome 2 and risk of primary open-angle glaucoma in the Afro-Caribbean population of Barbados. *Proc Natl Acad Sci USA*. 2009;**106**:17105–10.
47. Noecker RJ, Earl ML, Mundorf TK, Silverstein SM, Phillips MP. *Curr Med Res Opin* 2006;**22**:2175–80.
48. Sakurai M, Higashide T, Takahashi M, Sugiyama K. Association between genetic polymorphisms of the prostaglandin F2alpha receptor gene and response to latanoprost. *Ophthalmology* 2007;**114**:2012.
49. MacDonald IM. Pharmacogenetics – getting closer. *Open Ophthalmol J* 2009;**3**:46–9.
50. Ederer F, Gaasterland DA, Dally LG *et al*. AGIS Investigators. The Advanced Glaucoma Intervention Study (AGIS): 13. Comparison of treatment outcomes within race: 10-year results. *Ophthalmology* 2004;**11**:651–64.
51. WuDunn D. Genetic basis of glaucoma. *Curr Opin Ophthalmol* 2002;**13**:55–60.
52. AAO PPP (American Academy of Ophthalmology Preferred Practice Pattern). *Primary Open Angle Glaucoma*, 2003, http://one.aao.org/CE/PracticeGuidelines/PPP.aspx (last accessed 22 November 2011).
53. Bowman DM, Allen RC. Erbium:YAG laser in cataract extraction. *J Long Term Eff Med Implants* 2003;**13**:503–8.
54. Dobelle WH. Artificial vision for the blind by connecting a television camera to the visual cortex. *ASAIO J* 2000;**46**:1–7.

CHAPTER 86

The ageing auditory system – pathology and epidemiology of age-related hearing loss

Mathieu Marx and Olivier Deguine

Hôpital Purpan and Université Toulouse III, CNRS, Toulouse, France

Age-related hearing loss (ARHL), improperly assimilated into presbycusis, is one of the most prevalent chronic conditions in elderly and its social impact is progressively increasing with the global ageing of the population. This particular handicap has traditionally been underestimated, since in many people's minds, hearing deterioration with ageing is a normal evolution. However, accidents related to hearing loss are not uncommon and inability to communicate generates frustration and isolation that can contribute to depressive syndromes or cognitive impairment. Prevention of these adverse consequences is necessary and possible through rehabilitative measures, which have been shown to improve quality of life. Improvement of screening and rehabilitation should therefore become a public health priority. The first part of this chapter is dedicated to the auditory system, its disorders and their diagnosis. The second objective is to provide an overview of hearing impairment epidemiology in the elderly population, based upon large cross-sectional and longitudinal studies and to consider the management of hearing loss in the elderly population.

The auditory system

Physiology of hearing

Sound

Sound is an aerial variation of pressure, producing an acoustic vibration. It is characterized by its frequency – measured in hertz (Hz)–perceived as the *pitch*, and its pressure – measured in decibels (dB)–perceived as the *loudness*.

A normal human ear perceives a pitch between 20 (low pitch) and 20 000 Hz (high pitch).and is able to perceive loudness from 0 to 120 dB. Sounds louder than 120 dB elicit a painful sensation. The scale of loudness is logarithmic, providing the human ear with a very wide dynamic range (Table 86.1). Further, the sensitivity of the ear is better for frequencies around 1000 Hz, covering the voice frequencies range.

The human ear

The human ear is divided into three segments

1 The external ear is composed of the external auditory meatus and the pinna. Its role is to gather the environmental sounds, to amplify them in the 2–5 kHz range and to drive them to the eardrum. It protects the delicate middle ear structures from external trauma.

2 The middle ear is composed of the tympanic membrane (eardrum), the ossicular chain (malleus, uncus, stapes) and the middle ear cavities (tympanic cavity, mastoid, Eustachian tube). It transforms the acoustic energy of sound into mechanical movement transmitted to the inner ear. It protects the inner ear from external (atmospheric) or endogenous pressure variations.

3 The inner ear includes the auditory organ, called the cochlea, and the balance organ. The cochlea is embedded in a solid bone structure, the otic capsule, which contains liquids (perilymphatic and endolymphatic fluids) and the sensory hearing organ, called the organ of Corti. Vibrations of the stapes through the oval window impulse a fluid circulation into the three ramps, that stimulate hair cells contained in the organ of Corti. Hair cells are organized according to the sound frequency, that is, tonotopically, in a spiral shape. The base of the cochlea responds to high-frequency sounds and the apex responds to low-frequency sounds. Inner hair cells represent the transducer, that is, the sensory cells, whereas outer hair cells are devoted to frequency selectivity, improving speech intelligibility.

Auditory pathways

Inner hair cells synapse with a rich array of dendrite that converge to the spiral ganglion, from where the auditory

Principles and Practice of Geriatric Medicine, Fifth Edition. Edited by Alan J. Sinclair, John E. Morley and Bruno Vellas.

Table 86.1 Dynamic scale of sound pressure level.

Pressure (dB)	Hearing sensation	Communication type	Noise type
130	Protection necessary		
120		No possible discrimination	
110	Painful		Airplane during take-off
90	Painful	No possible conversation	Car horn at 4 m
80		Conversation possible but difficult	Noisy traffic
70	Loud but bearable	Loud voice	Normal traffic
60	Common noise	Conversation with background noise	Supermarket
50	Moderate noise	Quiet conversation	Office
30	Quiet	Whispered voice	Quiet room
20	Very quiet		Sound of a mild wind
10	Unusual silence		Double-walled soundproof room
0	Normal hearing threshold		

nerve starts. The auditory nerve crosses the cerebellopontine angle to the cochlear nucleus, inside the brainstem. Afterwards, auditory fibres are divided in bilateral folds; the main auditory pathway crosses the middle line to the opposite side and reaches the temporal lobe to the primary auditory area. From this primary auditory area, different networks of neurons go towards secondary auditory and cognitive areas, integrating a multisensorial network.

Assessment of hearing function

Subjective measurements

The Rinne test and Weber test are common *tuning fork tests* that can help in differentiating conductive from sensorineural deafness. In the Rinne test, the tuning fork is placed on the mastoid and the skull transmits the sound to the cochlea until the subject's hearing threshold. The tuning fork is then placed next to the external auditory canal, the perception of the sound indicating a normal conductive mechanism. In cases of conductive deafness, the sound is perceived louder by bone conduction than by air conduction. In the Weber test, the tuning fork is placed centrally on the skull. Under normal conditions, the sound is transmitted to both ears equally. In the presence of conductive deafness, the sound is lateralized in the affected ear because the middle ear acts as a resonating drum. In sensorineural deafness, lateralization is observed in the healthy ear as the cochlea does not perceive transmitted sound.

Table 86.2 Degree of hearing loss according to the average hearing loss.

Mild	From 21 to 40 dB
Moderate	From 41 to 70 dB
Severe	From 71 to 90 dB
Profound	From 91 to 110 dB
Total (= deafness)	Above 110 dB

Pure-tone audiometry measures the subjective hearing threshold in various pure-tone frequencies for air conduction (through headphones) and for bone conduction (through a vibrator). The results are presented graphically and the average hearing loss is calculated by averaging hearing thresholds into 500, 1000, 2000 and 4000 Hz. Based on the average hearing loss, hearing impairment can be categorized from mild to total (Table 86.2). Under normal conditions, air conduction is similar to bone conduction. In the presence of conductive deafness, air conduction is at least 15 dB poorer than bone conduction. In sensorineural hearing loss, both air and bone conduction are affected. Mixed hearing loss is a combination of air and bone hearing loss.

Speech audiometry yields a better evaluation of the subject's functional status. This examination is usually performed using headphones and the subject is asked to repeat words from a standardized list, at various intensities. The percentage of correct answers is reported graphically according to the corresponding intensity. The speech reception threshold is the intensity for which 50% of words are correctly repeated. The optimal discrimination score is the highest score that can be achieved. Under normal conditions, it is obtained using a loudness level about 30 dB above the pure-tone threshold. Pure-tone audiometry and speech audiometry are the main evaluation criteria in the assessment of a rehabilitative measure (surgery or hearing aid), before and after intervention.

Suprasegmental tests are not used in current clinical practice. Speech perception in noise (SPIN) evaluates central auditory function.[1] Stereoaudiometry is useful for evaluating the impact of unilateral hearing loss. Gap detection and decay tests are used to diagnose auditory neuropathies.

Questionnaires and screening tests for hearing impairment are recommended by several national institutions for public health, but no standardized procedure has been shown to improve long-term hearing outcomes. However, routine screening would certainly be helpful since the psychosocial impact of hearing loss is significant and effective rehabilitative measures for hearing impairment are available. There are many simple tests for hearing that have been used as

Table 86.3 Hearing Handicap Inventory for the Elderly – Screening.

		Yes	Sometimes	No
E1	Does a hearing problem cause you to feel embarrassed when you meet new people?	4	2	0
E2	Does a hearing problem cause you to feel frustrated when talking to a member of your family?	4	2	0
S1	Do you have difficulty hearing when someone speaks in a whisper?	4	2	0
E3	Do you feel handicapped by a hearing problem?	4	2	0
S2	Does a hearing problem cause you difficulty when visiting friends, relatives, or neighbours?	4	2	0
S3	Does a hearing problem cause you to attend religious services less often than you would like?	4	2	0
E4	Does a hearing problem cause you to have arguments with family members?	4	2	0
S4	Does a hearing problem cause you difficulty when listening to the TV or radio?	4	2	0
E5	Do you feel that any difficulty with your hearing limits or hampers your personal or social life?	4	2	0
S5	Does a hearing problem cause you difficulty when in a restaurant with relatives or friends?	4	2	0
Totals for each column				
Grand total (add all Totals above) [a]				

[a]If the grand total score is greater than 10, an audiological evaluation is recommended.
Adapted from Ventry and Weinstein.[2]

Box 86.1

The minimum assessment in case of hearing loss should include an otoscopy, a pure-tone audiometry and a speech audiometry.

part of the physical examination, such as the whispered voice test. The degree of hearing loss is related to the furthest distance at which patients correctly discriminate words that have been whispered. This method may be used as a screening test but its reproducibility appears erratic. Screening hearing loss with a vibrating tuning fork has also been evaluated, but again, this method provides insufficient objective and reproducible outcomes.

The same self-administered questionnaire, the Hearing Handicap Inventory for the Elderly – Screening (HHIE-S), has been used in several cross-sectional studies and showed significant value in screening for hearing impairment[2] (Table 86.3). This instrument is a 10-item, 5 min questionnaire that measures the degree of social and emotional handicap due to hearing loss. The patient respond 'yes' (4 points), 'sometimes' (2 points) or 'no' (0 points) to each question concerning a particular handicap (Box 86.1). The total score ranges from 0 (no handicap) to 40 (maximum handicap). A total score of 0–8 indicates a 13% probability of hearing impairment, a score of 10–24 indicates a 50% probability of hearing impairment and a score of 26–40 indicates an 84% probability of a hearing impairment.[3] Scores of 10 and above provide a sensitivity between 63 and 80%[4] and a specificity between 69 and 77%. These levels seem acceptable since HHIE-S measures a functional but not audiometric hearing loss.

The Glasgow Benefit Inventory (GBI) is a measure of patient benefit developed especially for otorhinolaryngological interventions. Patient benefit is the change in health status resulting from this intervention. The GBI was developed to be maximally sensitive to ORL interventions, such as hearings aids, middle ear surgery or cochlear implantation. The change in quality of life is categorized between 'much worse' and 'much better' in three domains, physical, social and general, and is reported as a score ranging from −100 to +100.[5]

The Abbreviated Profile of Hearing Aid Benefit (APHAB) is a 24-item assessment inventory in which patients report the amount of trouble they experience with communication or noises in various everyday situations. Benefit is calculated by comparing the patients' reported difficulty in the unaided condition with their amount of difficulty when using amplification. The APHAB produces scores for four subscales: ease of communication, reverberation, background noise and aversiveness.[6]

The audioscope represents another screening instrument that can be used and is recommended by the Canadian Task Force on Preventive Health Care. It is a hand-held combination of an otoscope and an audiometer that delivers a pure tone from 25 to 40 dB at frequencies of 0,5, 1, 2 and 4 kHz. The audioscope is positioned directly in the external auditory canal with a probe tip sealing the canal. Tones are presented at each frequency and the listener's threshold is determined according to his/her responses. The probe is also used for direct inspection of the ear canal and the tympanic membrane. Patients with abnormal otoscopy and/or elevated hearing thresholds may then be referred for specialized evaluation. The sensitivity of audioscope testing exceeds 90%[4,7] and its specificity is estimated to be between 69 and 80%.

Objective measurements

Tympanometry is a measure of acoustic admittance, which depends on tympanic membrane integrity or stiffness, or the presence of a middle ear effusion. Thus, tympanometry is an additional tool in the diagnosis of the cause in

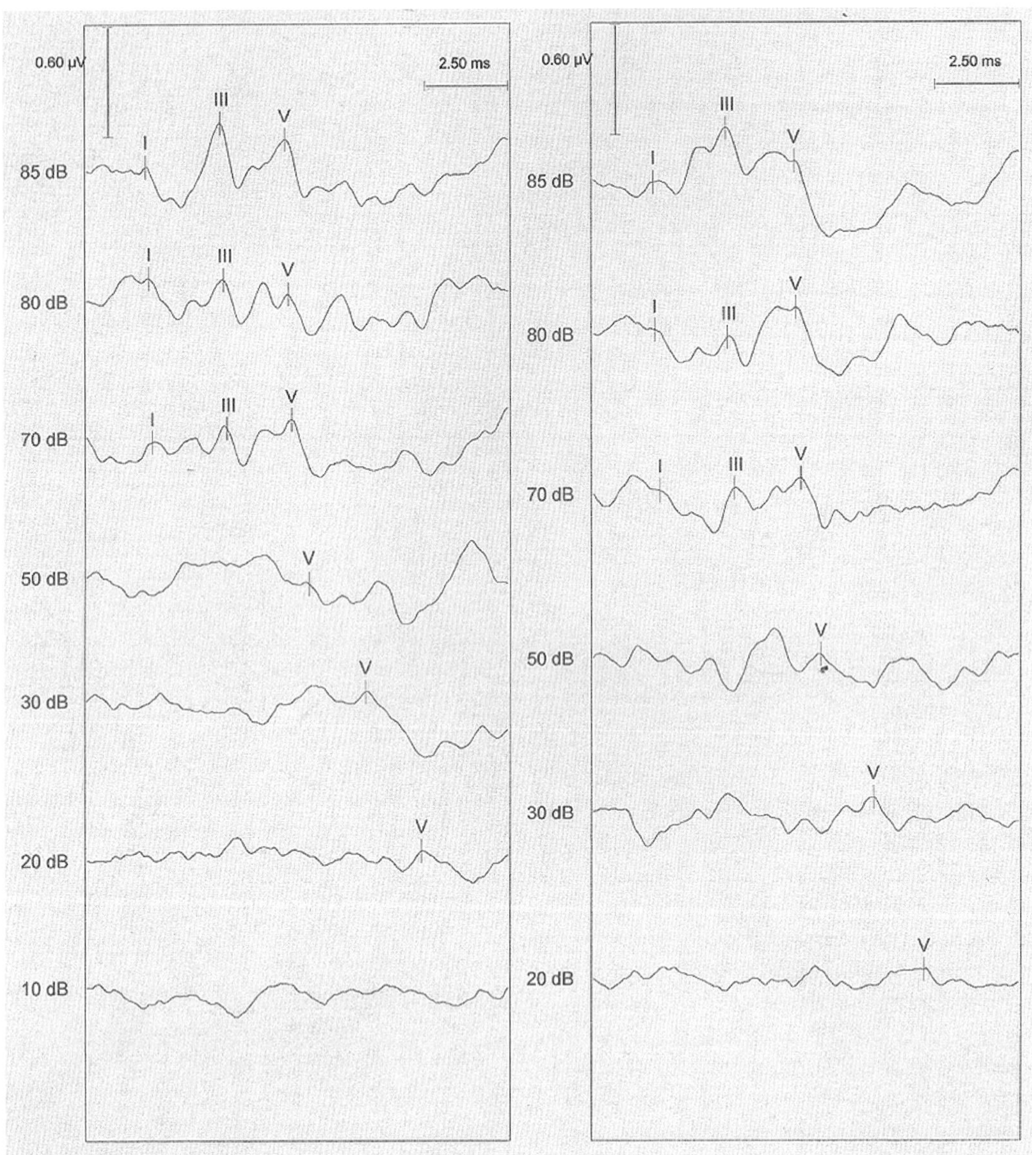

Figure 86.1 Auditory brainstem responses (right ear and left ear). Wave I, distal portion of cochlear nerve; wave II, proximal portion of cochlear nerve; wave III, cochlear nucleus; wave IV, superior olivary complex, nucleus of lateral lemniscus; wave V, inferior colliculus.

some cases of conductive deafness. It is also used to assess functioning of the muscle of the stapes, which reflects the integrity of the ossicular chain and of the facial and the cochleovestibular nerves.

Auditory evoked brainstem responses (Figure 86.1) are an electrophysiological examination that provides an objective assessment of auditory pathways function, from the external ear to the brainstem. Analysis of latency and delay between the recorded waves provides an objective threshold of hearing above 2 kHz and helps in localization of hearing loss cause (external or middle ear, inner ear, nerve lesion).

Evoked otoacoustic emissions are an acoustic response that is produced by the outer hair cells in the cochlea and which bounces back out of the cochlea in response to a sound stimulus. The test is performed by placing a probe that contains a microphone and a speaker into the external auditory canal. The sound stimulus is generated in the probe and, while the sound is processed by the cochlea, a second and separate sound is emitted by outer hair cells and comes back into the external auditory canal. This response is recorded and represented graphically.

Imaging may be used as an additional tool in the aetiological diagnosis or in the preoperative assessment.

High-resolution computed tomographic (CT) scanning provides an accurate representation of the mastoid, the middle ear cavities and the otic capsule that contains the cochlea and vestibular end organs. In chronic otitis media, it may specify a cholesteatoma extension and more particularly to the facial nerve, to the tegmen tympani or to the inner ear. It confirms otosclerosis, showing a hypodensity of the otic capsule, anterior to the oval window.

Magnetic resonance imaging (MRI) is mandatory in cases of asymmetric sensorineural hearing loss to rule out a cerebellopontine angle tumour and ventricular system dilatation. A vestibular schwannoma appears as a tumour enhanced after gadolinium injection during T1 sequence. MRI is also performed in the cochlear implant preoperative assessment to confirm the presence of auditory nerve and labyrinthine fluids.

fMRI and PET scanning are still research investigations and not used currently for isolated hearing disorders.

Pathology

The ageing auditory system

External and middle ear

With age, external ear skin shows various changes in its physical properties, such as atrophy, dehydration and decrease in elasticity. Combined with reduced self-cleaning abilities of the external auditory meatus and increase in cerumen (wax) production, older adults have a tendency to impact cerumen. Elderly people fitted with hearing aids are more exposed to this cerumen impaction. Further, they may experience dermatitis due to intolerance to hard materials.[8]

The tympanic membrane becomes thinner and its vascularization decreases. Arthritic changes can affect ossicle joints. Atrophy and degeneration progressively affect middle ear muscles and ligaments. Nevertheless, the changing conditions of the middle ear with age do not affect hearing significantly and inner ear changes with age account for most age-related hearing losses.

Inner ear

Biological ageing of the inner ear has been studied through many reports concerning temporal bones histopathology. Schucknecht has been one of the most active contributors to anatomical and histological studies of presbycusis.[9] He described six distinct categories of presbycusis according to their histopathological features: sensory, neural, strial, cochlear conductive, mixed and intermediate presbycusis. In sensory presbycusis, histology shows typically a loss of sensory hair cells that first occurs at the extreme basal end of the cochlea (high-frequencies region) and a degeneration of supporting cells, such as Deiters and Hensen cells. Noise exposure might play an important role in this type of age-related hearing loss as it usually affects outer hair cells. Age-related neural hearing loss is characterized by a loss of spiral ganglion cells and a discrepancy between speech and pure-tone audiometry, speech discrimination being poorer than pure-tone audiometry thresholds would lead one to expect. Histopathology of age-related strial hearing loss involves a loss of strial tissue and strial cells, resulting in an atrophy of stria vascularis, primarily in the apical and middle turns of the cochlea. Strial atrophy might be the most prominent histological finding in age-related hearing loss[10] and affects all frequency regions. Age-related mixed hearing loss represents an association of two or more inner ear histological changes and age-related intermediates characterized by submicroscopic alterations to intracellular organelles in hair and supportive cells. Cochlear conductive hearing loss is due to loss of elasticity of the basilar membrane and/or diminished attachment of the spiral ligament.

Auditory pathways and auditory brain

In addition to biological ageing of neurons, the decrease in peripheral input from ears may lead to a central auditory hearing loss that account for specific auditory deficiencies, such as temporal resolution and binaural processing. Age-related changes in the auditory brain are neither well documented nor specific. Neuronal alterations with age are characterized by shrinkage of neuronal stromas, which tend to accumulate lipofuscin more than in younger neurons and a reduced volume of central structures. Changes in sensory input resulting from age-related peripheral auditory pathology induce a functional and possibly structural reorganization of auditory brain. For instance, the central frequency map (i.e. central tonotopy) may be modified in the brainstem (inferior colliculus) and in the auditory cortex, by occurrence of a progressive high-frequency hearing loss, that leads to an over-representation of neurons responding to lower frequencies.[11] Connections between auditory cortices and higher levels areas, such as language processing sites, might also be altered secondarily to attenuation of auditory peripheral input.[12]

Types of hearing loss (HL)

Recent advances in the knowledge of HL suggest a modern classification of hearing impairment, as described by Zeng and Djallilian.[13]

Conductive HL

Conductive HL usually involves abnormalities of the external and/or the middle ear, due to mechanical or inflammatory causes, accessible to physical examination.

Cerumen accumulation is the most frequent cause of conductive HL; deafness occurs when the occlusion of the ear canal is complete or the cerumen impinges against the tympanic membrane.

In *acute otitis media*, hypoacusia appears behind pain and hyperthermia.

Chronic otitis media can impair hearing through different mechanisms: a perforation in the tympanic membrane, a lysis of the ossicular chain, a fixation of the ossicular chain by tympanosclerosis or a reduced vibration due to middle ear effusion. Several forms of chronic otitis media must be distinguished. Middle ear effusion and tympanic membrane perforations are the more benign conditions. Retraction pocket is an evolutive chronic otitis media due to a dysfunction of gas exchange in the middle ear. The retraction pocket is potentially dangerous; it progressively erodes the incus and the stapes and extends to the different cavities of the middle ear. Its ultimate evolution stage is the cholesteatoma, which is an abnormal and growing mass of keratin debris. Cholesteatoma has a lytic potential and can destroy ossicles, tegmen tympani or the inner ear. Therefore, cholesteatoma can lead to severe complications such as total deafness, vertigo, mastoiditis, facial nerve palsies, lateral sinus thrombosis, meningitis or temporal abscesses. As it is painless, its evolution is insidious in elderly persons. The diagnosis of chronic otitis media is based on HL associated with chronic or intermittent otorrhoea.

Otosclerosis is the most common cause of conductive deafness with normal tympanic membrane. Although it is known to occur in younger persons, aged patients may also be concerned, especially if otosclerosis worsens a concomitant presbycusis. It is characterized by a fixation of the stapes due to a focal osteodystrophy.

Cochlear HL

The most common cause of cochlear hearing loss in elderly is presbycusis. Typically, this deafness is characterized by a bilateral, symmetrical and progressive high-frequencies hearing loss. An early symptom is speech discrimination impairment in background noise or several speakers' conversations, which makes communication challenging in most social settings. The highest frequencies (6–10 kHz) are initially affected but once the loss progresses to the 2–4 kHz range, discrimination of consonants can be affected with frequent confusion of phonemes that requires repetition of utterances.

Idiopathic unilateral sudden hearing loss is not uncommon. Several pathophysiological factors have been proposed but the aetiology is not yet clear. Viral infections, immune disorders and microvascular injuries have been implicated but the viral hypothesis seems to be the most robust.[14]

Neural HL

Neural HL is also called 'auditory neuropathy' or 'auditory dyssynchrony'. It is due to dysfunctional synapse between inner hair cells or to lesions of the auditory nerve itself. The cochlear function is normal. The most significant characteristic is a temporal processing deficit, leading to a speech perception difficulty whereas the degree of HL is low.

Unilateral sensorineural deafness can appear suddenly or progressively. In both cases, complementary explorations (auditory brainstem responses associated with vestibular caloric testing and/or MRI) must be performed to search for a vestibular schwannoma, a benign tumour affecting the cochleovestibular nerve and developing in the cerebellopontine angle.

Central HL

Hearing impairment due to central lesions is usually defined as a central auditory processing disorder. Cochlear and nerve functions are considered normal. This type of HL is often associated with language impairment, learning disability and attention deficits. Although it is essentially observed in children, it may be associated with cognitive disabilities in the elderly population.

Epidemiology of hearing

Prevalence of hearing disorders in the elderly

In the next 10 years, the number of individuals over the age of 65 years is set to outnumber those under the age of 5 years for the first time in history and by 2040, those over 65 years old will make up 14% of the total world population.[15] Public health policies have to be reshaped regarding new needs that will emerge from this demographic shift. Hearing impairment requires considerable attention because the prevalence of age-related hearing loss (i.e. presbycusis) is increasing dramatically. At the same time, as old adults live healthier and longer, their lifestyle is changing and most of them experience an active retirement. Communication skills are therefore expected to remain normal or near-normal even if natural evolution of presbycusis is worsening hearing.

According to the Royal National Institute for Deaf People,[16] there are already 300 million people in the world with presbycusis and by 2050 it is projected that there will be 900 million. Prevalence studies of hearing impairment in the elderly find varying results according to the age range considered and the definition of hearing impairment that is used. Hence there may be a potential discrepancy between audiometric hearing thresholds and self-reported hearing impairment, due to under- or overestimation of the hearing handicap. The study of the Framingham cohort,[14] consisting of 1475 patients over a 6 year period, established that hearing loss is the third most prevalent condition in older Americans after hypertension and arthritis; between 25 and 40% of the population aged 65 years or older is hearing impaired. This prevalence increases with age, ranging from 40 to 66% in patients older than 75 years and more than 80% in patients older than 85 years. Hearing deterioration appears different according to the frequency that is considered. For instance, in the same study, hearing threshold worsening was more important in high frequencies (between 10 and 15 dB at 8 kHz over 6 years) than in low frequencies (between 1 and 8 dB at 250 kHz). The right ear advantage, that is, better thresholds in the right ear for pure-tone audiometry and speech perception, that exists in young normal hearing subjects tends to increase with ageing. In the UK, presbycusis is estimated to affect 40% of people aged 61–80 years in its mild form (hearing loss >25 dB) and a further 20% if the hearing loss is >35 dB.[17] A recent UK Health Technology Assessment report[18] revealed lower but still significant proportions regarding the range for age: 12% of people aged between 55 and 74 years have hearing problems and 14% present a hearing loss exceeding 35 dB on pure-tone audiometry. Even though the results differ slightly from one study to another, all of them highlight the growing number of hearing-impaired people and the effect of age on the prevalence of presbycusis.

Risk factors

Age-related hearing loss (ARHL) is the result of interaction between physiological degeneration and environmental factors, medical disorders and associated treatments and individual susceptibility.

Non-genetic risk factors (Box 86.2)

Noise exposure is the best documented risk factor for HL. The primary lesion is the loss of outer hair cells. At this stage, speech intelligibility is altered, whereas pure tone audiometry may be preserved. Noise exposure has a cumulative effect: duration of exposure and natural degeneration of the inner hair cells due to age will increase the sensorial deficit.[19]

The effect of smoking has been proved to be a strong risk factor for HL. Based on a meta-analysis, Nomura *et al.*[20] suggested that minimizing exposure to smoking maintains healthy hearing acuity and smoking cessation may be a cost-effective strategy in a hearing health programme.

Alcohol abuse and repetition of head traumas have also been implicated.[21] Arterial hypertension[22] and more particularly elevated systolic blood pressure is a recognized risk factor for hearing loss, whose detection and treatment are common in a general practice. Thus, several studies have shown that stroke, myocardial infarction, high body mass index and diabetes mellitus were all associated with excessive hearing loss.[10] Maintenance of a healthy general status would then prevent hearing worsening.

Box 86.2

The main non-genetic risk factors for age-related hearing loss are arterial hypertension, noise exposure and ototoxic drugs. They should be treated or prevented. Associated conditions such as cognitive impairment or depressive symptoms should also be investigated.

Table 86.4 Ototoxic drugs.

Antibiotics	Aminoglycosides, erythromycin, vancomycin, streptomycin
Antineoplastics	Cisplatin, carboplatin, vincristine sulfate
Loop diuretics	Furosemide, ethacrynic acid
Anti-inflammatory	Salicylates, quinine

Special attention must be paid to the medication in the ageing population and the iatrogenic potential also exists in otology, since a considerable amount of drugs can have ototoxic side effects (Table 86.4) The ototoxic effects of aminoglycosides and platinum compounds are well documented but one should also assess the risk of using high doses of aspirin or furosemide.

Genetic factors

Familial history is not uncommon in ARHL. According to Gates *et al.*,[23] heritability estimates indicate that 35–55% of the variance of ARHL is attributable to the effects of genes. The study of the Framingham cohort[24] shows that heritability would especially interfere in strial age-related hearing loss, where all frequencies are affected (flat audiogram). Genetic inheritance of ARHL should be distinguished from genetic HL, which is diagnosed from infancy to adult age and is now well documented. In contrast, most of the candidate genes for presbycusis are still under investigation.[25] As genome-wide association studies are expensive and time consuming, most current genetic linkage researchers use genotyping of pooled samples or target candidate genes in large populations of hearing-impaired elders. To date, GRHL2,[26] a transcription factor in a variety of epithelial tissues that is expressed in cells of the cochlear duct, and GRM7,[27] a metabotropic glutamate receptor expressed in inner ear hair cells and spiral ganglions, have shown a significant association with ARHL. Further, some genetic mutations have been shown to interact with environmental factors and enhance the risk of HL. For instance, the 1555G mitochondrial DNA mutation sensitizes the inner ear to aminoglycoside antibiotics.[28]

Associated pathologies and influence of hearing on behaviour

Poor hearing has been identified as a significant risk factor for mortality in elderly people, via increased disability for walking and cognitive impairment,[29] and its coexistence with several medical conditions is now well documented. Hearing impairment favours isolation and dependence in socioenvironmental interactions, which may negatively influence self-esteem and relationships with others. A recent review of the literature concerning risk factors for depression in the elderly[30] highlighted the role of sensory degeneration and more particularly hearing loss.

In patients with hearing loss, the mean odds ratio (OR) for depression across reviewed studies was 1.71 [95% confidence interval (CI), 1.28–2.27]. In another study of 580 patients over 65 years of age, Saito *et al.*[31] compared one group of hearing-impaired subjects with a group of normal hearing subjects. Incidence of depressive symptoms was 19.4% in the first group versus 8% in the group without a hearing handicap; the OR for depression was 2.45 (95% CI, 1.26–4.77). This strong association between hearing loss and depression emphasizes the altered quality of life in hearing-impaired elderly persons.

Quality of life measurements are necessary because they reflect the burden that represents hearing handicap in a patient's daily life and because they may estimate effects of rehabilitative measures. Furthermore, quality of life studies may assist in the allocation of public resources, such as finance and delivery of healthcare services. As previously mentioned, the effects of hearing impairment may be measured based on generic questionnaires or scores more specific to hearing, such as the HHIE-S. A correlation between hearing impairment (determined using HHIE-S scores) and independence for daily life activities (measured via the Katz index) was found to be significant in a study by López-Torres Hidalgo *et al.*[32] which emphasized the influence of hearing status on autonomy. A study of 2431 subjects aged >48 years by Chia *et al.*[33] evaluated the relationship between hearing thresholds and generic quality of life indices from the 36-item Short Form Health Survey. In this study, half of all participants reported hearing problems and the rate of hearing-impaired individuals increased from 16% in 50–59-year-olds to 65% in 70–79-year-olds. The authors found an adverse association between hearing thresholds and social or emotional dimensions of the questionnaire. For example, hearing impairment negatively impacted on emotional withdrawal, intimate relationships and family distress. Effects of hearing impairment on the physical dimension were also found, although this probably reflected a more general decline that can occur with ageing. Activities such as walking or preparing meals were found to be difficult by hearing-impaired elders. They then evaluated the use of hearing aids and its effects on quality of life measurements. Among people with hearing impairment, 33.3% owned a hearing aid and only 25.5% used it habitually, with physical scores that tended to be better than for subjects not using their hearing aid.

Cognitive status and relationship with hearing loss

As mentioned previously, elderly persons must deal with global ageing of hearing structures, from the external ear to auditory cortex, and a global decline of the auditory system is probably a current condition. More than a co-occurrence, peripheral hearing loss and cognitive decline interact and enhance the hearing handicap. Thus, oral communication relies not only on normal auditory structures and pathways, but also on basic cognitive processes. For instance, attention facilitates speech reception and the listening working memory provides a mental system for storage and processing of information: the elderly have to recognize incoming words and to integrate them with just previously heard words in order to give a meaning to the discourse to which they are listening. If the listener has to focus his/her mental energy to perform the first operation due to hearing impairment,[34] processing of speech by the listening working memory may be disrupted, with limited speech comprehension as consequence.

Interactions between hearing impairment and cognitive status exist but their nature is still under investigation. Poor auditory thresholds are common in patients with cognitive decline, and a higher prevalence of hearing loss in populations of adults with a diagnosis of dementia than in comparable population free of such a diagnosis is regularly shown.[35] However, the reasons underlying this association remain unclear and under discussion: a primary central auditory processing disorder due to Alzheimer's temporal lesions is a valuable hypothesis, but the psychosocial consequences of hearing loss just emphasized are recognized risk factors for dementia. Further, hearing impairment may interfere as a bias in neuropsychological assessments of patients. In a study of 82 elderly persons categorized into three groups according to their clinical dementia rating scale scores, central auditory testing using a dichotic sentences discrimination test revealed a strong deficit in patients with mild cognitive impairment or Alzheimer's disease, whereas peripheral testing using pure-tone audiometry and auditory brainstem responses did not show a difference between groups.[36] On the other hand, Acar *et al.*,[37] in a study of 34 hearing-impaired patients, showed an improvement of scores in the Mini Mental State Examination after 3 months of peripheral rehabilitation via hearing aids, associated with significant positive changes regarding daily life and social activities.

In summary, hearing and cognitive functions are closely related and interdependent. To specify the characteristics of this relation, future studies will have to confront results of central auditory processing tests, audiometric tests and validated neuropsychological measures in patients with various degrees of cognitive impairment.

Tinnitus

Tinnitus is a conscious perception of a sound in the absence of an acoustic stimulus. Objective and subjective tinnitus must be differentiated (Table 86.5). Patients with objective tinnitus are hearing real sounds, whether pulsatile or clicking, which are normally inaudible. Usually, pulsatile tinnitus is related to turbulent blood flow that reaches

Table 86.5 Aetiology of tinnitus.

Type	Cause
Subjective	
Otological	Noise-induced hearing loss, presbycusis, sudden deafness, labyrinthitis, otitis media, otosclerosis, impacted cerumen
Neurological	Head trauma, multiple sclerosis, vestibular schwannoma
Drug-related	Salicylates, loop diuretics, platinum-derived, aminoglycosides
Objective	
Pulsatile	Vascular tumours (glomus), arteriovenous malformations, carotid stenosis, severe hypertension, high cardiac output (anaemia)
Muscular	Palatal myoclonus, temporo-mandibular joint dysfunction, spasm of stapedius or tensor tympani muscle

the vicinity of the cochlea and clicking sounds are linked with an abnormal muscular contraction in the middle ear. Pulsatile tinnitus should alert the practitioner to use a stethoscope on the head, looking for an arteriovenous malformation or a glomus jugular tumour.

The pathophysiology of subjective tinnitus remains unclear, but cochlear damage seems to be the cause in most cases. The cochlear injury leads to reorganization of central auditory pathways, as evidenced by neuroimaging studies that have shown hyperactivation of auditory cortices and the limbic system in patients with tinnitus. Tinnitus may be characterized by different features: lasting, lateralization, loudness, pitch. Transient tinnitus, typically after exposure to a loud sound, is a common experience, but many people, and especially those over 65 years old, suffer from a continuous or repetitive tinnitus. Physical examination of the external ear and the tympanic membrane eliminates obvious causes of tinnitus and/or hearing loss, such as cerumen impaction or otitis media. The impact of tinnitus on hearing function must be evaluated with pure-tone audiometry and speech audiometry. As unilateral hearing loss, persistent unilateral tinnitus necessitates the search for a retro-cochlear pathology as a vestibular schwannoma. Quality of life questionnaires, such as the Tinnitus Questionnaire, allow the effects of tinnitus on sleep, emotional status and social activities to be quantified.

Management of ARHL

Medical and surgical treatments

Family and personal otological priors can help in the aetiological investigation of the deafness. The physical examination includes a complete cardiovascular and neurological systems examination. Otoscopy is the main step in the diagnosis of external or middle ear abnormalities causing conductive deafness and the practitioner should keep in mind that cerumen accumulation is a trivial but common cause of hearing loss (up to 30% in the elderly).

Conductive hearing loss

Cerumen impaction can be revealed by simple physical inspection of the external auditory canal. Small hooks and curettes can be used to remove cerumen, and ear canal irrigation with warm water can be applied. Hydrogen peroxide-containing solutions may be used to loosen firm cerumen accumulation. In cases of tympanic membrane perforation or prior ear surgery, the patient can be referred to an otolaryngologist for safe removal or microsuction under microscopic examination.

Middle ear effusion can be diagnosed by otoscopy. The inspection of the tympanic membrane reveals the presence of serous fluid (i.e. serous otitis) or seromucuous secretions behind the membrane. There is no evidence of any medication efficiency but steroid inhalers are commonly used. In cases where effusion persist for several weeks, patients should be referred to an otolaryngologist for surgical treatment (transtympanic tube) and a complete ENT examination, as nasopharyngeal carcinoma may be revealed by a unilateral serous otitis.

Other chronic otitis media must be referred for a complete audiological and anatomical evaluation. The otolaryngologist may propose surgical treatment in cases of cholesteatoma or tympanic membrane perforation with iterative infections. In contrast, they may propose a regular follow-up for a retraction pocket without any auditory or infective consequences.

Otosclerosis also requires treatment by a hearing specialist. Surgical treatment (stapedotomy or stapedectomy) or rehabilitation with a hearing aid may be considered.

Sensorineural hearing loss

Patients with unilateral hearing loss must be referred to an otolaryngologist for a complete assessment of the hearing loss and an aetiological investigation (including a specific search for a vestibular schwannoma). Sudden hearing loss is a controversial topic in many respects. We have already discussed the various pathogenic factors that have been implicated and studied. Conflicting reports concerning the treatment approach have also generated uncertainty. So far, systemic glucocorticoids are the only treatment whose efficiency has been demonstrated in a placebo-controlled trial.[38] Additional use of antiviral agents or hyperbaric oxygenation has been proposed but no evidence for its efficacy has been provided. Most recent studies have assessed the use of transtympanic drug delivery, with particular interest in local administration of steroids.

Prevention plays an important role in hearing impairment care. For instance, hearing must be regularly evaluated when known ototoxic agents need to be administered. Early detection of a high-frequencies hearing loss may help to adapt drugs and doses in order to prevent a secondary deterioration. The use of earplugs provides a 15–25 dB attenuation of sounds and can prevent noise-induced hearing loss. Screening and treatment of systemic cofactors, such as arterial hypertension or smoking, would logically reduce the risk of hearing loss.

The environment may be adapted to the hearing disability through simple measures (turning off the television or radio during a conversation, speaking more slowly) or with the use of an assistive hearing device (telephone amplifier, infrared system for television). Most of these systems may be tested and prescribed in audiology services. For patients wearing hearing aids, frequency-modulated systems, consisting of a microphone placed near the source of sound, a transmitter and a receiver worn by the patient can be used in difficult hearing conditions.

Acoustic amplification via a hearing aid is indicated when the average hearing threshold reach 40 dB on the pure-tone audiogram and can be proposed for smaller losses according to the professional or occupational needs. There are various types of hearing aids, according to the size and shape, including the traditional behind-the-ear, in-the-ear and open-fit models. The audiologist plays a major role in the selection and fitting of the hearing aid, adapted to the patient. Many factors, such as severity of deafness, anatomical configuration of the external ear, social conditions and fine motor skills must be considered. Analogue hearing aids are usually less expensive than digital ones, but the latest provide multiple programmes that operate adaptively and can reduce a noisy background or acoustic feedback. Improvement of quality of life has been shown for a long time in patients wearing hearing aids. Mulrow *et al.*[39] conducted a randomized clinical trial comparing 95 deaf patients fitted with hearing aids with 99 patients without a hearing aid. The first group showed significant improvements in social life, emotional status and cognitive functions whereas these parameters had not been modified in the second group. The size and shape of hearing aids may influence satisfaction. In various studies,[40,41] the in-the-ear type has been identified as the easiest to manipulate and the most often used (45.4 versus 19.5 h per week for the behind-the-ear type). In both studies, patients with a behind-the-ear hearing aid reported significantly more 'undesirable' experiences (ear discomfort, negative sound experience), but the emergence of open fit behind-the-ear aids has significantly decreased these manifestations.

Unfortunately, it is estimated that only 3–20% of potential hearing aid users actually purchase them and most elderly persons are reluctant to do so because of hearing aids' social standing.[41] Moreover, only 60–75% of people will continue wearing their hearing aid once they have been fitted with it.[42] The reasons for dissatisfaction or non-use are cosmetic, unconsciousness of hearing disability, intolerance to amplification and local trauma.

Tinnitus

Patients with tinnitus should be referred to the otolaryngologist for several conditions:

- tinnitus associated with a hearing loss and/or an abnormal ear condition
- persistent (>3 months) unilateral tinnitus
- persistent intrusive tinnitus
- pulsatile tinnitus unless associated with acute otitis media.

The impact of tinnitus on quality of life can be major and associated depressive symptoms must be taken into account. Unfortunately, medical treatment of tinnitus is challenging and the doctor–patient relationship is strongly involved. Many drugs (benzodiazepines, tricyclics, peripheral vasoactives) have been tested but no evidence for their efficacy has been found. As in drug-induced hearing loss, ototoxic medication must be known and eventually adapted in cases of tinnitus. For instance, salicylates can provoke only temporary tinnitus and hearing loss[43] if the cessation is early enough.

Masking devices cover up the tinnitus and provide relief for some patients who have a response to masking during the audiological evaluation. Hearing aids may be proposed if there is an associated hearing loss and some programmes implement masking sounds in the frequency range where tinnitus is most prominent.

Auditory implants

Middle ear implants and bone-anchored hearing aids (BAHAs)

Some elderly people cannot wear hearing aids for medical (chronic external otitis, external auditory canal stenosis) or cosmetic reasons and present a hearing loss that is not severe enough to match cochlear implantation criteria. They may be good candidates for active middle ear implants that may be used to treat mild to severe sensorineural, conductive or mixed hearing losses. A middle ear implant requires a surgical intervention and consists of an audio processor that encodes acoustic signals to mechanical vibrations of a transducer positioned against an element of the ossicular chain. BAHAs require a simpler surgery under local anaesthesia and it relies on bone conduction of sound vibration. Outcomes of middle ear implants in the elderly population as a subgroup have not been specifically documented but most studies report an audiometric gain and an improvement of speech comprehension in quiet or in challenging conditions.[44] Middle ear implants would be particularly indicated in elderly persons who experience difficulty in manipulating hearing aid controls or suffer from recurrent inflammation of the external auditory canal due to the hearing aid.

Cochlear implants

Audiometric criteria for implantation have been progressively extended from total to severe hearing loss.

Cochlear implants are established as effective in elderly patients but there is a justified reticence to operate owing the fragile condition of many elderly patients. Actually, intra- or postoperative complication rates remain comparable to those in younger patients[45] and improvement in speech recognition scores has such a positive impact on quality of life that cochlear implantation has become a robust alternative in rehabilitation of severe to profound deafness.[46] Vermeire *et al.*[47] compared audiometric results and quality of life changes for three age groups (<55, 56–69 and 70+ years). Even though the oldest group had poorer speech recognition scores than the two younger groups, all groups experienced significant improvement of speech recognition and all had similar quality of life outcomes (Glasgow Benefit Inventory, Hearing Handicap Inventory for Adults). Shin *et al.*[48] studied gains after implantation in conversation with familiar or unfamiliar persons and in perception of environmental sounds in a group of elderly implanted patients compared with a control group of younger patients. The results between the two groups were comparable in all conditions. For instance, the gain in conversation with a familiar person was 59% in the elder group versus 58% in the younger group. Further, many patients retain residual hearing in at least one ear and are advised to use the cochlear implant in one side and their hearing aid in the contralateral ear (i.e. bimodal stimulation), if the latter still transmits acoustic information although not providing sufficient speech discrimination. The combination of residual hearing and cochlear implant has been widely evaluated and seems to improve auditory gain and comfort in challenging listening conditions (background noise, reverberant places, music perception).

Associated treatments (Box 86.3)

Speech therapy

Speech therapy may provide substantial help in rehabilitation of this communication handicap. Patients can be taught speech reading as lip movements and facial expressions provide assistance in semantic analysis of a sentence where unheard words are missing. Patients with severe hearing losses also perceive benefit from auditory training, which improves their recognition of key words and environmental noises.[49]

> **Box 86.3**
>
> Patients with age-related hearing loss may benefit from several rehabilitative measures, medical and surgical treatments, from hearing aids to cochlear implants, including speech therapy and environmental adaptations.

Correction of visual defects

Visual rehabilitation is an important part of global care of the elderly. Visuoauditive interactions play a prominent role in rehabilitation of severely hearing impaired subjects, which manifest particularly in lip-reading activity. A study by Rouger *et al.* showed that cochlear implanted subjects maintained their lip-reading abilities even 5 years after the cochlear implantation and that multisensorial integration facilitated their speech comprehension with speech recognition scores reaching 100% in audiovisual condition.[50]

Conclusion and the future

Hearing impairment is a common and potentially severe handicap among the elderly population. Although its adverse effects on quality of life and general medical condition are now well documented, age-related hearing loss remains underdiagnosed and insufficiently rehabilitated. Simple screening methods, such as the HHIE-S questionnaire, are available and effective and should be used in everyday geriatric exercise. In cases of mild to moderate hearing loss, various types of hearing aids may be proposed and are reasonably expected to improve quality of life. A cost reduction would probably encourage more people to search for audiology services expertise. If hearing loss is more severe, speech therapy may represent an additional help and cochlear implants have been shown to be safe and efficient in elderly people. Future directions for research include the evaluation of local interventions into the inner ear, such as cell- or gene-based therapies or drug delivery such as steroids or antioxidants. Atoh1-expressing viruses have been shown to produce some structural and functional recovery in the cochlea of deafened guinea pigs[51] and transtympanic dexamethasone[52] is regularly evaluated in tinnitus or sudden hearing loss treatment. The development of new cochlear implants, allowing local drug delivery, has already begun and seems to maintain the remaining hearing function. In the same field, cochlear implants have recently been evaluated in the treatment of unilateral tinnitus associated with deafness and would provide significant improvements in quality of life indices.[53] In the coming years, demographic shifts will make hearing loss one of the main challenges in public health. Substantial investments from governments and industry are especially needed to promote hearing research and to develop curative solutions for hearing loss.

Key points

- Age-related hearing loss is the third most prevalent chronic condition in the elderly and will affect a growing number of individuals.
- Presbycusis represents the main cause but may coexist with middle ear pathologies or central disorders.
- The main non-genetic risk factors for age-related hearing loss are arterial hypertension, noise exposure and ototoxic drugs and should be treated or prevented. Associate conditions such as cognitive impairment or depressive symptoms should also be investigated.
- The minimal assessment in case of hearing loss should include an otoscopy, a pure-tone audiometry and a speech audiometry.
- Effective rehabilitative measures and medical, surgical and instrumental treatments are available and must be applied to reduce the handicap provoked by age-related hearing loss. These treatments should be complemented by additional care, such as consideration of isolation, speech therapy and correction of visual and cognitive deficits.

References

1. Bilger RC, Nuetzel JM, Rabinowitz WM and Rzeczkowski C. Standardization of a test of speech perception in noise. *J Speech Hear Res* 1984;**27**:32–48.
2. Ventry IM and Weinstein BE. The Hearing Handicap Inventory for the Elderly – a new tool. *Ear Hear* 1982;**3**:128–34.
3. Lichtenstein MJ, Bess FH and Logan SA. Validation of screening tools for identifying hearing-impaired elderly in primary care. *JAMA* 1988;**259**:2875–8.
4. Ciurlia-Guy E, Cashman M and Lewsen B. Identifying hearing loss and hearing handicap among chronic care elderly people. *Gerontologist* 1993;**33**:644–9.
5. Robinson K, Gatehouse S and Browning GG. Measuring patient benefit from otorhinolaryngological surgery and therapy. *Ann Otol Rhinol Laryngol* 1996;**105**:415–22.
6. Cox RM and Alexander GC. The abbreviated profile of hearing aid benefit. *Ear Hear* 1995;**16**:176–86.
7. McBride WS, Mulrow CD, Aguilar C and Tuley MR. Methods for screening for hearing loss in older adults. *Am J Med Sci* 1994;**307**:40–2.
8. Weinstein B. *Geriatric Audiology*, Georg Thieme, New York, 2000.
9. Schuknecht HF and Gacek MR. Cochlear pathology in presbycusis. *Ann Otol Rhinol Laryngol* 1993;**102**(1Pt 2):1–16.
10. Gates GA and Mills JH. Presbycusis. *Lancet* 2005;**366**:1111–20.
11. Thai-Van H, Micheyl C, Norena A *et al*. Enhanced frequency discrimination in hearing-impaired individuals: a review of perceptual correlates of central neural plasticity induced by cochlear damage. *Hear Res* 2007;**233**:14–22.
12. Frisina R. Aging changes in the central auditory system. In: A Rees and A Palmer (eds), *The Oxford Handbook of Auditory Science: the Auditory Brain*, Oxford University Press, Oxford, 2010, pp. 417–38.
13. Zeng F and Djallilian H. Hearing impairment. In: C Plack (ed.), *The Oxford Handbook of Auditory Science: Hearing*, Oxford University Press, Oxford, 2010, pp. 325–47.
14. Tucci DL. Sudden sensorineural hearing loss: a viral etiology? *Arch Otolaryngol Head Neck Surg* 2000;**126**:1164–5.
15. Kinsella K and He W. *An Aging World: 2008. US Census Bureau International Population Reports*, P95/09-1, US Government Printing Office, Washington, DC, 2009.
16. Vio MM and Holme RH. Hearing loss and tinnitus: 250 million people and a US$10 billion potential market. *Drug Discov Today* 2005;10:1263–5.
17. Fletcher AE, Jones DA, Bulpitt CJ and Tulloch AJ. The MRC trial of assessment and management of older people in the community: objectives, design and interventions [ISRCTN23494848]. *BMC Health Serv Res* 2002;**2**:21.
18. Davis A, Smith P, Ferguson M *et al*. Acceptability, benefit and costs of early screening for hearing disability: a study of potential screening tests and models. *Health Technol Assess* 2007;**11**(42):1–294.
19. Mills JH, Dubno JR and Boettcher FA. Interaction of noise-induced hearing loss and presbyacusis. *Scand Audiol* 1998;**27**:117–22.
20. Nomura K, Nakao M and Morimoto T. Effect of smoking on hearing loss: quality assessment and meta-analysis. *Prev Med* 2005;**40**:138–44.
21. Rosenhall U, Sixt E, Sundh V and Svanborg A. Correlations between presbyacusis and extrinsic noxious factors. *Audiology* 1993;**32**:234–43.
22. Brant LJ, Gordon-Salant S, Pearson JD *et al*. Risk factors related to age-associated hearing loss in the speech frequencies. *J Am Acad Audiol* 1996;**7**:152–60.
23. Gates GA, Couropmitree NN and Myers RH. Genetic associations in age-related hearing thresholds. *Arch Otolaryngol Head Neck Surg* 1999;**125**:654–9.
24. Gates GA, Cooper JC Jr, Kannel WB and Miller NJ. Hearing in the elderly: the Framingham cohort, 1983–1985. Part I. Basic audiometric test results. *Ear Hear* 1990;**11**:247–56.
25. Liu XZ and Yan D. Ageing and hearing loss. *J Pathol* 2007;**211**:188–97.
26. Van Laer L, Van Eyken E, Fransen E *et al*. The grainyhead like 2 gene (GRHL2), alias TFCP2L3, is associated with age-related hearing impairment. *Hum Mol Genet* 2008;**17**:159–69.

27. Friedman RA, Van Laer L, Huentelman MJ *et al*. GRM7 variants confer susceptibility to age-related hearing impairment. *Hum Mol Genet* 2009;**18**:785–96.
28. Hutchin T. Sensorineural hearing loss and the 1555G mitochondrial DNA mutation. *Acta Otolaryngol* 1999;**119**:48–52.
29. Karpa MJ, Gopinath B, Beath K *et al*. Associations between hearing impairment and mortality risk in older persons: the Blue Mountains Hearing Study. *Ann Epidemiol* 2010;**20**:452–9.
30. Huang Q and Tang J. Age-related hearing loss or presbycusis. *Eur Arch Otorhinolaryngol* 2010;**267**:1179–91.
31. Saito H, Nishiwaki Y, Michikawa T *et al*. Hearing handicap predicts the development of depressive symptoms after 3 years in older community-dwelling Japanese. *J Am Geriatr Soc* 2010;**58**:93–7.
32. López-Torres Hidalgo J, Boix Gras C, Téllez Lapeira J *et al*. Functional status of elderly people with hearing loss. *Arch Gerontol Geriatr* 2009;**49**:88–92.
33. Chia EM, Wang JJ, Rochtchina E *et al*. Hearing impairment and health-related quality of life: the Blue Mountains Hearing Study. *Ear Hear* 2007;**28**:187–95.
34. Pichora-Fuller MK. Cognitive aging and auditory information processing. *Int J Audiol* 2003;**42**(Suppl 2):2S26–32.
35. Weinstein BE. Validity of a screening protocol for identifying elderly people with hearing problems. *ASHA* 1986;**28**:41–5.
36. Gates GA, Karzon RK, Garcia P *et al*. Auditory dysfunction in aging and senile dementia of the Alzheimer's type. *Arch Neurol* 1995;**52**:626–34.
37. Acar B, Yurekli MF, Babademez MA *et al*. Effects of hearing aids on cognitive functions and depressive signs in elderly people. *Arch Gerontol Geriatr* 2011;**52**:250–2.
38. Wilson WR, Byl FM and Laird N. The efficacy of steroids in the treatment of idiopathic sudden hearing loss. A double-blind clinical study. *Arch Otolaryngol* 1980;**106**:772–6.
39. Mulrow CD, Aguilar C, Endicott JE *et al*. Quality-of-life changes and hearing impairment. A randomized trial. *Ann Intern Med* 1990;**113**:188–94.
40. Tonning F, Warland A and Tonning K. Hearing instruments for the elderly hearing impaired. A comparison of in-the-canal and behind-the-ear hearing instruments in first-time users. *Scand Audiol* 1991;**20**:69–74.
41. Upfold LJ, May AE and Battaglia JA. Hearing aid manipulation skills in an elderly population: a comparison of ITE, BTE and ITC aids. *Br J Audiol* 1990;**24**:311–8.
42. Popelka MM, Cruickshanks KJ, Wiley TL *et al*. Low prevalence of hearing aid use among older adults with hearing loss: the Epidemiology of Hearing Loss Study. *J Am Geriatr Soc* 1998;**46**:1075–8.
43. Brien JA. Ototoxicity associated with salicylates. A brief review. *Drug Saf* 1993;**9**:143–8.
44. Uziel A, Mondain M, Hagen P *et al*. Rehabilitation for high-frequency sensorineural hearing impairment in adults with the symphonix vibrant soundbridge: a comparative study. *Otol Neurotol* 2003;**24**:775–83.
45. Kelsall DC, Shallop JK and Burnelli T. Cochlear implantation in the elderly. *Am J Otol* 1995;**16**:609–15.
46. Cohen SM, Labadie RF, Dietrich MS and Haynes DS. Quality of life in hearing-impaired adults: the role of cochlear implants and hearing aids. *Otolaryngol Head Neck Surg* 2004;**131**:413–22.
47. Vermeire K, Brokx JP, Wuyts FL *et al*. Quality-of-life benefit from cochlear implantation in the elderly. *Otol Neurotol* 2005;**26**:188–95.
48. Shin YJ, Fraysse B, Deguine O *et al*. Benefits of cochlear implantation in elderly patients. *Otolaryngol Head Neck Surg* 2000;**122**:602–6.
49. Hickson L and Scarinci N. Older adults with acquired hearing impairment: applying the ICF in rehabilitation. *Semin Speech Lang* 2007;**28**:283–90.
50. Rouger J, Lagleyre S, Fraysse B *et al*. Evidence that cochlear-implanted deaf patients are better multisensory integrators. *Proc Natl Acad Sci USA* 2007;**104**:7295–300.
51. Izumikawa M, Batts SA, Miyazawa T *et al*. Response of the flat cochlear epithelium to forced expression of Atoh1. *Hear Res* 2008;**240**:52–6.
52. Dodson KM and Sismanis A. Intratympanic perfusion for the treatment of tinnitus. *Otolaryngol Clin North Am* 2004;**37**:991–1000.
53. Jolly C, Garnham C, Mirzadeh H *et al*. Electrode features for hearing preservation and drug delivery strategies. *Adv Otorhinolaryngol* 2010;**67**:28–42.

CHAPTER 87

Disorders of the vestibular system

Charlotte Ågrup and Linda M. Luxon
University College of London Hospitals NHS Trust and University College London, London, UK

Introduction

Man has developed a sophisticated system for maintaining balance, which requires the integration and modulation of visual, vestibular and proprioceptive information within the central nervous system (CNS) (Figure 87.1). Pathology of any one of the three sensory inputs or of the central vestibular pathways may give rise to disequilibrium, as may many pathological processes that affect directly or indirectly the systems essential for perfect balance (Table 87.1). Dizziness is a frequent complaint in elderly people and the prevalence of balance problems at age 70 years has been reported in 36% of women and 29% of men, increasing with advanced age to 45–51% at ages 88–90 years.[1] Dizziness and vestibular abnormalities are reported to be a major risk factor predisposing to falls among the elderly[2] and the significance of this lies in the high morbidity and mortality associated with falls in this age group. In addition, fear of falling may constitute an independent risk factor for disability, leading older people to restrict their daily living activity unnecessarily.[3] However, with the correct diagnosis, many vestibular disorders are treatable, leading to improved quality of life. Therefore, for the geriatrician, an understanding of the pathophysiology of the vestibular system and its central connections is particularly important if the common complaint of disequilibrium is to be managed successfully.

Vestibular anatomy

The inner ear is a minute, complex, fluid-filled structure surrounded by a bony labyrinth located deep in the temporal bone. The cochlea corresponds to the acoustic end-organ, whereas the vestibular end-organs consist of the three semicircular canals, the saccule and the utricle. The semicircular canals are called the *horizontal* (or *lateral*), the *posterior* and the *superior canal*. The two ends of all semicircular canals open into the vestibule, near the utricle. One end of each semicircular canal has a dilated portion, called the ampulla, containing the sensory epithelium, that is, the hair cells. The *utricle* and the *saccule* correspond to the otolith organs and both contain a small area of sensory epithelium, called maculae. All vestibular sensory epithelium is covered with a gelatinous mass, which, in the saccule and the utricle, contains calcium carbonate-rich crystals termed *otoconia*. A force parallel to the surface of the sensory epithelium provides the maximum stimulus. The semicircular canals with their ampullary tissue sense angular acceleration, whereas the saccule and the utricle sense linear acceleration. The planes of the two otolith organs lie approximately at right-angles to each other. The utricular macula is oriented roughly horizontally and the saccular macula is roughly vertical. Accordingly, the saccule is well equipped to sense vertical head acceleration and the constant pull of gravity, whereas the utricle senses linear head motion in the horizontal plane. The utricle also plays an important role in signalling the spatial upright when the head is tilted with regard to gravity. The ampullae in the semicircular canals are insensitive to the static gravitational vector or position of the head in space. However, when an appropriate angular force is introduced, the fluid in the semicircular canal is displaced along the lumen of the canal leading to changed activity in the sensory epithelium of the ampullae.

Physiology and ageing of the vestibular apparatus

In a normal subject holding the head in the anatomical position, the sensory epithelium in each ear generates resting neural activity, which passes via the VIIIth cranial nerve and the vestibular nuclei within the brainstem to the cortex.

Head movements result in linear and/or angular accelerations, which stimulate the vestibular sensory epithelium and modulate the neural activity in an equal but opposite manner in each ear. Hence an asymmetry of information is generated, which passes into the CNS. This asymmetric vestibular input allows cortical awareness of head position in space and provides the stimulus for compensatory eye and body movement.[4]

Principles and Practice of Geriatric Medicine, Fifth Edition. Edited by Alan J. Sinclair, John E. Morley and Bruno Vellas.

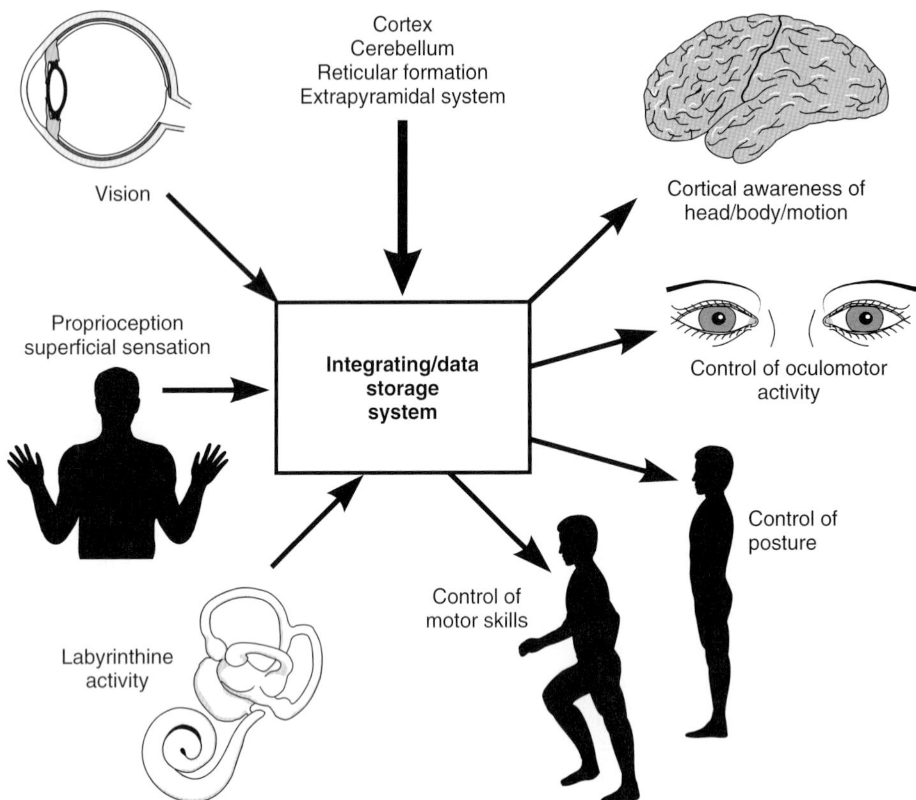

Figure 87.1 Mechanisms subserving balance in man. Reproduced from Savundra and Luxon,[4] Copyright 1997, with permission from Elsevier.

Pathology involving the peripheral labyrinth, VIIIth cranial nerve or central vestibular connections may result in an asymmetry of vestibular information, which is 'misinterpreted' by the brain and perceived as vertigo and instability. The incidence of vertigo has been reported to rise with advancing age, in parallel with the incidence of hearing loss.[5] Histopathological age-related changes reported in the human vestibular sensory organs include progressive hair-cell degeneration, otoconial degeneration in the otolith organs and decreasing number of vestibular nerve fibres.[6] In addition, age-dependent changes in both caloric and rotation test responses have been demonstrated.[5,7] However, vestibular symptoms result from an asymmetry of afferent information arising within the vestibular apparatus and degenerative changes tend to occur symmetrically. It is therefore unlikely that disequilibrium in the elderly is solely consequent upon vestibular degenerative changes and is more probably multifactorial in origin.[8] Accordingly, dizziness in the elderly is often the result of central pathology and/or sensory deficits: visual impairment (not correctable); neuropathy; vestibular deficits; cervical spondylosis; and orthopaedic disorders, interfering with joint mechanoreceptors.

Following an acute unilateral vestibular upset, the patient experiences vertigo, but usually the symptoms are relatively short lived and resolve in 6–12 weeks, as a result of processes collectively known as *cerebral compensation*. Functional recovery depends on the degree of vestibular loss and cerebral compensation. The restoration of perfect balance involves reduction or abolition of the asymmetry in postural and ocular motor tone and recalibration of the gain of dynamic vestibular reflexes, in order to ensure symmetrical compensatory vestibulospinal and vestibulo-ocular reflex action during movement of the head and body. However, in some patients recovery does not occur. The persisting symptoms are usually less dramatic and the vertigo may not be rotational, but may consist of more vague symptoms of floating, rocking or a sense of depersonalization. Such symptoms may be continuous, but may also present as episodic attacks of disequilibrium frequently triggered by an intercurrent illness or a psychological upset such as bereavement (Figure 87.2). It is well established that vestibular compensation is dependent on a variety of brainstem, cerebellar and cortical structures, together with sensory inputs including vision, somatosensory afferents and remaining labyrinthine input, which are

Table 87.1 Causes of dizziness in the elderly.

General medical	
Haematological	Anaemia
	Polycythaemia
	Hyperviscosity syndromes
Cardiovascular	Postural hypotension
	Carotid sinus syndrome
	Dysrhythmias
	Mechanical dysfunction
	Shock
Metabolic/endocrine	Hypo- and hyperglycaemia
	Thyroid disease
	Chronic renal failure
	Alcohol
Neurological	
Supratentorial	Trauma
	Neoplasia
	Epilepsy
	Cerebrovascular disease
	Syncope
	Psychogenic
Infratentorial	Vertebrobasilar insufficiency
	Subclavian steal syndrome
	Wallenberg's syndrome
	Anterior inferior cerebellar artery syndrome
	Degenerative disorders including neuropathy
	Tumour, including those of the vestibulocochlear nerves
Infective disorders	Ramsay–Hunt
	Neurosyphilis
	Tuberculosis
Foramen magnum abnormalities	
Cerebellar degeneration	
Basal ganglion disease	
Multiple sclerosis	
Otological	
Drug-induced/ototoxic	
Degenerative (e.g. positional vertigo)	
Posttraumatic syndrome	
Infection	
Vascular	
Tumours	
Menière's syndrome	
Otosclerosis and Paget's disease	
Autoimmune disorders	
Others	
Migraine	
Multisensory dizziness syndrome	

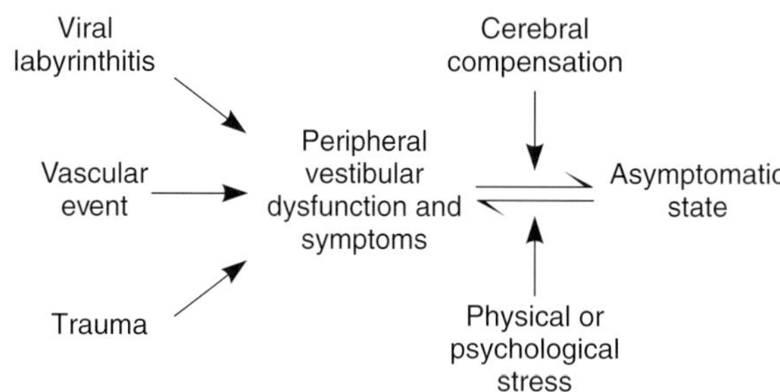

Figure 87.2 Diagram to illustrate normal sequence of events leading to recovery from a peripheral vestibular abnormality and factors relevant in decompensation.

involved in the normal perception of space, body posture and locomotion. The causes of failure of compensation or intermittent decompensation are not clear, but cerebellar damage, impairment of proprioception, visual impairment, mild cerebral dysfunction and psychological disorders have all been cited as possible contributing factors. Thus, the age-dependent changes in sensory inputs and CNS function noted above would suggest that central compensation for vestibular deficits in the elderly is likely to be less efficient.

Clinical aspects and diagnostic strategy

Vertigo, defined as 'an hallucination of movement', is a cardinal manifestation of a disordered vestibular system, whereas dizziness is a lay term, defined in the *Concise Oxford Dictionary* as 'a feeling of being in a whirl or in a daze or as if about to fall', associated commonly with a multiplicity of general medical disorders. This semantic distinction is rarely volunteered by the elderly patient, who more frequently complains of feeling faint, swimmy or lightheaded. Hence, for practical purposes, all complaints of disorientation are considered most easily within a single diagnostic approach.

History

In the history, the character, time course and associated symptoms of the dizziness/vertigo are valuable pointers in elucidating the underlying diagnosis.

Character of dizziness

Classically, the vertigo/dizziness of peripheral labyrinthine origin is manifested as acute, unprecipitated, short-lived attacks of rotational disequilibrium, associated with nausea and vomiting and more rarely diarrhoea, while the vertigo/dizziness of central vestibular origin is described as a more insidious, protracted sense of instability. Exceptions to the former include epilepsy and vertebrobasilar artery ischaemia, and exceptions to the latter include uncompensated peripheral vestibular disorders, bilateral vestibular failure and psychogenic disequilibrium. Additional common symptoms with peripheral vestibular dysfunction are a sensation of being pulled downward or sideways or of the room tilting and a sensation of swimming, floating and lightheadedness. However, if a clear description of subjective or objective motion is given, the suspicion of vestibular pathology is raised, whereas symptoms of lightheadedness, swimminess or faintness are more likely to be attributable to a general medical/neurological disorder.

Time course

Acute rotational vertigo of less than 1 min duration is most commonly associated with the diagnosis of benign positional vertigo of paroxysmal type (see the following text), whereas acute rotational vertigo of less than 1 h duration may suggest the diagnosis of vertebrobasilar insufficiency. Vertigo of several hours' duration (less than 24 h) is most commonly associated with migraine and Menière's disease (see the following text). Acute rotational vertigo of several days' duration, with gradual resolution of symptoms, points to a viral or vascular vestibular neuritis, although persistence of such symptoms in the elderly patient may indicate poor compensation from a peripheral vestibular insult or a fixed neurological deficit as a result of a vascular event within the brainstem. Apart from the duration of the vertigo, the time course of the episodes is also of diagnostic value. A single acute episode with gradual resolution over days or weeks would point to a peripheral vestibular pathology, such as a viral neuritis or an ischaemic event. In the elderly patient, cerebral plasticity is reduced, as noted previously, hence compensation from such a single insult may be protracted and intercurrent illness may result in an exacerbation of symptoms (decompensation). Repeated short episodes with complete and rapid recovery in between would suggest migraine, Menière's disease or, most commonly, benign positional vertigo. It should be emphasized that in these conditions, the episodes also tend to occur in clusters, with intervals of months or even years of freedom.

Associated symptoms

Within the labyrinth and VIIIth cranial nerve, the vestibular and cochlear elements are in close anatomical proximity. Hence pathology in these sites gives rise commonly to both cochlear and vestibular symptoms. Frequently, the elderly patient will not volunteer a complaint of tinnitus or hearing loss, as they attribute the symptoms to their age, and it is therefore important to enquire specifically. Within the CNS, the vestibular and auditory pathways diverge and vestibular symptoms of brainstem or cerebellar origin are rarely associated with cochlear symptoms, but commonly associated with neurological symptoms and signs. Loss of vestibular function leads to impaired gaze stabilization during fast head movements, that is, *oscillopsia*.[9] Typically, the patients complain of blurred vision or bouncing images while walking or riding in a car. The vestibular system is sensitive to fast, high-frequency head movements (1–10 Hz) and cortical–optokinetic reflexes are too slow to compensate for this functional loss above 2–3 Hz. Many patients with vestibular dysfunction report a worsening or triggering of dizziness with certain visual stimuli, such as rapidly changing images, fast-moving traffic, crowds and striped material. This symptom is called *visual vertigo*.[9] In addition, anxiety disorders, depression and panic attacks have been described in association with peripheral vestibular disease, and it is likely that in some patients vestibular dysfunction may play an important role in the aetiology of these disorders.[3]

Examination

A detailed medical examination is essential with special reference to the fundi, visual fields and acuity, a general neurological examination and examination of the cardiovascular and peripheral vascular systems. On the basis of a comprehensive history and a thorough examination, the diagnosis of many neurological and general medical disorders will be excluded. The diagnosis of vestibular disorders giving rise to vertigo/dizziness is based on a neuro-otological examination, which may be divided into the following:

- an examination of the external ear and otoscopy (to exclude infection, mass or perforated ear drum) together with clinical tests of auditory acuity/whispered voice tests and tuning-fork tests
- an assessment of vestibulo-ocular function
- an assessment of vestibulospinal function, as part of the overall balance.

Otological examination

In all patients with vertigo, particularly in ethnic minorities, immigrants and immunosuppressed patients, it is essential to exclude active, chronic middle-ear disease with labyrinthine erosion. A labyrinthine fistula should be suspected in all patients with vertigo and previous surgery for middle ear disease. Clinical tests of auditory function, including tuning-fork tests (Rinne and Weber test), are important when attempting to localize pathology, since the presence of an auditory deficit may suggest an underlying labyrinthine or VIIIth nerve pathology.

Vestibulo-ocular examination

A detailed account of vestibular physiology and pathophysiology is beyond the scope of this chapter, but a clear understanding of these subjects is essential if an informed assessment of vestibular function and vestibular investigations are to be made.[10] As has been outlined earlier, an asymmetry of vestibular activity may result from unilateral peripheral vestibular, VIIIth nerve or brainstem pathology. This asymmetry is 'monitored' by the brain and, via the pathways subserving the vestibulo-ocular reflex, results in a slow vestibular-induced drift of the eyes in the same direction as the peripheral labyrinthine lesion. For reasons that are not fully understood, this slow drift is interrupted by rapid saccadic eye movements, which are generated within the brainstem in the opposite direction. This combination of slow and fast eye movements is known as *spontaneous vestibular nystagmus* and is characteristic of acute peripheral vestibular lesions. Initially, the nystagmus present with fixation but is more prominent without fixation. As a general rule, nystagmus with fixation (nystagmus seen on routine neurological examination) disappears within 1–2 weeks after the acute lesion. By contrast, spontaneous nystagmus can be observed without optic fixation, using Frenzel's glasses, for as long as 5–10 years after the acute episode. Spontaneous vestibular nystagmus will usually beat away from the affected side, unless the lesion is irritative (infection or tumour). By definition, for clinical purposes, the direction of the nystagmus is defined by the fast phase. Thus, a right peripheral vestibular lesion gives rise to horizontal left beating nystagmus, which obeys Alexander's law. This states that the nystagmus is always in one direction irrespective of direction of gaze and that the intensity of the nystagmus is greatest when the eyes are deviated in the direction of the fast phase. For purposes of accurate review, nystagmus should be described in the following terms: primary nystagmus describes nystagmus which is beating in the same direction as gaze deviation; secondary nystagmus describes nystagmus in the midposition of gaze; and tertiary nystagmus describes nystagmus which is beating in the opposite direction to the direction of gaze (e.g. to the right, when the eyes are deviated to the left). Bidirectional nystagmus (e.g. first-degree nystagmus to the right on looking to the right and first-degree nystagmus to the left on looking to the left), vertical nystagmus (i.e. upbeat nystagmus and/or downbeat nystagmus) and dysconjugate nystagmus (a differing nystagmic response in each eye) indicate CNS disease, requiring further investigation. Clinically, *spontaneous nystagmus* should be sought in every patient complaining of dizziness/vertigo. The eyes should be examined in the midposition of gaze, with eyes 30° to the right and 30° to the left. Care must be taken that this angle is not exceeded, otherwise physiological end-point nystagmus may be observed and this may be confused with pathological nystagmus. In addition, vertical nystagmus with the eyes 30° upwards and 30° downwards should be sought.

The *head thrust test* is a quick and simple clinical test used to assess failure of the vestibulo-ocular reflex (Figure 87.3).[11] The head thrust test is positive for the side that causes the corrective saccades, indicating a vestibular hypofunction on the same side.

The presence of *positional nystagmus* is a most valuable and most frequently overlooked sign and should be sought by a briskly performed *Hallpike manoeuvre* (Figure 87.4). The patient is made to sit close to the top end of a flat examination couch. The head is held firmly between the examiner's hands and turned 30–45° to the right or left. The patient is then carried rapidly backwards with the head over the edge of the couch and the eyes are carefully observed. If nystagmus develops, it is observed until it disappears or for 2–3 min, until it is clear that the nystagmus is persistent. The patient is then returned to the upright position

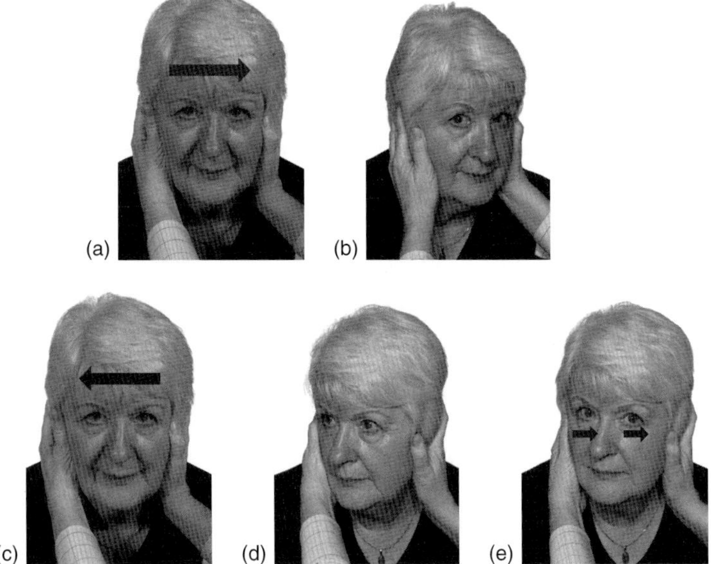

Figure 87.3 Head thrust test: normal to the left (a) and (b), abnormal to the right (c)–(e). (a), (c) Starting position with subject's head in mild cervical flexion and eye's focused on target; for example the examiner's nose. (b) On thrust of the head to the left; subject's eyes remain on target. (d) On thrust of the head to the right; the eyes move with the head and lose the target. (e) Saccadic corrections of the eyes required to bring visual focus back to target. Large arrows: direction of thrust of the head. Small arrows: direction of corrective eye saccades.

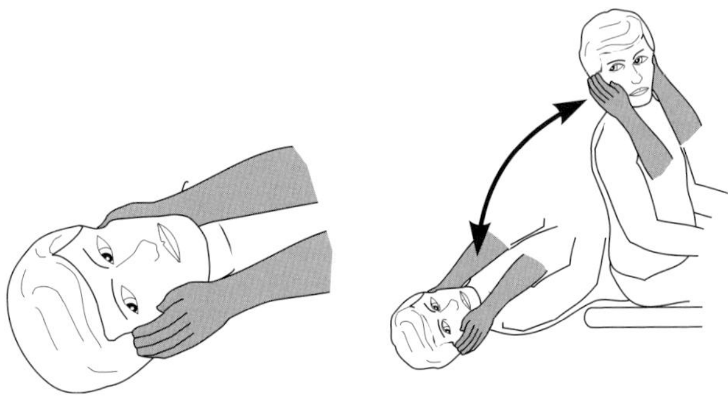

Figure 87.4 The Hallpike manoeuvre for inducing positional nystagmus.

Table 87.2 Characteristics of positional nystagmus.

	Benign paroxysmal type	Central type
Latent period	2–20 s	None
Adaptation	Disappears in 50 s	Persists
Fatigue ability	Disappears on repetition	Persists
Vertigo	Always present	Typically absent
Direction of nystagmus	To undermost ear	Variable
Incidence	Relatively common	Relatively uncommon

and the procedure repeated in the opposite direction. In broad clinical terms, the positional nystagmus which may develop can be divided into two main types, as identified in Table 87.2, although there are cases which do not clearly fit into either category and those should be investigated, as should the 'central' category, for neurological disease. If the positional nystagmus is of peripheral labyrinthine origin, after a latent period of a few seconds in the head-back position, severe vertigo develops which lasts for less than 1 min, but during which the patient may feel extremely distressed and nauseated. The nystagmus is rotatory in nature and directed towards the undermost ear. Symptoms and signs adapt and fatigue on repeated testing. Therefore, care must be taken that the procedure is carried out correctly at the first attempt. Moreover, it is important to establish this condition, as it is a troublesome cause of vertigo for which highly effective treatment is available (see the following text).

The vestibular system, via the vestibulo-ocular reflex (VOR), provides one system for the control of eye movements and gaze stability. Visual stimuli provide another mechanism for stabilizing gaze, that is, smooth pursuit and optokinetic reflexes and in general all three systems interact to produce precise and accurate eye movements. Under certain circumstances the visual and vestibular inputs to eye movement control may conflict. For example, watching a tennis tournament, as the head turns to the right to follow a ball flying through the air, the vestibulo-ocular reflex would tend to result in a compensatory eye movement to the left, whereas the subject wishes to keep the eyes fixed on the ball moving to the right. In this situation, the visual stimulus overrides the vestibular stimulus by modulation of neural activity at the level of the vestibular nuclei. This is known as *visual suppression of the vestibular responses* and clinical examination of this function allows assessment of central vestibular integrating ability. The simplest clinical means of assessing vestibulo-ocular reflex suppression is by observing the effect of optic fixation upon rotationally induced vestibular nystagmus. This may be simply accomplished in the clinic by observing the patient's eyes, while the patient is oscillated on an office chair while fixating his/her own thumbs.[9] If the eyes remain fixated on the target, VOR suppression is intact. In contrast, if clear nystagmus is elicited by the rotation, VOR suppression is abnormal, indicating CNS pathology.

Vestibulospinal assessment

Vestibulospinal function cannot be assessed in isolation and tests are non-specific and insensitive, compared with tests of vestibulo-ocular function, but tests of stance and gait may provide an indication of the extent of the patient's disability and interaction of vestibulospinal activities with other systems. The *Romberg test* is performed by asking the patient to stand in the upright position with feet together, arms by the side and eyes closed. A tendency to sway to one side usually suggests peripheral vestibular pathology, whereas an inability to stand with the feet together is more characteristic of cerebellar ataxia. Baloh *et al.*[12] demonstrated that there is a marked increase in postural sway in elderly patients with unilateral vestibular hypofunction, in comparison with younger patients with the same disorder. Anxious elderly patients frequently tend to fall backwards like a wooden soldier and this is indicative of a non-organic component to their symptoms, but it must be emphasized that this is almost always observed in the presence of an underlying abnormality, which will be elucidated on full examination. *Gait testing* is assessed by asking the patient to walk towards a fixed point in a normal manner, but with eyes closed. Again, a tendency to veer in one direction is most commonly the result of an ipsilateral peripheral vestibular disturbance, but may on occasions be observed with cerebellar disease. This latter diagnosis is most commonly associated with a broad-based, ataxic gait. Having briefly reviewed vestibular physiology and pathophysiology and outlined the aspects in the history and examination, which may enable the clinician to identify a vestibular abnormality, the remainder of this chapter will be devoted to a review of the more common causes of vestibular pathology in the elderly and the therapeutic options available.

Peripheral vestibular disorders

Viral vestibular neuritis

Single episodes of acute rotational vertigo associated with nausea and vomiting, with or without cochlear symptoms, occur in all age-groups. The attacks are usually unprecipitated, but may be preceded by an upper respiratory- tract infection, and are therefore presumed to be of viral origin, although there is little definitive evidence for this.[13] Additional possible causes of vestibular neuritis include other infectious agents and vascular or immune-mediated disorders. The vertigo may last for a few hours or several days and the patient may then be extremely unsteady for a period of weeks, during which time cerebral compensation produces a degree of symptomatic recovery. However, in the elderly patient, the plasticity of the CNS is compromised and recovery is often slower and is rarely complete.

Ramsay–Hunt syndrome (see Chapter 117, Infections of the central nervous system)

The Ramsay–Hunt syndrome or herpes zoster oticus is an example of a mononeuritis of the VIIth cranial nerve. The patient experiences a deep, burning pain in the ear, which is followed within a few days by a vesicular eruption in the external auditory canal and on the concha. The patient often develops facial paralysis. In addition, some patients present with hearing loss, tinnitus, vomiting, vertigo and nystagmus indicating VIIIth nerve involvement.

Bacterial infection

Chronic middle-ear disease is a prevalent condition in the elderly and it cannot be overemphasized that in any patient with vestibular symptoms in whom there is the slightest suspicion of middle-ear disease or history of previous middle-ear surgery, the presumptive diagnosis must be of labyrinthine erosion. *Perilymph fistulae* may result from bony erosion by cholesteatoma with the lateral semicircular canal being the most commonly affected site.[14] Rarely, perilymph fistulae may be caused by barotraumas, syphilitic osteitis, tuberculous otitis media, chronic perilabyrinthine osteomyelitis or glomus jugulare tumour. *Otitis externa* is a common benign disorder, but in debilitated elderly patients, particularly those with diabetes and other immunosuppressive conditions, it may present in a more malignant form. The causative organism is mainly *Pseudomonas aeruginosa*. The disease spreads rapidly, invading surrounding soft tissues, cartilage and bone structures, with occasional involvement of adjacent cranial nerves, causing hearing loss and vertigo. Prolonged treatment with effective antibiotics, carbenicillin or gentamicin, has improved the previously poor prognosis.

Neoplasia

Vestibular disorders as a direct result of neoplasia are uncommon, even in the elderly. The non-metastatic complications of carcinomatous encephalomyelitis may involve the vestibular nerve, while cochlear and vestibular symptoms have been reported in patients with carcinomatous meningitis.[15] Secondary tumour involvement of the inner ear by blood-borne metastases from hypernephroma and lung, prostate, breast and uterine carcinoma have been reported and direct extension of nasopharyngeal carcinoma may occur. Aural tumours are rare, with the exception of cholesteatoma, as outlined previously. Cochlear symptoms (tinnitus and hearing loss) are the most common presenting symptoms of *acoustic neurinoma* (vestibular Schwannoma), but 10% of patients complain of vertigo, dizziness and/or unsteadiness. A unilateral asymmetric hearing loss must be investigated and brainstem auditory-evoked responses provide the best screening technique. If these are abnormal, a computed tomography (CT) scan or, preferably, a magnetic resonance imaging (MRI) scan, should be obtained. The diagnosis and management of this condition in the elderly do not differ from those of any other patient and early diagnosis is essential, as excellent surgical results are achieved with small tumours (<20 mm in size). However, it has been shown that small tumours do not invariably enlarge with time and the high sensitivity of MRI may mean that clinically insignificant tumours may be detected. In the elderly patient, it is appropriate to monitor the growth of small acoustic neuromas (vestibular Schwannoma), but this must be balanced against the significantly decreased mortality/morbidity associated with surgery for smaller tumours.

Vascular disorders

Both the peripheral and central vestibular apparatus are supplied by the vertebrobasilar circulation and, as cerebrovascular disease is common in developed countries (the risk factors being diabetes mellitus, hypertension and a raised haematocrit), disequilibrium in the elderly is commonly ascribed to vascular pathology. Ischaemia of the internal auditory artery may give rise to three differing clinical syndromes: vestibular disorders alone, cochlear disorders alone or combined vestibulocochlear symptomatology. An isolated acute episode of rotational vertigo, as outlined in the description of viral vestibular neuritis, may be of vascular origin, but recurrent isolated vertigo is rarely of vascular origin. The diagnosis is usually presumptive and is based on evidence of vestibular dysfunction in a patient with other manifestations of vascular disease. Risk factors (diabetes mellitus, hyperlipidaemia, hypertension, myxoedema) should be sought and treated appropriately.

Trauma

The elderly are particularly prone to falls and vestibular abnormalities as a result of even trivial head injury are now well recognized.[16] Damage to the vestibular system may be the result of direct injury, for example, labyrinthine concussion and/or temporal bone fracture, or of secondary shearing forces in the brainstem and cerebellum. Falls may cause cervical trauma in the elderly, which may also give rise to vestibular disturbances.[16]

Two post-traumatic vestibular syndromes may be identified, as follows.

Unilateral auditory and vestibular failure

This is associated with transverse fractures of the temporal bone, in which severe vertigo and hearing loss are accompanied by bleeding from the ear, nausea and vomiting. The patient prefers to lie completely still with the affected ear uppermost. Over a period of 6–12 weeks there is marked improvement in the disequilibrium related to cerebral compensation, although in the elderly patient, as noted earlier, this may be slower and less complete than in a younger person. There is no recovery of the auditory deficit.

Benign positional vertigo of paroxysmal type

This is the most common clinical syndrome after head injury, but may also be seen in the elderly as an idiopathic disorder or secondary to vestibular neuritis. Recent work has led to the theory of canalithiasis (Figure 87.5), which explains the majority of the characteristic features of benign positional nystagmus.[17, 18] This theory proposes that debris from the otolith organ lies in the most dependent portion of the posterior canal and, upon assuming the critical head position, the clot moves in an ampullofugal direction and, thus, has a 'plunger' effect within the narrow posterior semicircular canal. This causes movement of the cupula in an ampullofugal direction, with a brief paroxysm of vertigo and nystagmus as a result.

The clinical course of post-traumatic benign positional vertigo is that some days or weeks after even a trivial head injury, momentary, short-lived episodes of vertigo occur on assuming specific head positions, particularly associated with neck extension and typically appearing when lying down on one ear, bending forwards or looking up. Frequently, the only abnormal clinical sign is benign positional nystagmus of paroxysmal type on performing the Hallpike manoeuvre (see above). The vertigo associated with this condition is particularly severe and the elderly patient is frequently extremely afraid, as the attacks are very sudden and may cause a drop to the ground and vomiting. This leads to anxiety, partly from fear of embarrassment if this should happen in a public place, and partly from fear of being incapacitated at home, unable to reach help. Not infrequently, this diagnosis is overlooked

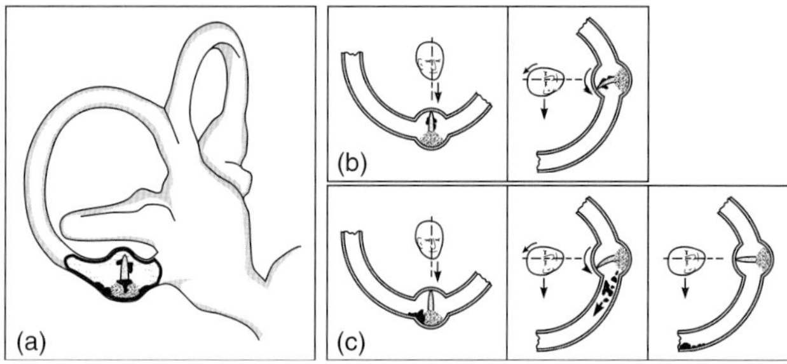

Figure 87.5 Diagram to illustrate the pathophysiological mechanisms of cupulolithiasis and canalithiasis. (a) Illustration of cupula in ampulla of posterior semicircular canal, with debris attached to and surrounding the cupula. (b) Illustration of the effect of gravity on the cupula and debris as proposed by the theory of cupulolithiasis. (c) Illustration of the effect of gravity on the cupula and debris as proposed by the theory of canalithiasis. Reproduced from *Vestibular Research*, vol. 3, Brandt T and Steddin S, pp. 373–82, Copyright 1993, with permission from IOS Press.

and the clinician merely observes an extremely anxious elderly patient, who finds difficulty explaining such brief yet severe symptoms. It is therefore extremely important that the Hallpike manoeuvre is performed and a clear explanation of the benign nature of the condition given. In 1980, Brandt and Daroff[19] reported complete relief of symptoms in 66 of 67 patients with benign positional vertigo as a result of precipitating head positions 'on a repeated and serial basis'. They suggested that the mechanism of improvement using this therapy lay in rapid and aggressive vertigo-provocative movements, which loosened and dispersed otholitic debris from the cupula of the posterior semicircular canal (cupulolithiasis) (Figure 87.5). However, on the basis of our current knowledge, it seems more likely that these manoeuvres cleared debris from the most dependent part of the posterior semicircular canal into the utricle, where they no longer interfered with semicircular canal dynamics. More recently, single positional manoeuvres[20] have been described in which specific movements of the head allow the offending debris in the posterior canal to be moved by gravitation into the utricle: the *Epley manoeuvre* (Figure 87.6). The patient is instructed to sit upright for 48 h after this procedure, which has been reported to be effective in 80–85% of patients in the first attempt at treatment and in a further 10% upon a second attempt. Relapses may occur, but the manoeuvre should then be repeated. Pretreatment sedation is not required except for the most anxious of patients and the manoeuvre is as effective in older people as in younger people. In a small percentage of patients, it would appear that the particle repositioning procedures are not effective and, in intractable cases, plugging of the posterior semicircular canal or section of the posterior and ampullary nerve should be considered.[21]

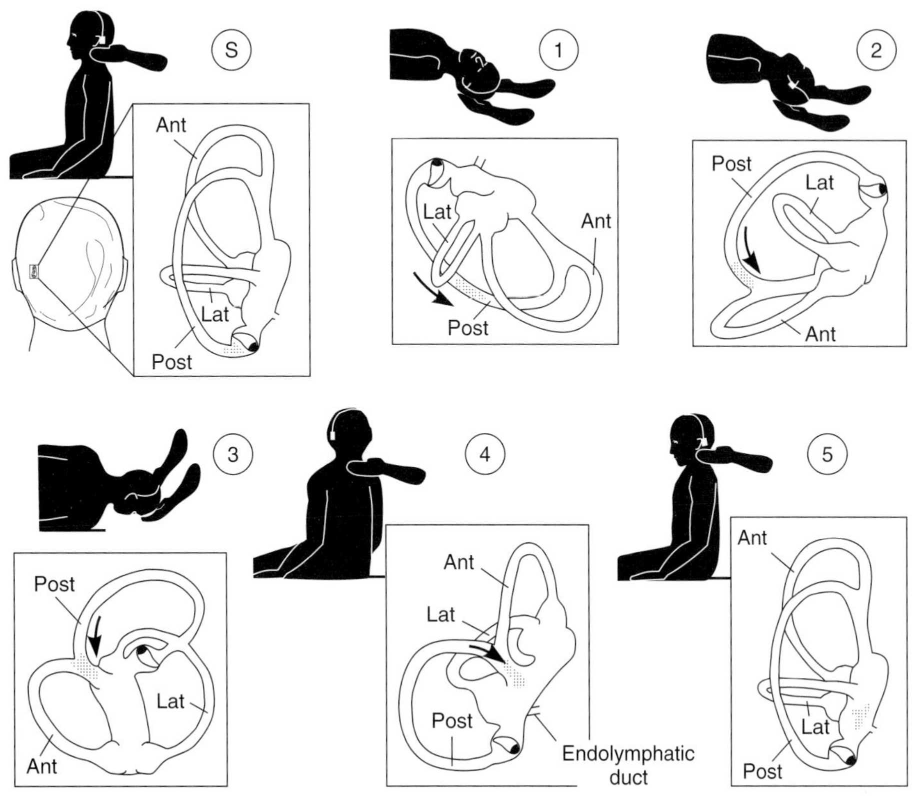

Figure 87.6 Diagram to illustrate particle repositioning procedure for canalithiasis of left posterior semicircular canal, as described by Epley.[20] S, sitting; 1 – 5, Stages of manoeuvre. Semicircular canals: Ant, anterior; Post, posterior; Lat, lateral. Reproduced from Epley,[20] Copyright 1992, with permission from Elsevier.

Menière's disease

Menière's disease was first described in 1861 by Prosper Menière and is characterized by episodic vertigo, low-frequency hearing loss with tinnitus and aural fullness. Menière's disease does occur in the elderly[22] and the pathological underlying process is thought to be due to an increase in endolymph volume, that is, endolymphatic hydrops. Treatment remains empirical but routinely consists of a salt-free diet and diuretics, which is effective in most patients. In intractable cases with incapacitating vertigo, intratympanic gentamicin injection or surgical intervention (e.g. vestibular neurectomy and labyrinthectomy) may be considered.

Iatrogenic vestibular dysfunction

Iatrogenic dizziness may be surgical or medical in origin and it is well established that otological surgery carries a risk of inducing dizziness/vertigo postoperatively. Moreover, vestibular disturbances after non-otological surgery have been documented. Drug-induced dizziness is a very significant problem in the elderly and many, if not all, drugs may produce dizziness, although it is often impossible to identify the underlying mechanism causing disequilibrium. Anaemia secondary to gastrointestinal bleeding, hypoglycaemia, cardiovascular effects including reduction in cardiac output, dysrhythmias and postural hypotension and ototoxicity should all be considered. The most common drugs giving rise to dizziness in the elderly are shown in Table 87.3.

Ototoxic damage is of particular importance, as it is irreversible. The vestibulotoxic effect of the aminoglycoside antibiotics is common knowledge and in the elderly they should be used only as a lifesaving measure. It is well established that age is an important factor in the susceptibility to aminoglycoside ototoxicity and for this reason blood levels of these drugs should be measured meticulously in the elderly, especially in the presence of concurrent diuretic therapy and/or any change in the overall medical state. However, the correlation between blood levels of the ototoxic drug and ototoxic effect can be poor, due to interindividual differences and a possible accumulation of the drug in the inner ear fluids. Although standard vestibular tests are not feasible in a severely ill patient, recent methods of assessing vestibular function at the bedside have been developed and are of particular value in potential ototoxicity.[9, 11, 23]

Table 87.3 Drugs causing dizziness/vertigo[a].

Psychotropic drugs	
Antidepressants	Tricyclics, MAOIs, SSRIs
Tranquilizers	Benzodiazepines, phenothiazines
Anticonvulsants	Phenytoin, carbamazepine, gabapentine, lamotrigine
Analgesics	Paracetamol, acetylsalicylate, NSAIDs, opioids
Cardiovascular drugs	
Antihypertensives	Diuretics (thiazides and loop), β-blockers, calcium-channel blockers, ACE inhibitors, methyldopa, hydralazine
Anti-arrhythmic	β-Blockers, verapamil, mexiletine, flecainide, amiodarone, disopyramide
Anti-angina	Nitrates, calcium-channel blockers, β-blockers, potassium-channel activators
Antimicrobials	Aminoglycosides, tetracyclines, macrolides, chloroquine, isoniazid
Anti-allergic drugs	Non-sedating and sedating antihistamines
Hormone replacement/ substitute	Hypoglycaemics, corticosteroids, HRT
Chemotherapeutic agents	Cisplatin, busulfan, cyclophosphamide, vinblastine, methotrexate

[a]MAOI, monoamine oxidase inhibitor; SSRI, selective serotonin reuptake inhibitor; NSAID, non-steroidal anti-inflammatory drug; ACE, angiotensin-converting enzyme inhibitors; HRT, hormone replacement therapy.

Central vestibular disorders

Cerebrovascular disease

Cerebrovascular disease is most commonly secondary to atheroma, although giant cell arteritis should be considered in the elderly. The vertebrobasilar circulation supplies the peripheral vestibular apparatus as described earlier, but also supplies the vestibular nuclei. These nuclei occupy a large area in the lateral zone of the brainstem and are particularly susceptible to a reduction in the blood flow of the main basilar artery and the cerebellum, which is extremely important in modulating information required for balance at the level of the vestibular nuclei. The vertebral and internal carotid arteries provide the brain with a rich blood supply and the terminal branches anastomose to form the circle of Willis. This forms an anatomical safeguard against ischaemia arising from narrowing of one vessel and, in addition, there are autoregulatory mechanisms within the cerebral circulation protecting it from fluctuations in the systemic blood pressure. Nonetheless, cerebrovascular disease is one of the most common causes of chronic disability and death. In addition, white-matter changes due to vascular ischaemic damage produce gait disorders and also cognitive impairment, both of which predispose to falls.

Vertebrobasilar artery ischaemia

Episodic vertigo in an elderly patient is commonly ascribed to vertebrobasilar insufficiency, in the knowledge that cerebrovascular disease is common in the elderly and also on the basis that vertigo and/or dizziness have been reported as the first and most frequent symptom of this condition.[24, 25] The classical symptoms of vertebrobasilar insufficiency include dizziness/vertigo, dysarthria, numbness of the face, hemiparesis, headache, dysphagia, sensory disturbance, cerebellar ataxia and visual disturbances. The diversity of symptoms and signs reflects the close proximity of cranial nerve nuclei and motor and sensory tracts, within the small confines of the brainstem. The duration of transient ischaemic attacks in the vertebrobasilar territory may be variable, but by definition must be without actual infarction and less than 24 h. They may recur at variable intervals and may or may not be stereotyped.

Classical attacks of vertebrobasilar artery ischaemia associated with vertigo do not present a diagnostic problem. In this context, it is important to emphasize that dizziness or vertigo, accompanied by only VIIIth nerve manifestations, is unlikely to be of vascular origin. Moreover, tinnitus and deafness are unusual manifestations of vertebrobasilar ischaemia and, if present, are almost always accompanied by other symptoms and signs of brainstem involvement. Despite the presence of vestibular and oculomotor abnormalities in vertebrobasilar ischaemia, no characteristic pattern of neuro-otological findings has emerged in this disorder. Hence isolated episodes of rotational vertigo in an elderly patient should not be ascribed to vertebrobasilar insufficiency, unless there is other neurological evidence to support this diagnosis.

Completed strokes (see Chapter 57, Acute stroke care and management of carotid artery stenosis)

Completed strokes in the vertebrobasilar territory may involve the vestibular nuclei and there are a number of well-recognized syndromes. The Wallenberg or lateral medullary syndrome may result from occlusion of the posterior inferior cerebellar artery or the vertebral artery.[24] The syndrome is characterized by acute rotational vertigo with nausea and vomiting and ipsilateral dissociated sensory loss in the distribution of the facial nerve, together with contralateral truncal loss and ipsilateral cerebellar ataxia, bulbar palsy and Horner syndrome. Specific visuo-vestibular abnormalities have been identified with Wallenberg syndrome, including spontaneous rotatory nystagmus, with the fast phase directed towards the normal side, tonic deviation of the eyes towards the side of the lesion, with loss of fixation, voluntary and involuntary saccades of larger amplitude in the direction of the lesion and asymmetry of smooth pursuit, optokinetic and vestibular responses as a result of the interaction between spontaneous nystagmus and/or slow eye movements. Pontine/medullary and cerebellar haemorrhages may involve the vestibular apparatus. In the former, there are multiple brainstem signs and vertigo is usually a fleeting event, although a common presenting symptom, before the patient becomes unconscious. Cerebellar haemorrhage presents with acute vertigo, vomiting and an inability to stand, in the presence of cerebellar signs. The importance of rapid diagnosis lies in the ability to correct this condition surgically. Without rapid intervention, the patient dies from brainstem compression.

Cervical vertigo

Cervical vertigo is defined as vertigo induced by changes of position of the neck in relation to the body.[26] There is much controversy as to the underlying pathophysiology of cervical vertigo, but sympathetic irritation resulting in vertebrobasilar ischaemia, intermittent vertebral artery compression by osteophytes caused by cervical spondylosis and deranged sensory input from the cervical kinaesthetic receptors have been postulated. It is a widely held belief, particularly in the elderly, that vertigo and nystagmus may result from vertebrobasilar ischaemia, secondary to compression of blood vessels, as a result of arthritic changes in the neck. This seems unlikely noting the observations that unilateral, or indeed bilateral, compression of the vertebral arteries in the presence of a normal circle of Willis and internal carotid arteries produces only minimal brainstem ischaemia. It should be emphasized that radiological findings may prove misleading, as osteoarthritic changes in the cervical vertebrae are common in the elderly and not directly related to symptomatology. Neuro-otological tests in patients suspected of having cervical vertigo are frequently normal and no specific assessment objectively defines the condition. The diagnosis will be facilitated with the development of a specific test defining specific abnormalities.

Neoplasia

Dizziness and/or vertigo are early or initial symptoms in 25% of brainstem tumours. In later life, metastases are the most common neoplasms involving the brainstem and/or cerebellum, which give rise to vestibular dysfunction. Brainstem lesions typically present with progressive cranial nerve palsies together with long tract signs, whereas midline cerebellar lesions give rise to truncal ataxia and oculomotor abnormalities, including impaired smooth pursuit, saccadic dysmetria and rebound nystagmus.[4] Hemispheric cerebellar lesions cause ataxia of the ipsilateral limbs with truncal ataxia. Temporal lobe tumours give rise to 'disequilibrium' more frequently than in any other cortical site. This is not surprising as the temporal lobes exert a modifying influence upon the vestibular nuclei. Cerebellopontine angle lesions and, in particular, acoustic neurinomas (vestibular schwannomas) have been mentioned above, but are a rare cause of vestibular symptoms. Acoustic neurinomas (vestibular schwannomas) arise mainly on the vestibular division of the VIIIth cranial nerve and as they expand in the cerebellopontine angle, there is involvement of the Vth and VIIth cranial nerves, together with ipsilateral cerebellar signs and ultimately lower cranial nerve involvement. If surgical intervention is not undertaken, brainstem compression results in death.

Infection

Although tuberculosis is no longer a common disorder in developed countries, the possibility of a tuberculoma in the brainstem, cerebellopontine angle or temporal lobe should be borne in mind, especially in elderly immigrants and in elderly, debilitated or alcoholic patients. Neurosyphilis may involve the vestibular apparatus at all stages of the disease.[27] A high index of suspicion is necessary if rare cases in the elderly are not to be missed.

Neurological conditions

Many neurological disorders may affect the central vestibular connections and a discussion of each is beyond the scope of this chapter. In the elderly, of special note are Parkinson's disease, cerebellar disease and multisystem atrophies. Migraine is an important cause of various forms of episodic vertigo and may occur at any time throughout life.[28] The vertigo may last a few minutes or several hours and in 32% of patients vertigo and headache are not contemporaneous. The symptoms often resolve with effective antimigrainous treatment. The importance of the cerebellar connections on the vestibular system in terms of maintaining balance and eye position has been emphasized. Neuro-otological abnormalities in cerebellar disease are well defined.[29] Cerebellar degeneration may be seen in the elderly in association with malignancy (paraneoplastic syndrome), phenytoin intoxication, hereditary ataxias, alcoholism and myxoedema. Early diagnosis may lead to effective treatment in these groups. Of importance in the elderly, Paget's disease may give rise to basilar impression which may be accompanied by vertigo. The neurological symptoms produced by spinal cord and cerebellar compression together with obstruction of the fourth ventricle usually overshadow the vestibular disorder.

This review of vestibular disorders in the elderly has concentrated on the more common vestibular pathologies affecting this age group, but it must be emphasized that any vestibular disorder may occur and conditions such as endolymphatic hydrops, migraine and multiple sclerosis should not be overlooked.

Management

The initial management of a patient must be directed at establishing the presence of an underlying diagnosis for which specific treatment may be instituted. A number of elderly patients will be found to have minor visual impairment, which should be corrected if possible. If there is proprioceptive impairment that is predominantly in the lower limbs, it may be helpful to provide a walking stick to obtain additional proprioceptive information through the upper limbs. In addition, assistive devices and interventions for preventing falls should be considered. The management of peripheral vestibular dysfunction consists in counselling and vestibular rehabilitation exercises.[30] Drug therapy may be of value in the management of acute vertigo, but has no place in the long-term management of chronic vestibular symptoms, as it delays compensation. Symptoms of disequilibrium are especially disturbing for the elderly, not only because they fear some sinister pathology but also because they are terrified of the consequences of repeated attacks of vertigo during which they may be unable to summon outside assistance. It is therefore extremely important to obtain a detailed history, carry out a full examination and appropriate investigations and give a simple and clear explanation of the underlying cause of symptoms of disequilibrium and the therapeutic options that are available. Chronic vestibular symptoms may be caused by central vestibular pathology or uncompensated peripheral vestibular disorders. The management of central vestibular dysfunction remains poorly understood, but a trial of cinnarizine, clonazepam, baclofen, gabapentin or carbamazepine may prove of value. The sedative side effects of these drugs should be recalled in the elderly and the dose titrated against sedation. In patients with a sense of instability and falls, which are frequently associated with basal ganglia disorders and cerebellar disease, physiotherapy to teach alternative gait strategies may prove invaluable in enabling the patient to regain a sense of confidence and improve their mobility.

Vertigo associated with peripheral vestibular disorders may either be attributable to specific conditions, for which there is a recognized treatment regime, or a specific aetiology may not be identified despite the evidence of peripheral vestibular dysfunction on standard vestibular tests. The treatment of specific otological disorders is no different in the elderly to any other age group and the reader is referred to standard otology texts. Persistent vestibular symptoms due to peripheral labyrinthine dysfunction are frequently amenable to vestibular rehabilitation and it cannot be overemphasized that destructive surgical procedures should not be considered, particularly in the elderly, until detailed neuro-otological investigations determining the site of lesion and exhaustive medical management have been tried. There is no reason to assume that a patient will compensate more efficiently from a total labyrinthine destruction than from a partial impairment of vestibular function, particularly when it is likely that the failure of compensation in the elderly may be due to mild central processing disorders or unsuspected psychological factors.

Acute vertigo associated with nausea and vomiting requires immediate treatment with an anti-emetic such as prochlorperazine, by buccal absorption, intramuscularly or by suppository, or metoclopramide intramuscularly, such that nausea and vomiting are alleviated. This allows the administration of a vestibular sedative, of which cinnarizine 15 mg every 8 h is the treatment of choice. Again, in the elderly patient, sedative side effects must be carefully monitored and the dose adjusted accordingly.

Chronic or recurrent vertigo, associated with poorly compensated peripheral pathology (Figure 87.7), is frequently accompanied by secondary symptoms of psychological distress (anxiety, depression and phobic symptoms), malaise, fatigue and cervical pain related to tension in neck muscles, as a result of conscious or subconscious limitation of neck movements, which are likely to precipitate an increase in vertiginous symptoms. The development of psychological symptoms in patients with disequilibrium is now well recognized,[3] and appropriate psychological support in the form of behavioural therapy or psychiatric care is essential for patients who manifest psychological symptoms if optimal vestibular compensation is to be achieved.

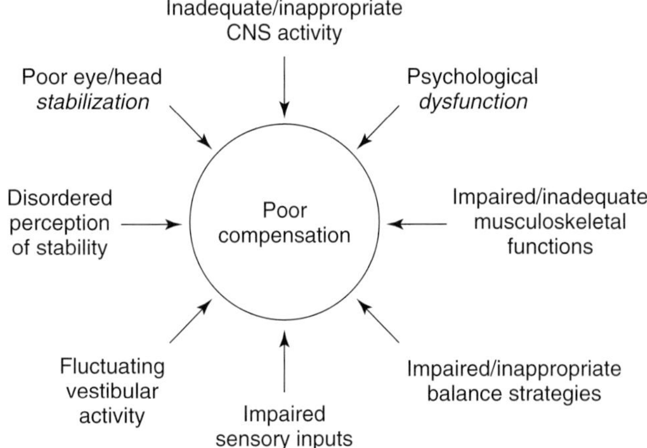

Figure 87.7 Factors predisposing to decompensation. After Shumway-Cook and Horak.[30]

This is particularly important in the elderly age group, who are more likely to be susceptible than their younger counterparts and are therefore deeply concerned by disorders that impair their physical abilities and threaten their independence.

As early as the mid-1940s, physical exercise regimes (the *Cawthorne–Cooksey exercises*) were introduced as a means of expediting recovery from peripheral vestibular disorders. These exercises are a graduated series of exercises aimed at encouraging head and eye movements, which provoke dizziness in a systematic manner and facilitate vestibular compensation. The exercises are not an endurance test and for the elderly patient it is important to modify the regime within the limits of the patient's physical abilities. The passage of time has supported the efficacy of these exercises and successful vestibular rehabilitation improves activities of daily living and reduces fall risk. Significant improvement has been shown in patients with peripheral vestibular dysfunction, but also in patients with central balance disorders. Moreover, there is no evidence that age is a negative prognostic factor. Recent work has suggested that 'customized' exercises, tailored to the individual patient, are equally effective. Specific positional manoeuvres for the management of benign positional vertigo (Epley and Semont manoeuvres) have been described earlier and form an important element of vestibular management.

A combination of canalith repositioning manoeuvre and vestibular rehabilitation has been shown to improve benign positional vertigo in the elderly. Although repositioning manoeuvre is the most effective treatment, vestibular rehabilitation can be added to improve the results in the treatment, particularly with regard to the high recurrence of positional vertigo. As noted previously, vestibular sedatives such as cinnarizine are of value in the management of acute vertigo, but have a very limited role in the management of chronic vestibular syndromes. In particular, anti-emetics such as prochlorperazine should be avoided, because of the rare but irreversible syndrome of extrapyramidal dysfunction. Moreover, psychotropic drugs should be administered only for specific psychiatric indications, as such medication may interfere with compensatory mechanisms for peripheral vestibular disorders. In the elderly, the indications for otological surgery for vestibular disorders must be carefully weighed against the general medical state of the patient and the likely extent of recovery postoperatively. Ludman's excellent review of the surgical treatment of vestibular disorders outlines the various techniques available.[21] As has already been noted, compensation may be prolonged or indeed incomplete as a result of dysfunction of the integrating ability of the CNS and/or other sensory modalities. The risk of a persisting imbalance after vestibular destruction must therefore be borne in mind.

Key points

- Do not attribute vertigo to 'age'.
- A thorough history and examination will often provide a clear direction as to diagnosis.
- Correct diagnosis allows the treatment of many of the peripheral and central vestibular disorders.
- Introduce vestibular rehabilitation/gait strategy exercises in the elderly early and aggressively.
- Destructive surgical procedures should not be considered until detailed neuro-otological investigation and medical management have been tried exhaustively.

References

1. Jonsson R, Sixt E, Landahl S and Rosenhall U. Prevalence of dizziness and vertigo in an urban elderly population. *J Vestib Res* 2004;**14**:47–52.
2. O'Loughlin JL, Robitaille Y, Boivin JF and Suissa S. Incidence of and risk factors for falls and injurious falls among the community dwelling elderly. *Am J Epidemiol* 1993;**1**:342–54.
3. Burker EJ, Wong H, Sloane PD *et al.* Predictors of fear of falling in dizzy and nondizzy elderly. *Psychol Aging* 1995;**10**:104–10.
4. Savundra P and Luxon LM. The physiology of equilibrium and its application in the dizzy patient. In: AG Kerr (ed.), *Scott-Brown's Otolaryngology*, vol. 1, 6th edn, Butterworth, London, 1997.
5. Enrietto JA, Jacobson KM and Baloh RW. Aging effects on auditory and vestibular responses: a longitudinal study. *Am J Otolaryngol* 1999;**20**:371–8.
6. Nadol JB Jr and Schuknecht HF. Pathology of peripheral vestibular disorders in the elderly. *Am J Otolaryngol* 1990;**11**,213–27.
7. Kazmierczak H, Pawlak-Osinska K and Osinski P. Visuoocular reflexes in presbyvertigo. *Int Tinnitus J* 2001;**7**:112–4.
8. Baloh RW. Dizziness in older people. *J Am Geriatr Soc* 1992;**40**:713–21.
9. Bronstein AM. Vision and vertigo; some visual aspects of vestibular disorders. *J Neurol* 2004;**251**:381–7.
10. Eggers SD and Zee DS. Evaluating the dizzy patient: bedside examination and laboratory assessment of the vestibular system. *Semin Neurol* 2003;**23**:47–58.
11. Schubert MC, Tusa RJ, Grine LE and Herdman SJ. Optimizing the sensitivity of the head thrust test for identifying vestibular hypofunction. *Phys Ther* 2004;**84**:151–8.
12. Baloh RW, Jacobson KM, Enrietto JA *et al.* Balance disorders in older persons: quantification with posturography. *Otolaryngol Head Neck Surg* 1998;**119**:89–92.
13. Strupp M and Brandt T. Vestibular neuritis. *Semin Neurol* 2009;**29**:509–19.

14. Minor LB. Labyrinthine fistulae: pathobiology and management. *Curr Opin Otolaryngol Head Neck Surg* 2003;**11**: 340–6.

15. Aparicio A and Chamberlain MC. Neoplastic meningitis. *Curr Neurol Neurosci Rep* 2002;**2**:225–35.

16. Luxon LM. Post-traumatic vertigo. In: RW Baloh and M Halmagyi (eds), *Handbook of Neuro-otology/Vestibular System*, Oxford University Press, New York, 1996, pp. 381–95.

17. Brandt T and Steddin S. Current view of the mechanism of benign paroxysmal positioning vertigo: cupulolithiasis or canalolithiasis. *J Vestib Res* 1993;**3**:373–82.

18. Baloh RW. Clinical features and pathophysiology of posterior canal benign positional vertigo. *Audiol Med* 2005;**3**:12–5.

19. Brandt T and Daroff RB. Physical therapy for benign positional vertigo. *Arch Otolaryngol* 1980;**106**:484–5.

20. Epley JM. The canalith repositioning procedure: for treatment of benign paroxysmal positional vertigo. *Otolaryngol Head Neck Surg* 1992;**107**:399–404.

21. Ludman H. Vestibular disorders. In: H Ludman and T Wright (eds), *Diseases of the Ear*, Oxford University Press, New York, 1998, pp. 516–34.

22. Ballester M, Liard P, Vibert D and Hausler R. Menière's disease in the elderly. *Otol Neurotol* 2002;**23**:73–8.

23. Schubert MC and Minor LB. Vestibulo-ocular physiology underlying vestibular hypofunction. *Phys Ther* 2004;**84**:373–85.

24. Brandt T. Vascular vertigo. In: T Brandt (ed.), *Vertigo: its Multisensory Syndromes*, Spinger, New York, 1999, pp. 301–24.

25. Caplan LR. Vertebrobasilar disease. *Adv Neurol* 2003; **92**:131–40.

26. Brandt T. Cervical vertigo-reality or fiction? *Audiol Neuro-Otol* 1996;**1**:187–96.

27. Marra CM. Update on neurosyphilis. *Curr Infect Dis Rep* 2009;**11**:127–34.

28. Haan J, Hollander J and Ferrari MD Migraine in the elderly: a review. *Cephalalgia* 2007;**27**:97–106.

29. Baloh RW, Yee RD and Honrubia V. Late cortical cerebellar atrophy. Clinical and oculographic features in 240 cases. *Neurology* 1986;**37**:371–8.

30. Shumway-Cook A and Horak FB. Rehabilitation strategies for patients with vestibular deficits. *Neurol Clin North Am* 1990;**8**:441–57.

CHAPTER 88

Smell and taste

Richard L. Doty
Smell & Taste Center, University of Pennsylvania School of Medicine, Philadelphia, PA, USA

Introduction

Since 1900, the percentage of Americans over the age of 65 years has more than tripled (4.1% in 1900 to over 12% in 2000) and their number has increased over eleven times (from 3.1 million to 34.9 million).[1] Given the fact that the ability to perceive odours and tastes decreases markedly with age,[2] it is not surprising that increasing numbers of elderly patients are seeking medical help for their chemosensory problem. Indeed, over half the population between the ages of 65 and 80 years, and over three-quarters beyond 80 years, have significant olfactory loss. The implications of such age-related chemosensory losses are far-reaching. Aside from being unable to appreciate fragrances, the taste of food, and the freshness of spring and the seashore, elderly persons suffering from chemosensory disorders are compromised in their ability to detect fire, leaking natural gas, toxic fumes and spoiled food. Many become depressed, and a disproportionate number die in accidental gas poisonings.[3] Others lose their lives or are severely burned in the hundreds of butane and propane gas explosions that occur each year.

It is now well documented that olfactory dysfunction is among the first, if not the first, clinical signs of Alzheimer's disease and sporadic Parkinson's disease (for review, see Hawkes and Doty[4]). Although, as described later in this chapter, smell loss has multiple determinants and is not always a harbinger for such diseases, it is incumbent upon the physician to be aware of this association. Given the dietary and safety consequences of chemosensory disturbances, it is also incumbent upon the physician to employ the most modern means available to evaluate, counsel and treat patients with chemosensory disturbances whenever possible.

This chapter provides the gerontologist with an up-to-date overview of the nature and cause of age-related chemosensory disturbances, means for evaluating such disturbances, and approaches useful for counselling patients and treating the underlying dysfunction.

Characterization of chemosensory problems

The general term for inability to smell is anosmia, and for lessened smell function hyposmia. The corresponding terms for taste are ageusia and hypogeusia. In the older medical literature, anosmia is sometimes referred to as olfactory anaesthesia or anosphrasia. In some nosological schemes, anosmia and hyposmia are classified under the general term dysosmia (distorted smell function), whereas ageusia and hypogeusia are classified under the term dysgeusia (distorted taste function). In this scheme, dysosmia includes forms of dysfunction in addition to anosmia, such as distorted smell sensations (parosmia, cacosmia) and smell hallucinations (phantosmia). Dysgeusia similarly includes both ageusia and distortions in taste function, such as strong salty or sour sensations in the absence of appropriate stimulation. Today, however, it is more common that anosmia, ageusia, dysosmia and dysgeusia are classified separately from one another, with the first two terms signifying losses, and the second two distortions, of smell and taste sensations, respectively.

Anatomy of the olfactory system

To be sensed, odorants must enter the nose and reach specialized receptors within the olfactory neuroepithelium, a patch of tissue a few square centimetres in size that lines the upper recesses of the nasal vault, including the cribriform plate and sectors of the nasal septum, middle turbinate and superior turbinate[5] (Figure 88.1). When activated, the odorant receptors open or close (e.g. via second-messenger systems) membrane channels on the cilia, resulting in a flux of ions and an alteration of the cell's resting potential that ultimate leads to an axonal action potential.[6] cAMP is the primary second messenger involved in the transduction process. cAMP amplifies the signal coming from the receptors and facilitates the release of glutamate, the main neurotransmitter of olfactory receptor cells, into the synapse.

Principles and Practice of Geriatric Medicine, Fifth Edition. Edited by Alan J. Sinclair, John E. Morley and Bruno Vellas.

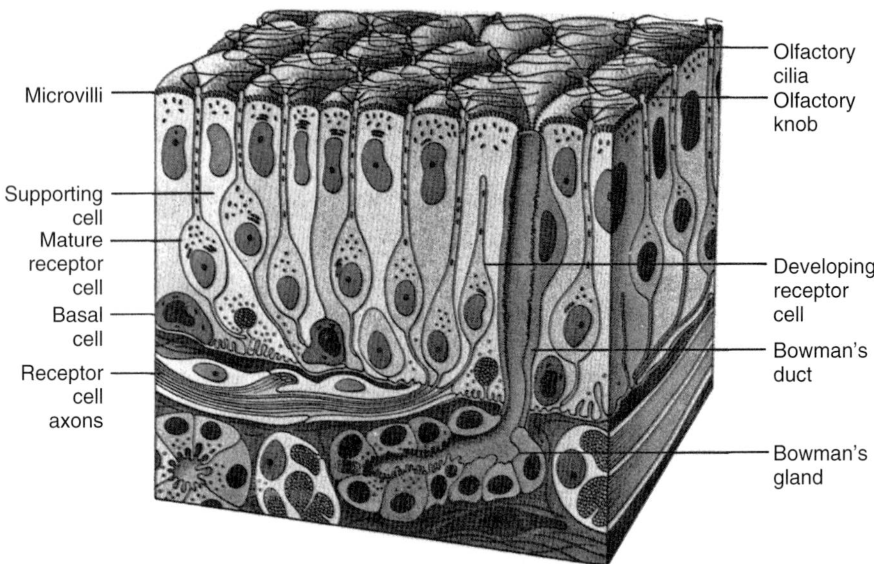

Figure 88.1 Schematic of the cellular organization of the human olfactory neuroepithelium. Not pictured are the microvillar cells, which are small goblet-shaped cells interspersed among the other cell types at the surface of the epithelium in a ratio to the mature receptor cells of 1:10. Reprinted from *Gray's Anatomy*, Warwick R and Williams PL, Copyright 1973, with permission from Elsevier.

Odorant receptor genes, whose discovery by Buck and Axel in 1991 led to the Nobel Prize for Medicine or Physiology in 2004,[7] represent the largest of all mammalian gene families, comprising nearly 3% of the more than 30 000 genes in the mouse and human genomes. Interestingly, only one type of receptor is expressed on the surface of the cilia of a given receptor cell, and odorants typically bind to more than one type of receptor. The olfactory receptor cells number 6–10 million in the adult human and are insulated from one another at the epithelial surface by sustentacular cells.[5] A blanket of mucus, which contains a number of enzymes (e.g. cytochrome P450), covers the olfactory neuroepithelium and deactivates or filters materials that absorb into the mucus, including some odorants.[8] This mucus also aids in protecting the epithelium from desiccation, heat and xenobiotic insult, and serves as a solvent and carrier for odorant binding proteins – proteins that facilitate the transport of some lipophilic molecules to the receptors through aqueous phases of the mucus.

The unmyelinated axons of the bipolar olfactory receptor cells collect into 15–20 fascicles (fila olfactoria) that collectively make up the olfactory nerve (cranial nerve (CN) I). These axons course through the cribriform plate and synapse within spherical masses of neuropile within the olfactory bulb termed glomeruli. Second order connections with the dendrites of mitral and tufted cells are made within these structures. The latter cells – the primary output cells of the olfactory bulb – project to the olfactory cortex, which includes the piriform, periamygdaloid and entorhinal cortices. These structures have extensive connections with the hippocampus, mediodorsal thalamus, hypothalamus and other brain regions, in addition to having efferent connections with cells within the olfactory bulb.[4]

Most odorants stimulate a broad range of receptor cells. Although limited sets of such cells respond to a given odorant, overlap is common and the pattern of neuronal activity across cells codes odour quality. Receptor cells that express the same receptor project to the same glomerulus, where information is further transformed. The second-order neurons – the mitral and tufted cells – send dendritic processes into the glomeruli, where they synapse with the axons of the incoming receptor cells. The axons of the mitral and tufted cell project, via the lateral olfactory tract, to the olfactory cortex, where further connections occur with structures in which perceptual elements of odours are formed; that is, perceived pleasantness and associations with environmental objects. It is noteworthy that the olfactory system differs from other sensory systems in sending projections first to the cortex rather than to the thalamus. It also is unique in the degree to which it exhibits plasticity – the olfactory receptor cells have the propensity to regenerate from stem cells within the basement membrane, and cells within the olfactory bulb, namely the periglomerular cells and the granule cells, are continuously repopulated by cells that migrate from periventricular regions along the rostral migratory stream. Because olfactory receptor cells directly project from the environment of the nasal cavity into the brain, they are a major conduit for viruses and a range of xenobiotic agents into the brain and may initiate neurodegenerative pathology in genetically susceptible individuals.[9]

In addition to the sensory innervation of the olfactory nerve, free nerve endings of the trigeminal nerve (CN V) are distributed throughout the nasal mucosa. The ophthalmic and maxillary divisions of CN V carry information regarding irritation, temperature and pungency. Sensations mediated by non-CN I nerves are those of the 'common chemical sense' and do not encode the qualitative perception of 'odour', *per se*.[10] Although humans possess a rudimentary vomeronasal (Jacobson's organ) pouch at the base of the nasal septum, the elements of this system are vestigial and humans lack an accessory olfactory bulb which would normally receive a projection from this structure. Despite fanfare to the contrary, it is questionable whether humans – indeed mammals in general – communicate by so-called pheromones.[11]

Anatomy of the gustatory system

Taste receptor cells are located within taste buds on the tongue, soft palate, uvula, epiglottis, rostral oesophagus and mucous membranes of the laryngeal cartilages. Most lingual taste buds are found imbedded in the surface of protuberances termed papillae. Fungiform papillae are prevalent on the anterior tongue, circumvallate papillae within the chevron of the posterior tongue, and foliate papillae within the lateral margins of the medial tongue separating the anterior and posterior sectors[12] (Figure 88.2).

The sense of taste is supplied by three cranial nerves: the facial nerve (CN VII), the glossopharyngeal nerve (CN IX), and vagus nerve (CN X). As shown in Figure 88.2, the taste buds on the fungiform papillae are supplied by the chorda tympani branch of CN VII, whereas the taste buds on the other types of taste papillae are supplied by the lingual branch of CN IX. Although it is generally believed that the innervation of CN IX is limited to the posterior third of the tongue, recent studies suggest that it may project afferent fibres beyond this posterior boundary.[13] Taste buds located on the soft palate send their projections centrally via the greater superficial petrosal branch of CN VII and those on the epiglottis, oesophagus and larynx transmit taste information by way of the superior laryngeal branch of CN X. As in the case of olfaction, trigeminal (CN V) free nerve endings, distributed throughout the oral cavity, mediate somatosensory sensations (e.g. pungency, burning, sharpness). All branches of the gustatory nerves enter the brainstem and terminate in the rostral part of the nucleus of the solitary tract. The subsequent projections are not thoroughly understood in humans; however, connections are made with the ventral posteriormedial thalamus and insular cortex. In rodents, fibres from the pons also travel to areas involved in feeding and autonomic regulation,

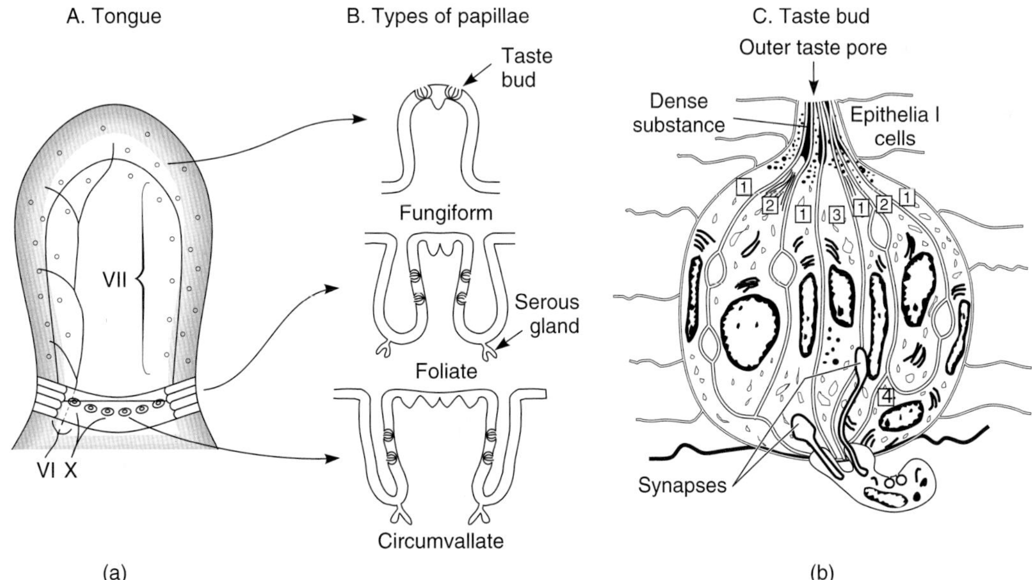

Figure 88.2 (a) and (b) Schematic of the distribution of taste buds on the human tongue. Taste buds of the fungiform and foliate papillae are innervated by CN VII. Those of the circumvallate papillae are innervated by CN IX. CN V carries non-taste somatosensory sensations. See text for details. (c) Schematic of fine structure of taste bud. (1) and (2) are presumably supporting cells that secrete materials into the lumen of the bud; (3) is a sensory receptor cell; and (4) a basal cell from which other cell types arise. Image courtesy of RG Murray, 1973. Copyright RG Murray.

including the lateral hypothalamus, central amygdala and stria terminalis.[14]

Clinical tests of olfactory and gustatory function

The physician of the past assessed the ability to smell by asking a patient to sniff vials containing one or two odorants such as coffee or tobacco, and to report whether or not an odour is perceived. The analogous taste test was to sprinkle grains of sugar or salt onto the tongue, and ask about the corresponding sensations. Unfortunately, such procedures are akin to testing vision by shining a flashlight into the eye, or audition by sounding a bull horn next to the ear. This problem is not corrected, in the case of olfaction, by having the patient attempt to identify the presented odorants, since without cuing even normal subjects have difficulty identifying most odorants. In the case of taste, non-solubilized tastants are often not recognized by patients whose mouths are dry, or who have little time to dissolve the tastants into saliva.

During the last 25 years remarkable progress has been made in the development of reliable, valid and clinically practical olfactory tests. Physicians and insurance carriers are now aware, more than ever, that objective chemosensory assessment is essential for (a) establishing the validity of a patient's complaint, (b) characterizing the specific nature of a chemosensory problem, (c) accurately monitoring medical or surgical interventions, (d) detecting malingering, (e) counselling patients to help cope with their problem, and (f) assigning disability compensation. Importantly, accurate assessment decreases the costs of continuing treatment seeking on the part of patients, who are usually assumed to have a problem even in the absence of objective data.

It should be noted that patients have difficulty ascribing the degree of their olfactory or gustatory dysfunction unless total or near-total loss is apparent. In the case of taste, for example, questionnaire statements such as 'I can detect salt in chips, pretzels, or salted nuts', 'I can detect sourness in vinegar, pickles, or lemon', 'I can detect sweetness in soda, cookies, or ice cream', and 'I can detect bitterness, in coffee, beer, or tonic water' are relatively insensitive in detecting true cases of dysfunction. However, such questions are sensitive in detecting persons without such problems (i.e. they exhibit low positive but high negative predictive value).[15]

Several commercially available tests of olfactory function are now available, including tests of odour detection and identification (for review, see Doty, 2001).[16] The most widely used of these tests (the University of Pennsylvania Smell Identification Test or UPSIT: commercially termed the Smell Identification Test™, Sensonics, Inc., Haddon Hts, NJ) was developed at our centre and evaluates the ability of patients to identify, from sets of four descriptors, each of 40 'scratch and sniff' odorants[2] (Figure 88.3). The number of items correctly identified out of 40 serves as the test score. This measure is compared to norms based upon data from a large number of individuals sampled from the community at large and a percentile rank is determined, depending upon the age and gender of the patient. This test, which correlates strongly with traditional threshold tests, is amenable to self-administration and provides a means for detecting malingering. Commercially available taste tests with high reliability, validity and practicality are now being developed for use by physicians,[17,18] and electrogustometry, which has been available for a number of years, provides quantitative assessments of taste function that are correlated with the number of underlying taste buds.[19]

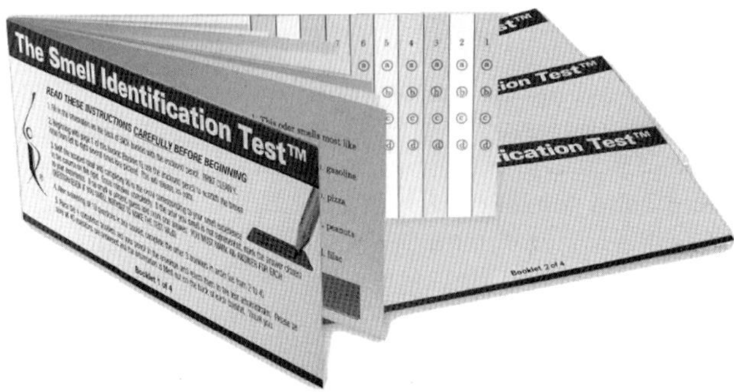

Figure 88.3 The 40-odorant, self-administered, University of Pennsylvania Smell Identification Test (UPSIT). Each page contains a microencapsulated odorant that is released by means of a pencil tip. Answers are marked on the columns on the last page of each booklet. Copyright 2004, Sensonics, Inc., Haddon Heights, NJ 08035.

Traditionally, physicians have assumed that if a patient presenting with the complaint of anosmia fails to report the presence of an irritating vapour via CN V, he or she is malingering. However, this test is not foolproof, as even the most ardent malingerer rarely denies not perceiving a strong irritating substance, particularly one which leads to reflexive mucous secretion or eye watering. Furthermore, trigeminal thresholds to chemicals can be quite variable among individuals. Thus, a more valid means for detecting malingering is to determine the percentage of responses to stimuli that are correct in a forced-choice situation where chance responding can be calculated. When significantly fewer correct responses than expected on the basis of chance responding are demonstrated, malingering is suspected.

Age-related changes in olfactory function

The now well-established age-related decline in olfactory function is exemplified in Figure 88.4.[2] As can be seen in this figure, considerable average decline occurs in the

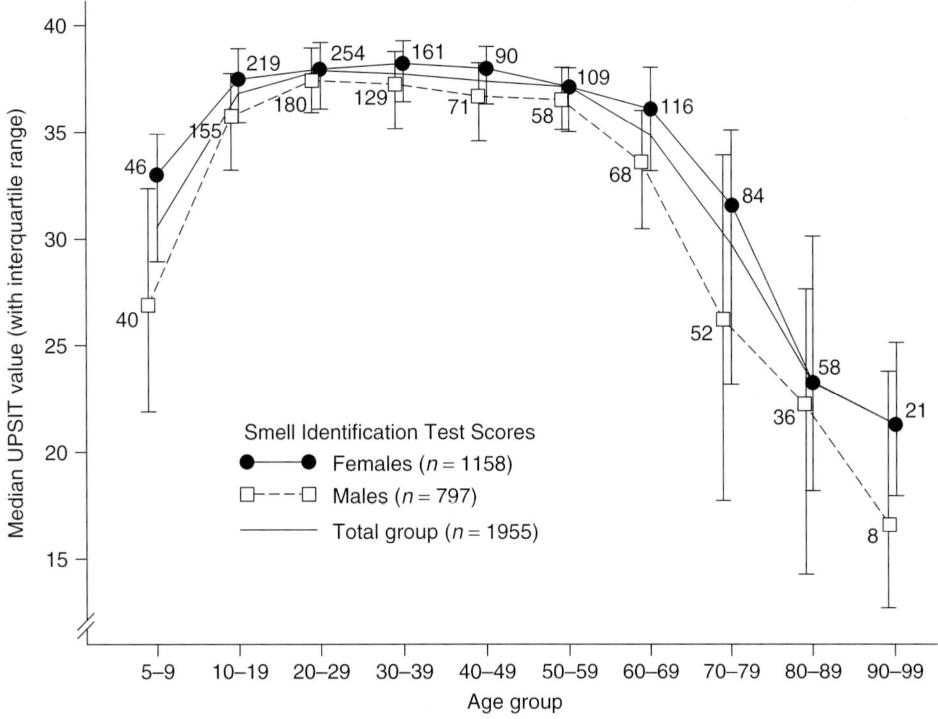

Figure 88.4 Scores on the University of Pennsylvania Smell Identification Test (UPSIT) as a function of age in a large heterogeneous group of subjects. Numbers by data points indicate sample sizes. Reprinted with permission from Doty RL et al., Smell identification ability: changes with age. *Science;***226**:1441–3. Copyright 1984 AAAS.

ability to identify odours in persons after the age of 60 years. In general, olfactory identification ability peaks, for both men and women, during the third to fifth decades of life and significantly declines in the seventh decade. Women outperform men at all ages, with the gender gap increasing in later years.[21]

It is not known to what extent such age-related changes in olfactory function represent the process of ageing, *per se*, or alterations in the chemosensory systems brought about by factors correlated with age (i.e. cumulative viral insults, repeated exposures to environmental agents and air pollutants, alterations in trophic factors, the early progression of neurodegenerative disease pathology, etc.). It is now clear that cumulative exposure to high levels of air pollution significantly alters the ability to smell and may well contribute to neurodegenerative disease pathology.[20] Age-related declines occurs, however, in all cultures, although large individual differences are present, and women, on average, maintain function later in life than men.

Age-related changes in gustatory function

Taste function, like olfactory function, also declines over the lifespan. Older persons show decreased ability to discern sweet, sour, bitter and salty tasting agents, including a number of amino acids at both threshold and suprathreshold levels. Functionally, however, such a decrease has much less impact on the individual than olfactory loss, since whole-mouth tests often show only moderate declines in age-related function.[22] This is due, in part, to the fact that the taste buds in different regions of the mouth are innervated by several different sets of cranial nerves. Such nerves are less susceptible to insult than the fine olfactory filaments. In the case of head trauma, for example, total ageusia, as measured by whole-mouth testing, is rare (<0.5 %), compared to total anosmia.[23] Nevertheless, studies that have tested well-defined localized regions of the tongue to brief presentations of stimuli report marked age-related dysfunction[24] (Figure 88.5). Such losses may be particularly significant for foodstuffs which minimally leach chemicals during mastication.

It is of interest that damage to the chorda tympani nerve, which innervates the anterior tongue, increases the sensitivity of the glossopharyngeal nerve, which innervates more posterior regions of the tongue.[25,26] This phenomenon likely ensures that limited lingual nerve damage does not place an individual at risk from an inability to taste toxic agents, particularly bitter tasting ones. Some dysgeusias seen in the elderly may reflect such release of inhibition.[27] Chorda tympani damage can occur from a number of factors, including

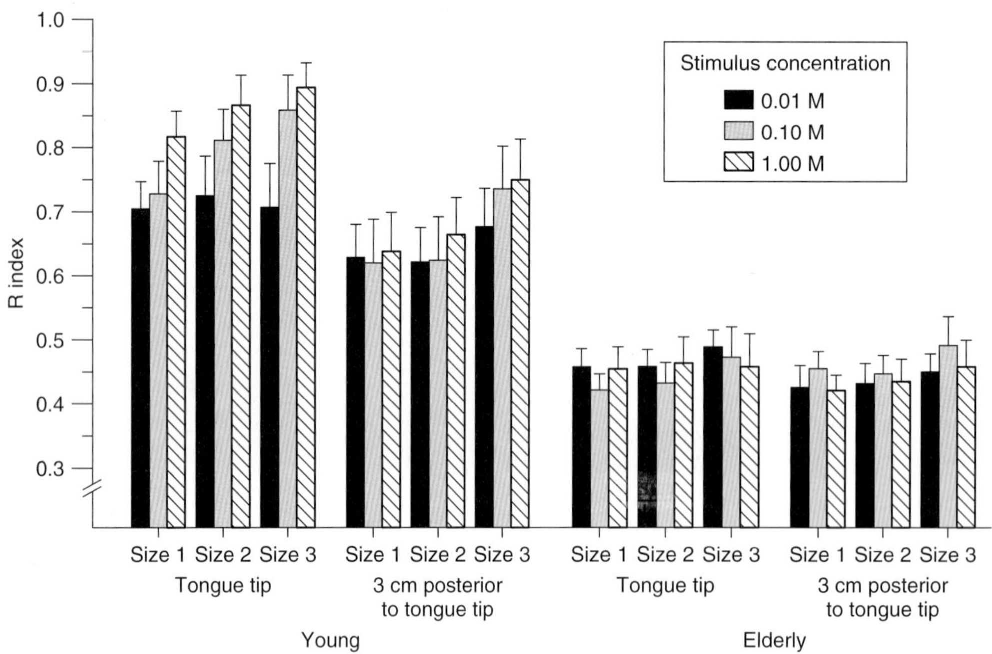

Figure 88.5 Mean (±SEM) sensitivity values (R index) obtained from 12 young and 12 elderly subjects for sodium chloride stimuli presented to the tongue tip and to a medial tongue region 3 cm posterior to the tongue tip for three stimulation areas (12.5, 25, 50 mm^2) and three stimulus concentrations. The sensitivity of the elderly subjects was at near-chance levels and the sensitivity did not increase as either a function of the stimulus area or concentration. Note also that, unlike the case with the young subjects, the tongue tip of the elderly subjects was no more sensitive than the tongue region 3 cm posterior to the tongue tip. Reproduced from Matsuda and Doty,[24] by permission of Oxford University Press.

wisdom tooth removal and ear infections, such as otitis media, experienced early in life.[28]

It is important for the clinician to be aware that complaints of loss of 'taste' usually reflect the loss of flavour sensations derived from retronasal stimulation of the olfactory receptors.[29,23] Thus, other than basic sweet, sour, salty and bitter sensations (or possibly metallic or 'Umami' sensations) or temperature or textural sensations (sharpness, pungency, burning, etc.), the rich experiences attributed to 'taste' are really due to molecules which enter the nose from the oral cavity via the nasal pharynx. Among the hundreds of 'tastes' which are really due to stimulation of CN I are banana, chocolate, strawberry, pizza sauce, vanilla, root beer, cola, liquorice, steak sauce, steak, fried chicken, apples and lemon.

Causes of smell dysfunction in the elderly

The olfactory receptors are rather directly exposed to the outside environment, making them susceptible to insult from bacteria, viruses, toxic agents and other nosogenic stimuli. For this reason, it is not surprising that environmentally induced damage to the olfactory epithelium appears to be the most common cause of age-related decrements in the ability to smell. Indeed, cumulative destruction of the olfactory epithelium occurs over the course of one's life with metaplasia from respiratory-like epithelium appearing as islands within the membrane.[30] However, age-related functional or structural changes may also directly damage the epithelium or predispose it to damage from environmental insults, such as from influenza. Potential changes include reduced protein synthesis or metabolic insufficiency (as in hypothyroidism), changes in the vascular elasticity of the epithelium, altered airway patency, decreased intramucosal blood flow, loss of neurotrophic factors, occlusion of cribriform plate foramina through which the olfactory nerve axons project, increased viscosity of the nasal mucus, atrophy of secretory glands and lymphatics, and, potentially, decreases in enzyme systems that deactivate xenobiotic materials within the olfactory mucosa.[31]

The vast majority of elderly patients complaining of a smell deficit can be classified into one of six proximal aetiologic categories: (i) nasal/paranasal sinus disease; (ii) prior upper respiratory infection (URI); (iii) head trauma; (iv) Alzheimer's disease; (v) Parkinson's disease; or (vi) idiopathic.

Nasal/paranasal sinus disease

Inflammation of the nasal cavity and sinuses (e.g. chronic sinusitis, allergic rhinitis, bacterial rhinitis, viral rhinitis) reduces upper airway patency, thereby restricting odorant access to the olfactory neuroepithelium. Additionally, structural abnormalities such as marked sepal deviation (particularly with adhesions to the turbinates), polyps and neoplasms can lead to decreased olfactory sensitivity. Even individuals with a moderate degree of ostiomeatal disease, without intranasal polyps, may complain of olfactory loss.[32] The loss of smell can be quite severe in patients with nasal sinus disease, with most being anosmic or profoundly hyposmic. These patients are more likely to describe a gradual onset of olfactory loss than are those patients whose loss is due to prior upper respiratory infections. Fluctuations in smell sensitivity are also characteristic of nasal sinus disease. For example, nasal decongestion from exercise, hot showers or medications may temporarily improve the sense of smell. Administration of corticosteroids (particularly systemic) typically improves smell function in this group of patients and can be used to diagnose olfactory loss due to nasal sinus disease when function is still present. Unfortunately, sustained corticosteroid treatment is not medically indicated in most cases and chronic nasal sinus disease can lead to damage to the olfactory mucosa.[33] Once such damage occurs, olfactory function is not improved by administration of an anti-inflammatory agent. It is encouraging, however, that olfactory dysfunction arising from nasal sinus disease is often amenable to treatment. Management of allergies, sinusitis and structural abnormalities through medication or endoscopic surgery can alleviate smell loss in a number of these patients.

Prior upper respiratory infections

Upper respiratory infections are the most common cause of permanent decreased olfaction in persons older than 50 years.[23] The diagnosis of viral-induced olfactory dysfunction is based upon a history of a viral illness prior to the onset of olfactory loss in combination with the absence of other aetiologic factors. Patients will often describe an olfactory deficit during a 'cold' that was more severe than usual. After recuperation from the illness, however, the sense of smell does not return. These patients are more likely to experience a non-fluctuating hyposmia in comparison with the fluctuating anosmia of patients with nasal sinus disease.

Whether viral-induced smell loss is reflective of the age-related resistance to viral insult or a culmination of repeated insults to the olfactory neuroepithelium (or both) is unknown. Olfactory biopsies in individuals with olfactory dysfunction secondary to tipper respiratory infections demonstrate a decrease in the number of olfactory receptor cells, extensive scarring and islands of metaplasia from respiratory-like epithelium.[5] These characteristics are frequently evidenced in the olfactory epithelium of elderly individuals, suggesting the possibility that cumulative viral insults over time may be one basis for their overall loss, even if a precipitating event cannot be identified or differs from a viral infection.

Currently, no well-established treatments are available for viral-induced chronic anosmia or hyposmia. Nevertheless, there is evidence that some slight improvement occurs over time in approximately half of individuals with this problem, although return to normal function is relatively rare. In one study, for example, 11.31% of anosmic and 23.31% of microsmic patients regained normal age-related function over time.[34]

Head trauma

Most studies have reported incidence rates of smell loss following head trauma between 5 and 15%, although such estimates are not available from random samples of head injury patients at large.[35] Injuries that involve rapid acceleration/deceleration of the brain are most commonly associated with smell loss. Such coup/contrecoup movements lead to shearing or tearing of the olfactory nerve filaments at the level of the cribriform plate. Interestingly, occipital blows are more likely to produce smell loss than frontal blows, presumably because less soft tissue is available for absorbing the impact. It is not presently known whether equivalent head injuries in young and older persons produce equivalent degrees of damage to the olfactory pathways, although it would seem reasonable to expect the elderly to be more susceptible to such loss.

Smell loss in head trauma patients tends to be severe, as most are anosmic rather than hyposmic under objective testing. As with the case of viral-induced smell loss, prognosis depends upon the degree of initial dysfunction, with microsmic patients being more likely than anosmic patients to regain some function over time.[34] In many cases, scar tissue forms at the level of the cribriform plate, blocking entry of axons from regenerating olfactory neurons through the cribriform plate into the central nervous system.

Alzheimer's disease

Most individuals with even mild Alzheimer's disease (AD) demonstrate decreased olfactory function relative to age-matched controls. Physiological changes associated with normal ageing may be responsible, in part, for some of the AD-related olfactory dysfunction. However, even relatively young and early-stage AD patients with mild dementia score markedly lower on olfactory tests than do age-matched controls. Thus, on the 40-item University of Pennsylvania Smell Identification Test, 50% of the items, on average, cannot be identified by early stage AD patients. In a picture identification test analogous to the odour identification test (except that pictures, rather than odours, need to be identified), only 5% of the items are similarly misidentified by the same AD patients.

It now appears that olfactory dysfunction – particularly in conjunction with other risk factors – may be a predictor of subsequent development of AD in older persons.[36–38] In one study, for example, a standardized 12-item odour identification test was administered to 1604 non-demented community-dwelling senior citizens 65 years of age or older.[37] The olfactory test scores were found to be a better predictor of cognitive decline over the following two years than scores on a global cognitive test. Persons who were anosmic and possessed at least one ApoE4 allele exhibited 4.9 times the risk of having cognitive decline than normosmic persons not possessing this allele. This was in contrast to a 1.23 times greater risk for cognitive decline in normosmic individuals possessing at least one such allele. A sex difference was noted. Thus, women who were anosmic and possessed at least one ApoE4 allele were 9.71 times more likely than their normosmic non-allele-possessing counterparts. This corresponding figure for men was 3.18. Women and men who were normosmic and possessed at least one allele were only 1.9 and 0.67 times more likely, respectively, than their normosmic non-allele-possessing counterparts.

Although the olfactory system-related neuropathology of AD may involve the neuroepithelium, most likely central structures are the most heavily involved.[39–43] There is evidence that AD pathology begins in olfactory regions within the medial temporal lobe, most notably layer II of the entorhinal cortex[44,45] and progresses from there to neocortical regions, although involvement of the olfactory bulbs early in the disease process has also been demonstrated.[46,47] A 40% decrease in cross-sectional area of the olfactory tract and a 52% loss of myelinated axons has been reported in AD. Neurofibrillary tangle formation occurs earlier than amyloid deposition within the olfactory bulb of AD patients, and the presence of more than 10 neurofibrillary tangles per olfactory bulb section is associated with a 93.3% AD diagnostic accuracy rate.[41]

Parkinson's disease

Idiopathic Parkinson's disease (PD) is another age-related neurodegenerative disorder characterized by olfactory dysfunction. Interestingly, the proportion of early-stage PD patients with olfactory dysfunction appears to be equal to or greater than the proportion of early-stage PD patients exhibiting a number of the cardinal signs of PD (e.g. tremor). The following general observations have been made: (a) PD-related smell loss is typically bilateral and presents very early in the disease process; (b) the magnitude of olfactory dysfunction is unrelated to disease stage, severity of motor dysfunction or use of antiparkinsonian medications; (c) the olfactory loss is stable over time, even when motor elements of the disease progress; (d) olfactory-evoked potentials are abnormal in PD patients, demonstrating a prolonged latency, or in most cases, an absent response; and (e) among the major motor disorders, the olfactory loss of PD is relatively specific.[48] Thus, decreased ability to smell is absent, or present infrequently or only to a minor degree, in progressive supranuclear palsy (a condition which shares a number of signs with PD), essential tremor, multiple system atrophy, amyotrophic lateral sclerosis, and parkinsonism induced by intravenous administration of the proneurotoxin 1-methyl-4-phenyl-1,2,3,6-tetrahydropyridine (MPTP).[49–51]

While the basis for the olfactory deficit in idiopathic PD is unknown, it appears to be indistinguishable from that observed in AD, suggesting the possibility that these two disorders may share a common neuropathological substrate.[52] As with AD, both olfactory vector and degenerative hypotheses could explain the dysfunction. Tangential support for the olfactory vector hypothesis comes from evidence that (a) certain viruses (e.g. encephalitis lethargica) have been epidemiologically associated with PD, (b) a number of xenobiotic agents, including viruses associated with encephalitis, enter the central nervous system via the primary olfactory neurons, and (c) patients whose parkinsonism is due to the intravenous administration of MPTP have relatively normal olfactory function.[9] The possibility exists that the common olfactory alterations observed in AD and PD are secondary to damage to the anterior olfactory nucleus. Thus, intraneuronal pathology related to the protein τ is clearly marked in the anterior olfactory nucleus of neurodegenerative diseases such as AD and PD which are associated with olfactory loss, but nearly absent in such disorders as progressive supranuclear palsy, corticobasal degeneration and frontal temporal dementia, disorders with little or no olfactory dysfunction.[43,53]

Idiopathic factors

A number of individuals presenting with an olfactory complaint lack a clear aetiology for their dysfunction. It is possible that subclinical manifestations of disorders that alter the sense of smell are responsible for some of these cases. For example, we have observed patients presenting to our clinic with complaints of distorted olfactory function of unknown origin who came down with influenza a week or two later. The olfactory losses of a disproportionate number of idiopathic cases occur during the influenza season; thus, some of these cases may reflect influenza that culminates in no other noticeable clinical manifestations.

Causes of taste dysfunction in the elderly

As discussed in detail earlier in this chapter, the subjective complaint of 'taste' loss, a common complaint of the elderly, is often not verified by whole-mouth taste testing. A number of such patients are undoubtedly confusing 'taste' with 'flavour', and upon careful testing exhibit major olfactory, rather than major gustatory, deficits.[23]

As with olfactory dysfunction, a broad array of age-related changes may predispose the taste system to damage from environmental insults or other factors, including reduced protein synthesis or metabolic insufficiency, changes in epithelial vascularity, decreased blood flow, loss of neurotrophic factors and atrophy of secretory glands and lymphatics.[31] Common conditions seen in the elderly that may interfere with the access of the tastant to the taste bud (transport loss) include inflammatory processes of the oral cavity, bacterial and fungal colonization of the taste pore, and xerostomia. Poor oral hygiene may also contribute to taste dysfunction.

Viral infections, medications and radiation therapy to the oral cavity and pharynx represent the most common causes of sensory gustatory loss. The chorda tympani is particularly susceptible to viral or bacterial insult as it courses through the middle ear. In turn, the middle ear is connected to the Eustachian tube and nasopharynx which provide a portal of entry for infectious agents. Thus, it is not surprising that taste loss or distortion has been associated with upper respiratory and middle ear infections. Numerous drugs have been suggested to alter the ability to taste, including antihypertensives and antilipidemics[54] and drugs affecting cell turnover, such as antineoplastic, antithyroid and antirheumatic agents.[55] Some medications, such as the sleeping agent Lunesta (eszopiclone), produce bitter taste sensations which correlate with their blood and saliva levels.[56]

Neural gustatory loss results from head trauma, neoplasms and a variety of dental and otologic operations that may damage the facial nerve or glossopharyngeal nerve. Injury in this patient population can be to the taste nerves or to more central structures.

In addition to the aforementioned causes of altered taste perception in the elderly, several other conditions are important. Diabetics often experience a loss in taste perception, especially for glucose. This loss can be progressive and eventually extend to other taste stimuli.[57] Burning mouth syndrome is a poorly characterized disorder in which patients describe an intraoral burning sensation that commonly occurs in combination with dysgeusia.[58] This problem is prevalent in postmenopausal women. Although no clear aetiologic factor has been identified, hormone replacement and tricyclic antidepressants are reportedly effective in alleviating the oral sensations in some cases. The degree to which neurological diseases such as Alzheimer's disease influence taste function is currently under study.

Evaluating and managing elderly patients with chemosensory dysfunction

In general, a thorough medical history will identify the proximal cause of most smell and taste problems. During this history, the clinician should question the patient as to whether there is loss (e.g. anosmia) or a decrease (e.g. hyposmia) in function and whether the symptoms are unchanging, progressive or fluctuant. The degree to which the loss or distortion is localized to one nostril or the other, or to one section of the tongue or the other, is useful in establishing whether a given nerve is involved. Antecedent events (i.e. prior upper respiratory infection, head trauma, medications, surgery) leading up to the dysfunction as well as the duration of symptoms are important pieces of information to be gathered from the history. For example, fluctuating olfactory deficits suggest interference with the transport of the odorant to the olfactory neuroepithelium (e.g. nasal sinus disease) rather than a sensorineural disorder.

After obtaining a thorough medical history, it is critical to evaluate the patient objectively, so as to characterize the nature of the dysfunction. In most cases, olfactory dysfunction is the problem. Thus, even when the patient reports that smell is all right and that taste is problematic, quantitative olfactory testing should be performed. If unilateral dysfunction is suspected, the olfactory test can be administered to each half of the nose separately while occluding the contralateral naris using a piece of Microfoam^{TM} tape (3M Corporation, Minneapolis, MN). Contemporaneously, a thorough upper airway examination, ideally using endoscopic procedures, should be performed along with appropriate imaging of the sinuses and higher brain structures. If nasal or intracranial disease is found, appropriate medical or surgical treatment should be initiated, and olfactory testing should be repeated some time after the completion of the treatment regimen to ascertain if improvement has occurred. Obviously, the basic diseases associated with ageing should be ruled out by the physician to preclude their possible association with the chemosensory dysfunction. Importantly, a review of the medications taken by the elderly should be undertaken, particularly if dysgeusia is the presenting symptom.

If the medical tests prove negative, it is likely that the dysfunction is due to neural damage for which no treatment is available (e.g. damage to the olfactory receptors proper). In this case, it is still prudent to assess the chemosensory function quantitatively and obtain a percentile score for the patient. While an older person may evidence, in an absolute sense, considerable olfactory loss, it is still important to characterize this person relative to his or her peer group. Thus, an 85-year-old man may have olfactory loss indicative of marked hyposmia; however, he may still be at the 75th percentile of his normative group, indicating that he is outperforming three-quarters of his peers. Simply telling him this fact is highly therapeutic as elderly persons expect some degree of decline in their function, but appreciate it when their decline is still not as great as that seen in most of their peers. This simple rule is very beneficial and ensures that at least half the patients complaining of chemosensory function can receive meaningful psychological benefit.

In cases where borderline dysfunction is present in menopausal women, the astute clinician can explore whether or not hormone or vitamin replacement therapy may be indicated in an attempt to return function. This is particularly the case in burning mouth syndrome, where such treatments have been found effective in some cases.[59] Although zinc therapy has been suggested in the literature, double-blind studies indicate that zinc is no more effective than placebo in helping patients with chemosensory disorders (unless, of course, frank zinc deficiency is present).[60] One study reporting effectiveness of the antioxidant α-lipoic acid had no controls and the number reporting resolution was of the same magnitude as would be expected from spontaneous resolution.[61] Some cases of taste dysfunction may represent age-related xerostomia, and therefore this condition should be addressed and, if present, treated as well as possible.

Acknowledgments

Supported, in part, by the following research grants: USAMRAAW81XWH-09-1-0467, RO1 DC 04278, RO1 DC 02974, and RO1 AG 17496. Disclosure: Dr Doty is a major shareholder in Sensonics, Inc., the manufacturer and distributor of tests of taste and smell function.

Key points

- Taste and smell are critical for determining the flavour of foods and beverages and for protection from leaking natural gas, fire, toxic agents, and spoiled beverages and foodstuffs.
- Smell dysfunction is the norm, not the exception, for persons over the age of 65 years.
- It is important for the physician and patient to have an accurate understanding of a patient's abilities to taste and smell, and sample quantitative tests of smell function are widely available.
- Smell loss is among the very earliest signs of Alzheimer's disease and idiopathic Parkinson's disease.
- The most common cause of *permanent* smell loss in the elderly is an upper respiratory infection.
- Some recovery can occur spontaneously over time. Factors that determine prognosis include age, time since onset of problem, and degree of dysfunction, with the latter being most important.

References

1. Anonymous. Facts for Features. In: US Census Bureau Report, Government Printing Office, Washington, DC, 2004.
2. Doty RL, Shaman P, Dann M. Development of the University of Pennsylvania Smell Identification Test: a standardized microencapsulated test of olfactory function. *Physiol Behav* 1984;**32**:489–502.
3. Chalke HD, Dewhurst JR, Ward CW. Loss of smell in old people. *Public Health (London)* 1958;**72**:223–30.
4. Hawkes CH, Doty RL. *The Neurology of Olfaction*, Cambridge University Press, Cambridge, 2009.
5. Menco BPM, Morrison EE. Morphology of the mammalian olfactory epithelium: form, fine structure, function, and pathology. In: Doty RL (ed.), *Handbook of Olfaction and Gustation*, Marcel Dekker, New York, 2003, pp. 17–49.
6. Moon C, Ronnett GV. Molecular neurobiology of olfactory transduction. In: Doty RL (ed.), *Handbook of Olfaction and Gustation*, Marcel Dekker, New York, 2003, pp. 75–91.
7. Buck L, Axel R. A novel multigene family may encode odorant receptors: a molecular basis for odor recognition. *Cell* 1991;**65**:175–87.
8. Ding X, Dahl AR. Olfactory mucosa: composition, enzymatic localization, and metabolism. In: Doty RL (ed.), *Handbook of Olfaction and Gustation*, Marcel Dekker, New York, 2003, pp. 51–73.
9. Doty RL. The olfactory vector hypothesis of neurodegenerative disease: is it viable? *Ann Neurol* 2008;**63**:7–15.
10. Doty RL, Cometto-Muniz JE, Jalowayski AA *et al.* Assessment of upper respiratory tract and ocular irritative effects of volatile chemicals in humans. *Crit Rev Toxicol* 2004;**34**: 85–142.
11. Doty RL. *The Great Pheromone Myth*, Johns Hopkins University Press, Baltimore, 2010.
12. Shepherd GM. *Neurobiology*, Oxford University Press, New York, 1994.
13. Doty RL, Cummins DM, Shibanova A, Sanders I, Mu L. Lingual distribution of the human glossopharyngeal nerve. *Acta Otolaryngol* 2009;**129**:52–6.
14. Pritchard TC. The primate gustatory system. In: Getchell TV, Doty RL, Bartoshuk LM, Snow JB, Jr (eds), *Smell and Taste in Health and Disease*, Raven Press, New York, 1991, pp. 109–25.
15. Soter A, Kim J, Jackman A *et al.* Accuracy of self-report in detecting taste dysfunction. *Laryngoscope* 2008;**118**:611–17.
16. Doty RL. Olfaction. *Ann Rev Psychol* 2001;**52**:423–52.
17. Smutzer G, Lam S, Hastings L *et al.* A test for measuring gustatory function. *Laryngoscope* 2008;**118**:1411–16.

18. Landis BN, Welge-Luessen A, Bramerson A *et al.* "Taste Strips" – a rapid, lateralized, gustatory bedside identification test based on impregnated filter papers. *J Neurol* 2009; **256**:242–8.
19. Miller SL, Mirza N, Doty RL. Electrogustometric thresholds: relationship to anterior tongue locus, area of stimulation, and number of fungiform papillae. *Physiol Behav* 2002;**75**:753–7.
20. Calderon-Garciduenas L, Franco-Lira M, Henriquez-Roldan C *et al.* Urban air pollution: Influences on olfactory function and pathology in exposed children and young adults. *Exp Toxicol Pathol* 2009; Mar 16. [Epub ahead of print].
21. Doty RL, Cameron EL. Sex differences and reproductive hormone influences on human odor perception. *Physiol Behav* 2009;**97**:213–28.
22. Weiffenbach JM, Cowart BJ, Baum BJ. Taste intensity perception in aging. *J Gerontol* 1986;**41**:460–8.
23. Deems DA, Doty RL, Settle RG *et al.* Smell and taste disorders, a study of 750 patients from the University of Pennsylvania Smell and Taste Center. *Arch Otolaryngol – Head Neck Surg* 1991;**117**:519–28.
24. Matsuda T, Doty RL. Regional taste sensitivity to NaCl: relationship to subject age, tongue locus and area of stimulation. *Chem Senses* 1995;**20**:283–90.
25. Bartoshuk LM, Snyder DJ, Grushka M *et al.* Taste damage: previously unsuspected consequences. *Chem Senses* 2005; **30**:I218–i219.
26. Kveton JF, Bartoshuk LM. The effect of unilateral chorda tympani damage on taste. *Laryngoscope* 1994;**104**:25–9.
27. Yanagisawa K, Bartoshuk LM, Catalanotto FA, Karrer TA, Kveton JF. Anesthesia of the chorda tympani nerve and taste phantoms. *Physiol Behav* 1998;**63**:329–35.
28. Bartoshuk LM, Duffy VB. Supertasting and earaches – Genetics and pathology alter our taste worlds. *Appetite* 1994; 23:292–3.
29. Burdach KJ, Doty RL. The effects of mouth movements, swallowing, and spitting on retronasal odor perception. *Physiol Behav* 1987; **41**:353–6.
30. Nakashima T, Kimmelman CP, Snow JB, Jr. Structure of human fetal and adult olfactory neuroepithelium. *Arch Otolaryngol* 1984;**110**:641–6.
31. Doty RL. Smell and taste in the elderly. In: Albert ML, Knoefel JE (eds), *Clinical Neurology of Aging*, Oxford University Press, New York, 1994.
32. Murphy C, Doty RL, Duncan HJ. Clinical disorders of olfaction. In: Doty RL (ed.), *Handbook of Olfaction and Gustation*, Marcel Dekker, New York, 2003, pp. 461–78.
33. Kern RC, Conley DB, Haines GK, III, Robinson AM. Pathology of the olfactory mucosa: implications for the treatment of olfactory dysfunction. *Laryngoscope* 2004;**114**:279–85.
34. London B, Nabet B, Fisher AR *et al.* Predictors of prognosis in patients with olfactory disturbance. *Ann Neurol* 2008;**63**: 159–66.
35. Doty RL, Yousem DM, Pham LT *et al.* Olfactory dysfunction in patients with head trauma. *Arch Neurol* 1997;**54**:1131–40.
36. Devanand DP, Michaels-Marston KS, Liu X *et al.* Olfactory deficits in patients with mild cognitive impairment predict Alzheimer's disease at follow-up. *Am J Psychiatry* 2000;**157**:1399–405.
37. Graves AB, Bowen JD, Rajaram L *et al.* Impaired olfaction as a marker for cognitive decline: interaction with apolipoprotein E epsilon4 status. *Neurology* 1999;**53**:1480–7.
38. Wilson RS, Arnold SE, Schneider JA *et al.* Olfactory impairment in presymptomatic Alzheimer's disease. *Ann N Y Acad Sci* 2009;**1170**:730–5.
39. Esiri MM, Wilcock GK. The olfactory bulbs of Alzheimer's disease. *J Neurol Neurosurg Psychiatry* 1984;**47**:56–60.
40. Hyman BT, Arriagada PV, van Hoesen GW. Pathologic changes in the olfactory system in aging and Alzheimer's disease. *Ann N Y Acad Sci* 1991;**640**:14–19.
41. Kovacs T, Cairns NJ, Lantos PL. beta-amyloid deposition and neurofibrillary tangle formation in the olfactory bulb in ageing and Alzheimer's disease. *Neuropathol Appl Neurobiol* 1999;**25**:481–91.
42. Davies DC, Brooks JW, Lewis DA. Axonal loss from the olfactory tracts in Alzheimer's disease. *Neurobiol Aging* 1993; **14**:353–7.
43. Tsuboi Y, Wszolek ZK, Graff-Radford NR, Cookson N, Dickson DW. Tau pathology in the olfactory bulb correlates with Braak stage, Lewy body pathology and apolipoprotein epsilon4. *Neuropathol App Neurobiol* 2003;**29**:503–10.
44. Brouillet E, Hyman BT, Jenkins BG *et al.* Systemic or local administration of azide produces striatal lesions by an energy impairment-induced excitotoxic mechanism. *Exp Neurol* 1994;**129**:175–82.
45. Gomez-Isla T, Price JL, McKeel DW, Jr *et al.* Profound loss of layer II entorhinal cortex neurons occurs in very mild Alzheimer's disease. *J Neurosci* 1996;**16**:4491–500.
46. Kovacs T, Cairns NJ, Lantos PL. Olfactory centres in Alzheimer's disease: olfactory bulb is involved in early Braak's stages. *Neuroreport* 2001;**12**:285–8.
47. Braak H, Braak E. Evolution of neuronal changes in the course of Alzheimer's disease. *J Neural Transm Suppl* 1998; **53**:127–40.
48. Doty RL. Odor perception in neurodegenerative diseases. In: Doty RL (ed.), *Handbook of Olfaction and Gustation*, Marcel Dekker, New York, 2003, pp. 479–502.
49. Doty RL, Golbe LI, McKeown DA *et al.* Olfactory testing differentiates between progressive supranuclear palsy and idiopathic Parkinson's disease. *Neurology* 1993;**43**:962–5.
50. Wenning GK, Shephard B, Hawkes C *et al.* Olfactory function in atypical parkinsonian syndromes. *Acta Neurologica Scandinavica* 1995;**91**:247–50.
51. Sajjadian A, Doty RL, Gutnick DN *et al.* Olfactory dysfunction in amyotrophic lateral sclerosis. *Neurodegeneration* 1994;**3**:153–7.
52. Doty RL, Perl DP, Steele JC, Chen KM, Pierce JD, Jr., Reyes P, Kurland LT. Olfactory dysfunction in three neurodegenerative diseases. *Geriatrics* 1991;**46** Suppl 1:47–51.
53. Doty RL. Olfactory dysfunction in neurogenerative disorders. In: Getchell TV, Doty RL, Bartoshuk LM, Snow JB, Jr (eds), *Smell and Taste in Health and Disease*, Raven Press, New York, 1991, pp. 735–51.
54. Doty RL, Philip S, Reddy K, Kerr KL. Influences of antihypertensive and antihyperlipidemic drugs on the senses of taste and smell: a review. *J Hypertens* 2003;**21**:1805–13.
55. Doty RL, Bromley SM. Effects of drugs on olfaction and taste. *Otolaryngol Clin North Am* 2004;**37**:1229–54.

56. Doty RL, Treem J, Tourbier I, Mirza N. A double-blind study of the influences of eszopiclone on dysgeusia and taste function. *Pharmacol Biochem Behav* 2009;**94**:312–8.
57. Settle RG. The chemical senses in diabetes mellitus. In: Getchell TV, Doty RL, Bartoshuk LM, Snow JB, Jr (eds), *Smell and Taste in Health and Disease*, Raven Press, New York, 1991, pp. 829–43.
58. Ship JA, Grushka M, Lipton JA et al. Burning mouth syndrome: an update. [Review] [65 refs]. *J Am Dent Assoc* 1995; **126**:842–53.
59. Grushka M, Sessle BJ. Burning Mouth Syndrome. In: Getchell TV (ed.), *Smell and Taste in Health and Disease*, Raven Press, New York, 1991, pp. 665–82.
60. Henkin RI, Schecter PJ, Friedewald WT, Demets DL, Raff M. A double-blind study of the effects of zinc sulfate on taste and smell dysfunction. *Am J Med Sci* 1976;**272**:285–99.
61. Hummel TM, Heilmann SM, Huttenbriuk KBM. Lipoic acid in the treatment of smell dysfunction following viral infection of the upper respiratory tract. [Article]. *Laryngoscope* 2002;**112**:2076–80.

Additional reading

Wilson DA & Stevenson RJ. *Learning to Smell*, Johns Hopkins University Press, Baltimore, 2006.

SECTION 9

Bone and Joint Health

CHAPTER 89

Paget's disease of bone

Horace M. Perry III
St Louis University School of Medicine, and Geriatric Research, Education and Clinical Center,
St Louis Veterans' Affairs Medical Center, St Louis, MO, USA

Introduction

Sir James Paget described the disease that bears his name as *osteitis deformans* in a series of monographs published in the latter half of the nineteenth century.[1] At this time, we understand much more about the disease, including how to treat it, but its aetiology remains uncertain, perhaps even mysterious.

Paget's disease occurs in monostotic or polyostotic forms. The monostotic form occurs in a single bone, most frequently in a small quarter to half-dollar size lesion in the pelvis or lumbar spine. The pathologic description given below describes both monostotic and polyostotic Paget's disease. Monostotic Paget's disease is usually asymptomatic, although unusual placement of monostotic disease in the higher vertebrae, for example, with pathologic fracture can become symptomatic. Polyostotic Paget's disease is generally described as involving more than one bone. It is worth noting that monostotic disease of a long bone, the femur for example, behaves more like polyostotic disease than monostotic disease, even if only one bone is involved. The rest of the presentation will describe polyostotic Paget's disease unless otherwise noted.

Pathology of Paget's disease

Microscopic

Pathology at the cellular level is frequently divided into three types that correspond to early, middle and late stages of Paget's disease (Table 89.1). These may all be found in a single bone, proceeding in an orderly manner from early to late.[2] The early descriptions of the stages were generally called osteoclastic (early), osteoblastic (mid) and mixed (late). One could occasionally run across a very late stage of the mixed phase that was described as 'burned out'. More modern descriptions combine the osteoblastic and mixed phases to one and include the 'burned-out' phase as the third. The early stage corresponds to increased osteoclastic activity without compensatory increase in osteoblastic activity. Examination of such areas of pagetic bone demonstrate large osteoclasts, frequently several times bigger than normal osteoclasts. All osteoclasts appear to have multiple nuclei, perhaps in the range of four to eight, but pagetic osteoclasts frequently have 20 to 40 nuclei. In the second phase (Table 89.1) osteoblastic activity in the area appears to be dramatically increased, but severely disorganized. Routine findings include disorganized matrix, woven bone and occasional areas of malacic or non-mineralizing osteoid. The characteristic order and architecture of cortical bone is lost and the cortical-trabecular boundary is lost. In this phase, both osteoclastic and osteoblastic activity is increased. Finally, in the 'burned-out' phase, activity of the pagetic bone appears to have returned to about normal, but the abnormal architecture remains. Most monostotic Paget's is found in either phase two (mixed) or in the 'burned-out' form. In the third phase the abnormal architecture remains despite the relative normalization of cellular activity. Normal bone in the same individual, from another skeletal site or from an uninvolved portion of the pagetic bone, appears perfectly normal. It has appropriately sized osteoclasts with normal activity as well as normal osteoblasts and osteoblastic activity.[3] This appears to be true even for areas that might be expected at some later date to become pagetic.

Macroscopic

Pagetic bone is larger than normal bone, but significantly weaker. The bone appears 'coarse' rather than with the smooth surface of normal bone. Although the origin of the bone remains recognizable, it is frequently misshapen or bent, virtually always in weight-bearing long bones. The bone is hypervascular and may have multiple arteriovenous shunts.[4] Paget's disease is one reported cause of high output congestive heart failure.

Principles and Practice of Geriatric Medicine, Fifth Edition. Edited by Alan J. Sinclair, John E. Morley and Bruno Vellas.

Table 89.1 Phases of Paget's disease.

Phase	Bone morphology	Activity
Osteoclastic	Normal, but increased osteoclastic size and activity	Osteoclast
Mixed	Changes of osteoclastic phase plus great increases in osteoblastic activity, poorly mineralized or osteomalacic bone, woven bone, large seams of osteoid, loss of cortical trabecular interface	Osteoclast and Osteoblast
Burned out	Activity returning to normal but may still appear somewhat increased	Osteoclast and Osteoblast

Pagetic involvement of bones occurs idiosyncratically within very specific parameters. Large bones are much more likely to be involved than small bones. Anyone who has treated multiple cases of Paget's will have seen some unusual small bone involvement in wrist, hand or foot, for example. A list of bones frequently involved is shown in Table 89.2. Involvement in long bones generally starts at one end and proceeds toward the other end over a period of years. The disease does not cross joint spaces for long bones. Similarly, involvement in the pelvis or skull begins at one location and gradually extends across the entire bone. Unlike long bones, Paget's disease does frequently seem to spread across sutures in the bones of the skull or pelvis. Involvement of one long bone, the left femur for example, does not determine the involvement of the other, in this example the right femur. Usually, it is not involved, but occasionally it is.

The sequelae of Paget's disease may generally be inferred from the observations of micro- and macroscopic changes in bone. Changes in measures of osteoclastic activity either in serum or urine occur first and remain elevated. Urinary hydroxyproline was the measurement first used, but required specific dietary restrictions to avoid gelatine and gelatine-containing foods to be used accurately. Serum acid phosphatase, a potential serum marker of osteoclast activity, was occasionally used in some studies, but suffered from a series of difficulties. It was only elevated in about 20% of cases of Paget's and was also a marker for prostatic disease, a fairly common finding in many male patients with Paget's. More recent measures of bone-specific collagen breakdown markers in serum or urine have obviated these difficulties. These markers include N-telopeptide and pyridinium cross-links and provide much better estimates of osteoclastic activity. Urine studies should always be accompanied by a measurement of urinary creatinine to ensure comparability of one specimen to the next. These measures are routinely elevated in all phases of Paget's disease.[5] Measures of osteoblastic activity, primarily in serum, are also routinely elevated in Paget's disease. Older measures of this activity include serum alkaline phosphatase and the heat-stable fraction of the serum alkaline phosphatase. Although the first measure is routinely available in chemistry panels, it is not terribly specific. The heat-stable fraction is more specific, but is relatively difficult to do. It is still not entirely specific for bone alkaline phosphatase as opposed to the enzyme from other sites. Additional tests assays of osteoblastic function including bone-specific alkaline phosphatase and other markers like osteocalcin are now available They are not reported to be as sensitive a marker for Paget's disease as the older assays despite the fact they are generally considered to be more specific.[6] Radiological changes can be seen from the earliest (osteoclastic) stages of the disease on both plain films and radionuclide scans. On plain films, the early lesions appear as lucencies. Depending on the site they frequently have specific names. The most common of these include 'osteoporosis circumscripta'. This describes an early lesion in the skull that appears as a circular lucency on plain film of the skull. Similarly, the 'blade of grass' lesion describes a chevron-shaped lucency in a long bone. Over time (years), this lesion may be observed to march down the length of the bone at an approximate rate of one centimetre per year followed by signs of the osteoblastic/mixed stages of the disease.[7] These signs include enlargement of the bone, irregular calcification and loss of the cortical trabecular demarcation in bone. Radionuclide scans of bone will also show significant changes. Affected areas are hot. In long bones or other large bones, clear demarcation can be seen between affected and unaffected. All of these radiological findings are generally considered pathognomonic for Paget's disease except that 'osteoporosis circumscripta' needs to be clearly delineated

Table 89.2 Bones commonly affected by Paget.

- Pelvis
- Femur
- Tibia
- Skull
- Vertebrae
- Clavicle

from the 'punched out' lesions observed in the skull with multiple myeloma. Further, very occasionally, lesions of the lower lumbar vertebra may be impossible to differentiate from metastatic (prostate) carcinoma without biopsy. Magnetic resonance imaging (MRI) has been a major boon in this regard, however.[8]

Sequelae of Paget's disease

Most of the sequelae of Paget's disease can be inferred from the knowledge of its effect on bone, that is the bone becomes larger, but weaker. The major exception to this is the most feared complication of Paget's disease, osteosarcoma. This tumour is a rare but deadly outcome arising from pagetic bone, usually decades after it was first affected. Estimates of its frequency are quite low perhaps 1–3% of individuals with Paget's disease.[9] Mortality in affected individuals is quite high, in some series 100%, even after the development of successful protocols for the treatment of childhood osteosarcomas. The reasons for the abysmal outcomes in osteosarcomas related to Paget's are at least twofold. First, the central location of Paget's disease prevents the common first-step treatment, excision/amputation. Secondly, the symptoms of osteosarcoma are very non-specific and therefore frequently missed. The major presenting complaint is a significant worsening of Paget's symptoms, particularly bone pain. Bone pain waxes and wanes spontaneously throughout the course of Paget's disease. After many years or decades of such spontaneous changes, patients frequently do not complain of them to their physicians until it has been present for several months. In this setting, the osteosarcoma has frequently progressed too far for successful treatment upon its initial discovery.

A second feared complication of Paget's is probably more unusual, platybasia, or basilar invagination. Individuals with severe Paget's disease of the skull will be noted to have a 'sharpening' or 'lipping' of the occiput on lateral skull films. Instead of the normal curve of the occiput noted on lateral film, the bone begins to protrude downwards or 'lip'. This is a radiological sign of a falling down of the skull around the spinal column. Essentially, the skull is too weak to hold its own weight and over a period of time it will collapse while the falxes hold the brain in place. This circumstance will cause hydrocephalus and eventual herniation of brain with death. This process extends over years. Neurosurgical intervention for the hydrocephalus can maintain normal pressure.[10]

Congestive heart failure is a reported complication of Paget's disease. Arteriovenous shunting of blood through affected bone is reported to produce high output congestive heart failure in individuals with more than 15% of their skeleton involved by the disease. Even in very active polyostotic Paget's disease, this complication is very rare in my experience and is only included for completeness and because the causes of high output failure are so limited. Urgent treatment to limit the activity of the pagetic bone is recommended. This reduces the arteriovenous shunting and decreases the need for the high output state. Altered blood supply ('steal syndrome') is suspected or reported in individuals with Paget's disease of the skull who complain of somnolence. Similarly, this 'steal syndrome' has been implicated in an individual with Paget's of a vertebra and paralysis below that level.[4,11]

Other complications are more common, but generally less severe. Fracture through weaker pagetic bone is relatively common. Considerable excess blood loss may occur because of the vastly increased vascularity of pagetic bone. Longitudinal fractures or fissures are described. Bowing of affected weight-bearing long bones is an integral part of the disease and is associated with gait abnormalities and/or unsteadiness, osteoarthritis in nearby or adjacent joints and in painful microfractures that occur in severely bowed lower extremities. Some of these microfractures extend through the bone and become full-blown displaced fractures. Such microfractures occur when weight placed on the bowed extremity increases the curvature (circumference) of the bone, stretching the bone beyond its endurance. Treatment of this type of fracture requires either bracing or osteotomy to straighten the bone in order to heal and prevent further fractures in that bone. In the case of osteotomy, patients should be treated prior to surgery to reduce the vascularity of the affected bone.

Any place a nerve passes through a bony foramen or through bone, the potential exists for Paget's disease to narrow the channel and impinge upon the nerve, causing pain and/or eventually loss of the nerve function.[12] The most common of these is probably seen in Paget's of the skull where approximately 70% of patients are reported to have mixed sensineural hearing loss. Other nerves pass through foramen in the skull. Blindness is an unusual but reported complication also. Facial nerve palsies can also be observed. Hypercementosis in teeth, an idiopathic condition of increased accretion of bone on one or more roots, causing tooth pain has also been reported in individuals with Paget's of the skull.[13]

Similar nerve palsies may be observed in effected peripheral locations. Certainly the most severe of these may be related to weakness/fracture, as is the case in (partial) spinal cord transaction related to thoracic or cervical vertebra collapse due to pagetic involvement. Spinal stenosis, related to involvement of one or more vertebra with Paget's resulting in critical narrowing of the spinal canal has also been reported, but is thought to be less common than the steal syndrome.[10,12]

A final important sequelae relates to the ongoing extended and accelerated bone resorption and formation. Paget's disease of the pelvis in an individual after hip replacement can result in an unstable position for the acetabulum, which over a period of years can move a significant distance. Similarly, Paget's disease of the skull or mandible can result in tooth migration. In the cases in which this was reported, dentures required constant attention over a period of years to ensure comfort and adequate mastication.

For the patient, aside from the unusual catastrophic sequelae, Paget's disease represents an almost constant chronic irritation. The symptoms of the disease are limited, but the symptoms of the sequelae have an almost constant effect depending on the bone(s) affected: arthritic complaints in the joints most nearly related to the affected bone are constant; partial deafness in individuals with Paget's of the skull; gait abnormalities and pain in individuals with long bone involvement. Many of these may be at least partially ameliorated by the use of braces, shoe lifts and other orthotic devices.[14]

Presentation of Paget's disease

Patient's with Paget's disease generally present in one of three ways. First, individuals discovered on a routine blood test with an alkaline phosphatase elevated several times above normal. While other obvious sources of pathology would need to be ruled out, the evaluation should include a more specific measure of osteoblast activity as described above, a serum bone specific alkaline phosphatase or osteocalcin. Measures of osteoclastic activity like N-telopeptide or pyridinium cross-links in serum or urine would be appropriate if readily available, but not necessary. If the serum alkaline phosphatase is elevated due to Paget's disease, one would expect that measures of osteoclast activity would surely also be elevated. If these measures were elevated more than 50%, then the next step would be to perform a radionuclide scan of bone and obtain X-rays of hot spots. If these tests showed an individual with Paget's disease outside of the lumbar spine or pelvis (that is a patient with polyostotic rather than monostotic disease) appropriate treatment would then be undertaken. Individuals with apparent monostotic Paget's disease in the pelvis should followed longitudinally over a period of years to make sure the Paget's disease is not extending.

The second major group will present either with chronic bone pain or deformity. In this group, pain may have been present for years, and the deformity has usually been slowly worsening. On physical exam, the indicated area is usually warm and erythematous, but not painful. It is without nodes or other indications of infection. The patient may have complaints specific to the pagetic involvement, loss of hearing and headaches for Paget's of the skull. They may have arthralgias as well as bone pain around the involved bone, or occasionally some distance from it. The laboratory evaluation for this patient should include the tests described above: a test of osteoblastic activity, a bone-specific alkaline phosphatase or osteocalcin, but again, not necessarily a measure of osteoclast activity. If these are elevated then the patient should get a radionuclide scan with X-rays of the hot spots. Pain suggesting microfracture or stress fracture should probably prompt referral to an orthopaedist for appropriate follow-up.

The third major group will be individuals who present with an established diagnosis. In these cases, review of the patient's record should demonstrate a radionuclide scan with appropriate X-rays of 'hot spots', serial serum measures of osteoblastic activity over the course of treatment and non-treatment intervals and finally appropriate follow-up exams, for example audiology evaluations in patients with Paget's disease of the skull or appropriate gait evaluations for individuals with lower limb involvement of their disease. Appropriate follow-up radionuclide scans should probably not be performed more frequently than annually, unless new or changed symptoms appear.

Epidemiology of Paget's disease

Autopsy series suggest a prevalence rate of about 4% for Paget's disease in individuals over the age of 40 years and about 7% for individuals over the age of 70 years.[2,12] The disease increases in prevalence with age. These numbers include both individuals with monostotic and polyostotic Paget's disease. It is generally thought that polyostotic disease makes up 5% or less of the combined numbers and is probably less common than that in the younger age group. The other caveat that needs to be considered in estimating the number of individuals with Paget's is the ethnic origin of the population. This factor plays a large role in the frequency of Paget's disease. Individuals of European descent, particularly northern Europe, excluding Scandinavia, are particularly likely to get Paget's disease.[15,16] Individuals of southern European descent are less likely, but the risk is still appreciable. Native African and Asian peoples have miniscule prevalence of Paget's disease. On the other hand, African-Americans are clearly noted to get Paget's disease. Thus the origin of the population studied determines in part the prevalence of Paget's disease.

Men are slightly more likely to get Paget's disease than women with a ratio that approximates three to two. Since the absolute number of women in the general population is about double that of men over the age of 65, the relative risk for Paget's disease is probably about three times greater in men.

Aetiology of Paget's disease

Even at this relatively late date, the aetiology of Paget's disease of bone remains somewhat obscure. There is a clearly positive family history in about 10–50% of patients with

Paget's disease of bone.[17] The effect of this observation is blunted by the fact that in everyday practice, the individuals affected seem most frequently to be cousins or uncles. Occasionally, the relationship is even more obscure. Two of the most severely affected individuals I have ever seen were related – as sisters-in-law. It seems relatively unusual for siblings to be involved or for a parent and child to be involved. As a measure of the rarity of this effect, there are reports of multiple generational involvements in several kindreds, but good documentation of the effect even recently is still reportable. Some of this effect can probably be accounted for by the relatively late onset of the disease. At the time a patient presents with Paget's, frequently his or her parents and their siblings will be unavailable for examination and their own children may still be years away from the potential to develop the disease. There is about a 15% chance of acquiring Paget's disease in one's lifetime if a first-degree relative has that diagnosis. Recent studies have reported genes associated with Paget's. The database, *Online Mendelian Inheritance in Man*, lists Paget's disease as a heritable trait with four different loci on three separate chromosomes being linked to Paget's (as of this writing).[18–22]

Despite the recognition of vertical transmission of Paget's within kindreds, several investigators believe that the disease is transmitted by a slow virus. They point to the fact that the disease is distributed in relatively temperate climates, as one might expect of a virus. Viruses, measles for example, cause giant cell formation (in the pneumonic form) that resembles the pagetic osteoclast. Lastly investigators have reported viral like particles in these pagetic osteoclasts using electron microscopy. There is some disagreement about which virus it is, but respiratory syncytial, canine distemper and paramyxo viruses have all been reported to be associated with it.[23–25] Recent reports have discounted the evidence for involvement of measles specifically, and a separate report has suggested that the evidence for virus particles in osteoclasts previously reported may be related to contamination, rather than as a causative agent.[26]

One potential issue that remains to be resolved is whether or not all Paget's disease is the same and therefore has the same aetiology. In particular, descriptions of Paget's disease in several generations frequently sound unlike the usual type of Paget's disease. Thus, kindreds are described with multiple recurrent fractures through clastic lesions in appendicular bone resulting in limb amputations in multiple members of the kindred. It is clear that the description falls in the range of Paget's disease and it would be difficult to call it anything else. Still, this is a very unusual outcome for the disease. These observations implicitly raise the question of whether or not *osteitis deformans* is a 'final common pathway for a series of diseases of hyperactive osteoclasts or a single specific disease'. In that vein, Paget's disease of bone has a series of puzzling qualities, which seem to make the latter possibility more likely. The frequent presence of the disease in large bones, rather than small bones, as well as the local presence of the disease in one femur rather than both, or one humerus rather than both would be hard to understand if a genetic defect were the cause, since all the bones would be affected. An infectious process would be easier to understand, since these are usually localized by definition. Recent reports suggest that a combination of genetic and infectious (viral) aetiologies combine to produce Paget's disease[18,27] working via disturbances in osteoclast and osteoblast physiology. This hypothesis suggests abnormalities even in normal bone, but still does not explain the observed self-limitations of the disease to pagetic versus non-pagetic bone.

In summary, the aetiology of Paget's disease is not conclusively known. Good evidence exists for both a viral and a genetic basis for the condition, although the specifics of how either would produce the syndrome observed remains uncertain.

Treatment of Paget's disease

The aims of treatment of Paget's disease of bone must be to decrease the deformities of bone and reduce the rate of fractures induced by the disease. Controlling the disease should, by definition control the risk for sequelae. That said, there is no evidence-based report of any drug decreasing deformities or reducing fractures in Paget's disease in a double-blind, placebo-controlled trial. On the other hand, decreasing the cellular activity of pagetic bone should limit all of the sequelae of the disease. Multiple drugs in multiple trials have been shown to decrease the activity of pagetic bone.

The earliest successful treatments of Paget's disease used calcitonin (Table 89.3). Calcitonin is a peptide hormone secreted from the thyroid. Thyroid tissue was readily available from slaughter houses to be extracted. Calcitonin acts directly on osteoclasts via receptors to decrease cellular activity. Its effect in man appears to be limited. Individuals with clear cell thyroid carcinoma may have levels of serum calcitonin of a magnitude higher than normal without apparent abnormalities of mineral metabolism. Fowl and fish calcitonins appear to be several times more potent than human calcitonin. In egg-laying animals, serum calcium rises in order to provide calcium to the egg. Osteoclast activity rises in order to mobilize this calcium from the skeleton. When the eggs require less calcium, calcitonin is secreted, osteoclastic activity declines rapidly, and the serum calcium returns to normal. The rationale for the use of calcitonin for the treatment of Paget's disease of bone is readily apparent. The earliest available calcitonin in wide usage was salmon calcitonin given by daily injection. It reduced serum alkaline phosphatase by about 40% within six months. The side effects were limited to local reaction at

Table 89.3 Calcitonin.

- Only injectable is approved
- Side effects – nausea in about 20%
- Flushing occasionally
- Not as powerful as bisphosphonates
- Useful only for people who cannot take bisphosphonates
- Tachyphylaxis develops within six months
- Dosage 50 or 100 IU daily or thrice weekly for 6–18 months can be reported after a rest period – usually at least three months

the injection site, about 20% of patients complained about flushing after the injection and about 20% complained of nausea. The injection was usually given immediately before retiring to avoid or minimize these complaints. Of more concern, however, was tachyphylaxis. By about six months, virtually all patients had reached the maximum benefit to be achieved from therapy. Stopping therapy for some period of time (3–6 months) then restored some additional sensitivity to the drug, but usually also allowed some escape from the drug during the rest period. The end result is that some resistance to therapy appears to supervene over a period of years. Lastly, it needs to be noted that although inhaled calcitonin has been approved for osteoporosis therapy, the FDA has only approved injectable salmon calcitonin for therapy of Paget's disease. Injectable calcitonin remains in limited use for treatment of Paget's disease.[28]

At about this time, an early bisphosphonate, etidronate also became available for use in treatment of Paget's disease (Table 89.4). Bisphosphonates block osteoclastic activity and in the case of etidronate and several other early variations of the class also interfere with osteoblastic activity. All oral forms of the drug are remarkably poorly absorbed. They require strict adherence to protocol for adequate absorption, usually first thing in the morning (i.e. nil per os (NPO)) taken only with 6–8 oz of water and nothing else by mouth for an extended period, usually about an hour. Still in its day, etidronate provided a relatively good response with serum alkaline phosphatase falling about 50% from pretreatment levels. The drug could only be used for six months at a time; it then required a 'rest period' of about 3–6 months. Failure to permit this rest period can be followed by symptomatic osteomalacia.[2,12,29] Newer bisphosphonates have generally supplanted etidronate for therapy of Paget's disease.

Table 89.4 Bisphosphonates.

Agent	Route	Dose and frequency
Etidronate	Oral	200 or 400 mg daily for 6 mos. May repeat after 6 mos. Rest between repetitions imperative
Alendronate	Oral	40 mg daily for 6 mos. May repeat if necessary
Risedronate	Oral	30 mg daily for 2 mos
Pamidronate	IV	30 mg over 4 hrs for 3 days or 60 mg over 4 hrs daily twice
Zoledronic acid	IV	5 mg over 15 min. Repeat after two years if necessary

The newer oral bisphosphonates, alendronate, risedronate, ibandronate and the injectable forms, pamidronate and zoledronic acid (Table 89.4) appear to target only the osteoclast. They are much more successful in reducing osteoclastic and therefore osteoblastic activity than the older drugs.[30–33] These drugs permit reduction of alkaline phosphatase to the normal range in about 80% of cases. There are a few open-label head-to-head trials in series that permit some stratification of effect. Thus, pamidronate probably works less well than the others and zoledronate may work best. Pamidronate and zoledronate are probably the most convenient in that they only require infusion over a relatively short period of time. Further, patient compliance is assured. They may be repeated if necessary. The oral forms are used for relatively short periods of time and may also be repeated if necessary. These therapies will reduce osteoclastic/osteoblastic activity to normal in most cases, although more than one round of therapy may be needed.

Non-prescription and non-pharmacological therapy

Individuals taking bisphosphonates should always assure adequate calcium intake. This will probably necessitate calcium supplementation. Depending on dietary intake, most patients will need an additional 1200 mg of supplemental calcium. Adequate vitamin D intake should be assured also. We routinely give 1000 IU per day to our patients with or without Paget's disease. The aim would be to maintain a serum vitamin D measure more than 35 ng dl^{-1}. To treat bone pain, arthralgia, or arthritis, non-steroidal anti-inflammatory agents are recommended.

Indications for treatment

The major indications for therapy are to ameliorate symptoms related to Paget's disease, including bone pain and headache. Most physicians would also like to prevent the sequelae, including nerve entrapment, bowing of weight bearing extremities and fractures. As mentioned previously, there is no double-blind, placebo-controlled study that demonstrates that this is possible, but it seems likely that reducing the effect of Paget's at a cellular level would have this outcome. 'Burned-out' disease or previously treated disease, notable for relatively normal serum studies of osteoblastic activity despite obvious bony abnormalities on X-ray or bone scan should be followed. All patients should have non-pharmacological interventions described above offered to them. Individuals with Paget's disease and renal disease should be treated with injectable salmon calcitonin rather than bisphosphonates.

Follow-up studies after treatment with injectable bisphosphonates are appropriate within weeks of the treatment and as the physician deems appropriate until the next date of potential treatment. Individuals whose serum tests normalize should be followed until their tests begin to rise or symptoms recur at which time therapy can be considered again (see below). Since oral bisphosphonates take longer to act, follow-up intervals may be spaced further apart. We tend to use an interval of 4–6 weeks for the first visit. At that visit it is important to ensure the patient is taking the drug as prescribed. Further visits usually occur at three and six months from the time the drug was started. The drug must be stopped by six months. Follow-up visits then occur at three-month intervals until the next date for available therapy, unless the patient's osteoblastic markers have normalized. In this case, we would move the follow-up visits out to about 4–6 months until evidence of disease reactivation recurred as described above. We would then treat again.

Final considerations in Paget's disease

In individuals without metabolic bone disease, bone turnover occurs slowly, such that the half-life of skeletal calcium is estimated to be about 10 years. In areas of active Paget's disease, the half-life of skeletal calcium is estimated to be about six months. This stark difference may be responsible for the reported increased incidence of hypercalcaemia or primary hyperparathyroidism reported with Paget's disease. In the older literature, the incidence of primary hyperparathyroidism was reported to be as high as 15%. On the other hand, much of this data was obtained prior to our present understanding of the inverse relationship between serum 25-hydroxyvitamin D and parathyroid hormone. Individuals with low serum 25-hydroxyvitamin D, high serum calcium and elevated parathyroid hormone can return serum calcium concentrations toward normal or into the normal range with appropriate vitamin D supplementation. The recommended dosage and duration of supplementation is the subject of some debate now, but raising serum vitamin D levels into the lower end of normal range should be adequate for this effect. This can probably be accomplished with a supplement of 1000 IU of vitamin D per day. It must also be remembered that the increased activity of the pagetic bone is releasing more calcium from the skeleton into serum. This calcium should suppress parathyroid hormone release. Finally, individuals lose renal function as they age and when enough renal function is lost, serum parathyroid hormone levels begin to rise. Patients with age-related (or unrelated) renal impairment with secondary hyperparathyroidism who develop Paget's disease (or in whom it progresses significantly) may then present with hypercalcaemia with elevated or not completely suppressed serum parathyroid hormone levels. These factors should be kept in mind when evaluating a patient with Paget's disease and hypercalcaemia.

The second issue to be considered is related to this first issue. The question of normal bone in Paget's disease has intrigued investigators for years. The majority of bone in a patient with Paget's disease is normal, at least as far as we can tell. Treating the pagetic bone necessarily exposes the normal bone to the same treatment. Therapies for Paget's are frequently used to treat normal (but osteoporotic bone), but the doses are usually greatly increased. In the old days, using etidronate (an early bisphosphonate) required a drug holiday of usually six months after six months of therapy to avoid the development of osteomalacia in normal bone. The newer bisphosphonates that are more osteoclastic specific should not require (as much) drug holiday. A potential cloud on this horizon, however, relates to recent reports of osteonecrosis or minimal trauma non-osteoporotic fracture after prolonged use of these bisphosphonates. The risk for developing this complication is about 5 in 10 000, when the drugs are used at 'osteoporotic' dosages, not at the higher doses used in Paget's disease. It is likely that bisphosphonates preferentially locate to the active bone of Paget's disease and initially the normal bone is relatively spared. As successful treatment progresses, however, the pagetic bone will become less active and the exposure to normal bone should become correspondingly greater. This type of fracture with minimal trauma or osteonecrosis in Paget's, have been associated.[34] This is certainly not a reason to not treat Paget's disease. It is a reason to carefully consider how long and how aggressively to continue to treat Paget's disease.

The last presently unanswered question about Paget's relates to recently reported declines in prevalence of the disease in areas where it was once greater.[35] These observations will have to be integrated with the theories of genetic versus (or combined with) viral aetiologies.

Key points

- Paget's disease produces large but weak bone.
- Paget's disease can develop into osteosarcoma.
- Side effects include platybasia, heart failure, deafness, fractures and deformity.
- Bisphosphonates are the treatment of choice for Paget's disease.

References

1. Paget J. Chronic inflammation of bones (osteitis deformans). *Trans Med-Chir Soc* 1877;**60**:37–63.
2. Altman R. Paget's disease of bone. In: Coe FL, Favus MJ (eds), *Disorders of Bone and Mineral Metabolism*, 2nd edn, Lippincott Williams & Wilkins, Philadelphia, 2002, pp. 985–1020.
3. Meunier PJ, Coindre JM, Edouard CM, Arlot ME. Bone histomorphometry in Paget's disease. Quantitative and dynamic analysis of pagetic and nonpagetic bone tissue. *Arthritis Rheum* 1980;**23**:1095.
4. Rongstad KM, Wheeler DL, Enneking WF. A comparison of the amount of vascularity in pagetic and normal human bone. *Clin Orthop Relat Res* 1994;**306**:247–9.
5. Blumsohn A, Naylor KE, Assiri AM, Eastell R. Different responses of biochemical markers of bone resorption to bisphosphonate therapy in Paget disease. *Clin Chem* 1995;**41**: 1592–8.
6. Kaddam IM, Iqbal SJ, Holland S, Wong M, Manning D, Comparison of serum osteocalcin with total and bone specific alkaline phosphatase and urinary hydroxyproline:creatinine ratio in patients with Paget's disease of bone. *Ann Clin Biochem* 1994;**31**(Pt 4):327–30.
7. Doyle FH, Banks LM, Pennock JM. Radiologic observations on bone resorption in Paget's disease. *Arthritis Rheum* 1980;**23**:1205–14.
8. Sundaram M, Khanna G, El-Khoury GY. T1-weighted MR imaging for distinguishing large osteolysis of Paget's disease from sarcomatous degeneration. *Skeletal Radiol* 2001; **30**:378–83.
9. Grimer RJ, Cannon SR, Taminiau AM *et al.* Osteosarcoma over the age of forty. *Eur J Cancer* 2003;**39**:157–63.
10. Poncelet A. The neurologic complications of Paget's disease. *J Bone Miner Res* 1999;**14**(Suppl 2):88–91.
11. Yost JH, Spencer-Green G, Krant JD. Vascular steal mimicking compression myelopathy in Paget's disease of bone: rapid reversal with calcitonin and systemic steroids. *Rheumatol* 1993;**20**:1064–5.
12. Whyte MP. Paget's disease of bone. *N Engl J Med* 2006;**355**: 593–600.
13. Rao VM, Karasick D. Hypercementosis - an important clue to Paget's disease of the maxilla. *Skel Radiol* 1982;**9**:126–8.
14. Hadjipavlou AG, Gaitanis IN, Kontakis GM. Paget's disease of the bone and its management. *J Bone Joint Surg Br* 2002;**84**:160–9.
15. Barker DJP. Epidemiology of Paget's disease of bone. *Brit Med Bull* 1984;**40**:396–400.
16. Altman RD. Epidemiology of Paget's disease of bone. *Clin Rev Bone Miner Metab* 2002;1:99–102.
17. Siris ES, Ottman R, Flaster E, Kelsey JL. Familial aggregation of Paget's disease of bone. *J Bone Miner Res* 1991;**6**:495–500.
18. Whyte MP. Paget's disease of bone and genetic disorders of RANKL/OPG/RANK/NF-kappaB signaling. *Ann N Y Acad Sci* 2006;**1068**:143–64.
19. Laurin N, Brown JP, Lemainque A *et al.* Paget disease of bone: mapping of two loci at 5q35-qter and 5q31. *Am J Hum Genet* 2001;**69**: 528–43.
20. Takata S, Yasui N, Nakatsuka K, Ralston SH. Evolution of understanding of genetics of Paget's disease of bone and related diseases. *J Bone Miner Metab* 2004;**22**:519–23.
21. Haslam SI, Van Hul W, Morales-Piga A *et al.* Paget's disease of bone: evidence for a susceptibility locus on chromosome 18q and for genetic heterogeneity. *J Bone Miner Res* 1998; **13**:911–7.
22. Good D, Busfield F, Duffy D *et al.* Familial Paget's disease of bone: nonlinkage to the PDB1 and PDB2 loci on chromosomes 6p and 18q in a large pedigree. *J Bone Miner Res* 2001;**16**:33–8.
23. Reddy SV, Singer FR, Mallette L, Roodman GD. Detection of measles virus nucleocapsid transcripts in circulating blood cells from patients with Paget disease. *J Bone Miner Res* 1996;**11**:1602–7.
24. Gordon MT, Mee AP, Anderson DC, Sharpe PT. Canine distemper virus transcripts sequenced from pagetic bone. *Bone Miner* 1992;**19**:159–74.
25. Mills BG, Frausto A, Singer FR *et al.* Multinucleated cells formed *in vitro* from Paget's bone marrow express viral antigens. *Bone* 1994;**15**:443–8.
26. Ralston SH, Afzal MA, Helfreigh MH *et al.* Multicenter blended analysis of RT-PCR detection methods for paramyxovirus in relation to Paget's disease of bone. *J Bone Miner Res* 2007;**4**:569–77.
27. Roodman GD. Insight into the pathogenesis of Paget's disease. *Ann N Y Acad Sci* 2010;**1192**:176–180.
28. Singer FR. Clinical efficacy of salmon calcitonin in Paget's disease of bone. *Calcif Tissue Int* 1991;**49**(Suppl 2): S7–8.
29. Gibbs CJ, Aaron JE, Peacock M. Osteomalacia in Paget's disease treated with short term, high dose sodium etidronate. *Br Med J* 1986;**292**:1227–9.
30. Walsh JP, Ward LC, Stewart GO *et al.* A randomized clinical trial comparing oral alendronate and intravenous pamidronate for the treatment of Paget's disease of bone. *Bone* 2004;**34**:747–54.
31. Reid IR, Miller P, Lyles K *et al.* Comparison of a single infusion of zoledronic acid with risedronate for Paget's disease. *N Engl J Med* 2005;**353**:898–908.
32. Merlotti D, Gennari L, Martini G *et al.* Comparison of different intravenous bisphosphonate regimens for Paget's disease of bone. *J Bone Miner Res* 2007;22:1510–7.
33. Seton M, Krane SM. Use of zoledronic acid in the treatment of Paget's disease. *Ther Clin Risk Manag* 2007;**3**:913–8.
34. Mavrokokki T, Cheng A, Stein B, Goss A. Nature and frequency of bisphosphonate-associated osteonecrosis of the jaws in Australia. *J Oral Maxillofac Surg* 2007;**65**:415–23.
35. Van Staa TP, Selby P, Leufkens HG *et al.* Incidence and natural history of Paget's disease of bone in England and Wales. *J Bone Miner Res* 2002;**17**:465–71.

CHAPTER 90

Management of osteoporosis; its consequences: a major threat to quality of life

Roger M. Francis
Institute for Ageing and Health, Newcastle University, Newcastle upon Tyne, UK

Introduction

Osteoporosis is a skeletal disorder, characterized by compromised bone strength, predisposing a person to an increased risk of fracture. The major fragility fractures are those of the forearm, vertebral body and hip, but fractures of the humerus, pelvis and tibia are not uncommon in patients with osteoporosis. Fragility fractures are a major cause of excess mortality, substantial morbidity and health and social service expenditure in older people.[1] It is therefore important that effective strategies are developed and implemented to prevent these fractures.

Epidemiology of osteoporosis and fractures

The World Health Organization (WHO) has quantitatively defined osteoporosis as a bone mineral density (BMD) 2.5 standard deviations or more below the mean value for young adults (T-Score ≤ -2.5).[2] The prevalence of osteoporosis at the hip increases in women from 8% in the seventh decade of life to 47.5% in the ninth decade. The incidence of fragility fractures also increases with advancing age, but is higher in women than men. The majority of these fractures occur in people above the age of 75 years, with a three- to fourfold higher rate in institutionalized older people than community-dwelling individuals of the same age. The lifetime risk of fragility fractures for a 50-year-old woman in the UK is 53.2%, compared with 20.7% for a 50-year-old man.[1]

Although forearm fractures may lead to deformity of the wrist and the development of osteoarthritis and the complex regional pain syndrome, there is no evidence of an increase in mortality. Nevertheless, forearm fractures are associated with an increased risk of vertebral and hip fractures in both men and women, so provide an opportunity for consideration of secondary prevention.

Only a third of vertebral fractures come to medical attention, but symptomatic vertebral fractures have a major impact on a patient's quality of life (QOL), because of back pain, loss of height and kyphosis. Vertebral fractures may also result in loss of energy, emotional problems, sleep disturbance, social isolation and reduced mobility. Studies suggest that the impairment of QOL increases with the number of vertebral fractures. The magnitude of the problems encountered by patients with symptomatic vertebral fractures is demonstrated by the fact that they visit their GP 14 times more often than control subjects in the year following fracture. Vertebral fracture is associated with an increased risk of further vertebral fractures, which may be as high as 20% in the following year. There is also an increased risk of hip and other non-vertebral fractures. Vertebral fractures are associated with an excess mortality of 17–20%, which is likely to be due to coexisting conditions associated with osteoporosis, rather than the fracture itself.[1,3]

Hip fractures are the most important fractures in older people, as they cause greater morbidity, higher mortality and more expenditure than all the other fragility fractures combined. Between 25% and 50% of patients become more immobile and dependent after hip fracture, but this is particularly apparent in men and women above the age of 75 years, those with a poor clinical outcome and those who were already dependent before fracture. The excess mortality following hip fractures has been reported to be about 17% over five years, but most deaths occur within six months, suggesting that this is due to complications arising from the fracture and subsequent surgery. Mortality after hip fracture also increases with the number of comorbid conditions. A number of studies show a higher mortality after hip fracture in men than women, but the reason for this is still unclear.[1] It has been estimated that fragility fractures are associated with health and social service costs of £2.3 billion in the UK, almost 90% of which is due tox hip fractures. It has estimated that the average cost of hip

Principles and Practice of Geriatric Medicine, Fifth Edition. Edited by Alan J. Sinclair, John E. Morley and Bruno Vellas.

fracture in the UK is £12 000, of which £4800 is due to the cost of acute hospital care. About 40% of all patients with hip fracture have experienced a prior fragility fracture, potentially representing a lost opportunity for secondary prevention. There is also rapid bone loss after hip fractures and an increased risk of fracture of the contralateral hip and at other sites.

Bone remodelling throughout life

Bone is a living tissue which constantly remodels throughout life, allowing the skeleton to grow during childhood, respond to the mechanical forces placed on it and repair damage due to structural fatigue or fracture. The three major bone cells involved in bone remodelling are osteoclasts, osteoblasts and osteocytes. Osteoclasts are multinucleate cells derived from macrophage-monocyte precursors which resorb bone. Osteoblasts are derived from fibroblast precursors and produce bone matrix or osteoid, which is then subsequently mineralized. Osteocytes are mature osteoblast trapped within calcified bone, which have long interconnecting dendritic processes, and which may serve as mechano-sensory receptors.[1]

Recent research has highlighted the major role of the receptor activator of nuclear factor kappa B (RANK) and RANK ligand (RANKL) system in the regulation of bone remodelling. RANKL is produced by osteoblasts and attaches to RANK on the surface of osteoclasts and osteoclast precursors, leading to osteoclast differentiation and proliferation. The action of RANKL on RANK is blocked by osteoprotegerin (OPG), a decoy receptor produced by osteoblasts and marrow stromal cells. It is now apparent that the beneficial effects of osteoporosis treatments may be mediated in part by changes in the RANK, RANKL and OPG system.[4]

Another regulator of bone turnover is sclerostin, which is produced by osteocyte, under the control of the SOST gene. Sclerostin binds to low density lipoprotein receptor-related protein 5 (LRP5) and inhibits the Wnt signalling pathway, leading to reduced bone formation. Mutations associated with loss of function of the SOST gene lead to sclerosteosis, characterized by increased bone formation, whereas mutations of the LRP5 gene cause the osteoporosis pseudoglioma syndrome.[5]

Pathogenesis of osteoporosis and fractures

BMD at any age is determined by the peak bone mass achieved at maturity, the age at which bone loss starts and the rate at which it progresses. Genetic factors account for up to 80% of the variance in peak bone mass, with the remainder being due to environmental factors, exercise, diet and age at puberty. Bone loss starts between the ages of 35 and 45 in both sexes, but this is accelerated in the decade after the menopause in women. Bone loss then continues until the end of life in men and women, aggravated by factors such as physical inactivity, smoking, alcohol consumption and vitamin D insufficiency, and secondary hyperparathyroidism. There are also a number of causes of secondary osteoporosis, including oral glucocorticoid therapy, male hypogonadism, hyperthyroidism, primary hyperparathyroidism and the use of anti-epileptic drugs.[6]

The risk of fractures is determined by skeletal and non-skeletal risk factors. There is an inverse relationship between bone density and fracture risk, with a two- to threefold increase in fracture incidence for each standard deviation reduction in BMD. The risk of fracture is also determined by other skeletal risk factors, such as bone turnover, cortical and trabecular bone architecture, skeletal geometry and the degree of mineralization of the skeleton. Non-skeletal risk factors for fracture include postural instability, impaired neuromuscular function, physical and mental frailty, and reduced fat and muscle bulk around the hip.[6]

Up to 30% of women and 55% of men with symptomatic vertebral fractures have an underlying cause of secondary osteoporosis, such as oral glucocorticoids, anti-epileptic medication, male hypogonadism, hyperthyroidism, alcohol abuse and myeloma. Risk factors for hip fracture include causes of secondary osteoporosis and conditions associated with falls, such as stroke, Parkinson's disease, dementia and visual impairment.[1,6]

Diagnosis of osteoporosis

Osteoporosis may be diagnosed by performing BMD measurements at the lumbar spine, total hip and femoral neck using dual energy X-ray absorptiometry (DXA). The WHO definition of osteoporosis (T-Score ≤ -2.5) was initially developed for epidemiological studies to assess the prevalence of the condition in different populations, but has increasingly been used as a threshold for diagnosis and therapeutic intervention. Although DXA measurements are generally accurate and precise, lumbar spine BMD may be spuriously elevated in the presence of vertebral fractures, degenerative changes and aortic calcification. Furthermore, only 50% of people with fragility fractures have osteoporosis on DXA scanning, suggesting that other skeletal and non-skeletal risk factors are important in determining fracture risk.

Fracture risk assessment

The WHO has developed a fracture risk assessment tool (FRAX®), which estimates the 10-year risk of fractures of the major fragility fractures (forearm, humerus, spine and hip) and of hip fracture in particular.[7] Country-specific algorithms use age, gender, weight, height and the presence or absence of appropriately weighted risk factors, with or without femoral neck BMD measurements, to estimate fracture risk. The clinical risk factors for fracture used in FRAX®, which are at least in part independent of BMD, comprise low body mass index (BMI), prior fracture after age of 50 years, parental history of hip fracture, current smoking, oral steroid therapy, alcohol intake >2 units/day and chronic conditions associated with bone loss such as rheumatoid arthritis.[7] Other fracture risk assessment tools are being developed, with a view to identifying people at the highest risk of treatment, in whom to target therapeutic intervention.

Guidance has been developed in the USA, UK and in other countries on the level of fracture risk at which treatment should be considered. This will depend not only on the health economy of the country and the cost of the available therapeutic options, but also individual patient factors such as age and the presence of other comorbid conditions. Most clinical trials of treatments to prevent fractures have recruited participants on the basis of documented osteoporosis or the presence of vertebral fractures. Some clinicians are therefore reluctant to use these treatments at patients at high risk of fracture who have a BMD T-Score > − 2.5, as there is no definite evidence that they will prevent fractures in this situation.

Investigation

In patients with documented osteoporosis, underlying causes of bone loss should be identified by careful history, physical examination and appropriate investigation (Table 90.1), particularly when the BMD is lower than expected for age (Z-Score <2.0). These investigations should also be considered in patients with fragility fractures, as specific treatment of underlying conditions such as hyperthyroidism, hypogonadism and primary hyperparathyroidism may increase BMD by up to 15%.[1,6] Investigations for hypogonadism in men may be less appropriate in older men, where the adverse effects of testosterone replacement on the prostate may outweigh the potential benefits. Serum 25-hydroxyvitamin D (25OHD) and parathyroid hormone (PTH) measurements may show vitamin D insufficiency and secondary hyperparathyroidism, but these measurements are probably unnecessary if calcium and vitamin D supplementation is planned. Nevertheless, serum 25OHD and PTH measurements should be considered in patients with possible vitamin D deficiency osteomalacia, which is particularly likely in housebound patients or those with previous gastric resection, malabsorption or the long-term use of anti-epileptic drugs. In patients with severe unexplained osteoporosis, low BMI or anaemia, investigations to exclude a diagnosis of coeliac disease should be performed, particularly if there are symptoms of possible malabsorption.

Table 90.1 Investigations in patients with fragility fractures or low BMD.

Investigation	Finding	Possible cause
Full blood count	Anaemia	Malignancy or malabsorption
	Macrocytosis	Alcohol abuse or malabsorption
ESR and CRP	Raised inflammatory markers	Malignancy
Biochemical profile	Hypercalcaemia	Hyperparathyroidism or malignancy
	Abnormal liver function tests	Alcohol abuse or liver disease
	Persistently high AP	Skeletal metastases
Thyroid function tests	Suppressed TSH; high T_4 or T_3	Hyperthyroidism
Testosterone, SHBG, LH, FSH (men)	Low total testosterone or calculated free testosterone with abnormal gonadotrophins	Hypogonadism
PSA (men with vertebral fractures)	Raised PSA	Metastatic prostate cancer
Serum and urine electrophoresis (Patients with vertebral fractures)	Paraprotein band	Myeloma
Serum 25OHD and PTH	Low 25OHD and raised PTH	Vitamin D insufficiency and secondary hyperparathyroidism.
IgA tissue transglutaminase antibodies (severe osteoporosis, low BMI, anaemia)	Raised antibody levels	Coeliac disease

ESR, erythrocyte sedimentation rate; CRP, C–reactive protein; AP, alkaline phosphatase; TSH, thyroid stimulating hormone; T_4, thyroxine; T_3, triiodothyronine; SHBG, sex hormone binding globulin; LH, luteinizing hormone; FSH, follicle stimulating hormone; PSA, prostate specific antigen; 25OHD, 25-hydroxyvitamin D; PTH, parathyroid hormone; BMI, body mass index.

Lifestyle measures

All patients with documented osteoporosis and/or fragility fractures should be given advice on lifestyle measures to decrease further bone loss, including regular physical activity, eating a balanced diet rich in calcium, smoking cessation, avoiding excess alcohol consumption and maintaining regular exposure to sunlight during the summer months. They should also be advised on measures to reduce the risk of falls. Multidisciplinary falls assessment should also be considered in patients with recurrent falls or abnormal gait and balance.

Drug treatment

The aim of drug treatment is to increase bone density, improve bone strength and reduce the risk of fragility fractures. As bone is a living tissue, treatments target the cells involved in bone remodelling. Most of the currently available treatments are anti-resorptive agents, which act on the osteoclast to decrease bone resorption. Although these treatments lead to a rapid suppression of bone resorption, there is a subsequent reduction in bone formation, because of the close coupling of bone turnover. This leads to a small improvement in BMD, which is then maintained with continuing treatment. In contrast, anabolic treatments act predominantly on the osteoblast to increase bone formation. There may also be a subsequent increase in bone resorption, but the relative imbalance between formation and resorption leads to a greater increase in BMD than that seen with anti-resorptive agents.

A number of treatments for osteoporosis have now been shown in large randomized controlled trials (RCTs) to improve BMD and reduce the risk of fractures (Table 90.2). The choice of treatment will depend on the individual's biological rather than chronological age, BMD, fracture risk, cost and other potential risks and benefits. As compliance and long-term persistence with medication for chronic disease is relatively poor, tolerability and patient preference is also important, as inadequate compliance with osteoporosis treatment is associated with less benefit in terms of BMD and fracture.

Table 90.2 The effect of osteoporosis treatments on the risk of vertebral, non-vertebral and hip fractures. A indicates that a significant reduction in fractures has been demonstrated in a randomized controlled trial, whereas (A) indicates that a beneficial effect on fractures risk was only found in *post hoc* subgroup analysis. ND indicates that fracture reduction has not been demonstrated.

	Vertebral fractures	Non-vertebral fractures	Hip fractures
HRT	A	A	A
Raloxifene	A	ND	ND
Alendronate	A	A	A
Risedronate	A	A	A
Zoledronate	A	A	A
Ibandronate	A	(A)	ND
Denosumab	A	A	A
Strontium ranelate	A	A	(A)
Teriparatide	A	A	ND
PTH 1–84	A	A	A
Calcium and vitamin D	ND	A	A

Hormone replacement therapy

Hormone replacement therapy (HRT) was previously used widely in the prevention and treatment of younger postmenopausal women with osteoporosis, but this changed with the publication of the results of the Women's Health Initiative Study.[8] Although this showed a reduction in colon cancer, vertebral, hip and other factures, overall the benefits were outweighed by the increased risk of breast cancer, coronary heart disease, stroke and venous thromboembolism. Nevertheless, subsequent subgroup analysis suggests that the adverse effects of HRT may be less in women below the age of 60 years, especially those with a previous hysterectomy who can be treated with unopposed estrogen.

Selective estrogen receptor modulators

Selective estrogen receptor modulators (SERMs) have estrogen-like actions on the bone, where they decrease bone resorption and bone loss, but have antagonist actions on the breast and endometrium, thereby decreasing the risk of breast cancer without stimulating endometrial proliferation. Raloxifene decreases the incidence of vertebral fractures, but has no effect on non-vertebral fractures.[9] It is therefore useful in younger postmenopausal women at high risk of vertebral fractures, but less appropriate in older women at significant risk of non-vertebral fractures. Newer SERMs such as lasofoxifene may decrease the incidence of vertebral and non-vertebral fractures, as well as reduce the risk of breast cancer, stroke and cardiovascular disease.[10] Like HRT and raloxifene, lasofoxifene is associated with an increased risk of venous thromboembolism. At the present time, lasofoxifene has not been licensed for the treatment of osteoporosis.

Bisphosphonates

Oral bisphosphonates are currently the treatment of choice for osteoporosis, as they improve BMD and decrease the risk of vertebral, non-vertebral and hip fractures by 35–50%.[11–13] Although these agents are available as daily (alendronate and risedronate), weekly (alendronate and risedronate) and monthly (ibandronate) preparations, they should be ingested in a fasting condition, to ensure adequate absorption from the bowel. They also need to be taken with water and subsequent recumbency avoided for between 30 and 60 minutes depending on the preparation, to decrease the potential risk of oesophageal side effects of treatment. Oral bisphosphonates are generally well tolerated, but the most common side effects include, acid reflux symptoms, heartburn and indigestions. These may be more likely with alendronate than risedronate, and the clinical studies of the latter included patients with upper gastrointestinal disorders.

The complex instructions for administration, upper gastrointestinal side effects and poor compliance and persistence may limit the use of oral bisphosphonates in some patients. Annual intravenous infusion of zoledronate or three-monthly intravenous injections of ibandronate provide a useful alternative option in this situation. Intravenous zoledronate has been shown to decrease the risk of vertebral fractures by 70% and hip fractures by 41% in women with osteoporosis.[14] A further study in patients with recent hip fracture demonstrated that intravenous zoledronate decreased the risk of vertebral and non-vertebral fractures, but also reduced mortality by 28%.[15] The improvement in mortality was not attributable to the prevention of hip fractures, but may reflect a reduction in deaths due to other conditions. Intravenous bisphosphonate treatment may lead to an acute phase reaction in about 15% of cases, associated with transient 'flu-like symptoms lasting for a few days. The severity of these symptoms can be reduced by the use of paracetamol 1 g four times daily for three days, starting on the day of treatment. As zoledronate has been reported to cause a decline in renal function in patients with pre-existing renal impairment, it should be avoided in the presence of dehydration or when the glomerular filtation rate is less than $35\,\mathrm{ml\,min^{-1}}$. As zoledronate is a potent inhibitor of bone resorption it may lead to symptomatic hypocalcaemia in patients with low serum calcium or vitamin D concentrations. If there is any doubt about a patient's vitamin D status, they should receive supplementation before zoledronate is administered.

There has been some concern about potential over-suppression of bone turnover with long-term bisphosphonate treatment. This may lead to structural fatigue and an inability to repair microdamage within the skeleton. Case-series of atypical subtrochanteric fractures of the femur have been reported in patients on long-term bisphosphonate treatment. These atypical fractures are rare and the potential risks appear to be outweighed by the benefits in hip fracture prevention. Nevertheless, the development of prodromal thigh pain in patients on bisphosphonate treatment should alert the clinician to the possible development of an atypical subtrochanteric fracture.

Prolonged bisphosphonate treatment has also been implicated in the development of osteonecrosis of the jaw (ONJ). In this condition, which can occur in the absence of bisphosphonate treatment, there is necrosis of bone in the maxilla or mandible, as a result of occlusion of the blood supply. This results in retraction of the overlying gum and exposure of the necrotic bone. Most cases occur after tooth extraction or other dental surgery, with the remainder occurring mainly in denture wearers, where local trauma and infection may have been implicated. There has been speculation that over-suppression of bone turnover with bisphosphonates may compromise the skeletal response to local trauma and infection, resulting in focal osteonecrosis. ONJ appears to be more common when frequent, high-dose intravenous bisphosphonates are used in the treatment of malignancy (1in 20 to 1 in 100), than with intravenous (1 in 1000 to 1 in 10 000) or oral bisphosphonates in osteoporosis (1 in 10 000 to 1 in 100 000).

Bisphosphonates persist in the skeleton beyond the period of administration, which may result in the maintenance of their beneficial effect on bone density and fracture incidence. As a result of this and concern about the potential adverse effects of long-term treatment, there is increasing debate about the optimal duration of treatment and the possible option of a 'drug holiday'. In the extension phase of the initial clinical trials of alendronate treatment, participants who had taken the bisphosphonate for five years, were randomized to continue treatment or receive placebo for a further five years. Although there was some bone loss and increase in bone resorption five years after stopping alendronate, the BMD was higher and bone turnover markers were lower than baseline values before treatment. Overall, 10 years' treatment with alendronate was not associated with a lower incidence of non-vertebral fractures than five years' treatment followed by placebo, but the risk of clinical vertebral fractures was lower with 10 years' alendronate treatment.[16] A subsequent subgroup analysis demonstrated that in women without a vertebral fracture, continuation of alendronate only decreased the risk of non-vertebral fractures in women whose femoral neck BMD T-Score was still ≤ -2.5 after five years' treatment.[16] Although the number of patients sustaining non-vertebral fractures in this study was relatively small, the results suggest that it may be reasonable to stop alendronate treatment after five years if the patient has a BMD T-Score above -2.5 or is at low risk of vertebral fractures.

Denosumab

Denosumab is a monoclonal antibody directed against RANK ligand. This leads to a marked reduction in bone resorption and an increase in BMD. A large randomized controlled trial in women with osteoporosis showed that six-monthly subcutaneous injections of denosumab 60 mg decreased vertebral fractures by 68%, non-vertebral fractures by 20% and hip fractures by 40%.[17] The drug appeared to be well tolerated, but there was an increase in eczema and cellulitis in participants treated with denosumab compared with those receiving placebo. There was no increase in cancer, infections or hypocalcaemia in women treated with denosumab over the three years of the study. Although denosumab leads to a substantial reduction in bone resorption, no cases of atypical fractures or ONJ were observed with denosumab, although the latter has now been reported in a patient treated with this drug. In contrast to the situation with bisphosphonates, there is a rapid increase in bone resorption when treatment with denosumab is discontinued. Although this should avoid the potential problem of persistent over-suppression of bone turnover, treatment withdrawal may lead to rapid reversal of any previous improvement in bone density.

Strontium ranelate

Strontium ranelate has been described as a dual-acting bone agent, which reduces bone resorption and increases bone formation. The effects of strontium ranelate on the biochemical markers of bone turnover suggest that the effect on bone resorption is less marked than that seen with bisphosphonates, whereas the effect on new bone formation is more modest than that with anabolic agents. Nevertheless, treatment leads to an improvement in bone strength, even if the underlying mechanism is not readily apparent.

A large clinical trial of three years' treatment with strontium ranelate in women with osteoporosis showed increases in BMD of 12.7% in the lumbar spine and 8.6% in the hip and a 41% reduction in new vertebral fractures.[18] About 50% of the apparent increase in BMD is spurious, due to the incorporation of strontium into the skeleton. Another large study in women with osteoporosis showed a 16% reduction in non-vertebral fractures with strontium ranelate, but a *post-hoc* subgroup analysis in older women with low BMD (T-Score <−3.0) demonstrated a 36% reduction in hip fractures.[19] Strontium ranelate has also been shown to decrease the incidence of vertebral and non-vertebral fractures in women above the age of 80 years, with the benefits extending over a five-year period of treatment.[20]

Strontium ranelate is available in powder form in sachets, the contents of which are dissolved in water. It should preferably be taken at bedtime, at least two hours after eating, to ensure adequate absorption from the bowel. Strontium has been generally well tolerated in clinical trials, but reported side effects have included diarrhoea and a small increased risk of venous thromboembolism, but the reason for the latter remains unclear. In post-marketing surveillance, a small number of cases of drug rash with eosinophilia and systemic symptoms (DRESS) have been reported. This occurred within 3 to 6 weeks of starting treatment, presenting with skin rash, accompanied by a fever and swollen glands.

Parathyroid hormone

Parathyroid hormone (PTH) stimulates bone turnover, with an increase in bone resorption and new bone formation. The continuously high circulating concentration of PTH found in primary and secondary hyperparathyroidism is associated with an increase in bone turnover, but bone resorption is stimulated more than bone formation, resulting in loss of bone from the skeleton. In contrast, intermittent administration of PTH stimulates bone formation more than resorption, resulting in an increase in bone mass and density. There are two licensed PTH preparations available, recombinant human PTH 1–34 (teriparatide) and PTH 1–84, both of which are administered by daily subcutaneous injection.

Clinical studies of PTH treatment show a larger increase in BMD than that observed with bisphosphonates. There is also a stimulation of periosteal new bone formation, leading to a small increase in the diameter of long bones, which may contribute to bone strength. Teriparatide decreases the incidence of vertebral and non-vertebral fractures, but no reduction in hip fractures has been demonstrated.[21] PTH 1–84 has also been shown to reduce the incidence of vertebral fractures.[22] Treatment with PTH is generally well tolerated, but may be associated with transient mild hypercalcaemia, nausea, dizzyness and headaches.[21,22] As these preparations are more expensive than bisphosphonates, their use is generally restricted to patients with severe osteoporosis, or those who fail to respond to bisphosphonate treatment. The anabolic effect of PTH treatment may be attenuated by concomitant administration of a bisphosphonate, but this has not been a consistent finding in clinical studies.

Vitamin D

Vitamin D is essential for musculoskeletal health, as it promotes calcium absorption from the bowel, enables the mineralization of newly formed osteoid tissue in bone and plays an important role in muscle function. There is no universal agreement on what constitutes optimal vitamin D status for musculoskeletal health. Nevertheless, vitamin D insufficiency is common in older people, especially in those who are housebound or living in residential and nursing homes. Vitamin D insufficiency leads to bone loss because of the associated secondary hyperparathyroidism and may also contribute to an increased risk of falls as a result of muscle weakness and impaired neuromuscular function.[23]

The results of studies of vitamin D supplementation on the risk falls have been inconsistent, but a recent meta-analysis which only included trials where falls were a major outcome measure, demonstrated a 19% reduction in falls with vitamin D in doses of 700–1000 IU daily.[24] The most convincing evidence for the benefit of vitamin D supplementation in fracture prevention was provided by a large study in 3270 women living in nursing homes or sheltered housing, where combined calcium and vitamin D supplementation decreased the risk of hip and other non-vertebral fractures by 43% and 32% respectively.[25] Subsequent studies of vitamin D supplementation, with or without additional calcium, on the risk of fracture have produced conflicting results. Recent meta-analyses suggest that combined calcium and vitamin D supplementation leads to a modest reduction in hip and other non-vertebral fractures, whereas vitamin D alone is ineffective.[26,27]

Although combined calcium and vitamin D supplementation leads to a small decrease in fracture risk, compliance and persistence with supplements containing calcium is relatively poor. Calcium and vitamin D supplementation should therefore be directed on those who are likely to have vitamin D insufficiency, such as care home residents and housebound people living in the community.[28] The use of calcium and vitamin D supplementation should also be considered in people on other osteoporosis treatments, in accordance with recommendations from the National Institute of Health and Clinical Excellence (NICE), unless the clinician is confident that they are calcium and vitamin D replete.[29]

Future treatments

Potential new treatments for osteoporosis which are currently being investigated include cathepsin K inhibitors, sclerostin inhibitors, selective androgen receptor modulators (SARMS) and calcium-sensing receptor antagonists. Cathepsin K is an important enzyme secreted by osteoclasts which resorbs bone. The importance of this enzyme is highlighted by the rare condition of pycnodysostosis (Toulouse-Lautrec syndrome), where a genetic mutation leads to cathepsin K deficiency, associated with the development of dense bones and short stature. The weekly administration of oral odanacatib has recently been shown to reduce the biochemical markers of bone resorption and increase spine and hip BMD in postmenopausal women with low bone density.[30]

Sclerostin is also an important target for the development of new treatments for osteoporosis, as it binds to LRP5 and inhibits the Wnt signalling pathway, leading to reduced bone formation. A recent study of a monoclonal antibody directed against sclerostin has shown an increase in bone formation, bone density and bone strength in cynomolgus monkeys.

SARMS offer the exciting prospect of a treatment which is anabolic for bone and muscle, without unwanted androgenic effects on the prostate in men or virilization in women. Nevertheless, developing a therapeutic agent with the appropriate spectrum of agonist and antagonist actions on the androgen receptor at different sites is likely to be challenging.

Calcium-sensing receptor antagonists or calcilytics are oral agents which lead to the endogenous production of PTH. As noted earlier, continuously raised PTH concentrations in hyperparathyroidism lead to bone loss, whereas pulsatile high concentrations achieved with daily subcutaneous administration of PTH increase bone density. Early work on the effect of calcilytics on bone density have been disappointing, possibly because of a failure to achieve the optimal pulsing of circulating PTH concentrations.

Key points

- Fragility fractures are an important cause of excess mortality, substantial morbidity and health and social service expenditure in older people.
- The risk of fracture is determined by skeletal factors influencing bone strength and by non-skeletal risk factors associated with falls.
- Strategies to prevent fractures should include measures to improve bone strength and reduce the risk of falls.
- A number of osteoporosis treatments have been shown to decrease the risk of fractures. The use of bone density measurements and clinical risk factors for fracture should identify people at the highest risk of fracture, in whom treatment should be considered.

References

1. Francis RM. Metabolic bone disease. In: Tallis RC, Fillit HM (eds), *Brocklehurst's Textbook of Geriatric Medicine and Gerontology*, 7th edn, WB Saunders, 2010, pp. 553–65.
2. World Health Organization (WHO). Assessment of fracture risk and its application to screening for postmenopausal osteoporosis. Report of a WHO Study Group, WHO, Geneva, 1994.
3. Francis RM, Baillie SP, Chuck AJ *et al.* Acute and long term management of patients with vertebral fractures. *Q J Med* 2004;**97**:63–74.
4. Kearns AE, Khosla S, Kostenuik PJ. Receptor activator of nuclear factor kappa β ligand and osteoprotegerin regulation of bone remodeling in health and disease. *Endocr Rev* 2008;**29**:155–192.

5. Rosen CJ. Exploiting new targets or old bone. *J Bone Miner Res* 2010;**25**:934–6.
6. Tuck SP, Francis RM. Best practice: osteoporosis. *Postgrad Med J* 2002;**78**:526–32.
7. Kanis JA on behalf of the World Health Organization Scientific Group. Assessment of osteoporosis at the primary health-care level. Technical Report. WHO Collaborating Centre, University of Sheffield, UK, 2008.
8. Rossouw JE, Anderson GL, Prentice RL *et al.*; Writing Group for the Women's Health Initiative Investigators. Risks and benefits of oestrogen plus progestin in healthy postmenopausal women: principal results from the Women's Health Initiative randomized controlled trial. *JAMA* 2002;**288**:321–33.
9. Ettinger B, Black DM, Mitlak BH *et al.* Reduction of vertebral fracture risk in postmenopausal women with osteoporosis treated with raloxifene. Results from a 3 year randomised clinical trial. *JAMA* 1999;**282**:637–45.
10. Cummings SR, Ensrud K, Delmas PD *et al.*; PEARL Study Investigators. Lasofoxifene in postmenopausal women with osteoporosis. *N Engl J Med* 2010;**362**:686–96.
11. Black DM, Cummings SR, Karpf DB *et al.* Randomised trial of effect of alendronate on risk of fracture in women with existing vertebral fractures. Lancet 1996;**348**:1535–41.
12. Harris ST, Watts NB, Genant HK *et al.*; for the Vertebral Efficacy With Risedronate Therapy (VERT) Study Group. Effects of risedronate treatment on vertebral and nonvertebral fractures in women with postmenopausal osteoporosis: a randomized controlled trial. *JAMA* 1999;**282**:1344–52.
13. McClung MR, Geusens P, Miller PD *et al.* Effect of risedronate on the risk of hip fracture in elderly women. Hip Intervention Program Study Group. *N Engl J Med* 2001;**344**:333–40.
14. Black DM, Delmas PD, Eastell R *et al.* HORIZON Pivotal Fracture Trial. Once-yearly zoledronic acid for treatment of postmenopausal osteoporosis. *N Engl J Med* 2007;**356**: 1809–22.
15. Lyles KW, Colón-Emeric CS, Magaziner JS *et al.* HORIZON Recurrent Fracture Trial. Zoledronic acid and clinical fractures and mortality after hip fracture. *N Engl J Med* 2007; **357**:1799–809.
16. Schwarz AV, Bauer DC, Cummings ST *et al.*; for the FLEX Research Group. Efficacy of continued alendronate for fractures in women with and without prevalent vertebral fracture: The FLEX Trial. *J Bone Miner Res* 2010;**25**:976–82.
17. Cummings SR, San Martin J, McClung MR *et al.*; for the FREEDOM Trial. Denosumab for prevention of fractures in postmenopausal women with osteoporosis. *N Engl J Med* 2009;**361**:756–65.
18. Meunier PJ, Roux C, Seeman E *et al.* The effects of strontium ranelate on the risk of vertebral fracture in women with postmenopausal osteoporosis. *N Engl J Med* 2004;**350**:459–68.
19. Reginster JY, Seeman E, De Vernejoul MC *et al.* Strontium ranelate reduces the risk of nonvertebral fractures in postmenopausal women with osteoporosis: Treatment of Peripheral Osteoporosis (TROPOS) study. *J Clin Endocrinol Metab* 2005;**90**:2816–22.
20. Seeman E, Boonen S, Borgström F *et al.* Five years treatment with strontium ranelate reduces vertebral and nonvertebral fractures and increases the number and quality of remaining life-years in women over 80 years of age. *Bone* 2010;**46**: 1038–42.
21. Neer RM, Arnaud CD, Zanchetta JR *et al.* Effect of parathyroid hormone (1-34) on fractures and bone mineral density in postmenopausal women with osteoporosis. *N Engl J Med* 2001;**344**:1434–41.
22. Greenspan SL, Bone HG, Ettinger MP *et al.*; Treatment of Osteoporosis with Parathyroid Hormone Study Group. Effect of recombinant human parathyroid hormone (1-84) on vertebral fracture and bone mineral density in postmenopausal women with osteoporosis: a randomized trial. *Ann Intern Med* 2007;**146**:326–39.
23. Francis RM, Anderson FH, Patel S, Sahota O, van Staa TP. Calcium and vitamin D in the prevention of osteoporotic fractures. *Q J Med* 2006;**99**:355–63.
24. Bischoff-Ferrari HA, Dawson-Hughes B, Staehelin HB *et al.* Fall prevention with supplemental and active forms of vitamin D: a meta-analysis of randomised controlled trials. *Br Med J* 2009;**339**:b3692.
25. Chapuy MC, Arlot ME, Duboeuf F *et al.* Vitamin D_3 and calcium to prevent hip fractures in elderly women. *N Engl J Med* 1992;**327**:1637–42.
26. Boonen S, Lips P, Bouillon R, Bischoff-Ferrari HA *et al.* Need for additional calcium to reduce the risk of hip fracture with vitamin D supplementation: evidence from a comparative meta-analysis of randomized controlled trials. *J Clin Endocrinol Metab* 2007;**92**:1415–23.
27. The DIPART (vitamin D Individual Patient Analysis of Randomized Trials) Group. Patient level pooled analysis of 68 500 patients from seven major vitamin D fracture trials in US and Europe. *Br Med J* 2010;**340**:b5463.
28. Aspray TJ, Francis RM. Vitamin D and fractures: where are we now ? *Maturitas* 2010;**66**:221–2.
29. National Institute for Health and Clinical Excellence (NICE). Alendronate, etidronate, risedronate, raloxifene and teriparatide for the secondary prevention of osteoporotic fragility fractures in postmenopausal women (amended). NICE Technology Appraisal 161, January 2010.
30. Bone HG, McClung MR, Roux C *et al.* Odanacatib, a cathepsin-K inhibitor: A two-year study in postmenopausal women with low bone density. *J Bone Miner Res* 2010;**25**: 937–47.

CHAPTER 91

Gait, balance and falls

Dulce M. Cruz-Oliver[1]
Saint Louis University, Saint Louis, MO, USA

Introduction

Falls and imbalance are important causes of disability, morbidity and mortality in an ageing population. More than one third of adults aged 65 years and older fall each year. Among nursing homes residents, as many as three out of four residents fall each year; 10–20% cause serious injuries. Falls are the leading cause of accidental deaths and account for most of non-fatal injuries and hospital admissions for trauma. The direct cost of fall injuries in 2000 ranged from US$0.2–19 billion.[1] Similar to many other conditions in the geriatric population, factors that can contribute to falls are multiple, and very often more than one of these factors plays an important role. For this reason risk factor assessment, prevention and therapeutic interventions will be the primary focus of this chapter.

Balance

Balance or equilibrium is an ability to maintain the centre of gravity (also known as the centre of mass-COM) of a body within the base of support with minimal postural sway. It is a complex process that depends on the integration of vision, vestibular and proprioception, central coordination and neuromuscular responses that control muscle actions. The senses must detect changes of body position with respect to the base, regardless of whether the body moves or the base moves. When standing, any changes in orientation are perceived by proprioceptive and cutaneous sensors in the feet. Vision detects linear and angular motion of the visual field and the vestibular apparatus detects sway-related linear and angular acceleration of the head. When the support surface is irregular or in motion, vestibular input becomes essential. When the surface is fixed and level, proprioception is predominant. An age-related decline in function can be demonstrated in all parts of this system.

Maintenance of this upright position is associated with postural sway mainly in the anterior/posterior (A/P) direction. Both A/P sway velocity and the area are seen to increase in normal older subjects. Increase in A/P sway has been correlated with spontaneous falls, but a better predictor is mediolateral (side to side) sway. Falls depend on the relationship between the COM and the base of support. In older people, postural reactions controlling the COM are slowed and there appears to be particular difficulty in controlling lateral instability. Moreover, unexpected perturbations require an adjustment of the base of support through compensatory stepping, and older fallers often have problems controlling these compensatory stepping movements. Experiments with a movable platform that can produce multidirectional perturbations show that younger controls react with a rapid compensatory abducting their arms uphill, and hinging at the hips and trunk, thus keeping their COM away from the direction of tilt. In older subjects, compensatory trunk movements are reduced (probably due to stiffening) and their arms are stretched in the direction of the fall.[2]

Peripheral sensation (proprioception and touch) is the most important afferent control mechanism of standing balance in healthy older people. Other factors that are highly correlated with increased sway are reduced muscle strength in the legs, poor near visual acuity, and slowed reaction time. Vision can partially compensate for loss of other sensory inputs, and with increasing age as the postural task gets harder so the reliance on vision becomes greater. Thus, patients with proprioceptive or vestibular impairments are easily upset if the visual field is faulty or misleading in any way. There is no doubt that some individuals maintain good postural control, even into extreme old age, indicating that age-related changes alone have only a minor effect and that imbalance is largely the result of pathology.

[1]This update is based on the excellent chapter by Peter W. Overstall and Thorsten Nikolaus in the previous edition of the book.

Principles and Practice of Geriatric Medicine, Fifth Edition. Edited by Alan J. Sinclair, John E. Morley and Bruno Vellas.

Disequilibrium syndromes are identified by inspection of arising, standing, turning and response to perturbation. There are four main syndromes: dysmetria, or lack of coordination of movement associated with cerebellar disorders; bradykinesia, or delayed postural responses associated with akinetic-rigid disorders (parkinsonism); sensory deprivation due to vestibular dysfunction, or loss of proprioception due to peripheral neuropathy; and apraxia, a central disorganization of learned motor programmes for standing and walking, mainly due to frontal lobe dysfunction.[3]

Disease-related balance disorders are also common, such as cerebrovascular, cognitive impairment and Parkinson's disease (PD). Of major importance is the slowing of central coordination due to cerebrovascular or Alzheimer's disease (AD). In its early stages, this is often unrecognized, and the diagnosis is not made until the patient is seen in a falls clinic. In cerebral multi-infarct states patients with few or any neurological signs may present with disequilibrium (during standing and with perturbations) and gait abnormalities (decreased hip and knee flexion during swing phase and instability during stance phase).[4] Minor and even major cognitive impairment is often not considered in the differential diagnosis among recurrent fallers. Balance depends on cognitive processes and attention, which may be affected by anxiety and depression as well as brain pathology. The ability to recover balance demands more attention even for healthy older people when compared with young adults. Older people appear less able to shift weight and select appropriate responses quickly when the environment changes suddenly. The ability to perform multiple or dual tasks is challenged with ageing and becomes diminished in cognitive impairment. One study on institutionalized patients with dementia showed a tendency to stop walking while talking. The difficulties increase as the tasks become more complex, and both the young and the old tend to prioritize gait performance over the secondary cognitive task.[5]

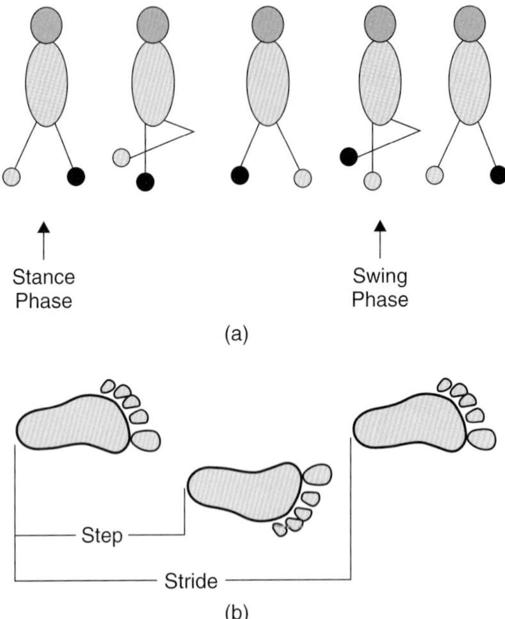

Figure 91.1 The walking gait cycle. (a) During double stance, the weight is transferred from one foot to the other; this is known as the stance phase. During single stance, the centre of mass of the body passes over the foot in preparation for shifting to the other limb, resulting in the swing phase. (b) Step versus Stride. Step is described as the period from initial contact of one limb to the initial contact of the contralateral limb. Stride or gait cycle is described as the period from the initial contact of a particular limb to the point of initial contact of the same limb and is equivalent to one gait cycle. Therefore, there are two steps in each stride.

Gait

Gait is defined as the pattern of movement of the limbs during locomotion over a solid surface, 'manner of walking' or 'sequence of foot movements'. Figure 91.1 illustrates the components of gait cycle.

Human locomotion depends on higher command and control centres in the brainstem and forebrain. Its physiological function depends on the origin of stimuli, either *internal or external cues*. In normal walking–an *internally cued*, well-learned motor act–the supplementary motor area (SMA) of the frontal cortex engages in significant firing just prior to gait ignition. This preparatory activity represents submovement programme selection, which is subsequently sent to the primary motor cortex area (M1). This SMA activity is switched off by phasic activity generated by the basal ganglia (BG), which provides a non-specific cue both to trigger the submovement and to instruct the SMA to prepare for the next. It is this interaction between phasic activity from the BG and SMA, which is responsible for smooth running of predictable, well-learned, automatic movement sequences that depend on internal cues. The sequence of activation, however, is different when movement occurs in response to *external cues*. In this situation the BG/SMA pathways could be bypassed with sensory information from the environment feeding directly into the pre-motor area (PMA) through visual, auditory and propioceptive pathways, with the PMA subsequently activating the M1.[4] The pedunculopontine nucleus (PPN), an area near to the nucleus cuneiformis below the cerebellar peduncle receives afferent connections from the BG, cerebellum and motor cortex and projects to the brainstem reticular nuclei. Then instructions for gait are passed along non-pyramidal pathways in the ventral spinal cord.[6]

Parkinson's disease affects gait by disordered cueing from the BG due to a disturbance in internal rhythm formation in the BG such that the SMA is not switched off on time. This leads to some of the clinical features of PD including bradykinesia, gait ignition failure and freezing. For this reason PD patients seem to rely heavily on intact sensory/PMA pathways to initiate movements (i.e. better walking while stepping over coloured patterns on the ground and drawing movements when they are aided by external cues). An analogous situation may exist among vascular higher-level gait disorders from infarcts to the aforementioned pathways.[4]

Changes in gait patterns associated with advanced age have been identified, such as slow walking speed due to shorter step length and increased time spent in double limb support. Gait speed declines 12–16% per decade for self-selected gait speed and up to 20% decline for maximum gait speed.[7] These age-related changes in walking patterns have been interpreted as indicating adoption of a more conservative or less destabilizing gait, suggesting that older people compensate for their reduced physical capabilities by being more cautious. Menz and colleagues compared a small sample of young and old subjects and found that old subjects exhibited changes in walking, sensory function and muscle strength. Authors concluded that the normal age-related decline in leg strength may be the primary limiting factor that prevents older people walking at an equivalent speed to younger people.[8]

Gait abnormalities are common in the elderly. An abnormal gait, defined by shuffling or degree of difficulty with turns, was observed in 31% of patients older than 67 years.[6] The factors that affect gait in the elderly may include physiological, medical and social aspects. Individually or in combination, these risk factors predispose elders to gait and balance abnormalities.

Physiological factors include neural control, muscle function and posture control, which are impaired by ageing and/or degenerative disease. Neuromuscular ageing changes are contributors of gait alterations, specifically, the loss of cross-sectional muscle mass (10–40%), decrease in type I and type II muscle fibres, prolonged contraction and relaxation time, and a decrease in conduction velocity in sensory and motor nerves with resultant loss of proprioception. Further, within the articular cartilage, there is formation of cross-links and loss of elastic fibres, resulting in stiffer joint capsules and ligaments that affect the quality of movement and gait. The resultant movement pattern will be slower, more uncertain and uncoordinated, and lacking full range of motion.[7]

Medical factors include the use of psychotropic medications, previous falls, cognitive and neurodegenerative diseases, cardiopulmonary, musculoskeletal, psychological (i.e. depression, anxiety), visual, vestibular and proprioceptive impairments. Along with these factors related to gait impairments the following *social factors* need to be considered as potential contributors to reduced mobility. They consist of self-efficacy or dependence in activities of daily living (ADL), motivation, lack of social support, use of assistive devices and low level of physical activity.[7]

Gait disorders are particularly important in older people because they threaten independence and contribute to falls and injury. A classification of gait disorders based on neural system affected has been proposed.[3,6] The lowest-level gait disorders include peripheral sensory dysfunction with peripheral neuropathy, vestibular, visual and propioceptive deficits; and peripheral motor dysfunction with arthritis and neuromuscular diseases (focal myopathic, neuropathic weakness). Middle-level gait disorders consist of hemiplegia/paraplegia (arm and leg weakness, spasticity, equinovarus), cerebellar ataxia (poor trunk control, lack of coordination) and extrapyramidal syndromes (rigidity, bradykinesia, trunk flexion). The highest-level gait disorders are: cautious gait, mild AD, cerebrovascular disease and normal pressure hydrocephalus (cognitive impairment, gait apraxia, and urinary incontinence). Nevertheless, a clinical approach seems more useful for physicians to address gait abnormalities. Sudarsky and Nutt present a clinical syndrome classification of seven gait abnormalities: cautious gait, gait limited by weakness, stiff gait, ataxic gait, veering, freezing and toppling gait, and bizarre gaits[3,6] (see Table 91.1).

Falls

A fall, defined by consensus statement as the 'unexpected event in which the patient comes to rest on the ground, floor or lower level',[9] is one of the most common events that threaten the independence of older persons. As with other geriatric syndromes, falls result from the accumulated effect of impairments in multiple domains. The causes of falling often involve a complex interaction among factors intrinsic (medical and neuropsychiatric conditions; impaired vision and hearing; and ageing changes in neuromuscular, gait and balance reflexes) and extrinsic (medications, improper use of assistive device and environmental hazards) to the individual. Rarely is a fall related to a single factor.

Age-related changes in postural control and gait probably play a major role in many falls among older persons. Increasing age is associated with diminished proprioceptive input: slower righting reflexes, diminished strength of muscles, and increase postural sway. All these changes can contribute to falling, especially the ability to avoid a fall after encountering an unexpected trip or hazard. Although ageing changes in gait may not be sufficiently prominent to be labelled truly pathological, they can increase susceptibility to falls. Elderly men tend to develop wide-based, short-stepped gaits; elderly women often walk with a narrow-based, waddling gait.[10]

Although not all elderly individuals with orthostatic hypotension (OH) are symptomatic, this could play a role in causing instability and precipitating falls. People

Table 91.1 Gait syndromes features and disease examples. Clinical syndrome classification of seven gait abnormalities with its features and disease examples.

Gait syndrome	Features	Disease example
Dysmetria	Imbalance with slow and halting gait with wide base of support and irregular progression	Cerebellar ataxia (Friedreich's ataxia), chorea, sensory ataxia
Stiff/rigid	Loss of fluidity, stiffness of legs and trunk with circumduction, scissoring and equinovarus gait.	Spasticity (cerebral palsy, spinal cord disorders), parkinsonism, dystonia, musculoskeletal
Weakness	Waddling, lateral path deviation with regular stride and foot drop	Myopathy, peripheral neuropathy (vincristine, cisplatin chemotherapy, paraproteinemia)
Veering	Deviation of gait or falls on one side	Vestibular disorders, thalamic astasia
Freezing	Start and turn hesitation, stepping movements with side to side shuffling	Multi-infarct, parkinsonism (PD, supranuclear palsy, Lewy body disease, multiple system atrophy)
Cautious	Slowing, short steps, en bloc turns, wider base, shorter swing base	Non-specific, multifactorial
Bizarre/ psychogenic	Embellished, inconsistent, distractible	Anxiety, conversion disorder, fear of falling or space phobia

with orthostatic and/or postprandial hypotension are at particular risk for near syncope and falls, especially when treated with diuretics and antihypertensive drugs. Ooi and colleagues measured supine and standing blood pressure four times in a single day in 844 nursing home residents, both before and after meals. The outcome measure was any subsequent fall over 1.2 years. Fifty percent had OH on at least one measurement. OH did not predict falls in those who had never fallen, but was predictive of recurrence in previous fallers (relative risk 2.6). The timing of OH before or after meals did not affect fall risk. They conclude that OH is an independent risk factor for recurrent falls in institutionalized elderly.[11]

Other pathological conditions, such as degenerative joint disease, can cause pain, unstable joints, muscle weakness and neurological disturbances. Healed fractures of the hip can cause an abnormal and less steady gait. Diminished sensory input, such as in diabetes and other peripheral neuropathies, impaired hearing and visual acuity diminish cues from the environment that normally contribute to stability and thus predispose to falls. Some studies have shown certain gait abnormalities characteristics of patients with dementia and mild cognitive impairment that may lead to falls. Foot deformities (bunions, calluses, nail disease, joint deformities, etc.) can also cause instability and falls.[10]

Across studies, many risk factors were found to be consistently associated with falls. These included age, cognitive impairment, female gender, past history of falls, lower extremity weakness, gait problems, foot disorders, balance problems, hypovitaminosis D, psychotropic drug use and use of four or more prescription medications, arthritis, and PD. The risk of falling consistently increases as the number of these risk factors increases. Among these, previous history of a fall is the strongest risk factor for future falls, with sensitivity of 50%, specificity of 80% and 55% absolute risk of falling during follow-up (RR of 2.4; 95% CI 2.1–2.8) across studies.[12] A history of stroke demonstrated an absolute risk of falling during follow-up of 34% and dementia demonstrated an absolute risk of falling of 47% across studies.

Risk factors might be easily remembered with the mnemonic 'AGAIN I'VE FALLEN' (see Table 91.2).[13] In this way a risk-based assessment can help the clinician approaching geriatric fallers as well as non-fallers.

Table 91.2 Fall risk factors. 'AGAIN I'VE FALLEN' is a mnemonic for risk-based assessment to approach geriatric fallers.

Fall risk factors
Again fallen (previous history of fall)
Gait and balance problems (arthritis, cerebellar disease)
Activities of Daily Living loss
Impaired mental status (cognitive impairment, dementia)
Number and type of drugs (more than four drugs and use of psychotropic, analgesic, diuretic and anti-hypertensive drugs)
Illness (new illness, delirium)
Vestibular disorders
Eyes (glaucoma, retinopathy, cataract), Ears
Foot disorders (bunions, calluses, nail disease, joint deformities)
Alcohol
Lower extremity weakness (stroke, myopathy, deconditioning)
Low blood pressure (orthostatic or postural hypotension)
Environmental hazards (loose rugs, clutter, poor lighting, wet floor, unstable furniture, patient restraints)
Neurological disorders (peripheral neuropathy, stroke, Parkinson's disease, slowed reflexes

Adapted from The Saint Louis University Geriatric Evaluation Mnemonics and Screening Tools (Flaherty and Tumosa[13]).

Clinical presentation of falls

More than half of all falls are related to medical conditions, emphasizing the importance of a careful medical assessment. There are multiple and often interacting causes of falls that include accidents, syncope, drop attacks, dizziness or vertigo, orthostatic hypotension, drug-related and specific disease process.

Accidental

Accidental or unintentional falls occur in less than half of all falls.[1] When people are asked why they fell, by far the most common explanation is that they tripped or slipped. Other causes include a misplaced step, such as stepping into a hole, loss of balance, their legs giving way, or being knocked over. Many attribute their fall to hurrying too much or not looking where they were going; however patients should be screened for poor balance that predisposes to future falls. Addressing the environmental hazards begins with a careful assessment of the environment, like identifying cluttered surroundings and hazards that need to be changed. This may be done by an occupational therapist.

Syncope

Discussion of the complete differential diagnosis of *syncope* is beyond the scope of this chapter. Report of loss of consciousness by the patient or informant helps distinguish syncope or near-syncope as the cause of fall but in most of them the cause for syncope remains unidentified. Common causes of falls associated with loss of consciousness include neurocardiogenic syncope and epilepsy. Neurocardiogenic syncope may be caused by OH, vasovagal syncope, carotid sinus sensitivity, arrhythmias and aortic stenosis. Syncope and seizure are commonly confused, in part because motor activity including clonic jerks frequently follows a syncopal attack. Lempert documented motor activity following syncope in over 90% of healthy volunteers.[14] The most reliable feature that distinguishes 'fit from faint' is the presence of a prolonged post-ictal state. Syncope is transient hypoperfusion, whereas generalized seizures result in slow wave depression of cortical activity, mediated by the thalamus. The slow wave activity persists for minutes to hours following a generalized tonic clonic seizure, whereas cortical activity returns to normal after syncope as soon as perfusion is restored. Tongue biting, incontinence and jerking can be seen in both syncope and epilepsy, so the history both before and after the event is critical to the diagnosis. Many patients with convulsive syncope are erroneously given a diagnosis of epilepsy, and are placed on anticonvulsants for years without a true indication. A reliable witness is invaluable. The patient should be queried about pre-ictal lightheadedness, visual blurring, muffled hearing–all premonitory symptoms of syncope. Patients with unexplained loss of consciousness should undergo tilt table testing to exclude OH, vasovagal syncope, or convulsive syncope (*see* **Chapter** 61, **Epilepsy**).

Drop attack

A *drop attack* is described as sudden collapse without loss of consciousness. There is no warning. One minute the patient is on his feet, the next he is on the ground without knowing why. Patients often remark on their feeling of helplessness, almost paralysis, when lying on the floor, with immediate recovery once they are helped back onto their feet. However, after any type of fall about a half of older fallers, especially if they are also frail, are unable to get up without help. Causes of drop attacks include medication-induced asterixis (gabapentin, others), OH, cervical cord impingement due to stenosis or other compressive lesions, cataplexy, Ménière's disease, and impaired postural feedback. Although often attributed to vertebrobasilar insufficiency, brainstem ischaemia is rarely proved. Vertebrobasilar ischaemia should only be considered in the presence of the 5 Ds – dizziness, diplopia, dysarthria, dysphagia, dysequilibrium.

Dizziness and vertigo

Dizziness and unsteadiness (described as a sense of imbalance and spinning of head) are common complaints among elders who fall and those who do not fall. In most patients dizziness is multifactorial and 85% of chronically dizzy patients have more than one diagnosis: vestibulopathy, OH, multiple medication effects, primary gait disorders, cerebrovascular and cardiovascular disease, cervical spondylosis, anxiety and poor vision are some of the commonest. Dizziness related to cervical spondylosis results from an imbalance in the flow of stimuli from damaged mechanoreceptors in the cervical spine.

Vertigo (a sensation of rotational movement of surroundings) is probably an uncommon precipitant of falls in the elderly and can be caused by central (brainstem, cerebellum) or peripheral (vestibular) vertigo. Vertigo is also recognized as a feature of migraine. Peripheral vertigo is most commonly associated with disorders of the inner ear, such as paroxysmal positional vertigo (BPPV), acute labyrinthitis and Ménière's disease). Benign paroxysmal positional vertigo should be considered in patients complaining of vertigo provoked by head movements (typically, sitting up or rolling over in bed) because it is one of the few disorders of balance for which there is a simple, safe and effective treatment (*see* **Chapter** 87, **Disorders of the Vestibular System**). Patients with symptoms suggestive of vertigo will benefit from a thorough otological examination including auditory testing, which may help clarify the symptoms and differentiate inner ear from CNS involvement.

Orthostatic hypotension

Alterations in blood pressure play a major role in the aetiology of falls. *Orthostatic hypotension* (OH) is identified by taking the blood pressure and heart rate in supine position, within 1 minute in the sitting position and within 3 minutes in the standing position. A drop of more than 20 mmHg in systolic blood pressure or a 10 mmHg drop in diastolic blood pressure is diagnostic of OH.[15] OH may be symptomatic or asymptomatic; however, several conditions can cause OH or worsen it precipitating a fall. For instance, hypovolaemia, heart failure, prolong bed rest, autonomic dysfunction, anaemia and medications. Anaemia is associated with an increase in falls in the nursing home because of orthostasis, but also because it causes decreased mobility, myocardial infarction and frailty. Postprandial hypotension may lead to falls and syncope within two hours following a meal. It appears to be related to an increased release from the gut of vasodilatory peptides. It can be attenuated by giving the antidiabetic drug, acarbose, prior to meals.

Drugs

Drugs that should be suspected of playing a role in falls include diuretics (hypovolaemia), hypoglycaemics, antihypertensives (hypotension), sedatives, antipsychotics (sedation, muscle rigidity, postural hypotension) anticholinergic effects from antidepressants and others.[10] Cardiovascular medications most associated with falls include nitrates, digoxin and type IA antiarrhythmics, calcium-channel blockers, beta-blockers and ACE inhibitors. Among psychotropic medications, consider selective serotonin-reuptake inhibitors (SSRI), tricyclic antidepressants, neuroleptic agents, benzodiazepines and anticonvulsants. A meta-analysis showed that there is a small but consistent association between most classes of psychotropic drugs and falls. The odds ratio for one or more falls with any psychotropic drug use is 1.73.[16] A more recent systematic review of one randomized control and 28 observational studies also showed that psychotropic drugs seem to be associated with an increased risk of falls. Antiepileptics and drugs that lower blood pressure were weakly associated with falls.[17] There is an increased risk of recurrent falls in old people taking more than three or four drugs of any type. In nursing home residents it has been found that three or more medications; having recent change in medication and the presence of antidepressants (SSRI) and anti-anxiety drugs were associated with increased fall risk.[18] For this reason one suggested strategy is to have a consultant pharmacist reviewing medications in all persons with falls in the nursing home.[19]

Disease process

Several *disease processes* are associated with falls, including cardiac arrhythmias, abnormal vision, cerebrovascular, neurodegenerative, cerebellar and spinal cord diseases. Dysrhythmia may manifest with syncope from aortic stenosis or carotid sinus sensitivity. The former indicates valve replacement and the latter indicates increased vagal tone with bradycardia and hypotension, requiring behavioural interventions. Visual loss (acuity 6/18 or worse) detected by standard test of visual acuity is associated with falls and hip fracture. But visual loss by itself requires other postural defects to induce falling, such as impaired limb propioception where patients depend on vision for depth perception.[20] The visual factors that are most strongly predictive of falls are impaired depth perception, contrast sensitivity and low-contrast visual acuity. Stroke does not usually cause loss of consciousness or syncope but falls, yes, and this should be considered only if there are accompanying focal neurological symptoms. Normal pressure hydrocephalus should be considered in patients who present gait instability and falls. The increased stiffness and loss of flexibility of the PD patient increases fall risk. The classic forward-pitched gait (marche de petit pas) reduces stability, and the reduced height of the forefoot from the ground during the swing phase increases the risk of tripping. Mild cognitive impairment (MCI) syndromes have gait abnormalities, such as reduced gait speed and stride length.[21] Patients with dementia have twice the annual incidence of falls compared with cognitively normal older people; their risk of fall-related injuries is high and they have a threefold increase in fractures. Patients are particularly vulnerable during dual tasking and even a simple additional task impairs postural control. This is particularly greater in vascular dementia (79%) and Lewy body dementia (75%) than in AD (25%).[7] Urinary incontinence, urgency and nocturia may cause a distraction, similar to the 'dual-tasking' studies mentioned above, and thereby predispose to falls.[10]

Consequences of falls

Falls in older people are a leading cause of disability, distress, admission to supervised care (like hospital or nursing home placement), and death; it is these consequences that make falls important. Approximately one in ten falls results in a serious injury such as hip fracture, other fractures, subdural haematoma, other serious soft tissue injury, or head injury. Falls are responsible for approximately 10% of visits to the emergency department and 6% of urgent admissions among elderly persons. Nearly 85% of deaths from falls in 2004 were among people older than 75 years. This age group has increase likelihood of admission to a long-term care facility for a year or longer after the fall. Fall fatality rate is higher in men (49%) but fall rate is higher in women. Twenty to 30% of people who fall suffer moderate to severe injuries such as bruises, hip fractures, or head trauma. These injuries can make it hard to get around and limit independent living, plus they increase the risk of early death. Most traumatic brain injury and fractures among older adults are caused by falls.[1]

Fear of falling (FoF), by itself is considered a risk factor for falls. It refers to the lack of self-confidence that normal activities can be performed without falling. This fear may cause older adults to limit their activities, leading to reduced mobility and physical fitness. The prevalence varies between 21–85% and correlates with female sex and older age.[22] A systematic review by Alarcon *et al.*, suggested using direct questions to the patients to assess for FoF.[23] It has been proposed that FoF may reduce the amount of cognitive resources available for gait and balance control.

Diagnostic assessment

Falls

Inquiry about falls is a vital part of the geriatric assessment. All older people should be asked about falls in the prior year and then those with a single prior fall should have a 'get up and go test'. Those with two or more falls should be given full assessment with history of fall circumstances, medications and medical conditions that might contribute. Then examination of vision, gait and balance, and lower extremity joint function should follow. Basic neurological (mental status, muscle strength, lower extremity sensation, reflexes, test of cortical, extra-pyramidal and cerebellar function) and cardiovascular (heart rate and rhythm, postural pulse and blood pressure, and carotid sinus stimulation test) examination should be included.[24] When evaluating the elderly patient who falls a multifactorial approach has been recommended (Figure 91.2).

Further work-up may be directed to the suspected underlying medical causes of falls. If the history suggests carotid sinus sensitivity, the carotid can be gently massaged for five seconds to observe whether this precipitates a drop (50% reduction) in heart rate or a long pause (two seconds). On the other hand, if gait and balance impairment is suspected the short physical performance battery may be used (see Appendix 91.1). It is a composite of three tests that evaluate balance, gait and lower extremity weakness: standing balance test includes tandem, semi-tandem and side-by-side stands; gait speed test includes two-timed gait speed; and finally the chair stand test with five-time standing and timing. This battery has shown to predict mortality and institutionalization at six years of follow-up in community-dwelling seniors. Along with self-reported activities of daily living (ADL) this tool complements information on elder's functional status and detection of disability.[25]

Brain imaging should be considered if a neurological disorder is suspected, especially high-level gait disorders. Electroencephalography is rarely helpful and is indicated only if there is a high degree of clinical suspicion of seizure. Magnetic resonance imaging (MRI) is frequently obtained to screen for cerebral infarcts, demyelinating disease, posterior fossa malformation, cerebellar degenerations, and hydrocephalus.

Gait

To assess for gait abnormalities, it is important to watch the patient stand from a chair and observe the gait while walking. Gait observation provides a direct assessment of the patient's disability and motor performance problem. There are three suggested screening assessments of mobility, gait and balance. Uniform gait protocols are lacking and diagnosis of gait abnormalities is highly dependent on examiners' expertise. Measuring gait speed is suggested as a simple way to assess health and function in seniors. Verghese showed that each 10 cm s^{-1} decrease in gait speed was associated with a 7% increased risk for falls.[26] In the United States, these techniques have been introduced as Pay-for-Performance measures by the Center for Medicare Services, giving the clinician an additional incentive to screen all elderly patients and document in the chart the results (www.cms.gov).

1 The timed Get Up and Go Test (GUGT) is a simple exam measuring the time it takes a person to rise from a standard arm chair, walk 3 meters (10 feet), turn around, walk back to the chair and sit down (see Appendix 91.2). Patients who require more than 20 s are at high risk for falls. It has a sensitivity of 77% and a positive predictive value of 93% among community-dwelling seniors across observational studies on GUGT's screening ability. In the inpatient setting the sensitivity was 91% but low specificity, 22%.[12] It is a functional measurement easy to perform and the older adult can use an assistive device.

2 Another assessment tool is the Tinetti's Mobility Scale where evaluation of dynamic balance and gait is performed through the performance of 14 tasks (see Appendix 91.3). It is used to identify fall risk in community-dwelling adults. A score less than 24 (score range 0–28) indicates risk for falls. Across observational studies this tool yielded a mean sensitivity of 82% and mean specificity of 65%.[12] This is a long assessment tool, and may be impractical in a busy clinic.

3 Standing unassisted from sitting position, which measures patient's ability to rise from sitting in a chair without using their arms, was found to have 31% of sensitivity and 90% of specificity.[12] The risk of falling increased if a person is unable to stand or requires more than 2 s to do so.

Balance

Doing two things at once ('dual tasking') becomes more difficult in old age; it has been reported that

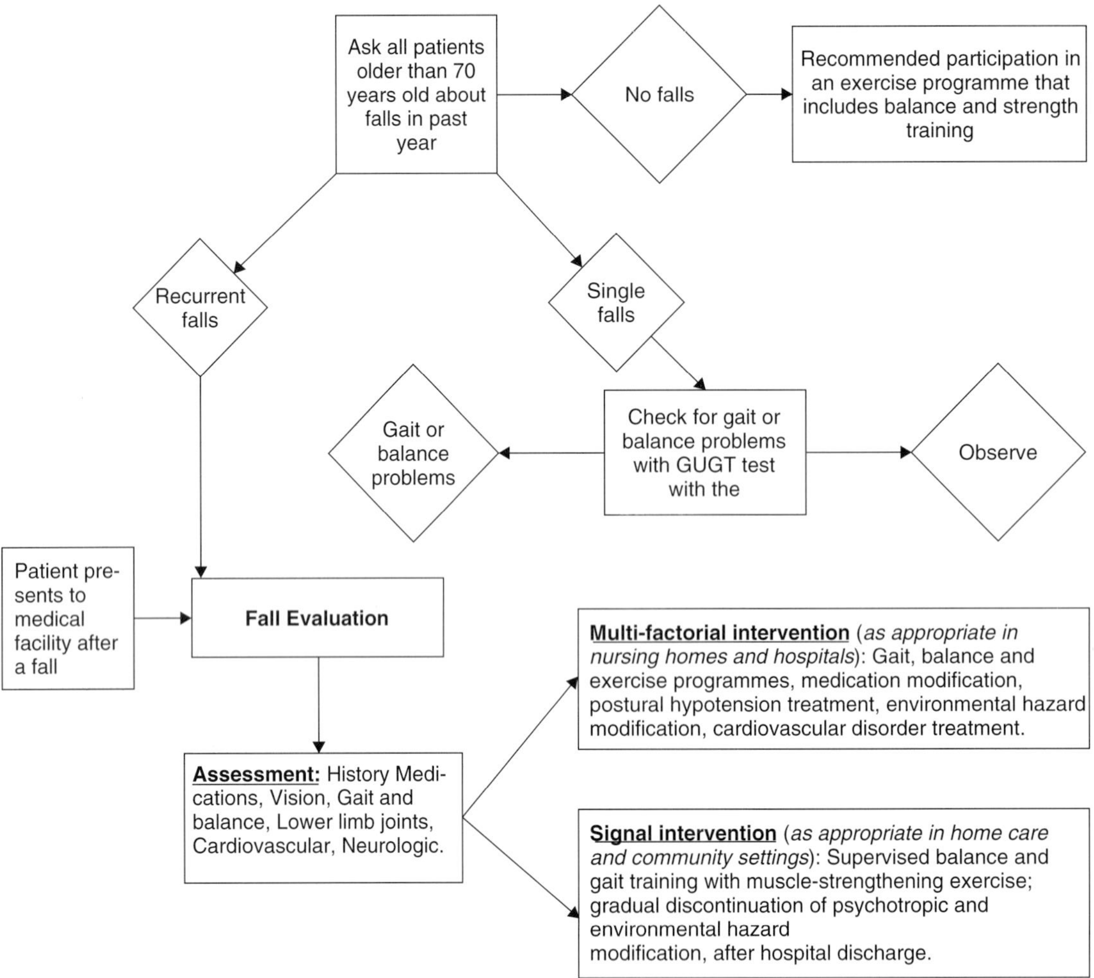

Figure 91.2 The assessment and management of falls. Adapted from AGS/BGS/AAOS Panel on Falls Prevention.[24]

institutionalized older people who were unable to keep up a conversation while walking had a high risk of falls ('stops walking when talking'). Subsequent investigations have shown that dual tasking impairs not only gait but also static and dynamic balance. The difficulties increase as the tasks become more complex, and both the young and the old tend to prioritize gait performance over the secondary cognitive task.[27] For this reason the Saint Louis University Department of Geriatrics has proposed a screening tool for fall risk called dual tasking. It consists of performing one or all of the following tasks: walking speed while counting backward from 100 by sevens; get up and go test while holding a full glass of water; dancing with turn while waltzing; and one leg stand with eyes closed. A gait that worsens when eyes are closed and improves when minor support is given by the examiner is a further clue to proprioceptive problems. Failure to perform either of the dual tasks suggests risk of falling and the patient should be treated with physical therapy. A mini-review by Zijlstra *et al.*[28] demonstrated that dual balance task correlated better with fall prediction than single balance task and had better sensitivity (49%) and specificity (85%) across studies. But no conclusion can be made due to incomplete comparisons among these two measures and variability across studies.

Dynamic standing balance can be measured by the functional reach (FR) test, where the subject stands behind a line and stretches arm as far forward as possible without taking a step. Then the evaluator measures the distance reached and presence of risk of falling is suspected if the patient is able to reach less than 10 inches. This has been shown to correlate with other methods of balance and mobility and also has a relationship with the risk of falls and performance in activities of daily living (ADL). Lin and authors reported that FR significantly predicted a decline in ADL, but it did not predict occurrence of falling (OR 1.00; AUC 0.59).[29]

Therapeutic approach

The American Geriatrics Society and The British Geriatric Society developed in 2001 a set of recommendations for assessing people who fall. Although this initiative may have contributed to a reduction in falls, some of the recommendations have been disproven, like the multifactorial approach and home safety interventions. They might decrease the number of falls but not the rate of falls or injurious falls. Its multifactorial approach makes it costly and less efficient due to less likelihood of compliance. This has led to recent research on single interventions. Furthermore, their application on different settings (community, nursing home and inpatient) has different results in their effectiveness to prevent falls. For this reason, we will discuss the interventions based upon clinical setting in the next section.

Intervention according to underlying disease or causes needs also to be considered. Foot problems can be addressed by podiatric consultation and by changing footwear. Treatment of PD with levodopa and shunting of patients with hydrocephalus remain the most dramatic therapeutic interventions for gait disorders. It is presently unclear to what degree pallidotomy and deep brain stimulation procedures improve gait in PD. Rehabilitation strategies have been explored for gait freezing in patients with PD and in patients with frontal gait disorder. Patients with sensory deficits, who are often at high risk for falls and injuries, often benefit from an intervention such as sensory balance training.[6]

Outpatient setting

Evidence-based guidelines suggested by AGS/BGS/AAOS Panel in 2001 for interventions to reduce risk of falls among community-dwelling populations include review and reduction of medications (specially psychotropics), gait training (with or without assistive devices), and exercise programmes with balance training.[24] Nonetheless, an updated systematic review reinforces and expands current guideline interventions.

A Cochrane Systematic Review on 111 randomized controlled trials, with a total of 55 303 participants revealed that among community-dwelling older people the only intervention that reduced both rate of falling and falling risk was exercise, either as a multiple-component group, Tai chi or individually prescribed home-based multicomponent exercise.[30] These exercise programmes may target strength, balance, flexibility and endurance. Programmes that contain two or more of these components reduced falls risk and rate. Psychotropic medication withdrawal and multifactorial interventions reduced rate of falls but not fall risk. Although drug withdrawal is a complicated intervention that requires the weighing of risks and benefits, its fall reduction effect was well demonstrated by Campbell *et al.*[31] A prescribing modification programme for primary care physicians that entailed ensuring medication review and adjustment reduced risk of falling.[32] Home safety interventions reduced risk of falls in high-risk patients, especially those with severe visual impairment. Common alterations include the installation of locks on cupboards and covers on electrical sockets, improvement of lighting in halls and stairways, and the removal of rugs and other falls hazards. An anti-slip shoe device worn in icy conditions can reduce falls. Similarly, vitamin D supplement reduced falls only in people with lower vitamin D levels. First eye cataract surgery as well as pacemakers in people with carotid sinus hypersensitivity reduced rate of falls.[30]

Results from several randomized controlled clinical trials involving multifaceted fall prevention programmes have yielded encouraging, if not uniform, results. The uneven efficacy could be explained by the variation in combinations of fall reduction interventions. A meta-analysis of multifactorial versus physical exercise-alone interventions revealed that among community-dwelling healthy individuals (without dementia), exercise (i.e. strength, balance training, coordination of movements) decreased fall risk by 55% compared to 10% by multifactorial intervention, and compared to 33% by both interventions (multifactorial and exercise).[33] Interventions were more effective if their duration was less than 12 months, in seniors older than 70 years of age and smaller groups. This may suggest that compliance is better in short-term group programmes as compared to longer-duration individualized programmes. This supports the Cochrane results that the impact of exercise is stronger than multifactorial interventions.

On the other hand, the weak effect on falls found in these two studies may be related to the poor or inefficient implementation of the multifactorial intervention. Therefore, education of physicians is needed. Training clinicians regarding referral to physical therapy or home care for balance and gait problems, performing medication review and reduction, and screening and treating postural hypotension, resulted in a reduction of fall-related injuries by 9% and less fall-related use of medical service by 11%.[32]

Falls have a psychological and social impact that put seniors at risk of disability and death. For this reason multiple studies focus on fear of falling (FoF) and have found effective interventions. A meta-analysis among six randomized control studies indicated that the intervention for more than four months with exercise and education combination was effective in reducing FoF.[34] This result suggests that a combination programme is better than exercise alone because the FoF is influenced not only by physical problems but also by psychological and cognitive issues. They also found that hip protectors did not reduced falls but reduced hip fractures and FoF. Hip protectors appear to improve confidence. The duration of intervention should be between 4–12 months to provide a programme that will ensure compliance.

Nursing homes

Interventions with demonstrated efficacy in long-term care include comprehensive assessments, staff education, use of and training in assistive devices, and reduction of medications. Preliminary data by Cochrane Systematic Review on interventions for preventing falls in older people in nursing home revealed that multifactorial interventions done by multidisciplinary teams decreased the rate of falls.[35] Further, the effect of multifactorial interventions vary by nursing home subgroups (better in patients with previous history of fall, MCI, urinary incontinence, but not in depressed patients). A review by Vu *et al.* revealed that multifaceted fall prevention programmes were effective in reducing falls by 20–45%. Although fall-risk assessment on admission to long-term care facilities and then quarterly has not been proven to be effective, it continues to be mandated as standard practice in nursing facilities. The authors note that current literature only assesses the effect of environmental assessment/modification, medication assessment/modification, hip protector use and exercise intervention programmes as individual interventions in nursing homes.[36]

Most of the evidence on environmental adjustment focused on restraint reduction as the main intervention. Reduction in restraint use will not decrease fall rate but is associated with reduced likelihood of severe injuries. A simple approach in patients with dementia would be to increase their time in the wander garden (a special care unit with specialized staff and facilities for patients with dementia).

Similarly, authors stressed that a clear association between the use of certain medications and increased fall rates, but no studies examine the effect of medication reduction or elimination on fall rate in nursing home residents.[7] Nevertheless, a systematic review by Sterke *et al.* among 17 observational studies revealed that there is strong evidence of increased fall risk with the use of antidepressants, anxiolytics and use of multiple drugs in nursing home residents with dementia. The evidence on fall risk with withdrawal of psychotropic medications is limited in this subgroup.[37] But there is evidence that among seniors that live in the community the withdrawal of psychotropics has beneficial effects on fall risk.[30] Hip protector use (which are believed to operate under the principle that deflection of forces away from the greater trochanteric process will result in fewer femoral fractures) in nursing homes showed a reduction in hip fractures but not in fall rate.[38]

Exercise programmes (involving strength, balance and flexibility training) for nursing home residents failed to demonstrate a similar effect on falls despite improvement in some objective measures of functional status. The reason for the inability of this intervention to prevent nursing home falls could be related to increased frailty among residents compared with community-dwelling counterparts. A frail nursing home resident offered an exercise regimen increases the risk for falling by becoming more mobile. There is vast evidence of the benefit of exercise in nursing home patients with dementia and cognitive impairment; it improves behaviour and gait. Regardless of this finding a systematic review on fall interventions in the nursing home among seven randomized controlled trials demonstrated inconsistent results on supervised exercise intervention. Vitamin D supplementation reduced fall rate but not risk of falls among nine trials.[35]

Hospital setting

Older adults account for a majority of acute hospitalizations. The risk of falling is certainly a concern in this setting because older people are particularly susceptible to falls during acute illness or exacerbation of chronic disease and one month after hospital discharge. Preliminary data by Cochrane Systematic Review on interventions for preventing falls in older people in hospitals among 10 randomized controlled trials revealed that multifactorial intervention decreased rate of falls as well as risk of falling. Supervised exercise interventions showed a significant reduction in risk of falling. A potential method of reducing falls during hospitalization is through the use of care partners. A large amount of patients at risk of falls in this setting are the patients that suffer stroke. Findings are consistent in stroke rehabilitation that these patients have better outcomes with more intense exercise.[39]

Prevention

From the public health perspective, fall prevention lies across the threshold between primary (avoid fall) and secondary (detect fall risk) prevention. Both preventions have been studied but the most efficient has been the secondary type as discussed in the following section. This is based upon the recognition that it may not be possible to prevent falls completely and what endangers patients is the recurrence of falls more than the risk of falls. Nevertheless, any reduction in fall rate would be expected to also reduce the risk of injurious falls. The US Preventive Services Task Force as well as the European Silver Paper on Health Promotion and Preventive Actions recommends that all persons older than 70 years of age who have known risk factors be counselled about specific measures to prevent falls, encourage physical activity and provide a range of exercise opportunities.

An efficient secondary prevention is education of patient and caregiver. The person at risk and the family should be educated about the multifactorial nature of most falls, specific risk factors and recommended interventions. Multifactorial assessment followed by interventions targeting the identified risk factors has been the most successful preventive approach. It includes the following components: review and reduction of medications; balance and gait training, muscle-strengthening exercise; evaluation of postural blood pressure; home-hazard modifications; and targeted medical and cardiovascular assessments and treatments. If living alone, the patient should be taught what to do if they fall and cannot get up. A personal emergency response system may be helpful.

Other strategies targeted to persons without history of falls or recent hospitalizations have proved ineffective, such as general exercise programmes, cognitive-behavioural approaches and home-hazard modifications.

There is increasing evidence that vitamin D may be helpful in preventing falls and fractures; even decrease mortality in older people. Therefore, it is appropriate to evaluate patients who fall recurrently for vitamin D deficiency and provide supplement with high dose vitamin D3 (800 IU per day).

Fall clinics

As a response to the importance of falls as a geriatric syndrome, fall clinics where created. They were established in several European countries, Australia, United States and Canada. Equipment and staff make an in-depth examination and assessment of fallers so that relevant physiological and pathological problems can be identified and appropriate interventions organized. In such units, the diagnostic accuracy and effect of interventions is considerably higher than in non-specialized clinics.

Exercise

There are several identified positive effects of exercise including decrease cognitive impairment, improve function, decrease dysphoria and behavioural disturbances, reduce falls, fall injuries and FoF, decrease frailty, reverse sarcopenia, slow bone loss, reduce pain, decrease constipation and incontinence, enhance sleep, improve glycaemic control and QOL. This favours the prescription of exercise by primary care physician no matter what setting they are or how much their patients fall or not. The criterion for a minimal effective exercise dose would equate to a twice-weekly programme running over 25 weeks (using a combining supervised group with interspersed home exercise programmes). Intensity and frequency depends on the patient's fitness. A high-fitness elder may perform 30–60 mins of moderate activity 5–7 days per week. Low-fitness elders should do moderate activity that will increase heart rate 55–69% (or 220-age in males; 220-[0.6 x age] in females). Activity less than 10 minutes may be permitted with gradual increase.[40] In view of the overwhelming evidence on the effectiveness of moderate-high intensity balance training, clinicians may recommend a simple balance exercise. For instance, join dancing or Tai chi group exercise or have the person stand on one leg holding on to a stable object and then shut their eyes four times on each leg.

Key points

DO'S

- Distinguish between falls, syncope and seizure.
- Distinguish between 'dizziness' and true vertigo.
- Assess for correctable underlying causes of falls by history and targeted physical examination.
- Pay particular attention to:
  - Uncorrected vision impairment
  - Orthostatic blood pressure and pulse supine and standing after 3 min
  - Psychotropic medication and quantity of prescribed drugs
  - Gait and balance abnormalities
  - Inappropriate footwear
  - Incorrect use of canes and other assistive devices
  - Environmental hazards
  - A simple 'get up and go' test on all patients who have fallen.
- Ensure safety in recurrent fallers by urgent interventions to prevent injury.
- Refer patients to rehab therapist (physical and occupational) whenever appropriate for detailed environmental and safety assessments, strengthening and proper prescription and use of assistive devices.

DON'TS

- Send all patients for extensive diagnostic studies or cardiac monitoring.
- Test all patients for vitamin D levels.

CONSIDER

- Referring selected patients for Tai chi if they have balance problems and classes available.
- Prescribe vitamin D 800–1200 IU daily.
- Recommending hip protectors in carefully selected nursing home patients who are at high risk for fracture and who are recurrently falling.

Adapted from Kane RL *et al.*[10], Ch. 9, p. 291.

Acknowledgment

The author thanks Mrs Valerie Tanner for administrative assistance and Dr Laurence J. Kinsella for chapter review.

Appendix 91.1

Short Physical Performance Battery

1. Repeated Chair Stands

Instructions: Do you think it is safe for you to try and stand up from a chair five times without using your arms? Please stand up straight as quickly as you can five times, without stopping in between. After standing up each time, sit down and then stand up again. Keep your arms folded across your chest. Please watch while I demonstrate. I'll be timing you with a stopwatch. Are you ready? Begin

Grading: Begin stop watch when subject begins to stand up. Count aloud each time subject arises. Stop the stopwatch when subject has straightened up completely for the fifth time. Also stop if the subject uses arms, or after 1 minute, if subject has not completed rises, and if concerned about the subject's safety.. Record the number of seconds and the presence of imbalance.. Then complete ordinal scoring.

Time: _____sec (if five stands are completed)

Number of Stands Completed: 1 2 3 4 5

Chair Stand Ordinal Score: _____

0 = unable

1 = > 16.7 sec

2 = 16.6-13.7 sec

3 = 13.6-11.2 sec

4 = < 11.1 sec

2. Balance Testing

Begin with a semitandem stand (heel of one foot placed by the big toe of the other foot). Individuals unable to hold this position should try the side-by-side position. Those able to stand in the semitandem position should be tested in the full tandem position. Once you have completed time measures, complete ordinal scoring.

a. Semitandem Stand

Instructions: Now I want you to try to stand with the side of the heel of one foot touching the big toe of the other foot for about 10 seconds. You may put either foot in front, whichever is more comfortable for you. Please watch while I demonstrate.

Grading: Stand next to the participant to help him or her into semitandem position. Allow participant to hold onto your arms to get balance. Begin timing when participant has the feet in position and lets go.

Circle one number

2. Held for 10 sec
1. Held for less than 10 sec; number of seconds held _____
0. Not attempted

b. Side-by-Side stand

Instructions: I want you to try to stand with your feet together, side by side, for about 10 sec. Please watch while I demonstrate. You may use your arms, bend your knees, or move your body to maintain your balance, but try not to move your feet. Try to hold this position until I tell you to stop.

Grading: Stand next to the participant to help him or her into the side-by-side position. Allow participant to hold onto your arms to get balance. Begin timing when participant has feet together and lets go.

Grading

2. Held of 10 sec
1. Held for less than 10 sec; number of seconds held_____
0. Not attempted

c. Tandem Stand

Instructions: Now I want you to try to stand with the heel of one foot in front of and touching the toes of the other foot for 10 sec. You may put either foot in front, whichever is more comfortable for you. Please watch while I demonstrate.

Grading: Stand next to the participant to help him or her into the side-by-side position. Allow participant to hold onto your arms to get balance. Begin timing when participant has feet together and lets go.

Grading

2. Held of 10 sec
1. Held for less than 10 sec; number of seconds held_____
0. Not attempted

Balance Ordinal Score: _____

0 = side by side 0-9 sec or unable

1 = side by side 10, <10 sec semitandem

2 = semitandem 10 sec, tandem 0-2 sec

3 = semitandem 10 sec, tandem 3-9 sec

4 = tandem 10 sec

3. 8' Walk (2.44 meters)

Instructions: This is our walking course. If you use a cane or other walking aid when walking outside your home, please use it for this test. I want you to walk at your usual pace to the other end of this course (a distance of 8'). Walk all the way past the other end of the tape before you stop. I will walk with you. Are you ready?

Grading: Press the start button to start the stopwatch as the participant begins walking. Measure the time take to walk 8'. Then complete ordinal scoring.

Time: _____ **sec**

Gait Ordinal Score: _____

0 = could not do

1 = >5.7 sec (<0.43 m/sec)

2 = 4.1-6.5 sec (0.44-0.60 m/sec)

3 = 3.2-4.0 (0.61-0.77 m/sec)

4 = <3.1 sec (>0.78 m/sec)

Summary Ordinal Score: _____

Range: 0 (worst performance) to 12 (best performance). Shown to have predictive validity showing a gradient of risk for mortality, nursing home admission, and disability.

Source: Guralnik JM *et al.* A short physical performance battery assessing lower extremity function: association with self-reported disability and prediction of mortality and nursing home admission. *J Gerontol Med Sci* 1994;**49**:M85–M94.

Appendix 91.2

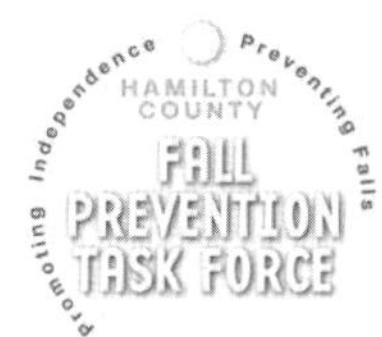

Timed Get Up and Go Test

Measures mobility in people who are able to walk on their own (assistive device permitted)

Name________________________

Date__________________________

Time to Complete________________**seconds**

Instructions:

The person may wear their usual footwear and can use any assistive device they normally use.

1. Have the person sit in the chair with their back to the chair and their arms resting on the arm rests.
2. Ask the person to stand up from a standard chair and walk a distance of 10 ft (3m).
3. Have the person turn around, walk back to the chair and sit down again.

Timing begins when the person starts to rise from the chair and ends when he or she returns to the chair and sits down.

The person should be given 1 practice trial and then 3 actual trial. The times from the three actual trials are averaged.

Predictive Results

Seconds	Rating
<10	Freely mobile
<20	Mostly independent
20-29	Variable mobility
>20	Impaired mobility

Source: Podsiadlo D., Richardson, S. The timed 'Up and Go' Test: a test of basic functional mobility for frail elderly persons. *J Am Geriatr Soc* 1991;**39**:142–8.

Appendix 91.3

Tinetti Assessment Tool: Description

Population:	Adult population, elderly patients
Description:	The Tinetti Assessment Tool is a simple, easily administered test that measures a patient's gait and balance. The test is scored on the patient's ability to perform specific tasks.
Mode of Administration:	The Tinetti Assessment Tool is a task performance exam.
Time to Complete:	10 to 15 minutes
Time to Score:	Time to score is included in time to complete
Scoring:	Scoring of the Tinetti Assessment Tool is done on a three point ordinal scale with a range of 0 to 2. A score of 0 represents the most impairment, while a 2 would represent independence of the patient. The individual scores are then combined to form three measures; an overall gait assessment score, an overall balance assessment score, and a gait and balance score.
Interpretation:	The maximum score for the gait component is 12 points. The maximum score for the balance component is 16 points. The maximum total score is 28 points. In general, patients who score below 19 are at a high risk for falls. Patients who score in the range of 19-24 indicate that the patient has a risk for falls.
Reliability:	Interrater reliability was measured in a study of 15 patients by having a physician and a nurse test the patients at the same time. Agreement was found on over 85% of the items and the items that differed never did so by more than 10%. These results indicate that the Tinetti Assessment Tool has good interrater reliability.
Validity:	Not reported
References:	Lewis C. Balance, gait test proves simple yet useful. *P.T. Bulletin* 1993;**2**:9, 40. Tinetti ME. Performance-oriented assessment of mobility problems in elderly patients. *J Am Geriatr Soc* 1986;**34**:119–26.

Tinetti Assessment Tool: Balance

Patient's Name: ____________________ **Date:** ______________________

Location: ________________________ **Rater:** ______________________

Initial Instructions: Subject is seated in a hard, armless chair. The following maneuvers are tested.

Task	Description of Balance	Possible	Score
1. Sitting Balance	Leans or slides in chair Steady, safe	= 0 = 1	
2. Arises	Unable without help Able, uses arms to help Able without using arms	= 0 = 1 = 2	
3. Attempts to arise	Unable without help Able, requires > 1 attempt Able to rise, 1 attempt	= 0 = 1 = 2	
4. Immediate standing balance (first 5 seconds)	Unsteady (swaggers, moves feet, trunk sway) Steady but uses walker or other support Steady without walker or other support	= 0 = 1 = 2	
5. Standing Balance	Unsteady Steady but wide stance (medial heels > 4 inches apart) and uses cane or other support Narrow stance without support	= 0 = 1 = 2	
6. Nudged (subject at max position with feet as close together as possible, examiner pushes lightly on subject's sternum with palm of hand 3 times.	Begins to fall Staggers, grabs, catches self Steady	= 0 = 1 = 2	
7. Eyes closed (at maximum position #6)	Unsteady Steady	= 0 = 1	
8. Turning 360 degrees	Discontinuous steps Continuous steps Unsteady (grabs, swaggers) Steady	= 0 = 1 = 0 = 1	
9. Sitting Down	Unsafe (misjudged distance, falls into chair) Uses arms or not a smooth motion Safe, smooth motion	= 0 = 1 = 2	
		Balance Score:	

Tinetti Assessment Tool: Gait

Patient's Name: ____________________ **Date:** ________________________

Location: __________________________ **Rater:** ________________________

Initial Instructions: Subject stands with examiner, walks down hallway or across the room, first at "usual" pace, then back at "rapid, but safe" pace (using usual walking aids).

Task	Description of Gait	Possible	Score
10. Initiation of gait (immediately after told to "go")	Any hesitancy or multiple attempts to start No hesitancy	= 0 = 1	
11. Step length and height	a. Right swing foot does not pass left stance foot with step b. Right foot passes left stance foot c. Right foot does not clear floor completely with step d. Right foot completely clears floor e. Left swing foot does not pass right stance foot with step f. Left foot passes right stance foot g. Left foot does not clear floor completely with step h. Left foot completely clears floor	= 0 = 1 = 0 = 1 = 0 = 1 = 0 = 1	
12. Step Symmetry	Right and left step length not equal (estimate) Right and left step appear equal	= 0 = 1	
13. Step Continuity	Stopping or discontinuity between steps Steps appear continuous	= 0 = 1	
14. Path (estimated in relation to floor tiles, 12-inch diameter; observe excursion of 1 foot over about 10 feet of the course).	Marked deviation Mild/moderate deviation or uses walking aid Straight without walking aid	= 0 = 1 = 2	
15. Trunk	Marked sway or uses walking aid No sway but flexion of knees or back, or spreads arms out while walking No sway, no flexion, no use of arms, and no use of walking aid	= 0 = 1 = 2	
16. Walking Stance	Heels apart Heels almost touching while walking	= 0 = 1	
	Gait Score:		
	Balance + Gait Score:		

Source: Tinetti ME. Performance-oriented assessment of mobility problems in elderly patients. *J Am Geriatr Soc* 1986;**34**: 119–26.

References

1. Falls among older adults. *Center for Disease Control and Prevention* (CDC), *National Center for Health Statistics*, 2005. Available at: http://www.cdc.gov/nchs/ (accessed 5 February 2010).
2. Allum JH, Carpenter MG, Honegger F *et al*. Age-dependent variations in the directional sensitivity of balance corrections and compensatory arm movements in man. *J Physiol* 2002; **542**(Pt 2):643–63.
3. Nutt JG. Classification of gait and balance disorders. *Adv Neurol* 2001;**87**:135–41.
4. Liston R, Mickleborough J, Bene J *et al*. (2003). A new classification of higher level gait disorders in patients with cerebral multi-infarct states. *Age and Aging* **32**:252–8.
5. Bloem BR, Valkenburg VV, Slabbekoorn M *et al*. The multiple tasks test: development and normal strategies. *Gait & Posture* 2001;**14**:191–202.
6. Sudarsky L. Neurologic disorders of gait. *Curr Neurol Neurosci* 2001;**1**:350–6.
7. Canavan PK, Cahalin LP, Lowe S *et al*. Managing gait disorders in older persons residing in nursing homes: a review of literature. *J Am Med Dir Assoc* 2009;**10**:230–237.
8. Menz HB, Lord SR, Fitzpatrick RC. Age-related differences in walking stability. *Age and Ageing* 2002;**32**:132–42.
9. Lamb SE, Jorstad-Stein EC, Hauer K *et al*. Development of a common outcome data set for fall injury prevention trials: The prevention of falls network Europe consensus. *J Am Geriatr Soc* 2005;**53**:1618–22.
10. Kane RL, Ouslander JG, Abrass IB. *Essentials of Clinical Geriatrics*, 6th edn, McGraw-Hill, Hightstown, NJ, 2009, pp. 265–95.
11. Ooi WL, Hossain M, Lipsitz LA. The association between orthostatic hypotension and recurrent falls in nursing home residents. *Am J Med* 2000;**108**:106–11.
12. Thurman DJ, Stevens JA, Rao JK. Practice parameter: Assessing patients in a neurology practice for risk of falls (evidence-based review). *Neurology* 2008;**70**:473–9.
13. Flaherty JH, Tumosa N. *Saint Louis University Geriatric Evaluation Mnemonics Screening Tools*, 2nd edn, 2008, p. 72.
14. Lempert T. Recognizing syncope: pitfalls and surprises. *J R Soc Med* 1996;**89**:372–5.
15. The Consensus Committee of the American Autonomic Society and the American Academy of Neurology. Consensus statement on the definition of orthostatic hypotension, pure autonomic failure, and multiple system atrophy. Neurology 1996;**46**:1470.
16. Leipzig RM, Cumming RG, Tinetti ME. Drugs and falls in older people: a systematic review and meta-analysis: I. Psychotropic drugs. II. Cardiac and analgesic drugs. *J Am Geriatr Soc* 1999;**47**:30–50.
17. Sterke CS, Verhagen AP, van Beeck EF *et al*. (2008). The influence of drug use on fall incidents among nursing home residents: a systematic review. *Int Psychogeriatr* 2008;**20**:890–910.
18. Lim KD, Ng KC, Ng SK, Ng LL. Falls amongst institutionalized psycho-geriatric patients. *Singapore Med J* 2001;**42**: 466–72.
19. Morley JE. Falls and fractures. *J Am Med Dir Assoc* 2007;**4**: 276–7.
20. Lord SR, Dayhew J. Visual risk factors for falls in older people. *J Am Geriatr Soc* 2001;**49**:508–15.
21. Verghese J, Robbins M, Holtzer R *et al*. Gait dysfunction in Mild Cognitive Impairment Syndromes. *J Am Geriatr Soc* 2008;**56**:1244–51.
22. Reelick MF, Van Iersel MB, Kessels RPC *et al*. The influence of fear of falling on gait and balance in older people. *Age and Aging* 2009;**38**:435–40.
23. Alarcon T, Gonzalez-Montalvo JI, Puime AO. Assessing patients with fear of falling: Does the method use change the results? A systematic review. *Aten Primaria* 2009;**41**:262–8.
24. AGS/BGS/AAOS. Panel on Falls Prevention. Guideline for the prevention of falls in older persons. *J Am Geriatr Soc* 2002; **49**:664–72.
25. Guralnik JM, Simonisick EM, Ferrucci L *et al*. A short physical performance battery assessing lower extremity function: Association with self reported disability and prediction of mortality and nursing home admission. *J Gerontol Med Sci* 1994;**49**:85–94.
26. Verghese J, Holtzer R, Lipton RB *et al*. Quantitative gait markers and incident fall risk in older adults. *J Gerontol A Biol Sci Med Sci* 2009;**64**:896–901.
27. Bloem BR, Valkenburg VV, Slabbekoorn M *et al*. The multiple tasks test: development and normal strategies. *Gait & Posture* 2001;**14**:191–202.
28. Zijlstra A, Ufkes T, Skelton DA *et al*. Do dual task have an added value over single tasks for balance assessment in fall prevention programs? A mini-review. *Gerontology* 2008; **54**:40–9.
29. Lin MR, Hwang HF, Hu MH *et al*. Psychometric comparisons of the timed up and go, one-leg stand, functional reach, and Tinetti balance measures in community-dwelling older people. *J Am Geriatr Soc* 2004;**52**:1343–8.
30. Gillespie LD, Robertson MC, Gillespie WJ *et al*. Interventions for preventing fall in older people living in the community. *Cochrane Database Syst Rev* 2009;**2**:CD007146.
31. Campbell AJ, Robertson MC, Gardner MM *et al*. Psychotropic medication withdrawal and a home-based exercise program to prevent falls: a randomized, controlled trial. *J Am Geriatr Soc* 1999;**47**:850–3.
32. Tinetti ME, Baker DI, King M *et al*. Effect of dissemination of evidence in reducing injuries from falls. *N Engl J Med* 2008; **359**:252–61.
33. Petridou ET, Manti EG, Ntinapogias AG *et al*. What works better for community-dwelling older people at risk to fall? A meta-analysis of multi-factorial versus physical exercise-alone interventions. *J Aging Health* 2009;**21**:713–29.
34. Jung D, Lee J, Lee SM. A meta-analysis of fear of falling treatment programs for elderly. *West J Nurs Res* 2009;**31**:6–16.
35. Cameron ID, Murray GR, Gillespie LD *et al*. Interventions for preventing falls in older people in nursing care facilities and hospitals. *Cochrane Database Syst Rev* 2010;**1**:CD005465. [Abstract only available]
36. Vu MQ, Weintraub N, Rubenstein LZ. Falls in the nursing home: are they preventable? *J Am Med Dr Assoc* 2004;**5**:401–6.
37. Sterke CS, Verhagen AP, van Beeck EF *et al*. The influence of drug use on fall incidents among nursing home residents: a systematic review. *Int Psychogeriatr* 2008;**20**:890–910.

38. Parker MJ, Gillespie WJ, Gillespie LD. Hip protectors preventing hip fractures in older people. *Cochrane Database Syst Rev* 2005;**3**:CD001255.

39. Sherrington C, Whitney JC, Lord SR *et al.* Effective exercise for the prevention of falls: a systematic review and meta-analysis. *J Am Geriatr Soc* 2008;**56**:2234–43.

40. Pompei P, Murphy JB (eds), *Geriatrics Review Syllabus: A Core Curriculum in Geriatric Medicine*, 6th edn, American Geriatrics Society, New York, 2006, pp. 59–62.

CHAPTER 92

Foot problems

Arthur E. Helfand[1] and Donald F. Jessett[2]

[1]Temple University, Philadelphia, Thomas Jefferson University Hospital, Philadelphia, and Philadelphia Corporation for Aging, Philadelphia, PA, USA

[2]Formerly of University of Wales Institute, Cardiff, UK

Introduction

Diseases and disorders of the foot and related anatomical structures affect the QOL (quality of life), dignity and the ability of individuals to remain independent and to live life, to the end of life. Foot problems in the older population result from disease, disability and deformity related to multiple chronic diseases as well as focal changes associated with repetitive use and trauma. Older people are at high risk of developing foot-related disease and should receive continuing assessment, education, surveillance and care. The foot is a mirror of health and disease.[1]

The human foot is unique. It evolved to serve as an interface between man and whatever territory he or she most commonly traverses, resulting in a wide range of adaptations to use. Those whose footwear is minimal because of climatic conditions or the nature of territory require little or no covering; have feet that are different from those in industrial civilizations and are related to the needs of society and custom. Feet are required to withstand variable repetitive stress imposed by activities and occupations. The forces of pressure, the adaptations required for ambulation, prior care and the effects of disease and ageing, present different problems in the elderly making comprehensive podogeriatric assessment an essential in patient evaluation and increasing the need for the continuing assessment and examination of the feet and related structures, followed by appropriate care, management, surveillance, education and preventive strategies. All health policies should include appropriate and proper podiatric services.[2]

At one extreme may be the long periods of limited movement that present particular occupational risks. At the other end of the scale may be those occupations, activities and/or interests involving great variability of movement that includes weight/stress-related involvements. All these leave their mark upon the foot in the form of a wide range of morbidities, which usually manifest in later life and produce residual disability in the elderly. Some may produce discomfort or temporary disability. Others will produce insidious but cumulative effects that cause podalgia, ambulatory dysfunction and limitation of activity. As age increases, problems that may have been tolerated in earlier years will limit the mobility of the individual and decrease the QOL. The focus in the management of the older patient may turn from cure to comfort and providing a means to maintain ambulation in order to retain one's independence and dignity.

The feet are covered with hosiery and then thrust into coverings that hide them from view for long periods of time. Footwear, either hosiery or shoes, does not always complement the size and/or shape or function of the foot. Extremes in width, length, last, or depth of the foot will complicate shoe fitting, even with a relatively wide range of mass-produced footwear. This potential functional incompatibility between anatomy and coverings potentiates problems, which become more evident and pronounced in later life. Congenital and/or acquired and disease processes may deform feet in a variety of ways which will result in difficulties throughout life and require proper care over long periods of time to manage these chronic diseases and impairments, such as changes in the circulatory and neurological systems. The primary treatment goals include the relief of pain, restoring the individual to a level of maximum function, and maintaining that function once achieved. Fashion in footwear cannot be disregarded. When style predominates over fit and function, foot problems are again initiated and/or exacerbated due to this functional incompatibility that is many times, with a foot to shoe last (model, design, or shape) incompatibility.[3–5]

Principles and Practice of Geriatric Medicine, Fifth Edition. Edited by Alan J. Sinclair, John E. Morley and Bruno Vellas.

Risk disorders with pedal manifestations

Foot problems and their management are not always regarded as an essential part of some general health programmes or even as being related to general health. The exception is usually related to the catastrophic effects of diabetes mellitus, such as amputation. It is significant but regrettable, that many believe that feet are a part of the body that is designed to hurt. This is true for patients and other elements of the healthcare systems. A majority of patients expect to be able to pursue their normal activities and occupations despite the presence of foot conditions that require rest, but not necessarily hospitalization. With advancing age and the changes in older adult lifestyle, including assisted living and long-term care, these concerns magnify and may be the difference between living life with some quality and sedentary institutionalization. In addition, because of age-related changes and disease, patients are frequently unable to reach their feet because of arthritis, failing eyesight, obesity, postural hypotension, or some other related disorder. Continuing assessment, evaluation and appropriate care is most essential for the 'at-risk' older patients. Tables 92.1 and 92.2 identify some of the primary risks associated with the development of foot problems in the older population (for an example, see also Figure 92.1).

The primary risk diseases that present with significant pedal manifestations as identified by Medicare are summarized in, but not limited to, Table 92.3 as follows:

On 16 June 2009, the Department of Veterans Affairs (VHA Directive 2009-030) expanded the Medicare primary risk categories to appropriately include those conditions listed in Table $^{92.3A}$.

A secondary list of systemic 'at-risk' conditions are summarized but not limited to Table 92.4. There are also specialized risks identified in, but not limited to Table 92.5.

Joint diseases such as arthroses, gout, rheumatoid arthritis and osteoarthritis are frequently manifested in the feet. Their primary clinical findings are noted but not limited to those listed in Table 92.6 (gout), Table 92.7 (rheumatoid arthritis), and Table 92.8 (osteoarthritis or degenerative joint diseases).

In the older patient, the consequences of these diseases usually result in deformity, swollen joints, impaired foot function, and an altered and potentially podalgic gait. In many cases, the foot may be the primary site of deformity, disability and limitation of activity that makes weight bearing difficult and causes significant problems in obtaining adequate footwear to compensate for the residuals of these diseases.

Variable and wide-ranging effects accompany endocrinopathies, such as diabetes mellitus, in the cardiovascular and neurological systems. Many of the symptoms and complications associated with the disease are manifested in the feet and produce potential and serious complications in the older patient. The changes involving the foot are the cause for a significant number of potentially life-threatening hospitalizations. In addition, it has been estimated in the

Table 92.1 Generalized risk.

- The process of ageing
- History of diabetes
- Poor glucose control
- History of prior amputation
- Impaired vision
- Inability to bend
- Patients who live alone
- Tobacco use (smoking)
- Dementia and Alzheimer's disease
- History of alcohol use
- Risk-taking behaviour
- Obesity
- Sensory loss, loss of protective sensation and neuropathy
- Altered biomechanics and pathomechanics
- Structural abnormalities including:
  - Limited joint mobility
  - Hallux Valgus
  - Digiti flexi (hammertoes)
  - Prominent metatarsal heads and prolapse (declination)
- Altered gait, ambulatory dysfunction, and fall risk
- Abnormal or excessive foot pressure
- Soft tissue and plantar fat pad atrophy
- Subkeratotic and/or subungual haematoma
- History of previous foot ulcers
- Peripheral arterial and venous disease
- Toenail pathology
- Xerosis and fissures
- Other related chronic diseases and complications
- Cardiovascular disease
- Renal disease
- Retinal disease
- Osteoarthritis
- Rheumatoid arthritis
- Gout

Table 92.2 Other related risks.

- The degree of ambulation
- The duration of prior hospitalization
- Limitation of activity
- Prior institutionalization
- Episodes of social segregation
- Prior care
- Emotional adjustments to disease and life in general
- Multiple medications and drug interactions
- Complications and residuals associated with risk diseases

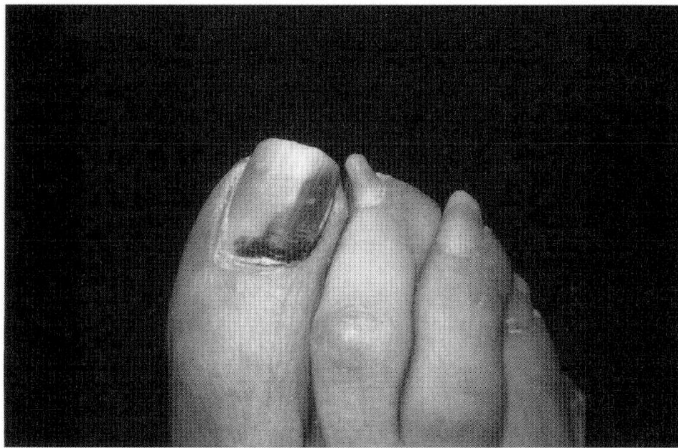

Figure 92.1 Subungual haematoma, onychodysplasia, hammertoes, trophic changes.

Table 92.3 Primary risk diseases.

- Amyotrophic lateral sclerosis (ALS)
- Arteriosclerosis obliterans (ASO, arteriosclerosis of the extremities, occlusive peripheral arteriosclerosis)
- Arteritis of the feet
- Buerger's disease (thromboangiitis obliterans)
- Chronic indurated cellulitis
- *Chronic thrombophlebitis
- Chronic venous insufficiency
- *Diabetes mellitus
- Intractable oedema – secondary to a specific disease (e.g. CHF, kidney disease, hypothyroidism)
- Lymphoedema – secondary to a specific disease (e.g. Milroy's disease, malignancy)
- Peripheral neuropathies involving the feet
- *Associated with malnutrition and vitamin deficiency
- Malnutrition (general, pellagra)
- Alcoholism
- Malabsorption (coeliac disease, tropical sprue)
- Pernicious anaemia
- *Associated with carcinoma
- *Associated with diabetes mellitus
- *Associated with drugs and toxins
- *Associated with multiple sclerosis
- *Associated with uraemia (chronic renal disease)
- Associated with traumatic injury
- Associated with leprosy or neurosyphilis
- Associated with hereditary disorders
- Hereditary sensory radically neuropathy
- Angiokeratoma corporis diffusum (Fabry's)
- Amyloid neuropathy
- Peripheral vascular disease (arterial and venous)
- Raynaud's disease

Note: Those conditions marked with an asterisk (*), require medical evaluation and care within 6 months of their primary foot care service.

Table 92.3A Primary risk categories.

- Documented peripheral arterial disease
- Documented sensory neuropathy
- Prior history of foot ulcer or amputation
- Visually impaired
- Physically impaired
- Neuromuscular disease, i.e. Parkinson's disease
- Severe arthritis and spinal disc disease
- Cognitive dysfunction
- Chronic anticoagulation therapy
- >70 years old without other risk factors
- Diabetes without foot complications
- Obesity

Table 92.4 Secondary risk conditions.

- Collagen vascular disease
- Malignancy
- Lymphoedema
- Postphlebitic syndrome
- Venous (peripheral) insufficiency
- Acromegaly
- Cerebral palsy
- Coagulopathies
- Post-stroke
- Sarcoidosis
- Sickle-cell anaemia
- Reflex sympathetic dystrophy
- Chronic obstructive pulmonary disease
- Hypertension
- Mental illness
- Mental retardation
- Haemophilia
- Patients on anticoagulant therapy
- Paralysis
- Ambulatory dysfunction
- Parkinson's disease
- Immunosuppressed states (HIV, AIDS)

Table 92.5 Specialized risks.

- Vascular grafts
- Joint implants
- Heart valve replacement
- Active chemotherapy
- Renal failure – dialysis
- Anticoagulant therapy
- Haemorrhagic disease
- Chronic steroid therapy

Table 92.6 Gout.

Acute

- Inflammation
- Painful
- Swelling
- Redness
- High uric acid levels
- Podalgia
- Limitation of motion
- Ambulatory dysfunction

Chronic tophaceous gout

- Deformity
- Pain
- Stiffness
- Soft tissue tophi
- Atrophy of soft tissue
- Loss of bone substance
- Gouty arthritis
- Joint deformity
- Excessive pain associated with the acute episodes and
- Exacerbations

United Kingdom and United States, that 50–75% of all amputations relating to the complications associated with diabetes mellitus could be prevented and reduced with an appropriate programme of preventive foot care and foot health education.

The most common clinical findings relating to the diabetic foot are listed but not limited to those in and Table 92.9 (for an example, see also Figure 92.2).

To these problems one must add the effects of repeated microtrauma from footwear, environmental surfaces, lifestyle, neglect and heat-reflecting surfaces, which produce hyperkeratosis and subkeratotic haemorrhage, a predisposing factor for ulceration. Diabetic foot problems in the elderly are characterized by paresthesias, numbness, sensory impairment, a loss of pain sensation, motor weakness, reflex loss, neurotrophic arthropathy, absence of pedal pulses, atrophy, infection, dermopathy, angiopathy, peripheral neuropathy, ulceration and necrosis/gangrene.[6]

Clinically, the most marked change perhaps for the elderly diabetic is sensory neuropathy. When combined with visual impairment, the elderly can be completely unaware of their feet. Paralysis of intrinsic foot muscles due to motor neuropathy will result in deformities of the toes, claw toes. The bony prominences thus formed on the dorsum of the toes and the plantar aspect of the metatarsophalangeal joints may be the site of skin lesions,

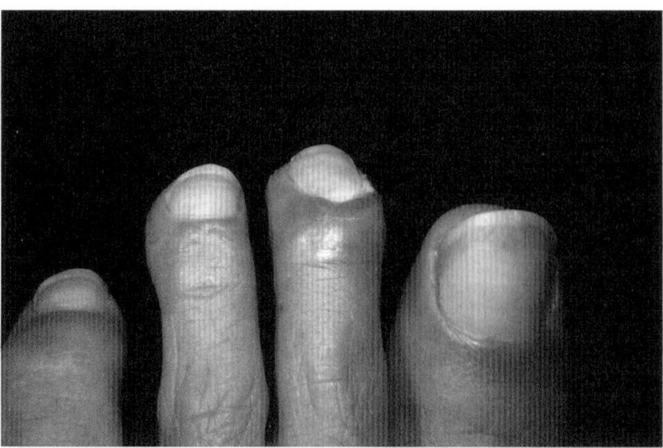

Figure 92.2 Onychia, peripheral arterial disease, early paronychia.

Table 92.7 Rheumatoid arthritis.

- Hallux limitus
- Hallux rigidus
- Hallux valgus
- Hallux abducto valgus
- Cystic erosion
- Sesamoid erosion
- Sesamoid displacement
- Metatarsophalangeal subluxation
- Metatarsophalangeal dislocation
- Interphalangeal subluxation
- Interphalangeal dislocation
- Digiti flexi (hammertoes)
- Ankylosis (fused joints)
- Phalangeal reabsorption
- Talonavicular arthritis
- Extensor tenosynovitis
- Rheumatoid nodules
- Bowstring extensor tendons
- Tendon displacement
- Ganglions
- Rigid pronation
- Subcalcaneal bursitis
- Retrocalcaneal bursitis
- Retroachillal bursitis
- Calcaneal ossifying enthesopathy (spur)
- Prolapsed metatarsal heads
- Atrophy of the plantar fat pad
- Soft tissue displacement
- Digiti quinti varus
- Tailor's bunion
- Early morning stiffness
- Pain
- Fibrosis
- Spurs
- Periostitis
- Bursitis
- Plantar fasciitis
- Nodules
- Contracture
- Deformity
- Impairment of function
- Loss or reduction of normal ambulation

Table 92.8 Degenerative joint diseases: osteoarthritis.

- Pain related to minimal trauma
- Inflammation
- Strain
- Plantar fasciitis
- Spur formation
- Periostitis
- Myofascitis
- Decalcification
- Stress fractures
- Tendonitis
- Tenosynovitis
- Residual deformities
- Pes planus
- Pes cavus
- Hallux valgus
- Digiti flexus (hammertoes)
- Rotational digital deformities
- Joint swelling
- Increase pain
- Limitation of motion
- Reduced ambulatory status

such as hyperkeratosis (tyloma and/or heloma, i.e. corns and calluses), and/or the sites of ulceration, due to pressure, residual subkeratotic haemorrhage and local tissue ischaemia.

The plantar surface of the foot has been the most common site for the development of diabetic ulceration, which is trophic in character. These ulcers develop underneath keratosis with pressure and thus the skilled and proper débridement of the keratosis is a prerequisite to the successful management of the diabetic ulcer and in the prevention of ulcer development (see Figure 92.3). Appropriate weight diffusion and dispersion procedures are also essential elements to management, particularly in the elderly.

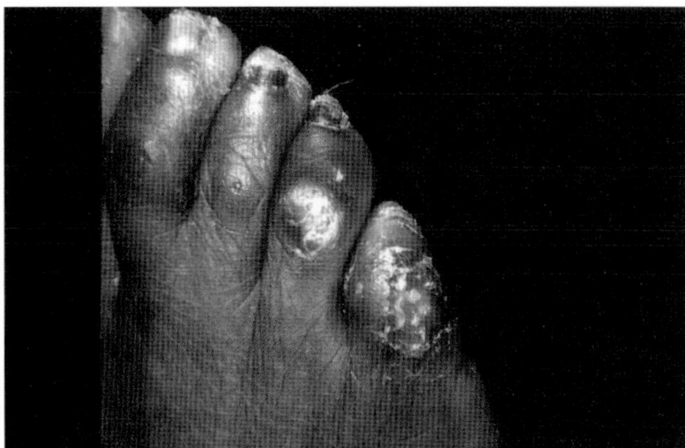

Figure 92.3 Multiple hammer toes, heloma, preulcerative keratosis, subungual haematoma, peripheral arterial disease, trophic changes.

Table 92.9 Diabetic foot changes.

- Vascular impairment
- Degenerative changes related to ageing
- Neuropathy
- Dermopathy
- Atrophy
- Deformity
- Insensitivity
- Podalgia
- Fatigue
- Paresthesia
- Sensory impairment to pain and temperature
- Motor weakness
- Pododynia Dysbasia
- Diminished or lost Achilles and patellar reflexes
- Decreased or vibratory sense (pallesthesia)
- Loss of proprioception
- Neuropathy
- Loss of protective sensation
- Blebs
- Excoriation
- Hair loss
- Xerosis
- Anhidrosis
- Neurotrophic arthropathy
- Neurotrophic ulcers
- Disparity in foot size and shape
- Higher prevalence of infection
- Necrosis
- Gangrene
- Pallor
- Absence or decrease in posterior tibial and dorsalis pedis pulses
- Dependent rubor
- Decreased venous filling time
- Coolness of the skin
- Trophic changes
- Numbness
- Tingling
- Claudication
- Pigmentation
- Cramps
- Pain
- Loss of the plantar metatarsal fat pad
- Hyperkeratotic lesions
- Tendon contractures
- Claw toes (hammertoes)
- Ulceration
- Foot drop
- Diabetic dermopathy (pretibial lesions – shin spots)
- Necrobiosis
- Arthropathy
- Deformity
- Radiographic
    - Thin trabecular patterns
    - Decalcification
    - Joint position change

(*continued overleaf*)

Table 92.9 (*continued*).

- Osteophytic formation
- Osteolysis
- Deformities
- Osteopenia
- Osteoporosis

- Pruritus
- Cutaneous infections
- Dehydration
- Trophic changes
- Fissures
- Onychial changes
- Onychodystrophy
- Diabetic onychopathy (nutritional and vascular changes)
- Onychorrhexis (longitudinal striations)
- Subungual hemorrhage (bleeding in the nail bed)
- Onychophosis (keratosis)
- Onychauxis (thickening with hypertrophy)
- Onychogryphosis (thickening with gross deformity)
- Onychia
- Paronychia
- Onychomycosis (fungal infection)
- Subungual ulceration (ulceration in the nail bed)
- Deformity
- Hypertrophy
- Incurvation or involution (onychodysplasia)
- Splinter haemorrhage (non-traumatic)
- Onycholysis (freeing from the distal segment)
- Onychomadesis (freeing from the proximal segment)
- Autoavulsion

Skin texture and sweating patterns are also markedly altered in the elderly diabetic, due to autonomic neuropathy and oedema. The consequent enlargement of the foot is another cause of epidermal abrasions of the skin from footwear and other forms of trauma and pressure. The management of infection becomes complicated unless appropriate metabolic management is instituted and maintained early in the disease process. The resulting sepsis can lead to necrosis, gangrene and amputation of the limb, which additionally complicates the management of the disease in the elderly as well as necessitating changes in the patient's lifestyle.[7]

Varicose veins are a common manifestation in the legs and feet of the elderly. Varices may be observed on the dorsum of the foot sometimes extending as far as the toes, and also along the medial plantar arch area. Haemosiderin deposited in the skin over the lower one-third of the leg and the foot, giving them a freckled appearance and sometimes imparting a coppery hue where the change becomes marked. Oedema of the foot and ankle also are a frequent accompaniment of varicose veins. Trauma to these vessels can produce haemorrhage. The diminished blood flow resulting from the presence of varicose veins impairs wound healing and causes trophic changes in the skin and nails. Adhesive dressings, even though they may be hypoallergenic, are not well tolerated by such skin for prolonged periods of time. Appropriate treatment may be required to improve both the appearance and function of the extremity.

Complicating factors of venous disease in the elderly include thrombophlebitis, deep venous thrombosis, and postphlebitic syndrome, which produce an 'at-risk' status for the patient with foot problems.

The more common arterial diseases that can be observed in the elderly include the residuals of vasospastic disease, such as Raynaud's disease or phenomenon, acrocyanosis, livedo reticulosis, pernio and erythromelalgia. Occlusive diseases such as arteriosclerosis obliterans, the residuals of thromboangiitis obliterans and related diseases, such as arteritis, periarteritis nodosa, polymyalgia rheumatica, systemic lupus erythematous, erythema nodosum, erythema induratum, nodular vasculitis and hypertensive arteriolar disease. The primary risk factors for the development of peripheral arterial diseases in older patients include smoking, diabetes mellitus, hypertension, Buerger's and Raynaud's diseases. With inadequate perfusion, non-healing wounds, infection, tissue loss and amputation are complications. The primary clinical findings associated with arterial insufficiency are summarized but not limited to those listed in Table 92.10.

In the geriatric patient, arterial insufficiency is heralded by rest pain or nocturnal cramps and/or intermittent claudication. Although it is usually brought on by exercise or use, it may also occur at rest in severe cases of arterial occlusion. Any muscle may claudicate and thus foot pain in the elderly may be related to arterial insufficiency rather than biomechanics or pathomechanics. Painful ulcerations may occur over bony prominences and result from minor trauma and/or pressure. Smoking must be prohibited. Appropriate vascular studies, such as: imaging (arteriography, digital subtraction angiography, MRI, CT arteriography and Doppler imaging), non-invasive studies (Doppler, oscillometric, ankle-brachial index, segmental pressure measurement, plethysmographic waveform analysis, pulse volume recording, skin perfusion pressure, laser Doppler pressure, colour Doppler, ultrasonography, transcutaneous oxygen content (TcPO3), cutaneous oximetry and treadmill exercise testing), and surgical consideration should be provided when pain is uncontrolled and/or when ulceration and infection are significant.

Because of the risk involved in the geriatric patient and the relationship to multiple chronic diseases, assessment, examination and evaluation of the feet and related structures, are essential. Elements of this process include needs, relationships to ambulation and activities of daily living (ADL), instrumental activities of daily living (IADL), and the fact that foot pain can result in functional disability, dysfunction and increased dependency.

Table 92.10 Primary clinical vascular findings.

Fatigue
Rest pain
Coldness
Decreased skin temperature
Burning
Colour changes
Absent or diminished digital hair
Tingling
Numbness
Ulceration
History of phlebitis
Cramps
Oedema
Claudication
History of repeated foot infections
Diminished or absent pedal pulses
Popliteal and/or femoral pulse change
Colour changes – rubor – erythema and/or cyanosis
Temperature changes – cool – gradient
Xerosis, atrophic and dry skin
Atrophy of soft tissue
Superficial infections
Onychial changes
Onychopathy
Onychodystrophy
Nutritional changes
Subungual haemorrhage
Discolouration
Onycholysis
Onychauxis (thickening)
Onychorrhexis (longitudinal striations)
Subungual keratosis
Deformity
Blebs
Varicosities
Delayed venous filling time
Prolonged capillary filling time
Femoral bruits
Ischaemia
Necrosis and gangrene

A Comprehensive Podogeriatric Assessment Protocol (Helfand Index), has been developed by the Pennsylvania Department of Health in cooperation with Temple University, School of Podiatric Medicine and is included as Table 92.11.

In addition, Medicare in the United States has three additional sets of criteria for Class Findings required to qualify for primary foot care (Table 92.12); Criteria for Therapeutic Shoes for Diabetics (Table 92.13); Criteria of the Loss of Protective Sensation (LOPS) (Table 92.14); Criteria for Onychomycosis (see Figure 92.4) (Table 92.15).

A systems review of known chronic and risk diseases is a key element in the assessment process. Conditions such as

Table 92.11 Podogeriatric assessment protocol developed under a contract to the Pennsylvania Department of Health as the 'Helfand Index' by Arthur E. Helfand, DPM. Reproduced with permission.

Date of visit MR#	
Patient's name Age	
Date of birth	Social Security #
Address	
City State Zip code	
Phone number	
Sex M F Race B W A L NA	
Weight in Pounds Height in Inches	
Social status M S W D SEP	
Name of primary physician/health-care facility	
Date of last visit	
History of Present Illness	
Swelling of feet Location	
Painful feet Quality	
Hyperkeratosis Severity	
Onychial Changes Duration	
Bunions Context	
Painful toe nails Modifying factors	
Infections Associated signs and symptoms	
Cold feet	
Other	
Past History	
Heart disease Diabetes mellitus	
High blood pressure * IDDM	
Arthritis * NIDDM	
* Circulatory disease Hypercholesterol	
Thyroid	
Gout	
Allergy	
History of Smoking – Alcohol – Substance Abuse	
Family – Social	
Systems Review	
Constitutional	
ENT	
Card/Vasc	
GU	
Eyes	
Musculo-Skeletal	
Neurologic	
Skin – Hair – Nails	
Skeletal Endocrine	
Respiratory	
GYN	
GI	
Psychiatric	
Allergic	
Immunologic	
Hematologic	
Lymphatic	
Medications	

(continued overleaf)

Table 92.11 (*continued*).

Dermatologic
* Hyperkeratosis
Xerosis
Onychauxis B-2-b
Tinea pedis
Infection
Verruca
* Ulceration Hematoma
Onychomycosis
Rubor
Onychodystrophy
* Preulcerative
* Cyanosis B-2-e
Discolored

Foot Orthopedic
* Hallux valgus
* Hallux rigidus-limitus
* Anterior imbalance
* Morton's syndrome
* Digiti flexus
Bursitis
* Pes planus
* Prominent Metatarsal Head
* Pes Valgoplanus
* Charcot joints
* Pes cavus
Other

Vascular Evaluation
* Coldness C-2
* Claudication C-1
* Trophic changes B-2-a
Varicosities
* DP absent B-3
* PT absent B-1
* Amputation
* Night cramps
* AKA BKA FF T A-1
* Edema C-3
Atrophy B-2-d
Other

Neurologic Evaluation
* Achilles
* Superficial plantar
* Vibratory
* Joint Position
* Sharp/Dull
* Burning C-5
* Paresthesia C-4
Other

Risk Category – Neurologic
0 = No Sensory Loss
* 1 = Sensory Loss
* 2 = Sensory Loss and Foot Deformity
* 3 = Sensory Loss, Hx Ulceration, and Deformity

Table 92.11 (*continued*).

Risk category – Vascular
0 – 0 No Change
* I – 1 Mild Claudication
* I – 2 Moderate Claudication
* I – 3 Severe Claudication
* II – 4 Ischemic Rest Pain
* III – 5 Minor Tissue Loss
* III – 6 Major Tissue Loss

Class Findings
A1 Nontraumatic Amputation
B1 Absent Posterior Tibial
B2 Advanced Trophic Changes
B2a Hair Growth (Decrease or Absent)
B2b Nail changes (Thickening)
B2c Pigmentary Changes (Discoloration)
B2d Skin Texture (Thin, Shiny)
B2e Skin Color (Rubor or Redness)
B3 Absent Dorsalis Pedis
C1 Claudication
C2 Temperature Changes (cold)
C3 Edema
C4 Paresthesia
C5 Burning

Onychomycosis: Documentation of mycosis/dystrophy causing secondary infection and/or pain, which results or would result in marked limitation of ambulation.
Discoloration
Hypertrophy
Subungual Debris
Onycholysis
Secondary Infection
Limitation of Ambulation and Pain

Classification of Mechanical or Pressure Hyperkeratosis – Grade
Description
0 No lesion
1 No specific tyloma plaque, but diffuse or pinch hyperkeratotic tissue present or in narrow bands
2 Circumscribed, punctate oval, or circular, well defined thickening of keratinized tissue
3 Heloma miliare or heloma durum with no associated tyloma
4 Well-defined tyloma plaque with a definite heloma within the lesion
extravasation, maceration, and early breakdown of structures under the tyloma or callus layer
5 Complete breakdown of structure of hyperkeratotic tissue, epidermis, extending to superficial dermal involvement

Plantar keratomata pattern
LT 5 4 3 2 1
RT 1 2 3 4 5

Ulcer classification
Grade – 0 – Absent skin lesions
Grade – 1 – Dense callus but not preulcer or ulcer
Grade – 2 – Preulcerative changes
Grade – 3 – Partial thickness (superficial ulcer)

(*continued overleaf*)

Table 92.11 (*continued*).

Grade – 4 – Full thickness (deep) ulcer but no involvement of tendon, bone, ligament or joint
Grade – 5 – Full thickness (deep) ulcer with involvement of tendon, bone, ligament or joint
Grade – 6 – Localized infection (abscess or osteomyelitis)
Grade – 7 – Proximal spread of infection (ascending cellulitis or lymphadenopathy)
Grade – 8 – Gangrene of forefoot only
Grade – 9 – Gangrene of majority of foot

Onychial Grades at Risk
- Grade I Normal
- Grade II Mild hypertrophy
- Grade III Hypertrophic
  - Dystrophic
  - Onychauxis
  - Mycotic
  - Infected
  - Onychodysplasia
- Grade IV Hypertrophic
  - Deformed
  - Onychogryphosis
  - Dystrophic
  - Mycotic
  - Infected

Footwear Satisfactory Hygiene satisfactory
- Yes
- No

Hygiene Satisfactory
- Yes
- No

Stockings
- Nylon
- Cotton
- Wool Other
- None

Assessment
Plan
Podiatric referral
Patient education
Medical referral
Special footwear
Vascular studies
Clinical lab
Imaging
Rx

Notes: B, Black; W, White, A, Asian; L, Latino/Hispanic; N/A, Native American; S, Single; M, Married; W, Widow/Widower; D, Divorced; S, Separated; DP, Dorsalis pedis pulse; PT, Posterior tibial pulse; AKA, Above the knee amputation; BKA, Below the knee amputation; FF, Forefoot amputation; T, Toe amputation; Hx, History of; Rx, Prescription for treatment as a part of the key to data analysis and risk stratification, the key notes of number and letter (i.e. 2-a) indicate Medicare class findings as risk factors and those noted with an asterisk (*) identify risk factors to qualify patients for therapeutic shoes under Medicare.

Table 92.12 Medicare Class Findings.

Class Findings

Class A findings
- Non-traumatic amputation of foot or integral skeletal portion thereof

Class B findings
- Absent posterior tibial pulse
- Absent dorsalis pedis pulse
- Advanced trophic changes as (three required)
  - Hair growth (decrease or absence)
  - Nail changes (thickening)
  - Pigmentary changes (discolouration)
  - Skin texture (thin, shiny)
  - Skin colour (rubor or redness)

Class C findings
- Claudication
- Temperature changes (e.g. cold feet)
- Oedema
- Paresthesias (abnormal spontaneous sensations in the feet)
- Burning

Table 92.13 Therapeutic shoe criteria.

- History of partial or complete amputation of the foot
- History of previous foot ulceration
- History of pre-ulcerative callus
- Peripheral neuropathy with evidence of callus formation
- Foot deformity
- Poor circulation

Table 92.14 Onychomycosis: Documentation of mycosis/dystrophy causing secondary infection and/or pain, which results or would result in marked limitation of ambulation.

- Discolouration
- Hypertrophy
- Subungual debris
- Onycholysis
- Secondary infection
- Limitation of ambulation and pain
- Dystrophic
- Onychodysplasia
- Onychauxis
- Onychogryphosis

diabetes mellitus, arteriosclerosis, anaemia, chronic renal disease, CHF, arthritis, stroke and neurological deficits are examples of these risk conditions. The patients' living conditions should also be noted as they are a relationship to care and needs. The chief complaint of the patient should be identified related to their daily lives in terms of activity

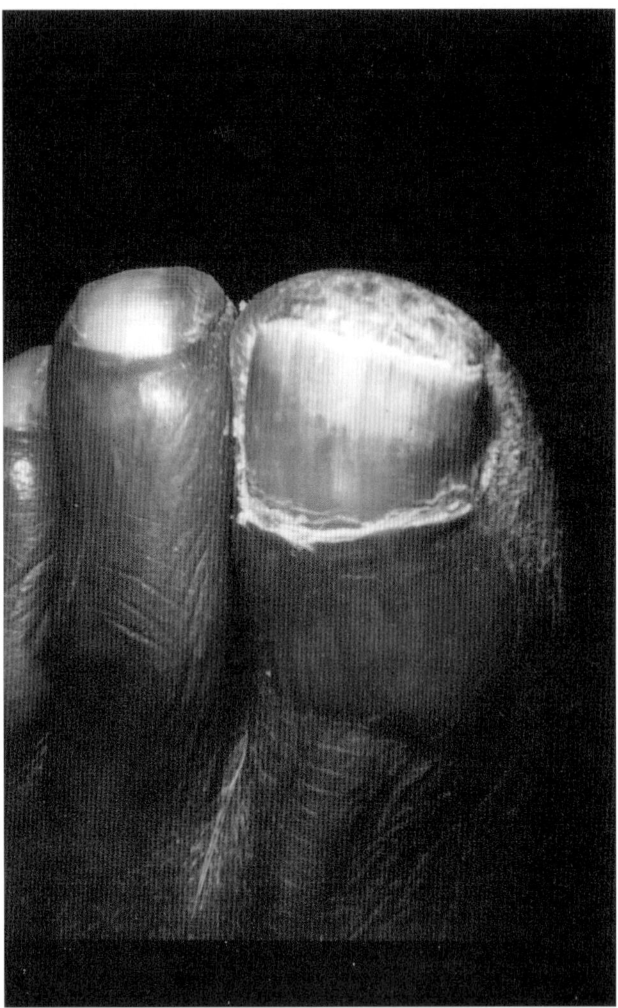

Figure 92.4 Onychomycosis, onychauxis, xerosis, onychorrhexis, and peripheral arterial disease.

and social needs. The duration, location, severity, prior treatment and results should also be identified in relation to the presented condition. A social history is also a part of this assessment process.

The dermatological symptoms and signs and the onychial findings are listed but not limited to Tables 92.16 (see also Figure 92.5) and 92.17.

The neurological symptoms and signs are included but not limited to Table 92.18. The vascular findings are noted in Table 92.10.

A drug history and summary of findings, clinical impressions and special notations for some of the primary basics for assessment, as anticoagulants, steroids and medications to control diabetes mellitus present additional risk.

The primary musculoskeletal clinical findings are noted but not limited to Table 92.19.

There are biomechanical and pathomechanical factors that combine with structural abnormalities and deformities to increase the risk for pedal ulceration. They are listed but not limited to Table 92.20.

The forefoot (metatarsals and phalanges) is the most mobile part of the foot and the majority of problems that develop occur in this area. Pressure from deformities and shoe to foot incompatibility, will give rise to keratotic lesions as an initial response to pressure and friction, but footwear is by no means the only cause of painful lesions in the feet or the prime aetiological factor. Congenital and acquired deformities will result in malfunction and dysfunction and give rise to secondary lesions as the body attempts to compensate for pain and deformity. Alteration in shape and function can arise from trauma, paralysis, changes in function as a result of surgical revision and/or diseases, such as arthritis, which embarrass normal function. The mobility of the foot has a great influence on the type and extent of painful secondary foot lesions.

Table 92.15 Loss of protective sensation (LOPS).

Services furnished for the evaluation and management of a diabetic patient with diabetic sensory neuropathy, resulting in a LOPS must include the following:

1 A diagnosis of LOPS
2 A patient history
3 A physical examination consisting of findings regarding at least the following elements:
   a Visual inspection of the forefoot, hindfoot and toe web spaces
   b Evaluation of protective sensation
   c Evaluation of foot structure and biomechanics
   d Evaluation of vascular status
   e Evaluation of skin integrity
   f Evaluation and recommendation of footwear
4 Patient education

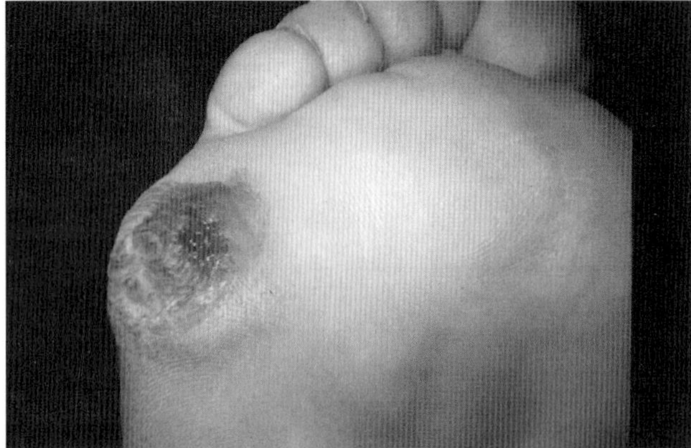

Figure 92.5 Preulcerative keratosis, subkeratotic haematoma, digiti quinti varus, metatarsal prolapse, anterior plantar fat pad displacement.

Table 92.16 Dermatological findings.

Exquisitely painful or painless wounds
Slow healing or non-healing wounds
Trophic ulceration
Necrosis
Skin colour changes such as cyanosis or redness
Changes in texture and turgor
Pigmentation
Haemosiderin deposition
Chronic itching – pruritus
Neurogenic, and/or emotional dermatoses
Contact dermatitis
Stasis dermatitis
Atopic dermatitis
Nummular eczema
Scaling
Xerosis or dryness
Excoriations
Recurrent infections
Paronychia
Tinea pedis
Onychomycosis
Pyoderma
Cellulitis
Keratotic dysfunction
Keratotic lesions without haemorrhage or haematoma
Tyloma (callus)
Heloma durum (hard corn)
Heloma miliare (seed corn)
Heloma molle (soft corn)
Heloma neurofibrosuum (neuritic)
Heloma vasculare (vascular)
Onychophosis (callus in the nail groove)
Intractable plantar keratosis
Keratotic lesions with haemorrhage or haematoma (pre-ulcerative)
Verruca
Psoriasis
Fissures
Hyperhidrosis
Bromidrosis
Maceration
Diminished or absent hair growth
Diabetic dermopathy
Necrobiosis lipoidica diabeticorum
Bullous diabeticorum
Poroma
Absence of hair
Ulceration

Table 92.17 Onychial findings.

Onychoatrophia (atrophy)
Onychia sicca (dryness)
Onycholysis (freeing from the free edge)
Subungual hyperkeratosis
Onychexallis (degeneration)
Diabetic onychopathy
Onychauxis (hypertrophy)
Onychogryphosis (hypertrophy and deformity)
Onychomycosis (fungal infection)
Onychia
Paronychia
Onychitis (inflammation)
Onychalgia (pain)
Subungual abscess
Subungual heloma (keratosis)
Subungual exostosis
Periungual verruca
Onychophyma (painful degeneration with hypertrophy)
Onychomadesis (freeing from the proximal portion)
Onychoschizia (splitting)
Onychyphemia (haemorrhagic)
Onychoclasis (cracking)
Onychomalacia (softening)
Onychoptosis (shedding)
Subungual spur
Onychophosis (hyperkeratosis in the nail groove)
Subungual haematoma
Splinter haemorrhage
Onychocryptosis (ingrown toenail)
Periungual ulcerative granulation tissue
Onychodysplasia (involuted or pincer nails)
Onychodystrophy (trophic changes)
Onychorrhexis (longitudinal ridging)
Beau's lines (transverse growth cessation)
Pterygium (hypertrophy of eponychium)
Onychoclasis (breaking of the nail)
Diabetic onychopathy (trophic diabetic changes)
Hypertrophic onychodystrophy

Rigid feet usually have circumscribed areas of hyperkeratosis. Mobile feet have more extensive areas of keratotic development. Where the foot is deficient in fibro-fatty padding or where the stress is chronic, constant and severe, the so-called neurovascular heloma or tyloma may develop, creating a disruption in the normal dermal–epidermal relationship. Small blood vessels and nerve endings then extend into the epidermis and are enveloped in the keratotic lesion, creating excessive pain and complicating management. Such lesions may be completely disabling and in some patients, result in distressing hyperaesthesia that is difficult to manage.

Footwear can also reveal a great deal about disease and dynamic foot function. Neglected footwear generally demonstrates neglected foot care and may indicate social poverty. It may also demonstrate poor eyesight. Urine splashes that have dried on the uppers of shoes are sometimes the first indication of occult diabetes mellitus.

Table 92.18 Neurological findings.

Sensory changes
Burning
Tingling
Clawing sensations
Pain and hyperactivity
Two-point discrimination
Motor changes
Weakness
Foot drop
Autonomic
Diminished sweating
Hyperhidrosis
Sensory deficits
Vibratory
Proprioceptive
Loss of protective sensation
Changes in pain and temperature perception
Hyperaesthesia
Diminished to absent deep tendon reflexes (Achilles and Patellar)
Hypohidrosis with perfusion
Diabetic dermopathy or pretibial lesions (shin spots)
Thickened skin with calluses under high-pressure areas, demonstrating an intrinsic minus foot (marked digital contractures, metatarsal prolapse, prominent metatarsal heads, and plantar fat pad atrophy and displacement)
Bowstring tendons
Charcot foot

Table 92.19 Musculoskeletal findings.

Gradual change in shape or size of the foot
A sudden and painless change in foot shape with swelling and no history of trauma
Cavus feet with claw toe
Drop foot
'Rocker bottom foot' or Charcot foot
Neuropathic arthropathy
Elevated plantar pressure
Decreased muscle strength
Decreased ranges of motion
Multiple foot deformities
Limited joint mobility
Abnormal foot pressure and subsequent ulceration
Structural abnormalities or foot deformities
Hammertoes
Claw toes
Prominent metatarsal heads
Atrophy of plantar fat pad
Plantar fat pad displacement
Foot muscle atrophy
Hallux valgus
Hallux limitus
Hallux rigidus
Tailor's bunion
Plantar Fasciitis
Spur formation
Calcaneal spurs
Bursitis
Periostitis
Decalcification
Stress fractures
Tendonitis
Tenosynovitis
Metatarsalgia
Morton's syndrome
Joint swelling
Bursitis
Haglund's deformity
Neuritis
Entrapment syndrome
Neuroma
Sesamoid erosion
Sesamoid displacement
Tendo-Achilles contracture
Digital amputation
Partial foot amputation
Charcot's joints
Phalangeal reabsorption
Functional abnormalities
Pes cavus
Equinus
Pes planus
Residuals of arthritis (degenerative, rheumatoid and gouty)
Biomechanical and pathomechanical variations
Gait evaluation

(*continued overleaf*)

Keratotic lesions

The presence of hyperkeratotic lesions, such as tyloma and/or heloma (callous or corns) on the foot is associated with some degree of malfunction of the foot, especially in the elderly. Elimination and/or management of the underlying causes are the principle objective of therapy. There are a wider range of treatment options to be considered including continuing surveillance, monitoring and primary management including débridement, pressure reduction, orthotics, shoe modification and surgical revision of deformities, usually when conservative measures are unresponsive. It is the same approach as utilized for any other chronic condition.[8]

The normal response of the epidermis to intermittent, chronic pressure and/or stress is to increase in thickness. The resulting hyperkeratosis may be both hyperplastic and hypertrophic. These lesions commonly occur on the plantar aspect of the metatarsophalangeal joints, the hallux, the margins of the heel, the dorsum of the toes, especially with contracture, and in the nail grooves. Atrophy of the adjacent dermis and soft tissue is common especially in the

Table 92.19 (*continued*).

Shoe evaluation
Type of shoe
Fit and size
Shoe wear and patters of wear
Shoe lining wear
Foreign bodies
Insoles
Orthoses

Table 92.20 Factors leading to ulceration.

- Body mass
- Gait
- Ambulatory speed
- Tissue trauma
- Weight diffusion
- Weight dispersion
- Pathomechanics, defined as structural change in relation to function
- Biomechanics, defined as forces that change and affect the foot in relation to function
- Imbalance, defined as the inability to adapt to alterations of stress
- Force – alteration in physical condition, either shape or position
- Compression stress – one force moves toward another
- Tensile stress – a pulling away of one part against another
- Shearing stress – a sliding of one part on the other
- Friction – the force needed to overcome resistance and usually associated with a sheering stress
- Elasticity – weight diffusion and weight dispersion
- Fluid pressure – soft tissue adaptation and conformity to stress

patient demonstrating a LOPS. With continuing pressure and neurovascular involvement, fibrous tissue may develop to bind the skin to the underlying joint capsule and/or tissues.

Patients with diabetic peripheral neuropathy involving the lower extremities also present with reported numbness or a reduced ability to feel pain and/or temperature changes; tingling, burning, or prickling sensations; sharp, jabbing, or electric shock like pain that is magnified at night; extreme sensitivity to light touch; loss of balance and/or coordination; muscle weakness, pain and ambulatory dysfunction (pododynia dysbasia); and serious complications, such as ulceration, infection, Charcot's deformity, and significant risk of amputation.[9]

Subkeratotic haematomas indicate areas where blood has been forced from vessels and are indicative of extensive pressure and/or a complication of an associated systemic disease, such as diabetes mellitus. Occasionally, this makes a 'lake' in the area and produces a moist, shallow ulceration, which usually dries and heals when the area is débrided of keratosis and appropriately managed.

The characteristic of a heloma durum (hard corn) is the presence of a nucleus. Heloma represent a reaction to more localized stress than is the case with tyloma (callosity). Heloma may also present as a central area in a tyloma. The nucleus is small and may be circular or even crescentic in shape. It is harder due to increased density than the surrounding hyperkeratosis. The nucleus may represent parakeratotic changes histologically, similar to that which occurs in psoriasis.

Like tyloma, heloma are essentially epidermal in origin but may become more complex because of alteration in the dermis and a source of considerable intractable chronic pain. This is due to the imbalance created in the normal chemo-epidermal function and the development of hyperkeratotic lesions with neural and vascular components, many times encapsulated, giving rise to significant pain and discomfort. The resulting neurovascular lesion, heloma neurovarsculare signifies a long-standing lesion. They result from improper and inappropriate treatment, repeated self-treatment, resulting in haemorrhage and inadequate follow-up care.

Heloma (corn) may arise anywhere on the skin where a bony prominence provides resistance to external pressure. The resulting intermittent stress – a combination of pressure, friction, and shearing – provokes changes in the skin. In the elderly, atrophy of soft tissue and a reduction in the fluidity and elasticity of the soft tissues predispose the elderly to the development of these lesions.

Bursae may occur in the tissues adjacent to a heloma. Localized pinpoint lesions, heloma miliare, or seed corns, occur with extreme localization of pressure, joint deformity, spur formation and/or a protruding irregularity in a shoe. Heloma molle or soft corns are located between the toes, and are macerated due to excessive moisture. Their aetiology is usually due to digital compression accompanied by bony abnormality and/or digital deformities, such as hammertoes and/or rotational deformities. Management in the elderly is essential to prevent infection, particularly from improper débridement. Atrophy of soft tissue and localized pressure lead to keratotic lesions that become chronic and intractable.

Management includes initial débridement, the use of emollients such as 20% urea or 12% ammonium lactate, and procedures and materials to reduce pressure. Silicone moulds to compensate for deformity, padding materials to provide weight diffusion, orthotics to provide stability and weight dispersion, and shoe modifications as needed are also considerations in a long-range approach to the management of these lesions in the elderly. Surgical repair should be considered when indicated.[10]

Ulcers

Diabetes mellitus, peripheral vascular insufficiency, and repetitive trauma are the primary aetiologies in the development of ulcerations in feet. A resolution of the ulcer can be maintained with periodic assessment and management and addressing the underlying cause.[11]

Diabetic ulceration commonly occurs on weight-bearing areas of the foot. The tissues overlying any bony prominence exposed to repetitive pressure may also breakdown and ulcerate. Even bed-ridden patients may develop ulcers due to the weight of bedclothes or that of one limb upon another. Diabetic ulcers may involve deeper structures. Surgical intervention may be required; débridement, drainage and possible skin grafting. The use of contact casts or removable cast walkers can be considered, but the patient's ability to adapt to these ambulatory changes must be part of the consideration for their use.[12,13]

Ulcers that are due to arterial insufficiency are usually very painful and present with pending necrosis and gangrene. The ulcer is usually dry and at some point, the decision to manage and/or amputate will require consideration. The decision should be based on the clinical presentation and the needs of the patient.

Ulcer aetiology and assessment are initial considerations. Location, wound size and shape, wound bed, colour, drainage, wound edges, pain, periwound area, odour, oedema and the signs of infection are important issues. Management includes removing devitalized tissue by débridement (mechanical and/or chemical), autolytic enzymes and appropriate dressings. The potential for infection is a critical issue, requiring early management. Preventing local injury and supporting the repair process are equally important. Vascular complications require indicated consultations and possible surgical intervention. Topical recombinant platelet-derived growth factors can assist in wound care. Continuing evaluation, local wound care, management and prevention are continuing issues, particularly in the older patient.[14]

Management should also include relief of pressure, control of infection and appropriate débridement. Note should be made of the duration of the ulcer, size of the ulcer, depth of the ulcer, and the amount of necrotic tissue present. Treatment parameters also include assessment of the patient's mental status, mobility, infection, tissue oxygenation, chronic pressure, arterial insufficiency (small vessel ischaemia), venous stasis, oedema, type of dressings and chronic illnesses such as diabetes mellitus, uraemia, COPD (chronic obstructive pulmonary disease), malnutrition, CHF (congestive heart failure), anaemia, iron deficiency and immune deficiency disorders. In addition, signs and symptoms, other medical conditions, the wound status, the patient's response to treatment, and early consultation are also important factors to preserve the patient's limb and life.[15]

Toenails

As appendages of the skin, toenails very readily reflect its state, becoming hard, dry and brittle as age advances. Not infrequently, the nail plate is thinner than usual due to atrophy. In other instances, the toenails become so thickened and deformed that the patient cannot cut them and they are ashamed to show their nails to another person. The resulting discomfort may prevent them from wearing any other footwear than a house slipper, making the patient housebound. In addition, the deformity may present a podalgic gait and produce a degree of ambulatory dysfunction, making the patient partially functionally disabled and at risk for a fall.

Trauma is a precipitating factor in the development of thickening of the nail plate. The trauma may have been acute and marked or may be chronic and minimal, such as the constant friction or impaction of the toenail against the inner portion of the toe box of the shoe. The nail plate may grow and twist across the foot (onychogryphosis or 'Ram's horn nail') (see Figure 92.6). It also presents as a residual of inappropriate or no treatment. The danger of this condition is that the nail may penetrate the skin and provide a portal of entry for pathogens, resulting in infection.

Toenails sometimes assume a claw-like appearance due to a dramatic increase in the transverse curvature (involution, convolution, or onychodysplasia). They may also become thickened (onychauxis). Unskilled and inappropriate attempts to 'dig out' the corners of this so-called ingrown toenail, because it is painful, very often lead to inflammation (onychia) and infection (paronychia). Temporary relief may be obtained but skin retraction usually

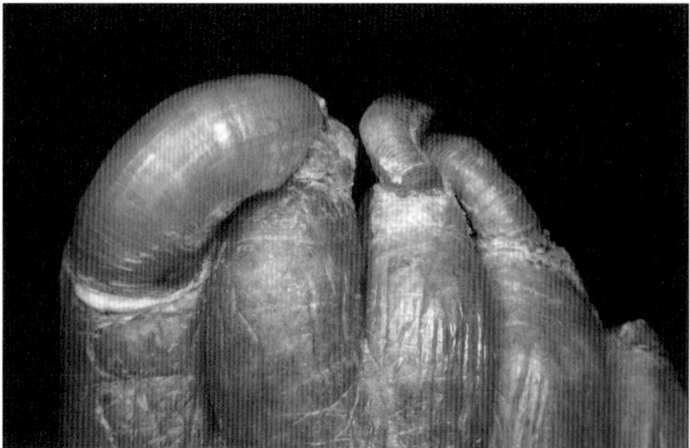

Figure 92.6 Onychogryphosis, onychomycosis, onychodystrophy, multiple hammertoes, soft tissue atrophy, peripheral arterial disease.

results in increased pain and infection a short time after this attempt. Patients who have poor peripheral arterial supply may face serious consequences from the improper management of this condition. Very thin nail plates may also penetrate the skin of adjacent toes, with similar results.[16]

Hyperkeratosis in the nail grooves (onychophosis) or under the free edge of the nail also creates pain. Periodic débridement of the thickness and length of the toe nail then permits débridement of the keratotic tissue. This is achieved with the use of a nail forceps, curette, and drill, and an appropriate burr. Suitable dressings of chamois, leather, ointments, or silicones, such as Viscogel can be utilized as nail packing under the nail plate to prevent it from digging into the surrounding tissue. The use of emollients such as 20% urea or 12% ammonium lactate also helps as a preventive measure. Depending on the patient's general health and the pain and deformity, avulsion of the whole nail or part of the nail plate, under local or regional anaesthesia may be considered.

Another relatively common cause of thickening of the nail plate is mycotic infection. Streaks of yellow or brown discolouration may extend from the free edge, proximally to the lunula. One or more nails are usually involved, become thickened, brittle and produce a characteristic musty odour. The patient's concern may be the unsightly nail that makes a hole in hosiery and sometimes the uppers of their footwear. Pain is associated with deformity. However, this chronic infection may produce a mycotic onychia and may serve as a focus of infection.[17]

The most common organism producing these changes is *Trichophyton rubrum*. Although it is generally confined to the nails, the surrounding skin and interdigital spaces may become scaly and itch intensely. Sometimes the infection spreads more extensively over the so-called moccasin area. Miconazole nitrate is an example of an antifungal agent that is effective in the treatment of mycotic infections of the skin. Oral terbinafine hydrochloride, itraconazole and topical ciclopirox are available for the management of onychomycosis. Forty percent urea gel is also utilized as a topical application to assist in local onychial débridement. The appearance of the nail plate can be improved and the patient's comfort increased by reducing the thickness of the nail plate and providing a smooth surface to the plate.[18–20] Laser application is also being utilized as a part of overall management.

Bursitis

Bursae are found in a number of situations in the foot. The adventitious bursa over the medial aspect of the first metatarsophalangeal joint frequently becomes inflamed when the joint it overlies is deformed and enlarged, as in hallux valgus. Bursae are also found superficial and deep to the Achilles tendon, the plantar aspect of the heel and the lateral aspect of the fifth metatarsophalangeal joint (tailor's bunion). If for any reason, a superficial bursa is ruptured, secondary infection can ensue. A sinus may be formed and chronic subacute bursitis is then a persistent problem.[21]

Enforced rest for long periods due to debilitating illness or accidental injury may lead to laxity and atrophy of the plantar calcaneal fibro-fatty padding, associated with dehydration. The plantar calcaneal bursa is then vulnerable due to overuse. Plantar calcaneal spurs and plantar myofascitis may also become troublesome in these circumstances.[22]

The immediate treatment for bursitis is to reduce the inflammation and to manage any secondary infection that may be present. Pressure on the areas can be reduced with padding and shoe modifications. Physical modalities, such as heat and ultrasound can be of assistance if properly utilized. Local steroid injections and the use of non-steroidal anti-inflammatory drugs are indicated, when appropriate, in the elderly.[23]

In the long term, stress on the bursae has to be reduced to minimize an exacerbation of the condition, once the acute symptoms are resolved. This may involve modification to footwear and/or the wearing of an appropriate shield (orthotic), such as a silicone mould. Plantar bursitis, with fasciitis and calcaneal spurs, can be improved with the use of heel cups, silicone heel pads, and/or orthosis that provide weight diffusion and modify the weight/pressure relationships in a superior, lateral and posterior direction. Insoles from Plastazote, PPT and other similar materials can aid in weight diffusion and dispersion. The normal warmth of the foot, even in the geriatric patient, will help mould the Plastazote. The resulting wear marks can be a good guide when constructing a more durable orthotic from materials such as Vitrathane. Plastazote as an insole or lining material in combination with Vitrathane will relieve the patient of the feeling that they are walking on pebbles, which is the result of soft tissue atrophy and atrophy of the plantar fat pad.

Scarring

Scarring of the plantar surface of the foot may result from accidental injury, for example, penetration of a foreign body, when walking barefoot. It is not infrequently iatrogenic in origin, that is, following surgery. The plantar metatarsal is the most common site for painful scars on the foot, which in the geriatric, is already deficient in fibrofatty padding. This can be completely disabling. Patients will require primary podiatric care to débride the keratotic lesions that usually develop within the scar tissue. Appropriate orthotics and insoles as noted above, should be employed to reduce friction and pressure by weight diffusion and dispersion.

Fissures

Fissures will frequently penetrate the underlying dermis and provide a portal of entry for pathogens. Soft tissue haematoma is also a pre-ulcerative state. In the geriatric, stress marks along the outer portion of the heel also serve as an aetiological factor and form the initial stages of pressure ulcerations. Fissures around the heel are usually dry and vertically oriented. Secondary infection is always an added risk. Interdigitally, fissures are usually moist and follow the flexures of the skin. Infection of the interdigital fissures may penetrate the fascial planes and require surgical drainage. The edges of the fissures usually become hyperkeratotic and indurated in the elderly patient, which prevents healing and can be extremely painful.

Moist fissures respond well to antiseptic dressings and if required, antifungal agents. When healed, follow-up skin care is essential. The hard edges of the dry fissures should be débrided. This may be aided by the use of 12.5% salicylic acid in collodion. Its action is to soften the hyperkeratosis and make débridement easier and less painful for the patient. Tissue stimulants can also be employed, once débridement is completed. Bland emollients that help soften keratosis and maintain skin integrity can also be suggested, such as 20% urea creams and 12% ammonium lactate lotion, in addition to daily hygiene.

Management considerations

Since healthy feet are essential for mobility and independence, as well as a catalyst to maintain patient dignity, none who are concerned with health and well-being of older persons should disregard foot care. The particular knowledge and skills of the podiatrist are vital for the multidisciplinary team caring for the geriatric patient. Regular assessment and inspection of the feet are an effective means of monitoring the preventive aspects of the complications of diabetes mellitus and arthritis for example. Other symptoms and overt abnormalities are many times detected during a foot evaluation, with appropriate referral for care to justify the secondary preventive aspects of chronic disease. Periodic evaluation also provides an appropriate time for health education.[24–26]

The following elements are suggested delivery of podiatric care in ambulatory settings, hospitals, long-term care facilities and related programmes:

- Pain should be explored to its fullest extent with all appropriate diagnostic modalities utilized.
- Appropriate, specialized medical consultation is to be employed when indicated. When the diagnosis is in doubt, systemic disease is present and contributing as a complicating factor, then clinical care should be interdisciplinary in approach and based on total patient need.
- Appropriate diagnostic tests should be available and employed when indicated.
- Débridement, pathomechanical, foot orthopaedic, biomechanical, radiographic, orthotic, dermatological and surgical procedures must be applied as elements of total patient care.
- Appropriate pharmacology must be utilized in accordance to local policies and privileges, and the provisions and Drug Enforcement Administration.
- Corrected footwear and orthotics are to be programme components.
- Biopsy and guidelines for follow-up of potential malignancies must be considered and provided.
- Onychial care is to be provided in a suitable manner with consideration of the diagnosis and patient outcome projections.
- At-risk patients who have concomitant systemic disease, such as diabetes, are to receive patient instruction and education as part of the patient education programmes.
- Appropriate physical modalities and procedures for primary inflammation of the foot are to be available, and a component of patient management to complement mechanical and orthotic procedures.
- Health education should be utilized for individual patients, in-group educational settings, and as a part of a total interdisciplinary approach to preventive care.
- Podiatric surgical care is to be in accordance to individual delineation, local facility admitting privileges, and performed in the appropriate setting, utilizing suitable anaesthesia services for patient care.

Foot care

Advice regarding foot care for patients will benefit all elderly people whatever their state of general health. There are a number of excellent publications, available on the Internet, which can be duplicated for patients. Examples include the following:

Nation Institute on Aging – Age Page – Foot Care
American Podiatric Medical Association – Foot Health and Aging
The British Chiropody and Podiatry Association – Foot Care for the Elderly
Public Health Agency of Canada – Foot Care Info-sheet for Seniors
American Geriatrics Society – Aging in the Know – Foot Problems and The Diabetic Foot
American Diabetes Association – Preventive Foot Care in Diabetes
Merck Manual of Geriatrics – Foot Disorders
Pennsylvania Department of Health – Feet First, If the Shoe Fits, and
Assessing the Older Diabetic Foot

These documents plus those listed in the references of this chapter provide a significant amount of information for professionals and patients which can be applied to the care of older patients for ambulatory care, hospitals, long-term care facilities as well as community and public health programmes.[27]

Footwear

The treatment and long-term management of foot morbidities requires consideration that the foot must be adequately accommodated in proper footwear. The shoe or boot must have adequate width, depth, last and length, especially in the region of the toes. A lace-up shoe reasonably ensures that the foot and shoe are held in the correct relationship as well as having the added virtue that the lace is infinitely adjustable – important where the foot may enlarge because of oedema. The extra depth or super depth shoe is such an example. A surgical shoe or walker is ideal when specific dressing changes are required. High arched feet do sometimes have difficulty with a high lacing shoe. Here a slip-on shoe with an elasticized gusset may be more acceptable. An alternative may be a Velcro and loop closure or elastic laces. This is also useful when the patient is unable to tie his/her shoes. A broad heel with a maximum height of 1.5 in (38 mm) will provide stability. The flaring of the heel on one side or the other to further enhance stability and balance.[28]

The upper of boots or shoes should be plain – devoid of fancy stitching or designs, which involve the overlapping of several pieces of the upper material. These all limit the 'give' of the material and the footwear fails to mould and accommodate minor foot deformities, such as hammer toes and bunion deformities (Figure 92.7).

Traditionally, leather has been the best material for the uppers of footwear, but very satisfactory manmade materials can provide lighter and economical made-to-measure footwear for patients with feet deformed by disease or altered in shape as a result of surgical intervention.

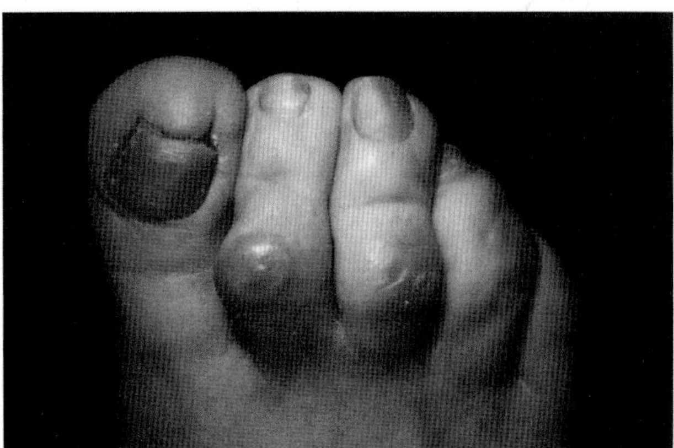

Figure 92.7 Multiple hammer toes, heloma durum, onychodysplasia, onychauxis, onychophosis.

Synthetic materials used for the sole and heels of modern footwear have good wearing qualities. Their thickness provides a surface that is shock-absorbing and insulating. Modern manufacturing processes easily produce shoes that are relatively waterproof. Flexion of the first metatarsophalangeal joint can be limited by the addition of a steel splint or rocker sole. This can also be helpful in the management of osteoarthrosis of the first metatarsophalangeal joint or in incipient rigidity of this joint. Patients should be encouraged to keep all footwear in good repair. Serious injuries to the ligaments of the ankle and subtalar joints are frequently the result of badly worn heels.[29–31]

Orthotics

The prolonged application to the foot of adhesive pads and dressings is undesirable, even with modern hypoallergenic adhesives. It is also aesthetically unacceptable. The warmth and moisture resulting from occlusion of the skin may provoke contact dermatitis or infection, particularly in the elderly. Because of the fact that for many elderly patients, correction or cure is not possible, comfort becomes a primary goal. Deformities may need to remain but care should be directed to relieving pain, restoring a maximum level of function, and maintaining that restored degree of pain-free activity. Many forms of orthotics are available including silicone moulds, soft, rigid or semi-rigid devices. Others include devices that can be made to prescription and fabricated from manmade materials of varying thickness and density. Thermoplastic materials may be combined in one orthotic to give cushioning or support or redistribute the pressure load. These are all fabricated to meet the individual needs of individual patients and the presenting condition. The resulting appliance is more desirable and aesthetically more pleasing since it can be removed, cleaned and utilized in many pairs of footwear.

Where patients are unable to fit and remove these devices themselves, relatives or neighbours can help. A moulded shoe, made from light microcellular material and able to accommodate the most bizarre deformities is the only other alternative, if need be. Sandals or a surgical shoe may be a satisfactory alternative also, where the condition and climate are suitable.

Gels

Whilst podiatrists are familiar with silicone pastes which, by the addition of an activator can be moulded to the unique requirements of individual patients, the resulting orthosis can be bulky and not very resilient. An alternative is to use pre-moulded props, toe separators and toe caps incorporating gels, all of which are washable. Gels are medical-grade mineral oil thermoplastic elastomers from which mineral oil is continually exuded, thus improving the condition of the skin.

Knitted tubing of various diameters, lined with a gel coating is available. This can be cut to the required size. There are also toe caps of various sizes without the knitted cover. Sheet material, 2 mm thick, may be cut to size. Gels may also be incorporated into heel cups and wedges and other types of orthotic to provide 'soft spots' to relieve heel spurs for example. Socks and anklets incorporating gels are also available. These can help in moisturizing atrophic skin and compensating for the loss of subcutaneous soft tissue. They may also be helpful in the treatment of heel fissures and bed sores.

Key points

- Podogeriatrics is that special area of podiatric medical practice that focuses on health promotion, prevention and the treatment and management of foot and related problems, disability, deformity and the pedal complications of chronic diseases in later life. The reasons to refer patients for podiatric care include as examples, the following:
  - –Signs suggesting generalized disease that include neuropathy, vascular disease infection, etc. and focal neoplastic disease;
  - –In those cases where concomitant therapy is indicated;
  - –Where initial management is not effective;
  - –In the presence of skin, nail, postural and joint deformities of the foot and related structures;
  - –In the presence of diabetes mellitus, neurosensory, peripheral
  - –vascular and other risk diseases;
  - –In the presence of foot problems combined with walking problems and/or a history of falls;
  - –Where orthotics are indicated;
  - –If the patient is unable to obtain and/or provide foot care;
  - –If the patient complains of a foot problems or has specific questions about care including information on footwear.
- Foot problems are common in the older population as a result of disease, disability, deformity and complications related to multiple chronic diseases. They also result from neglect and a lack of preventive service, at the primary, secondary and tertiary levels. Foot problems contribute to disability and can reduce an older person's independence and quality of life.
- Because of the risk involved in the geriatric patient and the relationship to multiple chronic diseases, assessment, examination and evaluation of the feet of the elderly is critical. Essential as elements of this process include needs, relationships to ambulation and activities of daily living, instrumental activities of daily living, and the fact that foot pain can result in functional disability, dysfunction, increased dependency, limit mobility and prevent older individuals to live life to the end of life.

References

1. Helfand AE. Disorders and diseases of the foot. In: EL Cobbs, ED Duthie, JB Murphy (eds), *Geriatric Review Syllabus: A Core Curriculum in Geriatric Medicine*, 6th edn, Blackwell Publishing, Oxford, 2006.
2. Arenson C, Busby-Whitehead J, Brummel-Smith K *et al. Reichel's Care of the Elderly: Clinical Aspects of Aging*, 6th edn, Cambridge University Press, New York, NY, 2009.
3. Birrer RB, Dellacorte MP, Grisafi PJ. *Common Foot Problems in Primary Care*, 2nd edn, Henley & Belfus, Inc., Philadelphia, PA, 1998.
4. Helfand AE. Clinical podogeriatrics: Assessment, education, and prevention. In: *Clinics in Podiatric Medicine and Surgery*, Vol. 20, No. 3, WB Saunders Co., Philadelphia, PA, 2003.
5. Ham RJ, Sloane PD, Warshaw GA, Bernard MA, Flaherty R. *Primary Care Geriatrics: A Case Based Approach*, 5th edn, Mosby/Elsevier, Philadelphia PA, 2007.
6. Capezuti EA, Siegler EL, Mezey MD. *The Encyclopedia of Elder Care: A Comprehensive Resource on Geriatric and Social Care*, 2nd edn, Springer, New York, NY, 2008.
7. Dauber R, Bristow I, Turner W. *Text Atlas of Podiatric Dermatology*, Martin Dunitz, London, 2001.
8. Gabel LL, Haines DJ, Papp KK. *The Aging Foot, An Interdisciplinary Perspective*, The Ohio State University, College of Medicine and Public Health, Department of Family Medicine, Columbus, OH, 2004.
9. Helfand AE. Assessing the Older Diabetic Patient [CD-ROM], Pennsylvania Diabetes Academy, Pennsylvania Department of Health, Temple University, School of Medicine, Office for Continuing Medical Education, Temple University, School of Podiatric Medicine, Harrisburg, PA, December 2001.
10. Yates B. *Merriman's Assessment of the Lower Limb*, 3rd edn, Churchill Livingstone/Elsevier, Edinburgh, 2009.
11. Armstrong DG, Lavery LA. *Clinical Care of the Diabetic Foot*, American Diabetes Association, Alexandria, VA, 2005.
12. Edmonds ME, Foster AVM, Sanders LJA. *Practical Manual of Diabetic Footcare*, Blackwell Publishing, Oxford, 2004.
13. International Diabetes Federation. International Consensus on the Diabetic Foot and Practical Guidelines on the Management and Prevention of the Diabetic Foot, Amsterdam, the Netherlands, 2007.
14. Foster AVM. *Podiatric Assessment and Management of the Diabetic Foot*, Churchill Livingstone/Elsevier, Edinburgh, 2006.
15. Bowker JH, Pfeifer MA. *Levin and O'Neal's The Diabetic Foot*, 7th edn, Mosby Elsevier, Philadelphia, PA, 2008.

16. Baran R, Haneke E. *The Nail in Differential Diagnosis*, Informa Healthcare, Oxford, 2007.

17. Turner WA, Merriman LM. *Clinical Skills in Treating the Foot*, 2nd edn, Churchill Livingstone/Elsevier, Edinburgh, 2005.

18. Lorimer D, French G, O'Donnell M, Burrow JG. *Neale's Disorders of the Foot: Diagnosis and Management*, 6th edn, Churchill Livingstone, New York, NY, 2002.

19. Menz HB. *Foot Problems in Older People: Assessment and Management*, Churchill Livingstone/Elsevier, Edinburgh, 2008.

20. Robbins JM. *Primary Podiatric Medicine*, WB Saunders Co., Philadelphia, PA. 1994.

21. Levy LA, Hetherington VJ. *Principles and Practice of Geriatric Medicine*, 2nd edn, Data Trace Publishing Co., Brooklandville, MD, 2006.

22. Helliwell P, Woodburn A, Redmond A, Turner D, Davys H. *The Foot and Ankle in Rheumatoid Arthritis: A Comprehensive Guide*, Churchill Livingstone/Elsevier, Edinburgh, 2007.

23. Banks A, Downey MS, Martin DE, Miller SJ. *McGlamry's Forefoot Surgery*, Lippincott, Williams & Wilkins, Philadelphia, PA, 2004.

24. Halter JB, Ouslander JG, Tinetti ME *et al. Hazzard's Geriatric Medicine and Gerontology*, McGraw-Hill, New York, NY, 2009.

25. Helfand AE (ed.). The geriatric patient and considerations of aging. In: *Clinics in Podiatric Medicine and Surgery*, WB Saunders Co., Philadelphia, PA, Vol. I, January 1993; Vol. II, April 1993.

26. Helfand AE, Jessett DF. Foot problems. In: MSJ Pathy, AS Sinclair JE Morley (eds), *Principles and Practice of Geriatric Medicine*, 4th edn, John Wiley & Sons, Ltd., Chichester, 2006.

27. Evans JG, Williams FT, Beattie BL, Michel JP, Wilcock GK. *Oxford Textbook of Geriatric Medicine*, 2nd edn, Oxford University Press, Oxford, 2000.

28. Tyrrell W, Carter G. *Therapeutic Footwear: A Comprehensive Guide*, Churchill Livingstone/Elsevier, Edinburgh, 2009.

29. Helfand AE (ed). *Foot Health Training Guide for Long-Term Care Personnel*, Health Professions Press, Baltimore, MD, 2007.

30. Helfand AE (ed.) *Public Health and Podiatric Medicine: Principles and Practice*, 2nd edn, APHA Press, American Public Health Association, Washington DC, 2006.

31. Helfand AE. An overview of shoe modifications and orthoses in the management of adult foot and ankle pathology. *Turkiye Klinikleri Journal of Physical Medicine and Rehabilitation – Special Topics* 2010; 3: 107–14.

CHAPTER 93

Hip fracture and orthogeriatrics

Christine Lafont

Toulouse University Hospital and Centre of Geriatric Medicine, Toulouse, France

Background

In the elderly population, hip fracture is the most common cause of unplanned admission to an acute orthopaedic ward[1] and the second cause of hospital admission in general. The incidence of such fractures has been constantly increasing over the last 70 years and, if we are to believe the demographic projections, it will increase even further. The overall number of fractures, which was 1.6 million per year in 1990, should reach 4 million in 2025 and 7–21 million in 2050.[2] This 'orthopaedic epidemic' raises major medical, economic and social problems and is a challenge in terms of public health, if we wish to promote prevention and develop the least costly and most effective mode of management.

The risk of hip fracture increases exponentially from the age of 60 and 75% of these fractures occur in women, who are at greater risk because of their longer lifespan and high prevalence of osteoporosis. Femoral neck fracture has many causal factors, associating osteoporosis and falls, the prerogative of 'frail'» subjects. It is a hallmark of ageing, as it primarily affects persons with the highest comorbidity (29% have respiratory disorders, 55% have dementia and 68% have cardiorespiratory diseases), who make the greatest demands on home care structures and the most use of walking aids. Nursing home residents are three to four times more likely to be affected as they combine several risk factors (advanced age, low bone mass, impaired mobility, cognitive disorders).

In spite of advances in surgery, anaesthesia and rehabilitative management, hip fracture still has a poor vital and functional prognosis. Depending on the studies, mortality ranges from 5 to 10% in the first month and one-third of elderly patients die within 1 year of fracture, whereas the expected annual mortality in a population of the same age is 10%.[3] These figures have not changed for over 20 years. However, only one-third of these deaths are directly attributable to the fracture and in the remaining cases comorbid disorders are the explanatory factor. The criteria of poor prognosis are advanced age, male gender, poorly controlled comorbid conditions, cognitive disorders, low autonomy and institutionalization.

Proximal femoral fracture is a turning point for the worse in the life of the elderly person and it often leads to loss of independence and social decline, marked by admission to an institution. Only half of patients regain their earlier walking ability. The factors of a good functional prognosis are the absence of cognitive disturbances, the ability to walk unaided with a device prior to fracture, rich social contacts and pursuit of an activity outside the home. About 10–20% of patients remain dependent for their activities of daily living (ADL) and must be placed in a nursing home.

The costs relating to management of femoral neck fracture are high because of the length of hospital stay (2–5 weeks) and the costs incurred for subsequent care due to dependence. According to Dolan and Torgerson,[4] they reach £20 000 for the first 2 years.

It therefore seems necessary to reflect on multidisciplinary management as soon as the patient is admitted and on the implementation of surgical and rehabilitative strategies that are adapted to the elderly person's specific needs if we wish to improve the outcome of these patients, who will be increasingly numerous due to lengthening life expectancy.

Diagnosis and classification

Usually, the diagnosis of hip fracture poses few problems. After a fall from a standing position, the patient complains of pain causing functional disability. A characteristic deformity is observed, associating shortening and external rotation of the leg. Inability to raise the heel above the bed surface with the leg extended is a suggestive sign.

Diagnosis is confirmed by radiography. Anterior images of the pelvis should be obtained with the lower limbs in 10° internal rotation, with a lateral view and sometimes a third anteroposterior view centred on the affected hip in 10° internal rotation.[3] However, it is often not easy to obtain

Principles and Practice of Geriatric Medicine, Fifth Edition. Edited by Alan J. Sinclair, John E. Morley and Bruno Vellas.

satisfactory images because of the patient's pain. In difficult cases, where there is a discrepancy between X-ray and clinical findings, fracture can only be excluded by radioisotope bone scan or magnetic resonance imaging (MRI) (the investigation of choice for non-displaced fractures). Bone scan seems to be less informative in this context, but it is easier to obtain within the short time needed for rapid initiation of treatment.

The radiological investigations allow the classification of the fractures according to the location of the fracture line and the degree of displacement, on which the choice of treatment depends. An anatomical and pathophysiological distinction is made between intra- and extracapsular fractures, whose prognoses differ (Figure 93.1).

Intracapsular fractures (45%) lie between the femoral head and the trochanters within the capsule, whether this is intact or not. They can lead to high-pressure haemarthrosis if the capsule remains intact after injury. These fractures may be displaced or non-displaced. The predominant risk is necrosis of the femoral head, secondary to vascular damage. The arterial branches that feed the femoral head are at risk of being lacerated or stretched by the displacement or may also collapse because of the increased pressure due to accumulation of blood caused by haemarthrosis in an intact capsule.

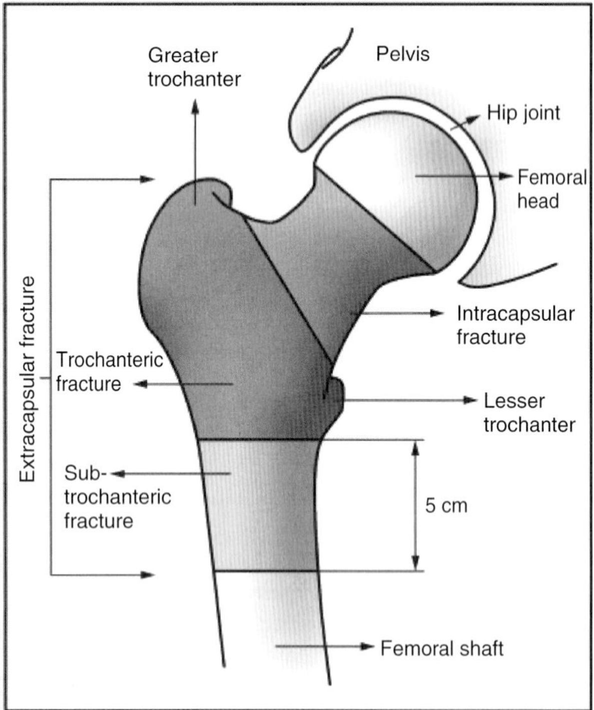

Figure 93.1 Classification of hip fractures by Parker and Johansen. Reproduced from Parker and Johansen,[1] with permission from BMJ Publishing Group Ltd.

Extracapsular fractures are metaphyseal fractures that always heal. They often lead to major bleeding. They are divided into two groups:

- fractures of the greater trochanter (45%), which are stable if there is a single fracture line and unstable if there are several lines
- subtrochanteric fractures (5–10%), which lie within 5 cm distal to the lesser trochanter.

Preoperative care

Analgesia

There is now a general consensus that pain needs to be managed in the emergency situation. Relief of pain reduces the neuroendocrine disturbances that follow the trauma, decreases the patient's agitation that can lead to secondary displacement of the fracture site and makes preoperative investigations easier. Pain is judged by repeated self-assessment. A simple verbal scale (from 0, no pain, to 4, extreme pain) is preferable to the visual analogue scale in the elderly person, who may find it difficult to cooperate.

In general, level 1 analgesics (paracetamol) used alone do not adequately relieve pain. They should be prescribed in association with a level 2 analgesic (codeine) or a morphine derivative. As a parenteral approach is often necessary, the dose of morphine derivatives must be carefully titrated in these frail patients. Non-steroidal anti-inflammatory drugs (NSAIDs) are inadvisable in the elderly patient as the risk of haemorrhage is increased by stress and because of pre-existing renal failure.

Peripheral blocks have considerably improved pain management in femoral neck fractures. An iliac fascia block carried out as soon as the patient has been admitted to the emergency department allows them to be mobilized and prepared for surgery.

Preoperative traction

Both skin and skeletal traction have been proposed in order to reduce pain and to facilitate fracture reduction. However, the studies available[5] have not provided sufficient evidence of sedation of pain in the first 2 days after surgery {relative risk (RR) = 1.14 [95% confidence interval (CI), 0.89–1.46]} and RR = 1.02 (95% CI, 0.74–1.41)] or of easier fracture reduction at the time of surgery.

Electrolyte balance and blood transfusion

In the elderly person with hip fracture, *electrolyte imbalance* is frequent and due to a variety of causes, such as renal failure, diabetes and diuretic medications. Patients are often dehydrated, either because they lay on the ground for several hours or because of preoperative fasting.

These imbalances should be corrected, while taking into account the borderline tolerance of volume restoration in elderly patients.

Anaemia, particularly frequent in fractures of the greater trochanter, increases the mortality rate at 6 and 12 months, lengthens the duration of hospital stay and compromises the functional prognosis.[6] The transfusion threshold is still difficult to establish, but it is generally accepted as 8–9 g dl^{-1} for elderly patients with no cardiovascular history and 10 g dl^{-1} for patients with poor tolerance or severe cardiovascular involvement.

Thromboembolic prophylaxis

Following proximal femoral fracture, the risk of thromboembolism is increased. The incidence of proximal thrombosis is 27% and mortality due to pulmonary embolism is 1.4–7% in the first 3 months after surgery.[7] In view of these figures, the absence of thromboprophylaxis may be considered as negligence. A Cochrane review of 31 studies (2858 participants) clearly demonstrated the efficacy of prophylactic treatment in reducing the incidence of deep venous thrombosis (DVT) and pulmonary embolism.[8] The modalities of management, however, still remain to be defined: the respective roles of pharmacological and physical methods, optimal duration of treatment. Several therapeutic protocols are under discussion:

- Administration of unfractionated heparin or low molecular weight heparin versus placebo (15 trials, 1199 participants) significantly reduced the risk of DVT [RR = 0.60 (95% CI, 0.50–0.71)], but evidence regarding pulmonary embolism was inadequate. Low molecular weight heparins were not more effective than fractionated heparins.
- Low-dose aspirin appears likely to decrease the incidence of DVT and pulmonary embolism.
- Antivitamin K agents may also be given during the first 10 days after surgery if a target international normalized ratio (INR) of 2.5 (min.–max. 2.0–3.0) is maintained.

However, we need to be aware that use of anticoagulants or antiplatelet agents increases the number of haemorrhagic complications.

The optimal duration of treatment[9] is still unclear. In general, it is continued for 14 days after surgery. The Seventh American College of Chest Physicians Conference on Antithrombotic and Thrombolytic Therapy[10] recommended that heparin should be given for at least 10 days after surgery. However, it has been demonstrated that even with anticoagulation treatment, thrombosis occurs in 15–30% of patients at discharge and that 10–25% of patients develop thrombosis 3–4 weeks later; these thromboses are symptomatic in less than 10% of cases. Eriksson and Lassen[11] showed that 4 weeks of heparin treatment reduced the incidence of pulmonary embolism compared with 1 week of treatment.

When surgery is deferred, initiation of anticoagulation treatment is recommended between admission and the surgical procedure.

Physical treatments have also been proposed. Mechanical pumping devices are more effective than no treatment [RR = 0.31 (95% CI, 0.12–0.51)] and they significantly reduce the risk of DVT and pulmonary embolism, but skin abrasions have been reported.[8] As for compression stockings, it is difficult to reach a conclusion regarding their efficacy.

Lastly, it is important to note that no method makes it possible to reduce the number of fatal pulmonary embolisms, or the mortality after hip fracture.

In addition to specific treatments, it is therefore important to give a considerable place to general measures[1] such as:

- combat against dehydration and excessive transfusion
- minimization of surgical delay and duration of the procedure
- early mobilization of the patient.

Minimizing surgical delay

The Royal College of Physicians' guidelines[12] recommend early surgery (within 24 h of admission). However, after analysis of 10 studies with a satisfactory level of proof, Beaupre *et al.*[7] emphasized that divergent results were obtained when surgical delay was taken into account. With regard to post-surgical mortality, Grimes *et al.*,[13] after adjustment for comorbid conditions, observed no differences between patients operated on after more that 96 h and those operated on within 48 h [HR = 1.01 (95% CI, 0.95–1.21)]. Conversely, Shiga *et al.*[14] carried out a meta-analysis of five prospective and 11 retrospective studies which showed that operative delays of more than 48 h increase 30 day mortality by 41% and mortality at 1 year by 32%. Excess mortality is particularly high in patients aged <70 years with no comorbid conditions. Most authors[15,16] agree that early surgery decreases the risk of postoperative complications such as pressure ulcers, urinary infections, thromboses and pneumonia, but that it sometimes increases the risk of postoperative bleeding and prosthesis-related complications.[16] Several authors also report that early surgery shortens hospital stay,[15] encourages earlier resumption of walking and reduces pain.

These arguments favour early surgery for younger, clinically stable patients. In other cases, it is important that existing comorbidities should be rapidly controlled before considering surgery.

Prevention of pressure ulcers

Following hip surgery, 10–40% of patients develop a pressure ulcer. This complication increases the burden of care, risk of nosocomial infection and duration of hospital stay. The heel is particularly at risk due to increased pressure on the operated side (immobility of the patient) and on the uninvolved side, because the patient uses the heel as a pivot to move in bed. These mechanical factors are augmented by haemodynamic factors: decreased local blood flow due to elevation of the operated limb during the procedure, fluctuations in blood volume due to anaesthesia and blood loss and sometimes episodes of low blood flow rate related to the cement used in total hip replacement. In these circumstances, bilateral pressure ulcers are observed.[17]

Two studies[7] assessed the preventive efficacy, in orthopaedic surgery, of foam or dynamic air mattresses and showed that their use reduced the incidence of pressure ulcers [RR = 0.34 (95% CI, 0.14–0.85) and RR = 0.20 (95% CI, 0.009–0.45)]. These means of prevention are effective above all for the sacrum and trochanter. A meta-analysis[18] exclusively centred on the prevention of heel ulcers showed that special foam or dynamic air mattresses were superior to standard hospital mattresses. With regard to heel pads and mattress overlays, the evidence was inadequate to reach a conclusion regarding their efficacy.

Overall, rational use of preventive aids (mattresses, heel supports, mattress overlays) is recommended based on evaluation of the patient's risk level using specific scales (see Chapter 126, The prevention and management of pressure ulcers).

Fracture repair and perioperative care

Surgical management

The majority of hip fractures are treated surgically, although conservative treatment, used before the advent of the first prostheses, may still be debated.

Conservative or operative treatment

Handoll and Parker, in a Cochrane review of five randomized trials (428 elderly subjects), compared surgical treatment and conservative treatment (traction and bed rest).[19] A study of 23 patients with non-displaced intracapsular fractures showed a lower risk of non-union in surgically treated patients. The other trials relating to extracapsular fractures found no difference in mortality, medical complications or pain between the two treatment modalities, whatever the prosthesis or surgical technique used. However, deformity and limb shortening were less frequently observed with surgical treatment (better anatomical reduction), duration of hospital stay was shorter and functional results were better. Conservative treatment should be the exception today, reserved for patients with formal contraindications to surgery, those who refuse it or those who are at the end of life.

Operative treatment

Undisplaced intracapsular fractures

Only internal fixation is recommended, as it reduces the risk of displacement. The surgical procedure is simple and can be carried out by a percutaneous approach under local anaesthesia or peripheral block. Two or three screws are used in parallel (Figure 93.2) or a sliding hip screw (SHS). This technique has the advantages of being conservative and of making nursing care easier. Active mobilization of the hip and knee can rapidly be started.

Displaced intracapsular fractures

Two options are possible: internal fixation or prosthetic replacement. Each treatment carries specific complications.

Internal fixation is a shorter procedure, with less blood loss and less risk of infection; the main complications are non-union and avascular necrosis of the femoral head, requiring revision in 35–50% of cases.

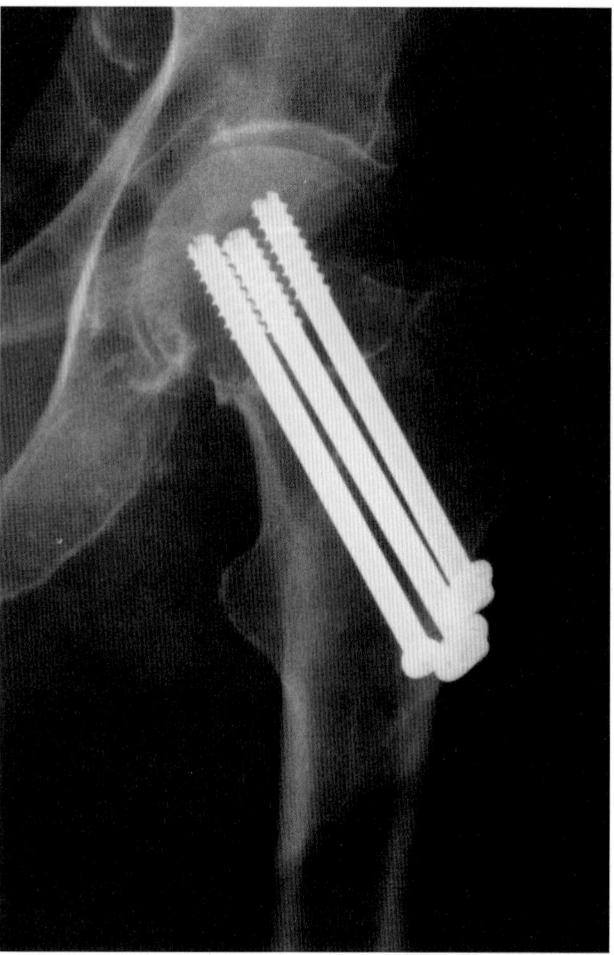

Figure 93.2 Intracapsular fracture fixed with three screws.

Several types of prostheses may be used:

- Cervicocephalic hemiarthroplasty prostheses (Figure 93.3) of Moore or Thompson type replace only the femoral head. They are non-cemented and are inserted as a press-fit in cancellous bone.
- Bipolar hemiarthroplasty prostheses (Figure 93.4) have a femoral part with a mobile acetabular socket joint which is intended to protect the acetabulum and to delay the development of mechanical complications.
- Total prostheses (Figure 93.5), very widely used in the surgical treatment of coxarthrosis, replace the entire coxofemoral joint.

Prostheses may be cemented or uncemented. Randomized trials comparing cement with cementless devices are summarized in a Cochrane review.[20] Cemented prostheses are less painful and the functional results are better, but with the drawback of a more lengthy and major surgical procedure (risk of cardiovascular collapse, toxic effects of cement). Mortality is not increased at 1 year.

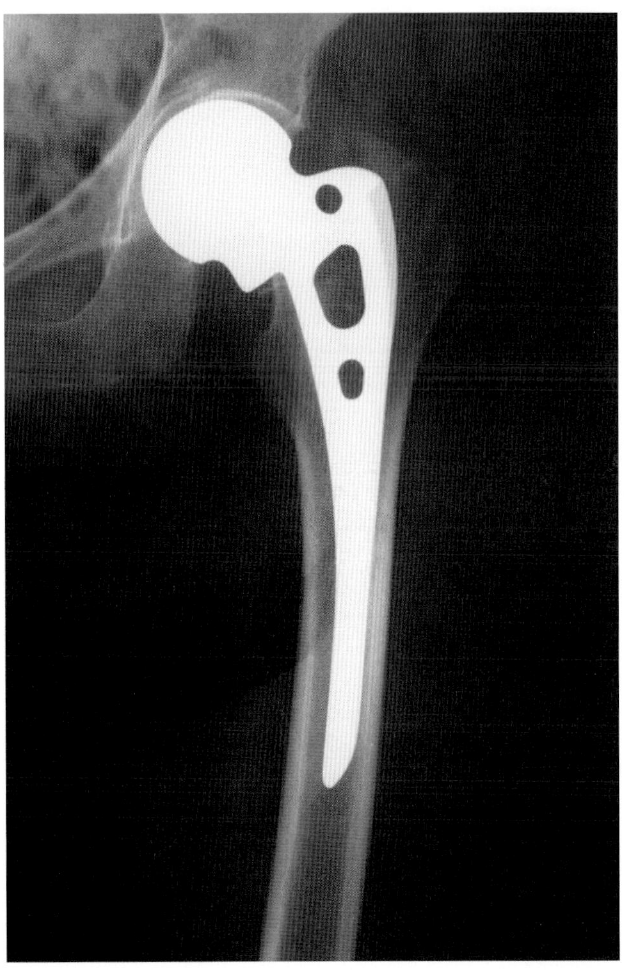

Figure 93.3 Fracture treated with an uncemented Moore hemiarthroplasty.

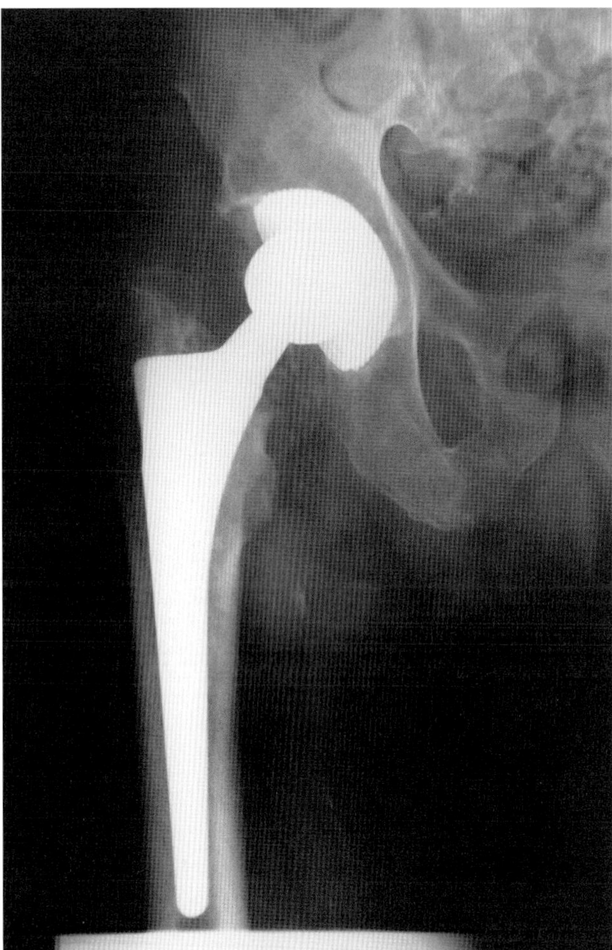

Figure 93.4 Fracture treated with a cemented total arthroplasty.

A Cochrane review compared the two operative techniques (internal fixation and hip replacement) in the adult.[21] The results did not differ in terms of mortality, but postoperative pain was less and the functional results were better after hip replacement. An observational study,[22] based on the Norwegian register of hip fractures and including 1569 subjects aged over 70 years operated on for femoral neck fracture, stressed that patients who underwent bipolar arthroplasty had a better quality of life at 4 months than those treated by internal fixation. They had less pain and were more satisfied with the intervention. Arthroplasty also gives better results in severely demented patients. however, the superiority of prostheses is apparent essentially for the most modern bipolar prostheses (hydroxyapatite) and for cemented prostheses.

In view of these considerations, the choice of operative technique must take into account the age of the patient, risk factors, cognitive state and level of mobility before the accident. It seems advantageous to propose total hip arthroplasty for subjects aged over 70 years who are active and in

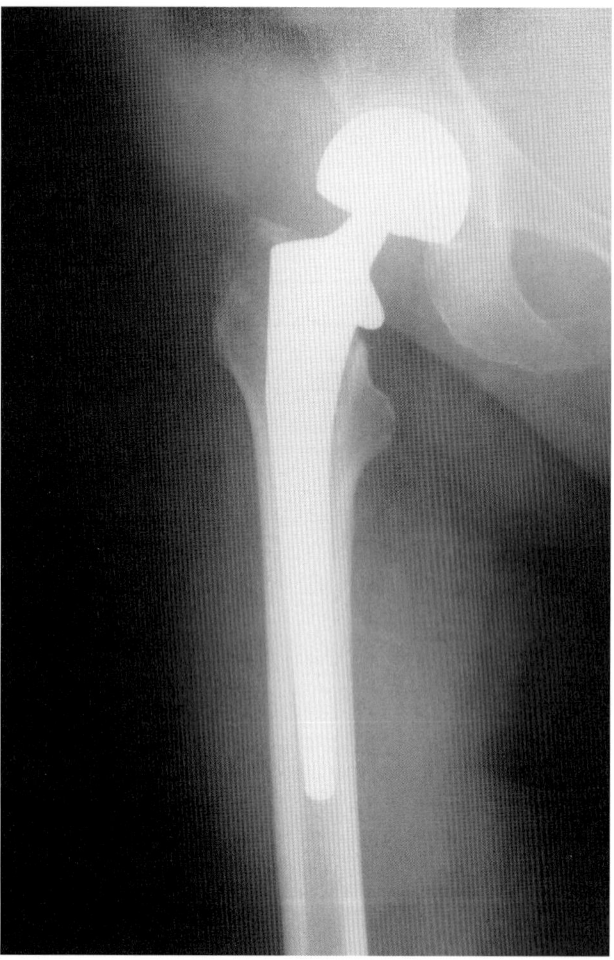

Figure 93.5 Bipolar hemiarthroplasty.

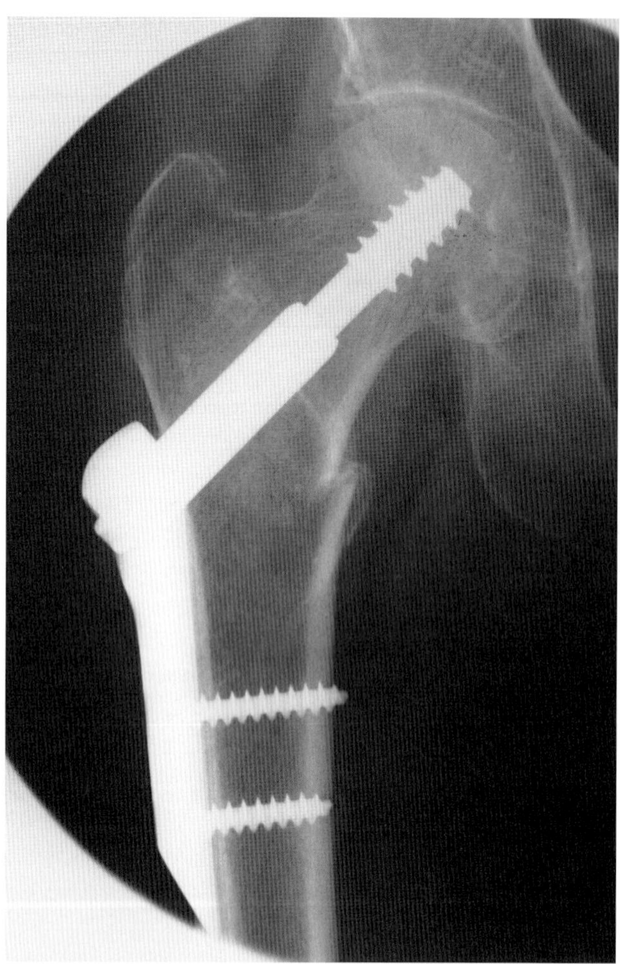

Figure 93.6 Trochanteric fracture fixed by dynamic hip screw.

good health and who still have a long life expectancy.[23] Total hip arthroplasty does not carry a higher risk of displacement.

Trochanteric fractures

Numerous surgical possibilities are available for this type of fracture, although SHS is the gold standard. The implants proposed are dynamic hip screws (DHS) (Figure 93.6), compression hip screws and Ambi screws. Among the more recent alternatives are the gamma nail (Figure 93.7), the intramedullary hip screw (IMHS), the proximal femoral nail (PFN), the Holland nail and the Targon nail. Compared with SHS, they seem to be accompanied by more frequent redisplacement and an increased number of reinterventions.[3] Hip replacement has also been proposed for particularly unstable fractures. A Cochrane review found no difference between hip replacement and SHS for surgical complications, mortality rate or functional results at 1 year.[24]

Subtrochanteric fractures

Stabilization is the main problem with these fractures. The prostheses proposed are SHS or centromedullary nails, with a risk of fracture in the vicinity of the nail stem.

Type of anaesthesia

General anaesthesia increases the risk of postoperative delirium in elderly subjects. A Cochrane review of 22 trials (2567 participants) showed decreased mortality at 1 month with regional anaesthesia (6.9 versus 10%), but these results were of borderline significance, with RR = 0.69 (95% CI, 0.5–0.95). The risk of DVT was also decreased, with RR = 0.64 (95% CI, 0.49–0.92).[25] Another systematic review of 141 studies (9559 participants) also showed lower mortality with regional anaesthesia.[26] Forty-four of these studies (31%) specifically involved elderly subjects and they confirmed that regional anaesthesia reduced the

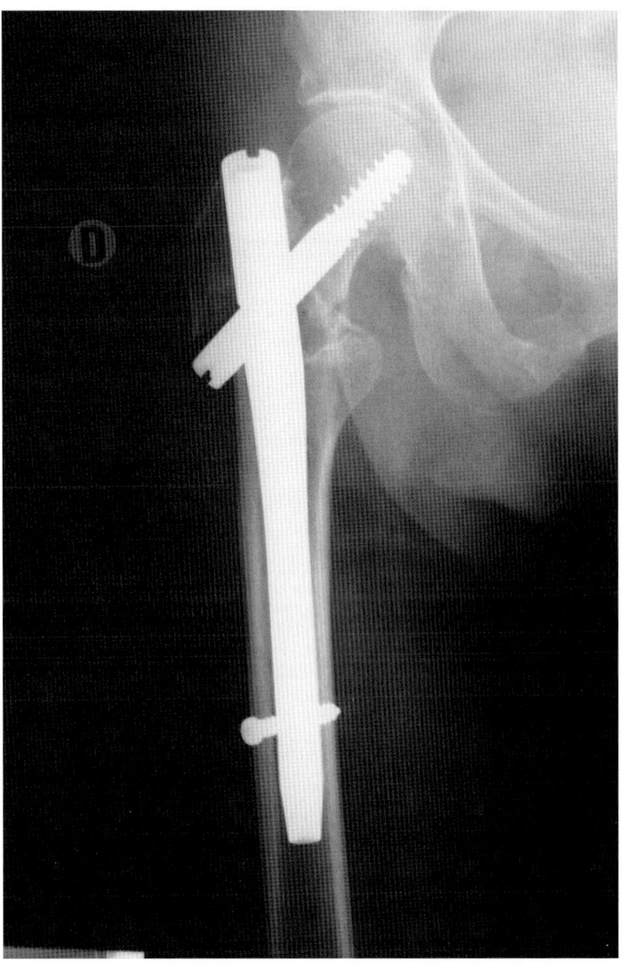

Figure 93.7 Trochanteric fracture fixed by gamma nail.

risk of DVT [odds ratio (OR) = 0.56 (95% CI, 0.43–0.72)], pulmonary embolism [OR = 0.45 (95% CI, 0.29–0.69)], transfusion requirements [OR = 0.50 (95% CI, 0.39–0.66)] and pneumonia [OR = 0.61 (95% CI, 0.48–0.76)]. However, the choice made by the anaesthetist must take into account the preferences of the patient and their family, and also imperatives related to the patient's clinical condition and the operative procedure.

Antibiotic prophylaxis

A meta-analysis of 22 randomized controlled trials (RCTs) (8307 subjects surgically treated for fracture), including 16 RCTs concerning surgical treatment of proximal femoral fractures, showed that antibiotic prophylaxis reduced the incidence of deep infections, with RR = 0.36 (95% CI, 0.21–0.65), and urinary infections, with RR = 0.66 (95% CI, 0.43–1). Results were identical with a single injection of an antibiotic with a long half-life (>12 h, such as cefazolin 1 g) or with multiple injections of antibiotics with a short half-life.[7]

Postoperative wound drainage

Insertion of a drain to prevent haematomas is usual practice in hip surgery, but can also create a portal of entry for infection. In a systematic review of three RCTs (333 participants), it was observed that infections and surgical revisions were not more numerous when a postoperative drain was placed and that the drain did not increase the risk of bleeding.[7]

Urinary tract catheterization

Following hip surgery, the incidence of urinary infections is 23–25%. In spite of the frequency of this complication, there have been few studies of the modalities and the consequences of catheterization during the perioperative period. Cumming and Parker[27] emphasized a possible relationship between deep infections and prolonged urinary catheterization. In this study, infected patients had been catheterized on average for 6.9 days, compared with 3.5 days for those who did not present this complication. The number of patients who had required a long-term catheter (>21 days) was higher in the infected group ($p = 0.01$). Lastly, multiple catheter insertions were also identified as a risk factor for infection.

It therefore seems reasonable to use long-term catheterization only if the patient has urine retention and to ensure meticulous technique during insertion and care of the catheter (see Chapter 104, The ageing bladder).

Prevention of delirium

Delirium in the elderly person with a proximal femoral fracture is a complication whose prevalence is difficult to determine (5–54.3% depending on the series). The available studies come up against an absence of consensus on evaluation tools and against the difficulty of diagnosis, since fluctuation of the signs is a diagnostic criterion. Delirium is a marker of poor prognosis and is associated with increased morbidity and mortality, longer hospital stay and the risk of institutionalization. It also increases the cost of management.

Juliebo *et al.*[28] identified the risk factors for preoperative delirium as cognitive impairment, indoor injury, fever and operative delay, and for postoperative delirium as cognitive impairment, body mass index <20 and indoor injury. The pathophysiological mechanisms of delirium in this setting are poorly known, but either cholinergic deficiency or an inflammatory process have been suggested. Patients treated with statins appear to be protected to some extent, perhaps because of the anti-inflammatory action of these drugs. The prognosis is worse if delirium is associated with dementia or a depressive syndrome. Reliable studies on means of prevention are lacking. A Cochrane review analysed six studies (833 participants) on postoperative delirium, of which five related to orthopaedic surgery.[29] A single study (126 patients) involved elderly subjects who had had surgical treatment for hip fracture. It found that a preoperative geriatric consultation effectively reduced the incidence of episodes of delirium and suggested that treating 5.6 patients resulted in the prevention of one case of delirium. This type of intervention seems particularly effective in preventing severe forms, but it does not influence duration of delirium or duration of hospital stay, cognitive status or rate of institutionalization at discharge. Another study emphasized the efficacy of low-dose haloperidol in reducing the severity and duration of these episodes and in shortening hospital stay.

Postoperative care

Early mobilization and weight bearing

Postoperatively, when the patient's clinical condition has been stabilized, all efforts are directed towards rehabilitation. Early mobilization of the patient is generally recommended to prevent the complications of bed rest. However, in a Cochrane review that included seven trials, Handoll *et al.*[30] did not find a sufficient level of proof to affirm that this approach improved results. With regard to time to resumption of weight bearing, there are no strict rules. After prosthesis insertion, weight bearing is permitted as soon as the patient's clinical condition allows it. For subjects who have had internal fixation, the assembly is in general sufficiently stable to allow partial weight bearing almost immediately, but in elderly subjects this recommendation is purely theoretical and weight bearing is guided above all by pain; there is no significant difference in outcome between subjects who resume weight bearing early or late.

Rehabilitation

Various modalities of rehabilitation have been described in the literature, but the trials are heterogeneous both in the techniques used and in the context and duration of care. The respective efficacy of the protocols is therefore difficult to assess, whether in terms of functional results or of cost.

Multidisciplinary rehabilitation

Multidisciplinary rehabilitation involving physical therapists, occupational therapists, psychologists and social workers, organized by a physician around a common objective, was the basis of several studies discussed in a Cochrane review.[31] The cumulative results of 11 trials showed no superiority of this mode of management in terms of medium-term mortality, patient outcome or number of hospital readmissions. However, some studies taken in isolation show that this method improves functional recovery. Results diverge with regard to duration of hospital stay.

Some authors have looked at the possibility of *rehabilitation at home* and have assessed its efficacy. According to Beaupre *et al.*,[7] multidisciplinary management at home did not lead to greater gains in ADL or IADL than conventional physical therapy, although walking ability appeared better in the intervention group. The intensity of exercise was not specified. Giusti *et al.*,[32] in a prospective 12 month study in an unselected population, showed that such an approach was feasible and reported more rapid recovery and better functional results in the group receiving rehabilitation at home.

Intensive rehabilitation

Intensive rehabilitation pursued for a long period after hospitalization has beneficial effects. Mangione *et al.*[33] showed that a 12 week programme after discharge, consisting of either aerobic endurance training or progressive resistance training to strengthen lower limb muscles, resulted in increased walking speed and muscle strength. The increase in strength, however, was greater in the group that underwent high-intensity resistance training. Adherence was 98%.

In a study by Host *et al.*,[34] patients underwent 6 months of rehabilitation (three sessions per week). For the first 3 months the subjects carried out a variety of exercises (suppleness, balance, coordination) and low-resistance muscle strengthening. For the following 3 months, work against resistance was intensified, first to 65% of 1 RM (repetition maximum), then to 85% of 1 RM. This method resulted in significantly increased lower limb muscle strength. The injured limb developed similar strength to the contralateral limb. Functional capacity, walking speed and stair-climbing speed all improved. Two-thirds of patients walked without a cane.

As yet, no method of rehabilitation has really provided evidence of its superiority and so we are unable to propose standardized protocols after treatment for hip fracture. The results largely depend on the patient's abilities and the social context. A personalized approach must therefore be envisaged, while taking into account established prognostic factors such as cognitive status, depression, nutritional status and previous level of autonomy. Based on these criteria, the modalities of rehabilitation may be determined: generally, the most disabled patients are treated in an institutional setting and receive care for a longer period.

Optimizing nutrition

About 30–50% of elderly victims of proximal femoral fracture are malnourished at admission to hospital and this is an independent risk factor of morbidity and mortality. This situation worsens during the perioperative period due to the hypercatabolism related to the stress of injury and surgery. Hypercatabolism persists for 3 months after surgery and protein and energy intakes are seen to be less than requirements, leading to weight loss to the detriment of lean mass. Interventional studies with the aim of improving the nutritional intake of these patients are numerous, but their methodology is often mediocre.[35] Eight trials assessed the efficacy of protein, energy, vitamin and mineral supplementation and showed that this type of intervention, even if it does not decrease mortality, improves the quality of survival, with RR = 0.52 (95% CI, 0.32–0.84). High-protein diets are likely to decrease long-term complications and to encourage progress in rehabilitation. However, intravenous administration of vitamin B_1 or vitamin D was of no benefit. Recourse to feeding by nasogastric tube must be avoided because of poor tolerance and unproven efficacy.

Conversely, a randomized trial yielded evidence that providing the patient with assistance in order to eat better tended to decrease mortality.[35] This type of approach ensures better compliance and greater patient satisfaction.

Lastly, a randomized double-blind study showed that an intravenous supplement given for 3 days followed by an oral nutritional supplement twice per day for 7 days reduced the number of infectious complications and decreased mortality 3 months postoperatively.[36] However, this is an unusual nutritional protocol whose results need to be confirmed (see Chapter 15, Epidemiology of nutrition and ageing).

Surgical complications

Wound healing complications

The most frequent complication is haematoma (2–10%). The haematoma is generally not abundant and regresses spontaneously, although some cases may require surgical drainage. Superficial infections generally respond favourably to appropriate antibiotics according to bacteriological findings.

Deep infections after hip replacement occur in 0.3–2% of first-time surgical procedures and in as many as 5% of hemiarthroplasties. These complications are severe in frail elderly subjects, leading to loss of mobility and even death (11% at 3 months and 33% at 12 months). The prosthesis has to be removed, definitively compromising walking for the frailest elderly. Deep infection is rare after internal fixation.

Internal fixation of intracapsular fractures

In the weeks following surgery or on weight bearing, redisplacement of the fracture site may be observed or at a later stage delayed union or even non-union. However, the most frequent complication is vascular osteonecrosis of the femoral head. This generally occurs in the first 2 years after fracture and requires insertion of a prosthesis.

Sliding hip screw and intramedullary nail: fixation of extracapsular fractures

This type of internal fixation may be complicated by redisplacement, which requires surgical revision to stabilize the fracture site or by displacement of the cephalic screw, which may perforate the femoral head and impinge on the acetabulum. Some patients complain of pain of the outer thigh due to irritation of soft tissue by the surgical material. This may need to be removed once the fracture is consolidated.

Arthroplasty complications

Dislocation represents 13–22% of early complications, depending on the series, and 32% in patients with cognitive impairment. The incidence can be reduced by training care teams to avoid movements that put the hip at risk of dislocating (Table 93.1) during transfers and by using abduction cushions.

Some time after surgery, pain may develop which restricts walking. It is generally related to acetabular erosion (particularly frequent after Moore hemiarthroplasty), to stem impaction or loosening of the prosthesis. The prosthesis is replaced whenever the patient's condition allows.

Secondary fracture prevention

After proximal femoral fracture, in spite of rehabilitation measures the majority of elderly patients complain of weakness and loss of strength that is greater in the operated leg. This worsens pre-existing disturbances of balance and gait and increases patients' frailty. During the first year after fracture, 56% of subjects have a fall, 28% have repeated falls, 12% present with a new fracture and 5% fracture the opposite hip.[37] The occurrence of a hip fracture therefore necessitates a specific management approach with the aim of reducing the incidence of new fractures. As fracture is the result of the fall impact on bone fragilized by ageing, prevention should centre round three points:

- assessment of risk of falls and development of preventive interventions
- protection of the trochanteric region with hip protectors
- management of osteoporosis.

Table 93.1 Recommendations for avoiding dislocation of a hip prosthesis.

- Avoid movements that increase the risk of dislocation:
  - hip flexion with abduction and external rotation
  - hip flexion with adduction and internal rotation
- Get out of bed on the replacement side
- Do not cross the legs
- Do not squat or sit on too low a chair
- Do not rotate the trunk with the foot on the ground

Falls risk assessment and intervention

In the elderly person, falls are generally the consequence of multiple risk factors and/or risk situations, which can very often be corrected (see Chapter 91, Gait, balance and falls). The modalities of evaluation of fall risk in subjects who have already had a fall are defined in the guidelines of the American Geriatrics Society[38] and the National Institute for Health and Clinical Excellence (NICE)[39] (Table 93.2). It must be stressed that risk increases exponentially when several factors are associated and this has led to the development of multifactorial interventions. In a Cochrane review, Gillespie *et al*. analyzed 62 trials (21 668 participants) and showed, for example, that interventions acting on the environment and state of health are effective in unselected populations [four trials, RR = 0.73 (95% CI, 0.63–0.85)] and also in subjects who have already had falls [five trials, RR = 0.86 (95% CI, 0.76–0.98)] or those living in sheltered housing [one trial, RR = 0.60 (95% CI, 0.50–0.73)].[40] Among the single-factor interventions that have demonstrated their efficacy, we may mention some personalized home-based programmes that combine muscle strengthening and balance training [three trials, RR = 0.80 (95% CI, 0.66–0.98)], the practice of tai chi for 15 weeks, customized safety measures in the home, reduction in psychotropic treatments and pacemaker implants (cardiac pacing) in patients with carotid sinus hypersensitivity. Other interventions, such as adaptation of footwear, prescription of walking aids or correction of visual impairments, have not provided sufficient evidence of their effectiveness.

Table 93.2 Summary of fall risk assessment and appropriate interventions.

Fall risk assessment	Intervention (as appropriate)
Identification of falls history	
Assessment of gait, balance and mobility and muscle weakness	Strength and balance training
Assessment of osteoporosis risk	
Assessment of the older person's perceived functional ability and fear relating to falling	Hazard and safety home intervention
Assessment of visual impairment	Visual correction
Assessment of cognitive impairment and neurological examination	
Assessment of urinary incontinence	
Assessment of home hazards	
Cardiovascular examination and medication review	Medication review and modifications/ withdrawal Cardiovascular disorder treatment

Falls may also be secondary to a malaise and so a medical cause should systematically be sought: postural hypotension, vasovagal syncope, carotid sinus hypersensitivity. The minimum investigations in a patient who falls should include measurement of arterial blood pressure in lying and standing positions and a 12-lead electrocardiogram (see **Chapter** 35, **Cardiac ageing and systemic disorder**).

Hip protectors

The majority of fractures of the upper femoral extremity follow a sideways fall directly on to the greater trochanter. One of the means of prevention proposed is the use of a hip protector, which consists of two rigid shells or foam padding, held in position over the trochanters by pants. The aim of this device is to absorb the shock and disperse the energy to the soft tissues. Numerous designs exist and, in the absence of manufacturing standards, we may suppose that their efficacy varies. Three reviews of the literature were published in 2005–2006, including a Cochrane review.[41] Their conclusions differed little. Hip protectors appear to result in marginally lower fracture incidence in institutions but are found to be ineffective in the elderly living at home. Patient adherence is low owing to the discomfort caused by some devices and also perhaps owing to caregivers' lack of motivation, as their workload is increased by the need to adjust the protector.

A multicentre study cast further doubt on the efficacy of this type of device in an institutional setting.[42] This study included 1042 retirement home residents, mean age 85 years, with a follow-up of 20 months. Each patient wore the hip protector on one hip only, the side being selected at random, and was under their own control. Although adherence was much higher than in previous studies, it was not possible to demonstrate the preventive value of hip protectors in this population.

Osteoporosis assessment and treatment

In the elderly subject, only 3% of hip fractures are pathological (metastasis, myeloma, bone cysts, Paget's disease, etc.), but over half of patients are osteoporotic and almost all have osteopenia. After the age of 80 years, a woman with bone mineral density that is normal for her age has a T-score of–2.5 SD (the definition of osteoporosis). Osteodensitometry for diagnostic purposes alone is thus only indicated in women aged <75 years.

Based on a review of 590 trials, the Division of Rheumatology, University of California at Los Angeles, developed quality indicators for the care of osteoporosis in vulnerable elders, a definition which corresponds to elderly victims of hip fracture.[43]

Hence in a patient who has presented a fragility fracture, it is recommended to obtain a full history of medications taken (corticosteroids) and alcohol consumption and to request laboratory tests (blood count, liver and kidney function tests, phosphorus and calcium levels, vitamin D, thyroid-stimulating hormone) in order to exclude curable secondary osteoporosis and avoid bone loss. In this population, secondary osteoporosis is infrequent and the dominant cause is hyperthyroidism. Malnutrition, low weight, hypogonadism and hyperparathyroid disorders must also be borne in mind.

Every vulnerable elderly person who has had a proximal femoral fracture should receive treatment to prevent a new fracture.

Pharmacological prevention of hip fracture is debated. Several treatments have been proposed and discussed:

• *Calcium and vitamin D in combination* had a beneficial effect in elderly women living in nursing homes, but in a single study carried out nearly 20 years ago.[44]

• *Bisphosphonates*, which have undergone many randomized trials, all led to a demonstrable gain in bone mass. A reduced number of hip fractures was observed with risedronate, pamidronate and zoledronic acid. These drugs were initially administered daily under stringent conditions so as to obtain optimal absorption of the agent, then weekly or monthly formulae were later introduced which made treatment easier. With this therapeutic class, infrequent gastrointestinal side effects have been described and rare cases of osteonecrosis of the jaw. A once-yearly infusion of zoledronic acid was recently introduced that allows the treatment of patients with poor compliance. This treatment reduces the risk of clinical fracture by 33%, of vertebral fracture by 77% and the incidence of peripheral fracture by 25%.[45] Supplemental vitamin D must be given beforehand. Adverse events have been described: influenza-like syndrome at the first infusion (one in three cases) and a higher incidence of atrial fibrillation than in the placebo group.

• *Teriparatide* decreases in osteoporotic women the risk of a new vertebral or non-vertebral fracture independently of the initial T-score, age and number of fractures. The gain in bone mass is dose dependent.

• *Raloxifene* has not been found to decrease the incidence of femoral neck fractures.

• *Hormone replacement treatment* for the menopause has been judged effective in preserving bone mass and decreasing the risk of fracture in several meta-analyses, in numerous controlled trials and in prospective studies. Some trials report adverse events: breast cancer, cardioembolic disease, cerebrovascular accident, coronary failure.

• *Selective estrogen receptor antagonists* must be avoided after femoral neck fracture because of the increased risk of thromboembolic complications.

• *Strontium ranelate* increased lumbar and femoral neck bone mineral density (BMD) compared with placebo after 5 years of treatment.[46] In a subgroup of women aged >80 years, a decreased number of non-vertebral fractures was observed, of femoral head fractures in particular. Two fatal cases of drug rash with eosinophilia systemic symptoms have been reported with this medication. In addition, precautionary measures must be taken if administered to subjects at risk of thromboembolic disease.

Whatever the treatment chosen, it must be combined with an adequate intake of calcium and vitamin D.

In addition to pharmacological treatments, general measures such as a calcium-rich diet, adequate exposure to the sun and regular physical activity should be encouraged.

Orthogeriatric collaboration and orthogeriatric models

Many practitioners consider that femoral neck fracture is a geriatric rather than an orthopaedic condition. However, these elderly patients often stay for at least a week in orthopaedic departments where the care teams have little awareness of geriatric problems. The National Service Framework for Older People in England recommends that every hospital should have at least one orthogeriatric ward,[1] whose ideal model in terms of efficacy, and also of cost-efficacy, remains to be defined. Orthogeriatric care must be not only a multidisciplinary activity but also a radical alternative to the traditional model, where all strategies that have demonstrated their efficacy in improving the prognosis of proximal femoral fracture are applied. From a review of the literature of the last 10 years, five existing models of collaboration between geriatricians and orthopaedic surgeons may be described:

1 *The traditional model* in which the patient is managed in the orthopaedic department, then transferred to the rehabilitation department and has access to geriatric consultations as required.

2 *A variant of this model*, in which a geriatric team intervenes at admission and at discharge from the orthopaedic department, thus sharing in the management of geriatric problems and in referring patients to the various rehabilitation services.

3 *The integrated model*, where orthopaedists and geriatricians share the management of medical and surgical problems, with the aim of rapid transfer to a geriatric rehabilitation unit.

4 A more *geriatric model*, where the patient is followed preoperatively by a geriatric team and is transferred immediately after surgery to a geriatric unit and then to a rehabilitation facility.

5 Lastly, a *comprehensive orthogeriatric approach* with uninterrupted geriatric management from admission to discharge and daily follow-up of the operated patient by the orthopaedist.

The 2009 update of the Cochrane review by Cameron *et al.*,[47] including two supplementary trials, was not able to demonstrate the superior efficacy of any one of these models, but emphasized a trend in favour of systems which strengthened genuine links between geriatricians and orthopaedists instead of juxtaposing their interventions. Cost studies are not in favour of this mode of functioning, which, however, should avoid the loss of time related to the various transfers, make it easier for the patient to adjust by doing away with changes of care team and relieve the pressure on the orthopaedic services.

This raises the question of whether it would not be legitimate to change our strategy and develop new models of orthogeriatric care, with early supported discharge or hospital at home and the intervention of a multidisciplinary team to organize rehabilitation.

Key points

- Femoral neck fracture is a 'condition of age' with a severe vital and functional prognosis.
- Current treatment is surgical: internal fixation or hip replacement.
- This condition demands multidisciplinary reflection bringing together the anaesthetist, surgeon, geriatrician and physiatrist.
- Each patient must receive individualized management in order to prevent new fractures.

References

1. Parker MJ and Johansen A. Hip fracture. *BMJ* 2006;**333**: 27–30.
2. Gullberg B, Johnell O and Kanis JA. World-wide projections for hip fracture. *Osteoporos Int* 1997;**7**:407–13.
3. Johansen A and Parker M. Hip fracture and orthogeriatrics. In: MSJ Pathy, AJ Sinclair and JE Morley (eds), *Principles and Practice of Geriatric Medicine*, 4th edn, John Wiley & Sons, Ltd, Chichester, 2006, pp.1329–45.
4. Dolan P and Torgerson DJ.. The cost of treating osteoporotic fractures in the United Kingdom female population. *Osteoporos Int* 1998;**8**:611–7.
5. Parker MJ and Handoll HH. Pre-operative traction for fractures of the proximal femur in adults. *Cochrane Database Syst Rev* 2006;(3): CD000168.
6. Foss NB, Kristensen MT and Kehlet H. Anaemia impedes functional mobility after hip fracture surgery. *Age Ageing* 2008;**37**:173–8.
7. Beaupre LA, Jones CA, Saunders LD *et al.* Best practices for elderly hip fracture patients. A systematic overview of the evidence. *J Gen Intern Med* 2005;**20**:1019–25.
8. Handoll HH, Farrar MJ, McBirnie J *et al.* Heparin, low molecular weight heparin and physical methods for preventing deep vein thrombosis and pulmonary embolism following surgery for hip fractures. *Cochrane Database Syst Rev* 2002;(4): CD000305.
9. Quinlan DJ, Eikelboom JW and Douketis JD. Anticoagulant (extended duration) for prevention of venous thromboembolism following total hip or knee replacement or hip fractures repair (protocol). *Cochrane Database Syst Rev* 2009;(4): CD 004179.
10. Geerts VH, Pineo GF, Heit JA *et al.* Prevention of venous thromboembolism. The 7th ACCP Conference on Antithrombotic and Thrombolytic Therapy. *Chest* 2004;**126**: 338S–400S.
11. Eriksson BI and Lassen MR. Duration of prophylaxis against venous thromboembolism with fondaparinux after hip fracture surgery: a multicenter, randomized, placebo-controlled double-blind study. *Arch Int Med* 2003;**163**:1337–42.
12. Bottle A and Aylin P. Mortality associated with delay in operation after hip fracture: observational study. *BMJ* 2006;**332**:947–51.
13. Grimes JP, Gregory PM, Noveck H *et al.* The effects of time-to-surgery on mortality and morbidity in patients following hip fracture. *Am J Med* 2002;**112**:702–9.
14. Shiga T, Wajima Z and Ohe Y. Is operative delay associated with increased mortality of hip fracture patients? Systematic review, meta-analysis and meta-regression. *Can J Anesth* 2008;**55**:146–54.
15. Verbeek DO, Ponsen KJ, Goslings JC *et al.* Effect of surgical delay on outcome in hip fracture patients: a retrospective multivariate analysis of 192 patients. *Int Orthop* 2008;**32**:13–8.
16. Lefaivre KA, Macadam SA, Davidson DJ *et al.* Length of stay, mortality, morbidity and delay to surgery in hip fractures. *J Bone Joint Surg Br* 2009;**91**:922–7.
17. Baumgarten M, Margolis D, Berlin JA *et al.* Risk factors for pressure ulcers among elderly hip fracture patients. *Wound Repair Regen* 2003;**11**:96–103.
18. Nicosia G, Gliatta AE, Woodbury MG *et al.* The effect of pressure-relieving surfaces on the prevention of heel ulcers in a variety of settings: a meta-analysis. *Int Wound J* 2007;**4**:197–207.
19. Handoll HH and Parker MJ. Conservative versus operative treatment for hip fractures in adults. *Cochrane Database Syst Rev* 2008;(2): CD000337.
20. Parker MJ and Gurusamy KS. Arthroplasties (with and without bone cement) for proximal femoral fractures in adults. *Cochrane Database Syst Rev* 2007;(2): CD001706.
21. Parker MJ and Gurusamy KS. Internal fixation versus arthroplasty for intracapsular proximal femoral fractures in adults. *Cochrane Database Syst Rev* 2006;(3): CD001708.
22. Gjertsen JE, Vinje T, Lie SA *et al.* Patient satisfaction, pain and quality of life 4 months after displaced femoral neck fractures: a comparison of 663 fractures treated with internal fixation and 906 with bipolar hemiarthroplasty reported to the Norwegian Hip Fracture Register. *Acta Orthop Scand* 2008;**79**:594–601.
23. Rogmark C and Johnell O. Primary arthroplasty is better than internal fixation of displaced femoral neck fractures: a meta-analysis of 14 randomised studies with 2,289 patients. *Acta Orthop Scand* 2006;**77**:359–67.
24. Parker MJ and Handoll HH. Replacement arthroplasty versus internal fixation for extracapsular hip fractures in adults. *Cochrane Database Syst Rev* 2006;(1): CD000086.

25. Parker MJ, Handoll HH and Griffiths R. Anaesthesia for hip fracture surgery in adults. *Cochrane Database Syst Rev* 2004;(4): CD000521.
26. Rodgers A, Walker N, Schug S *et al.* Reduction of post-operative mortality and morbidity with epidural or spinal anaesthesia: results from overview of randomised trials. *BMJ* 2000;**321**:1493–7.
27. Cumming D and Parker MJ. Urinary catheterisation and deep wound infection after hip fracture surgery. *Int Orthop* 2007;**31**:483–5.
28. Juliebo V, Bjoro K, Krogseth M *et al.* Risk factors for preoperative and postoperative delirium in elderly patients with hip fracture. *J Am Geriatr Soc* 2009;**57**:1354–61.
29. Siddiqui N, Holt R, Britton AM *et al.* Intervention for preventing delirium in hospitalised patients. *Cochrane Database Syst Rev* 2007;(2): CD005563.
30. Handoll HH, Sherington C and Parker MJ. Mobilisation strategies after hip fracture surgery in adults. *Cochrane Database Syst Rev* 2007;(1): CD001704.
31. Handoll HH, Cameron ID, Mark JC *et al.* Multidisciplinary rehabilitation for older people with hip fractures. *Cochrane Database Syst Rev* 2009;(4): CD007125.
32. Giusti A, Barone A, Oliveri M *et al.* An analysis of the feasibility of home rehabilitation among elderly people with proximal femoral fractures. *Arch Phys Med Rehabil* 2006;**87**:826–31.
33. Mangione KK, Craik RL, Tomlinson SS *et al.* Can elderly patients who have had a hip fracture perform moderate- to high-intensity exercise at home? *Phys Ther* 2005;**85**: 727–39.
34. Host HH, Sinacore DR, Bohnert KL *et al.* Training-induced strength and functional adaptations after hip fracture. *Phys Ther* 2007;**87**:292–303.
35. Avenell A and Handoll HH. Nutritional supplementation for hip fracture aftercare in older people. *Cochrane Database Syst Rev* 2010;(4): CD001880.
36. Eneroth M, Olsson UB and Thorngren KG Nutritional supplementation decreases hip fracture-related complications. *Clin Orthop Res* 2006;**451**:212–7.
37. Lloyd BD, Williamson DA, Singh NA *et al.* Recurrent and injurious falls in the year following hip fracture: a prospective study of incidence and risk factors from sarcopenia and hip fracture study. *J Gerontol A Biol Sci Med Sci* 2009;**64**:599–609.
38. American Geriatrics Society, British Geriatrics Society and American Academy of Orthopaedic Surgeons Panel on Falls Prevention. Guidelines for the prevention of falls in older persons. *J Am Geriat Soc* 2001;**49**:664–72.
39. National Institute for Health and Clinical Excellence. *Clinical Practice Guideline for the Assessment and Prevention of Falls in Older People*. NICE, London, 2004.
40. Gillespie LD, Robertson MC, Gillespie WJ *et al.* Interventions for preventing falls in older people living in the community. *Cochrane Database Syst Rev* 2009;(2): CD007146.
41. Parker MJ, Gillespie LD and Gillespie WJ. Effectiveness of hip protectors for preventing hip fractures in elderly people: a systematic review. *BMJ* 2006;**332**:571–3.
42. Kiel DP, Magaziner J, Zimmerman S *et al.* Efficacy of a hip protector to prevent hip fracture in nursing home residents: the HIP PRO randomized controlled trial. *JAMA* 2007;**298**:413–22.
43. Grossman J and MacLean CH. Quality indicators for the care of osteoporosis in vulnerable elders. *J Am Geriatr Soc* 2007;**55**: S392–402.
44. Chapuy MC, Arlot ME, Delmas PD *et al.* Effect of calcium and cholecalciferol treatment for three years on hip fractures in elderly women. *BMJ* 1994;**308**:1081–2.
45. Lyles KW, Colon-Emeric CS, Magaziner JS *et al.* Zoledronic acid and mortality after hip fracture. *N Engl J Med* 2007;**357**-1799–809.
46. Reginster JY, Felsenberg D, Boonen S *et al.* Effects of long-term strontium ranelate treatment on the risk of nonvertebral and vertebral fractures in postmenopausal osteoporosis. Results of a five-year, randomized, placebo-controlled trial. *Arthritis Rheum* 2008;**58**:1687–95.
47. Cameron ID, Handoll HH, Finnegan TP *et al.* Co-ordinated multidisciplinary approaches for inpatient rehabilitation of older patients with proximal femoral fractures. *Cochrane Database Syst Rev* 2009;(4): CD000106.

CHAPTER 94

Diseases of the joints

Terry L. Moore
Saint Louis University Medical Center, St Louis, MO, USA

Introduction

The clinical presentation of arthritis is one of joint pain, swelling, morning stiffness and limitation of motion. These are symptoms common to all types of arthritis. Different diseases of the joint can present with signs and symptoms that appear quite similar. There are over 100 types of arthritis that can affect the elderly with osteoarthritis and rheumatoid arthritis being the most common entities. Nevertheless, a thorough medical history and physical examination, together with radiographic and laboratory testing, will identify the correct diagnosis in most cases of diseases of the joints. Arthritis has to be differentiated from periarticular or other musculoskeletal pain syndromes that commonly occur in the aged.

Osteoarthritis

Osteoarthritis (OA) or degenerative joint disease is a chronic disorder characterized by softening and disintegration of articular cartilage with secondary changes in underlying bone, new growth of cartilage and bone (osteophytes) at the joint margins, and capsular fibrosis.[1] It is by far the most common form of chronic arthritis among the elderly. Its prevalence increases with age, occurring in greater than 50% of individuals older than 60.[2] OA is particularly common in elderly people, affecting more than 80% of those older than 75 years.[1] Susceptibility to OA involves systemic factors affecting joint vulnerability including age, gender and genetic susceptibility, nutritional factors, intrinsic joint vulnerabilities including previous damage, muscle weakness and malalignment, and extrinsic factors including obesity and physical activity.[1,3] The most common joints involved are those of weight-bearing including the knees, hips, cervical and lumbosacral spine, proximal (PIP) and distal (DIP) interphalangeal joints of the hands, first carpometacarpal joints (CMC), and metatarsophalangeal joints (MTP).[1] Involvement is typically symmetric, although it can be unilateral at first depending on previous trauma or unusual stress. The pain may be insidious and relieved by rest initially, but as the disease progresses it becomes persistent and more severe with activity. Stiffness following periods of inactivity may also become common. The patient may complain of problems such as knee locking, unsteadiness, or giving away. Some patients, especially women, experience inflammatory OA or erosive OA, which involves particularly the PIPs and DIPs of the hands. These may exhibit inflammatory manifestations such as redness, tenderness and local heat. Knees are often swollen with synovial fluid produced. Cervical and lumbosacral pain is a result of arthritis of hypophyseal joints, bony spur formation, pressure on ligaments or other surrounding tissues, or reactive muscle spasm. Impingement on nerve roots by osteophytes can cause radicular symptoms. Cord compression may result in spinal stenosis. In the cervical area, it causes localized pain and gait unsteadiness. In lumbar areas, it may result in spinal claudication, consisting of pain in the buttocks or legs while walking that is relieved after 10–15 mins of rest. Lumbar flexion and sitting usually relieve these symptoms, as opposed to aggravation of radicular disc symptoms by these positions.[4]

Examination of the joints may detect crepitus, deformities, subluxation, swelling, bony overgrowths such as Heberden's nodes of the DIPs, Bouchard's nodes of the PIPs, or CMC joints, and limitation of motion. Neurological evaluations may detect a radicular pattern of motor or sensory abnormalities, lower motor neuron or upper motor neuron signs in spinal stenosis, and sphincter abnormalities.[5]

No diagnostic laboratory tests are currently available (Table 94.1). The synovial fluid, when present, is noninflammatory with a white count less than 1000 cells/mm^3. Radiological abnormalities may lag behind symptoms. Typical findings are joint space narrowing, subchondral sclerosis, osteophytes and periarticular bone cysts. Oblique films of the spine must be obtained to evaluate the neuroforamina. Computerized tomography (CT) or magnetic

Principles and Practice of Geriatric Medicine, Fifth Edition. Edited by Alan J. Sinclair, John E. Morley and Bruno Vellas.

Table 94.1 Studies to screen for arthritis.

Complete blood count (CBC)
Urinalysis
Erythrocyte sedimentation rate (ESR)
C-reactive protein (CRP)
Chemistry panel including studies for kidney, liver, muscle, and uric acid
Rheumatoid Factor (RF), Anti-cyclic citrullinated peptide antibodies (αCCPAb)
Antinuclear antibody (ANA) and profile if indicated
Synovial fluid analysis if indicated (white count, crystal analysis, cultures)
X-rays of appropriate joints or spinal areas

resonance imaging (MRI) give better evaluation of the spinal pathology and can differentiate OA changes from discopathy, another common problem in older persons.[4]

Rheumatoid arthritis

Rheumatoid arthritis (RA) is a chronic inflammatory symmetrical disease of joints of unknown aetiology, affecting about 1% of the general population worldwide and about 2% of persons 60 years of age and older in the United States.[6,7] Extra-articular manifestations may also contribute to disease symptomatology.[8] Most elderly patients with RA have the disease onset before age 60 and commonly present with additional therapeutic problems when older because of the long duration of the disease and other illnesses. Older persons are more likely to develop joint deformities. Involvement of the cervical spine may result in pain, decreased range of motion and neurological deficits. Extra-articular manifestations, such as rheumatoid nodules, secondary Sjögren's syndrome (SS), and vasculitis are more frequent in this group of patients.[8]

Patients with elderly onset RA (EORA) are those in whom RA develops after age 60. Most patients present with a gradual onset of pain, swelling and stiffness in symmetrical joints, while in others the onset may be more acute. Fatigue, malaise and weight loss may be present. Joint symptoms are characteristically symmetric, although asymmetric presentation may occur. In the aged, asymmetric involvement may be seen in hemiplegic patients with sparing of the paralysed side. All peripheral joints may be involved, but the most common are the PIPs and metacarpophalangeal (MCPs) of the hands involved in 90% as are the wrists, MTPs and ankles. Knees, hips, elbows and shoulders are present to a lesser extent. DIPs of the hands are usually spared. Large joints are commonly involved in EORA, the shoulders more often than in younger patients.[8,9]

The majority of patients experience intermittent periods of active disease alternating with periods of relative or complete remission. A minority will suffer no more than a few months of symptoms followed by complete remission, whereas a small group will have severe, progressive disease. EORA is considered by many to be milder than RA developing at a younger age, which may be related to the lower incidence of rheumatoid factor (RF) positivity in the elderly.[9] RF-positive EORA patients are likely to have more severe disease.[6] Anti-cyclic citrullinated peptide antibodies (αCCPAb) are also found in patients with more severe EORA, but overall to a much lesser extent than younger patients with RA. Most laboratory abnormalities are not specific for RA, with the possible exception of high-titer 19S IgM RF and αCCPAb (Table 94.1). It should be noted that RF in low titers may occur in a small percentage of healthy older individuals, so a positive RF test itself may be not diagnostic. The erythrocyte sedimentation rate (ESR) and C-reactive protein (CRP) are usually increased in RA, often correlating with disease activity. Radiological evaluation of involved joints in early stages is likely to show only soft tissue swelling. Later, the typical findings of symmetric joint space narrowing and erosions can support the clinical diagnosis (Table 94.1).[5,6,8]

Gout

Gout is an inflammatory arthropathy caused by deposition of sodium monourate crystals in the joint and occurs in an overall prevalence from less than 1–15%.[10] Its prevalence increases with age.[10] The typical presentation is that of an acute monoarthritis in 85–90% of first attacks, most commonly occurring in the first MTP joint. The joint is usually extremely tender because it is associated with swelling and overlying erythema that sometimes mimics cellulitis or septic arthritis. Patients may be febrile and attacks can be precipitated by alcohol intake, use of diuretics and stress, such as that occurring with surgical procedures or acute medical illness. Gout occurs more readily in joints damaged by other conditions such as OA. Polyarticular involvement of gout is not uncommon in older persons. It sometimes resembles RA. Such attacks tend to have smouldering onset and longer course with a duration as long as three weeks. Chronic tophaceous gout is characterized by episodes of acute arthritis, chronic polyarthritis, joint deformities and tophi. Radiographic findings are non-specific in early stages. Punched out lesions or periarticular bone with overhanging borders are typically seen in chronic gout.[5,10]

Laboratory findings include hyperuricaemia in most cases.[10] Most individuals with hyperuricaemia never experience acute or chronic gout. About 10% have normal serum levels during the attack. Therefore, the diagnosis should be established by the identification of typical sodium monourate crystals in synovial fluid, preferably with the use of a polarized microscope. This is accompanied by evaluating serum uric acid level and also performing a 24-hour urine for total serum urate spillage to define if the patient is an over-producer or under-secreter of uric acid.

Calcium pyrophosphate deposition disease

Calcium pyrophosphate deposition disease (CPDD) is also a crystalline deposition arthropathy.[11] Women may be more commonly affected by CPPD crystal deposition than men.[12] Its prevalence increases with age, being 10% in age 60–75 years and 30% in those 80 years of age or older.[13] Most cases are primary, but in some people it is associated with certain conditions such as hypothyroidism, hyperparathyroidism and haemochromatosis. Many patients merely have asymptomatic chondrocalcinosis, commonly noted by X-rays in the knees and wrists where linear punctate radiodensities are found within the cartilage.[11]

Typical presentation is usually of two types, chronic arthropathy, which is sometimes polyarticular and presents with or without acute attacks with the knees most predominantly affected. Clinically, it may resemble OA or RA. Radiography may show features of both OA and CPDD, so it is not clear whether CPDD is primary or secondary. The second presentation is pseudogout, which is an acute monoarthritis, affecting mainly the knees and other large joints primarily and these resolve spontaneously within three weeks. It may infrequently affect a few articulations. Attack of pseudogout can be precipitated by stress or local trauma and fever is common.[12]

Connective tissue disease

Connective tissue disease, primary SS and systemic lupus erythematosus (SLE), may present in the older population. Fifteen percent of cases of SLE may begin after age 55.[14] It may present with arthralgias or symmetric polyarthritis involving primarily finger joints, best resembling RA at this stage. Previous studies indicated older onset SLE tended to be milder than the disease in younger patients with a lower incidence of nephropathy, neuropsychiatric manifestations, fever and Raynaud's symptoms.[15] However, a recent study suggested that older age-onset SLE is not benign.[16] There is an increased frequency of serositis, interstitial lung disease, myalgias and sicca symptoms.[14] Primary SS also often presents in the aged.[17] Patients complain of dryness of their eyes and also dryness in their mouth with swallowing difficulty. Nasal dryness, hoarseness, bronchitis, and skin and vaginal dryness may occur. The parotid glands may be swollen. Sicca symptoms (dry eyes and dry mouth) may be subtle and not obvious to the patients. Individual patients commonly have polyarthritis or arthralgias. Other features of the disease are myalgias, low-grade fever and fatigue. Most have hypergammaglobulinemia and the frequency of developing lymphoproliferative disease is increased.[17]

Antinuclear antibodies are present in most SS and SLE patients, with antibodies to SS-A (Ro) and SS-B (La) occurring in the SS patients and SLE patients; and SLE patients having antibodies alone to double-stranded DNA, Sm and RNP.[18] Other laboratory studies for evaluation include complement levels, antiphospholipid antibody studies, and other specific tests that may be helpful in diagnosing a particular connective tissue disease that is involved in the elderly patient.[19,20]

Drug-induced lupus (DIL) is also a disease of older patients because inciting drugs are prescribed more frequently in the elderly. Symptoms are mild in most patients and resemble those of older onset SLE. The diagnosis is suggested by a history of administration of drugs like procainamide, hydralazine, alpha-methyldopa, propylthiouracil, or minocycline.[21] Most of these patients have positive ANA tests and antibodies to histones or chromatin in 70–95% of the cases and occasionally antibodies to myeloperoxidase. Other antibodies occur infrequently.[22]

Infectious arthritis

Infectious arthritis typically presents as an acute monoarthritis of a large joint in more than 80% of cases with the knee involved in more than 50% of cases.[23] It is associated with systemic signs of infection such as high fever, chills and leukocytosis. Several factors predispose to an infected joint, including pre-existing joint disease, a prosthetic joint, an infectious process elsewhere, or an immunocompromised state, such as diabetes mellitus or treatment with corticosteroids or immunosuppressives.[24] Infectious arthritis has to be entertained in all elderly patients with arthritic complaints. The presentation may be atypical in the aged because normal leukocyte counts and a normal temperature are not uncommon.[24] In all cases of monoarthritis, synovial fluid should be aspirated, a Gram stain and culture performed, and a leukocyte count and differential determined. The leukocytes counts are usually >50 000 cells/mm^3, primarily neutrophils; however, the initial count may be less than 10 000 cells/mm^3.[25] The most common pathogen is *Staphylococcus aureus*, followed by streptococci and gram-negative bacilli.[23] *Staphylococcus epidermidis* is common in a prosthetic joint infection. Early diagnosis is mandatory to prevent the high rate of complications; a 19% mortality rate has been reported, and 38% of patients may develop osteomyelitis.[24] Treatment of infectious arthritis is determined by the organism isolated and then appropriate therapy.

Treatment

Effective treatment of elderly arthritic patients combines physical therapy, medications and in some cases, surgical intervention (Table 94.2).

Table 94.2 Treatment modalities for arthritis in the aged.

Physical therapy
Medications
• (Non-inflammatory arthritis)
–Analgesics
–Non-steroidal anti-inflammatories
• (Inflammatory arthritis)
–Non-steroidal anti-inflammatories
–Disease-modifying agents
–Biologics
–Corticosteroids
Surgery

Physical therapy

The value of physical therapy in improving the QOL of the elderly patients with arthritis cannot be overemphasized. The main goals are pain relief, prevention of deformities and maintaining mobility and independence.[5] Pain is relieved by periodic rest, splinting of affected joints and locally applied heat. Although rest decreases joint pain and swelling, it may contribute to the development of contractures, disuse atrophy of muscles and osteoporosis. In the aged, even brief periods of rest can result in loss of muscle strength and difficulty in resuming activities. An individual must maintain a certain level of activity even in the presence of active disease. Initial periods of relative rest should be followed by a programme of passive and then active exercises designed to maintain range of motion and muscle strength. The patients should be encouraged to participate in body toning exercise programmes such as regular swimming, walking, or water aerobics-type programmes. Foot, hand and cervical spine involvement can be helped with proper individualized footwear, paraffin baths and cervical collars, respectively. Fabricated orthoses can help maintain alignment and support mechanically deranged joints. Assistive devices for walking, dressing, eating and bathing can greatly improve the QOL of these patients.[5,26,27]

Medications

Treatment decisions should consider several age-related changes that may affect drug absorption, distribution, metabolism and elimination. The possibility exists that various treatments will have altered efficacy and be potentially more hazardous. Also, many elderly patients with arthritis have other diseases requiring other medications that could cause drug–drug interactions with the arthritis preparations.

Analgesic medications are given for mild arthralgias, especially for OA. Acetaminophen is commonly prescribed at a daily dose of 650 mg three to four times a day as needed. It has been shown to have equal efficacy to other anti-inflammatory agents for pain relief. It is a safe drug when used in therapeutic doses. It appears to be safe for patients with renal dysfunction or peptic ulcers; however, liver function studies must be followed to be sure there are no problems with hepatic toxicity.[28] Other analgesics and opioid receptor agonists are effective in pain management, but their use should be limited to short term, because abuse can lead to adverse effects, such as respiratory depression, drowsiness, constipation and addiction. The recent use of glucosamine and chondroitin sulfate for OA have been investigated and may be efficacious, especially glucosamine in some patients with OA of the hips and knees.[28] Diabetics and patients allergic to shellfish should not use these compounds. Also, the use of intra-articular injections of hyaluronic acid have been helpful to preserve knee cartilage and hip cartilage in some cases.[29,30] Topical agents such as capsaicin and 1% diclofenac gel can also be helpful.[28] Lastly, obesity is also an important risk factor in OA; therefore, regimens of weight loss and exercise can decrease pain and disability, especially of the knees and hips.[28]

Non-steroid anti-inflammatory drugs (NSAIDs) are the most frequently prescribed medications for arthritis.[5] In many cases, they are alone sufficient to induce the desired effect. The use of NSAIDs as primary therapy for older patients with OA and RA is not without problems.[27,31] Advanced age has been identified as a primary risk factor for adverse gastrointestinal (GI) events in users of NSAIDs.[32] Hospitalization for bleeding of the stomach or oesophagus occurs far more frequently in older patients who use NSAIDs than those who do not. However, patients are often asymptomatic. The risk factors for such events are advanced age, a history of GI problems, and the simultaneous use of corticosteroids, anticoagulants, alcohol, or tobacco. These factors should be documented in individual patients and treated accordingly.[32] Adverse events such as epigastric pain, mental changes, fluid retention, changes in blood pressure, and occult or gross blood loss should be monitored closely. A complete blood count (CBC), urinalysis, and liver and kidney function tests should be drawn initially for baseline, then in one month, and every three months thereafter to monitor toxicity in the elderly population. NSAIDs such as naproxen, meloxicam, sulindac and diclofenac have proved very effective in the treatment of OA or RA in patients. A concern about peptic ulcer disease has been relieved considerably by the availability of cyclooxygenase-2 (COX-2) inhibitors.[33] However, caution is still needed in older patients who have a history of ulcer disease. Some physicians still add proton pump inhibitors to this therapy when it is used in high-risk patients. Also, the use of H2 blockers such as famotidine, can also be helpful. Both the older NSAIDs and COX-2 selective NSAIDs have the potential for decreasing renal blood flow causing fluid retention, creating abnormal salt and water metabolism, and interfering with drug excretion, so they are not without their toxicity in the elderly population.[34] The COX-2 antagonists celecoxib and etoricoxib have been used extensively and have other advantages beyond decreased gastric acidity.[35] Clinical trials of these drugs have shown no effect on platelet aggregation or bleeding time at therapeutic doses and do not alter the anticoagulant effect of warfarin. However, the possibility of increased blood pressure, peripheral oedema, or predisposal to myocardial infarctions or strokes because of their effect on thromboxane A2 levels may be a contraindication to using some COX-2 inhibitors in the elderly population.[33]

The nephrotoxic effect of NSAIDs are well documented. The most common mechanism leading to renal dysfunction is inhibition of renal prostaglandin synthesis, which may adversely affect renal blood flow in certain situations, leading to acute insufficiency.[34] At special risk are patients with pre-existing changes in renal function, such as those changes related to ageing, diabetes mellitus, hypertension, congestive heart failure, or use of concomitant diuretics. Preferably, NSAIDs should not be prescribed to patients with these conditions or anybody with a creatinine of 1.5 or higher. NSAID-related psychotic reactions and depression occur more commonly in the aged. Also, NSAIDs can interact with several medications commonly used in older persons, mainly anticoagulants, oral hypoglycaemics, digoxin, seizure medications and lithium.[31] Combining NSAIDs with potassium-sparing diuretics increase the risk of hyperkalaemia.

In RA, the baseline therapy is the use of an NSAID and two remittive agents usually hydroxychloroquine and methotrexate or sulfasalazine to reduce erosions and joint space narrowing which generally occur in the first two years.[6] Hydroxychloroquine in doses of 200 mg once to twice daily is begun. It is considered to be effective in mild-to-moderate cases of RA. It is also effective in treating the arthritis and skin manifestations of SLE and SS and should be prescribed in all of these patients.[36] The third drug in the United States is usually methotrexate in doses of 10–25 mg weekly or in Europe sulfasalazine at doses of 2–3 g daily. These regimens appear to be effective for elderly patients with RA, as it is for younger ones. Methotrexate may have some toxicity in elderly, but is limited mainly to hepatotoxicity and in those with abnormal renal function. The lowest reasonable dose should be used.[32,36] CBC, urinalysis and comprehensive metabolic panel at baseline and in two weeks if changing dosages; otherwise, every six to eight weeks to monitor toxicity are recommended. Also, to reduce toxicity, the use of folic acid at 1–2 mg per day is very helpful. Sulfasalazine at 2–3 g daily should also be monitored at baseline and every two months by a CBC, urinalysis and comprehensive metabolic panel to reduce toxicity. Other remittive agents such as azathioprine at 50 mg bid or leflunomide at 20 mg qd, may be used in RA with efficacy.[37] The recent advent of biologics including etanercept, infliximab, adalimumab, anakinra, golimumab, certolizumab pegol and tocilizumab have been very helpful in bringing into remission elderly patients with RA.[38] These biologics inhibit tumour necrosis factor (TNF), interleukin-1 (IL-1), or IL-6. Etanercept, a TNF receptor antagonist, is given as 25 mg twice a week to 50 mg once a week subcutaneously. It has been shown to be very effective in decreasing sedimentation rate, joint activity, arthralgias, and in reducing erosions and joint space narrowing. The same can also be said for the other new biologics which are monoclonal antibodies directed toward TNF. The fully-humanized antibody, adalimumab, is given at 40 mg subcutaneously every two weeks and the chimeric molecule, infliximab, an intravenous preparation, is given at dosages from 3–10 mg kg^{-1} at baseline, two and six weeks, and then every four to eight weeks thereafter. A newer agent, also fully humanized, golimumab, has a longer half-life and can be given at 50 to 100 mg subcutaneously every 4 weeks with methotrexate. The pegylated TNF antagonist, certolizumab pegol, is given in combination with methotrexate at 400 mg subcutaneously initially and at 2 and 4 weeks, and then 200 mg every other week. Tocilizumab, the IL-6 blocking agent, has recently been approved for RA. It is given with methotrexate at 4 to 8 mg kg^{-1} every 4 weeks. Liver enzymes and lipid levels need to be monitored in patients on Tocilizumab.[38] All have been shown to have long-term efficacy and little toxicity. Injection site reactions may occur and are usually managed with local antihistamine or steroid cremes, or antihistamines. The only other common toxicity noted is the possible development of exacerbating an indolent tuberculosis infection. Therefore, a tuberculosis skin test and chest X-ray should be performed at baseline and yearly. Also, the possibility of aggravating any new infection has to be entertained. Therefore, a dose should be held if a viral or bacterial infection occurs. Caution, also should be maintained in giving a biologic to any patient with an artificial joint. A nidus of infection around the metallic implant could be exacerbated. Also, the long-term effect of blocking TNF is not well understood.[39] They should not be used for any patient with a demyelinating disorder[40] and monitoring for any type of lymphoproliferative processes to develop should they occur.[41] IL-1 blocking therapy, anakinra, can also be used in patients with RA, but may also be used in patients with gout. It is given at 100 mg subcutaneously daily, but a high incidence of injection site reactions may occur.[38] T-cell blocker agents have been developed for use in RA. Abatacept, a human immunoglobulin receptor fusion protein of IgG1 and CTLA4, is the first to be approved. CTLA4Ig binds to CD80 and CD86 on antigen-presenting cells, thereby preventing these molecules from engaging CD28 on T cells. Thus, blocking the T cell from proliferating and producing inflammatory cytokines which can activate other inflammatory cells. Abatacept is given at 10 mg kg^{-1}

intravenously on days 1, 15 and 30 and then monthly, but never over 1000 mg at one infusion. Abatacept is now available weekly as a subcutaneous injection. The safety profile is very good.[42] B-cell agents have also been developed. Rituximab is an ant-CD20 monoclonal antibody that binds the CD20 antigen on pre-B and mature B lymphocytes. Dosages of 1000 mg intravenously at base line and day 15 and the possible retreatment at 6 months can be effective in patients failing other biologic regimens. Side effects including infusion reactions, increased infections and mutifocal leukoencephalopathy developing have been reported.[43]

Corticosteroids can be used in low doses of 5–10 mg of prednisone daily in some elderly seronegative RA patients or in patients with remittive seronegative symmetrical synovitis with pitting oedema (RS3PE).[36] However, higher doses predispose the patient to the multiple side effects of steroids in the elderly including sodium and fluid retention, hypertension, hyperglycaemia, osteoporosis, infections and skin changes.[32,36] With the advent of the new remittive agents and biologics, the use of steroids should be diminished to only those who are unresponsive or cannot afford the other agents. If steroids are used, the use of calcium and vitamin D with that therapy should be included to prevent osteoporosis as much as possible. Intra-articular injections of steroid preparations are commonly employed in RA and OA in conjunction with other treatment modalities, especially when symptoms are limited to one or fewer joints.[36]

The treatment of acute gout in the elderly is still the use of colchicine, but at lower doses than in the past.[32] Generally, the dosage for long-term use of colchicine is one or two 0.6 mg tablets per day depending on the patient's renal function; however, only 0.3 mg in patients aged 70 years or older. When parental colchicine is used, the maximum dose used for an acute episode, in or out of the hospital, should be 1 mg per day intravenously. In renal compromised patients, the use of colchicine has resulted in neuromyopathy.[44] Allopurinol, a xanthine oxidase inhibitor, is another gout medication which can lower serum urate levels. It is best started slowly at 100 mg per day. If the hyperuricaemia is not responding, the dosage should be advanced to 100 mg twice a day and then finally up to 300 mg per day or higher depending on creatinine and uric acid response.[5] Platelet counts and hypersensitivity reactions should be monitored. A new medication, febuxostat, also a selective xanthine oxidase inhibitor in doses of 40–80 mg per day has been shown to be effective in controlling hyperuricaemia and gouty flares.[45,46] Anti-inflammatory agents in acute gout can be used, such as naproxen or the COX-2 inhibitor, etoricoxib.[10] In general, uric acid-lowering therapy should be administered when there are tophi, frequent attacks of gouty arthritis over three per year, or evidence of uric acid overproduction is documented. Baseline 24-hour urine of uric acid spillage over 750 mg per 24 hours or uric acid levels over 6.5 mg dl^{-1} may indicate the need for therapy.[10] Lastly, in refractory gout it has become clear that the inflammasome plays a role in the initiation of acute gout. IL-1β is released. In such patients, IL-1 blockade with anakinra at 100 mg subcutaneously daily till the flare resolves may be effective.[47]

In the treatment for pseudogout in adult patients, it has been shown that colchicine is less effective and is usually being managed by NSAIDs. The dosage of naproxen 500 mg bid, etoricoxib 60 mg once to twice a day, or diclofenac 50 mg tid can be very effective in the long-term management of patients with pseudogout.[13]

Surgery

The major goals of various orthopaedic procedures are to relieve pain and to improve function.[5] Joint replacement, tendon repair, carpal tunnel release and synovectomy are some of the frequently employed measures in RA.[48] In OA, treatments include bunion resection, decompression of spinal roots, and total knee and hip replacements. Arthroscopic lavage of knees has been reported to improve symptoms, but has not been widely employed as a therapeutic measure. Age itself is neither a contraindication to surgery nor a predictor of poor results. Rather, the presence of concurrent medical problems such as heart failure and pulmonary disease contribute more to perioperative morbidity and outcome. The goals, indications and timing of surgery should be individualized depending on the patient's general health status, function impairment, degree of pain and rehabilitation potential.[49]

In summary, arthritis is a common condition among the aged. The most common type is OA and the most common inflammatory process is RA. Optimal management includes physical therapy and medication, possibly combined with surgery, if necessary. Treatment modalities should be offered sometimes to accommodate age-related changes, and body mechanics and function. The long-term medical management of arthritis in the elderly requires close monitoring for potential adverse effects of medications.

Key points

- Arthritis is a common chronic condition among the aged.
- Osteoarthritis is the most common type.
- Rheumatoid arthritis is the most common inflammatory arthritis and can produce long-term morbidity if not treated aggressively.
- There are more than one hundred types of arthritis affecting the elderly.
- Gout, pseudogout, or infectious arthritis can present as red, hot, swollen joints and only synovial fluid aspiration can differentiate.

References

1. DiCesare PE, Abramson SB, Samuels J. Pathogenesis of osteoarthritis. In: GS Firestein, RC Budd, ED Harris *et al.* (eds.), *Kelley's Textbook of Rheumatology*, 8th edn, Saunders Elsevier, Philadelphia, 2009, pp. 1525–46.
2. Felson DT. The epidemiology of osteoarthritis: Results from the Framingham Osteoarthritis Study. *Seminars in Arthritis and Rheumatism* 1990;**20**(Suppl):42–9.
3. Felson DT. Obesity and vocational and avocational overload of the joint as risk factors for osteoarthritis. *J Rheumatol* 2004; **31**(Suppl):2–5.
4. Sellam J, Bernbaum F. Clinical features of osteoarthritis. In: GS Firestein, RC Budd, ED Harris *et al.* (eds), *Kelley's Textbook of Rheumatology*, 8th edn, Saunders Elsevier, Philadelphia, 2009, pp. 1547–61.
5. Nesher G, Moore TL. Clinical presentation and treatment of arthritis in the aged. *Clin Geriatr Med* 1994;**10**:659–75.
6. Firestein GS. Etiology and pathogenesis of rheumatoid arthritis. In: GS Firestein, RC Budd, ED Harris *et al.* (eds), *Kelley's Textbook of Rheumatology*, 8th edn, Saunders Elsevier, Philadelphia, 2009, pp. 1035–86.
7. Rasch EK, Hirsch R. Paulose-Ram R, Hochberg MC. Prevalence of rheumatoid arthritis in persons 60 years of age and older in the United States. *Arthritis Rheum* 2003;**48**:917–26.
8. Nesher G, Moore TL, Zuckner J. Rheumatoid arthritis in the elderly. *J Am Geriatr Soc* 1991;**39**:284–94.
9. Deal CL, Meenan RF, Goldenberg DL. The clinical features of elderly-onset rheumatoid arthritis: A comparison with younger-onset disease of similar duration. *Arthritis Rheum* 1985;**28**:987–94.
10. Wortman RL. Gout and hyperuricemia. In: GS Firestein, RC Budd, ED Harris *et al.* (eds), *Kelley's Textbook of Rheumatology*, 8th edn, Saunders Elsevier, Philadelphia, 2009, pp. 1481–506.
11. Gohr C. In vitro models of calcium crystal formation. *Curr Opin Rheumatol* 2004;**16**:263–7.
12. Terkeltaub R. Diseases associated with articular deposition of calcium pyrophosphate dehydrate and basic calcium phosphate crystals. In: GS Firestein, RC Budd, ED Harris *et al.* (eds), *Kelley's Textbook of Rheumatology*, 8th edn, Saunders Elsevier, Philadelphia, 2009, pp. 1507–24.
13. Reginato AJ, Schumacher HR. Crystal associated arthritis. *Clin Geriatr Med* 1988;**4**:295–301.
14. Tassiulas IO, Boumpas DT. Clinical features and treatment of systemic lupus erythematosus. In: GS Firestein, RC Budd, ED Harris *et al.* (eds), *Kelley's Textbook of Rheumatology*, 8th edn, Saunders Elsevier, Philadelphia, 2009, pp. 1263–300.
15. Boddaert J, Huong DL, Amaura Z. Late-onset systemic lupus erythematosus: A personal series of 47 patients and pooled analysis of 714 cases in the literature. *Medicine (Balt)* 2004;**83**:327–34.
16. Lalani S, Pope J, deLeon F *et al.* Clinical features and prognosis of late-onset systemic lupus erythematosus: Results from the 1000 faces of lupus study. *J Rheumatol* 2010;**37**:38–44.
17. Theander E, Manthorpe R, Jacobsson LTH. Mortality and causes of death in primary Sjögren's syndrome. *Arthritis Rheum* 2004;**50**:1262–9.
18. von Mühlen CA, Tan EM. Autoantibodies in the diagnosis of systemic rheumatic diseases. *Seminars in Arthritis and Rheumatism* 1995;**24**:323–58.
19. Illei GG, Tackey E, Lapteva L, Lipsky PE. Biomarkers in systemic lupus erythematosus. I. General overview of biomarkers and their applicability. *Arthritis Rheum* 2004;**50**:1709–20.
20. Illei GG, Tackey E, Lapteva L, Lipsky PE. Biomarkers in systemic lupus erythematosus. II. Markers of disease activity. *Arthritis Rheum* 2004;**50**:2048–65.
21. Rubin RL. Etiology and mechanisms of drug-induced lupus. *Curr Opin Rheumatol* 1999;**11**:357–63.
22. Brogan BL, Olsen NJ. Drug-induced rheumatic syndromes. *Curr Opin Rheumatol* 2003;**15**:76–80.
23. Ho GH, Siraj DS, Cook PP. Bacterial arthritis. In: GS Firestein, RC Budd, ED Harris *et al.* (eds), *Kelley's Textbook of Rheumatology*, 8th edn, Saunders Elsevier, Philadelphia, 2009, pp. 1701–14.
24. Vincent GM, Amirault JD. Septic arthritis in the elderly. *Clin Orthop Relat Res* 1990;**251**:241–60.
25. Coutlakis PH, Roberts WN, Wise CM. Another look at synovial fluid leukocytosis and infection. *J Clin Rheumatol* 2002;**8**, 67–71.
26. Calkins E. Arthritis in the elderly. *Bull Rheum Dis* 1991; **40**:15–18.
27. Brandt KD, Doherty M, Raffa BB *et al.* Controversies and practical issues in management of osteoarthritis. *J Clin Rheumatol* 2003;**9**(Suppl 2):1–39.
28. Lozada CJ. Management of osteoarthritis. In: GS Firestein, RC Budd, ED Harris *et al.* (eds), *Kelley's Textbook of Rheumatology*, 8th edn, Saunders Elsevier, Philadelphia, 2009, pp. 1563–77.
29. Day R, Brooks P, Conaghan PG, Peterson M. Double blind, randomized, multicenter, parallel group study of the effectiveness and tolerance of intraarticular hyaluronan in osteoarthritis of the knee. *J Rheumatol* 2004;**31**:775–82.
30. Berg P, Olsson U. Intra-articular injection of hyaluronic acid of osteoarthritis of the hip: A pilot study. *Clin Exp Rheumatol* 2004;**22**:300–6.
31. Johnson AG, Day RO. The problems and pitfalls of NSAID therapy on the elderly. *Drugs and Aging* 1991;**1**:130–51.
32. Willkens RF. Making the most of antirheumatic drugs in older patients. *Musculoskel Med* 2004;**21**:317–32.
33. Baigent C, Patrono C. Selective cyclooxygenase 2 inhibitors, aspirin, and cardiovascular disease. *Arthritis Rheum* 2003; **48**:12–20.
34. Perazella MA, Tray K. Selective cyclooxygenase-2 inhibitors: a pattern of nephrotoxicity similar to traditional non-steroidal anti-inflammatory drugs. *Am J Med* 2001;**111**: 64–7.
35. Brune K, Hinz B. Selective cyclooxygenase-2 inhibitors: similarities and differences. *Scan J Rheumatol* 2004;**33**:1–6.
36. Nesher G, Moore TL. Recommendations for drug therapy of rheumatoid arthritis in the elderly patients. *Clinical Immunotherapeutics* 1996;**5**:341–50.
37. Smolen J. Practical management of rheumatoid arthritis patients treated with leflunomide. *J Rheumatol* 2004;**31**(Suppl 71):1–30.
38. Furst DE, Keystone EC, Fleischmann R *et al.* Updated consensus statement on biological agents for the treatment of rheumatic diseases. *Ann Rheum Dis* 2010;**61**(Suppl 1):2–29.

39. Ellerin T, Rubin RH, Weinblatt ME. Infections and anti-tumor necrosis factor α therapy. *Arthritis Rheum* 2003;**48**:3013–22.
40. Robinson WH, Genovese MC, Moreland MW. Demyelinating and neurologic events reported in association with tumor necrosis factor α antagonism. *Arthritis Rheum* 2001;**44**: 1977–83.
41. Brown SL, Green MH, Gershon SK, Edwards ET, Braun MM. Tumor necrosis factor antagonist therapy and lymphoma development. *Arthritis Rheum* 2002;**46**:3151–8.
42. Kremer JM, Westhovens R, Leon M *et al.* Treatment of rheumatoid arthritis by selective inhibition of T-cell activation with fusion protein CTLA4 Ig. *N Engl J Med* 2003;**349**: 1907–11.
43. Edwards JC, Szcecpanski L, Szechinski J, *et al.* Efficacy of B-cell-targeted therapy with rituximab in patients with rheumatoid arthritis. *N Engl J Med* 2004;**350**:2572–8.
44. Kuncl RW, Duncan G, Watson D. Colchicine myopathy and neuropathy. *N Engl J Med* 1987;**316**:1562–8.
45. Becker MA, Schumacher HR, MacDonald PA *et al.* Clinical efficacy and safety of successful long-term urate lowering with febuxostat or allopurinol in subjects with gout . *J Rheumatol* 2009;**36**:1273–82.
46. Chohan S, Becker MA. Update on emerging urate-lowering therapies . *Curr Opin Rheumatol* 2009;**21**:143–9.
47. Grattan SB, Scalopino KJ, Fye KH. Case of anakinra as a steroid sparing agent for gout inflammation . *Arthritis Care and Research* 2009;**61**:1268–70.
48. Sledge CB. Principles of reconstructive surgery. In: S Ruddy, ED Harris, CB Sledge (eds), *Kelley's Textbook of Rheumatology* , WB Saunders Co., Philadelphia, 2001, pp. 1699–788.
49. Rosandrich PA, Kelley JT, Conn DL. Perioperative management of patients with rheumatoid arthritis in the era of biologic response modifiers . *Curr Opin Rheumatol* 2004;**16**: 192–8.

SECTION 10

Endocrine and Metabolic Disorders

CHAPTER 95

Endocrinology of ageing

John E. Morley and Kim J. Moon

Saint Louis University School of Medicine and St Louis Veterans' Affairs Medical Center, St Louis, MO, USA

Introduction

Hormones flow from the ductless glands into the circulation and regulate the metabolism of the body, and with ageing there is a decline in the circulating levels of a number of hormones. Deficiency of some of these hormones produces symptoms and signs similar to the changes seen with ageing. This has led different authorities to suggest that ageing is due to an endocrinopause and that replacement of one or more hormones will result in a reversal of the ageing process. Thus, it has been claimed that the ageing process is due to the somatopause, adrenopause, menopause or andropause. However, hormonal replacement has been as likely to produce negative effects as it has to lead to rejuvenation. Ageing is also associated with changes at the receptor or postreceptor level that can alter hormonal responsiveness.

Hormonal regulation and ageing

Hormones are regulated by a classical negative feedback system. Each peripheral hormone is regulated by a central system consisting of the hypothalamic–pituitary unit. The hypothalamus produces releasing hormones (and occasionally inhibitory hormones) that create a feedforward system that regulates the pulsatility and the circadian rhythm of hormone release. These releasing hormones regulate the release of anterior pituitary hormones, which in return result in the release of endorgan hormones. The endorgan hormones then feed back at the pituitary and the hypothalamic level to inhibit further release of pituitary hormones (Figure 95.1). When disease occurs in the endorgan hormone, it leads to failure of the endorgan and, therefore, negative feedback with an increase in the pituitary hormone (HYPO-disease) or increased activity of the endorgan with suppression of pituitary hormone release (HYPER-disease). When this occurs, the disease is considered to be primary endorgan disease, for example, primary hypothyroidism. Alternatively, failure can occur in the hypothalamic–pituitary unit, leading to a decrease in both the pituitary and the endorgan hormone, and this is known as *secondary disease*, for example, secondary hypogonadism. Finally, excess production of either a hypothalamic releasing hormone or pituitary hormone can occur. An example of this central form of HYPER-disease would be Cushing syndrome.

Ageing has effects on all levels of the hypothalamic–pituitary–gonadal axis. The circadian rhythm is controlled by the suprachiasmatic nucleus, which feeds information to the hypothalamus. The hypothalamic releasing hormones are responsible for maintaining the pulsatility of hormone release, which is essential for optimal hormonal action. With ageing, the pulse generator leads not only to a decline in maximal hormone production, but also to an irregular or 'chaotic' production of hypothalamic releasing hormones. This is amplified at the pituitary level where there is a decrease in the ability to respond to the hypothalamic signal. In addition, the endorgan itself has decreased responsiveness to the stimulus from the pituitary hormone[1-4] (Figure 95.2).

In addition, changes in hormonal binding to its receptor and postreceptor responsiveness can also occur with ageing. An example is the posterior pituitary hormone, arginine vasopressin (AVP) or antidiuretic hormone (ADH). There is a decline in the renal responsiveness to AVP with ageing, which leads to an increase in basal secretion of AVP. A small further increase in AVP then puts the older person at high risk of developing hyponatraemia and syndrome of inappropriate ADH.[5] There is also an attenuation of the normal increase in AVP that occurs at night. This increase is important for reabsorption of fluid during sleep and, therefore, its attenuation with ageing leads to increasing nocturia.[6]

Classically, endocrinologists have interpreted circulating hormone levels in the absence of an understanding of the functioning of the receptor. This is becoming less acceptable, as was shown recently by the example of the

Principles and Practice of Geriatric Medicine, Fifth Edition. Edited by Alan J. Sinclair, John E. Morley and Bruno Vellas.

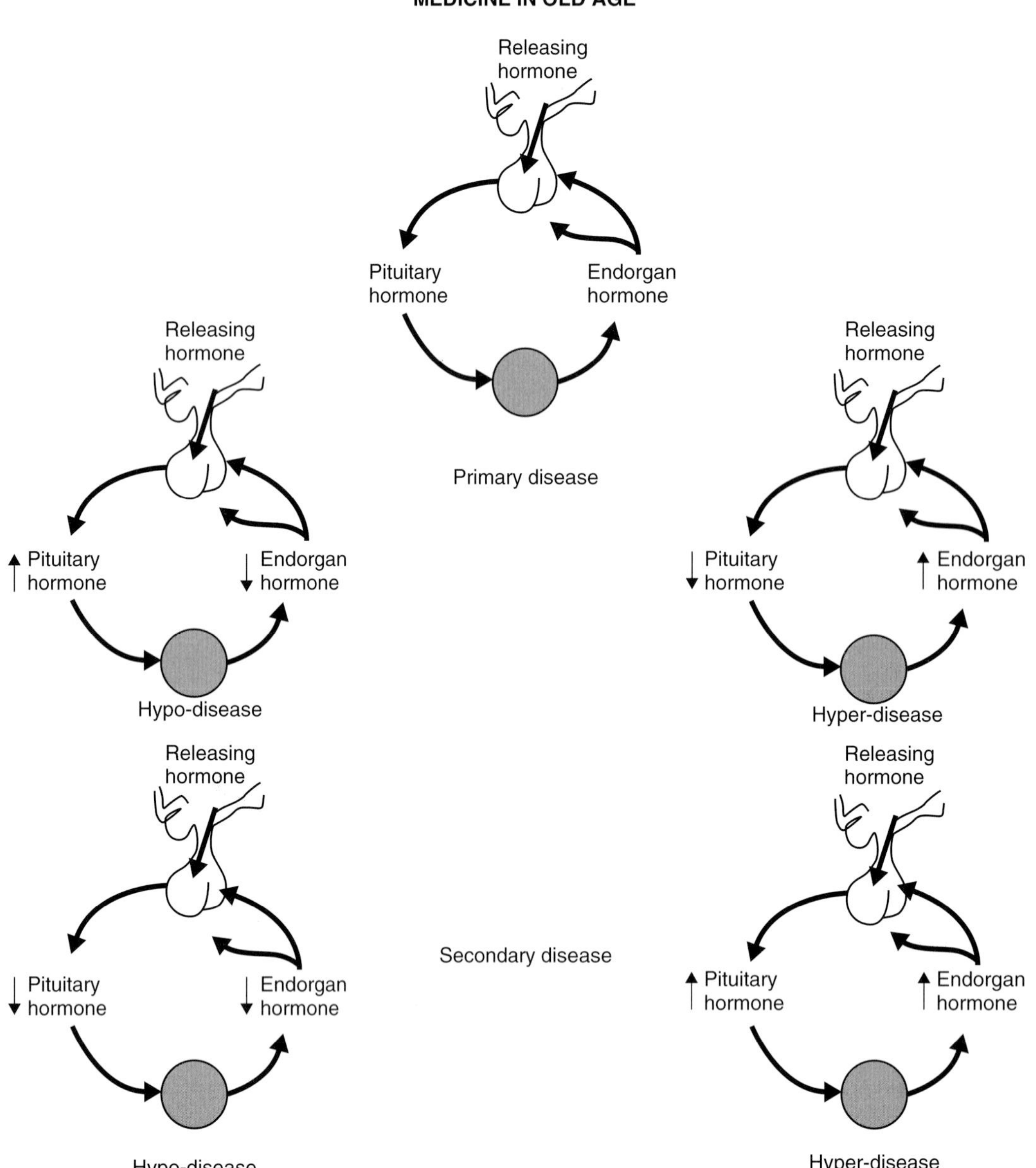

Figure 95.1 The normal hypothalamic–pituitary–endorgan and the effects of disease processes on it.

testosterone receptor and prostate cancer. The testosterone receptor contains a number of CAG repeats. The more the repeats, the less responsive the receptor is to testosterone. Prostate cancer occurs less often in males with a higher number of CAG repeats.[7]

Table 95.1 lists the hormonal changes seen with ageing. The levels of circulating hormones are determined by their production and clearance rates. Thus, the level of thyroxine remains normal because both the production and clearance rates decrease equally. Cortisol levels are slightly increased as there is a greater decrease in clearance rates. Cholecystokinin levels increase markedly due to the decline in clearance rate.[8]

It is generally believed that free hormone or tissue-available hormone levels determine the effectiveness of the hormone. Thus, in the case of testosterone in males, there is a marked increase in sex hormone binding globulin (SHBG) with ageing. The testosterone bound to SHBG is thought not to be available to tissues (Figure 95.3). The rest of the testosterone is free or bound to albumin, which is thought to be tissue available. Hence measurement of the bioavailable testosterone gives a more accurate reflection

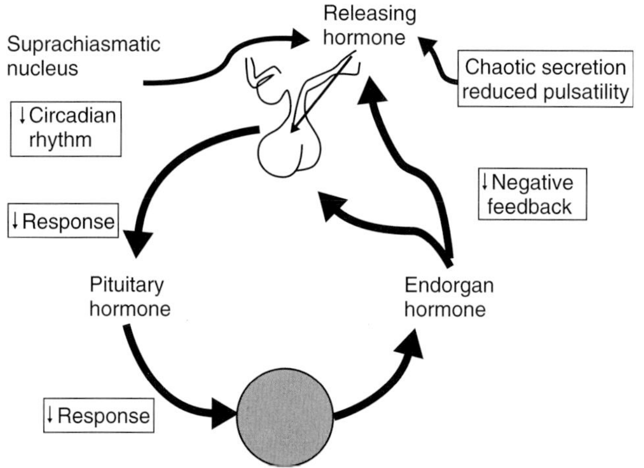

Figure 95.2 Effects of ageing on the hypothalamic–pituitary–endorgan axis.

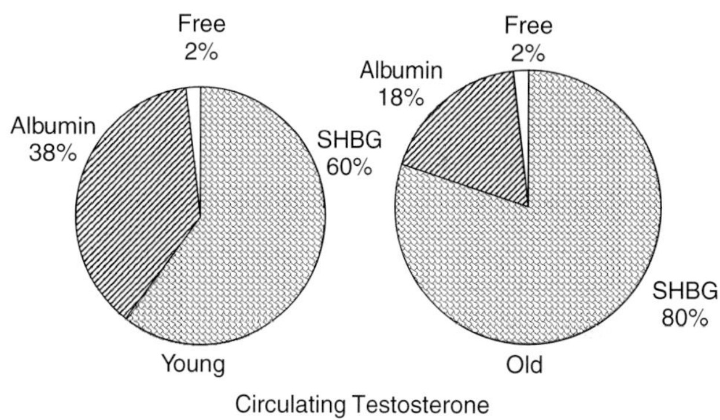

Figure 95.3 Effect of altered binding proteins with ageing on the effect of tissue-available hormones: the example of testosterone.

of the true testosterone level than does a total testosterone measurement.[9] Similarly, a number of growth hormone-binding proteins can produce marked changes in the ability of growth hormone to access its receptor.

Effects of ageing and related diseases on endocrine diseases

With ageing, there is a blurring of the boundaries between health and disease. The age-related decline in many hormone levels results in difficulties in making the biochemical diagnoses of endocrine disorders. The decreased functional reserve of endocrine organs that occurs with ageing increases the propensity for older persons to develop endocrine deficiency disorders. With ageing there is a decrease in T-suppressor lymphocytes and an increase in autoantibodies. Many endocrine disorders are due to autoimmune disease and these changes amplify the possibility of an older person developing hypoendocrine disease in old age. There is also an increased likelihood of the development of polyglandular failure syndromes.

The decline in receptor and postreceptor responsiveness that occurs with ageing often leads to atypical presentations. Apathetic thyrotoxicosis is due, in part, to the decreased postreceptor responsiveness for β-adrenergic receptors that occurs with ageing. The classical changes of apathetic thyrotoxicosis include depression, weight loss, atrial fibrillation, heart failure, blepharatosis and proximal myopathy. Apathetic thyrotoxicosis occurs only in about 7% of older persons with hyperthyroidism. The presentations of endocrine disease in older persons are further confused by the fact that they often present with non-specific symptoms, for example, delirium, fatigue, falls, weight loss, cognitive decline or depression. These symptoms are common in older persons and can lead to delayed diagnosis. For example, Addison's disease can present with weight loss, fatigue, abdominal pain, diarrhoea and hyponatraemia. The increase in cancer with ageing can lead to ectopic hormone production with an increase in endocrine disorders such as the syndrome of inappropriate ADH.

Table 95.1 Hormonal changes associated with ageing.

Decreased	Normal	Increased
Growth hormone	Estrogen (men)	ACTH
Insulin growth factor-1	Luteinizing hormone (men)	Cholecystokinin
Testosterone	Thyroxine	Insulin
Estrogen (women)	Pancreatic polypeptide	Amylin
Dehydroepiandrosterone	Gastric inhibitory peptide	Luteinizing hormone (women)
Pregnenolone	TSH	FSH
Triiodothyronine	Glucagon-releasing peptide	Vasoactive intestinal peptide
25-(OH)-vitamin D	Epinephrine	Cortisol
1,25-$(OH)_2$-vitamin D	Prolactin	Parathyroid hormone
Aldosterone		Norepinephrine
Calcitonin		Glucagon

Polypharmacy is common among older persons. This can lead to (1) interference with hormonal and metabolic measurements, for example, vitamin C interferes with the measurement of glucose; (2) altered circulating hormone levels, for example, phenytoin and thyroxine; (3) decreased hormonal responsiveness, for example, spironolactone and aldosterone; (4) altered requirement for appropriate hormonal replacement dose, for example, rifampin increases the thyroxine replacement dose; (5) precipitation of latent disease, for example, thyrotoxicosis by iodine-containing medicines; (6) drug–hormone interaction, for example, coumadin and oral hypoglycaemics to produce hypoglycaemia; (7) production of metabolic abnormalities, for example, vitamin A in megadoses produces hypercalcaemia; (8) poor compliance with endocrine replacement therapies; and (9) adverse drug reactions.

Hypothyroidism represents a classical example of an endocrine condition that has major overlap with symptoms commonly seen in older persons. These include cold intolerance, slowed pulse, constipation, fatigue, cognitive changes, erectile dysfunction, dry skin, dry, brittle hair and high blood pressure.

There are a number of endocrine disorders that occur virtually exclusively in older persons. These include osteoporosis, andropause, Paget's disease and endothelin-induced hypertension.

Insulin resistance syndrome and ageing

There is increasing awareness that insulin resistance syndrome is a cause of an accelerated ageing process.[10] This condition is produced by a genetic propensity interacting with overeating and lack of exercise, that is, the couch potato syndrome (Figure 95.4). It is classically associated with visceral obesity, that is, an increase in intra-abdominal fat. This leads to an increased production of tumour necrosis factor α and leptin and a decrease in adiponectin (a hormone that decreases insulin resistance). The insulin resistance syndrome consists of hyperinsulinaemia, diabetes mellitus, hypertension, hyperuricaemia, hypertriglyceridaemia, hypercholesterolaemia, increased small, dense low-density lipoprotein (LDL) molecules, alterations in coagulation status, myosteatosis (fat infiltration into muscle), cognitive decline and non-alcoholic steatohepatitis. Hypertriglyceridaemia is a key in the development of the myosteatosis and the cognitive decline. Persons with insulin resistance have an increased incidence of myocardial infarction and stroke. The insulin resistance syndrome is associated with frailty, disability and increased mortality.

Recent studies have suggested that a major component of the pathogenesis of the insulin resistance syndrome is accumulation of triglycerides and free fatty acids within muscle cells. This can occur either because of a failure of mitochondria leading to decreased utilization of intracellular fatty acids (primary syndrome) or because of excess circulating triglycerides and fatty acids (secondary syndrome). Accumulation of fatty acids within the cell leads to decreased activity of the insulin receptor substrate and, therefore, a decrease in GLUT-transporter activity.[13]

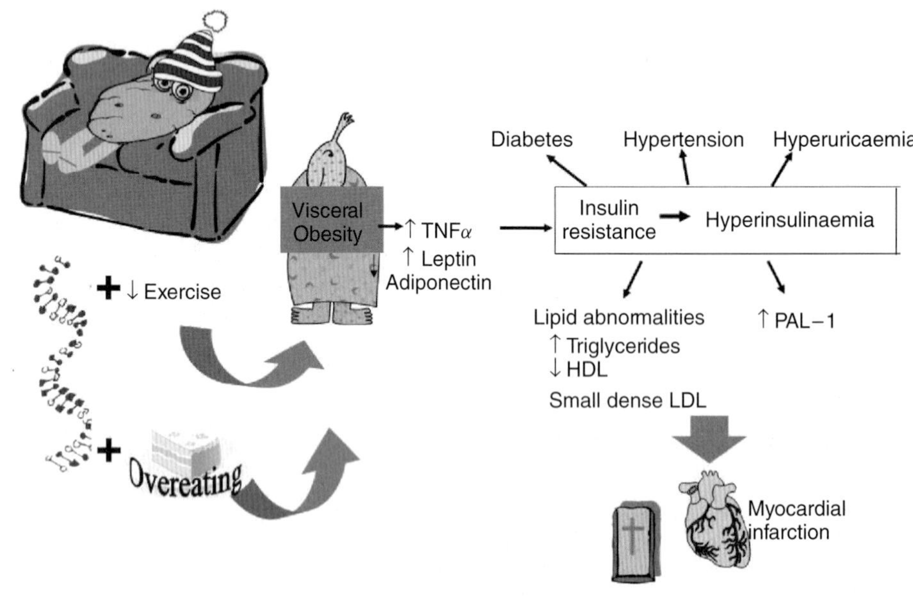

Figure 95.4 Metabolic syndrome: the deadly quintet.[11,12]

The hormonal fountain of youth

The parallel decline of many hormones with ageing and age-related symptoms has led to the suggestion that the hormonal decline may be a central component in the pathogenesis of ageing.[14] Unfortunately, with the exception of the role of vitamin D in age-related loss of bone mineral density, there is little evidence to support this premise. In this section, each of the hormones that have been suggested to play a role in the ageing process will be briefly discussed.

Vitamin D

Vitamin D has been shown in a longitudinal study to decline with ageing.[15] There is clear evidence that vitamin D (800 IU) together with calcium decreases the rate of hip fracture in older persons.[16] This is associated with a decline in mortality. Vitamin D replacement in persons who have clear vitamin D deficiency improves muscle strength and decreases falls.[17,18] Vitamin D deficiency is associated with increased mortality. Vitamin D deficiency should be suspected in any older person with a borderline low calcium level and an elevated alkaline phosphatase. Increased exposure to sunlight may be as efficacious as vitamin D replacement in increasing vitamin D levels. However, there is some evidence that old skin when exposed to ultraviolet light is less effective than young skin at manufacturing cholecalciferol. Ideally, vitamin D levels should be 30 ng dl^{-1} or greater.

Testosterone

Testosterone levels decline in both males and females with ageing. The effects of testosterone replacement in males and females with ageing is shown in Table 95.2. Testosterone replacement at relatively high doses in older males has been shown to increase muscle mass, strength, functional status and bone mineral density.[4,19] Testosterone increases libido in both males and females. In males, testosterone increases erectile strength, volume of ejaculation and visuospatial cognition. The major side effect is an excessive increase in haematocrit. The effects of long-term testosterone replacement on benign prostate hypertrophy and prostate cancer are unclear at present. Testosterone can cause gynaecomastia, produce water retention and may worsen sleep apnoea in a few individuals. The lack of long-term safety data for testosterone is a major concern. At present, testosterone should be considered a quality of life drug in both men and perhaps women (see Chapter 9, Sexuality and ageing; Chapters 99 and 100, Ovarian and testicular function). The development of selective androgen receptor modulators (SARMs) is under way in an attempt to avoid some of the potential side effects of testosterone. Nandrolone has been shown to be a potent anabolic agent in older persons.

Table 95.2 Effects of testosterone in older males and in postmenopausal females.

Older males	Postmenopausal females
Increased muscle mass	Increased muscle mass
Increased strength	Increased bone mineral density
Increased function	Increased libido
Increased bone mineral density	Decreased mastalgia
Increased haematocrit	
Increased visuospatial cognition	
Increased libido	
Increased strength of erection	
Increased volume of ejaculation	

Table 95.3 Lessons from growth hormone studies in older persons.

Growth hormone increases nitrogen retention
Growth hormone produces weight gain
Growth hormone increases muscle mass
Growth hormone possibly increases type-II muscle fibres
Growth hormone does not increase strength
Growth hormone is associated with multiple side effects
Growth hormone may improve function in malnourished older persons

Growth hormone

The concept that growth hormone may be able to rejuvenate older men was given impetus by a publication by Rudman *et al.*[20] in the *New England Journal of Medicine*. Unfortunately, since this original publication, numerous studies have failed to demonstrate any major positive effects of growth hormone (Table 95.3).[21] In addition, growth hormone has been shown to have a variety of side effects when administered for more than 3 months to older persons. There is some evidence that growth hormone may improve weight gain and function in malnourished older persons.[22,23]

Studies in animals have suggested that growth hormone-deficient animals live longer than growth hormone-sufficient animals.[24] Administration of a growth hormone-releasing hormone antagonist increased lifespan in older animals. In addition, in a human study, persons with the highest levels of growth hormone had the highest mortality rate. At present, there is no evidence to support the use of growth hormone to slow ageing or improve the quality of life of older persons.

Insulin growth factor-1 (IGF-1)

Insulin growth factor-1 (IGF-1) is produced in peripheral tissues in response to growth hormone. In human studies, it has tended to produce hypoglycaemia and minimal positive effects. In animals, it accelerates the growth of tumour cells.

Table 95.4 Ghrelin and ageing.

Ghrelin is produced in the fundus of the stomach
Ghrelin is slightly decreased with ageing
Ghrelin increases food intake
Ghrelin releases growth hormone from pituitary
Ghrelin increases body mass
Ghrelin enhances memory
Ghrelin produces its food and growth hormone effects through nitric oxide synthase stimulation
MK-771 (a ghrelin agonist) had minimal effects in older humans

In muscle, three different forms of IGF are produced, one of which is mechanogrowth factor (MGF). MGF levels increase in response to resistance exercise. Stem cell replacement of MGF has reversed the muscle atrophy seen in older rats.

Ghrelin

Ghrelin is produced in the fundus of the stomach and released into the circulation. It causes the release of growth hormone and increases food intake (Table 95.4). MK-771, a ghrelin analogue, while increasing growth hormone, has failed to produce major positive effects in older humans. Some studies have suggested that ghrelin agonists may be effective in frail older persons.

Dehydroepiandrosterone (DHEA)

Dehydroepiandrosterone (DHEA) is an adrenal hormone whose levels decline markedly with ageing. It has been touted as the 'mother hormone' by anti-ageing charlatans. DHEA has remarkable effects on the immune system and cognition in rodents. Unfortunately, a year-long study of 50 mg showed no effects on muscle mass or strength and only a small increase in libido in women over 70 years of age and some positive effects on the skin.[25-27] It may have some small effects on insulin resistance. At doses of 100 mg, it has been reported to have effects on humans, but at this dose it is converted into substantial amounts of circulating testosterone.

Pregnenolone

Pregnenolone is produced by the adrenals from cholesterol. It is the true 'mother hormone' as it is the precursor of DHEA. In mice, it is the most potent memory enhancer yet to be discovered.[28] Unfortunately, it has not been shown to have positive effects in humans.

Estrogen

Estrogens were originally touted as hormones that would make women 'feminine forever'. The Women's Health Initiative (WHI) has shown that premarin in older postmenopausal women increases breast cancer, pulmonary embolism, heart disease and Alzheimer's disease while decreasing hip fracture and colon cancer.[29-31] Although there are still scientists pursuing a better (safer) estrogen which will have the positive effects in women without the negative effects, estrogens should be avoided in women over the age of 60 years at present. The use at the time of the menopause represents a quality of life decision. Women with premature menopause should be given hormone replacement therapy.

Melatonin

Melatonin is synthesized from tryptophan in the pineal gland. Melatonin levels increase at night and fall to very low levels during the day. Melatonin has been used with minor success to enhance sleep in older persons. It does not alter the normal sleep structure. It may have a role in the treatment of seasonal affective disorder. Extravagant claims for the utility of melatonin have been based primarily on animal studies and include life extension, enhanced immune function and decreased tumour growth. Studies in humans to support these claims are virtually non-existent. The rate of decline of melatonin with age is less than was originally thought.

Key points

- It has been suggested that multiple hormonal changes occur with ageing which may play a role in the pathophysiological process associated with ageing.
- Many hormones decline with ageing but their replacement does not necessarily reverse ageing effects.
- The role of melatonin and dehydroepiandrosterone in ageing is unknown.
- The insulin resistance syndrome can be considered a cause of the accelerated ageing process.
- Testosterone and other hormones may play a role in the treatment of sarcopenia, which is an important proximate occurrence in the development of functional decline in older persons.

References

1. Harman SM and Tsitouras PD. Reproductive hormones in aging men. I. Measurement of sex steroids, nasal luteinizing hormone and Leydig cell response to human chorionic gonadotropin. *J Clin Endocrinol Metab* 1980;**51**:35–40.

2. Veldhuis JD. Recent insights into neuroendocrine mechanisms of aging of the human male hypothalamic–pituitary gonadal axis. *J Androl* 1999;**20**:1–17.
3. Veldhuis JD and Bowers CY. Human GH pulsatility: an ensemble property regulated by age and gender. *J Endocrinol Invest* 2003;**26**:799–813.
4. Matsumoto AM. Andropause: clinical implications of the decline in serum testosterone levels with aging in men. *J Gerontol A Biol Sci Med Sci* 2002;**57**: M76–99.
5. Miller M, Morley JE and Rubenstein LZ. Hyponatremia in a nursing home population. *J Am Geriatr Soc* 1995;**43**:1410–3.
6. Moon G, Jin MH, Lee JG *et al.* Antidiuretic hormone in elderly male patients with severe nocturia: a circadian study. *BJU Int* 2004;**94**:571–5.
7. Linja MJ and Visakorpi T. Alterations of androgen receptor in prostate cancer. *J Steroid Biochem Mol Biol* 2004;**92**:255–64.
8. MacIntosh CG, Morely JE, Wishart J *et al.* Effect of exogenous cholecystokinin (CCK)-8 on food intake and plasma CCK, leptin and insulin concentrations in older and young adults: evidence for increased CCK activity as a cause of the anorexia of aging. *J Clin Endocrinol Metab* 2001;**86**:5830–7.
9. Morley JE, Patrick P and Perry HM III. Evaluation of assays available to measure free testosterone. *Metab Clin Exp* 2002;**51**:554–9.
10. Morley JE. The metabolic syndrome and aging. *J Gerontol A Biol Sci Med Sci* 2004;**59**:139–42.
11. Camus JP. Gout, diabetes, hyperlipemia: a metabolic trisyndrome. *Rev Rhum Mal Osteoartic* 1966;**33**:10–4 (in French).
12. Reaven GM. Role of insulin resistance in human disease (syndrome X): an expanded definition. *Annu Rev Med* 1993; **44**:121–31.
13. Lowell BB and Shulman GI. Mitochondrial dysfunction and type 2 diabetes. *Science* 2005;**307**:384–7.
14. Morley JE. Is the hormonal fountain of youth drying up ? *J Gerontol A Biol Sci Med Sci* 2004;**59**:458–60.
15. Perry HM III, Horowitz M, Morley JE *et al.* Longitudinal changes in serum 25-hydroxyvitamin D in older people. *Metab Clin Exp* 1999;**48**:1028–32.
16. Chapuy MC, Arlot ME, Delmas PD and Meunier PJ. Effect of calcium and cholecalciferol treatment for three years on hip fractures in elderly women. *BMJ* 1994;**308**:1081–2.
17. Bischoff-Ferrari HA, Dawson-Hughes B, Willett WC *et al.* Effect of vitamin D on falls: a meta-analysis. *JAMA* 2004;**291**:1999–2006.
18. Bischoff-Ferrari HA, Willett WC, Wong JB *et al.* Fracture preventions with vitamin D supplementation: a meta-analysis of randomized controlled trials. *JAMA* 2005;**293**:2257–64.
19. Page ST, Amory JK, Bowman FD *et al.* Exogenous testosterone (T) alone or with finasteride increases physical performance, grip strength and lean body mass in older men with low serum T. *J Clin Endocrinol Metab* 2005;**90**: 1502–10.
20. Rudman D, Feller AG, Nagraj HS *et al.* Effects of human growth hormone in men over 60 years. *N Engl J Med* 1990; **323**:1–6.
21. Morley JE. Growth hormone: fountain of youth or death hormone ? *J Am Geriatr Soc* 1999;**47**:1475–6.
22. Chu LW, Lam KS, Tam SC *et al.* A randomized controlled trial of low-dose recombinant human growth hormone in the treatment of malnourished elderly medical patients. *J Clin Endocrinol Metab* 2001;**86**:1913–20.
23. Kaiser FE, Silver AJ and Morley JE. The effect of recombinant human growth hormone on malnourished older individuals. *J Am Geriatr Soc* 1991;**39**:235–40.
24. Bartke A. Insulin resistance and cognitive aging in long-lived and short-lived mice. *J Gerontol A Biol Sci Med Sci* 2005; **60**:133–4.
25. Percheron G, Hogrel JY, Denot-Ledunois S *et al.* Double-blind placebo-controlled trial. Effect of 1-year oral administration of dehydroepiandrosterone to 60- to 80-year-old individuals on muscle function and cross-sectional area: a double-blind placebo-controlled trial. *Arch Intern Med* 2003; **163**:720–7.
26. Baulieu EE, Thomas G, Legrain S *et al.* Dehydroepiandrosterone (DHEA), DHEA sulfate and aging: contribution of the DHEAge study to a sociobiomedical issue. *Proc Natl Acad Sci USA* 2000;**97**:4279–84.
27. Berr C, Lafont S, Debuire B *et al.* Relationships of dehydroepiandrosterone sulfate in the elderly with functional, psychological and mental status and short-term mortality: a French community-based study. *Proc Natl Acad Sci USA* 1996;**93**:13410–5.
28. Flood JF, Morley JE, Roberts E *et al.* Memory-enhancing effects in male mice of pregnenolone and steroids metabolically derived from it. *Proc Natl Acad Sci USA* 1992;**89**:1567–71.
29. Sherwin BB. Estrogen and memory in women: how can we reconcile the findings ? *Horm Behav* 2005;**47**:371–5.
30. Goldzieher JW. Hormone replacement therapy and the women's health initiative: the emperor has no clothes. *Endocr Pract* 2004;**10**:448–9.
31. Seelig MS, Altura BM and Altura BT. Benefits and risks of sex hormone replacement in postmenopausal women. *J Am Coll Nutr* 2004;**23**: 482S–96S.

CHAPTER 96

Water and electrolyte balances in ageing

Stewart G. Albert
Saint Louis University School of Medicine, St Louis, MO, USA

Introduction

Water and volume homeostasis are under meticulous control through a complex interrelationship of the hypothalamus–posterior pituitary and the renin–angiotensin–adrenal axis.[1] The elderly, however, are at increased risk for both syndromes of hyponatraemia and hypernatraemia and these disorders are associated with further clinical complications.[2–4] It is therefore important to understand the physiology involved in normal water homeostasis, the potential problems associated with ageing and the possible therapeutic modalities to correct these disorders.

Normal physiology

There is dual control of water and serum osmolality.[1] The hypothalamus and posterior pituitary are involved in water retention and the renin–angiotensin–aldosterone axis is involved in sodium retention.

The supraoptic and paraventricular nuclei of the hypothalamus respond primarily to increases in serum osmolality with the release of vasopressin [antidiuretic hormone (ADH)] Figure 96.1a. The release of ADH is mediated through changes in an electrochemical gradient in these magnocellular neurons to maintain serum osmolality at $285 \pm 2\,\mathrm{mOsm\,kg^{-1}}$. These neurons are also under the influence of neurotransmitters, such as acetylcholine (i.e. through the vagus nerve, as described below), catecholamines, opioids and angiotensin. Small changes in osmolality allow for acute adjustment of serum ADH levels with resulting water retention or free water clearance in the kidney.[1]

There is also a parallel autonomic nervous system regulation of water retention in which vascular receptors respond to decreases in total body water and changes in organ perfusion. There are high-pressure (blood pressure) baroreceptors in the carotid sinus and aortic arch and low-pressure stretch receptors in the cardiac atria and pulmonary venous systems. Both types of receptors transmit regulatory impulses via the vagus nerve to the hypothalamic neurons to stimulate ADH in the event of low effective arterial blood volume (EABV).[1] Pathophysiological states of diminished EABV will stimulate the release of ADH above that due to osmolality. Thus ADH may be 'appropriate' for the diminished EABV, but appears inappropriate for serum osmolality. Conditions which may increase ADH release are shown in Figure 96.1b. The baroreceptors may respond to changes in blood pressure associated with volume loss (gastrointestinal losses or diuretic-induced volume loss), decreased intravascular volume in hypoalbuminaemic oedema-forming states (ascites or nephrotic syndrome), orthostatic hypotension (due to adrenal cortical insufficiency, mineralocorticoid insufficiency or autonomic neuropathy) and decreased arterial perfusion (due to reduced cardiac output such as cardiac tamponade, cardiomyopathy or severe hypothyroidism). Decreased stretch of the volume receptors in the cardiac left atrium may occur in states of low EABV as described above. Diminished stretch in these receptors may also 'appear' as low pressure due to restrictions in pulmonary vascular return to the heart, as a result of increased intra-thoracic pulmonary pressure in severe reactive airway disease or with mechanical ventilation.[1]

Vasopressin activates V2 receptors in the distal collecting tubule of the kidney (Figure 96.2). In the absence of ADH, the tubule is impermeable to water transport. As shown in Figure 96.2, 15–30 l per day of free water may reach the distal collecting tubule. The entire volume may potentially be lost through the urine in central diabetes insipidus (lack of renal concentration ability due to either partial or complete ADH deficiency). In the presence of ADH, water is transported from the intraluminal collecting duct through aquaphorin-2 channels, across a concentration gradient to the intra-renal capillaries to reabsorb free water. The concentration gradient is derived at the loop of Henle through the medullary urea countercurrent system. The urea is freely permeable into the collecting duct. In the presence

Principles and Practice of Geriatric Medicine, Fifth Edition. Edited by Alan J. Sinclair, John E. Morley and Bruno Vellas.

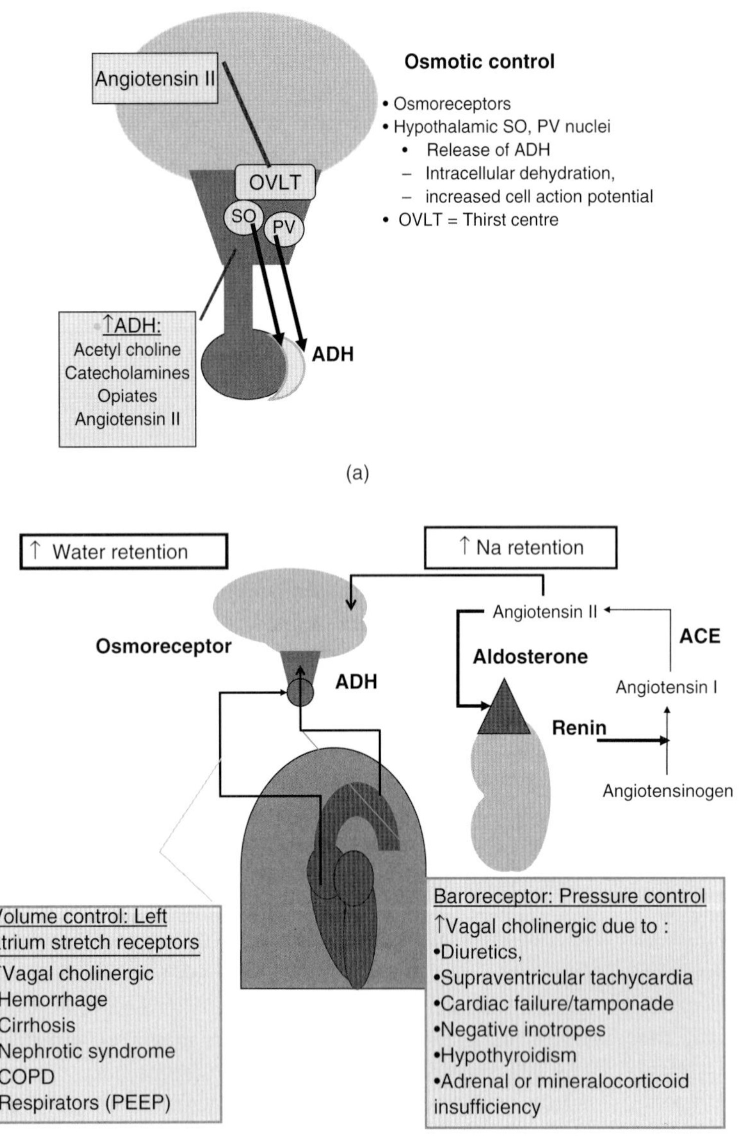

Figure 96.1 (a) Osmotic control of water balance. The hypothalamus supraoptic (SO) and paraventricular (PV) nuclei release antidiuretic hormone (ADH) through neural tracts to the posterior pituitary. Thirst is under control of a closely located series of hypothalamic neurons in the organum vasculosum of the lamina terminalis (OVLT). (b) Pressure–volume control of water and sodium balance. Baroreceptors (systemic blood pressure) in the aortic arch and volume receptors in the atria respond to changes in effective arterial blood volume (EABV) to induce release of ADH through vagal stimuli. Decreased intrarenal perfusion induces renin activation of the renin–angiotensin-aldosterone system to increase sodium retention.

of ADH, the kidney may concentrate the urine to a volume of 0.7 l per day with an osmolality of 600–1200 mOsm kg^{-1}, made up primarily of the secreted urea.

Thirst, the conscious desire to drink, is another active component of water retention.[1,5] Thirst is under control of a closely located series of hypothalamic neurons in the organum vasculosum of the lamina terminalis (OVLT). This area is independent of the blood–brain barrier. These neurons, like the ADH-secreting neurons, are under a similar influence of serum osmolality, neurotransmitters and angiotensin. Normally thirst lags ADH release in response to increases in serum osmolality. The threshold of thirst, as measured on a visual analogue scale or the volume of water ingested, is ~10 mOsm kg^{-1} greater than the ADH threshold.[5] There are pathological conditions in which thirst may be independent of ADH release. Thirst is inappropriately diminished in response to serum osmolality in central nervous system conditions characterized by a reset or diminished thirst response to serum osmolality (essential hypernatraemia) or in complete lack of thirst response to severe hypernatraemia (adipsia) (Figure 96.3).[5]

Whereas ADH is the main hormone involved in water homeostasis, the renin–angiotensin–aldosterone system is the main factor in sodium retention and systemic blood pressure/volume control. Renin is released from the juxtaglomerular apparatus of the kidney in response to low perfusion, low intravascular volume and low tubular sodium. Renin is an enzyme which converts liver-derived angiotensinogen to angiotensin 1 and lung-derived angiotensin-converting enzyme further metabolizes conversion

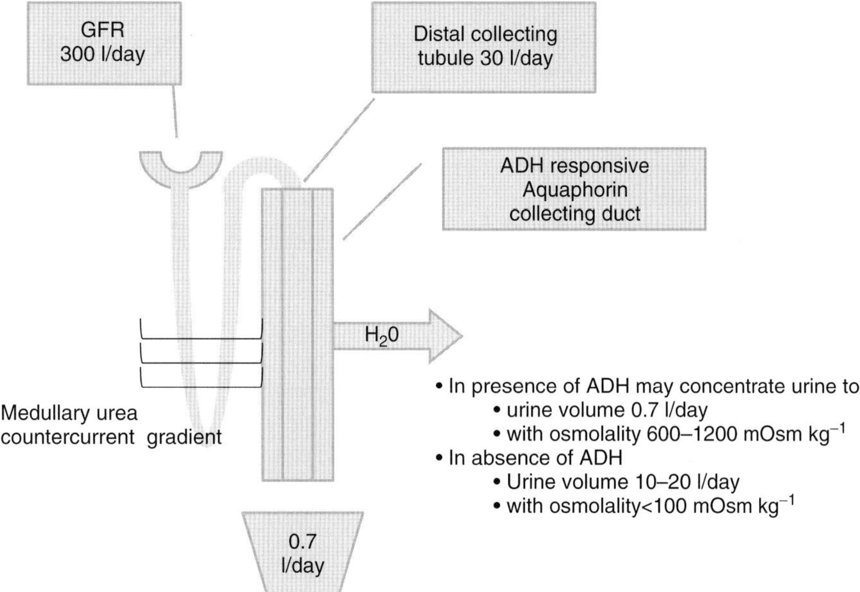

Figure 96.2 Renal action of ADH in water conservation.

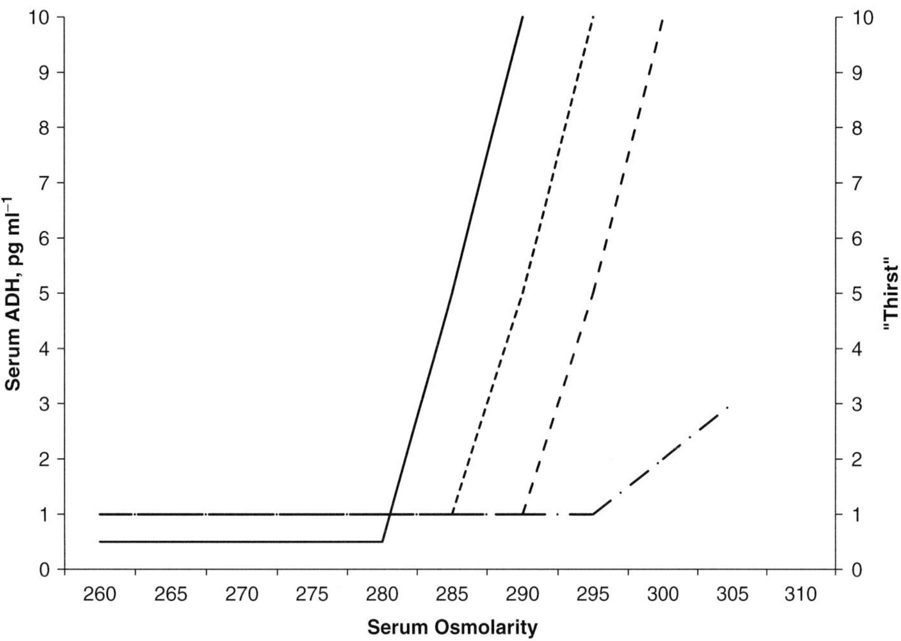

Figure 96.3 Comparisons of disorders of thirst. Serum ADH increases with serum osmolality at a threshold of 280 mOsm kg^{-1} (solid line). Thirst responses increase at approximately 5–10 mOsm kg^{-1} higher than that of ADH release (dotted line). Abnormally decreased thirst responses are found in essential hypernatreamia (dashed line) and severely impeded thirst responses are found in adipsia (dashed-dotted line).

to angiotensin 2. Angiotensin 2 both stimulates the release of the mineralocorticoid aldosterone to retain sodium and stimulates the hypothalamic neurons to release ADH and provoke thirst (Figure 96.1b).

Syndromes of hyponatraemia may reflect physiological 'appropriate' release of ADH in response to vagal stimuli due to decreased perfusion pressure or decreased plasma volume (decreased EABV). In these situations, the elevated ADH is inappropriate for the serum osmolality. The syndrome of inappropriate ADH secretion (SIADH) is a research definition which eliminates appropriate physiological ADH responses. The discussion of hyponatraemia includes both 'appropriate' and SIADH syndromes.

Hyponatraemia may be defined as a serum sodium level <135 mequiv l^{-1} and for clinically significant hyponatraemia <130 mequiv l^{-1}.[1] Aside from water intoxication associated with excessive water intake during exercise, most causes of hyponatraemia are associated with imbalances in ADH levels.[2–4,6] Clinical syndromes of hyponatraemia (and true hypo-osmolality) are associated with decreased effective serum osmolality,[7,8] where

$$\text{serum osmolarity} = (2 \times [\text{Na}], \text{mequiv l}^{-1}) + \frac{[\text{glucose}], \text{mg dl}^{-1}}{18} + \frac{[\text{BUN}], \text{mg dl}^{-1}}{2.8}$$

Serum concentrations of urea, which are included in the calculation of plasma osmolality, are not considered as part of the calculation of effective extracellular osmolality, since urea is freely permeable through cell membranes.

$$\text{effective serum osmolarity} = (2 \times [\text{Na}]) + \frac{[\text{glucose}]}{18}$$

Therefore, the major component of extracellular osmolality in the non-hyperglycaemic state is serum sodium with its corresponding anions. Severe clinically significant hyponatraemia is usually associated with serum sodium in the range <120 mequiv l^{-1} or with the rapid decline of serum sodium as in water intoxication or post-anaesthesiology hyponatraemia.[1,6] The major toxicities are due to changes in neurological functions (defined as hyponatraemic encephalopathy).[1,6] Symptoms may range from headache, nausea, disorientation and confusion to more severe symptoms of cerebral oedema with seizures, coma and, in extreme cases, cerebral tentorial herniation and death. Chronic hyponatraemia (which has developed over a time course of >48 h) usually results in central nervous system intracellular adaptation, with the extrusion of intra-neuronal organic and inorganic osmoles. During the treatment of symptomatic hyponatraemia, the concern therefore is that overly rapid correction of hyponatraemia (defined as an increase of >12 mequiv l^{-1} over 24 h or >18 mequiv l^{-1} over 48 h) may result in cerebral dehydration and pontine and extrapontine osmotic demyelination syndromes (ODS). These ODS may be delayed in onset and associated with severe neurological morbidity and mortality.[1,6]

Water homeostasis in the elderly

The elderly are prone to disorders of both hyper- and hyponatraemia.[1-6] These abnormalities may be due to the normal physiological changes in the ageing process, intercurrent illnesses or side effects of medications. Normal physiological changes due to ageing may result in a tendency towards hypernatraemia (sodium >145 mequiv l^{-1}).[4,5,9] Although renal function declines with age, fluid homeostasis is not affected by this decline until glomerular filtration rates are as low as 30–50 ml min^{-1}.[4] Compared with younger individuals subjected to water deprivation, healthy older adults have decreased thirst responses and increased serum ADH levels, but decreased urinary concentration and ability to excrete free water.[10,11] The decreased responsiveness of aquaporin-2 to ADH may be due to a physiological decreased aquaporin-2 receptor expression associated with ageing.[12] Also, after age 75 years there is a decrease in total body water from 60 to 50%, potentiating the risk for dehydration over short periods of time.[4]

The institutionalized elderly may be more prone to hypernatraemia.[9,13] Whereas normal elderly patients subjected to fluid restriction may have a decrease in thirst response compared with younger subjects, they retain their ability to secrete ADH. Those with Alzheimer's disease may be more severely compromised by having a more pronounced decrease in both thirst and ADH responses compared with even age-matched controls.[14] In patients with Alzheimer's disease, these thirst responses may fall in the range compatible with essential hypernatraemia[5] and the ADH levels may be inappropriately low for the degree of dehydration and comparable to levels found in states of partial central diabetes insipidus.[14] Unless patients are monitored, elderly institutionalized individuals dependent on caregivers for fluid intake (due to previous stroke or degenerative brain diseases) may not receive adequate fluids at or between meals.[13] These groups of people may have an 18% incidence of hypernatraemia.[5] The incidence of hypernatraemia may be exacerbated during acute intercurrent febrile upper respiratory illness to levels as high as 63%.[9] They may also have concurrent illnesses (such as hypercalcaemia or hypokalaemia) or be prescribed medications (such as lithium), all of which are associated with nephrogenic diabetes insipidus (renal insensitivity to ADH action) and inability to retain water.

Hyponatraemia is also very common in the elderly, as outpatients, inpatients and those in long-term care.[15,16] The prevalence of hyponatraemia among elderly outpatients is 7–11%[4] and for those in long-term care 11–53%.[2,3,15] The causes of hyponatraemia are less clearly defined than for hypernatraemia. There are physiological changes in the kidneys with ageing resulting in a decreased ability to concentrate urine and to excrete free water.[11,17] However, the onset of hyponatraemia may be associated with medication or responses to concomitant illnesses.[15,16] Many medications involved in central nervous system modulation and opioid transmission are associated with ADH secretion. Common agents associated with hyponatraemia in all people include antidepressants (both tri- and tetracyclics), antipsychotic drugs (phenothiazines, butyrophenones), antiepileptic drugs (carbamazepine, oxcarbazepine, sodium valproate) and opioids.[18] The elderly appear to be more sensitive to the hyponatraemic effects of selective serotonin reuptake inhibitors (SSRIs).[19] Diuretics, owing to their frequent use, are probably the most common medication associated with hyponatraemia, with a prevalence as high as 11% in the geriatric population.[18] Less commonly, other antihypertensive agents such as angiotensin-converting enzyme inhibitors and calcium channel antagonists produce a decrease in effective arterial blood volume (EABV) with physiologically 'appropriate' increases in ADH.[18] True SIADH syndromes, due to ectopic ADH production by cancer or inappropriate ADH due to neurological lesions, are less likely to be the cause of hyponatraemia unless there are positive clinical features. Among 50 elderly hospitalized patients with mild to moderate hyponatraemia, an exhaustive evaluation did not reveal these causes of inappropriate ADH syndrome. The investigators found that the hyponatraemia was associated with pneumonia and medication, although 60% remained idiopathic.[16]

Many patients may have primary orthostatic hypotension, for example, due to autonomic neuropathy in Parkinson's disease and multiple system atrophy or associated with low renin–low aldosterone mineralocorticoid deficiency. Older patients may have excessive treatment of their hypertension. The elderly should be monitored for orthostatic blood pressure changes and have more moderate adjustment of systolic hypertension than younger individuals.[20]

Other medications, not specifically used in the elderly, are associated with hyponatraemia. Antineoplastic agents include vincristine and cyclophosphamide. Vincristine may cause a hypothalamic neuropathy and cyclophosphamide treatment may potentiate an ADH effect at the renal tubule and requires patients to drink large volumes of water to prevent cystitis.[18] Uncommon causes of hyponatraemia associated with common drugs include non-steroidal anti-inflammatory drugs (NSAIDs), which may lower the levels of prostaglandins. Prostaglandins have an anti-ADH effect on the renal tubules, so lowered levels result in potentiated ADH action. Trimethoprim sulfamethoxazole may act as a mild diuretic and cause hyponatraemia if given in high doses or when given to a patient with renal impairment.[18]

Hyponatraemia is associated with a poor overall prognosis.[21] In a retrospective analysis of outpatient community subjects, there was a higher risk of death from cardiovascular disease associated with hyponatraemia.[21] It is not clear whether the hyponatraemia was causative of the increased mortality or whether the hyponatraemia was a comorbidity associated with an underlying congestive heart failure. Similarly, hyponatraemia was associated with gait disturbances, falls and bone fractures.[2,22] In a retrospective study of patients with bone fracture admitted after incidental falls, hyponatraemia was found in 13% of cases versus 4% of controls, $p < 0.0001$.[23] However, this study does not resolve the issue of assigning causality of the hyponatraemia with adverse events. Many of the patients with falls and hyponatraemia had higher incidences of underlying reasons for falls compared with controls. Those with hyponatraemia also were more frequently taking SSRIs (21% vs 15%, $p = 0.006$), benzodiazepines (39% vs 31%, $p = 0.007$) or other CNS class drugs (59% vs 49%, $p = 0.0004$), and had cognitive impairment (17% vs 7%, $p < 0.0001$) or orthostatic hypotension (6% vs 2%, $p = 0.003$). The simultaneous use of medications associated with neurocognitive impairment and hyponatraemia may explain the association of concurrence of hyponatraemia with the high rate of falls.

Therefore, it is important to assess the role of hyponatraemia within the context of a cause and effect relationship and to determine if the neurocognitive symptoms are reversible with correction of the hyponatraemia independent of correction of the underlying illness or of removal of potentially causative medications. Renneboog *et al.*[24] performed a retrospective analysis of patients admitted to an acute care hospital with serum sodium levels between 115 and 132 mequiv l^{-1}. Subjects were excluded from the analysis if they had heart failure, cirrhosis, nephrotic syndrome, acute polydipsic hyponatraemia or seizures and were compared with age- and sex-matched controls. In those with hyponatraemia there was a 21% incidence of falls compared with 5% in the controls ($p < 0.001$). The researchers then prospectively assessed eight subjects with hyponatraemia by tests for abnormalities in gait and cognition. The tests were compared prospectively when they had hyponatraemia (serum sodium $128 \pm 3\,\text{mequiv l}^{-1}$) and after correction of hyponatraemia ($138 \pm 2\,\text{mequiv l}^{-1}$). There were significant improvements after correction of hyponatraemia in abnormalities in gait (as determined through a standardized test of distance travelled by tandem gait on a pressure-sensitive calibrated platform). Direct linear gait improved (measured as a decrease in the total distance covered including erratic gait) from 1336 ± 320 mm vs 1047 ± 172 mm, $p = 0.003$. There were improvements in cognitive tests. determined by a decrease in reaction time on attention tests (from 673 ± 182 ms vs. 615 ± 184 ms, $p < 0.001$). Whether these improvements in neurocognitive functions were due to the correction of the hyponatraemia itself, the correction of the underlying illness or removal of the offending medication causing the hyponatraemia, was not determined.

It was therefore hoped that the issue of causation of mental status changes with hyponatraemia would be resolved by the correction of the hyponatraemia independent of modifications of either the underlying disease or medication adjustment. Prospective studies using vasopressin antagonists (see the discussion of vaptans below) have shown modest clinical benefits with correction of hyponatraemia. Tolvaptan, a specific vasopressin receptor antagonist, was assessed in a combined randomized prospective international multicentre study of 448 subjects, the SALT-1 (US cohort) and SALT-2 (international cohort). There was a statistically significant change in one component of a psychological profile test.[25] A planned analysis of scores on the Mental Component of the Medical Outcomes Study 12-item Short Form of the General Health Survey (SF-12) showed improvement. The SF-12, with a range of scores between 7 and 83 (with higher scores indicating better functioning), improved in the combined study, $p = 0.02$. However the changes were significant in the SALT-1 sub-study (US, baseline score 42.3 ± 11.7, treatment effect 3.9, $p = 0.04$) but not in the SALT-2 sub-study (international, baseline score 44.7 ± 12.0, treatment effect 2.2, $p = 0.15$). There were no changes in the physical component summary of the SF-12. The benefits in the SF-12 were more relevant in those with marked hyponatraemia (baseline serum sodium $<130\,\text{mequiv}\,l^{-1}$, $p = 0.04$).[25] Changes in the SF-12 were not considered in the primary outcome analysis and predesigned assessments of gait, balance or cognitive functions were not performed.

Workup and treatment of hyponatraemia

There may be a recognized history of excessive water intake which overwhelms the ability of the kidneys to clear free water, such as primary polydipsia (purposeful intake of 16–20 l of water per day), so-called beer potomania (beer intake of similar volumes) or excessive water intake during prolonged exercise (e.g. in long-distance runners). However, without that history, the usual cause of hyponatraemia is increased water retention, although there may be also a component of solute loss. Tests should be made on the serum for basal metabolic profile (BMP) and measured serum osmolality and on the urine for osmolality and sodium concentration. The BMP will help in the evaluation of acute renal disease (hyponatraemia due to acute tubular necrosis, renal obstruction) and in hyperosmolar pseudo-hyponatraemia due to hyperglycaemia. The serum osmolality will confirm hypo-osmolality (defined as $<275\,\text{mOsm}\,\text{kg}^{-1}$) and exclude conditions of pseudo-hyponatraemia due to excess lipids (triglycerides) or hyperosmolar hyponatraemia due to excess circulating osmoles from hyperglycaemia or elevated proteins (macroglobulinaemia). The urine osmolality is usually inappropriately elevated, namely $>100\,\text{mOsm}\,\text{kg}^{-1}$, and in many cases higher than the serum osmolality. The urine sodium is usually paradoxically elevated for the apparent serum sodium and is $>30\,\text{mequiv}\,l^{-1}$ and in many cases close to $100\,\text{mequiv}\,l^{-1}$. The cause of the paradoxical natriuresis is not completely understood and may be due to other factors such as elevations in cardiac derived atrial natriuretic peptide (ANP), cardiac or brain-derived brain natriuretic peptide (BNP) or may be due to a direct renal compensatory effect to maintain constant intravascular volume despite hyponatraemia.[1]

The evaluation of hypo-osmolar hyponatraemia should then focus on secondary causes of elevated ADH levels. Decreased effective arterial blood volume (EABV) may be associated with physiologically appropriate elevations in ADH levels which may be inappropriate for serum osmolality. These elevated ADH levels may be corrected by treating the underlying condition. The history and physical examination will help in the determination of volume depletion states (gastrointestinal losses, diuretic losses), low effective arterial blood volume states (orthostatic hypotension due to either primary or secondary adrenocortical insufficiency, hypo-reninaemic hypoaldosteronism), autonomic neuropathic hypotension (Parkinson's disease, multiple system atrophy) or drug-induced states (diuretics, angiotensin-converting enzyme inhibitors, calcium channel blockers). In diuretic-induced hyponatraemia, the urinary sodium is usually in a lower range ($<20\,\text{mequiv}\,l^{-1}$) due to the sodium-retaining effect of secondary hyperaldosteronism. Oedema states are those with decreased EABV with hypoalbuminaemia (e.g. cirrhosis, nephrotic syndrome) or decreased perfusion to the carotid baroreceptors resulting from congestive heart failure, cardiac tamponade, negative cardiac inotrophic medications and possibly poor cardiac contractility associated with hypothyroidism. All medications should be reviewed for their potential to cause hyponatraemia (Figure 96.4). Further workup should include evaluation for hypothyroidism (serum TSH) and for both primary and secondary adrenal insufficiency (by cosyntropin stimulation testing).

Other causes of hyponatraemia and more specifically SIADH syndrome include tumours: bronchogenic carcinoma, thymoma; central nervous system lesions: tumours, subarachnoid haemorrhage, neurosurgical procedures; cerebral salt wasting (a possible variant of SIADH syndrome due to acute central nervous system trauma or surgery, associated with hyponatraemia, hypotension and urinary sodium loss); pulmonary disease associated with increased intrathoracic pressure, COPD, positive pressure ventilation; and HIV–AIDS syndromes (which may be associated with relative adrenal or mineralocorticoid insufficiency).

The decision to treat the hyponatraemia depends on the symptoms of neurocognitive dysfunction. Those with serum sodium between 130 and $135\,\text{mequiv}\,l^{-1}$ are usually asymptomatic. If chronic, the hyponatraemia may have allowed time for the development of central nervous system compensation and may not require any therapy. Symptoms of gait disturbances and cognitive impairment found in patients with serum sodium between 125 and $130\,\text{mequiv}\,l^{-1}$ have been shown to improve with correction of hyponatraemia.[24,25] Review and withholding of possible

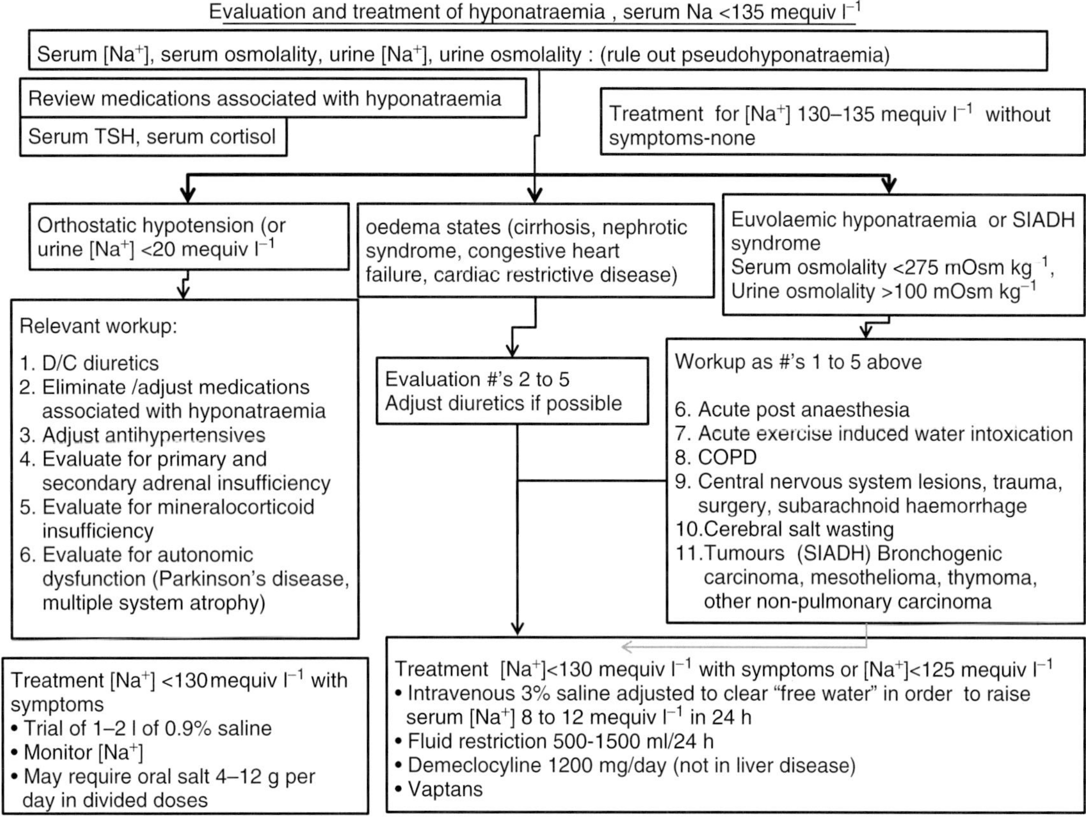

Figure 96.4 Algorithm of workup and therapy for hyponatraemia.

causative medications may be of benefit. Correction of hypothyroidism and hypoadrenalism is mandatory.

If there is orthostatic hypotension or low urine sodium (<20 mequiv l^{-1}), it is presumed that the hyponatraemia is secondary to 'appropriate' physiological vagal stimulation due to low EABV. If the hyponatraemia is diuretic induced, withholding of diuretics or a trial of 1–2 l of intravenous 0.9% saline may partially reverse the hyponatraemia. Usually 0.9% saline will have no effect on a true SIADH syndrome, as the sodium infused is quantitatively lost and the water is retained. If the orthostatic hypotension is due to antihypertensive treatment with excessive blood pressure reduction beyond requirements for the elderly, readjustment of the medication should be performed. If the orthostasis is due to autonomic neuropathy (Parkinson's disease, multiple system atrophy), then cautious use of oral salt 4–8 g per day along with antigravity support stockings may help to correct the underlying low EABV.

Those with serum sodium levels <125 mequiv l^{-1} or with symptoms will need therapy. There are controversies regarding the various protocols for correction of the hyponatraemia as none have been validated in comparative studies.[8] It is agreed that there are two major complications which should be avoided: (1) cerebral oedema due to the delay in correction of hyponatraemia and (2) osmotic demyelination syndrome due to overly rapid correction of the hyponatraemia. The former may occur during states of acute hyponatraemia, that is, in rare occurrences in women or children after general anaesthesia, in athletes with exercise-associated hyponatraemia (over ingestion of water relative to salt loss associated with sweating during prolonged running) or in patients after neurological surgery or subarachnoid haemorrhage.[6] In these situations, delayed correction of serum sodium of only 3–4 mequiv l^{-1} over 24 h has been associated with deteriorating mental state due to cerebral oedema.[6] The osmotic demyelination syndrome, however, occurs due to overly rapid correction of serum sodium, defined as >12 mequiv l^{-1} over 24 h or >18 mequiv l^{-1} over 48 h.

Fluid restriction is indicated for symptomatic euvolaemic and hypervolaemic hyponatraemia and contraindicated in hypovolaemic hyponatraemia. In hypovolaemic hyponatraemia, for example when the hypo-osmolality is due to diuretic or gastrointestinal volume losses, the serum aldosterone and ADH levels are elevated due to physiological responses to the decreased EABV. Infusion of 0.9% saline or the addition of oral salt will correct the serum sodium, since the elevated aldosterone will retain sodium and the increased EABV will lower ADH levels. Infusion of 0.9% saline solution is usually ineffective for euvolaemic and hypervolaemic hyponatraemia because the hyponatraemia may actually worsen as the infused sodium is quantitatively lost in the urine and the elevated levels of ADH will cause water retention.

In euvolaemic or hypervolaemic hyponatraemia, total fluid restriction between 500 and 1500 ml per day may be required. Symptomatic hyponatraemia with serum sodium $<120\,\text{mequiv}\,l^{-1}$ usually requires correction with intravenous sodium. The concept is to eliminate presumed excess water and restore fluid balance (assuming non-solute losses).[7,8] The treatment plan is to remove a calculated proportion of the free water excess over 24 h to accommodate an increase in serum sodium of $8–12\,\text{mequiv}\,l^{-1}$ and not to correct the serum sodium completely to normal. The formula uses an approximation of for total body water (TBW):

$$\frac{\text{change in free water}}{24\,\text{h}} = TBW \times \left(\frac{[\text{Na}]_{\text{goal}}}{[\text{Na}]_{\text{current}}} - 1\right)$$

where

$$TBW = 0.6 \times (\text{body weight, kg}) \text{ for individuals } < 75\text{years old}$$

or

$$TBW = 0.5 \times (\text{body weight, kg}) \text{ for individuals } > 75 \text{ years old}$$

and

$$[\text{Na}]_{\text{goal}} = [\text{Na}]_{\text{current}} + 10\,\text{mequiv}\,l^{-1}$$

Recommendations for the correction of symptomatic hyponatraemia are therefore made using 3% ($513\,\text{mequiv}\,l^{-1}$) saline solutions. Various protocols have been described,[7,8] although none have been validated or compared with the others. One method is to measure an hourly urine sodium loss in $\text{mequiv}\,h^{-1}$:

$$\frac{\text{urine volume }(\text{ml}\,h^{-1}) \times \text{urine }[\text{Na}^+]\,(\text{mequiv}\,l^{-1})}{1000\,\text{ml}\,l^{-1}}$$

and replace the sodium loss with the equivalent amount of hypertonic intravenous sodium to maintain a constant intravascular volume. For example, in a 70 kg patient less than 75 years old with a serum sodium of $110\,\text{mequiv}\,l^{-1}$ and with a goal of an increase in serum sodium to $120\,\text{mequiv}\,l^{-1}$ over 24 h, we would attempt to clear free water of $421 \times [(120/110) - 1)] = 3.8\,l$ per 24 h. If that person excretes $200\,\text{ml}\,h^{-1}$ of urine with a urine $[\text{Na}^+]$ concentration of $100\,\text{mequiv}\,l^{-1}$, then urine sodium losses per hour $= (200\,\text{ml} \times 100\,\text{mequiv}\,l^{-1})/(1000\,\text{ml}\,l^{-1}) = 20\,\text{mequiv}\,h^{-1}$. We would infuse 20 mequiv $[\text{Na}^+]$ per hour as 3% saline (40 ml of $513\,\text{mequiv}\,l^{-1}$ solution) with a net hourly loss of free water of (200 ml urine – 40 ml infused) of $-160\,\text{ml}\,h^{-1} = 3.8\,l$ per 24 h.

Alternatively, the 'traditional' correction method has been to calculate the 'theoretical' serum sodium deficit and replace that amount of sodium over 24 h using 3% saline, with the assumption that the infused sodium will re-equilibrate with intracellular water:

$$[\text{Na}]_{\text{required}},\ \text{mequiv} = TBW \times ([\text{Na}]_{\text{goal}} - [\text{Na}]_{\text{current}})$$

and

$$\text{volume of 3\% saline infused over 24 h} = \frac{[\text{Na}]_{\text{required}},\ \text{mequiv}}{513\,\text{mequiv}\,l^{-1}}$$

The 'traditional' method described above is independent of the urinary losses, although that method may very infrequently require the use of furosemide to promote urinary free water excretion.[7,8]

Medications have been used to assist in free water clearance and may be used in patients with mild symptomatic hyponatraemia in place of fluid restriction or may be used as adjuvants to hypertonic saline infusions in cases of symptomatic euvolaemic or hypervolaemic hyponatraemia. Demeclocycline, in doses as high as 1200 mg per day, may induce nephrogenic diabetes insipidus. Other agents such as lithium, diphenylhydantoin and urea have not been as reproducible or effective.[6]

The newer vaptans allow a further dimension in the therapy of mild symptomatic hyponatraemia. Two vasopressin receptor antagonists are currently approved for use in the correction of euvolaemic and hypervolaemic hyponatraemia[25-27] and two others are under experimental evaluation.[6] The vaptans are non-peptide low molecular weight antagonists of the vasopressin receptor. They bind to an internal domain in the receptor molecule and alter the configuration for normal vasopressin binding and coupling to the internal G protein.[28] Conivaptan is a combined V1a receptor and V2 receptor antagonist and tolvaptan is a selective V2 receptor antagonist. Conivaptan is approved for intravenous administration and tolvaptan is an oral antagonist, but both are to be started in hospitalized patients.[25-27] Conivaptan is administered by intravenous infusion of 20 mg over 30 min followed by 20 mg over 24 h, with the subsequent dose increased to 40 mg per 24 h if required. It is approved only for 4 days. Tolvaptan may be given at 15 mg once daily and may be titrated up as needed once daily to a maximum dose of 60 mg per day. Both drugs are metabolized by the hepatic cytochrome P-450 system of CYP3A and are contraindicated for use with other drugs which are CYP3A inhibitors (clarithromycin, itraconazole, fluconazole, ritonovir and ciclosporin).[27,28] Both drugs have been shown to improved serum sodium with rare increases in the level above the desired $12\,\text{mequiv}\,l^{-1}$ over 24 h. Tolvaptan has been shown to have modest clinical benefits as determined by a quality of life questionnaire in hyponatraemic subjects with serum sodium less than $130\,\text{mequiv}\,l^{-1}$,[25] and in patients with acute congestive heart failure by alleviating feelings of fatigue and dyspnea.[29] Clinical treatment indications for the outpatient management of hyponatraemia with tolvaptan are not well defined and the cost is ~\$3000 for 10 tablets.[27]

Workup and treatment of hypernatraemia

Chronic hypernatraemia ($[Na^+] > 145$ mequiv l^{-1}) is associated with extravascular hypertonicity with resultant intracellular dehydration. Clinical presentations may include altered mental status, irritability, hyper-reflexia, tachycardia, orthostasis and dry mucous membranes.[5,7,11] The most clinically significant symptoms are associated with central nervous system dysfunction, ranging from confusion to coma. In extreme cases, the brain dehydration may be associated with vascular rupture and subarachnoid haemorrhage. Chronic dehydration will result in adaptive responses by intracellular generation of organic osmoles. Correction of chronic hypernatraemia must take into account that the overly rapid correction of the hyponatraemia may result in cerebral oedema. Acute management therefore must follow the serum sodium on a regular basis (every 4 h) to adjust the regimen.

Treatment should reverse the underlying causes, such as treating pyrexia, managing gastrointestinal fluid losses and withholding diuretics or lactulose. Correction of the hyperosmolality should then proceed with a goal to decrease serum osmolality incrementally by ~10 mOsm kg^{-1} over 24 h rather than full correction of serum sodium to normal levels.[30] There are various formulas for correction which are usually based on the correction of total body water. The formula for calculating total body water is described above.[7,8,30] One must also supplement for anticipated continuing obligatory water losses (insensible, urinary and gastrointestinal water loss). Obligatory water loss may range from 0.5 to 1.5 l per day of free water. Replacement fluids may include 0.9% saline, 0.45% saline and 5% dextrose in water. If the dehydration is due purely to water without solute loss, the regimen for D5% water may be the easiest to calculate. The concept is similar to treatment of hyponatraemia as described above, except the calculated water deficit is to be added. The calculated free water should reduce the current serum sodium by 10 mOsm kg^{-1} over 24 h.

$$\frac{\text{water replacement}}{24\,\text{h}} = TBW \times \left(1 - \frac{[\text{Na}]_{\text{goal}}}{[\text{Na}]_{\text{current}}}\right) + (\text{insensible, gastrointestinal and urinary losses})$$

where

$$[\text{Na}]_{\text{goal}} = [\text{Na}]_{\text{current}} - 10\ \text{mequiv l}^{-1}$$

In situations where solute is lost in addition to pure water, then 0.45% saline may be a more appropriate intravenous infusion. The infused sodium will stay in the intravascular space to raise the blood pressure. However, the 0.45% saline will correct the osmolality by the 'free water' component, that is, the change in serum sodium per litre of infusate ($\Delta[Na^+]\,l^{-1}$ infusate):[30]

$$\Delta[\text{Na}]\,\text{l}^{-1}\text{of infusate} = \frac{[\text{Na}]_{\text{infusate}} - [\text{Na}]_{\text{serum}}}{TBW + 1}$$

and

$$\frac{\text{volume infused}}{24\,\text{h}} = \frac{\text{desired}\,\Delta[\text{Na}]}{\Delta[\text{Na}]\,\text{l}^{-1}\text{of infusate}}$$

Hence the replacement with 0.45% saline will require approximately twice the rate (or volume) of infusion compared with that calculated for D5% water. Because of the fear that overly rapid correction of the hypernatraemia will cause hyponatraemic cerebral oedema, clinicians are prone to use 0.9% saline for the correction. However, infusion of 0.9% saline, although hypotonic to the existing serum sodium, will not reduce the serum osmolality and may not supply sufficient free water to keep up with obligatory losses. This is explained in detail in the review by Adrogue and Madias.[30] For example, at a serum $[Na^+]$ of 162 mequiv l^{-1} and infusion of 1 l of 0.9% saline (154 mequiv l^{-1}) in a 70 kg person <75 years old, the change in serum sodium per litre ($\Delta[Na^+]_{serum}\,l^{-1}$) of infusate would only be (-8 mequiv l^{-1})/42 l) $= -0.2$ mequiv l^{-1} of infusate. It should be noted that there are many assumptions in the calculations for rehydration: that there are no solute losses either before or after the infusion (i.e. the water changes are due to changes in pure water; that the total body water is either 50 or 60%; and that the insensible water losses are between 500 and 1500 ml over 24 h, depending on the underlying illness, such as fever or diarrhoea. It is therefore mandatory to maintain close clinical and laboratory monitoring in order to allow for the large range of assumptions to remain within the desired correction range.

Conclusion

Disorders of water imbalance, hyper- and hyponatraemia, are common in a geriatric population. Among frail elderly patients in long-term care, the incidence of these abnormalities may be as high as 18–63%. Elderly persons, after fluid restriction, have diminished thirst and renal responsiveness to antidiuretic hormone (ADH), but retain their ability to secrete ADH. Hypernatraemia is prevalent in those with Alzheimer's dementia, who have further compromises in both thirst and ADH secretion. Institutionalized frail elderly individuals are often dependent on caregivers for water intake, especially during times of inter-current or febrile illness. Hyponatraemia may be associated with an age-related limitation of renal concentration ability. ADH may be inappropriately elevated due to medications or physiologically increased due to diminished effective arterial blood volume. Hyponatraemia may be associated with comorbidities of falls, bone fractures and death from heart disease, although causality has not been proven. Correction of hypo- and hypernatraemia should be guided by neurocognitive symptoms. In seriously symptomatic persons or for hyponatraemia ([Na$^+$]<125 mequiv l^{-1}) or hypernatraemia ([Na$^+$]>165 mequiv l^{-1}), adjustments of serum over the ensuing 24 h should be designed to increase the [Na$^+$] by 8–12 mequiv l^{-1} in hyponatraemia (to avoid osmotic demyelination syndromes) or to decrease the [Na$^+$] by ~10 mequiv l^{-1} in hypernatraemia (to avoid cerebral oedema). Vaptans are vasopressin antagonists that have been shown to improve serum [Na$^+$] in hyponatraemia, allow discontinuation of fluid restriction and have exhibited modest effects on quality of life testing. Further studies are necessary to demonstrate the effectiveness of vaptans in the correction of hyponatraemia to improve clinical parameters of gait and neurocognitive function.

Key points

- Older persons have abnormalities in thirst and vasopressin secretion.
- Hyponatraemia is associated with falls and delirium.
- Vasopressin antagonists, vaptans. can be used to treat symptoms of hyponatraemia.

References

1. Robinson AG and Verbalis JG. Posterior pituitary. In: HM Kronenberg, S Melmed, KS Polonsky and PR Larsen (eds), *Williams Textbook of Endocrinology*, 11th edn, Saunders, Philadelphia, PA, 2008, pp. 263–95.
2. Miller M. Role of arginine vasopressin receptor antagonist in hyponatremia in the elderly. *Geriatrics* 2007;**62**:20–6.
3. Miller M. Hyponatremia and arginine vasopressin dysregulation: mechanisms, clinical consequences and management. *J Am Geriatr Soc* 2006;**54**:345–53.
4. Luckey AE and Parsa CJ. Fluid and electrolytes in the aged. *Arch Surg* 2003;**138**:1055–60.
5. McKenna K and Thompson C. Osmoregulation in clinical disorders of thirst appreciation. *Clin Endocrinol* 1998; **49**:139–52.
6. Verbalis JG, Goldsmith SR, Greenberg A *et al.* Hyponatremia treatment guidelines 2007: expert panel recommendations. *Am J Med* 2007;**120**: S1–21.
7. Adrogue HJ and Madias NE. Hyponatremia. *N Engl J Med* 2000;**342**:1581–9.
8. Ellison DH and Berl T. The syndrome of inappropriate antidiuresis. *N Engl J Med* 2007;**356**:2064–72.
9. Arinzon Z, Feldman J, Peisakh A *et al.* Water and sodium disturbances predict prognosis of acute disease in long term cared frail elderly. *Arch Gerontol Geriatr* 2005;**40**:317–26.
10. Phillips PA, Rolls BJ, Ledingham JGG *et al.* Reduced thirst after water deprivation in healthy elderly men. *N Engl J Med* 1984;**311**:753–9.
11. Davis PJ and Davis FB. Water excretion in the elderly. *Endocrinol Metab Clin North Am* 1987;**16**:867–75.
12. Tian Y, Serino R and Verbalis JG. Downregulation of renal vasopressin V2 receptor and aquaporin-2 expression parallels age-associated defects in urine concentration *Am J Physiol Renal Physiol* 2004;**287**: F797–805.
13. Kayser-Jones J, Schell ES, Porter C *et al.* Factors contributing to dehydration in nursing homes: inadequate staffing and lack of professional supervision. *J Am Geriatr Soc* 1999; **47**:1187–94.
14. Albert SG, Nakra BRS, Grossberg GT and Caminal ER. Vasopressin response to dehydration in Alzheimer's disease. *J Am Geriatr Soc* 1989;**37**:843–7.
15. Miller M, Morley JE and Rubenstein LZ. Hyponatremia in a nursing home population. *J Am Geriatr Soc* 1995;**43**:1410–3.
16. Hirshberg B and Ben-Yehuda A. The syndrome of inappropriate antidiuretic hormone secretion in the elderly. *Am J Med* 1997;**10**:270–3.
17. Crowe MJ, Forsling ML, Rolls BJ *et al.* Altered water excretion in healthy elderly men. *Age Ageing* 1987;**16**:285–93.
18. Liamis G, Milionis H and Elisaf M. A review of drug induced hyponatremia. *Am J Kidney Dis* 2008;**52**:144–53.
19. Jacob S and Spinler SA. Hyponatremia associated with selective serotonin-reuptake inhibitors in older adults. *Ann Pharmacother* 2006;**40**:1618–22.
20. Beckett NS, Peters R, Fletcher AE *et al.* Treatment of hypertension in patients 80 years of age or older. *N Engl J Med* 2008; **358**:1887–98.
21. Sajadieh A, Binici Z, Mouridsen MR *et al.* Mild hyponatremia carries a poor prognosis in community subjects. *Am J Med* 2009;**122**:679–86.
22. Kinsella S, Moran S, Sullivan MO *et al.* Hyponatremia independent of osteoporosis is associated with fracture occurrence. *Clin J Am Soc Nephrol* 2010;**5**:275–80.
23. Gankam Kengne F, Andres C, Sattar L *et al.* Mild hyponatremia and risk of fracture in the ambulatory elderly. *Q J Med* 2008;**101**:583–8.
24. Renneboog B, Musch W, Vandemergel X *et al.* Mild chronic hyponatremia is associated with falls, unsteadiness and attention deficits. *Am J Med* 2006;**119**: 71.e1–8.
25. Schrier RW, Gross P, Gheorghiade M *et al.* for the SALT Investigators Tolvaptan, a selective oral vasopressin V2-receptor antagonist, for hyponatremia. *N Engl J Med* 2006; **355**:2099–112.
26. Anonymous. Conivaptan (Vaprisol) for hyponatremia. *Med Lett Drugs Ther* 2006;**48**:51–2.
27. Anonymous. Tolvaptan (Samsca) for hyponatremia. *Med Lett Drugs Ther* 2006;**51**:95–6.
28. Macion-Dazard R, Callahan N, Xu Z *et al.* Mapping the site of six nonpeptide antagonists to the human V2-renal vasopressin receptor. *J Pharmacol Exp Ther* 2006;**316**:564–71.
29. Gheorghiade M, Konstam MA, Burnett JC Jr *et al.* for the Efficacy of Vasopressin Antagonism in Heart Failure Outcome Study With Tolvaptan (EVEREST) Investigators. Short-term clinical effects of tolvaptan, an oral vasopressin antagonist, in patients hospitalized for heart failure: The EVEREST Clinical Status Trials *JAMA* 2007;**297**:1332–43.
30. Adrogue HJ and Madias NE. Hypernatremia. *N Engl J Med* 2000;**342**:1493–9.

CHAPTER 97

The pituitary gland

James F. Lamb[1] and John E. Morley[2]

[1]Ohio State University College of Medicine and Public Health, Columbus, OH, USA

[2]Saint Louis University School of Medicine and St Louis Veterans' Affairs Medical Center, St Louis, MO, USA

Introduction

The pituitary gland is the master endocrine gland as it detects and integrates multiple sources of information to regulate physiologic functions (Figure 97.1). The name 'pituitary' originated from the Latin *pituita*, which means mucus; it was believed that the pituitary excreted mucus from the brain through the nose. Understanding age-related changes in this gland and the manifestations of pituitary disease in the elderly is becoming increasingly important as the population ages. The magnitude of these age-related changes is highly variable and the confounding effect of illness on these changes must be appreciated. Interpreting age-associated changes in pituitary function must also take into account the rates and pulsatile secretion of hormones, the rapid changes in the levels of some hormones due to physiological states such as stress, the binding of hormones to plasma proteins, the hormone clearance rates from the plasma and the altered target tissue sensitivity to hormones. The comorbidity often seen in older persons can mask the usual presentation of pituitary disease and make the diagnosis and treatment of these disorders challenging.

This chapter reviews the pertinent changes in the pituitary gland that occur with ageing and the diseases that affect this gland and are relevant to the care of the older individual.

Anatomy

The pituitary gland is functionally divided into an anterior lobe, a posterior lobe and an intermediate lobe. It is located at the base of the brain within the sella turcica and is covered by the diaphragm sella. The pituitary stalk exits through the diaphragm sella to connect with the hypothalamus. The adult pituitary gland weighs 600 mg and measures 13 mm (transverse) × 6–9 mm (vertical) × 9 mm (anteroposteriorly).[1] The optic chiasm is located anterior to the pituitary stalk and is directly above the diaphragm sella, making the optic tracts vulnerable to compression by an expanding pituitary mass. The hypothalamus contains neurons that synthesize releasing and inhibiting hormones and also the hormones arginine vasopressin and oxytocin of the posterior pituitary. The five cell types that secrete hormone in the anterior pituitary gland are listed in Table 97.1.

In the elderly, the pituitary gland is moderately decreased in size and contains areas of patchy fibrosis, local necrosis, vascular alterations and cyst formation. Extensive cellular deposits of lipofuscin and regional deposits of amyloid are also seen. There are no prominent age-associated alterations in the relative proportions of different types of pituitary secretory cells. The LH and FSH contents are somewhat increased in older people, but there are no age-related changes in the pituitary content of GH, PRL and TSH.[2]

Blood supply

The blood supply to the anterior pituitary is through a rich vascular network. The superior hypophyseal arteries (from the internal carotid arteries) supply the hypothalamus and form a capillary network and portal vessels from this network supply the anterior pituitary. These vessels form the conduit for the releasing and inhibiting hormones of the hypothalamus to the anterior pituitary cells. Inferior hypophyseal arteries from the posterior communicating and internal carotid arteries supply the posterior pituitary. Drainage is into the cavernous sinus and internal jugular veins.

Anterior pituitary disorders – clinical manifestations

Pituitary tumours are very common, occurring at postmortem in 20–25% of persons.[3] Microadenomas are more common in men than in women and over half of the tumours in older persons have immunoreactive prolactin

Principles and Practice of Geriatric Medicine, Fifth Edition. Edited by Alan J. Sinclair, John E. Morley and Bruno Vellas.

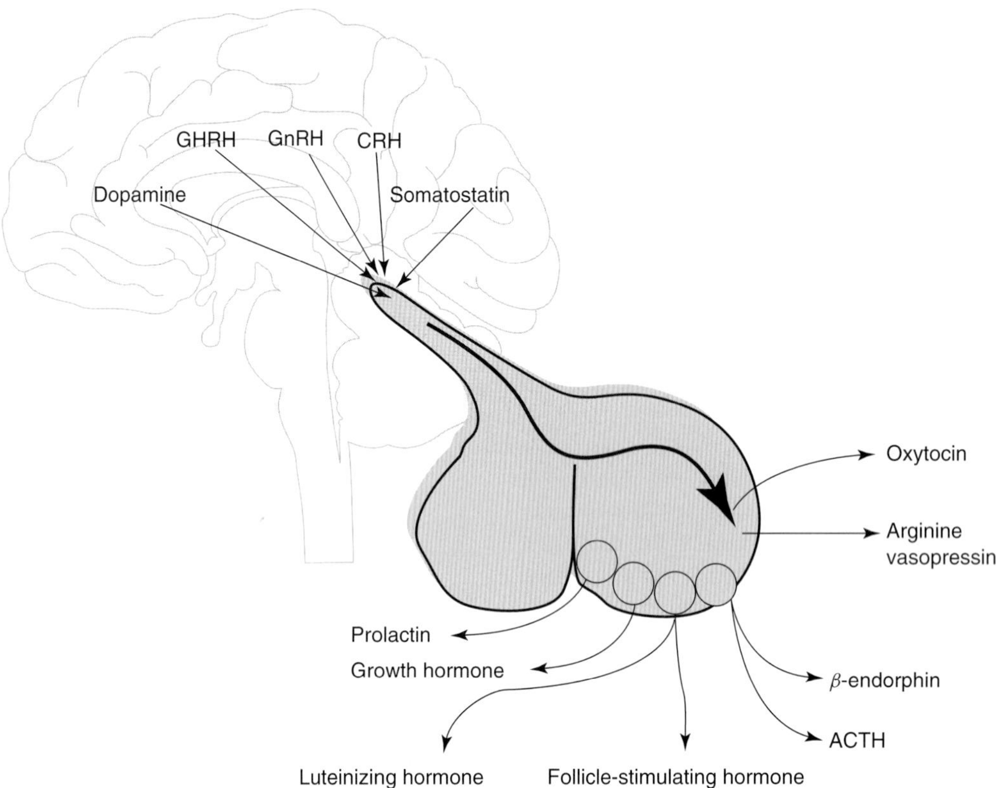

Figure 97.1 Hormones produced by the anterior pituitary and its hypothalamic controlling factors.

Table 97.1 Pituitary cell types, their hormones and their percentages[a].

Cell type	Hormone	Stimulators	Inhibitors	Percentage of anterior pituitary cells
Corticotroph	POMC including ACTH	Corticotropin-releasing hormone, vasopressin, cytokines	Glucocorticoids	15–20
Somatotroph	GH	GH-releasing hormone, GH secretagogues	Somatostatin, IGF	50
Thyrotroph	Alpha subunit and beta subunit (thyrotropin)	TRH	T3, T4, dopamine, somatostatin, glucocorticoids	<10
Gonadotroph	FSH and LH	Gonadotropin-releasing hormone	Sex steroids, inhibin	10–15
Lactotroph	PRL	Estrogen, TRH	Dopamine	10–25

[a]POMC, pro-opiomelanocortin peptides; ACTH, adrenocorticotrophic hormone; GH, growth hormone; FSH, follicle-stimulating hormone; LH, leuteinizing hormone; PRL, prolactin; TRH, thyrotropin-releasing hormone; IGF, insulin-like growth factor; T3, triode thyronine; T4, thyroxine.

staining in their cytoplasm. Despite the frequency of this occurrence, pituitary tumours in the elderly are a neglected subject in the literature. Outcome studies on the prevalence and treatment of the various types of pituitary adenomas are confounded by lack of long-term follow-up, comorbidity and a referral bias towards younger patients.[4] Pituitary tumours in persons over 60 years of age account for 3–13.4% of all brain tumours.[5] Pituitary lesions present with a variety of manifestations, including pituitary hormone hyper- and hyposecretion, enlargement of the sella turcica and visual loss. In the general adult population, hypersecreting pituitary adenomas are the most common cause of pituitary dysfunction and the earliest symptoms are due to endocrinological abnormalities. Visual loss and headache are later manifestations and are due to sellar enlargement. These later symptoms are seen only in patients with large tumours on extension above the sella.[6] Early visual symptoms include the hemifield slide phenomenon, that is, images floating apart from one another and the inability to focus on two points at the same time, for example, the inability to do needlework. The classical visual sign of pituitary tumours is bitemporal hemianopsia. In older persons, this sign can be difficult to detect as some degree of bitemporal hemianopsia occurs as a normal part of the ageing process.

In contrast, most clinically relevant pituitary tumours in the elderly are non-functioning and do not present with features of hormonal hypersecretion. Patients are more likely to be diagnosed with visual field deficits or as incidentalomas.[4] In a study by Cohen *et al.*,[7] 73% of 22 pituitary tumours diagnosed in patients over 70 years of age were non-functioning. Cushing's disease was diagnosed in one, prolactinoma in one and acromegaly in three. In the series by Kleinschmidt-DeMasters *et al.*,[5] of the 13 tumours one was a prolactinoma with subarachnoid haemorrhage and apoplexy and two secreted growth hormone. The other 10 were non-functioning.

Of the hormones hypersecreted by pituitary adenomas, prolactin (PRL) is the most common. Measuring PRL is an important part of the evaluation of patients with suspected pituitary disorders and should be performed in older patients presenting with gonadal dysfunction, secondary gonadotropin deficiency or sella turcica enlargement. The characteristic syndromes of acromegaly and Cushing's disease are due to the hypersecretion of GH and ACTH, respectively, but are rare presentations of pituitary disease in the older population. The characteristic symptoms of acromegaly are given in Table 97.2. Even more rarely, ectopic GH-releasing hormone causing somatotroph hyperplasia leading to acromegaly and corticotropin-releasing hormone to Cushing's disease can be due to abdominal or chest tumours.

Table 97.2 Symptoms of acromegaly in older persons with pituitary secreting. tumours[a].

Fatigue
Weakness
Swelling of hands and feet
Coarse facial features
Increased head size
Increased perspiration
Deepening of voice
Enlargement of lip, nose and tongue
Joint pain
Snoring
Cardiomyopathy
Headaches
Visual loss

[a]The diagnosis can often be made by looking at serial photographs taken over the lifetime to detect the physical changes that occurred.

Hypopituitarism is another manifestation of a pituitary adenoma. The clinical presentation of hypopituitarism depends on which hormones are affected, the acuteness or chronicity of the disorder and the severity of the hormone deficiencies (Table 97.3).

In adults, hypogonadism is the earliest clinical manifestation of an adenoma and is secondary to elevated PRL, ACTH and cortisol or GH. The hypogonadism is due to impaired secretion of gonadotropin-releasing hormone rather than anterior pituitary distinction. Older persons with hypopituitarism may present with recurrent falls,[8] hyponatraemia,[9] postural hypotension and hypothyroidism with an inappropriately suppressed TSH.[10] Tayal *et al.* reported pituitary adenomas as the most common cause of hypopituitarism in 12 patients aged 63–89 years.[11] The presenting features in this series were lethargy, hypotension, weakness, falls, weight loss, drowsiness, confusion, immobility and urinary incontinence. Other symptoms of hypopituitarism in older adults include changes in body composition (abdominal obesity and loss of muscle leading to decreased exercise tolerance and fatigue – due to GH loss), decreased sexual function (owing to gonadotropin loss), hypoglycaemia and hypocortisolism (caused by loss of ACTH), polyuria and polydipsia (due to deficits in vasopressin). Other causes of hypopituitarism are given in Table 97.4.

Pituitary apoplexy, resulting from haemorrhage or infarction of the pituitary gland, usually occurs as a

Table 97.3 Symptoms of hypopituitarism in older adults.

Insufficient thyroid-stimulating hormone production
- Confusion
- Cold intolerance
- Weight gain
- Dry skin
- Constipation
- Hypertension
- Fatigue

Insufficient growth hormone production
- Fatigue
- Decreased strength

Insufficient gonadotropin production
- Fine wrinkled skin
- In males, worsening libido

Insufficient corticotropin production (very rare)
- Fatigue
- Hypoglycaemia
- Hypotension
- Intolerance of stress

Table 97.4 Causes of hypopituitarism.

Primary hypopituitarism
- Pituitary tumours
- Hemosiderosis
- Infections
- Sarcoidosis
- Radiation therapy
- Tuberculosis
- Hypophysitis (autoimmune disease)
- Surgery
- Impaired vascular supply

Secondary hypopituitarism
- Hypothalamic tumours
- Head injuries
- Multiple sclerosis
- Inflammatory disease

sudden crisis in a patient with a known or previously unrecognized pituitary tumour, but may occur in a normal gland. The risk factors for this condition are common in the elderly. Symptoms at presentation include the sudden onset of headache, stiff neck, oculomotor disturbances and confusion.[4]

An enlarged sella turcica is another presentation of pituitary disease. The enlargement is usually noted on X rays performed for other indications such as trauma, sinusitis or mental status changes. Patients with an enlarged sella usually have a pituitary adenoma or empty sella syndrome as the cause.[6] In the elderly, carotid artery aneurysms would also be in the differential diagnosis, whereas craniopharyngiomas and lymphocytic hypophysitis seen in younger populations would be less likely. Pituitary function in the empty sella syndrome is usually normal, although some patients have hyperprolactinaemia. MRI confirms the diagnosis.

An increased suspicion of a pituitary/hypothalamic disorder should occur if patients present with unexplained unilateral or bilateral visual field deficits including bitemporal hemianopsia or visual loss. Vision changes were the most common presentation of pituitary adenomas in Cohen *et al.*'s series of 22 patients aged 70 years and over.[7] These patients should have a neuro-ophthalmological evaluation, MRI and a serum prolactin, and also an assessment for hypopituitarism. Additional concerns for large pituitary lesions are that they may have lateral extension into the cavernous sinus, leading to diplopia caused by dysfunction of the third, fourth or sixth cranial nerve. These large tumours may also extend in an inferior direction through the sphenoid sinus and roof of the palate and lead to cerebrospinal fluid leakage. Seizures and personality changes can result from invasion of the temporal or frontal lobe. Hypothalamic encroachment can lead to hypogonadism, diabetes insipidus and disorders of temperature regulation, appetite and sleep. Headaches can be due to stretching of the dural plate and do not necessarily correlate with size or extension of the mass.

Anterior pituitary disorders – treatment

Non-functioning pituitary tumours

The clinical features of these tumours are usually due to mass effects. Hypopituitary and hyperprolactinaemia (caused by impingement on the pituitary stalk and interference with tonic inhibition of lactotroph cells by dopamine secreted by the hypothalamus) are usually present in varying degrees. Less than one-third of the time there is an elevation of follicle-stimulating hormone (FSH), LH or their subunits. In one series of 27 patients, aged 65–81 years, there was global anterior hypopituitarism in 33% and partial hypopituitarism in 37% of patients.[12]

There is no effective medical therapy. Non-functioning microadenomas ($\leq$ 10 mm) have a benign natural history and can be followed with annual visual acuity and visual field testing and neuroimaging in the asymptomatic patient. Surgery and radiotherapy appear to be very effective in producing control of symptomatic non-functioning pituitary tumours. In Cohen *et al.*'s series,[7] transsphenoidal surgery was performed in 64% of the 16 patients and was well tolerated with few postoperative complications. Vision was significantly improved in seven and unchanged in one. Temporary visual deterioration occurred in one patient and permanent deterioration occurred in another. In Brada *et al.*'s population aged 60 years and over, 79% of patients treated with radiotherapy had a diagnosis of non-functioning pituitary adenoma and, after 10 years of follow-up, only one showed evidence of tumour progression.[13] In one series of macroadenomas, only 31% faced total removal of the tumour.[12] One-third required radiotherapy.

In the USA, 5497 pituitary surgery operations were performed between 1996 and 2000. There was a 0.6% death rate and a 3% discharge to long-term care. Age was a significant predictor of mortality and a worse outcome at hospital discharge.[14] Surgeons with a higher case load had much better outcomes.

Prolactinomas

In addition to symptoms caused by mass effects, post-menopausal women may present with galactorrhoea and men can present with hypogonadism including decreased libido. Excluding medications, hypothyroidism and other causes of hyperprolactinaemia is an important step in the initial approach to this problem. In general, treatment consists of medical therapy with a dopamine agonist. The available dopamine agonists include bromocriptine, lisuride, pergolide and cabergoline. Dopamine agonists can produce orthostans and delirium with hallucinations and delusions. Surgery is used for those intolerant or resistant to dopamine agonist therapy. Surgery is also indicated for those patients who require urgent decompression of the sella turcica for visual field deficits. Treatment is recommended for microprolactinoma ($\leq$ 10 mm) to prevent osteoporosis, the infrequent occurrence of tumour progression and the effects of prolonged hypogonadism.

The management of prolactinomas in the elderly is hindered by a lack of data. Several reviews included no elderly patients,[15–17] so extrapolation from data in younger populations and individualizing treatment decisions are necessary.

Cushing's disease

The diagnosis of Cushing's disease may be more challenging in the elderly because symptoms [weight gain, hypertension (HTN), diabetes mellitus (DM)] may be non-specific and because elevated urinary cortisol excrtion can be seen with Alzheimer's disease and multi-infarct dementia.[18] Lack of cortisol suppression after low-dose dexamethasone is seen with depression and Alzheimer's disease in addition to Cushing's disease and further complicates the diagnosis. In addition, up to 50% of ACTH tumours are not visible on MRI and require inferior petrosal sinus sampling and CRH-provocative testing.

Treatment of ACTH-producing tumours is by transsphenoidal resection. A higher relapse rate has been seen in younger than older patients.[19,20] Metyrapone has also been used to treat Cushing's disease in the elderly.[21]

Acromegaly

The predominant cause of acromegaly is GH-producing tumours and the effects of GH are medicated by insulin growth factor-1 (IGF-1) (produced by the liver). Symptoms are those of acromegaly plus those caused by mass effects of the tumour. The best screening test for this disease is an IGF-1 level. Because of secretion of GH is pulsatile, random levels are not helpful with the diagnosis. The treatment of choice for a GH-secreting tumour is excision. Pharmacological therapy with octreotide or radiotherapy can be considered if the disease persists after excision. Pegvisomant, which blocks the effect of growth hormone on its receptor, may be appropriate in some persons with oversecretion of growth hormone.

Acromegaly in older patients appears to be a milder disease than in younger patients,[22] and it has been suggested that treatment can be more conservative in this group.[23] It appears that elderly individuals respond well to both transsphenoidal surgery and medical treatment with somatostatin agonists.[4]

Thyrotropin (TSH)-secreting tumours

About 2% of all pituitary tumours are TSH-secreting. They can present with symptoms of thyrotoxicosis. Among 25 patients with TSH-producing tumours, one was 60, one 63 and one 80 years old.[24] There are few data on treatment in any age groups for this rare tumour. Octreotide appears to be a safe and effective treatment.[25] However, in older patients tumours tend to be large, requiring surgery and radiation. Often some tumour remnant remains in these patients.

Gamma-knife radiosurgery

Gamma-knife radiosurgery is a recent option for the management of pituitary tumours. The gamma-knife is a device that allows radiation to be delivered from outside the head to a precise position within the brain. It requires no incision. Multiple radiation beams are aimed at the pituitary. Each individual beam is too weak to damage the brain tissue through which it passed, with the tissue destruction happening only at the place in the pituitary where the beams meet. Accuracy is to within a fraction of a millimetre. Occasionally, gamma-knife therapy can cause local swelling 2–12 months following the procedure. Otherwise, it is relatively free of side effects.

Empty sella turcica

Empty sella turcica has been diagnosed in men and women in their 60s and 70s. It is characterized by enlargement of the bony structure enclosing the pituitary together with loss of pituitary tissue. It occurs most commonly in overweight women with high blood pressure. Symptoms include cephalgia, hypopituitarism or a runny nose. Most empty sellas are diagnosed incidentally during a radiological procedure of the head.

Anterior pituitary hormone secretion – functional changes with age

Functional changes in anterior pituitary hormone secretion occur with increasing age. Table 97.5 summarizes some of the changes that have been reported in these hormone.[26] Older persons with traumatic brain injury due to motor vehicle accidents or falls can lead to pituitary insufficiency.[27,28] Hypopituitarism in older persons is most commonly associated with macroadenomas and less commonly with an empty sella or pituitary hyperplasia.[29] Presenting symptoms included visual field defects, asthenia, memory or gait impairment, nausea and depression. Surgery and radiation are safe in this population.

Table 97.5 Changes reported in hormones.

Hormone	Increase	Decrease	None
Adrenocorticotrophin hormone	–	+	–
Follicle-stimulating hormone	+	+	–
Luteinizing hormone	+	+	–
Growth hormone	–	+	–
Thyroid-stimulating hormone	–	+	+
Prolactin	+	+	+

Gonadotropins (LH and FSH)

Blood concentrations if both LH and FSH increase abruptly and universally in about the sixth decade in women as ovarian secretion of estrogens decreases. These values gradually decline after age 75 years.[30] Serum FSH and LH rise approximately twofold in men aged 75–85 years and then decline gradually, as pituitary gonadotropic secretory capacity is reduced with advancing age. This is suggested by a decrease in the amplitude of LH and/or FSH responses to gonadotropin-releasing hormone.[31] There is a wide spread of values at these ages, suggesting primary hypogonadism in some men and secondary (central) hypogonadism in others. Secondary hypogonadism may be the rule rather than the exception with ageing.[32] The mean LH pulse amplitude and the maximum pulse amplitude are lower in elderly than in younger males.[33]

The changes in the LH response to ageing may be due to the effects of ageing on the catecholamine responses in the hypothalamus. The oestrous cycle in old female rats is reinstated by drugs that stimulate brain catecholamine neurotransmitters.[34] Naloxone administered to old rats partially restores the LH surge. This suggests that opiates from the hypothalamus may be partly responsible for reduction in LH secretion.[36]

Prolactin (PRL)

Unlike other pituitary hormones, hypothalamic control of prolactin is mainly inhibitory through dopamine. Other than simulating lactation in the post-partum period, prolactin has no significant physiological function. Hyperprolactinaemia suppresses sex steroid production.

There is no consensus on the effects of ageing on prolactin secretion. Investigators have reported decreases, increases or no change in prolactin changes.[2] Sawin *et al.*'s analysis of prolactin levels from the Framingham cohort showed no significant difference in the prolactin levels between the age-matched genders.[36] The mean prolactin level in men for ages 40–49 years was 6.4 ± 3.1 mg ml^{-1} compared with 8.4 ± 3.8 mg ml^{-1} for ages 80–89 years. In age-matched women, the values of 6.9 ± 3.1 and 8.8 ± 5.3 mg ml^{-1} corresponded to the same age groups as described for the men. Alterations of PRL in humans are probably of small magnitude and unlikely to affect sexual function in the older adult, but more likely the cause of hyperprolactinaemia in this population are medications and prolactinomas, which should be evaluated.[37]

Growth hormone

Both ageing and gender affect growth hormone secretory dynamics. Young women have twice as high daily growth hormone production as young men. The fall in growth hormone over the life span is from 1200 μg m^{-2} in adolescents to 60 μg m^{-2} in older individuals.[38] The fall in growth hormone secretion with ageing is due both to a decrease in the orderly production of growth hormone releasing hormone from the hypothalamus and to an increase in somatostatin production from the hypothalamus. The fall in growth hormone secretion leads to a decline in IGF-1.

Circulating growth hormone is bound to growth hormone-binding proteins. With ageing there is a decline in growth hormone-binding proteins. The level of growth hormone-binding proteins is approximately half that in nonagenarians compared with 60-year-olds.[39]

In older women, estrogen increases growth hormone secretion. In older men, only high doses of an aromatizable form of testosterone (200 mg) increased basal and the mytohemeral growth hormone production.[40]

Overall ageing is associated with multiple changes of the hypothalamic growth hormone–IGF-1 axis and their binding proteins. Interactions with sex hormones further complicate these effects. However, studies with growth hormone or ghrelin analogue replacement have failed to demonstrate physiologically important effects of these changes on the ageing process.

Posterior pituitary gland

The posterior pituitary gland is neural tissue and consists only of the distal axons of the hypothalamic magnocellular neurons. The cell bodies of these axons are located in the supraoptic and paraventricular nuclei of the hypothalamus. The axon terminals contain neurosecretory granules

Table 97.6 Causes of diabetes insipidus.

Hypothalamic malfunction or damage
Brain injury including cerebrovascular accidents
Tumours
Meningitis and encephalitis
Sarcoidosis
Tuberculosis

in which are stored the hormones oxytocin and vasopressin [antidiuretic hormone (ADH)]. Diseases of the posterior pituitary (diabetes insipidus, syndrome of inappropriate ADH) modulate water homeostasis. Persons with diabetes insipidus (insufficient production of vasopressin) present with excessive thirst, polyuria and dehydration. The major causes of diabetes insipidus are listed in Table 97.6.

Water excretion in the elderly is affected by physiological changes of the ageing process and leads to an increased risk of both hyponatraemia and hypernatraemia.[41,42] Multiple diseases common in elderly persons and the treatments for these diseases can further affect water balance. In addition, body water is reduced in the elderly. By age 75–80 years, total body water declines to 50% of the level in young adults and complicates studies of responses to dehydration, volume stimulation and osmolar stimulation.[43]

There is a reduced responsiveness of the renal collecting duct to vasopressin in older than younger individuals, the consequence of which is an increased vulnerability to water deprivation.[44] This decreased renal sensitivity to ADH is thought to be due to a decreased ability of vasopressin to stimulate aquaphorin-2 levels in the kidney and results in a chronic increase in vasopressin secretion and an eventual depletion of posterior pituitary hormone stores. This may cause a decreased visualization of the bright spot on T1-weighted MRI scans in elderly people.[45] The bright spot in the sella on MRI is due to stored hormone in neurosecretory granules in the posterior pituitary.

Vasopressin levels have a greater range of normal in older persons and do not correlate as directly with plasma osmolality.[46,47] Changes in vasopressin levels in response to osmotic stimulation are either normal[48] or increased,[48,49] while the vasopressin response to volume depletion (mediated by baroreceptors) is increased.[50]

Older persons also have a decrease in thirst in response to osmotic stimulation. As a result of the decrease in thirst and in the responsiveness of the kidney to vasopressin, it is easy for older patients to become dehydrated and hypernatraemic despite an increase in vasopressin secretion.[51] Even when recovering from dehydration, older people drink less fluid to return their volume to normal.[52]

Excreting a water load is also limited in the elderly. Decreases in glomerular filtration rate and a decreased suppression of vasopressin contribute to this phenomenon. Vasopressin is not shut off in the elderly as well as in the young in response to drinking and oral–pharyngeal receptor stimulation. Those older patients with increased levels of ADH secretion in response to a particular osmotic level have a downward alteration in their osmotic set point. This inability to execute a water load can lead to an increased tendency towards hyponatraemia in the elderly. Almost 75% of patients with the syndrome of inappropriate ADH secretion are over 65 years of age.[37]

Given the issues raised above by numerous studies, healthy older adults probably exhibit normal secretion of vasopressin but do have a decreased thirst appreciation and a decreased ability to maximally concentrate the urine to retain water or to maximally dilute the urine to excrete water. Both hyponatraemia[53] and hypernatraemia,[54] to which older people are susceptible due to the physiological changes noted above, can cause increased morbidity and mortality, especially in the frail elderly, and therefore warrant vigilance for their occurrence.

Key points

- Non-functioning pituitary tumours are extremely common in older persons.
- With ageing there is a decline in anterior pituitary function.
- Diabetes insipidus is due to insufficient production of vasopressin and leads to excessive thirst and polyuria.
- Treatment for pituitary tumours includes medical, surgery and most recently gamma-knife radiation.

References

1. Melmed S and Kleinberg D. Anterior pituitary. In: PR Larsen, HM Kronenberg, S Melmed and KS Polonsky (eds), *Williams Textbook of Endocrinology*, 10th edn, Saunders, Philadelphia, PA, 2003, pp. 177–260.
2. Blackman MR. Pituitary hormones and aging. *Clin Endocrinol Metab* 1987;**16**:981–94.
3. Costello RT. Subclinical adenoma of the pituitary gland. *Am J Pathol* 1936;**12**:205–14.
4. Turner HE and Wass JAH. Pituitary tumors in the elderly. *Balliere's Clin Endocrinol and Metab* 1997;**11**:407–22.
5. Kleinschmidt-DeMasters BK, Lillehei KO and Breeze RE. Neoplasms involving the central nervous system in the older old. *Hum Pathol* 2003;**34**:1137–47.
6. Aron DC, Findling JW and Tyrrel JB. Hypothalamus and pituitary gland. In: FS Greenspan and DG Gardner (eds), *Basic and Clinical Endocrinology*, 7th edn, McGraw-Hill, New York, 2004, pp. 106–175.
7. Cohen DL, Bevan JS and Adams BT. The presentation and management of pituitary tumors of the elderly. *Age Aging* 1989;**18**:247–52.

8. Johnston S, Hoult S and Chan CA. Falling again. *Lancet* 1996;**349**:26.
9. Mansell P, Scott VL, Logan RF and Reckless JPD. Secondary adrenocortical insufficiency. *BMJ* 1993;**307**:253–4.
10. Belchetz PE. Idiopathic hypopituitarism in the elderly. *BMJ* 1985;**291**:247–8.
11. Tayal SC, Bansal SK and Chandra DK. Hypopituitarism. *Age Ageing* 1994;**23**:320–2.
12. Del Monte P, Foppiani L, Ruelle A *et al*. Clinically non-functioning pituitary macroadenomas in the elderly. *Aging Clin Exp Res* 2007;**19**:34–40.
13. Brada M, Rajan B, Traish D *et al*. The long-term efficacy of conservative surgery and radiotherapy in the control of pituitary adenomas. *Clin Endocrinol* 1993;**38**:571–8.
14. Barker FG II, Klibanski A and Swearingen B. Transsphenoidal surgery for pituitary tumors in the United States 1996–2000: mortality, morbidity, and the effects of hospital and surgeon volume. *J Clin Endocrinol Metab* 2003;**88**: 4709–19.
15. Ciccarelli E, Ghigo E, Miola C *et al*. Long-term follow-up of 'cured' prolactinoma patients after successful adenomectomy. *Clin Endocrinol* 1990;**32**:583–602.
16. Soule SG, Farhi J, Conway GS *et al*. The outcome of hypophysectomy for prolactinomas in the era of dopamine agonist therapy. *Clin Endocrinol* 1996;**44**:711–6.
17. Bevan JS, Webster J, Binke CW and Scanlon MF. Dopamine agonist and pituitary tumor shrinkage. *Endocrine Rev* 1992;**13**:220–40.
18. Maeda T, Tanimoto K, Terada T *et al*. Elevated urinary free cortisol in patients with dementia. *Neurobiol Aging* 1991; **12**:161–71.
19. Bochicchio D, Losa M, Buchfelder M *et al*. Factors influencing the immediate and late outcome of Cushing's disease treated by transsphenoidal surgery. *J Clin Endocrinol Metab* 1995;**80**:3114–20.
20. Robert F and Hardy J. Cushing's disease: a correlation of radiological surgical and pathological findings with therapeutic results. *Pathol Res Pract* 1991;**187**:617–21.
21. Donckier J, Borrin JM, Ramsey ID and Joplin GF. Successful control of Cushing's disease in the elderly with long term metyrapone. *Postgrad Med J* 1986;**62**:727–30.
22. Klijn JGM, Lamberts SWJ, de Jong FH *et al*. Interrelationships between tumor size, age, plasma growth hormone and incidence of extrasellar extension in acromegalic patients. *Acta Endocrinol* 1980;**95**:289–97.
23. Clayton RN. Modern management of acromegaly. *Q J Med* 1993;**86**:285–7.
24. Brucker-Davis F, Oldfield EH, Skarulis MC *et al*. Thyrotropin-secreting pituitary tumors: diagnostic criteria, thyroid hormone sensitivity and treatment outcome in 25 patients followed at the National Institutes of Health. *J Clin Endocrinol Metab* 1999;**84**:476–87.
25. Charson P, Weintroub BD and Harrn AG. Octreotide therapy for thyroid-stimulating hormone-secreting pituitary adenomas. *Ann Intern Med* 1993;**119**:236.
26. Rehman HU and Masson EA. Neuroendocrinology of aging. *Age Ageing* 2001;**30**:279–87.
27. Wachter D, Gundling K, Oertel MF *et al*. Pituitary insufficiency after traumatic brain injury. *J Clin Neurosci* 2009;**16**: 202–8.
28. Berg C, Oeffner A, Schumm-Draeger PM, *et al*. Prevalence of anterior pituitary dysfunction in patient following traumatic brain injury in a German multi-centre screening program. *Exp Clin Endocrinol Diabetes* 2010;**118**:139–44.
29. Foppiani L, Ruelle A, Bandelloni R *et al*. Hypopituitarism in the elderly: multifaceted clinical and biochemical presentation. *Curr Aging Sci* 2008;**1**:42–50.
30. Vaninetti S, Baccarelli A, Romoli R *et al*. Effect of aging on serum gonadotropin levels in healthy subjects and patients with nonfunctioning pituitary adenomas. *Eur J Endocrinol* 2000;**142**:144–9.
31. Harman SM, Tsitouras PD, Costa PT *et al*. Reproductive hormones in aging men. *J Clin Endocrinol Metab* 1982;**54**:547–51.
32. Kaiser FE and Morley JE. Gonadotropins, testosterone and the aging male. *Neurobiol Aging* 1994;**15**:559–63.
33. Vermeulen A. Clinical problems in reproductive neuroendocrinology of men. *Neurobiol Aging* 1994;**15**:489–93.
34. Quadri SK, Kledzite GS and Meties J. Reinitiation of estrous cycles in old constant-estrous rats by central-acting drugs. *Neuroendocrinology* 1973;**11**:248–55.
35. Allen LG and Kalra SP. Evidence that a decrease in opioid tone may evoke preovulatory leuteinizing hormone release in rats. *Endocrinology* 1986;**118**:2375–81.
36. Sawin CT, Carlson HE, Geller A *et al*. Serum prolactin and aging. *J Gerontol* 1989;**44**:M131–5.
37. Harman SM and Blackman MR. The hypothalamic pituitary axes. In: JG Evans and TF Williams (eds), *Oxford Textbook of Geriatric Medicine* 2nd edn, Oxford University Press, 2000, Chapter 7.4.
38. Veldhuis JD and Bowers CY. Human GH pulsatility: an ensemble property regulated by age and gender. *J Endocrinol Invest* 2003;**26**:799–813.
39. Maheshwari H, Sharma L and Baumann G. Decline of plasma growth hormone binding protein in old age. *J Clin Endocrinol Metab* 1996;**81**:995–7.
40. Gentili A, Mulligan T, Godschalk M *et al*. Unequal impact of short-term testosterone repletion on the somatotropic axis of young and older men. *J Clin Endocrinol Metab* 2002;**87**:825–34.
41. Stout NR, Kenny RA and Baylis PH. A review of water balance in aging in health and disease. *Gerontology* 1999;**45**:61.
42. Davies I. Aging in the hypothalamo-neurohypophyseal-renal system. *Compr Gerontol* 1987;**1**:12.
43. Fulop T, Worum I and Csogne J. Body composition in elderly people. *Gerontology* 1985;**31**:150.
44. Davis PJ and Davis FB. Water excretion in the elderly. *Endocrinol Metabol Clin North Am* 1987;**16**:867.
45. Terano T, Seya A, Tamura Y *et al*. Characteristics of the pituitary gland in elderly subjects from MRI. *Clin Endocrinol* 1996;**45**:273.
46. Johnson AG, Grawford GA, Kelly D *et al*. Arginine vasopressin and osmolality in the elderly. *J Am Geriatr Soc* 1994;**42**:399.
47. Faull CM, Holmes C and Baylis PH. Water balance in elderly people. *Age Aging* 1993;**22**:114.

48. Stachenfeld NS, Mack GW, Takamata A *et al.* Thirst and fluid regulatory responses to hypertonicity in older adults. *Am J Physiol* 1996;**271**:R757.

49. Ayos JC and Arieff AI. Abnormalities of water metabolism in the elderly. *Semin Nephrol* 1996;**16**:277.

50. Phillips PA, Rolls BJ, Ledingham JG *et al.* Reduced thirst after water deprivation in healthy elderly men. *N Engl J Med* 1984;**311**:753.

51. Weinberg AD and Minaker KL. Dehydration. Evaluation and management in older adults. *JAMA* 1995;**274**:1552.

52. Phillips PA, Bretherton M, Johnston CI *et al.* Reduced osmotic thirst in healthy elderly men. *Am J Physiol* 1991; **261**:R166.

53. Roberts MM. Hyponatremia in the elderly. *Geriatr Nephrol Urol* 1993;**3**:43.

54. Hoffman NB. Dehydration in the elderly. *Geriatrics* 1991;**46**(6): 35.

CHAPTER 98

Thyroid disorders

Ligia J. Dominguez, Mario Belvedere and Mario Barbagallo
University of Palermo, Palermo, Italy

Introduction

Thyroid disorders are more common in older than in younger people, especially in women, and they are frequently undiagnosed.[1–3] Several changes in the thyroid function and laboratory tests arise with ageing. The understanding of these modifications may help to differentiate age-related physiological changes, subclinical dysfunction and overt disease, especially in the difficult decision of whether to start treatment or avoid it in subclinical dysfunction, which has long been a matter of controversy. In the past years, several reports have linked subclinical dysfunction with changes in cognition and cardiovascular risk, hence it is key to know how to identify correctly the subjects at true risk.[4–6] It is also possible that subtle thyroid alterations in younger people may evolve to overt clinical manifestation during ageing. For example, non-toxic goitre starting as a diffuse thyroid enlargement during early life may acquire nodularity and autonomous function with ageing and may progress, although not frequently, to toxic nodular goitre. Before becoming clinically apparent, chronic thyroiditis and toxic goitre may exhibit only slight laboratory modifications corresponding to subclinical states of hypothyroidism or hyperthyroidism. Nevertheless, only a portion of patients with subclinical laboratory dysfunction progresses to overt disease, hence it is essential to identify the patients at risk who merit treatment.

Even if thyroid dysfunction is more common in older than younger populations, it is frequently overlooked. The main reason why thyroid disorders in older persons often escape clinical detection is because their signs and symptoms often mimic age-associated functional changes or disease of other organs. For example, hypothyroidism may induce or worsen cognitive and physical decreased functions, constipation, cold intolerance, body weight gain, anaemia or lipid disorders, all frequently observed in euthyroid elders. Similarly, thyroid hyperfunction may be manifested as arrhythmia and congestive heart failure, which may well be interpreted as the manifestation of cardiac disease, very frequent at this age. Body weight loss associated with thyroid hyperfunction may be interpreted as part of the normal ageing process, undernutrition or neoplasia, also frequent in old age. In addition, thyroid hyperfunction may be asymptomatic or 'apathetic', presenting merely with subtle signs, again frequently misinterpreted as normal age-associated changes in different organ systems or as a reduced thyroid function.[1,3,5,6] In fact, older people may have similar manifestations that correspond to increased or decreased function, such as mental confusion, depression, falling, walking disturbances, urinary incontinence from immobility, congestive heart failure, constipation or diarrhoea. These signs also correspond to other disorders commonly observed in older people. The correct identification of thyroid disorders is critical in older persons, since they can significantly impact the quality of life, either because of the thyroid disorder itself or because of worsening of an underlying disease or impaired function. The existence of other diseases and the use of multiple medications may further mask or mimic the presentation of thyroid disease.

The lack of evident clinical manifestations of thyroid dysfunction in the elderly calls for a detailed clinical evaluation and a high index of suspicion to identify their presence, with the appropriate confirmation by means of reliable laboratory testing. Nevertheless, thyroid tests may also have minimal changes with age and caution in the interpretation of such changes is warranted.

This chapter explores the changes in thyroid function and disease in older age, highlighting the most common thyroid problems in this period of life, including overt and subclinical hypothyroidism and hyperthyroidism, nonthyroidal illness and the approach to thyroid nodules.

Age-related modifications in thyroid function

Several subtle changes occur in the thyroid function with advancing age, but the interpretation of the altered

Principles and Practice of Geriatric Medicine, Fifth Edition. Edited by Alan J. Sinclair, John E. Morley and Bruno Vellas.

findings in laboratory parameters is not easy because they are modified by several factors. Studying age-related changes in old age without confounders is cumbersome because an adequate sample of healthy elders is difficult to find. The variability of modifications reported in different studies is probably due to selection bias.[1] The main confounders include chronic non-thyroidal illness (NTI, see below), polypharmacy (Tables 98.1–98.3) and the increased prevalence of autoimmune subclinical hypothyroidism. It seems that the modifications that persist after taking into account these confounders include an age-dependent decrease in TSH, a decreased triiodothyronine (T3) and an increase in the inactive metabolite reversed T3 (rT3) with an apparent unchanged circulating concentration of total and free thyroxine (T4). Deiodination in the outer ring, responsible for the conversion of T4 into T3, decreases with age and seems to be a plausible explanation for the decreased concentration of T3 and the increase in rT3.[1,7,8] Recently, an increased inner ring deiodination, resulting in an elevated clearance of T4 and T3 and an augmented production of rT3, was proposed to contribute to these changes and mediate NTI.[9]

Table 98.1 Agents that inhibit thyroid hormone synthesis and secretion.

Block iodide transport into the thyroid gland
Monovalent anions (SCN^-, ClO_4^-, NO_3^-)
Complex anions (monofluorosulfonate, difluorophosphate, fluoroborate)
Minerals (bromine, fluorine)
Lithium
Ethionamide
Impair TG iodination and iodotyrosine coupling
Propylthiouracil, methimazole, carbimazole
Sulfonamides
Sulfonylureas
Salicylamides
Resorcinol
Aminoglutethimide
Amphenone
Thiocyanate
Antipyrine
Aminotriazole
Amphenidone
2,3-Dimercaptopropanol
Ketoconozole
Inhibitors of thyroid hormone secretion
Iodide (in large doses)
Lithium
Mechanism unknown
p-Bromdylamine maleate
Phenylbutazone
Minerals (calcium, rubidium, cobalt)
Interleukin II
γ-Interferon

Source: adapted from L. DeGroot, http://www.thyroidmanager.org.

Table 98.2 Compounds that affect thyroid hormone transport proteins in serum.

Increase TBG concentration	*Decrease TBG concentration*
Estrogens	Androgens and anabolic steroids
Heroin and methadone	Glucocorticoids
Clofibrate	L-Asparaginase
5-Fluorouracil	Nicotinic acid
Perphenazine	
Interfere with thyroid hormone binding to TBG and/or TTR	
Salicylates and salsalate	
Diphenylhydantoin and analogues	
Furosemide	
Sulfonylureas	
Heparin	
Dinitrophenol	
Free fatty acids	
Phenylbutazone	
Halofenate	
Fenclofenac	
Orphenadrine	
Thyroid hormone analogues	

Source: adapted from L. DeGroot, http://www.thyroidmanager.org.

The age-related decrease in TSH and thyroid hormones indicates the presence of a partial central hypothyroidism. However, Hollowell *et al.* reported an increased TSH with ageing in a large population including persons without circulating thyroid autoantibodies and without other risk factors for thyroid dysfunction.[10] Another possible confounder of the uneven results of different studies is the dissimilar iodine intake and diverse prevalence of subclinical thyroid disease in the examined populations. Whether age-associated changes in thyroid function contribute to the ageing process itself is not yet established.

The high prevalence of NTI (discussed below) among older people due to the presence of chronic illness and/or malnutrition is a major confounder in the evaluation of thyroid function in old age.[1] In a recent study evaluating ambulatory men, those with NTI – low serum T3 and a high serum rT3 – were older and had more comorbidity (i.e. diabetes, osteoarthritis, hypertension, congestive heart failure and chronic obstructive pulmonary disease) compared to subjects without NTI.[11] High rT3 was associated with a low performance score independent of the presence of disease.

The use of multiple medications, a hallmark in old populations, may also influence thyroid function tests. Drugs can inhibit thyroid hormone synthesis and secretion (Table 98.1), affect thyroid hormone transport proteins in serum (Table 98.2) and alter the extrathyroidal metabolism of thyroid hormone (Table 98.3). Pharmacological agents can induce hypothyroidism (e.g.. lithium, amiodarone),

Table 98.3 Agents that alter the extrathyroidal metabolism of thyroid hormone.

Inhibit conversion of T4 to T3
Propylthiouracil
Glucocorticoids
Propranolol
Iodinated contrast agents
Amiodarone
Clomipramine
Stimulators of hormone degradation or faecal excretion
Diphenylhydantoin
Carbamazepine
Phenobarbital
Cholestyramine and colestipol
Soybeans
Rifampin
Ferrous sulfate
Aluminium hydroxide
Sucralfate
Increase serum TSH concentration and/or its response to TRH
Iodine and iodide-containing compounds (i.e. expectorants, anti-arrhythmic and anti-anginal agents)
Lithium
Dopamine receptor blockers (metoclopramide, domperidone)
Dopamine-blocking agent (sulpiride)
Decarboxylase inhibitor (benserazide)
Dopamine-depleting agent (monoiodotyrosine)
L-Dopa inhibitors (chloropromazine, biperidine, haloperidol)
Cimetidine
Clomifene
Spironolactone
Amphetamines
Decrease serum TSH concentration and/or its response to TRH
Thyroid hormones (T4 and T3)
Thyroid hormone analogues (D-T4, 3,3′,5-Triac, etiroxate·HCl, 3,5-dimethyl-3-isopropyl-L-thyronine)
Dopaminergic agents (piribedil, apomorphine, lisuride)
Dopamine antagonist (pimozide)
Dopamine
L-Dopa
2-Bromo-α-ergocryptine
Fusaric acid (inhibitor of dopamine β-hydroxylase)
Pyridoxine (coenzyme of dopamine synthesis)
α-Noradrenergic blockers (phentolamine, thioridazine)
Serotonin antagonists (metergoline, cyproheptadine, methysergide)
Serotonin agonist (5-hydroxytryptophan)
Glucocorticoids
Acetylsalicylic acid
Growth hormone
Somatostatin
Octreotide
Opiates
Clofibrate
Fenclofenac

Source: adapted from L. DeGroot, http://www.thyroidmanager.org.

hyperthyroidism (e.g. amiodarone, iodine) and abnormal thyroid function tests by affecting thyroid-binding globulin (TBG) status (e.g. estrogens, glucocorticoids) or the binding of T4 to TBG (e.g. heparin); they can suppress T4 to T3 conversion (e.g. amiodarone, glucocorticoids, propranolol) or suppress TSH secretion (e.g. dopamine, glucocorticoids). The use of multiple medicaments is the rule in older patients and interactions among the different agents may have unknown effects on thyroid function.

Thyroid autoantibodies, including anti-thyroperoxidase and anti-thyroglobulin autoantibodies, increase with age, particularly in females over 60 years of age.[1,10] In the Whickham survey, the incidence of anti-thyroglobulin and anti-microsomial autoantibodies was 7 and 9% in females over 75 years of age compared with 2 and 5% in total population, respectively.[12] However, the prevalence of clinically overt autoimmune thyroid disease is not greater in older than younger groups. The increased TSH levels in elders shown in some studies[12,13] is probably due to the inclusion of women with a high titre of thyroid antibodies and/or subclinical hypothyroidism. The prevalence of thyroid autoantibodies was shown to be higher in subjects aged 70–85 years compared with people younger than 50 years, with centenarians having a similar prevalence to that of young subjects (<50 years old).[14] The prevalence of thyroid autoantibodies was higher in unselected or hospitalized elderly patients than centenarians, suggesting that the appearance of thyroid autoantibodies might be related to age-associated disease, rather than to the ageing process *per se*. Healthy, exceptionally long-lived persons may possibly represent a selected population with an unusually efficient immune system.[1] Moreover, thyroid autoimmunity is often associated with other autoimmune diseases, hence it was suggested that there may be a link between circulating thyroid autoantibodies and other diseases, such as atherosclerosis. However, the minor increase in coronary heart disease related to positive serum thyroid autoantibodies, reported in some epidemiological studies,[1] has not been confirmed by other reports.[1,15,16]

Other parameters, such as genetic polymorphisms in thyroid hormone pathway genes[17,18] and psychological factors,[19] have been proposed in recent years as factors influencing thyroid function tests in the elderly.

Prevalence of thyroid disease in older populations

The prevalence of thyroid disease varies widely according to age, gender and the environment. In large epidemiological studies conducted in older populations, the prevalence of hypothyroidism varies widely, from 1 to 20% of subjects, with women being more commonly affected than men and subclinical being more frequent than overt hypothyroidism. Hyperthyroidism is less common than hypothyroidism, but it is not infrequent, occurring in 0.5–3% of all elderly patients.[1–3] In iodine-sufficient areas, hypothyroidism has been reported to occur in 4–9.5% of the general population and hyperthyroidism in 0.4–3.2%.[4,10,12,20] The most frequent disorders of thyroid function in older persons are subclinical, thanks to newly devised methods for measuring serum TSH by ultrasensitive methods and free fractions of thyroid hormones, which have improved the early detection of thyroid dysfunction in the elderly. Subclinical hypothyroidism and subclinical hyperthyroidism are 2–4-fold more common than the corresponding overt conditions and are more prevalent in the elderly and in women. Hypothyroidism is more common in iodine-sufficient areas, whereas hyperthyroidism occurs more frequently in iodine-deficient areas.[21] In the latter, toxic nodular goitre is fairly frequent.[22–25] Subclinical hyperthyroidism was present in 15% of over 75-year-old persons living in an Italian iodine-deficient area[23] and in 6.5% of over 85-year-old persons living in an iodine-sufficient area of the USA.[10] The prevalence according to gender was also different in these two studies: it was equal for both genders in the Italian survey,[23] whereas in the USA it was more frequent in women.[10] The prevalence of hypothyroidism increases with ageing in up to 20% of females and 3–16% of over 75-year-old men in iodine-sufficient areas.[12,20] The prevalence in men and women is similar in hospitalized older patients.[1]

A survey in the UK found that overt hyperthyroidism and hypothyroidism were infrequent in the community (0.3 and 0.4%, respectively). Subclinical thyroid dysfunction was present in 5% of the studied population (subclinical hyperthyroidism in 2.1% and subclinical hypothyroidism in 2.9%).[26]

The prevalence of thyroid disease is higher in hospitalized elders and in long-term facility residents, although data available in these settings come from limited number of patients.[27–32] A study conducted in four nursing homes in Cape Town reported abnormal TSH in 15.6% of residents, with only 0.5% newly diagnosed cases of overt hyperthyroidism and 1% new cases of overt hypothyroidism. Subclinical thyroid disease was present in 6% of residents.[27] In a study conducted in Spain, there were 3.7% cases of previously undiagnosed subclinical hypothyroidism, 1.65% cases of overt hypothyroidism, 0.82% cases of subclinical hyperthyroidism and 10.3% cases of autoimmune thyroid disorders.[28] Another survey in Spain reported 7.9% cases of elevated TSH at admission to a nursing home and 13% cases of NTI, suggesting that TSH measurements should be performed regularly at admission.[29] In the USA, a study in nursing homes reported overt hypothyroidism in 0.7% of men and 1.5% of women and subclinical hypothyroidism in 9.7% of men and 14.6% of women.[30] The authors suggested the screening of all institutionalized elders since those with subclinical hypothyroidism are at risk for further decline in thyroid function. Nevertheless, the progression of subclinical hypothyroidism to overt disease has been estimated in only 5% of patients.[4,5] A survey conducted in two nursing homes in Georgia, USA, aimed to determine the sensitivity of clinical determinants for hypothyroidism during withdrawal of thyroid hormone therapy. Among 129 residents, the prevalence of hypothyroidism ranged from 6.2 to 7.8%; unnecessary therapy was given to 5.4% of the studied subjects.[31] Likewise, for half of nursing home residents receiving thyroid hormone, the prescription was found unnecessary in a survey conducted in the USA.[33] A survey conducted in Eastern Europe confirmed a higher prevalence of positive antithyroid antibodies in old age that was independent of iodine supply; in the same study, iodine supply was associated with the development of autoimmune hypothyroidism in older patients.[32]

Hypothyroidism

Overt hypothyroidism is characterized by low levels of thyroid hormones and increased levels of TSH. Decreased thyroid function is not uncommon in over 60-year-old persons, it increases with age and is higher in women than men.[2,5,34–36] Hypothyroidism (overt and subclinical) is found in 5–20% of women and 3–8% of men.[34] Undiagnosed hypothyroidism can be found in as many as 25% of nursing homes residents.[31,34] Overt hypothyroidism is 5–8 times more common in women than men, with an increased prevalence (up to 5%) in persons over 60 years of age.[37] Diverse medications, such as amiodarone and lithium, may induce hypothyroidism (see Tables 98.1–98.3). The most frequent cause of hypothyroidism in old age is autoimmune thyroiditis, followed by earlier thyroid surgery or radiation therapy for previous thyrotoxicosis.[2,3,5,38]

Symptoms of hypothyroidism are often atypical, specially in the oldest elders, and lack the classic presentation seen in younger patients.[1] They include memory loss, lethargy, constipation, cold intolerance, fatigue, congestive heart failure, depression and weight gain, all of them often attributed to old age or other causes. Furthermore, lack of these symptoms does not rule out the presence of hypothyroidism, hence a high index of suspicion is needed in formulating the diagnosis. The atypical presentation is due to a more insidious onset, the concurrence of several age-associated diseases and the notion that signs and symptoms are attributable to the ageing process. An elevated serum TSH level should be confirmed and supplemented with measurements of serum thyroxine (T4) and with thyroid antibodies (Figure 98.1).

Although hypothyroidism is common in older persons, it may not necessarily be associated with adverse outcomes in the oldest individuals when detected by screening alone, as illustrated by a population-based, prospective study of 558 individuals in The Netherlands. In this study, participants were screened for hypothyroidism during the month of

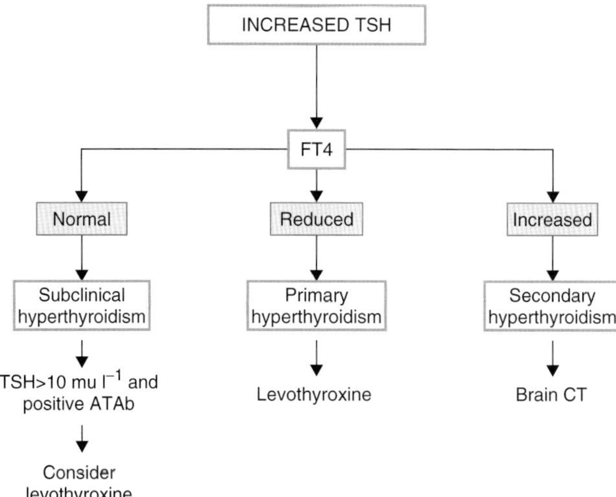

Figure 98.1 Algorithm for the diagnosis of thyroid disorders in the presence of an increased TSH. ATAb, anti-thyroid antibodies; FT3, free triiodothyronine; FT4, free thyroxine; rT3, reverse triiodothyronine; TSH, thyroid-stimulating hormone. Data from references 3, 5 and 6.

their 85th birthday and again 3 years later.[39] Annual evaluation included assessment of activities of daily living (ADLs), cognitive performance and depression scales. About 12% had hypothyroidism at baseline (7% overt and 5% subclinical). None of the patients with subclinical hypothyroidism had progressed to overt hypothyroidism when retested at age 88 years. There was no association of baseline TSH levels and cognitive function, depressive symptoms or ADLs disability. All these parameters declined over time, but the decline was not accelerated in those with subclinical or overt hypothyroidism. Conversely, increased TSH at baseline was associated with a slower decline in instrumental ADLs ability, and also with lower all-cause cardiovascular mortality despite higher serum cholesterol concentrations.[39]

In 1966, Brain *et al.* described a patient with Hashimoto's autoimmune thyroiditis under treatment with levothyroxine, who developed several episodes of cerebral disorders.[40] After this first report, the association of thyroid autoantibodies with encephalopathy (incorrectly called 'Hashimoto's encephalopathy') has been reported by a few other authors.[41,42] Nevertheless, chronic lymphocytic thyroiditis is rarely associated with serious neurological manifestations and the number of reported cases of 'Hashimoto's encephalopathy' is very small compared with the high prevalence of thyroid autoimmunity in the general population. Hence the disorder may not be caused by antithyroid antibodies or thyroid dysfunction but may represent an association of an uncommon autoimmune encephalopathy with a common autoimmune thyroid disease. Another study found a high number of perfusion defects in euthyroid patients with autoimmune thyroiditis, suggesting that cerebral vasculitis might be implicated in this condition.[43] Even if 'Hashimoto's encephalopathy' is rare, it is life-threatening and responds to therapy with corticosteroids (up to 83% of patients); for this reason, it should better be called 'corticosteroid-responsive encephalopathy'.[44] The awareness of this treatable condition is important considering the possible association of hypothyroidism symptoms and encephalopathy in an older subjects.

The decision to treat a patient with overt hypothyroidism is usually straightforward, in contrast with the decision to treat subclinical hypothyroidism (see below) that may depend on the individual presentation and on an accurate evaluation of the possible benefit to be gained with the therapy. Treatment of overt hypothyroidism in older persons should be started and monitored carefully in order to maintain TSH and FT4 within the normal range. Thyroid hormone increases myocardial oxygen consumption, which may induce angina pectoris, myocardial infarction or cardiac arrhythmias in older patients. Hence in older patients, and even more so in older patients with heart disease or multiple coronary risk factors, thyroid hormone replacement should be initiated conservatively. The initial dose of levothyroxine should be very low (12.5–50 μg per day) and should be increased slowly every 4–6 weeks, with the purpose of reaching the replacement dose after 3–4 months.[1,2,34,45] The replacement dose of levothyroxine in older people is usually lower than 1.6 μg/kg per day, which is the dose usually employed in younger patients.[46] This reduction appears to be dependent on a relative decrease in lean body mass with ageing and the physiological age-associated reduction in T4 production.[47] In older hypothyroid patients there is a narrow range between TSH suppression and substitution dose, which may be due to an increased sensitivity of the thyrotrophes to the negative feedback by T4.[1] Another good reason for giving a lower dose in the oldest patients is that two studies (in subjects >73 and >85 years of age) have shown that high TSH and/or low FT4 levels are associated with a lower mortality rate.[11,39] It is essential to examine TSH measurements carefully every 3 months and to complete hormone replacement gradually, so as to avoid over-treatment and heart and central nervous system problems, which may be seen if the replacement is accomplished too quickly. In selected patients, in particular those with heart failure or alterations of heart rhythm, a dose of levothyroxine lower than substitutive is necessary to prevent ischaemic heart symptoms. The patient and the caregiver must be warned of the possible increase in angina, dyspnea, confusion and insomnia and notify these symptoms to the prescribing physician. Over-replacement may induce osteoporosis, anxiety, muscle wasting and atrial fibrillation as adverse effects. In older patients on chronic replacement therapy with levothyroxine sodium, estimation of serum TSH level once or twice per year is recommended, with small dosage adjustments to keep the serum TSH level within the normal range.

It is worth remembering that many older patients began taking thyroid hormone therapy when younger either for inappropriate reasons or for transient hypothyroidism, and they continue to take it without control. A study of nursing home residents reported that thyroid hormone therapy was successfully withdrawn from half of the residents studied.[33]

Subclinical hypothyroidism

The current widespread availability of greatly sensitive assays and more frequent assessment of serum TSH concentrations has lead to a more frequent finding of subclinical thyroid disorders, which are particularly frequent in older people.[4–6] The overall prevalence of subclinical hypothyroidism is 4–10% in the general population and up to 20% in women older than 60 years.[4,5,10] Progression to overt hypothyroidism is reported to vary from 3 to 20%, the risks being greater in those patients with goitre or thyroid antibodies, or both, but it is generally around 5%. Hence patients with subclinical hypothyroidism should be followed and eventually treated.[4,5,12] (Figure 98.1).

This disorder is defined as an elevated serum TSH level in the face of normal or normal-low free thyroid hormone values. The finding of a TSH measurement over 4.5 $mU\,l^{-1}$ should be confirmed within 1–3 months and repeated every 6–12 months in asymptomatic patients. If the value is confirmed, the possibility of past radioiodine administration, previous thyroid surgery, the presence of thyroid enlargement and history of thyroid dysfunctions in the family should be considered. In addition, exploration of subtle clinical signs of hypothyroidism and evaluation of lipid profile are suggested. Antithyroid antibodies are useful for improving the prognosis of progression to overt hypothyroidism but they may not change the management of the patient. If during follow-up TSH increases to over 10 $mU\,l^{-1}$, the patient should be treated with levothyroxine. When TSH is between 4.5 and 10 $mU\,l^{-1}$, an *ex adjuvantibus* administration of levothyroxine may be considered in an individual basis to help improve subtle clinical symptoms (Figure 98.1). A consistent association of subclinical hypothyroidism with cardiovascular problems, increased LDL cholesterol or other cardiovascular problems present in overt hypothyroidism (e.g. hypertension, impaired diastolic relaxation) and to neuropsychiatric problems, is still a matter of debate.[4,5,48,49] For example, recent reports show an attenuated CHD-related morbidity and mortality in patients with subclinical hypothyroidism treated with levothyroxine,[48] but patients with acute ischaemic stroke and subclinical hypothyroidism show more favourable outcomes than those without subclinical hypothyroidism.[49]

There is still no consensus on the potential benefits and risks of therapy for subclinical hypothyroidism. Possible mechanisms proposed to explain the potential benefit include modifications in lipid profiles, coagulation parameters and low-grade chronic inflammation. Early clinical and autopsy studies had suggested an association between subclinical hypothyroidism and coronary heart disease (CHD), which was later confirmed by some,[48–52] but not all,[53–56] large cross-sectional and prospective studies. A cross-sectional study in Western Australia, with a follow-up of 20 years, examined the prevalence of CHD in 2108 subjects with and without subclinical thyroid dysfunction. There were 21 cardiovascular deaths observed compared with 9.5 expected and 33 CHD events observed compared with 14.7 expected among patients with subclinical hypothyroidism, which remained significant after further adjustment for standard cardiovascular risk factors.[57] There is evidence that restoration of euthyroidism with levothyroxine can improve LDL cholesterol levels in most patients with subclinical hypothyroidism,[52,58,59] but the reduction of cardiovascular events remains to be elucidated, even though a recent reanalysis of the Whickham survey reported an association between incident CHD events and CHD-related mortality with subclinical hypothyroidism over a 20 year follow-up.[48] Treatment of subclinical hypothyroidism seemed to attenuate CHD-related morbidity and mortality, which may help to explain why different longitudinal studies, which did not take into account the presence of replacement therapy, are not homogeneous. Nevertheless, a definitive answer is not yet available. The decision to treat a patient might depend on the presence of other cardiovascular risk factors, rather than on a TSH threshold. Even if levothyroxine replacement therapy is usually safe with adequate titration and monitoring of serum TSH levels, in the oldest old (>85 years of age) thyroid hormone substitution is not likely to be beneficial.[60] In effect, it may even be harmful according to two studies in subjects over 73 and over 85 years of age which showed that high TSH and/or low free T4 levels are associated with a lower mortality rate.[11,39] Perhaps the discrepant results reported in the above-mentioned studies can be explained by the fact that subclinical hypothyroidism seems to be detrimental in young to middle-aged subjects, whereas it may be harmless or perhaps beneficial at advanced age.[60] Prospective randomized studies are still needed to establish definitely whether early treatment with levothyroxine will be of any benefit in reversing CHD risk in patients with subclinical hypothyroidism.

There is still a great deal of debate concerning the possible impact of mild or subclinical thyroid disorders on cognitive function, performance and survival in older people. A prospective, observational study conducted in individuals older than 85 years in Leiden, The Netherlands, with a mean follow-up of 3.7 years reported that neither TSH nor free T4 was associated with disability in daily life, depressive symptoms and cognitive impairment at baseline or during follow-up. Moreover, elevated TSH levels were associated with a lower mortality rate that remained significant after adjustment for baseline disability and health status, favouring no treatment for subclinical hypothyroidism.[39] Likewise, a recent study showed that well-functioning 70–79-year-old individuals with subclinical hypothyroidism do not demonstrate increased risk for mobility problems and those with mild elevations in TSH level show a slight functional advantage.[61] A cross-sectional survey, conducted in a primary care setting in England on 5865 patients older than 65 years, including 295 patients with subclinical thyroid dysfunction, reported no association of mild thyroid dysfunction with cognition, depression and anxiety, after adjustment for comorbid conditions and use of medications.[62] However, other studies have shown an association of subclinical hypothyroidism with depression in older subjects.[63,64]

Hyperthyroidism

Overt hyperthyroidism is characterized by high levels of thyroid hormones and a low TSH. The most common causes of hyperthyroidism in the elderly are Graves' disease in iodine-sufficient areas and nodular goitre (Plummer's disease or multinodular toxic goitre) and functioning follicular thyroid adenoma in iodine-deficient areas.[6,22,23,65] Transient thyrotoxicosis may occur in subacute thyroiditis and during treatment with amiodarone (particularly in iodine-deficient areas), which may represent a major therapeutic challenge.[66] Transient thyrotoxicosis during treatment with levothyroxine and interferon are self-limited and remit with drug withdrawal.

Whereas in younger patients there are multiple emblematic symptoms related to an overactive thyroid, the older patient may have few symptoms and they are frequently atypical. Patients often lack the hyperdynamic symptomatology (tremor, heat intolerance, ocular signs, nervousness or tachycardia) typical of the young hyperthyroid patient and instead have a more sedated, apathetic presentation. However, the frequency of atrial fibrillation is higher. Weight loss and cardiac symptoms frequently predominate and goitre is frequently absent, making the diagnosis less obvious than in the younger patient.[1–3] In addition, depression and mania can be manifestations of hyperthyroidism in the elderly.

Treatment of older patients with hyperthyroidism includes antithyroid drugs and radioactive iodine (^{131}I). ^{131}I is the treatment of choice, especially when concomitant cardiovascular diseases are present, while surgery may be considered if obstructive symptoms caused by large goitres are present, even if it is rarely indicated because of the high operative risk in older subjects with comorbidity.[1,3,65] Nevertheless, radioiodine may be also successfully used in large compressive goitres.[67] Treatment with beta-blockers may prevent symptoms of thyrotoxicosis following ^{131}I treatment and in general atrial fibrillation reverts to sinus rhythm within a few months after restoration of euthyroidism. Antithyroid drugs (methimazole or propylthiouracil) may be the treatment of choice for controlling hyperfunction before a definitive treatment with ^{131}I. Beta-adrenergic blockers (propranolol, metoprolol) may be used with prudence and, when needed, the dosage should be the lowest possible.[3,65] Treatment of an underactive thyroid after definitive treatment with ^{131}I is simpler than recurrence of hyperthyroidism in an older patient.

Subclinical hyperthyroidism

The finding of TSH levels below 0.45 mU l^{-1} in the presence of thyroid hormones in the normal or high borderline range is indicative of subclinical hyperthyroidism. As with hypothyroidism, the prevalence of overt hyperthyroidism is much lower than the subclinical dysfunction (3.2%, which decreases to 2% after exclusion of subjects with known thyroid disease).[4,10] In most cases, the cause is recognized: initial Graves' disease, initial nodular toxic goitre, excessive TSH suppressive therapy with levothyroxine for benign thyroid nodular disease or differentiated thyroid cancer or hormone over-replacement in patients with hypothyroidism. However, other causes of a low TSH, such as NTI, fasting and the use of drugs (e.g. glucocorticoids), should be excluded before making the diagnosis. Subclinical hyperthyroidism in older people may be associated with relevant signs and symptoms of excessive thyroid hormone action leading to an important reduction in the quality of life.[6,35,68]

Subclinical hyperthyroidism is usually associated with a higher heart rate and a higher risk of supraventricular arrhythmias, especially atrial fibrillation (three times the risk compared with controls)[69] and with an increased left ventricular mass, often associated with impaired diastolic function.[70,71]

It is becoming increasingly apparent that subclinical hyperthyroidism may decrease bone mineral mass and accelerate the development of osteoporosis and fragility fractures, particularly in postmenopausal women with a pre-existing predisposition,[35,72,73] hence patients with subclinical hyperthyroidism should be carefully evaluated. TSH measurement should be repeated and, if the low value is confirmed in a patient with atrial fibrillation or cardiovascular or other medical problems, a thyroid scintigraphy may help to consider the presence of a toxic goitre, Graves' disease or thyroiditis (in the destructive phase) (Figure 98.2).

A retrospective study investigating nursing home residents with low TSH and normal total T4 levels showed that only three out of 40 patients with subclinical

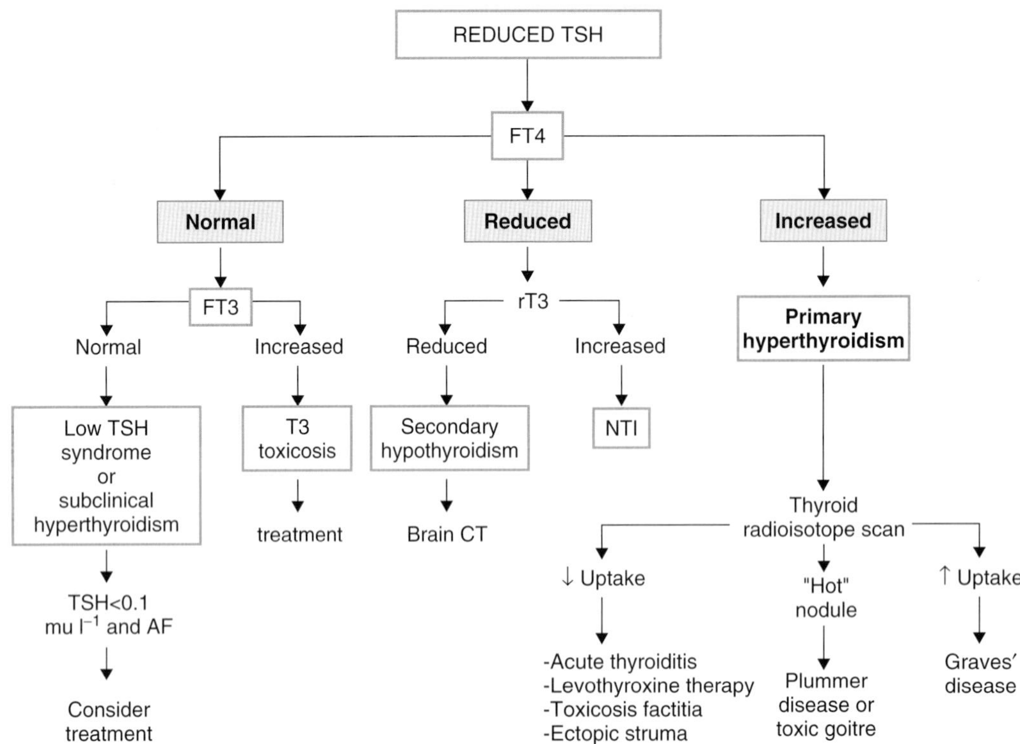

Figure 98.2 Algorithm for the diagnosis of thyroid disorders in the presence of a reduced TSH. AF, atrial fibrillation; ATAb, anti-thyroid antibodies; FT3, free triiodothyronine; FT4, free thyroxine; NTI, non-thyroidal illness; rT3, reverse triiodothyronine; TSH, thyroid-stimulating hormone. Data from references 3, 5 and 6.

hyperthyroidism became overt hyperthyroid. However, 17.5% of subjects with subclinical hyperthyroidism died during the first 4 months of follow-up compared with 7.5% in a control group, and 22.5% of subjects with subclinical hyperthyroidism had a history of or current atrial fibrillation, confirming the importance of identification of subjects at risk.[74] Regarding cognition, a recent study reported a higher risk (hazard ratio 2.26) of having cognitive dysfunction among participants with subclinical hyperthyroidism compared with those with normal thyroid function.[75]

The Cardiovascular Health Study of 3233 US community-dwelling individuals older than 65 years enrolled in 1989–1990 and reassessed through 2002 reported an incidence of subclinical hyperthyroidism of 1.5%. After exclusion of those with prevalent atrial fibrillation, persons with subclinical hyperthyroidism had a greater incidence of atrial fibrillation than those with normal thyroid function, with no differences for incident CHD, cerebrovascular disease, cardiovascular death or all-cause death.[54] Conversely, a population-based study in a cohort of 1191 individuals older than 60 years evaluated after 10 years in England and Wales revealed a significantly increased total and cardiovascular mortality in the first 5 years after first measurement in those with low TSH.[56] In fact, the association of endogenous subclinical hyperthyroidism with cardiovascular mortality is still controversial,[76] perhaps due to a lack of homogeneity among the diverse studies published on the subject, even meta-analyses giving conflicting results. Two studies with similar characteristics in terms of selection criteria and duration of follow-up but conducted in different populations (German and Japanese-Brazilian) reported opposite results.[77,78] Therefore, it remains controversial whether or not to treat middle-aged patients with low serum TSH levels until large prospective randomized controlled double-blind studies of young and old patients with subclinical hyperthyroidism and without underlying cardiac disease are available.

In view of the fact that subclinical hyperthyroidism and its related clinical manifestations are reversible, may in some cases cause significant morbidity and mortality and may be prevented by timely treatment,[35] it is important to consider the possible benefit of treatment on an individual basis. At present, most authors are in agreement regarding the treatment of elderly patients with subclinical hyperthyroidism and a clearly suppressed TSH level ($<0.1\,mU\,l^{-1}$) and follow-up for patients with TSH levels between 0.1 and $0.4\,mU\,l^{-1}$.[4,79,80] Beta-blockers have been proposed to reduce the cardiac effects of levothyroxine suppressive treatment.[35]

Another important issue is the cardiac and skeletal effects of long-term TSH suppression used to reduce thyroid cancer recurrence. According to recent guidelines from the American Thyroid Association, it is necessary to consider age, the presence of pre-existing cardiovascular and skeletal risk factors and the aggressiveness of thyroid cancer to decide the TSH target and to balance better the benefit against the potential adverse effects of long-term TSH suppression. In addition, adequate intake of calcium and vitamin D to prevent osteoporosis should be encouraged.[81]

Non-thyroidal illness (NTI)

Age-related diseases, both acute and chronic, and also malnutrition may modify thyroid tests either to mask existing thyroid dysfunction or to induce changes which simulate abnormal results by spuriously increasing or decreasing circulating concentrations of thyroid hormone and levels of pituitary TSH and transport proteins. In mild illness, a decrease in serum T3 levels can be found. However, as the severity and duration of the illness increase, both serum T3 and T4 decrease, without an elevation of TSH. The decrease in hormone levels is seen in starvation, sepsis, surgery, myocardial infarction, bypass, bone marrow transplantation and in fact probably any severe illness. This is often referred to as NTI,[82–84] which is also called 'euthyroid-sick syndrome'; however, in some sick patients it is possible that an acquired transient central hypothyroidism is present,[82,84] hence they may not be 'euthyroid', but this is still a controversial area.[84–86] Recently, evidence has accumulated that central hypothyroidism and altered peripheral metabolism of T4 and T3 combine to produce a state characterized by diminished serum and tissue supplies of thyroid hormones. The high prevalence of NTI in older populations is an important confounder in the assessment of thyroid function. For example, in a study including 403 healthy ambulatory men (aged 73–94 years), excluding subjects with systemic infectious, inflammatory and malignant disorders, 63 men met the criteria for NTI (low T3 and high rT3).[11] The subjects with NTI were older and more frequently had diseases such as hypertension, atherosclerosis, diabetes, chronic obstructive pulmonary disease, congestive heart failure and/or arthritis. Of note, high rT3 was associated with a low performance score independent of disease, probably due to the nutritional status, since caloric deprivation is known to result in an increase in serum rT3 levels.[87]

Systemic illnesses have multiple effects on thyroid hormone metabolism and on serum thyroid hormone concentrations, even in the absence of specific hypothalamic, pituitary or thyroid diseases. These changes seem to be primarily related to the severity and chronicity of illnesses,[88] rather to the specific disease states. Malnutrition and/or increased catabolism related to chronicity, which result in progressive declines in thyroid-binding protein concentrations, may play a key role in NTI. In addition, the ageing process itself is associated with decreased serum levels of T3 and TSH concentrations that are to some extent independent of NTI.[1] Despite these abnormalities, treatment of NTI patients with thyroid hormone, although controversial, appears to be of little benefit and it may even be harmful.[89] It has long been proposed that the changes in thyroid function during severe illness are protective in preventing excessive tissue catabolism.

The mechanisms proposed to mediate NTI are listed in Table 98.4.[84,90–96] These mechanisms include an induction of central hypothyroidism due to reduced hypothalamic TRH, probably signalled by a decrease in leptin caused by malnutrition and possibly a localized increase in hypothalamic T3 catalysed by altered expression of hypothalamic T3 deiodinases D2 and D3. In acute illness, a fall in T3 and T4 precedes the fall in hepatic D1, hence decreased thyroid hormones may be attributable to an acute phase response inducing a reduction in thyroid-hormone binding capacity of plasma.[84]

Measurement of serum rT3, the product of 5-monodeiodination of T4, may occasionally be helpful in distinguishing between NTI and central hypothyroidism, since rT3 concentrations are usually high in patients with NTI and low in patients with central hypothyroidism.[86,89] Thyroid hormones are low largely because of reductions in thyroid hormone-binding proteins. Not often, free T3 and free T4 are decreased because circulating substances may inhibit binding to thyroid hormone-binding proteins, such as free fatty acids or cytokines.[90] Almost all patients with subnormal but detectable TSH levels (<0.3 and $>0.05\,\mathrm{mU\,l^{-1}}$) will be euthyroid when reassessed after recovery from the acute illness. On the other hand, most patients with undetectable serum TSH levels ($<0.01\,\mathrm{mU\,l^{-1}}$) have hyperthyroidism.[65] Numerous drugs have important effects on thyroid function and/or on thyroid function test (Tables 98.1–98.3) and polypharmacy is very frequent in older patients, hence this non-thyroidal factor should be considered. A study evaluating 1153 determinations of T4 in nursing homes identified 22 individuals with low T4 and normal TSH, of whom 36% were treated with high-dose salicylates, 18% with phenytoin, 14% with carbamazepine and 9% with prednisone. Six of the 22 were placed on levothyroxine replacement without documentation of hypothyroidism, although in five of them, low T4 could be attributed to a medication effect.[97]

There is even greater uncertainly about hormone replacement therapy in ill patients with low serum T4 or T3 concentrations. It has been repeatedly recommended not to start replacement treatment, even if there is no factual support for that observation. Hence controlled clinical trials are needed to establish an evidenced-based recommendation. However, if there is evidence to support a diagnosis of hypothyroidism (e.g. a TSH $>20\,\mathrm{mU\,l^{-1}}$

Table 98.4 Possible mechanism of non-thyroidal illness (NTI)[a].[84,90–96]

	Low T3	Low T4	Low TSH	Low TRH
Albumin	Reduced	–	–	–
TBPA	Reduced	–	–	–
TBG	Reduced	Reduced	–	–
TRH	Reduced	Reduced	Reduced	Reduced
Dopamine	–	–	Increased	–
Glucocorticoids	–	–	Increased	–
NEFA	Increased	–	–	–
INF	–	Increased	Increased	–
Leptin	–	Reduced	–	Reduced
IL1	Increased	Increased	Increased	–
IL6	Increased	Increased	Increased	–
TNFα	Increased	Increased	Increased	–
D2, D3	–	–	–	Increased
Competitors for TH binding	Increased	Increased	–	–

[a]D2, D3, deiodinases 2 and 3; IL, interleukin; INF, interferons; NEFA, non-esterified fatty acids; TBG, thyronine-binding globulin; TBPA, thyroxine-binding prealbumin; TH, thyroid hormone; TNF, tumour necrosis factor; TRH, thyrotropin-releasing hormone

with low free T4 and/or history, symptoms and signs of hypothyroidism), prudent administration of thyroid hormone is appropriate.[85]

Thyroid nodules and nodular goitre

Most thyroid nodules (~95%), which occur with increasing frequency in older people, are benign. Nonetheless, clinical evaluation should be considered for all thyroid nodules given a 5–13% risk of evolving into thyroid malignancy.[98] The risk of malignancy is similar for solitary nodules and multinodular goitres; urgent referral to secondary care is necessary only if the nodule is growing rapidly (over a few weeks) or associated with stridor, hoarseness or cervical lymphadenopathy.[99] Goitre is more common in women than in men.[100] The American Association of Clinical Endocrinologists (AACE) reports a prevalence of palpable thyroid nodules in 3–7% in North America; however, the prevalence increases to ~50% based on ultrasound (US) or autopsy data.[98] Generally, goitre size increases with ageing and thyroid nodularity develops, with the largest goitres observed in the oldest age groups living in iodine-deficient areas. The prevalence of diffuse and nodular goitre in young adults participating in an iodine-deficient area survey (Pescopagano study) was 30% in young adults and increased to 75% in the age group 55–65 years, with nodular goitre accounting for about one-third of the total.[23]

Fine-needle aspiration biopsy (FNAB) is the most accurate method in the evaluation of a thyroid nodule, helping to determine which patients should be referred for surgery. Its accuracy is improved by high-resolution US guidance, which can also add useful information. Nonetheless, none of the US findings are diagnostic and FNAB remains the cornerstone of thyroid cancer diagnosis.[99] Thyroid cancer in old age is generally well differentiated, but its course is frequently less predictable than in younger patients. Lymphoma of the thyroid and undifferentiated cancers occur with increasing frequency in the elderly. Multinodular goitre, usually longstanding, is frequently seen in old age and thyroid hormone suppressive therapy not only is not indicated but also may contribute to exogenous hyperthyroidism with heart and bone adverse effects.[2] The physical examination of women with goitre may be complicated by hyperkyphosis and changes in posture associated with osteoporosis; if the thyroid gland can be palpated in an older woman, it is probably enlarged. Calcification of large goitres may be associated with dyspnea, dysphagia or dysphonia and can be misdiagnosed as cancer metastases to lymphoid nodes, hence FNAB is recommended to determine the nature of calcified lesions.[101] According to AACE guidelines, thyroid US should not be performed as a screening test; however, patients with a palpable thyroid nodule should undergo US examination. Management depends mainly on the results of needle aspiration but should also take into consideration the clinical and US features. FNAB (with or without US guidance) is recommended for nodules 10 mm or larger in diameter, with one or more of the following US characteristics: irregular margins, chaotic intranodular vascular spots, a more tall than wide shape and microcalcifications.[98] US–FNAB is suggested for nodules smaller than 10 mm only if clinical information or US features are suspicious. In general, FNAB is highly accurate.

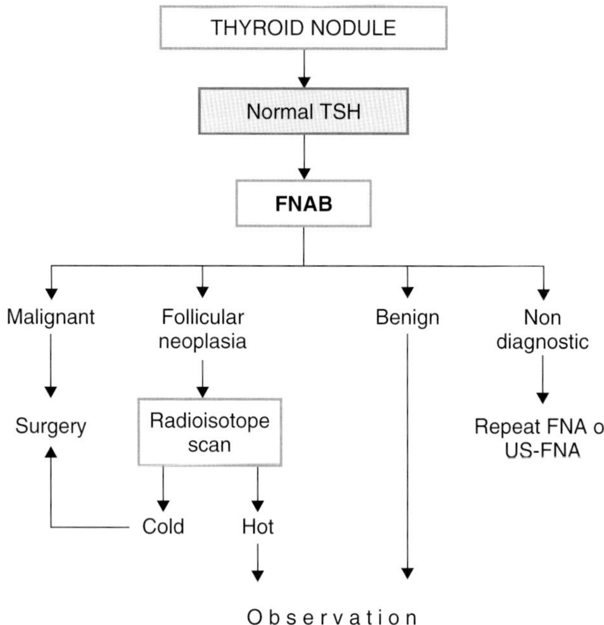

Figure 98.3 Algorithm for the diagnosis and management of thyroid nodules in the presence of normal TSH. FNAB, fine-needle aspiration biopsy; TSH, thyroid-stimulating hormone; US, ultrasound. Data from references 98–100.

However, a major limitation of FNAB is inadequate or indeterminate results, which occur in 10–25% of cases. In such cases, surgery is usually recommended for diagnosis, with the majority of these nodules proving to be benign.[98,100]

Benign thyroid nodules revealed by FNAB should undergo follow-up and malignant or suspicious nodules should be treated surgically. A thyroid radioisotope scan is useful if the TSH level is low or suppressed. Large, symptomatic goitres may be treated surgically or with radioiodine. Routine measurement of serum calcitonin is not recommended.[98] Figures 98.3 and 98.4 illustrate a suggested algorithm for the diagnosis and management of thyroid nodule.

A nodule(s) in multinodular goitre may become autonomous with ageing and progress to overt thyrotoxicosis, while large goitres may cause obstructive symptoms. When a goitre is asymptomatic, follow-up is the choice, whereas treatment is necessary in the case of toxic goitre or compressive symptoms. Suppressive levothyroxine treatment is generally not recommended in old age. ^{131}I is the first-choice treatment for thyroid autonomy and hyperthyroidism, whereas surgery is advised for large, non-toxic goitres causing significant compressive symptoms. ^{131}I therapy has been proposed in order to reduce thyroid volume in non-toxic goitres,

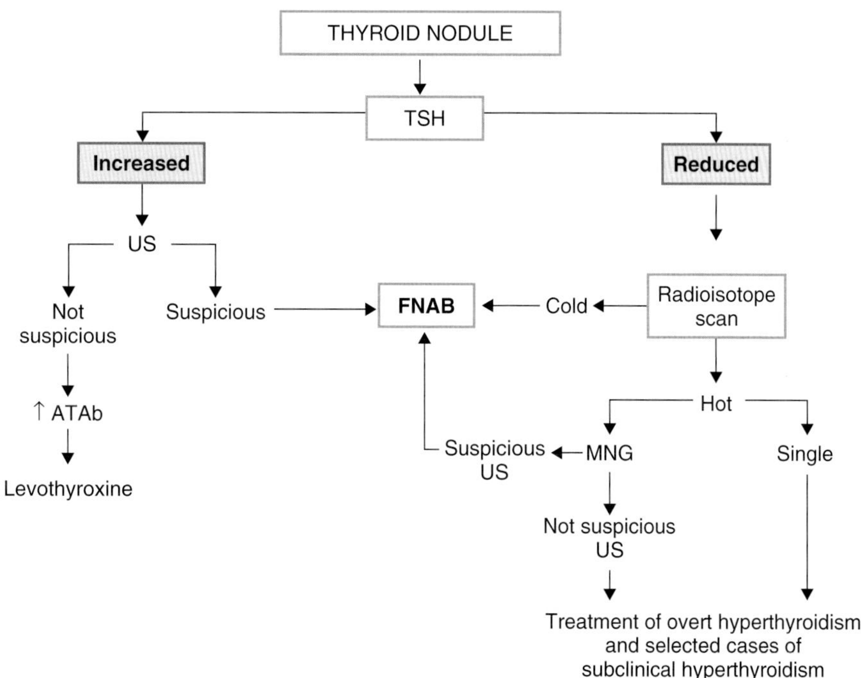

Figure 98.4 Algorithm for the diagnosis and management of thyroid nodules in the presence of an increased or reduced TSH. ATAb, anti-thyroid antibodies; FNAB, fine-needle aspiration biopsy; MNG, multinodular goitre; TSH, thyroid-stimulating hormone; US, ultrasound. Data from references 98–100.

with satisfactory results, even in the presence of structural and functional heterogeneity and large variability in ^{131}I dose. Pretreatment with recombinant TSH (rhTSH) may increase the efficacy of ^{131}I therapy.[102] However, since these strategies have been reported in relatively small studies with different thyroid size and function, definitive conclusions and recommendation cannot be drawn. Furthermore, severe acute adverse effects caused by radiation-induced thyroiditis and oesophagitis after rhTSH pretreatment have been reported, hence appropriate management protocols need to be defined.[103]

Conclusion

Ageing is associated with a number of thyroid function modifications. However, it is not simple to discern whether and to what extent these changes are an expression of the ageing process *per se* or of an age-associated thyroidal and/or non-thyroidal illness. Ageing is frequently associated with an increased prevalence of thyroid autoantibodies, which may be an expression of age-associated disease rather than a consequence of the ageing process itself. Thyroid diseases in older patients differ from those observed in younger patients in their prevalence, which is higher especially among women, and clinical expression. Their treatment often deserves special attention because of the increased risk for complications (e.g. cardiac arrhythmia, cognitive decline, bone loss). The thyroid hormone replacement dose in older people with overt hypothyroidism is usually lower than that in younger people and should be increased slowly every 4–6 weeks. Definitive treatment with ^{131}I is the treatment of choice for overt hyperthyroidism, especially when concomitant cardiovascular diseases are present, whereas surgery may be considered if important obstructive symptoms are present.

There is often significant delay and difficulty in the diagnosis of thyroid disorders in old age because clinical presentation is paucisymptomatic and attributed to normal ageing and because atypical presentations are not uncommon. Routine screening of asymptomatic, healthy adults is not recommended; however, physicians should maintain a high index of suspicion for testing thyroid function in subjects at risk. The interpretation of thyroid function tests may be complex in old individuals because of age-associated changes in thyroid function and also because of frequent alterations secondary to NTI, malnutrition and/or drugs. Subclinical abnormalities of thyroid function are more prevalent than overt disease in old populations. Subclinical hyperthyroidism appears to be a significant risk factor for cardiac arrhythmia, especially atrial fibrillation and fragility fractures in old age. The benefits of treatment of subclinical disease are not completely elucidated. Nonetheless, subclinical hypothyroidism has been linked to increased mortality in middle-aged and young elderly subjects, possibly via its atherogenic potential, but mild thyroid dysfunction appears to be devoid of unfavourable effects and possibly even be protective in the oldest-old persons. Hence the decision to treat subclinical conditions should be individualized and restricted to high-risk patients to avoid side effects of unnecessary thyroid replacement and antithyroid medications in vulnerable elderly, in whom appropriate caution and careful dose adjustments are needed. Treatment of thyroid disease deserves especial attention in the oldest patients because of the increased risk for complications and the lack of evidence-based data in this population.

Even if most of thyroid nodules in older persons are benign, clinical evaluation should be considered for timely identification of thyroid malignancy. FNAB remains the cornerstone of thyroid cancer diagnosis, and its accuracy may be improved by high-resolution US evaluation. Nonetheless, none of the US findings are fully diagnostic.

Key points

- Although thyroid disorders in older persons are frequent, they are difficult to suspect and diagnose (similar to ageing itself or other diseases and confounded by polypharmacy, malnutrition and comorbidity).
- Thyroid disorders have an important effect on quality of life, hence overt clinical disease should be identified in a timely manner and be adequately treated.
- Although no consensus regarding the wide treatment of subclinical thyroid disorders has been achieved, identification of subjects at highest risk is warranted, especially for subclinical hyperthyroidism.

References

1. Mariotti S, Franceschi C, Cossarizza A and Pinchera A. The aging thyroid. *Endocr Rev* 1995;**16**:686–715.
2. Levy EG. Thyroid disease in the elderly. *Med Clin North Am* 1991;**75**:151–67.
3. Mohandas R, Gupta KL. Managing thyroid dysfunction in the elderly. Answers to seven common questions. *Postgrad Med* 2003;**113**:54–6, 65–8, 100.
4. Surks MI, Ortiz E, Daniels GH *et al*. Subclinical thyroid disease: scientific review and guidelines for diagnosis and management. *JAMA* 2004;**291**:228–38.
5. Cooper DS. Clinical practice. Subclinical hypothyroidism. *N Engl J Med* 2001;**345**:260–5.
6. Toft AD. Clinical practice. Subclinical hyperthyroidism. *N Engl J Med* 2001;**345**:512–6.

7. Mariotti S, Barbesino G, Caturegli P *et al.* Complex alteration of thyroid function in healthy centenarians. *J Clin Endocrinol Metab* 1993;**77**:1130–4.
8. Chiovato L, Mariotti S and Pinchera A. Thyroid diseases in the elderly. *Bailliere's Clin Endocrinol Metab* 1997;**11**:251–70.
9. Peeters RP, Wouters PJ, van Toor H *et al.* Serum 3,3′,5′-triiodothyronine (rT3) and 3,5,3′-triiodothyronine/rT3 are prognostic markers in critically ill patients and are associated with postmortem tissue deiodinase activities. *J Clin Endocrinol Metab* 2005;**90**:4559–65.
10. Hollowell JG, Staehling NW, Flanders WD *et al.* Serum TSH, T(4) and thyroid antibodies in the United States population (1988 to 1994): National Health and Nutrition Examination Survey (NHANES III). *J Clin Endocrinol Metab* 2002; **87**:489–99.
11. van den Beld AW, Visser TJ, Feelders RA *et al.* Thyroid hormone concentrations, disease, physical function and mortality in elderly men. *J Clin Endocrinol Metab* 2005;**90**: 6403–9.
12. Tunbridge WM, Evered DC, Hall R *et al.* The spectrum of thyroid disease in a community: the Whickham survey. *Clin Endocrinol (Oxf)* 1977;**7**:481–93.
13. Sawin CT, Chopra D, Azizi F *et al.* The aging thyroid. Increased prevalence of elevated serum thyrotropin levels in the elderly. *JAMA* 1979;**242**:247–50.
14. Mariotti S, Chiovato L, Franceschi C and Pinchera A. Thyroid autoimmunity and aging. *Exp Gerontol* 1998;**33**:535–41.
15. Hak AE, Pols HA, Visser TJ *et al.* Subclinical hypothyroidism is an independent risk factor for atherosclerosis and myocardial infarction in elderly women: the Rotterdam study. *Ann Intern Med* 2000;**132**:270–8.
16. Imaizumi M, Akahoshi M, Ichimaru S *et al.* Risk for ischemic heart disease and all-cause mortality in subclinical hypothyroidism. *J Clin Endocrinol Metab* 2004;**89**:3365–70.
17. Peeters RP, van der Deure WM and Visser TJ. Genetic variation in thyroid hormone pathway genes; polymorphisms in the TSH receptor and the iodothyronine deiodinases. *Eur J Endocrinol* **1** 2006;**55**:655–62.
18. Hansen PS, van der Deure WM, Peeters RP *et al.* The impact of a TSH receptor gene polymorphism on thyroid-related phenotypes in a healthy Danish twin population. *Clin Endocrinol (Oxf)* 2007;**66**:827–32.
19. Kritz-Silverstein D, Schultz ST, Palinska LA *et al.* The association of thyroid stimulating hormone levels with cognitive function and depressed mood: the Rancho Bernardo study. *J Nutr Health Aging* 2009;**13**:317–21.
20. Canaris GJ, Manowitz NR, Mayor G and Ridgway EC. The Colorado thyroid disease prevalence study. *Arch Intern Med* 2000;**160**:526–34.
21. Bulow Pedersen I, Knudsen N, Jorgensen T *et al.* Large differences in incidences of overt hyper- and hypothyroidism associated with a small difference in iodine intake: a prospective comparative register-based population survey. *J Clin Endocrinol Metab* 2002;**87**:4462–9.
22. Laurberg P, Pedersen KM, Vestergaard H and Sigurdsson G. High incidence of multinodular toxic goitre in the elderly population in a low iodine intake area vs. high incidence of Graves' disease in the young in a high iodine intake area: comparative surveys of thyrotoxicosis epidemiology in East-Jutland Denmark and Iceland. *J Intern Med* 1991;**229**:415–20.
23. Aghini-Lombardi F, Antonangeli L, Martino E *et al.* The spectrum of thyroid disorders in an iodine-deficient community: the Pescopagano survey. *J Clin Endocrinol Metab* 1999;**84**:561–6.
24. Knudsen N, Bulow I, Jorgensen T *et al.* Comparative study of thyroid function and types of thyroid dysfunction in two areas in Denmark with slightly different iodine status. *Eur J Endocrinol* 2000;**143**:485–91.
25. Laurberg P, Bulow Pedersen I, Knudsen N *et al.* Environmental iodine intake affects the type of nonmalignant thyroid disease. *Thyroid* 2001;**11**:457–69.
26. Wilson S, Parle JV, Roberts LM *et al.* Prevalence of subclinical thyroid dysfunction and its relation to socioeconomic deprivation in the elderly: a community-based cross-sectional survey. *J Clin Endocrinol Metab* 2006;**91**:4809–16.
27. Muller GM, Levitt NS and Louw SJ. Thyroid dysfunction in the elderly. *S Afr Med J* 1997;**87**:1119–23.
28. Ayala C, Cozar MV, Rodriguez JR *et al.* Subclinical thyroid disease in institutionalised healthy geriatric population. *Med Clin (Barc)* 2001;**117**:534–55 (in Spanish).
29. Ania Lafuente BJ, Suarez Almenara JL, Fernandez-Burriel Tercero M *et al.* Thyroid function in the aged admitted to a nursing home. *An Med Interna* 2000;**17**:5–8 (in Spanish).
30. Drinka PJ and Nolten WE. Prevalence of previously undiagnosed hypothyroidism in residents of a midwestern nursing home. *South Med J* 1990;**83**:1259–61, 1265.
31. Thong H and Rahimi AR. Prevalence of hypothyroidism in a southeastern nursing home. *J Am Med Dir Assoc* 2000;**1**:25–8.
32. Szabolcs I, Podoba J, Feldkamp J *et al.* Comparative screening for thyroid disorders in old age in areas of iodine deficiency, long-term iodine prophylaxis and abundant iodine intake. *Clin Endocrinol (Oxf)* 1997;**47**:87–92.
33. Coll PP and Abourizk NN. Successful withdrawal of thyroid hormone therapy in nursing home patients. *J Am Board Fam Pract* 2000;**13**:403–7.
34. Laurberg P, Andersen S, Bulow Pedersen I and Carle A. Hypothyroidism in the elderly: pathophysiology, diagnosis and treatment. *Drugs Aging* 2005;**22**:23–38.
35. Biondi B, Palmieri EA, Klain M *et al.* Subclinical hyperthyroidism: clinical features and treatment options. *Eur J Endocrinol* 2005;**152**:1–9.
36. Drinka PJ, Nolten WE, Voeks SK and Langer EH. Follow-up of mild hypothyroidism in a nursing home. *J Am Geriatr Soc* 1991;**39**:264–6.
37. Vanderpump MP, Tunbridge WM, French JM *et al.* The incidence of thyroid disorders in the community: a twenty-year follow-up of the Whickham Survey. *Clin Endocrinol (Oxf)* 1995;**43**:55–68.
38. Diez JJ. Hypothyroidism in patients older than 55 years: an analysis of the etiology and assessment of the effectiveness of therapy. *J Gerontol A Biol Sci Med Sci* 2002;**57**:M315–20.
39. Gussekloo J, van Exel E, de Craen AJ *et al.* Thyroid status, disability and cognitive function and survival in old age. *JAMA* 2004;**292**:2591–9.
40. Brain L, Jellinek EH and Ball K. Hashimoto's disease and encephalopathy. *Lancet* 1966;**ii**:512–4.

41. Chong JY, Rowland LP and Utiger RD. Hashimoto encephalopathy: syndrome or myth? *Arch Neurol* 2003;**60**: 164–71.
42. Sawka AM, Fatourechi V, Boeve BF and Mokri B. Rarity of encephalopathy associated with autoimmune thyroiditis: a case series from Mayo Clinic from 1950 to 1996. *Thyroid* 2002;**12**:393–8.
43. Zettinig G, Asenbaum S, Fueger BJ *et al.* Increased prevalence of sublinical brain perfusion abnormalities in patients with autoimmune thyroiditis: evidence of Hashimoto's encephalitis? *Clin Endocrinol (Oxf)* 2003;**59**:637–43.
44. Fatourechi V. Hashimoto's encephalopathy: myth or reality? An endocrinologist's perspective. *Best Pract Res Clin Endocrinol Metab* 2005;**19**:53–66.
45. Wartofsky L. Levothyroxine therapy for hypothyroidism: should we abandon conservative dosage titration? *Arch Intern Med* 2005;**165**:1683–4.
46. Santini F, Pinchera A, Marsili A *et al.* Lean body mass is a major determinant of levothyroxine dosage in the treatment of thyroid diseases. *J Clin Endocrinol Metab* 2005;**90**:124–7.
47. Davis FB, LaMantia RS, Spaulding SW *et al.* Estimation of a physiologic replacement dose of levothyroxine in elderly patients with hypothyroidism. *Arch Intern Med* 1984; **144**:1752–4.
48. Razvi S, Weaver JU, Vanderpump MP and Pearce SH. The incidence of ischemic heart disease and mortality in people with subclinical hypothyroidism: reanalysis of the Whickham survey cohort. *J Clin Endocrinol Metab* 2010;**95**:1734–40.
49. Baek JH, Chung PW, Kim YB *et al.* Favorable influence of subclinical hypothyroidism on the functional outcomes in stroke patients. *Endocr J* 2010;**57**:23–29.
50. Singh S, Duggal J, Molnar J *et al.* Impact of subclinical thyroid disorders on coronary heart disease, cardiovascular and all-cause mortality: a meta-analysis. *Int J Cardiol* 2008;**125**, 41–8.
51. Rodondi N, Aujesky D, Vittinghoff E *et al.* Subclinical hypothyroidism and the risk of coronary heart disease: a meta-analysis. *Am J Med* 2006;**119**:541–51.
52. Biondi B, Palmieri EA, Lombardi G and Fazio S. Effects of subclinical thyroid dysfunction on the heart. *Ann Intern Med* 2002;**137**:904–14.
53. Yun KH, Jeong MH, Oh SK *et al.* Relationship of thyroid stimulating hormone with coronary atherosclerosis in angina patients. *Int J Cardiol* 2007;**122**:56–60.
54. Cappola AR, Fried LP, Arnold AM *et al.* Thyroid status, cardiovascular risk and mortality in older adults. *JAMA* 2006;**295**:1033–41.
55. Rodondi N, Newman AB, Vittinghoff E *et al.* Subclinical hypothyroidism and the risk of heart failure, other cardiovascular events and death. *Arch Intern Med* 2005;**165**:2460–6.
56. Parle JV, Maisonneuve P, Sheppard MC *et al.* Prediction of all-cause and cardiovascular mortality in elderly people from one low serum thyrotropin result: a 10-year cohort study. *Lancet* 2001;**358**:861–5.
57. Walsh JP, Bremner AP, Bulsara MK *et al.* Subclinical thyroid dysfunction as a risk factor for cardiovascular disease. *Arch Intern Med* 2005;**165**:2467–72.
58. Arem R and Patsch W. Lipoprotein and apolipoprotein levels in subclinical hypothyroidism. Effect of levothyroxine therapy. *Arch Intern Med* 1990;**150**:2097–100.
59. Kung AW, Pang RW and Janus ED. Elevated serum lipoprotein(a) in subclinical hypothyroidism. *Clin Endocrinol (Oxf)* 1995;**43**:445–9.
60. Mariotti S. Mild hypothyroidism and ischemic heart disease: is age the answer? *J Clin Endocrinol Metab* 2008;**93**:2969–71.
61. Simonsick EM, Newman AB, Ferrucci L *et al.* Subclinical hypothyroidism and functional mobility in older adults. *Arch Intern Med* 2009;**169**:2011–7.
62. Roberts LM, Pattison H, Roalfe A *et al.* Is subclinical thyroid dysfunction in the elderly associated with depression or cognitive dysfunction? *Ann Intern Med* 2006;**145**: 573–81.
63. Chueire VB, Silva ET, Perotta E *et al.* High serum TSH levels are associated with depression in the elderly. *Arch Gerontol Geriatr* 2003;**36**:281–8.
64. Fountoulakis KN, Kantartzis S, Siamouli M *et al.* Peripheral thyroid dysfunction in depression. *World J Biol Psychiatry* 2006;**7**:131–7.
65. Nayak B, Hodak SP. Hyperthyroidism. *Endocrinology and Metabolism Clinics of North America* 2007;**36**:617–56.
66. Martino E, Bartalena L, Bogazzi F and Braverman LE. The effects of amiodarone on the thyroid. *Endocr Rev* 2001;**22**:240–54.
67. Huysmans DA, Hermus AR, Corstens FH *et al.* Large, compressive goiters treated with radioiodine. *Ann Intern Med* 1994;**121**:757–62.
68. Auer J, Berent R, Weber T *et al.* Thyroid function is associated with presence and severity of coronary atherosclerosis. *Clin Cardiol* 2003;**26**:569–73.
69. Helfand M. Screening for subclinical thyroid dysfunction in nonpregnant adults: a summary of the evidence for the U.S. Preventive Services Task Force. *Ann Intern Med* 2004;**140**:128–41.
70. Sawin CT, Geller A, Wolf PA *et al.* Low serum thyrotropin concentrations as a risk factor for atrial fibrillation in older persons. *N Engl J Med* 1994;**331**:1249–52.
71. Biondi B, Palmieri EA, Fazio S *et al.* Endogenous subclinical hyperthyroidism affects quality of life and cardiac morphology and function in young and middle-aged patients. *J Clin Endocrinol Metab* 2000;**85**:4701–5.
72. Foldes J, Tarjan G, Szathmari M *et al.* Bone mineral density in patients with endogenous subclinical hyperthyroidism: is this thyroid status a risk factor for osteoporosis? *Clin Endocrinol (Oxf)* 1993;**39**:521–7.
73. Kumeda Y, Inaba M, Tahara H *et al.* Persistent increase in bone turnover in Graves' patients with subclinical hyperthyroidism. *J Clin Endocrinol Metab* 2000;**85**: 4157–61.
74. Drinka PJ, Amberson J, Voeks SK *et al.* Low TSH levels in nursing home residents not taking thyroid hormone. *J Am Geriatr Soc* 1996;**44**:573–7.
75. Ceresini G, Lauretani F, Maggio M *et al.* Thyroid function abnormalities and cognitive impairment in elderly people: results of the Invecchiare in Chianti study. *J Am Geriatr Soc* 2009;**57**:89–93.

76. Biondi B. Invited commentary. Cardiovascular mortality in subclinical hyperthyroidism: an ongoing dilemma. *Eur J Endocrinol* 2010;**162**:587–9.
77. Ittermann T, Haring R, Sauer S *et al*. Decreased serum TSH levels are not associated with mortality in the adult northeast German population. *Eur J Endocrinol* 2010;**162**: 579–85.
78. Sgarbi JA, Matsumura LK, Kasamatsu TS *et al*. Subclinical thyroid dysfunctions are independent risk factors for mortality in a 7.5-year follow-up: the Japanese-Brazilian thyroid study. *Eur J Endocrinol* 2010;**162**:569–77.
79. Gharib H, Tuttle RM, Baskin HJ *et al*. Subclinical thyroid dysfunction: a joint statement on management from the American Association of Clinical Endocrinologists, the American Thyroid Association and the Endocrine Society. *J Clin Endocrinol Metab* 2005;**90**:581–5; discussion 586–7.
80. Diez JJ and Iglesias P. An analysis of the natural course of subclinical hyperthyroidism. *Am J Med Sci* 2009;**337**:225–32.
81. Biondi B and Cooper DS. Benefits of thyrotropin suppression versus the risks of adverse effects in differentiated thyroid cancer. *Thyroid* 2010;**20**:135–46.
82. Chopra IJ. Clinical review 86. Euthyroid sick syndrome: is it a misnomer? *J Clin Endocrinol Metab* 1997;**82**:329–34.
83. De Groot LJ. Dangerous dogmas in medicine: the nonthyroidal illness syndrome. *J Clin Endocrinol Metab* 1999;**84**: 151–64.
84. Warner M and Beckett G. Mechanisms behind the nonthyroidal illness syndrome: an update. *J Endocrinol* 2010;**205**: 1–13.
85. DeGroot LJ. 'Non-thyroidal illness syndrome' is functional central hypothyroidism and if severe, hormone replacement is appropriate in light of present knowledge. *J Endocrinol Invest* 2003;**26**:1163–70.
86. Fliers E, Alkemade A and Wiersinga WM. The hypothalamic–pituitary–thyroid axis in critical illness. *Best Pract Res Clin Endocrinol Metab* 2001;**15**:453–64.
87. Peeters RP, Debaveye Y, Fliers E and Visser TJ. Changes within the thyroid axis during critical illness. *Crit Care Clin* 2006;**22**:41–55.
88. Van den Berghe GH. Acute and prolonged critical illness are two distinct neuroendocrine paradigms. *Verh K Acad Geneeskd Belg* 1998;**60**:487–518; discussion 518–20.
89. Utiger RD. Altered thyroid function in nonthyroidal illness and surgery. To treat or not to treat? *N Engl J Med* 1995;**333**:1562–3.
90. Boelen A, Platvoet-ter Schiphorst MC, Bakker O *et al*. The role of cytokines in the lipopolysaccharide-induced sick euthyroid syndrome in mice. *J Endocrinol* 1995;**146**: 475–83.
91. Davies PH, Black EG, Sheppard MC and Franklyn JA. Relation between serum interleukin-6 and thyroid hormone concentrations in 270 hospital in-patients with non-thyroidal illness. *Clin Endocrinol (Oxf)* 1996;**44**:199–205.
92. Heinen E, Herrmann J, Konigshausen T and Kruskemper HL. Secondary hypothyroidism in severe non thyroidal illness? *Horm Metab Res* 1981;**13**:284–8.
93. Kabadi UM. Thyrotropin dysregulation during a nonthyroidal illness: transient hypothalamic hypothyroidism? *J Endocrinol Invest* 2001;**24**:178–82.
94. Karga H, Papaioannou P, Venetsanou K *et al*. The role of cytokines and cortisol in the non-thyroidal illness syndrome following acute myocardial infarction. *Eur J Endocrinol* 2000;**142**:236–42.
95. Lim CF, Docter R, Krenning EP *et al*. Transport of thyroxine into cultured hepatocytes: effects of mild non-thyroidal illness and calorie restriction in obese subjects. *Clin Endocrinol (Oxf)* 1994;**40**:79–85.
96. Young R and Worthley LI. Diagnosis and management of thyroid disease and the critically ill patient. *Crit Care Resusc* 2004;**6**:295–305.
97. Amberson J and Drinka PJ. Medication and low serum thyroxine values in nursing home residents. *South Med J* 1998;**91**:437–40.
98. American Association of Clinical Endocrinologists and Associazione Medici Endocrinologi. Medical guidelines for clinical practice for the diagnosis and management of thyroid nodules. *Endocr Pract* 2006;**12**:63–102.
99. Mehanna HM, Jain A, Morton RP *et al*. Investigating the thyroid nodule. *BMJ* 2009;**338**:b733.
100. Hegedus L, Bonnema SJ and Bennedbaek FN. Management of simple nodular goiter: current status and future perspectives. *Endocr Rev* 2003;**24**:102–32.
101. Castro MR and Gharib H. Thyroid fine-needle aspiration biopsy: progress, practice and pitfalls. *Endocr Pract* 2003;**9**:128–36.
102. Nieuwlaat WA, Huysmans DA, van den Bosch HC *et al*. Pretreatment with a single, low dose of recombinant human thyrotropin allows dose reduction of radioiodine therapy in patients with nodular goiter. *J Clin Endocrinol Metab* 2003;**88**:3121–9.
103. Huysmans DA, Nieuwlaat WA and Hermus AR. Towards larger volume reduction of nodular goitres by radioiodine therapy: a role for pretreatment with recombinant human thyrotropin? *Clin Endocrinol (Oxf)* 2004;**60**:297–9.

CHAPTER 99

Ovarian function and menopause

Nicola Pluchino, Tommaso Simoncini and Andrea R. Genazzani
University of Pisa, Pisa, Italy

Introduction and definitions

As life expectancy increases beyond the eighth decade worldwide, particularly in developed countries, an increasing proportion of the female population is postmenopausal. With the average age of menopause being 51 years, more than one-third of a woman's life is now spent after menopause. Here symptoms and signs of estrogen deficiency merge with issues encountered with natural aging. As the world population increases and a larger proportion of this population is made up of individuals over 50, medical care specifically directed at postmenopausal women becomes an important aspect of modern medicine.

In an attempt to define the stages of reproductive aging and its clinical and biochemical markers, the Stages of Reproductive Aging Workshop was held in 2001 to develop a useful staging system and to revise the nomenclature. This system provides useful clinical definitions of the menopausal transition, perimenopause, menopause and postmenopause as follows:

- *Menopausal transition.* The menopausal transition begins with variation in menstrual cycle length and an elevated serum follicle-stimulating hormone (FSH) concentration and ends with the final menstrual period (not recognized until after 12 months of amenorrhoea). Stage − 2 (early) is characterized by variable cycle length (>7 days different from normal menstrual cycle length, which is 21–35 days). Stage − 1 (late) is characterized by two or more skipped cycles and an interval of amenorrhoea of ≥60 days; women at this stage often also have hot flushes.
- *Perimenopause.* Perimenopause means 'around the menopause', and begins in stage − 2 of the menopausal transition and ends 12 months after the last menstrual period.
- *Menopause.* Menopause is defined by 12 months of amenorrhoea after the final menstrual period. It reflects complete, or near-complete, ovarian follicular depletion and absence of ovarian estrogen secretion.
- *Postmenopause.* Stage +1 (early) is defined as the first 5 years after the final menstrual period. It is characterized by further and complete damping of ovarian function. The majority of women in this stage have symptoms. Stage +2 (late) begins 5 years after the final menstrual period and encompasses the ageing process until death.

Epidemiology

Menopause occurs secondary to a genetically programmed loss of ovarian follicles.

Although the average age at menopause is approximately 51 years, for 5% of women it occurs after age 55 years (late menopause) and for another 5% between ages 40 and 45 years (early menopause). Menopause occurring prior to age 40 years is considered to be premature ovarian failure. Unlike the average age of menarche, which has been affected over time by trends in nutritional status and general health, the average age of menopause has not changed much over time. A number of factors are thought to play a role in determining an individual woman's age of menopause, including genetics, ethnicity, smoking and reproductive history.

- *Genetics.* Based on family studies, heritability for age of menopause averaged 0.87, suggesting that genetics explain up to 87% of the variance in menopausal age. Other than gene mutations that cause premature ovarian failure (explained later in this chapter), no specific genes have been discovered to date that account for this genetic influence. However, several genes are likely involved, including genes coding telomerase, which is involved in ageing.
- *Ethnicity.* Ethnicity and race may also affect the age of menopause. Natural menopause occurs earlier among Hispanic women and later in Japanese-American women, compared with Caucasian women.
- *Smoking.* The age of menopause is reduced by about 2 years in women who smoke.
- *Reproductive history.* There is a tendency for women who never had children or who had shorter cycle length

Principles and Practice of Geriatric Medicine, Fifth Edition. Edited by Alan J. Sinclair, John E. Morley and Bruno Vellas.

during adolescence (a predictor of high basal FSH) to have earlier menopause.

Endocrinology and neuroendocrinology of menopause

Menopause is associated with a marked decline in oocyte number that is attributable to progressive atresia of the original complement of oocytes. However, the evidence for absolute oocyte depletion is limited. Residual oocytes and differentiating follicles have been identified in the ovaries of some postmenopausal women, although the follicles are frequently atretic.

Late reproductive stage

A decline in fertility begins in the third to fourth decade of life but accelerates rapidly after the age of 35 years in association with a well-documented decrease in the pool of ovarian follicles. This age-related decrease in follicle number and fertility is marked by a rise in FSH in the early follicular phase before increases in luteinizing hormone (LH) or decreases in estradiol. The presence of regular menstrual cycles and an increase in follicular-phase FSH define the late reproductive stage. In older ovulatory women, the early follicular phase peak in FSH occurs earlier with reference to the onset of menses than in their younger counterparts and the day 3 FSH value is widely used as an indicator of reproductive ageing in clinical settings.

Studies of reproductive ageing have provided important insights into the physiology of inhibin in humans and the role of the inhibins in the selective negative feedback regulation of FSH. Inhibin A and B are secreted differentially during the normal menstrual cycle (for a review, see the key references at the end of this chapter). The pattern of inhibin B secretion suggests that it is primarily secreted from small antral follicles; inhibin B increases across the luteal–follicular transition, reaching a peak in the mid-follicular phase, and is not correlated with the size of the dominant follicle. Inhibin B expression in the ovary is confined to the granulosa cells and is absent from the theca. In the quiescent ovary, inhibin B levels in serum increase in response to FSH administration, preceding secretion of estradiol and inhibin A. Secretion of inhibin B from human granulosa cells is not stimulated directly by FSH or cyclic adenosine monophosphate (AMP), however, but rather its secretion is constitutive.

Thus, the increase in inhibin B in response to endogenous or exogenous FSH is secondary to the recruitment of a cohort of follicles into the growing pool accompanied by a dramatic increase in granulosa cell number. During folliculogenesis, peak levels of inhibin A occur in the late follicular phase and inhibin A is correlated with the size of the dominant follicle in normal cycles, as is estradiol. Inhibin A is produced by granulosa cells in response to stimulation by FSH in small follicles and both LH and FSH at later stages of follicle development. Inhibin A is also secreted from the corpus luteum, its secretion paralleling that of progesterone.

The decrease in developing follicles is reflected in a parallel decrease in the serum concentration of inhibin B, which is probably the earliest easily measurable marker of follicular decline. The rise in the serum concentration of FSH in early menopause is also closely related to the fall in inhibin B; this suggests that inhibin B plays an important role in the normal control of FSH secretion. Serum concentrations of Müllerian-inhibiting substance (MIS) [also known as anti-Müllerian hormone (AMH)] may be a useful marker reflecting reproductive ageing. Low serum AMH concentrations were predictive of a poor ovarian response to exogenous gonadotropin stimulation and may mark a critical juncture in the timing of the menopausal transition.

Menopause transition

The onset of irregular cycles defines the transition from the late reproductive years to the menopausal transition. Variable cycle length is defined as cycle lengths that are more than 7 days different from an individual's normal cycle length and may therefore include cycles with both abnormally long and abnormally short intermenstrual intervals.

The menopausal transition is characterized by a dynamic period of markedly changing hypothalamic–pituitary feedback from the ageing ovary. There is a progressive decrease in menstrual cycle regularity and dramatic swings in estradiol from undetectable to levels that are several times higher than those observed in the ovulatory cycles of younger women. Levels of inhibin A and B are further decreased and FSH levels are generally much higher than during the regular cycles of the late reproductive years. FSH levels may occasionally decrease to near the normal range in association with prolonged increases in estradiol, however. The majority of longitudinal studies indicate that the menopausal transition is not a low-estrogen state but is characterized by widely fluctuating levels of estrogen that are often increased in comparison with earlier stages of reproductive life. These fluctuations in estrogen levels in particular are likely to account for many of the symptoms of the transition to menopause.

In addition to the decline in follicular number, there may be a decrease in hypothalamic–pituitary sensitivity to estrogen-positive feedback during perimenopause.

Postmenopause

Later, with the final menstrual period, levels of inhibin A and estradiol decrease dramatically and there is a further increase in FSH and LH. In particular, the loss of estradiol feedback on LH and FSH and inhibin feedback on FSH associated with menopause results in a 15-fold increase in FSH levels and a 10-fold increase in LH levels in comparison with the early follicular phase in healthy women in whom estradiol levels are at their nadir in the menstrual cycle. The loss of ovarian function at menopause is also associated with marked changes in hypothalamic and pituitary function. There is now evidence, however, that age-related neuroendocrine changes occur that are independent of those caused by the loss of ovarian feedback on the hypothalamic and pituitary components of the reproductive axis. There is an increase in the overall amount of gonadotropin-releasing hormone (GnRH) secreted despite a decrease in GnRH pulse frequency with ageing.

In addition, following menopause, gonadotropin levels decrease progressively with age. Studies in postmenopausal women indicate that between the ages of 45–55 and 70–80 years, there is a decrease of approximately 30% in mean levels of FSH from 148.6 ± 8.4 IU l^{-1} in younger postmenopausal women to 107.0 ± 5.4 IU l^{-1} in older women. There is a similar degree of change in LH from 95.8 ± 7.3 to 60.4 ± 3.9 IU l^{-1} in younger and older postmenopausal women, respectively. Whether the decline in gonadotropin secretion with age is caused by hypothalamic or pituitary effects has been an area of active recent investigation.

Ovarian ageing and sex steroids changes

Hormonal integration of the reproductive system is dramatically affected by reproductive ageing. At the menopause, the final menstrual cycle, a dramatic decline in plasma estradiol level occurs and the postmenopausal ovary will cease to contribute to estradiol levels in blood. Instead, peripheral conversion of androstenedione into estrone becomes prominent. Only 5% of the thus formed estrone is converted to estradiol through the action of 17-hydroxysteroid dehydrogenase. The activity of this enzyme is in a reversible reaction converting estrone to estradiol and back, depending on the oxido-reductive state that prevails in the cell. Further, the amount of estrone generated and the associated conversion to estradiol continue to decline during the first year after menopause and stabilizes thereafter. The amount of estrone generated is a function of the abundance of androstenedione and age. The corpus luteum synthesizes progesterone and in the absence of ovulation only basal levels derived from the adrenal glands are detected. In postmenopausal women, administration of adrenocorticotrophic hormone (ACTH) dramatically increases whereas human chorionic gonadotrophin has no effect on progesterone levels, attesting to the negligible role of postmenopausal ovaries in progesterone production.

Dehydroepiandrosterone (DHEA) is produced in both the ovaries and the adrenal glands under the influence of LH and ACTH, respectively. DHEA sulfate (DHEAS) is exclusively produced by the adrenal glands and is converted to DHEA by steroid sulfatase. Their declining plasma levels are due to age-related reduced steroid synthesizing capacity of the zona reticularis and due to ovarian ageing. During the reproductive years, both the adrenal glands and the ovaries share equally in androstenedione production. Bilateral oophorectomy in premenopausal women results in a 50% reduction in serum androstenedione levels while postmenopausal ovaries contribute only 20% of its total circulating levels. Since the metabolic clearance of androstenedione is not affected by ovarian function or age, the 30% drop represents the effect of ovarian senescence.

In premenopausal women, 50% of circulating testosterone is derived from peripheral conversion of androstenedione, while the remaining testosterone production is shared between the ovaries and the adrenal glands. In postmenopausal women, testosterone levels decrease compared with young women, although ovarian synthesis after the menopause appears to contribute a higher proportion of circulating testosterone. This may be due to higher LH levels and their effect on ovarian stromal steroidogenesis. In a recent cross-sectional study, a different aspect of ovarian ageing was reported. The circulating levels of DHEA, androstenedione and total and free testosterone were found to be highest during the third decade of life and to decline afterwards in the remaining reproductive years. Around the age of 50 years, free and total testosterone levels decrease by about 50%. Testosterone exists in circulation as free testosterone (1–2% of the total), loosely bound to albumin (31%) and tightly bound to sex hormone binding globulin (SHBG) (66%). It is the free and albumin-bound testosterone that is available to cells. Many clinicians and clinical investigators use the ratio of total testosterone to SHBG to derive the free testosterone index.

SHBG is a protein synthesized in the liver. Estrogen stimulates its synthesis whereas all androgens suppress its hepatic synthesis. Obesity, particularly with upper abdominal distribution, also suppresses SHBG levels. In the postmenopausal period, SHBG levels decline and that may account for the higher bioavailability of testosterone. A decrease in bioavailable testosterone level may result from impaired testosterone production or from increased SHBG levels in the presence of normal testosterone production. It is therefore necessary to consider SHBG levels in the assessment of bioavailable testosterone in women.

Surgical menopause

As can be expected, the removal of both ovaries in a premenopausal woman results in an abrupt decline in estrogen to undetectable levels, a 50% reduction in androstenedione and about a 70% drop in DHEA and testosterone levels. These women experience a sudden onset of the menopausal transition. In at least 30–50% of cases, symptoms of androgen deficiency are experienced despite 'adequate' estrogen replacement.

Specific healthcare problems in relation to the menopause

As many as 80% of women experience one or more physical or psychological symptoms of estrogen deficiency as ovarian function declines during the menopause, with almost one half of sufferers finding their symptoms distressing.

Short-term consequences of estrogen deficiency

The change in hormone levels that occurs during the climacterium, particularly the decline of estrogen, can cause acute menopausal symptoms.

Brain symptoms

Symptoms include the following:

- vasomotor symptoms (hot flushes and night sweats)
- sleep problems
- mood changes (depression and anxiety)
- sexual dysfunction
- impaired concentration and memory.

Sex steroids play pivotal neuroactive and brain region-specific roles on the central nervous system through genomic and non-genomic mechanisms. Therefore, their protective effects are multifaceted and brain region dependent. They encompass systems that range from chemical to biochemical and genomic mechanisms, protecting against a wide range of neurotoxic insults. Consequently, gonadal steroid withdrawal, during the reproductive senescence, dramatically impacts brain function, negatively affecting mood, anxiety behaviour and cognitive vitality.

The hallmark feature of declining estrogen status in the brain is the hot flush, which is more generically referred to as a vasomotor episode. Hot flushes occurs in up to 75% of women in some cultures. Hot flushes are most common in the late menopausal transition and early postmenopausal periods. They are self-limited, usually resolving without treatment within 1–5 years, although some women will continue to have hot flushes until after age 70 years. Hot flushes typically begin with a sudden sensation of heat centred on the upper chest and face that rapidly becomes generalized. The sensation of heat lasts from 2 to 4 min, is often associated with profuse perspiration and occasionally palpitations and is often followed by chills and shivering and sometimes a feeling of anxiety. Physiological studies have determined that hot flushes represent thermoregulatory dysfunction; there is inappropriate peripheral vasodilatation with increased digital and cutaneous blood flow and perspiration, resulting in rapid heat loss and a decrease in core body temperature below normal. Hot flushes usually occur several times per day, although the range may be from only one or two each day to as many as one per hour during the day and night. Hot flushes are particularly common at night. The fall in estrogen levels precipitates the vasomotor symptoms. Although the proximate cause of the flush remains elusive, the episodes result from a hypothalamic response (probably mediated by catecholamines) to the change in estrogen status. A speculative mechanism for the initiation of hot flushes is endogenous opioid peptide withdrawal. Estrogen increases central opioid peptide activity and estrogen deficiency may be associated with decreased or absent endogenous central opioid activity.

A distressing feature of hot flushes is that they are often associated with arousal from sleep. This association has been well documented by EEG studies, although, primary sleep disorders are common in this population, even in the absence of hot flushes. This disturbed sleep often leads to fatigue and irritability during the day and deficit of memory is often reported.

Psychological symptoms have been associated with the menopause, including depressed mood, anxiety, irritability, lethargy and lack of energy. Women with a longer menopausal transition and/or with more intense climacteric symptoms, surgical menopause, a history of depression, menstrual cycle-related and postpartum mood changes (premenstrual syndrome, postpartum depression), thyroid disease and unfavourable socio-environmental conditions are at greater risk of developing depression and mood disorder. Observational studies have demonstrated that, in women with a history of depression, the menopausal transition is accompanied by a significant risk of relapse.

The menopausal transition impacts a women's sexual life. Low libido is the main cause of female sexual dysfunction after the menopause. Estrogen deficiency leads to a decrease in blood flow to the vagina and vulva, which also causes decreased vaginal lubrication. Vaginal atrophy frequently determines dyspareunia. From a sexological point of view, dyspareunia in a postmenopausal patient must be treated in a timely fashion to avoid triggering a vicious circle by which dyspareunia leads to sexual dissatisfaction and therefore a further decrease in libido.

Urogenital symptoms

Vaginal dryness

The epithelial lining of the vagina and urethra are very sensitive to estrogen, and estrogen deficiency leads to thinning of the vaginal epithelium. This results in vaginal atrophy (atrophic vaginitis), causing symptoms of vaginal dryness and itching. The prevalence of vaginal dryness in one longitudinal study was 3, 4, 21 and 47% of women in the reproductive, early menopausal transition, late menopausal transition and 3 years postmenopausal stages, respectively. On examination, the vagina typically appears pale, with lack of the normal rugae, and often has visible blood vessels or petechial haemorrhages. Vaginal pH, which is usually <4.5 in the reproductive years, increases to the 6.0–7.5 range in postmenopausal women not taking estrogen. The increase in pH and vaginal atrophy may lead to impaired protection against vaginal and urinary tract infection.

Other urinary symptoms

Low estrogen production after the menopause results in atrophy of the superficial and intermediate layers of the urethral epithelium with subsequent atrophic urethritis, diminished urethral mucosal seal, loss of compliance and irritation; these changes predispose to both stress and urge urinary incontinence.

Recurrent urinary tract infections

These are also a problem for many postmenopausal women. In addition to epithelial atrophy, estrogen deficiency can increase vaginal pH and alter the vaginal flora, changes which may predispose to urinary tract infection.

Long-term consequences of estrogen deficiency

There are a number of long-term effects of estrogen, including osteoporosis, cardiovascular disease, cognitive impairment and dementia.

Osteoporosis is a common disease that is characterized by low bone mass with microarchitectural disruption and skeletal fragility, resulting in an increased risk of fracture. Osteoporosis occurs most commonly in postmenopausal women. Estrogen deficiency has been well established as a cause of bone loss. This loss can be noted for the first time when menstrual cycles become irregular in the perimenopause. From 1.5 years before to 1.5 years after the menopause, spine bone mineral density has been shown to decrease by 2.5% per year, compared with a premenopausal loss rate of 0.13% per year. Loss of trabecular bone (spine) is greater with estrogen deficiency than is loss of cortical bone. Postmenopausal bone loss leading to osteoporosis is a substantial healthcare problem. In white women, 35% of all postmenopausal women have been estimated to have osteoporosis based on bone mineral density. Further, the lifetime fracture risk for these women is 40%. The morbidity rate and economic burden of osteoporosis are well documented. Interestingly, there are data to suggest that up to 19% of white men also have osteoporosis. Bone mass is substantially affected by sex steroids through classic mechanisms to be described later in this chapter. Attainment of peak bone mass in the late second decade is key to ensuring that the subsequent loss of bone mass with ageing and estrogen deficiency does not lead to early osteoporosis. Estrogens suppress bone turnover and maintain a certain rate of bone formation. Bone is remodelled in functional units, called bone multicentre units (BMUs), where resorption and formation should be in balance. Multiple sites of bone go through this turnover process over time. Estrogen decreases osteoclasts by increasing apoptosis and thus reduces their lifespan. The effect on the osteoblast is less consistent, but E_2 antagonizes glucocorticoid-induced osteoblast apoptosis. Estrogen deficiency increases the activities of remodelling units, prolongs resorption and shortens the phase of bone formation. The molecular mechanisms of estrogen action on bone involve the inhibition of production of proinflammatory cytokines including interleukin 1, interleukin 6, tumour necrosis factor-α (TGF-α), colony-stimulating factor-1, macrophage colony-stimulating factor and prostaglandin E_2, which lead to increased resorption. Estradiol also upregulates TGF-β in bone, which inhibits bone resorption. Receptor activation of NF-κB ligand (RANKL) is responsible for osteoclast differentiation and action.

Ageing women undergo two phases of bone loss, whereas ageing men undergo only one. In women, the menopause initiates an accelerated phase of predominantly cancellous bone loss that declines rapidly over 4–8 years to become asymptotic with a subsequent slow phase that continues indefinitely. The accelerated phase results from the loss of the direct restraining effects of estrogen on bone turnover, an action mediated by estrogen receptors (ERs) in both osteoblasts and osteoclasts. In the ensuing slow phase, the rate of cancellous bone loss is reduced, but the rate of cortical bone loss is unchanged or increased. This phase is mediated largely by secondary hyperparathyroidism that results from the loss of estrogen actions on extraskeletal calcium metabolism.

Osteoporosis has no clinical manifestations until there is a fracture. *Vertebral fracture* is the most common clinical manifestation of osteoporosis. Most of these fractures (about two-thirds) are asymptomatic; they are diagnosed as an incidental finding on chest or abdominal x-ray. *Hip fractures* are relatively common in osteoporosis, affecting 15% of women and 4% of men by 80 years of age. *Distal radius fractures (Colles fractures)* are more common in women shortly after menopause, whereas the risk of hip fracture rises exponentially with age.

Cardiovascular diseases

The clinical phenomenon that premenopausal women experience lower rates of heart disease than men because of the presence of estrogen has been recognized for many years and initially formed part of the rationale for using hormone therapy (HT) in postmenopausal women.

The possible reasons for the increase in cardiovascular disease in postmenopausal women are the accelerated rise in total cholesterol in postmenopausal women [especially in levels of low-density lipoprotein cholesterol

(LDL-C)], changes of weight, blood pressure and blood glucose with ageing and menopausal status.

The abrupt fall in circulating estrogen levels might independently contribute to the rise in blood pressure, through partly unknown mechanisms, such as a direct effect on the arterial wall and the activation of the renin–angiotensin system and of the sympathetic nervous system. Postmenopausal hypertension fosters the development of left ventricular hypertrophy and is the main factor contributing to coronary artery disease, chronic heart failure and stroke in older women.

Premature menopause and bilateral oophorectomy in young women are associated with an increased incidence of cardiovascular disease, myocardial infarction and overall mortality. Observational studies suggest an interval of 5–10 years between loss of ovarian function and the increased risk of cardiovascular disease.

However, the cellular basis for the beneficial effects of estrogen on the cardiovascular system has been elucidated only in more recent times. Experimental studies in animal models of cardiovascular disease have demonstrated that the beneficial effects of estrogen are mediated via a number of mechanisms and involve a range of cell types, including endothelial, smooth muscle and cardiac muscle cells. At this level, estrogen triggers rapid vasodilatation, exerts anti-inflammatory effects, regulates vascular cell growth and migration and confers protection to cardiomyocytes. These so-called 'extranuclear actions' do not require gene expression or protein synthesis and are independent of the nuclear localization of ERs. Indeed, some of these actions are elicited by ERs residing at or near the plasma membrane. Through complex interactions with membrane-associated signalling molecules, such as ion channels, G proteins and the tyrosine kinase c-Src, liganded extranuclear ERs lead to the activation of downstream cascades such as mitogen-activated protein kinase (MAPK) and phosphatidylinositol 3-OH kinase (PI3K). These cascades are responsible for important cardiovascular actions of estrogen, for instance, the activation of nitric oxide synthesis or the remodelling of the endothelial actin cytoskeleton. Moreover, these cascades play crucial roles in regulating the expression of target proteins implicated in cell proliferation, apoptosis, differentiation, movement and homeostasis.

Cognitive impairment and dementia

The detection of early neural markers of brain ageing and cognitive dysfunction is one of the main challenges for the climacterium and the initial postmenopausal period; thus, the degree of cognitive vitality during the ageing process could also depend on early clinical interventions.

The evidence that estrogen has several neuroprotective effects brings new meaning to the potential impact of the prolonged postmenopausal hypoestrogenic state on learning and memory, and also to the possible increase of vulnerability in brain injury and neurodegenerative diseases in ageing women.

Results from the Mayo Clinic Cohort Study of Oophorectomy and Aging provide the level of the long-term influence that sex steroid deprivation has on cognitive vitality. In particular, women who underwent either unilateral or bilateral oophorectomy reported an increased risk of cognitive impairment or dementia compared with others with natural menopause [adjusted hazard ratio (HR), 1.46; 95% confidence interval (CI), 1.13–1.90]. In another study, the risk of Parkinson's disease was higher in women who underwent either unilateral or bilateral oophorectomy (adjusted HR, 1.68; 95% CI, 1.06–2.67). In both studies, a younger age at menopause was associated with increased risk of neurological impairment (i.e. the linear trend was significant). In this regard, significant linear trends of increasing risk for either outcome with younger age at oophorectomy were also observed.

As a conclusion, estrogen deficiency can be defined as the initial step in a chain of causality which determines the increased risk of cognitive impairment or dementia. In support of a neuroprotective effect of estrogen, women who underwent bilateral oophorectomy before age 49 years, but were given estrogen treatment until at least age 50 years, reported no increased risk.

Epidemiological surveys, prospectively monitoring women as they progress through the menopause transition, have suggested that self-reports of decreased concentration and poor memory are frequent accompaniments of this phase of life in addition to the postmenopausal period. In the Study of Women's Health Across the Nation (SWAN), more than 40% of perimenopausal and postmenopausal women endorsed forgetfulness on a symptom inventory compared with 31% of premenopausal women. In the Seattle Midlife Women's Health Study, ~62% of midlife women reported an undesirable change in memory.

In addition, the presence of objective hot flushes is a negative predictor of verbal memory in midlife women with moderate to severe vasomotor symptoms. This relationship appears to be primarily due to night- rather than daytime hot flushes, thus supporting the concept that hot flushes and sleep disturbances are a sign of brain vulnerability to sex steroid withdrawal, with a negative impact of cognition. Hypothalamic and hypothalamic–pituitary–gonadal (HPG) axis senescence induces vasomotor symptoms and hypogonadism that could trigger menopause-related mental decline in other brain areas, before deficits in learning and cognition start to become evident.

Hormone therapy in postmenopausal women

Much confusion has arisen among healthcare providers, the lay public and the media when general concepts of risk of hormone therapy in postmenopausal women are discussed. Understanding the benefits/risks of HT is critical to clinical decision-making around the menopause and beyond.

Hormone replacement therapy after the Women's Health Initiative (WHI)

After the publication of the randomized WHI trial in July 2002, the convictions regarding hormone replacement therapy (HRT) and menopause, which had been acquired over many years, started to waver. Beforehand, the majority of the preclinical and observational studies had demonstrated that HRT reduced the risk of coronary heart disease (CHD) and, possibly, decreased the risk or delayed the onset of cognitive deficits and senile dementia. The WHI results did not confirm these data. The disparity between these findings clearly lies in the selection of subjects and timing of HRT in relation to chronological age and menopausal age.

In the observational studies, replacement hormones had been prescribed to mostly symptomatic women during the menopausal transition, who generally were younger than 55 years upon initiation of the therapy. In contrast, in the WHI trial, HRT was started after age 55 years in 89% of subjects, often after a long period from the last menstruation and in the absence of menopausal symptoms. In the observational studies, a window of opportunity, by which early hormone replacement in younger symptomatic women is protective against the endocrine–metabolic effects of hypoestrogenism, was observed. This is in accordance with the physiopathology of age-related degenerative processes, such as atherosclerosis and neuronal degeneration, which develop over many years. Instead, in the WHI trial, treatment was begun in older women for whom a late hormonal replacement could not prevent the already present cardiovascular degenerative changes.

An early start on HRT, in terms of both age and years since menopause, may represent a determining factor to induce positive effects (CHD prevention and Alzheimer risk reduction) and to limit adverse events (venous thrombosis, stroke).

Pretreatment evaluation

HRT should not be recommended without a specific indication. Before prescribing HRT, a complete medical history of the patient should be taken and a thorough physical examination performed. A mammography should be carried out within 12 months prior to HRT initiation and should be repeated during treatment according to normal screening programmes. Other diagnostic examinations, such as bone densitometry, pelvic ultrasound and blood tests, should be recommended according to the characteristics of each subject. Menopausal women should be encouraged to follow the cancer screening programmes suggested for each age range.

Indications for hormone therapy and effects on various organ systems

Menopausal symptoms

The treatment of vasomotor symptoms is the primary indication for HRT. Replacement hormones are indeed the most efficient therapy for the treatment of symptoms due to estrogen deficiency (hot flushes, sweats, urogenital atrophy symptoms). Various preparations with equal pharmacological potency have comparable effects on hot flushes. Other menopause-related symptoms such as musculoskeletal pain, changes in mood, sleep disorders and libido reduction also benefit from HRT. Low dosages are efficient in resolving vasomotor symptoms in almost all symptomatic women. It is therefore appropriate to begin hormonal therapy at low dosages and increase them after some weeks if symptoms persist.

HRT improves quality of life in postmenopausal women, especially if symptoms are associated with estrogen deficiency.

Quality of life and sexuality must be taken into account in order to have a better view of the patient and treat her appropriately. An early individualized hormonal treatment (eventually associated with androgens where necessary) may prevent or reduce sexual disturbances, improving quality of life. HRT and vaginal estrogen therapy both reduce symptoms related to urogenital atrophy (vaginal dryness, vaginitis, dyspareunia). Estrogen therapy improves irritative bladder symptoms and urinary urgency. HRT is not indicated for the treatment and prevention of stress urinary incontinence. Hormonal (estrogen) vaginal therapy is the first choice if the only indication is urogenital atrophy.

Menopausal depression

HRT may be indicated to treat first-time mild to moderate depression, particularly if it is associated with hot flushes. The treatment of severe or recurring depression should always be instituted with antidepressive drugs or psychotherapy. HRT is not efficient and, therefore, is not indicated to treat postmenopausal major depression. According to some studies, HRT may enhance the effects of antidepressive drugs. Hence HRT is not contraindicated and can be added to antidepressive therapy, especially when climacteric symptoms are present.

Postmenopausal osteoporosis

HRT reduces the risk of osteoporosis, improves bone mineral density and restores normal bone turnover. Women who take HRT have better posture and a lower tendency to fall, with an important impact on fracture incidence. Moreover, HRT determines a lower fracture risk at all skeletal sites examined in the relative studies. In particular, the WHI trial subjects receiving active treatment showed a lower incidence of all fractures with respect to the placebo group: 8.6% in women treated with HRT versus 11.25% in the placebo group (HR, 0.76; 95% CI, 0.69–0.83). Total femoral bone mineral density increased by 3.7% after 3 years of estrogen–progestin therapy versus 0.14% recorded in the placebo group ($p > 0.01$). The WHI trial confirmed the importance of an adequate concomitant calcium supplementation to prevent fractures. Low-dose hormonal therapy associated with adequate calcium supplementation adds superimposable effects to the standard dose therapy on bone mineral density and metabolism. HRT initiation after the age of 60 years is not recommended at standard doses for the sole prevention of fractures. HRT continuation after age 60 years can be taken into consideration for osteoporosis prevention only if the route of administration and the dose are adequate and the risk/benefit ratio is comparable to those with other therapies. Finally, HRT seems to be protective against osteoarthritis, the incidence of which increases after the menopause.

Metabolic syndrome

Treatment of metabolic syndrome is mostly preventive and aimed at correcting lifestyle habits, controlling blood pressure and blood glucose levels. HRT prevents the increase in body weight and android fat distribution occurring at menopause. HRT may reduce the risk of metabolic syndrome and, if started early in menopause, it may diminish the risk of cardiovascular disease.

Diabetes mellitus

Observational and randomized studies have demonstrated that HRT reduces the risk of developing diabetes mellitus. The WHI trial confirmed this [HR, 0.79; 95% CI, 0.67–0.93 in the HRT group; HR, 0.88; 95% CI, 0.77–1.01 in the estrogen replacement therapy (ERT) group].

Arterial hypertension

The management of hypertension after the menopause requires modifications in lifestyle and antihypertensive therapy. No particular class of antihypertensive drugs is indicated for menopausal hypertension. HRT is not contraindicated in postmenopausal hypertensive women provided that the blood pressure is strictly controlled with treatment.

Coronary heart disease

The cardiovascular system is profoundly influenced by sex steroids. Estrogen, progesterone and androgen receptors are present in all of the cardiovascular system. As emphasized above, the WHI trial did not confirm the reduction in CHD reported in earlier studies. The discrepancy between these findings may be due to patient selection and timing of HRT relative to chronological and menopausal age. This view is supported by a review of the WHI data regarding the effects of HRT versus placebo in younger women (within 10 years from menopause), which evidenced a reduction in CHD [relative risk (RR) 0.76; 95% CI, 0.50–1.16) similar to that reported in observational studies. The potential role of HRT in primary prevention of CHD remains hypothetical and is supported by preclinical and observational studies and *post hoc* analyses of randomized studies.

Venous thromboembolism (VTE)

Both observational and randomized studies have demonstrated a significant risk increase (RR, 2–3) of VTE in postmenopausal women treated with HRT with respect to non-treated women. The risk seems to be correlated with the dosage, is evident in the first 2 years of treatment and tends to diminish with time. Moreover, it is greater in women aged over 60 years. The WHI results showed that the risk of VTE is age dependent. In the 50–59 year age group, an increase of 11 cases per 10 000 HRT-treated women and two cases per 10 000 ERT-treated women was recorded.

Stroke

HRT tends to increase the risk of stroke in postmenopausal women, but the data are not completely concordant. In the WHI trial, 8–12 additional cases of stroke per 10 000 women treated with HRT or ERT were recorded globally per year. However, in women aged between 50 and 59 years, within 5 years from menopause, the risk of stroke associated with HRT/ERT was lower and non-significant (1–3 additional cases per 10 000 women per year). Therefore, in the WHI trial, the younger women (aged 50–59 years) experienced a non-significant increase in stroke events with, in contrast, a significantly lower total mortality. However, HRT should not be used in patients with a high risk for stroke.

Cognitive decline and dementia

Many observational studies support the role of estrogens in preventing cognitive decline and reducing the risk of dementia.

Substantial biological evidence supports the importance of estrogen to cognitive function. ERs have been identified throughout the brain and appear particularly concentrated in the basal forebrain and cortex. The basal forebrain is of special interest since it is the major source of cholinergic innervation to the hippocampus. The cholinergic system is a neurotransmitter system important for regulation of memory and learning, and the hippocampus is the primary region of the brain mediating cognitive function. In experiments using animal models and cell lines, several mechanisms have been identified whereby estrogen may influence cognitive function:

- The cholinergic system is enhanced by estrogen. As an example, estrogen increases the synthesis of acetylcholine (the chemical that cholinergic neurons use to communicate with other nerve cells) by stimulating choline acetyltransferase activity and raises the concentration of hypothalamic nicotinic acetylcholine receptors.
- The glutamate system, a second neurotransmitter system involved in learning and memory, is also influenced by estrogen. Estrogen increases the expression of proteins from the NMDA (*N*-methyl D-aspartate) receptor, which is involved in glutamate activation and enhances long-term potentiation (the process by which we learn new things) in conditions that favour activation of NMDA receptors.
- Estrogen stimulates neurons and their ability to communicate with each other and may contribute to regulation of genes that influence neuron survival, differentiation, regeneration and plasticity.
- Estrogen may protect nerve cells from excitotoxins and may act as an antioxidant to shield nerve cells from free radical damage.
- Amyloid plaques are one of the pathological hallmarks of Alzheimer's disease and estrogen may be important in preventing amyloid deposition.

The ancillary study of the WHI on cognitive functions (WHIMS) did not show any positive effects related to HRT use. The WHIMS results are probably associated with vascular events, even at the subclinical level, in this population of advanced age. HRT initiation after age 65 years at standard dosages is not recommended for the prevention of senile dementia and cognitive decline. Although observational and preclinical studies have shown that estrogens have beneficial effects on the central nervous system and cognitive functions if treatment is begun early, before age 65 years, particularly in surgical menopausal women or if menopausal symptoms are present, available data are not sufficient to indicate or contraindicate HRT for the prevention of dementia.

Breast cancer

The risk of breast cancer represents the main impediment for HRT use. The risk of breast cancer is very fear-provoking, although the risk of dying from it is much lower than for other diseases such as lung cancer in female smokers or CHD. The lifetime risk of a woman developing breast cancer is one in eight. The slight increase in breast cancer incidence during HRT (from 30 to 36–38 cases per 10 000 women per year) has been known since the 1990s. The WHI trial confirmed this finding for long-term therapy. The risk increase for prolonged therapy (over 5 years) is smaller than for other risk factors, such as age at menarche or at first pregnancy or positive family history. The risk of breast cancer due to HRT is similar to that conferred by obesity and is not additive. In fact, HRT does not increase the risk of breast cancer in women with body mass index 42.5 $kg\,m^{-2}$, who already carry a higher risk than women with normal body weight. The risk of breast cancer tends to increase in women who take HRT for over 5 years. There is an absolute increase of six cases of breast cancer per 10 000 women per year in those treated with HRT for over 5 years with respect to the baseline incidence in non-users of 30 cases per 10 000 women per year.

The risk returns to baseline values after discontinuation of treatment. The WHI trial showed that, in hysterectomized women, ERT for over 7 years does not increase the incidence of breast cancer; on the contrary, eight fewer cases were reported per 10 000 women per year. Observational data from the Nurses Health Study have demonstrated that ERT is associated with an increase in breast cancer only after 15–20 years of treatment. Other European studies have shown that shorter periods of ERT can be associated with an increase in breast cancer. It is therefore reasonable to conclude that not all kinds of HRT determine the same modifications in breast cancer risk. It seems clear, from all the studies, that the addition of a progestin increases the risk of breast cancer with respect to the use of estrogens only or estrogens plus natural progesterone. Some data in the literature suggest that natural progesterone is associated with a lower risk of breast cancer than androgenic progestins. Breast cancer mortality is not increased in women treated with HRT. Recent data confirm that women surgically treated for breast cancer while using HRT have better survival and greater disease-free survival. HRT may cause an increase in mammographic density and this may alter the correct interpretation of the mammogram. In patients with a difficult mammographic interpretation due to an HRT-related increase in density, it is reasonable to interrupt the treatment and repeat a mammography after 30 days. Effecting HRT does not modify the optimal screening programme proposed by international scientific societies, which provides that an annual mammogram be performed.

Genital tumours

The risk of endometrial cancer increases with ERT. This risk increase has been annulled with the administration of HRT thanks to the addition of a progestin for at least 12 days per month. Endometrial cancers diagnosed during HRT are less aggressive. There is no proof compelling endometrial surveillance in patients under HRT without abnormal uterine bleeding. Cervical cancer, like adenocarcinoma of the vulva or vagina, is not influenced by sex steroids. The incidence of ovarian cancer is low. It is known that oral contraceptives reduce the risk of ovarian epithelial cancer but the impact of HRT is not clear. Although some evidence showed an increased risk, the WHI trial did not report any significant variation in ovarian cancer risk in HRT-treated women.

Progestin use

The use of a progestin, both continuously and sequentially, is necessary to contrast the endometrial effects of estrogens, which, if administered alone, would induce hyperplasia and cancer. If these recommendations are not followed, careful endometrial surveillance is advisable. Progestins are not usually needed in hysterectomized women nor are they indicated with a vaginal administration of low-dose estrogens. Different progestins have similar endometrial effects but exert different metabolic effects according to dosage, route of administration and combination with the estrogen preparation. Therefore, it is not correct to consider all progestins alike, and it is appropriate to keep in mind the different pharmacological properties.

Considerations

Several recent guidelines have endorsed the use of HT for control of symptoms (International Menopause Society, North American Menopause Society). These guidelines underline the relative safety in symptomatic women and that lower doses should be used with individualization regarding the dose and the type of hormones, the route of administration and the length of treatment.

The risk/benefit ratio must be evaluated according to the individual characteristics of each woman (age, medical history, clinical characteristics, type of menopause, years since menopause, prevalent symptoms) that can affect the absolute risk of osteoporosis, breast cancer, CHD, stroke, diabetes and VTE. Acceptance of HRT depends on the woman's perception and correct counselling. It seems appropriate to emphasize that the incidence of any disease depends on chronological age and menopausal age. Hypoestrogenism is an important risk factor for cardiovascular disease and osteoporosis. HRT has the best risk/benefit ratio in perimenopausal women, who are younger and symptomatic and who do not manifest the endocrine–metabolic disorders that lead to degenerative diseases. In contrast, the presence of clinically manifest or subclinical chronic degenerative diseases in women over the age of 65–70 years makes systemic HRT initiation at standard doses irrational and unacceptable considering the potential associated risks.

Indications for hormone replacement therapy/estrogen replacement therapy

Indications for HRT/ERT are:

- vasomotor symptoms
- atrophy-related urogenital symptoms
- prevention of osteoporosis and related fractures.

Ascertained benefits of hormone replacement therapy/estrogen replacement therapy

Benefits of HRT/ERT are:

- prevention of atrophic involution of
  - –epithelia
  - –skin
  - –connective tissue
- intervertebral discs
- improvement of mood changes
- improvement of low libido
- improvement of sleep disturbances
- reduction of colorectal cancer risk
- improvement of musculoskeletal pain
- improvement of stress urinary incontinence.

Potential benefits of hormone replacement therapy/estrogen replacement therapy

Potential benefits of HRT/ERT are:

- improvement of many aspects of metabolic syndrome
- diabetes risk reduction
- risk reduction of Alzheimer's dementia if HRT started at menopause
- risk reduction of CHD if HRT started at menopause.

Absolute contraindications for hormone replacement therapy/estrogen replacement therapy

Absolute contraindications of HRT/ERT are:

- undiagnosed vaginal bleeding
- history of breast or endometrial cancer
- thromboembolic disorders or history of recurrent VTE
- active or chronic liver disease
- CHD
- porphyria cutanea tarda
- refusal of informed consent on behalf of the patient.

Androgen therapy in postmenopausal women

Decreases in sex hormone levels with menopause may bring about a number of consequences for women's general health and sexual wellbeing, especially when levels decline suddenly and prematurely, as in surgical menopause. In addition to the well-established role of estrogens in preserving the biological basis of sexual response, there is emerging evidence that androgens are significant independent determinants affecting sexual desire, activity and satisfaction, and also mood, energy and other components of women's health. Hypoactive sexual desire disorder (HSDD), a persistent absence of sexual fantasies or thoughts and/or desire for and receptivity to sexual activity that causes personal distress, is experienced by some postmenopausal women. Even though conventional hormone therapy with estrogens or estrogens and progestogens may be effective for vaginal atrophy, increasing vaginal lubrication and reducing dyspareunia, it has not been shown to increase sexual desire or activity consistently and many women with sexual dysfunction remain unresponsive. Several recent, large, phase 3 studies have shown that transdermal testosterone in addition to conventional hormone therapy can be helpful in menopausal women presenting with HSDD. After 24 weeks of treatment in these studies, testosterone-treated women experienced significantly greater increases in satisfying sexual activity and sexual desire and greater decreases in distress than placebo-treated women. Accurate clinical assessment and individualized management of sexual symptoms are fundamentally important for all menopausal women with HSDD or other sexual problems.

In addition to testosterone, the marked age-related decline in serum DHEA and DHEAS has suggested that a deficiency of these steroids may be causally related to the development of a series of diseases which are generally associated with ageing. Postulated consequences of low DHEA include insulin resistance, obesity, cardiovascular disease, cancer, reduction of the immune defence and psychosocial problems such as depression and a general deterioration in the sensation of wellbeing and cognitive function. As a consequence, DHEA replacement (oral 25–50 mg per day) may be an attractive treatment opportunity and there are data that suggest that the use of oral DHEA in healthy postmenopausal women might improve condition evidenced with the ageing process, such as reduced sexual function and reduced wellbeing.

Androgen replacement therapy should be a primary choice especially in younger women with either premature ovarian or surgically induced menopause, suffering of loss of wellbeing, fatigue and loss of libido, that is not modified by estrogenic therapy. Among androgens, Δ^5-androgens such as DHEA and DHEAS, could be considered as an alternative choice to treat the androgen deficiency syndrome and/or symptomatic postmenopausal women.

Conclusion

Each phase of a woman's life is associated with specific issues related both to her reproductive health and to her general health. This is true for women globally and is specially relevant today as the majority of women (in developed countries) live for 20–30 years after the menopause.

Menopause is a clearly recognizable biological event, with a variety of potential health problems that can affect the quality and sometimes the duration of life. Deprivation of sex steroids at menopause can be defined as the initial step in a chain of causality, which determines the increased risk of several pathological conditions during the ageing process, years before their clinical manifestation.

On these bases, there is significant clinical interest in the potential long-term health effects of menopausal HT and the impact of treatment on women's health is debated.

It is becoming clear that the relative risks and benefits of treatment vary depending on a variety of factors, including age at initiation of HT, duration of therapy and the particular combination of hormones used in combined preparations. Thus, individualization of therapy is mandatory.

Changes attributed to the menopause need to be distinguished from those related to chronological ageing and HT represents an opportunity to be favourably considered in women's care, especially in the early postmenopausal period.

Key points

- The average age of menopause is 51 years.
- Estrogen deficiency has both short- and long- term consequences.
- HRT treatment requires a specific indication.
- Early HRT reduces cardiovascular disease.
- The Women's Health Initiative trial does not support the use of HRT after the age of 60 years.
- Testosterone can be used to treat hypoactive sexual desire disorder.

Further Reading

Genazzani AR (ed.). *Hormone Replacement Therapy and the Brain*, Taylor and Francis, London, 2003.

Genazzani AR, Pluchino N, Luisi S and Luisi M. Estrogen, cognition and female ageing. *Hum Reprod Update* 2007;**13**:175–87.

Hall JE. Neuroendocrine changes with reproductive aging in women. *Semin Reprod Med* 2007;**25**:344–51.

Lobo RA. Evidence-based medicine and the management of menopause. *Clin Obstet Gynecol* 2008;**51**:534–8.

Lobo RA (ed.). *Treatment of the Postmenopausal Woman*, 3rd edn, Academic Press, New York, 2007.

Manson JE, Allison MA, Rossouw JE *et al*. Estrogen therapy and coronary-artery calcification. *N Engl J Med* 2007;**356**:2591–602.

Mendelsohn ME and Karas RH. Molecular and cellular basis of cardiovascular gender differences. *Science* 2005;**308**:1583–7.

North American Menopause Society. Estrogen and progestogen use in postmenopausal women: 2010 position statement of the North American Menopause Society. *Menopause* 2010;**17**:242–55.

Practice Committee of the American Society for Reproductive Medicine. The menopausal transition. *Fertil Steril* 2008;**90**(5 Suppl):S61–5.

Rossouw JE, Prentice RL, Manson JE *et al*. Postmenopausal hormone therapy and cardiovascular disease by age and years since menopause. *JAMA* 2007;**297**:1465–77.

Simoncini T. Mechanisms of action of estrogen receptors in vascular cells: relevance for menopause and aging. *Climacteric* 2009; 12(Suppl 1): 6–11.

Sowers MF, Zheng H, Tomey K *et al*. Changes in body composition in women over six years at midlife: ovarian and chronological aging. *J Clin Endocrinol Metab* 2007;**92**:895–901.

Stefanick ML, Anderson GL, Margolis KL *et al*. Effects of conjugated equine estrogens on breast cancer and mammography screening in postmenopausal women with hysterectomy. *JAMA* 2006;**295**:1647–57.

Writing Group for the Women's Health Initiative Investigators. Risks and benefits of estrogen plus progestin in healthy postmenopausal women: principal results from the Women's Health Initiative randomized controlled trial. *JAMA* 2002; **288**:321–33.

Writing Group on behalf of Workshop Consensus Group. Aging, menopause, cardiovascular disease and HRT. International Menopause Society Consensus Statement. *Climacteric* 2009;**12**:368–77.

CHAPTER 100

Testicular function

Nazem Bassil
Saint Louis University Medical Center, St Louis, MO USA

Introduction

The percentage of the population in the older age group is increasing. With ageing, a significant percentage of men have a gradual and moderate decrease in testicular function. This decrease in either of the two major functions of the testes, sperm production and testosterone production, is known as hypogonadism. Hypogonadism in a male can result from disease of the testes (primary hypogonadism) or disease of the pituitary or hypothalamus (secondary hypogonadism). The main consequence is a decrease in the serum concentrations of testosterone known as late-onset hypogonadism (LOH), which is a clinical and biochemical syndrome. Testosterone deficiency is a common disorder in older men but it is underdiagnosed and often untreated. It has been estimated that only 5–35% of hypogonadal males actually receive treatment for their condition. The prevalence of hypogonadism was 3.1–7.0% in men aged 30–69 years and 18.4% in men over 70 years of age.[1] The most easily recognized clinical signs of relative androgen deficiency in older men are a decrease in muscle mass and strength, a decrease in bone mass and osteoporosis and an increase in central body fat. None of these symptoms are specific to the low androgen state but may raise suspicion of testosterone deficiency. In addition, symptoms such as a decrease in libido and sexual desire, forgetfulness, loss of memory, difficulty in concentration, insomnia and a decreased sense of wellbeing are more difficult to measure and differentiate from hormone-independent ageing. Clinicians tend to overlook it and the complaints of androgen-deficient men are merely considered part of ageing. This condition may result in significant detriment to quality of life and adversely affect the function of multiple organ systems. This LOH is important since it features many potentially serious consequences that can be readily avoided or treated. In men, endogenous testosterone concentrations are inversely related to mortality. However, this association could not be confirmed in the Massachusetts Male Aging Study (MMAS)[2] or the New Mexico Aging Study.[3]

Ageing and testicular function

As men age, the decrease in testicular function refers to a decline in either of the two major functions of the testes: testosterone production or sperm production.

Decline in serum testosterone

Both cross-sectional and longitudinal studies demonstrate a gradual decline in serum testosterone concentration starting after age 30 years. In older men, the changes in total testosterone are overshadowed by a more significant decline in free testosterone levels. This is a consequence of the age-associated increase in the levels of sex hormone-binding globulin (SHBG), which increases gradually as a function of age and binds testosterone with high affinity; less of the total testosterone is free.

In the European Male Ageing Study, a large cross-sectional study, the serum total testosterone concentration fell by 0.4% per year and the free testosterone concentration fell by 1.3% per year[4] between ages 40 and 79 years. Some of the effect of age was associated with obesity and comorbidities. In the Baltimore Longitudinal Study of Aging, the percentage of subjects with total testosterone concentrations in the hypogonadal range (total testosterone $<325\,\mathrm{ng\,dl^{-1}}$) was 20, 30 and 50% for men in their 60s, 70s and 80s, respectively.[5] The rate of age-related decline in serum testosterone levels varies in different individuals and is affected by chronic disease such as obesity, new illness, serious emotional stress and medications.[6] There is evidence that many of these men are not symptomatic. An interesting observation from the MMAS was that half of the men found to have symptomatic androgen deficiency at one stage were found to be eugonadal when retested at a later stage.[7] This is probably because there is subject-to-subject variation in testosterone secretion and in the testosterone threshold where symptoms become manifest. The measurement of low testosterone in a patient should be reconfirmed at a later stage before considering treatment.

Principles and Practice of Geriatric Medicine, Fifth Edition. Edited by Alan J. Sinclair, John E. Morley and Bruno Vellas.

Decline in spermatogenesis

Characteristic age-related morphological testicular alternations occurs with ageing, such as decreased numbers of Leydig cells paralleling decreased testosterone production, arteriosclerotic lesions, thickening and hernia-like protrusions of the basal membrane of the seminiferi tubules and fibrotic thickening of the tunica albuginea. Surprisingly, these alterations do not lead to dramatic change with increasing age. Testicular size was somewhat larger.[8] Ejaculated sperm density increase, slightly with age, but the percentage motility was slightly greater in younger people. However, children of elderly fathers have a higher risk for autosomal dominant diseases, presumably due to increasing numbers of germ cell meioses and mitoses.

Table 100.1 Androgen Deficiency in Aging Male (ADAM) questionnaire[a].

1	Do you have a decrease in libido or sex drive?
2	Do you have a lack of energy?
3	Do you have a decrease in strength and/or endurance?
4	Have you lost weight?
5	Have you noticed a decreased 'enjoyment of life'?
6	Are you sad and/or grumpy?
7	Are your erections less strong?
8	Have you noticed a recent deterioration in your ability to play sports?
9	Are you falling asleep after dinner?
10	Has there been a recent deterioration in your work performance?

[a]A positive ADAM questionnaire was defined as 'yes' for questions 1 and 7 and 2–4 for all other items.

Diagnosis of late-onset hypogonadism

The diagnosis of LOH requires the presence of symptoms and signs suggestive of testosterone deficiency.[1] The testosterone deficiency can be caused by a combination of both primary and secondary hypogonadism. The symptom most associated with hypogonadism is low libido. Other manifestations of hypogonadism include erectile dysfunction, decreased muscle mass and strength, increased body fat, decreased bone mineral density (BMD) and osteoporosis, mild anaemia, breast discomfort and gynaecomastia, hot flushes, sleep disturbance, body hair and skin alterations, decreased vitality and decreased intellectual capacity (poor concentration, depression, fatigue). The problem is that many of the symptoms of late-life hypogonadism are similar in other conditions or are physiologically associated with the ageing process. Depression, hypothyroidism and chronic alcoholism should be excluded, as should the use of medications such as corticosteroids, cimetidine, spironolactone, digoxin, opioid analgesics, antidepressants and antifungal drugs. Of course, diagnosis of LOH should never be undertaken during an acute illness, which is likely to result in temporarily low testosterone levels.

The Androgen Deficiency in Aging Male (ADAM) questionnaire (Table 100.1) and the Aging Male Symptoms Scale (AMS) may be sensitive markers of a low testosterone state (97 and 83%, respectively), but they are not tightly correlated with low testosterone (specificity 30 and 39%, respectively), particularly in the borderline low serum testosterone range. Therefore, questionnaires are not recommended for screening of androgen deficiency in men receiving healthcare for unrelated reasons. Moreover, healthy ambulatory elderly males over 70 years old, assessed by the AMS, had a high perception of sexual symptoms with mild psychological and mild to moderate somatovegetative symptoms. Note also that there is marked inter-individual variation of the testosterone level at which symptoms occur.

Hypogonadism in older men may be associated with chronic illnesses such as diabetes mellitus and renal disease. Systemic glucocorticoids can reduce testosterone biosynthesis in the testis and impact the hypothalamic–pituitary–gonadal (HPG) axis by inhibiting the release of luteinizing hormone (LH). Patients being treated with glucocorticoids for chronic conditions such as rheumatoid and osteoarthritic inflammation, skin inflammations, asthma, chronic obstructive pulmonary disease (COPD) and inflammatory bowel disease are at an increased risk for hypogonadism. COPD patients have a higher incidence of hypogonadism due to many factors, such as steroid treatment, chronic hypoxia and a systemic inflammatory response. Testosterone therapy can improve lean body mass, BMD and strength in hypogonadal men with COPD. Long-term use of opioids can lead to suppression of GnRH release by the hypothalamus, thereby inducing secondary hypogonadism, an entity called opioid-induced androgen deficiency (OPIAD). Androgen deficiency is strongly associated with AIDS wasting syndrome and testosterone therapy in HIV-positive hypogonadal men increases lean body and muscle mass and perceived wellbeing and decreases depression. Such chronic diseases should be investigated and treated.[9]

Laboratory diagnosis

Diagnosis of late-life hypogonadism requires both symptoms and low testosterone (Figure 100.1a). Careful clinical evaluations and repeated hormone measurements should be carried out to exclude transient decreases in serum testosterone levels such as those due to acute illnesses.

Serum testosterone has a diurnal variation; a serum sample should be obtained between 07.00 and 11.00 h. The most widely accepted parameter to establish the presence of hypogonadism is the measurement of serum total testosterone. The ISA/ISSAM/EAU/EAA/ASA guidelines suggest that subjects with total testosterone levels above 350 ng dl^{-1} do not require substitution. Patients with serum total testosterone levels below 230 ng dl^{-1} will usually benefit from testosterone treatment. If the serum total testosterone level lies between 230 and 350 ng dl^{-1} (8–12 nmol l^{-1}) the patient could benefit from having a repeat measurement of total testosterone together with a measurement of SHBG concentrations so as to calculate free testosterone levels or bioavailable testosterone (BT, free plus albumin-bound), particularly in obese men.[10] The gold standard for BT measurement is by sulfate precipitation and equilibrium dialysis for free testosterone. However, usually neither technique is available in most laboratories so that calculated values seem preferable. Salivary testosterone, a proxy for unbound testosterone, has also been shown to be a reliable substitute for free testosterone measurements.[11]

One can calculate free testosterone reliably by using total testosterone, albumin and SHBG concentrations using an online calculator (http://www.issam.ch/freetesto.htm) or measure free testosterone accurately in a laboratory by equilibrium dialysis. As with total testosterone measurements, there is no general agreement as to what constitutes the lower limit of normal free testosterone levels, but the Endocrine Society mentions 50 pg ml^{-1} for free testosterone measured by equilibrium dialysis and the ISA, ISSAM, EAU, EAA and ASA recommend 65 pg ml^{-1} for calculated free testosterone.

The final step in determining whether a patient has primary or secondary hypogonadism is to measure the serum LH and follicle-stimulating hormone (FSH) (Figure 100.1b) Elevated LH and FSH levels suggest primary hypogonadism, whereas low or low-normal LH and FSH levels suggest secondary hypogonadism. Normal LH or FSH levels with low testosterone suggest primary defects in the hypothalamus and/or the pituitary (secondary hypogonadism). However, in elderly males, the rise in serum gonadotropin, FSH more than LH, is not as great as one would expect from the fall in testosterone, suggesting that the fall in testosterone with ageing is due more to secondary than primary hypogonadism. Unless fertility is an issue, it is usually not necessary to measure FSH and determining LH levels alone is sufficient. If the total testosterone concentration is <150 ng dl^{-1}, pituitary imaging studies and prolactin level are recommended to evaluate for structural lesions in the hypothalamic–pituitary region. Also, in secondary hypogonadism, prolactin levels should be obtained to rule out prolactinoma in addition to screening for haemochromatosis. A karyotype should be considered in a young teenager or infertile man with primary hypogonadism to diagnose Klinefelter syndrome (Figure 100.1b).

Treatment of late-onset hypogonadism

The principal goal of testosterone therapy is to restore the serum testosterone concentration to the normal range to alleviate the symptoms suggestive of the hormone deficiency. However, the ultimate goals are to maintain or regain the highest quality of life, to reduce disability, to compress major illnesses into a narrow age range and to add years to life.

Delivery systems

Several different types of testosterone replacement exist, including tablets, injections, transdermal systems, oral, pellets and buccal preparations of testosterone. Selective androgen receptor modulators (SARMs) are under development but not yet clinically available. The selection of the preparation should be a joint decision of an informed patient and physician. Short-acting preparations may be preferred over long-acting depot preparations in the initial treatment of patients with LOH. It is important to keep in mind that the goal of testosterone replacement therapy (TRT) is to increase blood testosterone concentrations to the normal (eugonadal) range and to match the most appropriate treatment to the individual patient. However, older males need higher levels to obtain a therapeutic benefit.

Oral agents

The modified testosterone 17α-methyltestosterone is an effective oral androgen formulation for hypogonadism; however, it is not recommended because of its hepatotoxic side effects and its potential liver toxicity, including the development of benign and malignant neoplasms in addition to deleterious effects on levels of both low-density lipoprotein cholesterol (LDL-C) and high-density lipoprotein cholesterol (HDL-C). Oral testosterone undecanoate, however, bypasses first-pass metabolism through its preferential absorption into the lymphatic system. It is safe because of the lack of adverse liver side effects, but it is only available outside the USA.

Intramuscular injection

Testosterone cypionate and enanthate were frequently used for intramuscular injection of short-acting testosterone esters that usually produces supraphysiological peaks and hypogonadal troughs in testosterone levels, which result in fluctuations in energy, mood and libido in many patients corresponding to the fluctuations in serum testosterone levels. These fluctuations are more pronounced as the dosing interval is increased. The disadvantages are the need for deep intramuscular administration of an oily solution every 1–3 weeks and fluctuations in the serum

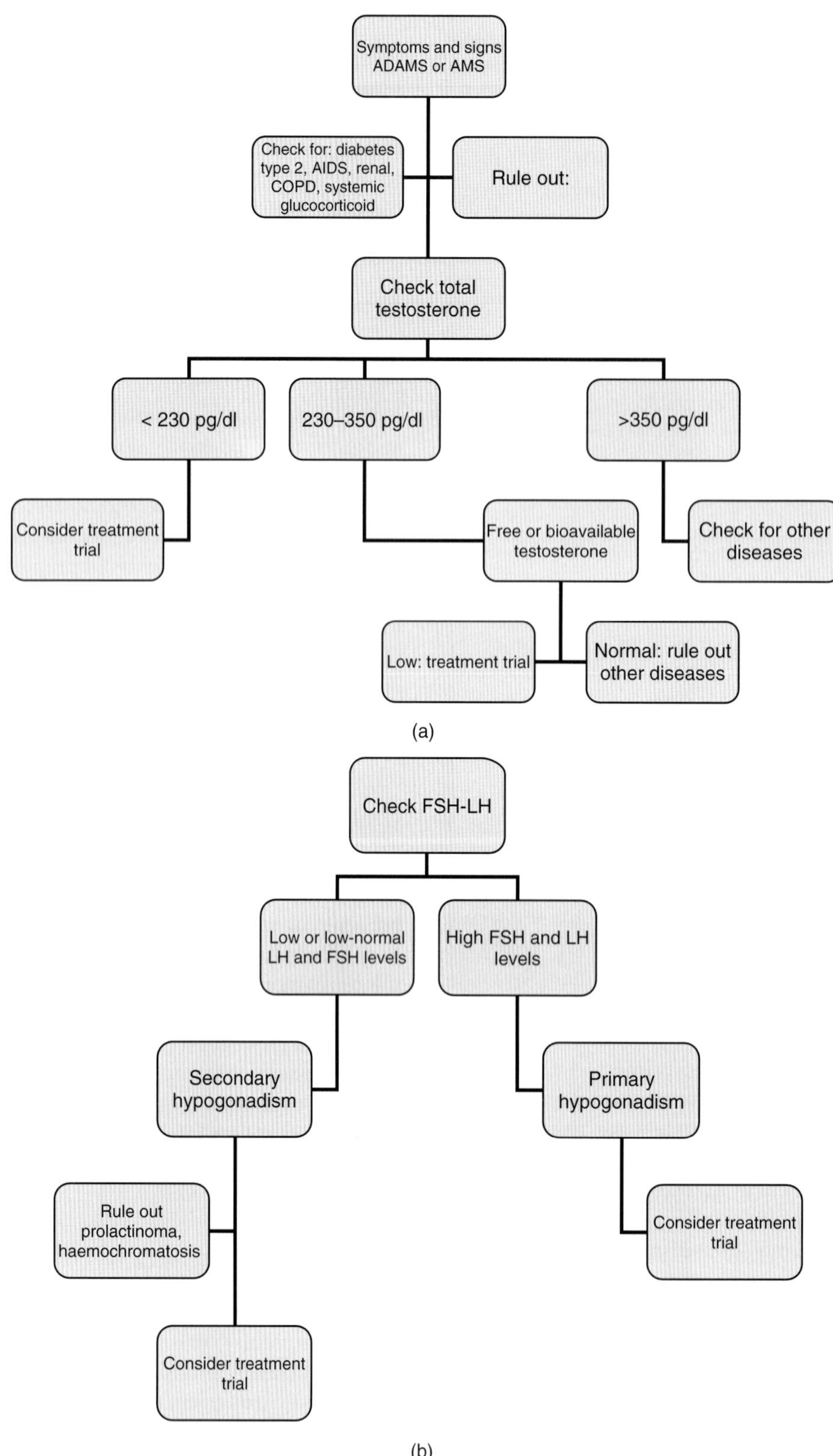

Figure 100.1 Diagnosis of hypogonadism.

testosterone concentration that result. A long-lasting formulation of testosterone undecanoate is available in the EU and other countries, but not yet in the USA. It consists of injections of 1000 mg of testosterone undecanoate at intervals of up to 3 months, offering an excellent alternative for substitution therapy of male hypogonadism. The serum testosterone concentration is maintained within the normal range.[12] However, the long duration of action creates a problem if there are complications of testosterone therapy. An oral formulation of this ester is also available in some countries, but it does not keep the serum testosterone concentration normal in hypogonadal men. Note that the intramuscular injections of testosterone can cause local pain, soreness, bruising, erythema, swelling, nodules or furuncles.

Transdermal systems

Transdermal testosterone is available in either a scrotal or a non-scrotal skin patch and more recently as a gel preparation, allowing a single application of this formulation to provide continuous transdermal delivery of testosterone for 24 h, producing circulating testosterone levels that approximate the normal levels (e.g. 300–1000 ng dl^{-1}) seen in healthy men. Daily application is required for each of these. They are designed to deliver 5–10 mg of testosterone per day and result in normal serum testosterone concentrations in the majority of hypogonadal men.[13] Scrotal patches produce high levels of circulating dihydrotestosterone (DHT) due to the high 5α-reductase enzyme activity of scrotal skin, but these are not so popular because the scrotum has to be shaved and the adherence is not good. Non-genital patches are applied once per day to the back, abdomen, thighs or upper arms. Skin irritation can occur and preapplication of a corticosteroid cream can help reduce this. The transdermal gels are colourless hydroalcoholic gels containing 1–2% testosterone. They are applied once per day to the skin. There is a lower incidence of skin irritation compared with the patch, but testosterone can be transferred from the patient to his partner or to children after skin contact. This risk can be minimized by covering the site of application with clothing after the gel has dried, by washing the application site when skin-to-skin contact is expected and by having patients wash their hands with soap and water after applying the gel. A reservoir-type transdermal delivery system for testosterone was developed using an ethanol–water (70:30) cosolvent system as the vehicle. This device is available in Europe as a body patch without reservoir and applied every 2 days. The advantages include ease of use and maintenance of relatively uniform serum testosterone levels over time, resulting in maintenance of relatively stable energy, mood and libido, in addition to the efficacy in providing adequate TRT.

Sublingual and buccal

Cyclodextrin-complexed testosterone sublingual formulation is absorbed rapidly into the circulation, where testosterone is released from the cyclodextrin shell. This formulation has been suggested to have good therapeutic potential, after adjustment of its kinetics, to produce physiological levels of testosterone.

A mucoadhesive buccal testosterone sustained-release tablet, delivering 30 mg, applied to the upper gum just above the incisor teeth, has been shown to restore serum testosterone concentrations to the physiological range within 4 h of application, with steady-state concentrations achieved within 24 h of twice-daily dosing and achieves testosterone levels within the normal range. Studies indicate that Striant is an effective, well-tolerated, convenient and discreet treatment for male hypogonadism. However, it has had minimal clinical uptake, owing to the difficulty of maintaining the buccal treatment in the mouth.[14] The incidence of adverse effects is low, although gum and buccal irritation and alterations in taste have been reported.

Subdermal implants

Subcutaneous pellets were among the earliest effective formulations for administering testosterone. Although not frequently used, they remain available. The testosterone pellets are usually implanted under the skin of the lower abdomen using a trochar and cannula or are inserted into the gluteus muscle. Six to ten pellets are implanted at one time and they last 4–6 months, when a new procedure is required to implant more. Testosterone pellets currently are the only long-acting testosterone treatment approved for use in the USA.

Subdermal testosterone implants still offer the longest duration of action with prolonged zero-order, steady-state delivery characteristics. The standard dosage is four 200 mg pellets (800 mg) implanted subdermally at intervals of 5–7 months.[15] However, the *in vivo* testosterone release rate of these testosterone pellets and its determinants have not been studied systematically. As a result of their long-lasting effect and the inconvenience of removing them, the risk of infection at the implant site and extrusion of the pellets which occurs in 5–10% of cases even with the most experienced, their use is limited only to men for whom the beneficial effects and tolerance of TRT have already been established.

Intranasal testosterone

Testosterone is well absorbed after nasal administration.[16] Application of MPP-10 results in a more pulse-like testosterone profile rather than the relatively sustained serum levels attained with transdermal administration. The intranasal drug delivery system represents a mechanism to proximate more closely the normal circadian variation of testosterone levels, in contrast to the abnormal steady-state levels seen with transdermal products or the large fluctuations over longer periods of time seen with injections. Further studies are necessary to determine the effect of nasal testosterone application in hypogonadal men over prolonged periods of time.

Benefits of testosterone replacement therapy

Restoring testosterone levels in older male patients to within the normal range by using TRT can improve many of the effects of hypogonadism. Most importantly, these include beneficial effects on mood, energy levels and patients' sense of wellbeing, sexual function, lean body mass and muscle strength, erythropoiesis, BMD, cognition and some benefits on cardiovascular risk factors. These are summarized in Table 100.2.

Improved sexual desire, function and performance

The prevalence of erectile dysfunction increases markedly with age. Sexual function, measured by frequency of orgasm or intercourse or by sexual satisfaction, is lower in elderly men than in young men. Men with hypogonadism due to known disease also have a decline in sexual function, as illustrated by an improvement after testosterone treatment. Serum free testosterone was significantly correlated with erectile and orgasmic function domains of the International Index of Erectile Function (IIEF) questionnaire. Men with greater sexual activity had higher bio-T levels than men with a lower frequency and androgen deficiency may contribute to the age-related decline in male sexuality; correspondingly low levels of bio-T were associated with low sexual activity. Compared with younger men, elderly men require higher levels of circulating testosterone for libido and erectile function. However, erectile dysfunction and/or diminished libido with or without a testosterone deficiency might be related to other comorbidities or medications.

Table 100.2 Potential benefits of TRT.

- Improved sexual desire and function
- Increased BMD
- Improved mood, energy and quality of life
- Changed body composition and improved muscle mass and strength
- Improved cognitive function

Men with erectile dysfunction and/or diminished libido and documented testosterone deficiency are candidates for testosterone therapy. Randomized controlled clinical trials indicate some benefits of testosterone therapy on sexual health-related outcomes in hypogonadal men.[17] Testosterone replacement has also been shown to enhance libido and the frequency of sexual acts and sleep-related erections. Transdermal TRT, in particular, has been linked to positive effects on fatigue and mood, which affect sexual activity.

A short therapeutic trial may be tried in the presence of a clinical picture of testosterone deficiency and borderline serum testosterone levels. An inadequate response to testosterone treatment requires reassessment of the causes of the erectile dysfunction. There is evidence that the combined use of testosterone and phosphodiesterase type 5 inhibitors in hypogonadal or borderline eugonadal men have a synergetic effect.[18] The combination treatment should be considered in hypogonadal patients with erectile dysfunction failing to respond to either treatment alone.

The role of testosterone supplementation in men with erectile dysfunction who are not androgen deficient or in the low-normal range needs further investigation to determine whether TRT will improve erectile function. Failure of improvement when the serum testosterone concentration has been restored to normal suggests another cause of the symptoms.

Bone mineral density

As men age, their BMD declines. Osteoporosis is an under-recognized problem in men. Testosterone plays a major role in BMD. Osteopenia, osteoporosis and fracture prevalence rates are greater in hypogonadal older men. In nursing homes, of elderly men who have experienced hip fractures, 66% are hypogonadal. Patients with prostate cancer treated with androgen deprivation therapy have an increased risk of osteoporotic fracture. Assessment of bone density at 2 year intervals is advisable in hypogonadal men and serum testosterone measurements should be obtained in all men with osteopenia. All persons with low testosterone should have their 25-hydroxyvitamin D levels measured and replaced if low.

Testosterone produces this effect by increasing osteoblastic activity and through aromatization to estrogen reducing osteoclastic activity. The role of the partial androgen deficiency in ageing males in bone fracture rate remains to be established. The correlation with bioestradiol, the levels of which decline in elderly males, was even stronger, suggesting that part of the androgen effects on bone are at least partially indirect, mediated via their aromatization.[19] An increase in osteocalcin levels, an index of osteoblast activity, was observed and a decrease in hydroxyproline excretion, an index of bone resorption, was also noted.

Trials of the effects of TRT on BMD yielded mixed results. Increases in spinal bone density have been realized in hypogonadal men, with most treated men maintaining bone density above the fracture threshold. An improvement in both trabecular and cortical BMD of the spine was seen, independent of age and type of hypogonadism; in addition, a significant increase in paraspinal muscle area has been observed, emphasizing the clinical benefit of adequate replacement therapy for the physical fitness of hypogonadal men. The pooled results of a meta-analysis suggest a beneficial effect on lumbar spine bone density and equivocal findings on femoral neck BMD. Trials of intramuscular testosterone reported significantly larger effects on lumbar bone density than trials of transdermal testosterone, particularly among patients receiving chronic glucocorticoids.[20] In eugonadal men with osteoporosis, testosterone esters (250 mg per 2 weeks) gave mixed results. Although there is significant evidence of an association between hypogonadism and osteoporosis, studies of TRT in men with osteoporosis are limited and none have used fractures as an end-point.

Improved body composition and muscle mass and strength

There is a significant change in body composition characterized by decreased fat free mass and increased and redistributed fat mass in elderly patients. These changes can impose functional limitations and increase morbidity. In men, declining testosterone levels that occur with ageing can be a contributing factor to these changes through a direct effect on muscle cells by testosterone or by stimulating IGF-1 expression directly and indirectly, leading to increased muscle protein synthesis and growth. Epidemiological studies have demonstrated a correlation between BT concentrations and fat-free mass; however, the correlation with grip strength is not clear.

Testosterone replacement may be effective in reversing age-dependent body composition changes and associated morbidity. Testosterone administration improves body composition with a decrease in fat mass and increase in lean body mass, but the body weight changes do not differ significantly.[21] Changes in lower-extremity muscle strength and measures of physical function were inconsistent among studies. Some studies showed a positive correlation between testosterone and muscle strength parameters of the upper and lower extremities, as measured by leg extensor strength and isometric hand grip strength, and also functional parameters, including the doors test, get up and go test and five-chair sit/stand test.[22] On the other hand, some reported an increase in lean body mass but no change in physical function or an increase in strength of knee extension or flexion.

It is not clear whether testosterone replacement in frail older men with low testosterone levels can improve physical function and other health-related outcomes or reduce the risk of disability, falls or fractures. A combination of testosterone and a nutritional supplement markedly reduced hospital admissions in older men and women.

Mood, energy and quality of life

Hypogonadal older men commonly complain of loss of libido, dysphoria, fatigue and irritability.[71] These symptoms overlap with signs and symptoms of major depression. There is significant correlation between BT, reduced feelings of wellbeing and a depression score in elderly men, independent of age and weight, but not with total testosterone levels.

TRT has variable effects on mood, energy, fatigue, irritability and sense of wellbeing. The results of placebo-controlled randomized trials on testosterone's effect on quality of life and depressive mood were inconsistent across trials and imprecise. Testosterone administered to non-depressed eugonadal men in physiological doses did not have effect on mood.[23] Administration of supraphysiological doses of testosterone to eugonadal men has been associated with mania in a small proportion of patients. Testosterone replacement of hypogonadal men with major depressive disorder might be an effective antidepressant or augmentation to partially effective antidepressant.[24] Testosterone gel had significantly greater improvement as augmentation therapy for depressive symptoms than subjects receiving placebo in hypogonadal men with selective serotonin reuptake inhibitor (SSRI) partial response. These significant correlations with testosterone levels were only observed when the levels were below the normal range, which suggests that once a minimally adequate testosterone/DHT level was achieved, further increase did not contribute further to improvement of mood. However, the studies reported tend to be of limited size and duration, with a lack of large-scale trials with extended long-term follow-up. This effect may be a direct effect of testosterone or related to positive effects of testosterone on weight and/or other anthropometric indices.

On the other hand, the testosterone–placebo difference distinguishable with respect to mood was not consistent. No relationship between testosterone level and depressive symptoms was found in the MMAS. This discrepancy in the results of the effects of TRT on mood may be explained by the genetic polymorphism in the androgen receptor which defines a vulnerable group in whom depression is expressed when testosterone levels fall below a particular threshold.

Finally, testosterone treatment must be considered experimental. More controlled studies using exogenous testosterone for depression in elderly men are needed. The best candidates for treatment may be hypogonadal men who are currently taking an existing antidepressant with inadequate response.

Cognitive function

Dementia is a major problem for older men. The decrease in serum testosterone concentrations that occurs with ageing in men may be associated with a decline in verbal and visual memory and visuospatial performance and a faster rate of decline in visual memory. Men with a higher ratio of total testosterone to SHBG predict a reduced incidence of Alzheimer's disease and patients with Alzheimer's disease had a lower ratio of total testosterone to SHBG compared with age-matched controls.[25] Low BT is strongly associated with amnestic mild cognitive impairment and higher bioavailable and free testosterone concentrations have each been associated with better performance in specific aspects of memory and cognitive function, with optimal processing capacity found in men ranging from 35 to 90 years of age even after adjustment for potential confounders including age, educational attainment and cardiovascular morbidity; whereas total testosterone was not.[26]

On the other hand, contradictory findings have also been reported between total or free testosterone and measures of working memory, speed/attention or spatial relations in older men. No association was found between lower free testosterone levels and higher performance on spatial visualization tasks and between higher free and total testosterone levels and poorer verbal memory and executive performance; however, there is a correlation with faster processing speed.[27] A possible source of conflicting results in these studies may stem from interactions between testosterone levels and other risk factors for cognitive impairment such as apolipoprotein E4 genotype and systemic illness that cause low testosterone.

In men undergoing hormonal therapy for prostate cancer, suppression of endogenous testosterone synthesis and blockade of the androgen receptor resulted in a beneficial effect on verbal memory but an adverse effect on spatial ability slowed reaction times in several attentional domains; plasma amyloid levels increased as T levels decreased. Discontinuation of treatment resulted in improved memory but not visuospatial abilities. One of the possible protective mechanisms of action of testosterone would be through its conversion into estradiol (E2), the most potent estrogen, which could exert protective effects on the brain structures in ageing patients.

Trials of TRT in men to evaluate its effects on measures of cognitive function and memory to date were all relatively small and of a relatively short duration and have shown mixed results. Androgen supplementation in elderly hypogonadal men improves spatial cognition and verbal fluency and in elderly men without dementia it may reduce working memory errors. Intramuscular testosterone improved verbal and spatial memory and constructional abilities in non-hypogonadal men with mild cognitive impairment and Alzheimer's disease. On the other hand, in Alzheimer's disease patients, testosterone treatment appeared to improve quality of life and verbal memory without imprecise effects on several dimensions of cognition.

Therefore, although the evidence from studies is not uniform, lower free testosterone appears to be associated with poorer outcomes on measures of cognitive function, particularly in older men, and TRT in hypogonadal men may have some benefit for cognitive performance.

Effect on metabolic syndrome and cardiovascular risk factors

Testosterone has a positive effect on reducing the risk factors for the metabolic syndrome and cardiovascular disease. The increased correlation between low testosterone levels and the severity of coronary artery disease may be related to the fact that low androgen levels are accompanied by an accumulation of abdominal visceral fat, which is known to be associated with increased cardiovascular risk factors,[28] impaired glucose tolerance and non-insulin-dependent diabetes mellitus (syndrome X). Low endogenous testosterone concentrations are related to mortality due to cardiovascular disease and all causes.

There is a relationship between testosterone levels and body mass index (BMI), waist circumference, waist–hip ratio, serum leptin, LDL-C, triglyceride and fibrinogen levels, hypertension, diabetes. At the same time, adipose tissue affects testosterone levels by increasing the aromatization of testosterone to estradiol, which provides negative feedback on the HPG axis and by decreasing testosterone levels via a decrease in SHBG levels. Thus, adiposity potentially leads to hypogonadism, which itself promote further adiposity.

Low testosterone concentrations are known to occur in association with type 2 diabetes. Prevalence in diabetic men has been estimated at 33–50%. There is no relation between the degree of hyperglycaemia and testosterone concentration. Prostate-specific antigen (PSA) is significantly lower in type 2 diabetics and this is related to their lower plasma testosterone concentrations.[29] Low testosterone concentrations predict the development of type 2 diabetes. Testosterone also may suppress insulin resistance independently of its effects on adiposity. In addition, diet and exercise increased testosterone levels in hypogonadal men with metabolic syndrome and newly diagnosed type 2 diabetes.

The effect of androgen replacement in elderly men on LDL-C and HDL-C is controversial. The relationship between testosterone and HDL is confounded by the fact that both HDL and testosterone are inversely related to BMI.

Data from the MMAS have demonstrated that low total or free testosterone correlates with low HDL-C. Testosterone replacement therapy in men with hypogonadism has little effect on serum concentrations of total cholesterol and LDL-C. HDL-C levels decrease in patients on oral testosterone therapy but not when given as a transdermal gel to hypogonadal men. In a meta-analysis of 10 studies of intramuscular testosterone esters and plasma lipids in hypogonadal men, a small, dose-dependent decrease was seen in total cholesterol, LDL-C and HDL-C.[30] The mechanism of the fall in lipids might be related to the decrease in the visceral abdominal fat mass under the influence of androgens, which inhibit lipoprotein lipase activity and increase lipolysis with improvement of insulin sensitivity and mobilization of triglycerides from abdominal fat tissue. Note that supraphysiological testosterone levels induce an increase in LDL-C and a decrease of HDL-C and may increase the risk of cardiovascular disease.

Testosterone treatment in elderly patients with chronic heart failure might improve insulin sensitivity and various cardio-respiratory and muscular outcomes. The administration of testosterone at physiological concentration increases coronary blood flow in patients with coronary heart disease. Transdermal TRT was found to be beneficial for men with chronic stable angina as they had greater angina-free exercise tolerance than placebo-treated controls. However, no consistent relationship between the levels of free or total testosterone and coronary atherosclerosis in men undergoing coronary angiography has been observed.

Improving anaemia

Endogenous androgens are known to stimulate erythropoiesis and increase reticulocyte count, blood haemoglobin levels and bone marrow erythropoietic activity in mammals, whereas castration has opposite effects. Testosterone deficiency results in a 10–20% decrease in the blood haemoglobin concentration, which can result in anaemia. The main androgen involvement in the mechanism of normal haematopoiesis is thought to be direct stimulation of renal production of erythropoietin by testosterone. Moreover, the latter may also act directly on erythropoietic stem cells.

Risks of testosterone replacement therapy

The risks of TRT depend upon age, life circumstances and other medical conditions. There is a risk for prostate cancer and worsening symptoms of benign prostatic hypertrophy, liver toxicity and tumour, worsening symptoms of sleep apnoea and congestive heart failure, gynaecomastia, infertility and skin diseases. TRT is not appropriate for men who are interested in fathering a child because exogenous testosterone will suppress the hypothalamic–pituitary–thyroid (HPT) axis. The risks of TRT are summarized in Table 100.3.

Table 100.3 Potential risks for TRT in elderly men.

- Stimulates growth of prostate cancer and breast cancer
- Worsens symptoms of benign prostatic hypertrophy
- Causes liver toxicity and liver tumour
- Causes gynaecomastia
- Causes erythrocytosis
- Causes testicular atrophy and infertility
- Causes skin diseases
- Causes or exacerbates sleep apnoea

The prostate and testosterone replacement therapy

In ageing men with LOH, TRT may normalize serum androgen levels but appears to have little effect on prostate tissue androgen levels and cellular functions and causes no significant adverse effects on the prostate. At present, there is no conclusive evidence that TRT increases the risk of prostate cancer or benign prostatic hyperplasia (BPH).

Benign prostatic hyperplasia

With ageing, some men experience an exacerbation of BPH symptoms; predominantly lower urinary tract symptoms (LUTS) due to urinary outflow obstruction. The testosterone dependence of BPH has been known for a long time. Testosterone supplements increase prostate volume with, eventually, a mild increase in PSA levels in old men. Although a meta-analysis showed that the total number of prostate events combined was significantly greater in testosterone-treated men than in placebo-treated men, the majority of events are due to prostate biopsy. At the same time, many studies have failed to show significant exacerbation of voiding symptoms attributable to BPH during testosterone supplementation and complications such as urinary retention have not occurred at higher rates than in controls receiving placebo, nor has there been any difference in the urine flow rates, post-voiding residual urine volumes and prostate voiding symptoms with patients receiving treatment in these studies. The poor correlation between prostate volume and urinary symptoms explains this illogicality. There are no compelling data to suggest that testosterone treatment exacerbates LUTS or promotes acute urinary retention. However, severe LUTS, due to BPH, represent a relative contraindication which is no longer applicable after successful treatment of lower urinary tract obstruction. The patient needs to be made aware that there might be increased voiding symptoms during treatment.

Prostate cancer

Prostate cancer is well known to be, in the majority of cases, an androgen-sensitive disease and prostate cancer has been treated in patterns designed to lower the testosterone level; androgen replacement therapy is an absolute contraindication. The prevalence of prostate cancer in many studies on patients receiving TRT was similar to that in the general population. So far, there is no compelling evidence that testosterone has a causative role in prostate cancer. There is, however, unequivocal evidence that testosterone can stimulate growth and aggravate symptoms in men with locally advanced and metastatic prostate cancer. A fuller explanation may be that prostate cancer is very sensitive to changes in serum testosterone when at low concentrations, but is insensitive at higher concentrations because of saturation of the androgen receptors. Men successfully treated for prostate cancer and diagnosed with hypogonadism are candidates for testosterone replacement after a prudent interval if there is no clinical or laboratory evidence of residual cancer.[31] In addition, no effect was found of TRT on PSA levels and the changes in PSA were not influenced by the mode of TRT, patient age or baseline levels of PSA or testosterone. It is important to mention that the occurrence of prostate cancer and PSA concentrations are lower in patients with type 2 diabetes and related to testosterone concentrations. It is not yet known if the normal PSA reference ranges should be lowered for men with type 2 diabetes.

In summary, there is no convincing evidence that the normalization of testosterone serum levels in men with prostate problems and low levels is deleterious. TRT can be cautiously considered in selected hypogonadal men treated with curative intent for prostate cancer and without evidence of active disease.

Liver problems

Benign and malignant hepatic tumours, intrahepatic cholestasis, hepatotoxicity and liver failure have been reported with TRT. These unfavourable hepatic effects do not appear to be associated with transdermal or intramuscular injections. For this reason, the oral forms of testosterone, with the exception of testosterone undecanoate, are discouraged. Other liver abnormalities associated with TRT include peliosis hepatis, hepatocellular adenoma and carcinoma.

Sleep apnoea

Sleep apnoea was worse in men with hypogonadism treated with testosterone. In contrast, in a recent meta-analysis, the frequency of sleep apnoea did not differ between testosterone and placebo-treated men. Physicians should inquire about symptoms, such as excessive daytime sleepiness and witnessed apnoea during sleep by a partner, and if indicated, polysomnography should be performed.

Erythrocytosis

There is a correlation between high testosterone levels and high haemoglobin. Erythrocytosis is a common adverse effect of testosterone administration. Testosterone-treated men were almost four times more likely to have a haematocrit >50%. Erythrocytosis can develop during testosterone treatment, especially in older men treated by injectable testosterone preparations. The elevation in haemoglobin above certain levels may have had a greater overall mortality and cardiovascular mortality, particularly in the elderly, because the increase in blood viscosity could exacerbate vascular disease in the coronary, cerebrovascular or peripheral vascular circulation, especially in people with other diseases that cause secondary polycythaemia, such as chronic obstructive pulmonary disease. Testosterone dosage correlates with the incidence of erythrocytosis and polycythaemia is related most of the time to supraphysiological levels.

Periodic haematological assessment is indicated (e.g. before treatment, then at 3–4 months and at 12 months in the first year of treatment and annually thereafter). Although it is not yet clear what critical threshold is desirable, dose adjustment and/or periodic phlebotomy may be necessary to keep the haematocrit below 52–55%.

Other side effects of TRT

Supraphysiological doses of androgens may cause decreased testicular size, acne and azoospermia. The decrease in testicular size and compromised fertility during TRT occur because of the down regulation of gonadotropins. It is related to aromatization of testosterone into estradiol in peripheral fat and muscle tissue. Even the ratio of estradiol to testosterone usually remains normal. It occurs especially with testosterone enanthate or cypionate. Dose adjustment may be necessary. Gynaecomastia is another benign complication of testosterone treatment.

TRT has been associated with exacerbation of sleep apnoea. The effect of testosterone is not on the dimensions of the upper airway, but it most likely contributes to sleep disorder breathing by central mechanisms. The development of signs and symptoms of obstructive sleep apnoea during testosterone therapy warrants a formal sleep study and treatment with continuous positive airway pressure (CPAP) if necessary. If the patient is unresponsive or cannot tolerate CPAP, the testosterone must be reduced or discontinued. Testosterone is anabolic and it will cause some nitrogen, sodium and water retention. Oedema may be worsened in patients with pre-existing cardiac, renal or hepatic disease. Hypertension has rarely been reported.

Symptom relief

The time course of the effects of testosterone replacement is variable. Once testosterone levels are restored to a stable normal range, there is an improvement in libido, sexual function, mood and energy levels, insulin resistance and fat-free mass relatively early in the course of treatment. The reduction in fat body mass, an increase in lean body mass and an improvement in BMD at the hip and spine started after a period between 6 and 24 months.

Monitoring patients on TRT

Patients who are treated with testosterone should be monitored to determine that normal serum testosterone concentrations are being achieved. If the patient has primary hypogonadism, normalization of the serum LH concentration should also be used to judge the adequacy of the testosterone dose, no matter which testosterone preparation is used. They should be monitored for both desirable and undesirable effects.

Once TRT has started, patients need to be carefully monitored. Patients should be monitored for signs of oedema, gynaecomastia, sleep apnoea, LUTS and low BMD. Laboratory parameters should be monitored before and during treatment. There are clinical practice guidelines from the Endocrine Society for monitoring patients receiving TRT. Testosterone level, digital rectal examination, PSA, haematocrit, BMD, lipids and liver function tests should be checked at baseline, then the patient should be evaluated 3 and 6 months after treatment starts and then annually to assess whether symptoms have responded to treatment and whether the patient is suffering from any adverse effects. If the haematocrit is more than 54%, therapy should be stopped until the haematocrit decreases to a safe level; the patient should be evaluated for hypoxia and sleep apnoea; therapy should then be reinitiated with a reduced dose. BMD of lumbar spine and/or femoral neck should be measured at baseline every 1–2 years of testosterone therapy in hypogonadal men with osteoporosis or low trauma fracture.

Testosterone levels should be monitored 3 months after initiation of TRT. A mid-morning total serum testosterone level should be obtained. A target range of 400–500 ng dl^{-1} (14.0–17.5 nmol l^{-1}) for older men is suggested. However, if there is no symptomatic response, higher levels may be necessary. For injectable testosterone, the serum level can be measured between injections. For men treated with a transdermal testosterone patch, the serum level should be measured 3–12 h after patch application. In patients receiving buccal testosterone tablets, the serum level should be measured immediately before application of a fresh system. Patients on testosterone gel may have levels checked any time after at least 1 week of therapy. In all cases, BT levels should also be monitored as testosterone therapy lowers SHBG.

For patients with BPH, LUTS should be assessed by the International Prostate Symptom Score (IPSS). For prostate cancer, digital rectal examination and measurement of serum PSA should be performed before initiating testosterone replacement, 3 months after initiation of treatment and then in accordance with evidence-based guidelines for prostate cancer screening, depending on the age and race of the patient. All men who present for TRT should undergo prostate biopsy if they have an abnormal PSA level or abnormal result on digital rectal examination with low threshold to do or repeat prostate biopsy if the PSA level or digital rectal examination changes. The American Urological Association (AUA) suggests a urological consultation for any of the following: if the patient has an abnormal digital rectal examination result, if the PSA levels exceed 2.5 ng ml^{-1} in males under 60 years or 4 ng ml^{-1} in men over 60 years, or a velocity change of 0.75 ng ml^{-1} or greater in a year.[32]

The use of testosterone preparations should be discussed with the patient, who should be closely monitored for efficacy and toxicities. Failure to benefit from clinical manifestations should result in discontinuation of treatment after 3 months for libido and sexual function, muscle function and improved body fat, and a longer interval for BMD. Further investigations for other causes of symptoms are then mandatory.

Precautions and contraindications for TRT

Healthcare providers must rule out contraindications to treatment before starting patients on TRT (Table 100.4). The presence of a clinical prostatic carcinoma is an absolute contraindication for TRT and should be carefully excluded by PSA, rectal examination and, eventually, biopsy before starting any therapy. There is also no clear recommendation for men successfully treated for prostate cancer who would be potential candidates for testosterone substitution after a 'prudent' interval if there is no clinical or laboratory evidence of residual cancer.

The presence of breast cancer is also a contraindication for TRT, and also a prolactinoma, as their growth may be stimulated by TRT. A very high risk of serious adverse outcomes, undiagnosed prostate nodules or indurations, unexplained PSA elevation, erythrocytosis (haematocrit $>50\%$), severe LUTS with benign prostatic hyperplasia with an IPSS >19, unstable congestive heart failure (class III or IV) and untreated obstructive sleep apnoea are

Table 100.4 Contraindications for TRT.

- Very high risk of serious adverse outcomes
- Prostatic carcinoma
- Breast cancer
- Prostate nodules or indurations
- Unexplained prostate-specific antigen (PSA) elevation
- Erythrocytosis (haematocrit >50%)
- Severe lower urinary tract symptoms with benign prostatic hyperplasia with an International Prostate Symptom Score (IPSS) >19
- Unstable congestive heart failure (class III or IV)
- Severe untreated sleep apnoea

considered as moderate to high risk factors for potential adverse outcomes.[33]

Conclusion and recommendations

The decrease in the major function of the testes, late-onset hypogonadism, is a common condition in the male population but it is still underdiagnosed and undertreated. The apparently increasing incidence and expanding range of treatment options may facilitate greater awareness of the condition. The symptoms in the elderly have a complex origin. It may be reasonably assumed that the age-associated decrease in testosterone levels is in part responsible for the symptoms of ageing. In the absence of known pituitary or testicular disease, we suggest TRT only for older men with low serum testosterone concentrations and clinically important symptoms of androgen deficiency. The benefits and risks of TRT must be clearly discussed with the patient and an assessment of the major risk factors made before commencing testosterone treatment. The major contraindication for androgen supplementation is the presence of a prostatic carcinoma. The response to testosterone treatment should be assessed. If treatment is undertaken, the patient should be screened before treatment and monitored during treatment for evidence of testosterone-dependent diseases. The target serum testosterone concentration in older men should be lower than that for younger men, for example, 300–400 rather than 500–600 ng dl^{-1}, to minimize the potential risk of testosterone-dependent diseases.[34]

If there is no improvement of symptoms and signs, treatment should be discontinued and the patient investigated for other possible causes of the clinical presentations. Many questions in the treatment of hypogonadism remain unanswered and there is a need for large clinical trials to assess the long-term benefits and risks of TRT in older men with LOH.

Key points

- Secondary hypogonadism occurs in at least 20% of older males.
- Testosterone replacement improves libido, potency, ejaculate volume, bone mineral density, erythropoiesis and cognition.
- Testosterone replacement increases muscle mass and decreases fat mass.
- Testosterone replacement techniques include patches, gels, injections and subdermal implants

References

1. Araujo AB, Esche GR, Kupelian V *et al.* Prevalence of symptomatic androgen deficiency in men. *J Clin Endocrinol Metab* 2007;**92**:4241–7.
2. Araujo A, Kupelian V, Page ST *et al.* Sex steroids and all-cause mortality and cause-specific mortality in men. *Arch Intern Med* 2007;**167**:1252–60.
3. Morley JE, Kaiser FE, Perry HM *et al.* Longitudinal changes in testosterone, luteinizing hormone and follicle-stimulating hormone in healthy older men. *Metabolism* 1997;**46**:410–3.
4. Wu FC, Tajar A, Pye SR *et al.* Hypothalamic–pituitary–testicular axis disruptions in older men are differentially linked to age and modifiable risk factors: the European Male Aging Study. *J Clin Endocrinol Metab* 2008;**93**:27–37.
5. Harman SM, Metter EJ, Tobin JD and Pearson, J. longitudinal effects of aging on serum total and free testosterone levels in healthy men. Baltimore Longitudinal Study of Aging. *J Clin Endocrinol Metab* 2001;**86**:724–31.
6. Gray A, Feldman HA, McKinlay JB and Longcope C. Age, disease and changing sex hormone levels in middle-aged men: results of the Massachusetts Male Aging Study. *J Clin Endocrinol Metab* 1991;**73**:1016–25.
7. Travison TG, Shackelton R, Araujo AB *et al.* The natural history of symptomatic androgen deficiency in men: onset, progression and spontaneous remission. *J Am Geriatr Soc* 2008;**56**:831–9.
8. Mahmoud AM, Goemaere S, El-Garem Y *et al.* Testicular volume in relation to hormonal indices of gonadal function in community-dwelling elderly men. *J Clin Endocrinol Metab* 2003;**88**:179–84.
9. Morley JE and Melmed S. Gonadal dysfunction in systematic disorders. *Metabolism* 1979;**28**:1051–73.
10. Wang C, Nieschlag E, Swerdloff R *et al.* Investigation, treatment and monitoring of late-onset hypogonadism in males: ISA, ISSAM, EAU, EAA and ASA recommendations. *J Androl* 2009;**30**:1–9.
11. Morley JE, Perry HM III, Patrick P *et al.* Validation of salivary testosterone as a screening test for male hypogonadism. *Aging Male* 2006;**9**:165–9.

12. Schubert M, Minnemann T, Hubler D *et al.* Intramuscular testosterone undecanoate: pharmacokinetic aspects of a novel testosterone formulation during long-term treatment of men with hypogonadism. *J Clin Endocrinol Metab* 2004;**89**:5429–34.

13. Dobs AS, Meikle AW, Arver S *et al.* Pharmacokinetics, efficacy and safety of a permeation-enhanced testosterone transdermal system in comparison with bi-weekly injections of testosterone enanthate for the treatment of hypogonadal men. *J Clin Endocrinol Metab* 1999;**84**:3469–78.

14. Wang C, Swerdloff R, Kipnes M and Matsumoto AM. New testosterone buccal system (Striant) delivers physiological testosterone levels: pharmacokinetics study in hypogonadal men. *J Clin Endocrinol Metab* 2004;**89**:3821–9.

15. Handelsman DJ. Clinical pharmacology of testosterone pellet implants. In: E Nieschlag, HM Behre (eds), *Testosterone Action Deficiency Substitution*, 2nd edn, Springer, Berlin, 1998, pp. 349–64.

16. Banks WA, Morley JE, Niehoff ML and Mattern C. Delivery of testosterone to the brain by intranasal administration: comparison to intravenous testosterone. *J Drug Target* 2009;**17**:91–7.

17. Hajjar RR, Kaiser FE and Morley JE. Outcomes of long-term testosterone replacement in older hypogonadal males: a retrospective analysis. *J Clin Endocrinol Metab* 1997;**82**:3793–6.

18. Greco EA, Spera G and Aversa A. Combining testosterone and PDE5 inhibitors in erectile dysfunction: basic rationale and clinical evidences. *Eur Urol* 2006;**50**:940–7.

19. Michael H, Härkönen PL, Väänänen HK and Hentunen TA. Estrogen and testosterone use different cellular pathways to inhibit osteoclastogenesis and bone resorption. *J Bone Miner Res* 2005;**20**:2224–32.

20. Michal J. Tracz, Sideras K and Bolon ERA. Clinical review: testosterone use in men and its effects on bone health. A systematic review and meta-analysis of randomized placebo-controlled trials. *J Clin Endocrinol Metab* 2006;**91**:2011–6.

21. Harman SM and Blackman MR. The effects of growth hormone and sex steroid on lean body mass, fat mass, muscle strength, cardiovascular endurance and adverse events in healthy elderly women and men. *Horm Res* 2003;**60**:121–4.

22. Breuer B, Trungold S, Martucci C *et al.* Relationship of sex hormone levels to dependence of daily living in the frail elderly. *Maturitas* 32001;**9**:147–59.

23. Haren MT, Wittert GA, Chapman IM *et al.* Effect of oral testosterone undecanoate on visuospatial cognition, mood and quality of life in elderly men with low–normal gonadal status. *Maturitas* 2005;**50**:124–33.

24. Seidman SN and Rabkin JG. Testosterone replacement therapy for hypogonadal men with SSRI-refractory depression. *J Affect Disord* 1998;**48**:157–61.

25. Hogervorst E, Bandelow S, Combrinck M and Smith AD. Low free testosterone is an independent risk factor for Alzheimer's disease. *Exp Gerontol* 2004;**39**:1633–9.

26. Thilers PP, MacDonald SWS and Herlitz A. The association between endogenous free testosterone and cognitive performance: a population-based study in 35–90year-old men and women. *Psychoneuroendocrinology* 2006;**31**:565–76.

27. Yonker JE, Eriksson E, Nilsson L-G and Herlitz A. Negative association of testosterone on spatial visualisation in 35 to 80year old men. *Cortex* 2006;**42**:376–86.

28. Kannell WB, Cupples LA, Ramaswami R *et al.* Regional obesity and the risk of coronary disease: the Framingham Study. *J Clin Epidemiol* 1991;**44**:183–90.

29. Dhindsa S, Upadhyay M, Viswanathan P *et al.* Relationship of prostate-specific antigen to age and testosterone in men with type 2 diabetes mellitus. *Endocr Pract* 2008;**14**:1000–5.

30. Whitsel EA, Boyko EJ, Matsumoto AM and Anawalt BD. Intramuscular testosterone esters and plasma lipids in hypogonadal men: a meta-analysis. *Am J Med* 2001; **111**:261–9.

31. Khera M and Lipshultz LI. The role of testosterone replacement therapy following radical prostatectomy. *Urol Clin North Am* 2007;**34**:549–53.

32. Carroll P, Albertsen PC, Babaian RJ *et al. Prostate-Specific Antigen Best Practice Statement: 2009; Update*. American Urological Association, Linthicum, MD, 2009.

33. Wang C, Nieschlag E, Swerdloff R *et al.* ISA, ISSAM, EAU, EAAS and ASA recommendations: investigation, treatment and monitoring of late-onset hypodonadism in males. *Int J Impot Res* 2009;**21**:1–8.

34. Bhasin S, Cunningham GR, Hayes FJ *et al.* Testosterone therapy in adult men with androgen deficiency syndromes: an Endocrine Society Clinical Practice Guideline. *J Clin Endocrinol Metab* 2006;**91**:1995–2010.

CHAPTER 101

Diabetes mellitus

Alan J. Sinclair[1] and Graydon S. Meneilly[2]
[1]Institute of Diabetes for Older People (IDOP), Luton, UK
[2]University of British Columbia, Vancouver, BC, Canada

Introduction

Diabetes care systems for older people require an integrated multidimensional approach involving general practitioners, hospital specialists and other members of the healthcare team. There should be an emphasis on diabetes prevention and its complications, early treatment for vascular disease and functional assessment of disability due to limb problems, eye disease and stroke.

Inequalities of care are common in many healthcare systems due to variations in clinical practice, particularly in relation to older people. This may be manifest as a lack of access to services, inadequate specialist provision, poorer clinical outcomes and patient and family dissatisfaction. The recent development of clinical guidelines that are responsive to the needs of older people with diabetes may be an important step to minimize deficits in care from country to country, worldwide.

Type 2 diabetes mellitus is a common disabling chronic cardiovascular and medical disorder that has a tremendous health, social and economic burden and has a high prevalence of 10–30% in subjects above 65 years of age across Europe. About 60% of total healthcare expenditure on diabetes in this special group can be accounted for by acute-care hospitalizations and compared with non-diabetic counterparts, the relative risk for admission to hospital is 5.0. At any one time, about one in 12 district hospital beds is occupied by older people who have diabetes and their length of stay is double that of non-diabetic inpatients. The introduction of insulin to their regimen results in a quadrupling of expenditure, presumably because of the additional resources required in both hospital and community settings to monitor and support the use of insulin.

A direct approach to the metabolic management of type 2 diabetes in older subjects is to concentrate on strategies designed to limit and ameliorate both defective insulin secretion and insulin resistance. Type 2 diabetes represents a cluster of cardiovascular risk factors that pose a significant vascular threat and, in ageing subjects, the added effects of ageing and renal impairment increase the impact of this syndrome, and some of the features may be present up to 10 years before the onset of overt hyperglycaemia, thus increasing the cardiovascular risk before the onset of diabetes. Since up to 50% of the variability in insulin action in insulin-resistant states may be associated with lifestyle differences such as obesity, physical activity levels and cigarette smoking, it becomes obvious that environmental, preventative and health promotional strategies are of vital importance in limiting the impact of this epidemic.

Management of diabetes in older people can be relatively straightforward, especially when patients have no other comorbidities and when vascular complications are absent. In many cases, however, special issues arise that increase the complexity of management and lead to difficult clinical decision-making. It is therefore not surprising that the present state of diabetes care for older patients varies throughout Europe and North America. Although *geriatric diabetes* is developing as a subspeciality interest in the UK, there is little evidence of its presence in other national diabetes care systems and virtually no specific provision for those who are housebound or in institutional care. This chapter can be considered to be a learning programme that aims to provide a succinct but comprehensive review of diabetes care for older people, focusing on special areas of concern.

We have identified two principal aims: (1) to develop and enhance the knowledge and application of the principles of diabetes and diabetes care in older persons and (2) to provide clinicians with the knowledge and skills and to influence attitudes to maximize their effectiveness in applying this learning within their own clinical setting. In addition, we have suggested that clinicians who study this chapter in depth should be able to demonstrate (1) an in-depth understanding of diabetes in older people and to analyze their own organization's provision and care, with

Principles and Practice of Geriatric Medicine, Fifth Edition. Edited by Alan J. Sinclair, John E. Morley and Bruno Vellas.

a view to enhancing local care; and (2) an understanding of the means by which the diabetes care team in their own organization and key players in their own community can be engaged in improving the quality of diabetes care for older people. Further goals might include the ability to (3) reflect on their personal learning and apply that learning to the approaches they take with team members, other care professionals, patients and carers, and (4) analyse and evaluate outcomes in the delivery of care to older people who have diabetes, taking into account the roles of other care professionals and the beliefs of people from different ethnic and cultural backgrounds.

Epidemiology, pathogenesis and modes of presentation

The WHO estimates that in 2011 there are around 350 million individuals with diabetes worldwide, and that number is projected to increase to over 450 million by 2030. Several important risk factors (Table 101.1) are likely to underpin this increase in prevalence, such as advancing age of the population, greater numbers of people from ethnic minority backgrounds adopting a 'transitional' lifestyle, greater levels of overweight and obesity and more sedentary lifestyles. From an epidemiological perspective, ageing is an important factor: in the USA, the number of people with diabetes aged 75 years and over doubled between 1980 and 1987. In most populations, peak rates are generally found in the sixth decade and subsequently, although in Pima Indians the peak rate is between the fourth and fifth decades.

Most developed countries have a prevalence rate of about 17% in white elderly subjects and 25% in non-white subjects. The prevalence in white British elderly is only around 9% although the prevalence in non-white British elderly is about 25% and the prevalence in British care homes is 25%.

There is an increasing view that diabetes in the elderly has a genetic basis.[1] Older people with a family history are often more likely to develop this illness as they age. In genetically susceptible people, various factors may increase the likelihood of type 2 diabetes developing. Elderly patients with diabetes have normal hepatic production of glucose, which is in contrast to younger subjects.[2] In lean elderly subjects, the principal defect appears to be impaired glucose-induced insulin release, whereas in the obese elderly, resistance to insulin-mediated glucose disposal is the major problem.[2]

Table 101.1 Risk factors for diabetes mellitus in older subjects.

- Aged 65 years and over
- People of Asian, Afro-Caribbean or African origin
- BMI >27 kg m^{-2} and/or large waist circumference
- Those with manifest cardiovascular disease or hypertension with or without hyperlipidaemia
- Presentation with a stroke
- Presentation with recurrent infections
- Use of diabetogenic drugs, e.g. corticosteroids, estrogens
- A family history of diabetes mellitus
- Those with IGT/IFG

Multiple drugs, reduced physical activity and a diet with low intake of complex carbohydrates also contribute to this increasing prevalence. Further research into discovering the molecular abnormalities in older people with diabetes is warranted.

Modes of presentation

Diabetes in older people has a varied presentation and may be insidious, which ultimately delays diagnosis[3] (Table 101.2). Detection of diabetes during hospital admissions for other comorbidities or acute illnesses is relatively common, although even when hyperglycaemia has been recognized initially, about half of the subjects receive no further evaluation for diabetes or treatment.[4] Some patients do not have the classic features of either diabetic ketoacidosis or hyperosmolar non-ketotic coma but present with a 'mixed' disturbance of hyperglycaemia (blood glucose levels 15–25 mmol l^{-1}), arterial blood pH of 7.2–7.3 (not particularly acidotic) and without marked dehydration or change in level of consciousness.

Impact of diabetes mellitus

Older patients with diabetes appear to burden the hospital care system two to three times more than the general

Table 101.2 Varying presentation of diabetes in older people.

Asymptomatic (coincidental finding)	
Classical osmotic symptoms	
Metabolic disturbances	Diabetic ketoacidosis Hyperosmolar non-ketotic coma 'Mixed' metabolic disturbance
Spectrum of vague symptoms	Depressed mood Apathy Mental confusion
Development of 'geriatric' syndromes	Falls or poor mobility: muscle weakness, poor vision, cognitive impairment Urinary incontinence Unexplained weight loss Memory disorder or cognitive impairment
Slow recovery from specific illnesses or increased vulnerability	Impaired recovery from stroke Repeated infections Poor wound healing

population[5] and use primary care services two to three times more than non-diabetic controls.[6] This latter primary care study from Denmark indicated that insulin-treated patients accounted for more than half of the service provision, mainly due to chronic vascular disease, with a correspondingly high number of hospital clinic visits.

Several UK-based studies have defined the prevalence of elderly patients in hospital diabetic populations. This has ranged from 4.6% (Edinburgh[7]) to 8.4% (Cardiff[8]).

Several important population-based and community studies have revealed that diabetes in older subjects is associated with considerable morbidity, mainly due to the long-term complications of diabetes. These include the Oxford Study,[9] the Poole Study,[10] the Nottingham Community Study[11] and the Welsh Community Diabetes Study.[12] In the last study, in subjects aged 65 years and over, one in three subjects with diabetes had been hospitalized in the previous 12 months (compared with one in six non-diabetic controls). One in four diabetic subjects required assistance with personal care and older people with diabetes had significantly lower levels of health status compared with non-diabetic counterparts. Visual acuity was impaired in 40% of diabetic subjects (compared with 31% of controls) and diabetes was found to be associated with an increased risk of visual impairment {odds ratio (OR) = 1.50 [95% confidence interval (CI) 1.09–2.05]}. Factors that were significantly associated with visual loss in diabetic subjects included advanced age, female gender, history of foot ulceration, duration of diabetes and treatment with insulin.

Diabetic foot disease

A study in The Netherlands[13] identified increasing age and a higher level of amputation as important factors leading to increases in both the period of hospitalization and the associated costs. The 3 year survival following lower extremity amputation is about 50%[14] and in about 70% of cases, amputation is precipitated by foot ulceration.[15] The principal antecedents include peripheral vascular disease, sensorimotor and autonomic neuropathy, limited joint mobility (which impairs the ability of older people to inspect their feet) and high foot pressures.[16]

The majority of the elderly diabetic population is at increased risk of developing foot ulcers and various risk factors have been identified (Table 101.3). Peripheral sensorimotor neuropathy, which is the primary cause or contributory factor in the vast majority of cases, may cause common symptoms of numbness, lancinating and burning pain, 'pins and needles' and hyperesthesia, which is typically worse at night and evidence of high foot pressures leading to gait disturbances, falls and other foot injuries. The presence of visual loss may exacerbate the consequences of this situation.[17]

Table 101.3 Risk factors for foot ulceration in the elderly.

- Peripheral sensorimotor neuropathy
- Automatic neuropathy
- Peripheral vascular disease
- Limited joint mobility
- Foot pressure abnormalities, including deformity
- Previous foot problems
- Visual loss
- History of alcohol abuse

Erectile dysfunction

After the age of 60 years, erectile dysfunction (ED) may affect 55–95% of diabetic men, while the corresponding figure for non-diabetic counterparts is 50%.[18] ED is defined as the inability to attain and maintain an erection satisfactory for sexual intercourse and is a complex problem involving several mechanisms: vasculopathy, autonomic neuropathy, hormonal dysregulation, endothelia dysfunction and psychogenic factors have all been implicated. Drug-related causes may be a particular problem in older patients, with thiazide diuretics, cimetidine, β-blockers and spironolactone especially being implicated. An alcohol history must be looked for. ED is evaluated initially with an interview with the patient and sexual partner where appropriate. A comprehensive history, full medical examination, blood testing for diabetes control, lipids, testosterone and thyroid function tests are necessary. Other more sophisticated tests are available through diabetes ED clinics in most large centres and may involve testing for prolactin, other gonadotrophins and nocturnal penile tumescence. For many older patients, extensive testing is often avoided. Type 5 phosphodiesterase inhibitors appear to be effective for the treatment of erectile dysfunction in carefully selected older people with diabetes.[19,20]

Metabolic comas

Older subjects with diabetes may present with either diabetic ketoacidosis (DKA) and hyperglycaemic hyperosmolar non-ketotic (HONK) coma. HONK occurs predominantly in subjects aged over 50 years. Compared with the young, older subjects with hyperglycaemic comas have a higher mortality, have a greater length of stay in hospital following admission, are less likely to have had diabetes diagnosed previously, are more likely to have renal impairment and require a greater amount of insulin as treatment.[21]

The tendency for hyperosmolarity in HONK comas may be worsened in elderly people, who may not appreciate thirst well, may have difficulty drinking enough to compensate for their osmotic diuresis and may also be on diuretics. It also appears that hyperosmolarity not only worsens insulin resistance but may also inhibit lipolysis.

Death may be due to the metabolic disturbance and to acute illnesses such as pneumonia and myocardial infarction. The cause of the hyperglycaemia may be infection, infarction, inadequate hypoglycaemic treatment or inappropriate drug treatment. Residents of care homes are also at increased risk of HONK coma associated with appreciable mortality.[22] Thiazide diuretics and steroids are known to increase blood glucose levels and may precipitate DKA; thiazide diuretics and frusemide may be particularly likely to precipitate HONK coma.

Diabetes-related disability, cognitive dysfunction and depression

Diabetes is associated with both functional impairment and disability. The wide spectrum of vascular complications, acute metabolic decompensation, adverse effects of medication and the effects of the condition on nutrition and lifestyle behaviour may all create varying levels of impairment and/or disability. These changes may have adverse rebound effects on vulnerability to other comorbidities, independence and quality of life.

In the 1998 *Health and Retirement Survey* (>6300 subjects aged 51–61 years at baseline), diabetes was identified as an important predictor of failing to recover from a mobility difficulty over a 2-year follow-up period.[23] In a systematic literature review of longitudinal studies examining the relationships between various risk factors and functional status outcomes,[24] diabetes was one of five conditions (others were hypertension, stroke or TIA, arthritis), which reported 10 or more studies showing a significant association between the risk factor and subsequent functional decline.

In a study examining the relationship between various chronic disease states and disability, a survey from Madrid, Spain,[25] of 1001 subjects aged 65 years and over living at home showed that diabetes was one of four chronic diseases (the others were cerebrovascular disease, depression/anxiety disorders) that had a strong association with disability [OR = 2.18 (95% CI, 1.24–3.83)].

The Welsh Community Diabetes Study[12] revealed significant excesses in physical {Barthel activities of daily living (ADL), $p < 0.0001$; extended ADL, $p < 0.0001$; cognitive [Mini Mental State Examination (MMSE)], $p < 0.001$; clock test, $p < 0.001$}, mobility (use of walking aid, $p < 0.01$) and visual disabilities [Snellen visual acuity (VA) chart, $p < 0.01$] in diabetic subjects assessed by objective measures.

In a cross-sectional survey of community-dwelling older Mexican Americans aged 65 years and over ($n = 2873$), the presence of diabetes predicted poorer performance on tests of lower limb function.[26]

The Third National Health and Nutrition Examination Survey (NHANES III) revealed that diabetes was a major cause of physical disability among subjects aged 60 years and over.[27] Disability in at least one of the physical tasks examined was reported in 63% of diabetic women (controls, 42%) and 39% of diabetic men (controls, 25%), with stronger associations between diabetes and more severe forms of disability. Diabetes was shown to have a 2–3-fold increased likelihood of a mobility disorder, with coronary heart disease being a major contributor to this excess disability in both sexes and stroke being an important contributor among men.

Other studies that have examined this relationship include the *Women's Health and Ageing Study* (2002)[28] and the *Study of Osteoporotic Fractures* (2002).[29] In the latter study, in community-dwelling white women aged 65–99 (mean 71.7) years, diabetes was associated with a 42% increased risk of any incident disability and a 53–98% increased risk of disability for specific tasks, for example, walking two to three blocks on level ground or doing housework.

Diabetes in the elderly is associated with an increased risk of falls and fractures.[30,31] This increased risk can be explained by many of factors noted above, including peripheral neuropathy, reduced vision and impaired strength and mobility. Insulin therapy is associated with increased falls. This is probably due in part to more severe disease and/or hypoglycaemic episodes. With regard to the latter, a low A1C in insulin users was associated with an increased risk of falls.[30]

Cognitive dysfunction

A decline in cognitive function has been demonstrated in older subjects with type 2 diabetes.[32] This can be demonstrated using relatively straightforward tests such as the Folstein MMSE[33] or the clock test.[34]

The Zutphen Study (1995)[35] and the Kuopio Study (1998)[36] showed that impaired glucose tolerance (IGT) is linked to cognitive dysfunction and increased serum insulin may be associated with decreased cognitive function and dementia in women. The Rotterdam Study (1996) showed that type 2 diabetes may be associated with both Alzheimer's disease and vascular dementia,[37] and the Rochester Study (1997) demonstrated that the risk of dementia is significantly increased for both men and women with type 2 diabetes.[38] In a 7 year follow-up study (the Hisayama Study, 1995), type 2 diabetes was associated with an increased risk of developing vascular dementia.[39] Poor glucose control may be associated with cognitive impairment that recovers following improvement in glycaemic control.[40] A prospective cohort study involving 682 women with self-reported diabetes (mean age of population sample 72 years) followed up for 6 years indicated a twofold increased risk of cognitive impairment and a 74% increased risk of cognitive decline.[41] Women who had had diabetes for longer than 15 years had a threefold increase of having cognitive impairment at baseline and a doubling of the risk of decline.

Table 101.4 Benefits of early recognition of cognitive impairment in diabetes.

- Prompts the clinician to consider the presence of cerebrovascular disease and to review other vascular risk factors
- May be an early indicator of Alzheimer's disease and provides early access to medication
- Allows patients and families to benefit early with social and financial planning and access to information about support groups and counselling
- Creates opportunities to consider interventions for diabetes-related cognitive impairment: optimizing glucose control; controlling blood pressure and lipids

In the Framingham Study (1997), type 2 diabetes and hypertension were found to be significant but independent risk factors for poor cognitive performance (on tests of visual organization and memory) in a large prospective cohort sample followed for over 20 years.[42] This relationship between cognitive decline and with the presence of either diabetes and hypertension was also observed in the Atherosclerosis Risk in Communities (ARIC) Study (2002) in a 6 year follow-up of nearly 11 000 individuals aged 47–70 years at initial assessment.[43] Hyperinsulinaemia in hypertension has also been shown to be associated with poorer cognitive performance.[44]

Various benefits may accrue from the early recognition of cognitive impairment in older people with diabetes (Table 101.4). Depending on its severity, cognitive dysfunction in older diabetic subjects may have considerable implications, which include increased hospitalization, less ability for self-care, less likelihood of specialist follow-up and increased risk of institutionalization.[45]

Cognitive dysfunction may result in poorer adherence to treatment, worsen glycaemic control due to erratic taking of diet and medication and increase the risk of hypoglycaemia if the patient forgets that they have taken the hypoglycaemic medication and repeat the dose.

Type 2 diabetes mellitus and depression

Diabetes was found to be significantly associated with depression, independent of age, gender or presence of chronic disease in one study;[46] also, the presence of diabetes appears to double the odds of developing depression.[47] The finding of depression was the single most important indicator of subsequent death in a group of diabetic patients admitted into hospital.[48] Failure to recognize depression can be serious since it is a long-term, life-threatening, disabling illness and has a significant impact on quality of life.[49] Depression may be associated with worsening diabetic control[50] and decreased treatment compliance. In the *Baltimore Epidemiological Project* (1996), a 13-year follow-up of more than 3400 household residents (about one in seven was aged 65 years and over), major depressive disorder had an adjusted OR of 2.23 for predicting the onset of type 2 diabetes.[51]

Importance of functional evaluation

Functional evaluation of older people with diabetes mellitus using well-validated assessment tools is an essential step in the initial assessment process. Evaluation of functional status should be a multidisciplinary approach and comprise at least three main areas for measurement: physical, mental and social functioning. However, further evaluation with measures of self-care abilities and independent living skills (generally assessed by ADL tools) are also required. The benefits of functional assessment in the context of diabetes are indicated in Table 101.5.

Functional assessment is a primary component of comprehensive geriatric assessment (CGA), which is an essential methodology for geriatric medical practice.[52] CGA is crucial at the initial assessment and helpful in planning care and rehabilitation and monitoring progress. CGA can be performed in many clinical and healthcare locations and not only involves a basic assessment of functional status but also includes various limited screening techniques, evaluation of social and medical problems, instigating initial treatment and ensuring follow-up. CGA and its variants (including in-home assessment packages) have been demonstrated to reduce mortality (by 14% at 12 months), increase the chance of remaining at home after referral (26% at 12 months), reduce hospital admissions (12% at 12 months), with gains in cognition and physical function having also been observed.[53] Not all patients gain from this approach and targeting is required. Criteria for older subjects with type 2 diabetes who may derive benefit from comprehensive assessment methods with a measure of functional status are given in Table 101.6. A summary of the various assessment methods in common use is given elsewhere in this book. The authors do not advocate that all practitioners in Europe should adopt CGA as a routine part of their assessment processes, but suggest that functional assessment become a routine measure in older

Table 101.5 Benefits of functional assessment: diabetes-related.

- Measures ability to comply with treatment goals and adherence to nutritional advice
- Assesses self-care ability and ability to apply sick-day rules
- Assesses the impact of vascular complications of diabetes, e.g. peripheral vascular disease or neuropathy
- Assesses likely ability to gain from educational interventions
- Assesses need for carer support
- Identifies any quality-of-life issues related to the disease or its treatment

Table 101.6 Criteria for targeting patients with type 2 diabetes for comprehensive geriatric assessment.

- Presence of a 'geriatric syndrome': confusional state, depression, falls, incontinence, immobility, pressure sores
- Those with several coexisting morbidities apart from diabetes with complex drug regimens
- Those with disabilities due to lower limb vascular disease or neuropathy requiring a rehabilitation programme
- Absence of a terminal illness or dementing syndrome

people with type 2 diabetes at diagnosis and at regular intervals thereafter.

Treatment and care issues: learning from the literature

The major aims in the management of older people with type 2 diabetes involve both medical and patient-oriented factors (Table 101.7). An initial plan for the early evaluation of patients is reflected in Table 101.8, which should form a framework for instigating the appropriate treatment pathway. An important aim of risk assessment in the general population is to identify subclinical cardiovascular risk, which may be the principal cause of undetected functional impairment or frailty in older people. Coronary risk charts are often based on Framingham data[54,55] and can be used to identify either 5 or 10 year event rates, but it is important to note that cardiovascular risk data are generally based on populations of individuals up to a maximum age of 74 years only. In a large proportion of older people with type 2 diabetes, excess cardiovascular risk is evident and active intervention should be considered.

A summary of the therapeutic areas for intervention and the relevant evidence base is provided in Table 101.9 and

Table 101.7 Major aims in managing older people with diabetes.

Medical	Patient-oriented
Freedom from hyperglycaemic symptoms	Maintain general wellbeing and good quality of life
Prevent undesirable weight loss	Acquire skills and knowledge to adapt to lifestyle changes
Avoid hypoglycaemia and other adverse drug reactions	Encourage diabetes self-care
Estimate cardiovascular risk as part of screening for and preventing vascular complications	
Detect cognitive impairment and depression at an early stage	
Achieve a normal life expectancy for patients where possible	

Table 101.8 Care plan for initial management of diabetes in an elderly person.

- Establish realistic glycaemic and blood pressure targets
- Ensure consensus with patient, spouse or family, general practitioner, informal carer, community nurse or hospital specialist
- Define the frequency and nature of diabetes follow-up
- Organize glycaemic monitoring by patient or carer
- Refer to social or community services as necessary
- Provide advice on stopping smoking, increasing exercise and decreasing alcohol intake

the main types of insulin regimes employed are indicated in Table 101.10. In the UK, the licence for pioglitazone has recently been modified to allow 'triple' therapy (pioglitazone and both a sulfonylurea and metformin to be coprescribed).

Glucose regulation

The management of blood glucose must form part of a multifaceted approach to dealing with the metabolic disorder of type 2 diabetes in older people since most patients have evidence of other cardiovascular risk factors and at least half are likely to satisfy the criteria for the metabolic syndrome proposed by a WHO Expert Committee in 1998[56] and more recently by the International Diabetes Federation.[57]

Although there is now overwhelming evidence that the level and duration of glycaemia influence the development of diabetes-related complications, specific studies in older subjects (>70 years) with type 2 diabetes are lacking.

The majority of the studies conducted in older populations have involved patients of Caucasian ancestry affected by type 2 diabetes. The applicability of these results to the elderly type 1 diabetic patient or to the non-Caucasian type 2 diabetic patient remains to be assessed. However, no randomized controlled trials assessing the impact of achieving optimal glucose control on primary prevention of cardiovascular outcomes in the elderly diabetic patient are available.

Recommendations

The following represent some of the more important recommendations on glucose regulation taken from the European Guidelines (Executive Summary, European Diabetes Working Party for Older People, 2011):[58]

1 At initial assessment, all patients with type 2 diabetes aged less than 85 years should have a cardiovascular-risk assessment. Evidence level 1+; Grade of recommendation A.

2 For older patients with type 2 diabetes, with single system involvement (free of other major comorbidities), a target HbA1c (DCCT aligned) range of 7.0–7.5% and a fasting glucose range of 6.5–7.5 mmol l^{-1} should be aimed for. Evidence level 2++; Grade of recommendation B.

Table 101.9 Treatment targets and intervention studies for elderly diabetic patients.

Blood glucose level	Blood pressure	Blood lipid level	Aspirin use
No specific studies in older people with diabetes	A 10 mmHg (systolic) and 5 mmHg (diastolic) fall in blood pressure in the intensive group resulted in a 24% decrease in risk of any diabetes-related endpoint, 44% reduction in risk of stroke and 37% risk reduction in macrovascular disease	Few studies in older people with diabetes	Antiplatelet Trialists Collaboration: 75–325 mg per day reduced major cardiovascular events in high-risk patients by 25%; NNT 26 (17–66)
UKPDS: HbA1c <7%; fasting blood glucose <7 mmol l^{-1}	HOT Study: diastolic lowering to ≤83 mmHg	PROSPER: pravastatin for 3.2 years resulted in a 1.0 mmol l^{-1} fall in LDL cholesterol and a modest relative risk (RR) of 15% for the primary composite outcome; no change in the decline of cognition was seen	HOT Study: 75 mg per day reduced major cardiovascular events by 15% and myocardial infarction by 36%; stroke was unaffected
A reduction in HbA1c of 0.9% between the study groups resulted in a 12% reduction in risk of any diabetes-related endpoint, but no significant reduction in major cardiovascular events	A systolic BP<80 mmHg resulted in a 51% reduction in major cardiovascular events compared with the target group of ≤90 mmHg		
	SHEP Study: systolic BP <150 mmHg A 34% reduction in risk of cardiovascular disease in the actively treated group was observed	Heart Protection Study: treatment with simvastatin for 5 years resulted in a fall of 1.0 mmol l^{-1} of HDL cholesterol and a 25% RR in incidence of first nonfatal or fatal stroke	
	A fall of 23/7 mmHg in the actively treated group was associated with a 55% decrease in mortality and a 69% reduction in cardiovascular endpoints	LIPID, CARE, 4S, VA-HIT Studies: total cholesterol <5 mmol l^{-1}, HDL cholesterol >1.0 mmol l^{-1} Triglycerides <2.0 mmol l^{-1}	
	MICRO-HOPE was not target driven but showed highly significant reductions in cardiovascular risk with ramipril for 4.5 years (22% RR in myocardial infarction; 33% RR in stroke). LIFE study: 24% RR in primary composite endpoint of cardiovascular mortality, stroke and all myocardial infarction after minimum 4 years of losartan treatment compared with atenolol. ALLHAT showed that after a mean of 4.9 years of follow-up, there were no significant differences in outcome between chlorthalidone, lisinopril or amlodipine	ALLHAT-LLT: 4.9 years of pravastatin showed modest reductions in cholesterol only and did not reduce mortality or coronary heart disease	
		ASCOT-LLA: study stopped after 3.3 years showing highly significant benefits of atorvastatin; a fall of 1.0 mmol l^{-1} of HDL cholesterol gave a 36% RR of primary end point but subgroup analysis of diabetic patients showed no benefit	

Table 101.10 Practice-orientated guidelines for insulin treatment in older people.

Treatment	Indications	Advantages	Disadvantages
Once-daily insulin	Frail subjects Very old (>80 years) Symptomatic control	Single injection Can be given by carer or district nurse	Control usually poor Hypoglycaemia common
Twice-daily insulin	Preferred if good glycaemic control Suitable for type 1 diabetes	Low risk of hypoglycaemia Easily managed by most older diabetic people	Normoglycaemia difficult to achieve Fixed meal times reduce flexibility Expensive
Basal/bolus insulin	Well-motivated individuals Can reduce microvascular complications	Allows tight control For acute illness in hospital Flexible meal times	Frequent monitoring required to avoid hypoglycaemia
Insulin plus oral agents	If glycaemic control is unsatisfactory with oral agents alone To limit weight gain in obese subjects	Limits weight gain by reducing total daily insulin Increased flexibility	May delay conversion to insulin in thin or type 1 patients

3 For frail (dependent; multisystem disease; care home residency including those with dementia) patients where the hypoglycaemia risk is high and symptom control and avoidance of metabolic decompensation are paramount, the target HbA1c range should be 7.6–8.5% and the fasting glucose range 7.0–9.0 mmol l^{-1}. Level of evidence 1+; Grade of recommendation A.

4 Glibenclamide should be avoided for newly diagnosed cases of type 2 diabetes in older adults (aged >70 years) because of the marked risk of hypoglycaemia. Level of evidence 1+; Grade of recommendation A.

5 In older adults with diabetes, the use of premixed insulin and prefilled insulin pens may lead to a reduction in dosage errors and an improvement in glycaemic control. Level of evidence 2++; Grade of recommendation B. *More recent data suggest that the clock test may be used to predict which elderly patients are likely to have trouble with insulin therapy.*[59] *Newer insulins such as glargine and insulin detemir may be associated with a lower frequency of hypoglycaemia than conventional insulin therapy in the elderly*[60,61] *and should be considered when problems arise with conventional insulin therapy.*

6 Where the risk of hypoglycaemia is considered moderate (renal impairment, recent hospital admission) to high (previous history, frail patient with multiple comorbidities, resident of a care home) and a sulfonylurea is considered, use an agent with a lower hypoglycaemic potential, for example, a DDP4 inhibitor, lower risk sulfonylurea. *Risk of hypoglycaemia: glibenclamide > glimepiride > gliclazide > tolbutamide.*[62] *Meglitinides are associated with a lower frequency of hypoglycaemia in the elderly than glyburide and may be preferred in subjects with irregular eating habits.*[63,64]

The thiazolidenediones pioglitazone and rosiglitazone are effective agents in the elderly, but the adverse cardiovascular effects reported with rosiglitazone use have led to its recent withdrawal in the European Union. Unfortunately, the incidence of fluid retention is greater in elderly patients treated with these drugs and concerns have been raised about an increased risk of fractures in elderly women and, potentially, an increased risk of cardiac events with rosiglitazone.[65–67]

It has been recognized for several years that the insulin response to oral glucose is greater than that to intravenous glucose, a phenomenon known as the incretin effect. The hormones responsible for this effect are GIP and GLP-1. Although patients with diabetes do not respond to GIP, the ability of GLP-1 to stimulate insulin secretion is preserved. Recently, drugs that act on the incretin pathway have attracted increasing interest because they do not cause weight gain and may even stimulate weight loss, rarely cause hypoglycaemia and suppress the high glucagon levels that are often seen in patients with diabetes. We have shown that GLP-1 is a very effective agent in elderly patients, but it is impractical for long-term use because it must be given by continuous infusion. The long-acting analogues of GLP-1, liraglutide and exenatide, have not yet been studied in the elderly. GLP-1 is broken down rapidly in the circulation by the enzyme DPPIV and inhibitors of this enzyme have recently been released for clinical use. Recent studies in the elderly have shown that these drugs can be very effective in this age group[68,69] and appear to safe. However, early reports have suggested that incretin analogues may be associated with an increased risk of pancreatitis. In addition, because DPPIV is a ubiquitous enzyme, especially in the immune system, concern has been raised about potential impacts on the risk of infection and cancer. For this reason, these drugs should be used with caution until more post-marketing surveillance has been conducted.

7 Optimal glucose regulation may help maintain cognitive performance, improve learning and memory and may help to minimize symptoms of mood disorder in

patients with depression. Level of evidence 1+; Grade of recommendation A.

Glucose targets

Four recent studies have had a major impact on our thinking about the benefits of tight glycaemic control. The ACCORD, ADVANCE and VADT studies[70–72] all evaluated the impact of tight glycaemic control on patients with a mean age in the 60s, many of whom were over 70 years of age. All patients had a diabetes duration of at least 5 years and at least one-third had evidence of complications at the outset of the study. The studies found no impact of tight glycaemic control on the risk of macrovascular events, but a potential impact on microvascular events. In the ACCORD study, the risk of death appeared to be increased in the group randomized to tight glycaemic control. The follow-up study of the UKPDS,[73] however, found that after 10 years, the benefits of glycaemic control on microvascular events persisted and a positive impact on macrovascular events and overall mortality became apparent. It is worth noting that patients in this study had new-onset diabetes, were substantially younger and were free from complications at the study onset. The results of these studies have been hotly debated. The consensus of opinion is that if a patient has new-onset diabetes and is free from complications, every effort should be made to control blood sugar rigorously. For patients with a longer duration of diabetes who have complications, glycaemic targets should be more modest and more emphasis should be placed on control of blood pressure and lipids.

Inpatient diabetes care

Early studies of critically ill patients suggested that tight control of blood sugar reduced mortality and improved other important outcomes.[74,75] However, more recent information suggests that tight control may do more harm than good[76,77] and experts are recommending that a glucose level of 7–10 mmol l^{-1} is an appropriate target in an intensive care setting. To date, there have been no studies evaluating the benefits or risks of tight glycaemic control for elderly inpatients outside the intensive care setting. Based on the concerns raised above, it would seem prudent to target preprandial sugars in the range 7–10 mmol l^{-1} in these patients pending the outcome of further studies.

Blood pressure regulation

Adverse cardiovascular outcomes (stroke and coronary heart disease) are clearly and directly related to increasing levels of blood pressure. In non-diabetic individuals, this is more pronounced in men than in women; antihypertensive treatment has been shown to produce worthwhile reductions in risk, especially in high-risk patients such as those with diabetes or the elderly, where the absolute benefit is greater.

Increasing age is also an independent risk factor for cardiovascular disease even in low-risk individuals with normal blood pressure.

There is an age-related increase in systolic blood pressure but diastolic blood pressure tends to peak at 66–69 years of age and then falls. A large percentage of older patients will have isolated systolic hypertension where the diastolic blood pressure is not raised. Hypertension is also associated with the insulin resistance syndrome in older subjects and in diabetic subjects who develop microalbuminuria, thus increasing the risk of nephropathy and end-stage renal failure.

Diagnosis of hypertension in diabetes

Established hypertension exists when blood pressure readings are persistently above 140/90 mmHg (Korotkov IV) over at least 1 month or when the diastolic blood pressure exceeds 110 mmHg or when there is evidence of target organ damage. As the presence of diabetes imposes a greater cardiovascular risk, it is reasonable to have lower blood pressure thresholds for treatment in these subjects, but most guidelines indicate 140/90 mmHg as the treatment threshold with lower target values for those with diabetes. Four national/international sets of guidelines for hypertension have been published and these can be downloaded from the relevant website or author address, for example, http://www.nhlbi.nih.gov/guidelines/hypertension/express.pdf. Each major guideline has a section on the management of hypertension in diabetes, but age modification of targets and thresholds is not detailed. In addition, there have been no specific randomized controlled trials in older subjects with type 2 diabetes and hypertension that have directly investigated the benefits and outcomes of treating blood pressure to target.

On the basis of an analysis of these sets of guidelines and the relevant clinical evidence base, the European Diabetes Working Party for Older People has developed an updated Executive Summary[58] of their 2004 guideline[78] and have set targets described in the clinical recommendations below.

Recommendations

1 The threshold for treatment of high blood pressure in older subjects with type 2 diabetes should be 140/80 mmHg or higher present for more than 3 months and measured on at least three separate occasions during a period of lifestyle management advice (behavioural: exercise, weight reduction, smoking advice, nutrition/dietary advice). Level of evidence 2++; Grade of recommendation B. *This decision is based on the likelihood of reducing cardiovascular risk in older subjects balanced with issues relating to tolerability, clinical* *factors and disease severity and targets likely to be achievable with monotherapy and/or combination therapy and with agreement with primary care colleagues. As most subjects aged 70 years and over with type 2 diabetes and hypertension will already by definition have a high CV risk, no additional weighting for extent of CV risk has been applied. A lower value of blood pressure should be aimed for in those who are able to tolerate the therapy and self-manage, and/or those with concomitant renal disease.*

2 For frail (dependent; multisystem disease; care home residency including those with dementia) patients, where avoidance of heart failure and stroke may be of greater relative importance than microvascular disease, an acceptable blood pressure is <150/<90 mmHg. Evidence level 2+; Grade of recommendation C – extrapolated data.

3 Optimal blood pressure regulation should be aimed for to help maintain cognitive performance and improve learning and memory – *Good Clinical Practice point.*

Guidelines on specific treatment strategy and medication

4 In older patients with a sustained blood pressure (≥140/80 mmHg) and in whom diabetic renal disease is absent, first-line therapies can include use of ACE inhibitors, angiotensin II receptor antagonists, long-acting calcium channel blockers or thiazide diuretics. Level of evidence 1+; Grade of recommendation A. *In terms of comparable efficacy, safety and cost-effectiveness, treatment with a thiazide diuretic may be preferred as the first-line therapy. Short-acting calcium channel blockers should not be used. β-Blockers are useful for patients with previous myocardial infarction, but are not particularly effective for the treatment of hypertension in the elderly patient with diabetes.*

The choice of antihypertensive agent should take into account metabolic factors, the presence or not of renal impairment or cardiovascular disease and the likelihood of causing postural hypotension, which may have particularly adverse consequences in older subjects. At the present time, α-adrenoreceptor blockers have no special indications in the treatment of hypertension in diabetes and may be harmful. The use of low-dose fixed combinations of two agents such as a thiazide diuretic plus an ACE inhibitor may also have additional advantages.

5 In older patients with a sustained blood pressure (≥140/80 mmHg) with microalbuminuria or proteinuria, treatment with an ACE inhibitor is recommended. Level of evidence 1+; Grade of recommendation B. *An angiotensin II receptor antagonist may be considered as an alternative to an ACE inhibitor where the latter class of drug is not tolerated or is contraindicated.*

Lipid regulation

Coronary heart disease (CHD) is the most common cause of mortality in type 2 diabetes and remains the principal challenge for older people with this metabolic disorder. Elevated levels of blood lipids are an independent risk factor for CHD and there is published evidence of cardiovascular benefit in using a lipid-lowering regimen, although this is limited in older subjects. As part of a multifaceted approach to the metabolic consequences of diabetes, effective management of blood lipids is essential to optimize vascular outcomes. Attention to risk factors such as smoking and other metabolic derangements such as blood pressure is also of paramount importance.

Cardiovascular risk assessment

Categories of risk based on lipoprotein levels in adults with diabetes mellitus according to most international recommendations are given without modification concerning age and duration of diabetes. Since general cardiovascular risk is increasing with both variables, especially age, cardiovascular risk in older diabetic patients is generally underestimated according to non-age-specific risk assessment. One approach is to calculate global risk in individuals without overt cardiovascular disease (primary prevention) using the Framingham Heart Study equation or the WHOISH risk table.[79,80] Another method relies on the calculation of individual risk on the basis of epidemiological data. For the purposes of this chapter, 'high' and 'low' cardiovascular risks are as described in Table 101.11.

Several large-scale clinical trials have shown benefit with statin therapy of high-risk (cardiovascular risk) individuals and these included a proportion of older subjects. They have also demonstrated that these agents are well tolerated and safe, with no consistent additional risk of cancer or non-vascular morbidity or mortality. Previous statin trials indicate that the absolute reduction in LDL cholesterol produces similar proportional risk reductions in older and younger people.

Table 101.11 High and low 10 year cardiovascular risk definitions.

High risk
Has manifest cardiovascular disease (history of symptoms of coronary heart disease, stroke or peripheral vascular disease) or a coronary (Risk Assessment Chart)[a] event risk of >15%;
Low risk
Does not manifest cardiovascular disease and whose coronary event risk[a] is ≤15%

[a]On the basis of joint British recommendations: British Cardiac Society, British Hyperlipidaemia Association, British Hypertension Society and British Diabetic Association. Joint British recommendations on prevention of coronary heart disease in clinical practice: summary. *BMJ* 2000;**320**:705–8. Adapted from NICE (UK).

Target values for total cholesterol and LDL cholesterol

Target values for treatment decisions based on total/LDL cholesterol level in adults with diabetes should be adopted without age limitation, especially in otherwise healthy and independent individuals ('single disease model'). Categories of risk are available depending on lipid levels (*American Diabetes Association criteria*), although treatment decisions based on an estimation of a 10 year cardiovascular risk may also be used (*National Institute for Health and Clinical Excellence* (*NICE*) guidelines]. Additional measurement of HDL cholesterol provides a more accurate assessment of cardiovascular risk because of the inverse relationship between cardiovascular risk and HDL cholesterol. These recommendations may not be directly applicable for old (>75 years of age) and very old (>85 years of age) patients because of the presence of multiple comorbidities, high dependency levels, care home residency and/or end-stage dementia ('frailty model').[81] In these situations, limited life expectancy or competing non-cardiovascular causes of mortality (e.g. cancer or infections), may mask or remove any benefit from lipid lowering and increase the likelihood of adverse drug reactions. Lipid regulation on an individual basis is required.

Initial assessment of the older patient

Initial assessment should include enquiry about alcohol consumption and presence or not of renal, thyroid or liver disease. An estimate of the level of physical activity is important and overweight (and obese) subjects should be encouraged to lose weight and be given exercise advice relative to their capability and overall functional status. Dietary modification may be of benefit as part of a revised lifestyle plan.

Assessments of total, HDL and LDL cholesterol and triglycerides are usually required as part of the annual review process (Grade of recommendation C) and should preferably be fasting samples at the start of treatment for those with abnormal profiles.

For these *Guidelines*, an abnormal lipid profile in older subjects can be regarded as total cholesterol $\geq$5.0 mmol l^{-1}, LDL cholesterol $\geq$3.0 mmol l^{-1} or triglycerides $\geq$2.3 mmol l^{-1}.

In general, pharmacological therapy of abnormal lipid levels should not be delayed or ignored because of the age of the individual and should be regarded as part of the routine interventions in managing older people with diabetes. In patients prescribed a statin, the clinician must always be alert to the potential side effects of treatment, including reversible myositis and myopathy.

Recommendations

Some of the principal recommendations related to the use of statins and fibrates in older people with diabetes can be summarized as follows:

1 Statin therapy is well tolerated and can be safely used in older subjects with diabetes.
2 Primary prevention: in subjects with no history of cardiovascular disease, a statin should be offered to patients with an abnormal lipid profile if their 10-year cardiovascular risk is >15%. *There is little evidence at present for primary preventative strategies for subjects aged >80 years.*
3 Secondary prevention: a statin should be offered to patients with an abnormal lipid profile who have proven cardiovascular disease.
4 A fibrate should be considered in patients with an abnormal lipid profile who have been treated with a statin for at least 6 months but in whom the triglyceride level remains elevated ($\geq$2.3 mmol l^{-1}).
5 A fibrate should be considered in patients with proven cardiovascular disease who have isolated high triglyceride levels ($\geq$2.3 mmol l^{-1}).
6 For patients with cardiovascular disease who have persistent raised fasting triglycerides >10 mmol l^{-1}, referral to a specialist lipid or diabetes clinic is recommended.

Care home diabetes

Within the European Union, the structure and provision of diabetes care within residential care homes are highly variable. High-quality diabetes care is unlikely to be present in the majority of care homes with many underlying reasons accounting for this rather dismal situation. These include organizational difficulties within the institutions, lack of clarity relating to medical and nursing roles and responsibilities, funding issues and a lack of a coherent professional framework for delivering diabetes care.

Several deficiencies of diabetes care within institutional settings have been identified (see Table 101.12). They represent a series of concerns that highlight the need for standards of diabetes care to be established.

A UK study highlighted problems in diabetes care delivery.[82] This study involved a medical examination of and semistructured interview with residents with

Table 101.12 Concerns and deficiencies in diabetes care – institutional facilities.

- Increasing number of institutionalized diabetic elderly
- Lack of specialist medical follow-up
- Inadequate dietary care and lack of structured health professional input
- Lack of individualized diabetes care plans
- Lack of educational and training programmes for care home staff
- No major intervention studies assessing the benefits of metabolic control and/or educational strategies
- Few national standards of diabetes care

diabetes in long-term care facilities in South Wales, which revealed a prevalence of known diabetes of 7.2%. One-third of residents with diabetes tested had a HbA1c >11.0%, 40% of those on oral hypoglycaemic agents were taking the long-acting sulfonylureas chlorpropamide or glibenclamide and none of the homes had a policy in place for recording hypoglycaemic events. Only eight out of 109 diabetic residents had a specialist follow-up arranged. Other health professional input was minimal.

More recently, a retrospective, cross-sectional study using the SAGE (Systematic Assessment of Geriatric Drug Use via Epidemiology) database reported that 47% of residents with diabetes were receiving no antidiabetic medication and that the presence of advanced age, being black, having a low ADL score, cognitive impairment and a low body mass index (BMI) (<21) increased the likelihood of not receiving antidiabetic medication.[83]

These and other studies indicate that diabetic residents of care homes appear to be a highly vulnerable and neglected group, characterized by a high prevalence of macrovascular complications, marked susceptibility to infections (especially skin and urinary tract), increased hospitalization rates and high levels of physical and cognitive disability. Communication difficulties (because of dementia and/or stroke) lead to unmet care needs and lack of self-care abilities and water and electrolyte disturbances increase the risk of metabolic decompensation. Many elderly residents in these institutions are treated with neuroleptic agents, which can have a major impact on patients with impaired glucose tolerance and diabetes,[84] and it is important to consider this fact when evaluating these patients.

Prevalence of diabetes mellitus in care homes

A number of prevalence surveys of diabetes within care homes provide estimates of between 7.2 and 26.7%, depending on the method used for identifying those with diabetes.

Additional information from the population-based SAGE database in the USA,[83] which involves five States and evaluation of all residents using the 350-item minimum data set (MDS), revealed a prevalence of diabetes of 18.1%, which decreased as age increased (e.g. 27% in those aged 65–74 years compared with 13% in those aged 85 years and over). The highest prevalence was recorded in Hispanics (28%) and black non-Hispanics (26%).

In a study screening care home residents for diabetes using two-point (fasting and 2 h postglucose challenge values) oral glucose tolerance tests, the overall prevalence rate (newly diagnosed + known diabetes) was calculated as 26.7%, with a rate of 30.2% for impaired glucose tolerance.[85] The majority of diagnoses were made according to the 2 h values rather than the fasting glucose levels, but it may be argued that these residents are at greater cardiovascular risk and may benefit from an intervention.

Intervention studies in care homes

Few intervention studies of diabetic residents of care homes have been reported. In Denver, CO, an educationally based intervention study in 29 nursing homes consisted of providing workshops and follow-up consultations to administrative staff designed to assist in developing and implementing diabetes care policies and procedures.[86] By 1 year, a significant increase in the adherence to previously published diabetes care plans was observed and although hospital admission rates had not changed, total bed days were smaller. Affiliation to a university-based academic faculty may also lead to an improvement in outcomes for nursing home residents with diabetes. In a study in California, significantly better glycaemic control was observed in a small group ($n = 47$) of nursing home diabetic residents (mean age 81 years; HbA1 8.9% on oral agents) compared with a group of ambulatory diabetic residents (mean age 66 years; 11.8% on oral agents), with only a small number of associated hypoglycaemic events.[87]

A small study (18 subjects) in Stanford, CA,[88] demonstrated that residents of care homes who are in good health and in good glycaemic control (mean fasting glucose of 7 mmol l^{-1}), that the introduction of a 'regular diet' compared with the standard 'diabetes diet' had minimal effects on glucose control, lipid levels and body weight over a 16 week period. In a small study of Italian nursing home residents with diabetes ($n = 30$; mean age 77 years), the substitution with insulin lispro treatment for 4 months as part of a series of treatment periods using regular insulin led to a significant decrease in mean daily blood glucose, HbA1c [7.6 versus 8.5% (regular), $p < 0.01$] and hypoglycaemic episodes.[89]

More recently, in an academic nursing home facility, a 5 month educational programme on dyslipidaemia treatment aimed at physicians and nurse practitioners led to an improvement in the frequency of prescribing lipid-lowering therapy.[90] This New York-based study demonstrated an increase from 26 to 67% for diabetic residents.

Rationale for early detection of diabetes mellitus in care homes

In view of the absence of clinical trial data, the rationale for early detection of diabetes mellitus has not been justified. However, each resident has a right to active investigation and intervention (where appropriate) and it is feasible that several benefits may accrue from such a policy (Table 101.13).

Aims of care for diabetic residents

Residents with diabetes in care homes should receive a level of comprehensive diabetes care commensurate with their health and social needs. The two most important

Table 101.13 Importance of early detection of diabetes mellitus in care homes.

- Improved metabolic control may improve cognition, decrease the risk of hyperosmolar coma and lessen osmotic symptoms
- Earlier treatment may delay vascular complications and reduce disability
- Knowledge of diagnosis of diabetes prompts the physician to be alert to diabetes-related complications, e.g. hyperosmolar coma
- Earlier dietary intervention may delay treatment (and therefore limit adverse drug reactions) with oral agents
- Treatment can reduce symptoms and may increase quality of life and functional wellbeing

aims of care according to the European Guidelines[78] (European Diabetes Working Party for Older People, 2001–2004) are as follows:

1 To maintain the highest degree of quality of life and wellbeing without subjecting residents to unnecessary and inappropriate medical and therapeutic interventions.

2 To provide support and opportunity to enable residents to manage their own diabetes condition where this is a feasible and worthwhile option.

Other crucial objectives of care include: (3) achieving a satisfactory (but optimal) level of metabolic control that reduces both hyperglycaemic lethargy and hypoglycaemia and allows the greatest level of physical and cognitive function; (4) optimizing foot care and visual health that promotes an increased level of mobility, reduced risk of falls and prevents unnecessary hospital admissions; (5) to provide a well-balanced nutritional and dietetic plan that prevents weight loss and maintains nutritional wellbeing; and (6) to screen effectively for diabetic complications regularly, especially eye disease, peripheral neuropathy and peripheral vascular disease that predispose to foot infection and ulceration.

Diabetes care home provision – modern approaches

Several important strategies to improve the quality and outcomes of diabetes care within these settings have been proposed[91] and more recently Diabetes UK has launched national guidance in this area. A series of recommendations have previously been proposed by the European Diabetes Working Party on Older People, as follows.

Recommendations

1 At the time of admission to a care home, each resident requires to be screened for the presence of diabetes.

2 Each resident with diabetes should have an individualized diabetes care plan with the following minimum details: dietary plan, medication list, glycaemic targets, weight and nursing plan.

3 Each resident with diabetes should have an annual review where the medical component is undertaken either by a general practitioner, geriatrician or hospital diabetes specialist.

4 If required, each resident with diabetes should have reasonable access to the following specialist services: podiatry, optometric services, hospital diabetes foot clinic, dietetic services and diabetes specialist nurse.

5 Each care home with diabetes residents should have an agreed Diabetes Care Policy or Protocol that is regularly audited.

Prevention

Impaired glucose tolerance occurs in ~25% of elderly patients and is a precursor for diabetes. The Diabetes Prevention Program showed that although metformin was not effective in the elderly, lifestyle interventions were beneficial in reducing the incidence of diabetes.[92] The Study To Prevent Non-Insulin-Dependent Diabetes Mellitus (STOP-NIDDM)[93] showed than α-glucosidase inhibitors reduced the incidence of diabetes and macrovascular events in elderly patients with impaired glucose tolerance. The DREAM study[94] demonstrated that rosiglitazone is also very effective in the prevention of diabetes in elderly subjects, but this agent has now been withdrawn from the European Union.

Conclusion

Diabetes mellitus in older subjects represents an often complex interplay between ageing, functional loss, vascular disease and the metabolic syndrome. Type 2 diabetes may be a potent cause of both premature and unsuccessful ageing. Functional assessment and estimation of disability levels form part of the important screening process in older adults with diabetes. There is increasing evidence that improving metabolic control will have important benefits even in older subjects. The recently published European Guidelines on managing older people with type 2 diabetes represents an important step forward in the provision of clinical guidance of this often neglected but highly prevalent group. We should encourage more research by randomized controlled design studies that examine the benefits of metabolic intervention and explore the value and cost-effectiveness of different diabetes care models for managing the frail elderly diabetic subject.

Key points

- Diabetes mellitus has a high prevalence in ageing populations and is associated with specific metabolic alterations.

- Cardiovascular disease is a major cause of morbidity and premature disability in older subjects with type 2 diabetes.
- Functional impairment remains a major challenge for clinicians managing older people with diabetes and a working knowledge of assessment methodology is helpful in planning therapies.
- Cognitive dysfunction, depressive illness and falls are important complications and strategies to prevent them require being included in the overall management plan.
- Further research (both basic science and clinical) into the pathogenesis and treatment of type 2 diabetes in senior citizens is urgently required.

References

1. Meneilly GS. Pathophysiology of diabetes in the elderly. In: AJ Sinclair and P Finucane (eds), *Diabetes in Old Age*, 2nd edn, John Wiley & Sons, Ltd, Chichester, 2001, pp. 17–23.
2. Meneilly GS and Ellitt T. Metabolic alterations in middle-aged and elderly obese patients with type 2 diabetes. *Diabetes Care* 1999;**22**:112–8.
3. Sinclair AJ. Issues in the initial management of type 2 diabetes. In: AJ Sinclair and P Finucane (eds), *Diabetes in Old Age*, 2nd edn, John Wiley & Sons, Ltd, Chichester, 2001, pp. 155–64.
4. Levetan CS, Passaro M, Jablonski K *et al*. Unrecognised diabetes among hospital patients. *Diabetes Care* 1998;**21**:246–9.
5. Damsgaard EM, Froland A and Green A. Use of hospital services by elderly diabetics: the Frederica Study of diabetic and fasting hyperglycaemic patients aged 60–74 years. *Diabet Med* 1987;**4**:317–22.
6. Damsgaard EM, Froland A and Holm A. Ambulatory medical care for elderly diabetics: the Fredericia survey of diabetic and fasting hyperglycaemic subjects aged 60–74 years. *Diabet Med* 1987;**4**:534–8.
7. Harrower ADB. Prevalence of elderly patients in a hospital diabetic population. *Br J Clin Pract* 1980;**34**:131–3.
8. Hudson CN, Lazarus J, Peters J *et al*. An audit of diabetic care in three district general hospitals in Cardiff. *Pract Diabetes Int* 1995;**13**(1):29–32.
9. Cohen DL, Neil HAW, Thorogood M *et al*. A population based study of the incidence of complications associated with type 2 diabetes in the elderly. *Diabet Med* 1991;**8**:928–33.
10. Walters DP, Gatling W, Mullee MA *et al*. The prevalence of diabetic distal sensory neuropathy in an English community. *Diabet Med* 1992;**9**:349–53.
11. Dornan TL, Peck GM, Dow JDC *et al*. A community survey of diabetes in the elderly. *Diabet Med* 1992;**9**:860–5.
12. Sinclair AJ and Bayer AJ. *All Wales Research in Elderly (AWARE) Diabetes Study*, Report 121/3040, Department of Health, London, 1998.
13. Van Houtum WH, Lavery LA and Harkless LB. The costs of diabetes-related lower extremity amputations in The Netherlands. *Diabet Med* 1995;**12**:777–81.
14. Palumbo PJ and Melton LJ. Peripheral vascular disease and diabetes. In: MI Harris and Mamman RF (eds), *Diabetes in America*, NIH Publication 85-1468, National Institutes of Health, Bethesda, MD, 1985, pp. 1–21.
15. Larsson J, Apelqvist J, Agardh DD and Stenstrom A. Decreasing incidence of major amputation in diabetic patients: a consequence of a multidisciplinary footcare team approach? *Diabet Med* 1995;**12**:770–6.
16. Young MJ and Boulton AJM. The diabetic foot. In: AJ Sinclair and P Finucane (eds), *Diabetes in Old Age*, 2nd edn, John Wiley & Sons, Ltd, Chichester, 2001, pp. 67–88.
17. Cavanagh PR, Simoneau GG and Ulbrecht JS. Ulceration, unsteadiness and uncertainty: the biomechanical consequences of diabetes mellitus. *J Biomech* 1993;**26** (Suppl 1):23–40.
18. Vinik A and Richardson D. Erectile dysfunction. In: AJ Sinclair and P Finucane (eds), *Diabetes in Old Age*, 2nd edn, John Wiley & Sons, Ltd, Chichester, 2001, pp. 89–102.
19. Wagner G, Montorsi F, Auerbach S *et al*. Sildenafil citrate (VIAGRA) improves erectile function in elderly patients with erectile dysfunction: a subgroup analysis. *J Gerontol A Biol Sci Med Sci* 2001;**56**: M1113–9.
20. Goldstein I, Young JM, Fischer J *et al*.; Vardenafil Diabetes Study Group. Vardenafil, a new phosphodiesterase type 5 inhibitor, in the treatment of erectile dysfunction in men with diabetes: a multicenter double-blind placebo-controlled fixed-dose study. *Diabetes Care* 2003;**26**:777–83.
21. Croxson SCM. Metabolic decompensation. In: AJ Sinclair and P Finucane (eds), *Diabetes in Olde Age*, 2nd edn, John Wiley & Sons, Ltd, Chichester, 2001, pp. 53–66.
22. Wachtel TJ, Tetu-Mouradjian LM, Goldman DL *et al*. Hyperosmolarity and acidosis in diabetes mellitus: a three-year experience in Rhode Island. *J Gen Intern Med* 1991;**6**:495–502.
23. Clark DO, Stump TE and Wolinsky FD. Predictors of onset of and recovery from mobility difficulty among adults aged 51–61 years. *Am J Epidemiol* 1998;**148**:63–71.
24. Stuck AE, Walthert JM, Nikolaus T *et al*. Risk factors for functional status decline in community-living elderly people: a systematic literature review. *Soc Sci Med* 1999;**48**:445–69.
25. Valderrama-Gama E, Damian J, Ruigomez A and Martin-Moreno JM. Chronic disease, functional status and self-ascribed causes of disabilities among noninstitutionalized older people in Spain. *J Gerontol A Biol Sci Med Sci* 2002;**57**: M716–21.
26. Perkowski LC, Stroup-Benham CA, Markides KS *et al*. Lower-extremity functioning in older Mexican Americans and its association with medical problems. *J Am Geriatr Soc* 1998;**46**:411–8.
27. Gregg EW, Beckles GL, Williamson DF *et al*. Diabetes and physical disability among older U.S. adults. *Diabetes Care* 2000;**23**:1272–7.
28. Volpato S, Blaum C, Resnick H *et al*. Comorbidities and impairments explaining the association between diabetes and lower extremity disability: the Women's Health and Aging Study. *Diabetes Care* 2002;**25**:678–83.

29. Gregg EW, Mangione CM, Cauley JA *et al.* Study of Osteoporotic Fractures Research Group. Diabetes and incidence of functional disability in older women. *Diabetes Care* 2002;**25**:61–7.
30. Schwartz AV, Vittinghoff E, Sellmeyer DE *et al.* Diabetes-related complications, glycemic control and falls in older adults. *Diabetes Care* 2008;**31**:391–6.
31. Lipscombe LL, Jamal SA, Booth GL and Hawker GA. The risk of hip fractures in older individuals with diabetes. *Diabetes Care* 2007;**30**:835–41.
32. Strachan MW, Deary IJ, Ewing FM and Frier BN. Is type II diabetes associated with an increased risk of cognitive dysfunction? A critical review of published studies. *Diabetes Care* 1997;**20**:438–45.
33. Folstein MF, Folstein SE and McHugh PR. 'Mini-mental state'. A practical method for grading the cognitive state of patients for the clinician. *J Psychiatr Res* 1975;**12**:189–98.
34. Shulman KI. Clock-drawing: is it the ideal cognitive screening test? *Int J Geriatr Psychiatry* 2000;**15**:548–61.
35. Kalmijn S, Feskens EJ, Launer LJ *et al.* Glucose intolerance, hyperinsulinaemia and cognitive function in a general population of elderly men. *Diabetologia* 1995;**38**:1096–102.
36. Stolk RP, Breteler MM, Ott A *et al.* The Rotterdam Study. Insulin and cognitive function in an elderly population. *Diabetes Care* 1997;**20**:792–5.
37. Ott A, Stolk RP, Hofman A *et al.* Association of diabetes mellitus and dementia: the Rotterdam Study. *Diabetologia* 1996;**39**:1392–7.
38. Leibson CL, Rocca WA, Hanson VA *et al.* Risk of dementia among persons with diabetes mellitus: a population-based cohort study. *Am J Epidemiol* 1997;**145**:301–8.
39. Yoshitake T, Kiyohara Y, Kato I *et al.* Incidence and risk factors of vascular dementia and Alzheimer's disease in a defined elderly Japanese population: the Hisayama Study. *Neurology* 1995;**45**:1161–8.
40. Gradman TJ, Laws A, Thompson LW and Reaven GM. Verbal learning and/or memory improves with glycemic control in older subjects with non-insulin-dependent diabetes mellitus. *J Amn Geriatr Soc* 1993;**41**:1305–12.
41. Gregg EW, Yaffe K, Cauley JA *et al.* Study of Osteoporotic Fractures Research Group. Is diabetes associated with cognitive impairment and cognitive decline among older women? *Arch Intern Med* 2000;**160**:174–80.
42. Elias PK, Elias MF, D'Agostino RB *et al.* The Framingham Study. NIDDM and blood pressure as risk factors for poor cognitive performance. *Diabetes Care* 1997;**20**:1399–5.
43. Knopman D, Boland LL, Mosley T *et al.* Atherosclerosis Risk in Communities (ARIC) Study Investigators. Cardiovascular risk factors and cognitive decline in middle-aged adults. *Neurology* 2001;**56**:42–8.
44. Kuusisto J, Koivisto K, Mykkanen L *et al.* Essential hypertension and cognitive function. The role of hyperinsulinemia. *Hypertension* 1993;**22**:771–9.
45. Sinclair AJ, Girling AJ and Bayer AJ. All Wales Research into Elderly (AWARE) Study. Cognitive dysfunction in older subjects with diabetes mellitus: impact on diabetes self-management and use of care services. *Diabetes Res Clin Pract* 2000;**50**:203–12.
46. Amato L, Paolisso G, Cacciatore F *et al.* The Osservatorio Geriatrico of Campania Region Group. Non-insulin-dependent diabetes mellitus is associated with a greater prevalence of depression in the elderly. *Diabetes Metab* 1996;**22**:314–8.
47. Anderson RJ, Freedland KE, Clouse RE and Lustman PJ. The prevalence of comorbid depression in adults with diabetes: a meta-analysis. *Diabetes Care* 2001;**24**:1069–78.
48. Rosenthal MJ, Fajardo M, Gilmore S *et al.* Hospitalization and mortality of diabetes in older adults. A 3-year prospective study. *Diabetes Care* 1998;**21**:231–5.
49. Egede LE, Zheng D and Simpson K. Comorbid depression is associated with increased health care use and expenditures in individuals with diabetes. *Diabetes Care* 2002;**25**:464–70.
50. Lustman PJ, Anderson RJ, Freedland KE *et al.* Depression and poor glycemic control: a meta-analytic review of the literature. *Diabetes Care* 2000;**23**:934–42.
51. Eaton WW, Armenian H, Gallo J *et al.* Depression and risk for onset of type II diabetes. A prospective population-based study. *Diabetes Care* 1996;**19**:1097–102.
52. Kane RA and Rubenstein LZ. Assessment of functional status. In: MSJ Pathy (ed.), *Principles and Practice of Geriatric Medicine*, 3rd edn, John Wiley & Sons, Ltd, Chichester, 1998, pp. 209–20.
53. Stuck AE, Siu AL, Wieland GD *et al.* Comprehensive geriatric assessment: a meta-analysis of controlled trials. *Lancet* 1993;**342**:1032–6.
54. Wilson PW, D'Agostino RB, Levy D *et al.* Prediction of coronary heart disease using risk factor categories. *Circulation* 1998;**97**:1837–47.
55. Menotti A, Puddu PE and Lanti M. Comparison of the Framingham risk function-based coronary chart with risk function from an Italian population study. *Eur Heart J* 2000;**21**:365–70.
56. Alberti KG and Zimmet PZ. Definition, diagnosis and classification of diabetes mellitus and its complications. Part 1: diagnosis and classification of diabetes mellitus provisional report of a WHO consultation. *Diabet Med* 1998;**15**:539–53.
57. Alberti KG and Zimmet PZ. *The IDF Consensus Worldwide Definition of the Metabolic Syndrome*. International Diabetes Federation, 2005, www.idf.org (last accessed 9 October 2011).
58. Institute of Diabetes for Older People. *Executive Summary, European Diabetes Working Party for Older People 2011. Clinical Guidelines for Type 2 Diabetes Mellitus*, www.instituteofdiabetes.org (last accessed 9 October 2011).
59. Trimble LA, Sundberg S, Markham L *et al.* Value of the clock drawing test to predict problems with insulin skills in older adults. *Can J Diabetes* 2005;**29**:102–4.
60. Garber AJ, Clauson P, Pedersen CB and Kølendorf K. Lower risk of hypoglycemia with insulin detemir than with neutral protamine hagedorn insulin in older persons with type 2 diabetes: a pooled analysis of phase III trials. *J Am Geriatr Soc* 2007;**55**:1735–40.
61. Janka HU, Plewe G and Busch K. Combination of oral antidiabetic agents with basal insulin versus premixed insulin alone in randomized elderly patients with type diabetes mellitus. *J Am Geriatr Soc* 2007;**55**:182–8.
62. Schernthaner G, Grimaldi A, Di Mario U *et al.* GUIDE study: double-blind comparison of once-daily gliclazide MR and

glimepiride in type 2 diabetic patients. *Eur J Clin Invest* 2004;**34**:535–42.

63. Del Prato S, Heine RJ, Keilson L *et al*. Treatment of patients over 64 years of age with type 2 diabetes: experience from nateglinide pooled database retrospective analysis. *Diabetes Care* 2003;**26**:2075–80.
64. Papa G, Fedele V, Rizzo MR *et al*. Safety of type 2 diabetes treatment with repaglinide compared with glibenclamide in elderly people: a randomized, open-label, two-period, cross-over trial. *Diabetes Care* 2006: **29**:1918–20.
65. Rajagopalan R, Perez A, Ye Z *et al*. Pioglitazone is effective therapy for elderly patients with type 2 diabetes mellitus. *Drugs Aging* 2004;**21**:259–71.
66. Kreider M and Heise M. Rosiglitazone in the management of older patients with type 2 diabetes mellitus. *Int J Clin Pract* 2002;**56**:538–41.
67. Solomon DH, Cadarette SM, Choudhry NK *et al*. A cohort study of thiazolidinediones and fractures in older adults with diabetes. *J Clin Endocrinol Metab* 2009;**94**:2792–8.
68. Pratley RE, Rosenstock J, Pi-Sunyer FX *et al*. Management of type 2 diabetes in treatment-naive elderly patients. *Diabetes Care* 2007;**30**:3017–22.
69. Pratley RE, McCall T, Fleck PR *et al*. Alogliptin use in elderly people: a pooled analysis from phase 2 and 3 studies. *J Am Geriatr Soc* 2009;**57**:2011–9.
70. The Action to Control Cardiovascular Risk in Diabetes Study Group. Effects of intensive glucose lowering in type 2 diabetes. *N Engl J Med* 2008;**358**:2545–59.
71. The ADVANCE Collaborative Group. Intensive blood glucose control and vascular outcomes in patients with type 2 diabetes. *N Engl J Med* 2008;**358**:2560–72.
72. Duckworth W, Abraira C, Moritz T *et al*. Effect of rosiglitazone on the frequency of diabetes in patients with impaired glucose tolerance or impaired fasting glucose: a randomised controlled trial. *N Engl J Med* 2009;**360**:129–39.
73. Holman R, Paul SK, Bethel MA *et al*. 10-year follow-up of intensive glucose control in type 2 diabetes. *N Engl J Med* 2008;**359**:1577–89.
74. Van den Berghe G, Wouters P, Weekers F *et al*. Intensive insulin therapy in critically ill patients. *N Engl J Med* 2001;**345**:1359–67.
75. Malmberg K, Rydén L, Efendic S *et al*. Randomized trial of insulin–glucose infusion followed by subcutaneous insulin treatment in diabetic patients with acute myocardial infarction (DIGAMI study): effects on mortality at 1 year. *J Am Coll Cardiol* 1995;**26**:57–65.
76. Van den Berghe G, Wilmer A, Hermans G *et al*. Intensive insulin therapy in the medical ICU. *N Engl J Med* 2006;**354**:449–61.
77. The NICE–SUGAR Study Investigators. Intensive versus conventional glucose control in critically ill patients *N Engl J Med* 2009;**360**:1283–97.
78. European Diabetes Working Party for Older People. *Clinical Guidelines for Type 2 Diabetes Mellitus 2001–2004*, www.eugms.org (last accessed 9 October 2011).
79. Kannel WB and McGee DL. Diabetes and cardiovascular disease: the Framingham Study. *JAMA* 1979;**241**:2035–8.
80. Winocour PH and Fisher M. Prediction of cardiovascular risk in people with diabetes. *Diabet Med* 2003;**20**:515–27.
81. Sinclair AJ. Diabetes in old age – changing concepts in the secondary care arena. *J R Coll Physicians Lond* 2000;**34**:240–4.
82. Sinclair AJ, Allard I and Bayer A. Observations of diabetes care in long-term institutional settings with measures of cognitive function and dependency. *Diabetes Care* 1997;**20**:778–84.
83. Spooner JJ, Lapane KL, Hume AL *et al*. Pharmacologic treatment of diabetes in long-term care. *J Clin Epidemiol* 2001;**54**:525–30.
84. Lipscombe LL, Lévesque L, Gruneir A *et al*. Antipsychotic drugs and hyperglycemia in older patients with diabetes. *Arch Intern Med* 2009;**169**:1282–9.
85. Sinclair AJ, Gadsby R, Penfold S *et al*. Prevalence of diabetes in care home residents. *Diabetes Care* 2001;**24**:1066–8.
86. Hamman RF, Michael SL, Keefer SM and Young WF. Impact of policy and procedure changes on hospital stays among diabetic nursing home residents – Colorado. *Morb Mortal Wkly Rep* 1984;**33**:621–9.
87. Mooradian AD, Osterweil D, Petrasek D and Morley JE. Diabetes mellitus in elderly nursing home patients. A survey of clinical characteristics and management. *J Am Geriatr Soc* 1988;**36**:391–6.
88. Coulston AM, Mandelbaum D and Reaven GM. Dietary management of nursing home residents with non-insulin-dependent diabetes mellitus. *Am J Clin Nutr* 1990;**51**:67–71.
89. Velussi M. Lispro insulin treatment in comparison with regular human insulin in type 2 diabetic patients living in nursing homes. *Diabetes Nutr Metab* 2002;**15**:96–100.
90. Ghosh S and Aronow WS. Utilization of lipid-lowering drugs in elderly persons with increased serum low-density lipoprotein cholesterol associated with coronary artery disease, symptomatic peripheral arterial disease, prior stroke or diabetes mellitus before and after an educational program on dyslipidemia treatment. *J Gerontol A Biol Sci Med Sci* 2003;**58**: M432–5.
91. BDA. *Guidelines of Practice for Residents with Diabetes in Care Homes*, British Diabetic Association, London, 1999.
92. Diabetes Prevention Program Research Group; Crandall J, Schade D, Ma Y *et al*. The influence of age on the effects of lifestyle modification and metformin in prevention of diabetes. *J Gerontol A Biol Sci Med Sci* 2006;**61**:1075–81.
93. Chiasson J-L, Josse RG, Gomis R *et al*. Acarbose for prevention of type 2 diabetes mellitus: the STOP-NIDDM randomised trial. *Lancet* 2002;**359**:2072–77.
94. The DREAM Investigators. Effect of rosiglitazone on the frequency of diabetes in patients with impaired glucose tolerance or impaired fasting glucose: a randomised controlled trial. *Lancet* 2006;**368**:1096–105.

CHAPTER 102

New therapies for diabetes mellitus

George T. Griffing
Saint Louis University Medical Center, St Louis, MO, USA

Why do we need new antiglycaemic medications and the 'diabetes conundrum'?

Everyone will agree that elevated blood glucose is bad, but why has it been so difficult to show that lowering blood glucose to normal is good? We have not had the same problem showing that lowering elevated levels of blood pressure and low-density lipoprotein (LDL) are beneficial. Hyperglycaemia leads to increases in mortality and cardiovascular disease, but antiglycaemic therapies have not alleviated this excess burden of disease. This is the 'diabetic conundrum' and it creates opportunities for new antiglycaemic therapies since the old ones have been lacking.

The purpose of this chapter is to discuss and evaluate new glucose-lowering (antiglycaemic) therapies for type 2 diabetes mellitus (T2DM). Although blood pressure- and LDL-lowering therapies are effective and important diabetic therapies, they will not be included in this discussion.

Definition of type 2 diabetes mellitus: disease or risk factor?

The American Diabetes Association (ADA) definition is a good place to start the discussion: *'Diabetes mellitus is a group of metabolic diseases characterized by hyperglycemia resulting from defects in insulin secretion, insulin action or both. The chronic hyperglycemia of diabetes is associated with long-term damage, dysfunction and failure of various organs, especially the eyes, kidneys, nerves, heart and blood vessels.'* Three points in this definition require emphasis, outlined below.[1]

'Hyperglycaemia', and when does T2DM start?

The difficulty in understanding T2DM is deciding where normoglycaemia leaves off and hyperglycaemia begins. The glycaemic risk for complications probably begins before the glucose level meets the current diagnostic threshold of T2DM. In this sense, hyperglycaemia is more like a risk factor with a continuous rather than dichotomous (i.e. the presence or absence of T2DM) threat to health.

That the therapeutic implications of hyperglycaemia present a graded rather than a dichotomous risk is emphasized by the new AACE treatment algorithm.[2] The AACE therapeutic approach emphasizes that increasing levels of hyperglycaemia require graded intensities of treatment. They divide hyperglycaemia into three tiers, recommending monotherapy for the first tier, duotherapy for the second tier and more complex strategies or consideration of insulin for the third tier. This tiered approach is similar to step therapy for different stages of hypertension in the JNC guidelines. In contrast, the ADA does not consider gradations of hyperglycaemia, but instead recommends a stepwise approach to intensification of therapy in T2DM.[3] The theoretical downside of ADA's stepwise versus AACE's tiered approach is the delay in reaching the desired glycaemic target.

'Defects in insulin secretion and action'

Halting the progression of these defects and worsening hyperglycaemia is one of the major therapeutic challenges in T2DM. With time, therapy must be intensified in both dose and numbers of medications to offset the steady decline in insulin secretion. One strategy is to use insulin sensitizers; another is to find drugs this increase β-cell function or mass or decrease apoptosis. Newer therapies with these characteristics will be reviewed.

'Long-term damage, dysfunction and failure of various organs'

Ultimately, it is the complications that we are most concerned about. They can be divided into microvascular, which responds well to antiglycaemic therapy, and macrovascular, for which it has been harder to show benefit.

Principles and Practice of Geriatric Medicine, Fifth Edition. Edited by Alan J. Sinclair, John E. Morley and Bruno Vellas.

Microvascular complications

Small-vessel disease in T2DM is responsible for blindness (retinopathy), renal failure (nephropathy) and lower limb amputations (neuropathy). Glucose-lowering therapy has been proved to reduce these complications (DCCT trial).

Macrovascular complications

Large-vessel disease includes coronary artery, cerebrovascular and peripheral vascular disease. All of the major antiglycaemic trials have failed to show benefits in large vessel disease or mortality in T2DM (ACCORD,[4] ADVANCE,[5] VADT,[6] UKPDS trials).

Cancer complications

Less well appreciated is the association of T2DM and cancer. T2DM patients have approximately twofold higher rates of cancer for a variety of organs, including liver, pancreas, endometrium, breast, colon and bladder, and non-Hodgkin's lymphoma. Potential explanations include the mitogenic effects of insulin (endogenous and exogenous) and underlying metabolic abnormalities such as increased oxidative stress, hyperglycaemia, hyperlipidaemia and obesity. Little is known about the impact of antiglycaemics and cancer, but metformin shows lower cancer rates than insulin and sulfonylurea (SU) therapies.[7]

Current adjunctive therapies for T2DM

Adjunctive therapy

The main focus of this chapter is antiglycaemic therapies, but the comprehensive treatment approach of T2DM is multi-factorial, as shown in the STENO-2 trial.[8] Drugs to control blood pressure and lipid levels are well-established treatments. Pushing these therapies too far, however, has shown their limits, particularly in T2DM with high risk for cardiovascular disease (CVD).[9,10] Even new aspirin guidelines call for tighter criteria for use in T2DM primary prevention.[11]

Medical nutrition and exercise therapy (MNET)

Medical nutrition and exercise therapy is unquestionably the foundation for T2DM prevention, antiglycaemia and CVD risk reduction. MNET should be prescribed to achieve treatment goals, preferably provided by a registered dietician familiar with diabetes education. The unresolved issue, however, is which target to use as a goal for MNET. Even though a body mass index (BMI) goal of <25 is recommended, this is not supported by the data. Based on BMI, over-weight and obese T2DM patients have the lowest rates of CVD and mortality compared with lower and higher BMI categories.[12] The 'U-shaped' relationship of BMI and CVD has been termed the 'obesity paradox' and probably reflects the fact that BMI does not accurately measure metabolically dangerous fat found in ectopic and intra-abdominal sites. Supine abdominal height, on the other hand, is a simple anthropometric measure and better predicts CVD risk and insulin sensitivity than BMI, waist girth and waist:hip ratio.[13]

Currently approved antiglycaemic therapies

Most physicians are feeling overwhelmed at the increasing number of antiglycaemics. If one of these drugs did the job, however, we wouldn't need so many (see Table 102.1). What the problems and needs are for approved and emerging antiglycaemics will be discussed.

Concerns about the benefits and harms of oral antiglycaemic medication have been with us since the UGDP (University Group Diabetes Program) study in 1970, which reported increased mortality and CVD risk with an SU (tolbutamide). Although in 1998 the UKPDS (United Kingdom Prospective Diabetes Study) was thought to have resolved this controversy, one arm in the study showed increased mortality and CVD risk when metformin was added to an SU (UKPDS34). In 2007, concern was again raised, this time for another drug, rosiglitazone, which was associated with excess mortality and CVD.[14]

Evaluating the safety and benefits of antiglycaemics is difficult because of the wide variability between classes and the number of drugs in each class. Furthermore, the hard outcomes data beyond glucose lowering are usually not available when making therapeutic decisions.

Even he US Congress is concerned. It directed the Agency for Healthcare Research and Quality (AHRQ), to evaluate the outcomes, comparative clinical effectiveness and appropriateness of prescription drugs, including antiglycaemics. Its report concluded that the evidence from clinical trials about drug efficacy on major clinical endpoints, such as cardiovascular mortality, is inconclusive.[15] Therefore, the whole area of T2DM therapeutics is filled with uncertainty. The US Food and Drug Administration (FDA) is making a small step in the right direction since it is requiring all new T2DM drug approvals to examine CVD endpoints and at least show no harm.

Metformin: life begins at 50

Metformin is on just about everyone's list of first-line antiglycaemics. Metformin been around for many years, beginning as *Galega officinalis* (French lilac) used in mediaeval Europe to treat many medical problems, including diabetes.[16] Fifty years ago, metformin was isolated from this plant and introduced for the treatment of T2DM. Since then, it has become the most widely prescribed diabetic therapy and with good reason. Metformin lowers glucose with

Table 102.1 Approved T2DM antiglycaemic therapies.

Class	Generic name	Trade name	Generic	Approved
Orals				
Sulfonylurea (SU)	Glipizide	Glucotrol	Yes	May 1984
		Glyburide DiaBeta, Glynase, Micronase		
	Glimepiride	Amaryl	Yes	November 1995
Biguanide	Metformin	Glucophage	Yes	March 1995
α-Glucosidase inhibitor	Acarbose	Precose	No	September 1995
	Miglitol	Glyset	No	December 1996
Thiazolidinedione (TZD)	Rosiglitazone	Avandia	No	June 1999
	Pioglitazone	Actos	No	July 1999
Meglitinide (glinide)	Repaglinide	Prandin	No	December 1997
	Nateglinide	Starlix	No	December 2000
DPP-4 inhibitor	Sitagliptin	Januvia	No	October 2006
	Saxagliptin	Onglyza	No	July 2009
Bile acid sequestrant	Colesevelam	Welchol	No	January 2008
Dopamine agonist	Bromocriptine	Cycloset	No	May 2010
SU and biguanide	Glyburide and metformin	Glucovance	Yes	July 2000
Biguanide and glitazone	Rosiglitazone and metformin	Avandamet	No	October 2002
Sulfonylurea and glitazone	Rosiglitazone and glimeriride	Avandaryl	No	November 2005
Biguanide and DPP-4 Inhib	Sitagliptin and metformin	Janumet	No	March 2007
Injectables				
Regular insulin	Human insulin (regular)	Humulin R, Novolin R	Yes	October 1982
Intermediate-acting insulin	Human insulin (NPH insulin)	Humulin N, Novolin N	Yes	October 1982
Human insulin combinations	Insulin regular and NPH insulin	Humulin 70/30	Yes	April 1989
Rapid-acting insulin analogues	Insulin lispro	Humalog	No	June 1996
	Insulin aspart	Novolog	No	June 2000
	Insulin glulisine	Apidra	No	April 2004
Long-acting basal insulin analogues	Insulin glargine	Lantus	No	April 2000
	Insulin detemir	Levemir	No	June 2005
Combinations (including analogues)	Insulin lispro/protamine	Humalog Mix 75/25 and 50/50	No	December 1999
	Insulin aspart-protamine	Novolog Mix 70/30	No	November 2001
Amylin analogue	Pramlintide	Symlin	No	March 2005
GLP-1 receptor agonist	Exenatide	Byetta	No	April 2005
	Liraglutide	Victoza	No	January 2010

negligible hypoglycaemia and measurable body weight loss. It decreases microvascular complications and one substudy of the UKPDS(34) showed a reduction in CVD and mortality as monotherapy in obese T2DM.

Metformin works by preventing hepatic gluconeogenesis through activation of AMP-activated protein kinase (AMPK), which in turn inhibits the expression of other hepatic gluconeogenic genes (e.g. PEPCK, phosphoenolpyruvate carboxykinase). Inhibition of gluconeogenesis lowers glucose production, but also reduces hepatic lactate uptake. Conditions which increase lactate production [alcohol intoxication, low-flow states, congestive heart failure (CHF), respiratory failure] combined with impaired renal clearance will potentially result in lactic acidosis. The most common adverse effects are diarrhoea and decreases in vitamin B_{12} levels.

Metformin has shown an anti-cancer effect compared with SU and insulin in observational studies.[7] The mechanism may be through activation of AMPK, which plays a role in tumour suppression. Beyond the cancer preventive effect, there is evidence that metformin may enhance chemotherapy for existing cancers.[17]

The bottom line is that this drug deserves to be first-line. It is cheap, effective and has outcomes data. Unfortunately, metformin does not halt T2DM progression and most patients will move on to need another drug; the big question is, which one?

Sulfonylureas (SUs)

'*Special warning on increased risk of cardiovascular mortality*' is how the SU class label reads resulting from the 1970 UGDP study. There is some biological plausibility because SUs block 'ischaemic preconditioning', which is a mechanism for protecting the myocardium during periods of ischaemia. SUs bind to the potassium (KATP) channel, leading to an increase in intracellular potassium ion concentrations, thereby opening voltage-gated calcium channels, resulting in an influx of calcium ions. In pancreatic β-cells, this calcium influx promotes insulin secretion, but in the heart it impairs 'ischaemic preconditioning'.

Most of the physicians who know about the package label warning are reassured by results of the UKPDS33 trial (but not the UKPDS34 trial) and the positive recommendations by the ADA, AACE and other experts. Also, SUs are inexpensive and effective at lowering both glucose and microvascular complications. The good news is that SUs are probably safe, but the bad news is that they do not work to lower CVD and mortality. SUs also do not halt the progression of T2DM, so should we still be using them?

Meglitinides (glinides): faster is not always better

This class of drugs can be thought of as a rapid-acting SUs. Although they are non-SUs chemically, they act through the same mechanism to stimulate insulin secretion. Because of the rapid onset and short duration of action, glinides are best used to lower postprandial glycaemia (PPG). This means that they have to be dosed before each meal several times per day, which makes them inconvenient. Other negative points include hypoglycaemia, measurable weight gain and lack of positive outcomes data.

The best hope for success for glinides was to show that targeting PPG would improve CVD and prevent progression of T2DM. Previous studies have suggested that PPG was an even greater risk for CVD than fasting plasma glycaemia (FPG) for people with glucose intolerance (DECODE study). Unfortunately, this hope was dashed when pre-meal glinide (nateglinide) therapy failed to show any CVD protection or slowing of the progression of hyperglycaemia.[18] Therefore, this appears to be another drug class that is lacking in efficacy.

Thiazolidinediones (TZDs): the bloom is off the rose and the pie is in the sky (rosiglitazone and pioglitazone) – downsizing expectations

At first, this class of drugs promised benefits beyond glucose reduction, as suggested by encouraging surrogate outcomes for CVD. Insulin resistance, interleukin-6 and VEGF-induced angiogenesis all decreased, adiponectin levels rose and visceral fat moved to the periphery. Among the positive attributes, TZDs do not produce hypoglycaemia and they slow the progression of β-cell loss. Compared with SUs and metformin, rosiglitazone has greater durability as monotherapy (ADOPT – A Diabetes Outcome Progression Trial).

The bloom fell off the rose, however, when a controversial meta-analysis for rosiglitazone changed the discussion from potential CVD efficacy to concerns over CVD safety. Subsequent CVD outcomes studies have not shown increased mortality, but neither have they shown much benefit (PROACTIVE and RECORD trials). The main safety concerns with this class is a fourfold increase in CHF and an acceleration of bone loss resulting in a doubling of fracture rates. TZDs' best benefits, however, may be prevention of T2DM, which is achieved at lower doses, thereby reducing these safety concerns.[19]

α-Glucosidase inhibitors (AGIs) – the drugs that get no respect

Drugs in this class are frequently the butt of jokes and no one takes them seriously. Like Rodney Dangerfield, these drugs 'don't get no respect', which is unfortunate given all of their positive attributes. Their mechanism of action is simple: they block the digestion and absorption of ingested polysaccharides, thus reducing the level of postprandial glucose and insulin excursions. Although the major impact is on postprandial glucose, they also reduce fasting glucose and HbA1c. This class of drugs has many positive features: no hypoglycaemia, consistent loss of body weight and the progression of T2DM is slowed. Blood pressure, triglycerides, inflammatory biomarkers and the development of hypertension are all reduced. Even better, these positive surrogate markers result in positive outcomes as measured by reduced progression of atherosclerosis (vascular intimal medial thickness) and cardiovascular events in an impaired glucose-tolerant (IGT) population (STOP-NIDDM trial). Even though this is a very safe drug class, almost half of the patients will have gastrointestinal complaints. Carbohydrate is usually absorbed in the upper intestine; upon initiation of AGIs, a large portion escapes digestion and is delivered to the colon causing excessive bacterial activity. To avoid this, AGIs should be titrated slowly over several months, giving time for the lower small intestine to acquire the ability to absorb carbohydrates.

AGIs are a good fit with metformin, although both have gastrointestinal side effects. AGIs are particularly effective in mild hyperglycaemia and in correcting postprandial hyperglycaemia. AGIs have CVD outcomes data and are very safe. These drugs should be thought of more often when prescribing antiglycaemics.

Colesevelam: LDL and A1c lowering – a match made in heaven

The bile-acid binding resin colesevelam was approved for LDL lowering in 2000 and 8 years later for glucose lowering in T2DM. This class of drugs has already been shown to reduce CVD and mortality, although not in a T2DM population.

The mechanism for colesevelam's antiglycaemic action is unknown, but the alteration in bile acid composition produces two possible antiglycaemic actions: (1) increased delivery of fatty acids to the distal intestine stimulating GLP-1 secretion and (2) activation of hepatic FXR (farnesoid X receptor), which inhibits gluconeogenesis. The combination of increased GLP-1 action and decreased hepatic gluconeogenesis is like combining a DPP4I (dipeptidyl-peptidase-4 inhibitor) with metformin (e.g., Janumet).

To date, colesevelam does not have micro- or macrovascular endpoint data, but it does lower both glucose and LDL with negligible hypoglycaemia and weight changes.[20] Colesevelam's LDL-lowering effects are additive with statins. The combination of colesevelam and a statin permits a reduction in the statin dose and risk of rhabdomyolysis and attenuates the rise in triglycerides observed with this class of drugs.

Because it is a bile acid-binding resin, it does not have systemic effects, but the main complaints are gastrointestinal. Recently, a convenient single dose packet dissolved in a glass of water has replaced the onerous six capsules daily.

Bromocriptine: born again

Physicians have been using this drug for many years to treat prolactin-secreting pituitary tumours, Parkinson's disease and many other off-label uses. Now it has been re-born as a quick-release formulation, Cycloset (0.8 mg tablets, VeroScience), to treat T2CM as an adjunct to diet and exercise.[21]

This is the only antiglycaemic believed to work through the central nervous system. Obese, insulin-resistant T2DM patients have twofold elevated plasma prolactin levels, indicating a hypothalamic dopamine deficiency. Administered as a single timed morning dose, this centrally acting dopamine D2 receptor agonist acts on circadian neuronal activities within the hypothalamus to reset abnormally elevated prolactin, plasma glucose, triglyceride and free fatty acid levels in fasting and postprandial states in insulin-resistant patients.

Bromocriptine may be used as monotherapy or combined with other oral antiglycaemics; use with insulin has not been studied. The recommended starting dose of bromocriptine is 0.8 mg daily and is increased in 0.8 mg increments weekly until the target range (1.6–4.8 mg) or until maximum tolerance is reached. Doses should be administered once daily within 2 h of waking in the morning and with food to reduce the risk for gastrointestinal tract adverse effects such as nausea.

Adverse events most commonly reported in clinical trials of bromocriptine included nausea, fatigue, vomiting, headache and dizziness. These events lasted a median of 14 days and were more likely to occur during initial titration of the drug. None of the reports of nausea or vomiting were described as serious.

Bromocriptine was the first diabetes drug to be approved under the FDA's new guidelines requiring clinical trials to demonstrate no increased cardiovascular risk. In a 52 week double-blind, placebo-controlled safety trial ($n = 3000$), treatment with bromocriptine did not increase the risk for a composite of myocardial infarction, stroke, hospitalization for unstable angina, CHF and revascularization surgery. In fact, the risk of this composite CVD endpoint was reduced (hazard ratio, 0.58; 95% confidence interval, 0.35–0.96). This drug appears also to be a good fit as a second agent with metformin and the positive (but preliminary) CVD data are encouraging.

Incretin therapies: the new kid on the block

Incretin therapy is the new class of antiglycaemic therapies which has generated the most excitement. Incretins are a group of gastrointestinal hormones including glucagon-like peptide-1 (GLP-1) which are secreted into the circulation when nutrients reach the small intestinal. Incretins (like GLP-1) travel to the pancreas, where they stimulate insulin and suppress glucagon secretion in a glucose-dependent manner. They also delay gastric emptying and promote satiety. GLP-1 is rapidly inactivated by the enzyme dipeptidylpeptidase-4 (DPP-4). Of the known incretins, GLP-1 has the greatest antiglycaemic activity and therapeutic GLP-1 analogues have been developed. The other incretin strategy is to inhibit DPP-4 and prolong the action of endogenous incretins. We will compare and contrast these drugs between and within classes.

Table 102.2 GLP-1 agonist and DPP4 inhibitor comparisons.

Item	GLP-1 agonists	DPP-4 inhibitors
Route of administration	Subcutaneous	Oral
Gastrointestinal side effects (fullness, nausea and vomiting)	Yes	No
Weight changes	Weight loss	Weight neutral
Selectivity	GLP-1 receptor only	Multiple substrates – GLP-2, NPY, SP, PACAP, others
Increase in GLP-1 activity	Supraphysiological	Near physiological and retained diurnal pattern
Gastric emptying	Delayed	Normal
Drug overdose	Problematic	Non-toxic
Plasma glucose	↓FPG (liraglutide only) and marked ↓PPG	↓FPG and slight ↓PPG
A1c reduction	1.0–2.0%	0.5–1.0%
Glucagon suppression	More	Less
Increased β-cell mass	Yes	Not known
Increased glucagon counter-regulation with hypoglycaemia	Yes	Not known
Severe renal failure	Not recommended	Dose adjustment

Comparing GLP1 agonist and DPP4 inhibitors

Both GLP-1 agonist and DPP4 inhibitors are antiglycaemic, with GLP-1s being more potent.[22] Both classes share the following attributes: (1) negligible hypoglycaemia because the insulin secretion is 'glucose dependent'; (2) neutral (DPP4I) or negative (GLP1) body weight changes; (3) suppression of pancreatic α-cell glucagon secretion; and based on animal data, incretin therapies may (4) potentially slow the progression of β-cell loss and (5) potentially reduce CVD through improved risk factor profile and direct CV protection.[23] (see Table 102.2).

GLP-1 agonists

Two GLP-1 agonists have been approved for use: exenatide and liraglutide; a comparison of their clinical characteristics is given in Table 102.3. Pharmacokinetics and immunological reactions are the main differences. Liraglutide has greater antiglycaemia effect and probably less gastrointestinal symptoms, probably because of a flatter and prolonged blood level. Future GLP-1 agonists will have even longer half-lives, allowing for once weekly dosing. The main concerns regarding GLP-1 agonists include medullary thyroid cancer and pancreatitis.

Medullary thyroid cancer

Rodent data show that GLP-1 agonist therapy increases calcitonin levels and produces c-cell hyperplasia and cancer. This is probably not a concern in humans, however, since calcitonin levels do not increase, there is no c-cell hyperplasia and there are no reports of medullary thyroid cancer in over one million patients exposed to exenatide.

Table 102.3 GLP-1 agonist comparisons: exenatide (Byetta) and liraglutide (Victoza).

Item Dose schedule	Exenatide Twice daily	Liraglutide Once daily
Blood levels	Peak and trough blood levels	Flat blood levels
Weight changes	Weight loss	Weight loss
Antiglycaemia	Lowers A1c and PPG	Lowers A1c, PPG and FPG
Antibodies	Antibodies	No antibodies
Skin reaction	Positive injection site reactions	No injection site reactions

Pancreatitis

Pancreatitis is more of a concern with incretin therapies (both GLP-1a and DPP4I), but still a rare occurrence. The connection was first suspected because of the overlap of the venoms from the scorpion, known to produce pancreatitis, and Gila monster, from which exendin 4 (exenatide) was isolated. It should be noted that T2DM itself has a threefold greater risk of pancreatitis (4.2 versus 1.5 per 1000 patient-years).

The precise risk and causality of pancreatitis with incretin therapy are unknown. Pancreatitis case reports for both exenatide and sitagliptin, however, have prompted new package labelling. Definitive data on the pancreatitis risk are lacking and the studies are mixed. Clinical trials of liraglutide showed about three times more pancreatitis than the comparator (2.2 versus 0.6 cases per 1000 patient-years). However, the numbers are very small, seven versus one. In addition, one study using an insurance claims database found no increase in pancreatitis with either exenatide (0.13%) or sitagliptin (0.12%) compared with metformin or glyburide users for up to 1 year. In conclusion, pancreatitis is a rare occurrence in incretin therapy users and the association is unclear. Nevertheless, caution dictates that one should avoid using incretin therapy in patients with chronic pancreatitis or at risk for this disease.

DPP4 inhibitors

One can think of DPP4 inhibitors as GLP-1's younger sibling – not quite as strong or as fast but safer and less likely to cause trouble. Compared with the GLP-1 agonists, DPP4Is have less antiglycaemia, glucagon suppression and weight loss effects, but they also are non-toxic, can be used in severe renal failure and have almost no adverse effects.[22] One potential advantage DPP4Is have as a class is that they increase levels of a wider range of incretins than just GLP-1. These additional incretins could have benefits above and beyond GLP-1, for example, β-cell neogenesis. Sitagliptin, the first DPP4I, was approved before FDA's CVD guidelines were in place. Saxagliptin, approved later, satisfied the FDA guidelines by demonstrating a 50% reduction in CVD endpoints.[23]

DPP4 inhibitors, ACE inhibitors and angioedema

One potential downside of DPP4Is is complications arising from inhibiting other non-incretin actions of this enzyme. For example, combining DPP4I with an acetylcholinesterase (ACE) inhibitor decreases the degradation and increases the levels of some of the vasoactive peptides linked to angioedema.[24] Angiotensin receptor blockers (ARBs) do not share the same risk and may be an alternative to ACE inhibition when there is concern about angioedema.

Amylin analogues – pramlintide

Amylin is co-secreted with insulin from pancreatic β-cells and acts centrally to slow gastric emptying, suppresses postprandial glucagon secretion and decreases food intake. Amylin is relatively deficient in patients with T2DM and essentially absent in T1DM. Pramlintide is an amylin analogue that has been shown to improve glycaemic control via reductions in postprandial glucose and to reduce bodyweight. Pramlitide is usually given as a meal-time subcutaneous injection bolus with the advantage of less hypoglycaemia and weight gain compared with bolus insulin.

Emerging but not yet approved antiglycaemics

If we had the perfect treatment for T2DM we would not need new therapies, and if lowering glucose were the only criteria then we could stop now. So what are the characteristics and unmet needs of the current antiglycaemics that new drugs should target? (see Tables 102.4 and 102.5).

Prevention and progression – too fat, too lazy and too little insulin

The pathophysiology of T2DM involves two hits: the first is that it starts with insulin resistance partly as a result of

Table 102.4 Approved antiglycaemics and their selected characteristics[a].

Drug	Insulin levels	Insulin sensitivity	β-Cell	PPG	Hypo	BW	RF	CVD
Metformin	↔	↑	↔	↔	↔	↓	↓	↓ *
TZD	↔	↑	↑	↔	↔	↑	↓	↔
AGI	↔	↔	↔	↓	↔	↓	↓	↓ **
SU	↑	↔	↔	↓	↑	↑	↔	↔
Glinide	↑	↔	↔	↓	↑	↑	↔	NR
Insulin	↑	↔	↔	↓	↑	↑	↔	↔
Amylin	↔	↔	↔	↓	↔	↓	↔	NR
GLP-1a	↑	↔	↑	↓	↔	↓	↓	NR
DPP4I	↑	↔	↑	↓	↔	↔	NR	↓ ***
Colesevelam	↔	↔	NR	0	↔	↔	↓	↓ ****
Bromocriptine	↔	↓	NR	↓	↔	↔	NR	↓ *****

[a]β-Cell = β-cell function or mass; Glucose = blood glucose levels; Hypo = hypoglycaemia; BW = body weight; RF = CVD risk factors; ↓* = UKPDS34 in obese T2DM as monotherapy, STOP-NIDDM in IGT reduced CVD and hypertension; ↓*** = saxagliptin in the FDA registration trials; ↓**** = class effect; ↓***** = in the FDA registration trials; NR = not reported.

Table 102.5 Antiglycaemic therapy's unmet needs.

1. *Prevention of T2DM–* improve insulin sensitivity
2. *Progression of insulin deficiency –* stop progressive β-cell loss
3. *Reduce postprandial glycaemia –* slow carbohydrate absorption or augment insulin secretion
4. *Prevent hypoglycaemia –* insulin secretion should be glucose dependent
5. *Prevent increasing body weight –* avoid increasing visceral or ectopic adiposity
6. *Improve CVD risk factors –* reduce blood pressure and LDL
7. *Reducing CVD and mortality –* the important but elusive goal

our lifestyle and the second is insulin deficiency from β-cell failure. Diet and exercise, although helpful, have not been the answer and we do not have a proven drug (although several candidates) which can restore β-cell function.

Postprandial glycaemia (PPG) – the stealth defect

In the early stages of T2DM, meal-related bolus insulin release is the first defect and in later stages it is the hardest defect to correct. In addition, PPG is a stealth defect and goes unnoticed because it is so difficult to detect.

Hypoglycaemia – the limiting factor

The closer T2DM glucose levels get to normoglycaemia, the greater is the risk of hypoglycaemia. There is hope, however. Newer insulin secretogogue therapies have the property of 'glucose dependency', meaning that insulin will not be secreted unless there are adequate levels of circulating glucose.

Weight gain

Insulin and SUs are noted for weight gain. The negative CVD consequences of weight gain, especially visceral and ectopic fat, may offset the positive effect of glucose lowering. It is encouraging that many of the newer antiglycaemics are either weight neutral or promote weight loss. The mechanisms are probably different for each class of medication but are generally thought to be related to reduced gastric emptying, enhanced metabolism or central appetite suppression.

Cardioprotection

Therapies are needed that will reverse the cardiovascular disease and mortality burden imposed by hyperglycaemia. This goal is arguably the most important, but also the most difficult, since very large and very long studies are required.

Developing antiglycaemic classes and their characteristics

A selection of developing antiglycaemic classes and their selected characteristics are described below (see Tables 102.6 and 102.7).

Dual and pan PPAR agonists: a fibrate, TZD, and exercise all in one pill

Peroxisome proliferator-activated receptors (PPARs) are a group of nuclear receptor proteins that function as transcription factors regulating the expression of genes involved in glucose, lipid and energy homeostasis.[25] The PPARs come in three types: α, γ and δ; α regulates triglyceride synthesis and energy homeostasis, γ regulates insulin sensitivity and glucose metabolism and δ enhances fatty acid metabolism.

Since T2DM is characterized by multiple metabolic defects, including dysglycaemia and dyslipidaemia, the PPARs are an attractive therapeutic target. Single PPAR agonists in the fibric acid drug class (PPAR-α agonists: clofibrate, gemfibrozil, ciprofibrate, bezafibrate and fenofibrate) and TZDs (PPAR-γ: rosiglitazone and pioglitazone) are already in use. Interest in dual and pan PPAR agonists (α–γ, α–δ, γ–δ and α–γ–δ) may lead to drugs that combine the actions of a TZD on hyperglycaemia and a fibrate drug on hypertriglyceridaemia and more.

However, the road for dual PPARs has been filled with potholes. Two of the most senior drugs in this class have been discontinued: tesiglitazar (Galidea) for decreasing glomerular filtration rate and muiraglitazar (Pargluva) for increasing cardiovascular events. Hope springs eternal, however, and another dual PPAR, aleglitazar, has shown a glucose-lowering effect, favourable lipid modifications and a good safety profile.

PPAR-δ agonists are perhaps the most interesting, and one of them has been termed the 'exercise pill'. Used alone, PPAR-δ can shift glucose utilization to fatty acid oxidation, which could reverse the metabolic abnormalities in obesity. When combined with an adenosine-augmenting agent, AICAR (aminoimidazole carboxamide ribonucleotide), the PPAR-δ agonist (GW1516) changes skeletal muscle phenotype to become more insulin sensitive, thus improving glucose homeostasis and mimicking the effects of exercise.[26]

SGLT2 inhibitors: now diabetics can eat that piece of cake without feeling guilty

Sodium glucose transport (SGLT) T2 inhibitors may lead to a paradigm shift of how we think about T2DM patients and their diets. With these drugs, T2DM patients can have their cake and eat it too, because the extra sugar can be excreted in the urine. The mode of action involves inhibiting SGLT2, which is responsible for 90% of renal glucose reabsorption. Inhibiting reabsorption results in glycosuria and blood

Table 102.6 Antiglycaemics in development.

Mechanism	Drug	Company	Target	Development (phase)
11BHSD inhibitor	11BHSD	Bristol-Myers Squibb	DM	Clinical trials
11BHSD inhibitor	AMG 221	Amgen	T2DM	P 1
11BHSD inhibitor	INCB-13739, 19602, 20817	Incyte	T2DM	P 2
11BHSD inhibitor	JTT 654	Japan Tobacco	T2DM	P 1
ACE inhibitor	Altace (ramipril)	King Pharmaceuticals	T2DM prevention	P 3
Adenosine receptor agonist	ATL-844 (Stedivaze, adenosine receptor agonist)	PGxHealth	T2DM	P 2
Anti-inflammatory	AMG 108 (IL-1 receptor antagonist)	Amgen	DM	P 2
	AVR 118 (chemokine/cytokine modulator)	Advanced Viral Research	T2DM	P 1
	BMS-741672 (CCR2 antagonist)	Bristol-Myers Squibb	DM	Clinical trials
	VGX-1027 (cytokine inhibitor)	VGX Pharmaceuticals	T1DM	P 1
	XOMA052 (interleukin inhibitor)	XOMA	T2DM	P 1
Anti-obesity	CE-326597 (CCK receptor antagonist)	Pfizer	T2DM	P 2
	Cetilistat (gut lipase inhibitor)	Alizyme	T2DM	P 2
Antioxidant	Succinobucol	AtheroGenics	T2DM	P 3
Antoimmune	Teplizumab	Eli Lilly	T1DM	P 2/3
	Autoimmune DM vaccine	Diamyd Medical	T1DM	P 3
	Canakinumab	Novartis Pharmaceuticals	T2DM	P 2/3
	DiaPep277	Andromeda Biotech	Latent autoimmune DM	P 2
	Larazotide	Alba Therapeutics	T1DM	P 1
	Lisofylline	DiaKine Therapeutics	T1DM	P 1
	NBI-6024	Neurocrine Biosciences	T1DM	P 2
	Otelixizumab	Tolerx	T1DM	P 2
	PEG-encapsulated islet cell	Novocell	T1DM	P 1/2
	Prochymal (stem cell Rx)	Osiris Therapeutics	T1DM	P 2 + A7
β-Cell regeneration	INGAP peptide	Kinexum Metabolics	T1DM	P 2
Biguanide	MetControl (metformin buccal)	Generex Biotechnology	T2DM	P 2
CFTR inhibitor	NP-500 (cystic fibrosis transmembrane conductance regulator inhibitor)	Napo Pharmaceuticals	T2DM	P 1
Cortisol Inhibitor	DIO-902 [(2*S*,4*R*)-ketoconazole, cortisol inhibitor]	DiObex	T2DM	P 2
DPP4 inhibitor	ABT-279, alogliptin	Abbott Laboratories	T2DM	P 1
	Alogliptin	Takeda Pharmaceuticals	T2DM	Clinical trials
	Alogliptin/pioglitazone	Takeda Pharmaceuticals	T2DM	Clinical trials
	AMG 222	Amgen	T2DM	P 2
	ARI-2243 (Arisaph)	Arisaph Pharmaceuticals	T2DM	P 1

(*continued overleaf*)

Table 102.6 (*continued*).

Mechanism	Drug	Company	Target	Development (phase)
	BI-1356 (Ondero)	Boehringer Ingelheim	T2DM	P 3
	Galvus (vildagliptin)	Novartis Pharmaceuticals	T2DM	Application
	KRP 104	ActivX Biosciences	T2DM	P 2
	MP-513	Mitsubishi Pharma	T2DM	P 1
	PF-734200	Pfizer	T2DM	P 2
	PHX-1149 (dutogliptin)	Forest Laboratories	T2DM	P 3
	R1579	Roche	T2DM	P 2
	Saxagliptin/metformin	AstraZeneca/BMS	T2DM	P 3
	SYR-472	Takeda Pharmaceuticals	T2DM	P 2
	TA-6666	Mitsubishi Pharma	T2DM	P 2
	Vildagliptin/metformin	Novartis Pharmaceuticals	T2DM	Clinical trials, resubmission?
FBPase inhibitor	MB07803	Metabasis Therapeutics	T2DM	P 2
Fibroblast growth factor	LP-10152 (FGF-21)	Eli Lilly	T2DM	P 1/2
Gastrin analogue	TT-223 and epidermal growth factor analogue	Eli Lilly	T1DM	P 2
	TT-223 and GLP-1 analogue	Eli Lilly	T1DM	P 1
	TT-223 and metformin	Eli Lilly	T1DM	P 2
Glucokinase agonist	AZD6370, 1656	AstraZeneca	T2DM	P 1
	Glucokinase activator	Bristol-Myers Squibb	DM	Clinical trials
	LY-2599506	Eli Lilly	T2DM	P 1
	LY-2121260	Eli Lilly	T2DM	P 1
	MK-0599	Merck	DM	P 1
	R1511	Roche	T2DM	P 1
	R4929	Roche	T2DM	P 1
	TTP355	TransTech Pharma	T2DM	P 1
Glinide	Metgluna (mitiglinide/metformin)	Elixir Pharmaceuticals	T2DM	P 3
GLP-1 agonist	756050 (albiglutide)	GlaxoSmithKline	T2DM	P 1
	AVE0010 (GLP-1a)	Sanofi-aventis	T2DM	P 2
	AVE0010 (GLP-1a XR)	Sanofi-aventis	T2DM	P 1
	Exenatide intranasal	Amylin Pharmaceuticals	T2DM	P 1
	LY-2189265	Eli Lilly	T2DM	P 2/3
	LY-2405319	Eli Lilly	T2DM	P 2
	R1583	Roche	T2DM	P 2
	SUN E7001	Asubio Pharma	T2DM	P 1
	Taspoglutide	Roche	T2DM	P 2
Glucagon receptor	AMG 477	Amgen	T2DM	P 1
antagonist	ISIS 32568	Isis Pharmaceuticals	T2DM	P 1
GPR-119 agonist	APD688	Arena/Ortho-McNeil-Janssen	T2DM	P 1
Guanidine	Pyrazolylguanidine	SuperGen	T2DM	P 2
Insulin	AI-401 (oral/nasal insulin)	AutoImmune	T1DM prevention	P 3
	Alveair (inhaled insulin)	Coremed	DM	P 1

Table 102.6 (*continued*).

Mechanism	Drug	Company	Target	Development (phase)
	AT1391 (insulin skin patch)	Altea Therapeutics	T1DM	P 1/2
	BHT-3021	Bayhill Therapeutics	T1DM	P 1/2
	Bydureon (exenatide XR)	Amylin Pharmaceuticals	T2DM	Submitted application
	HDV insulin (hepatic directed vesicle)	Diasome Pharmaceuticals	T2DM	P 2
	Insulin inhalation	Baxter Healthcare	DM	P 1
	Insulin inhalation	MicroDose Technologies	DM	P 1
	Insulin nasal spray	MDRNA	T2DM	P 2
	Insulin oral	Generex Biotechnology	DM	P 3
	Insulin transdermal	Dermisonics	T1DM	P 1
	Intesulin (oral insulin)	Coremed	DM	P 1
	Nasulin (intranasal insulin)	CPEX Pharmaceuticals	DM	P 2
	NN1250 (Degludec insulin)	Novo Nordisk	DM	Clinical trials
	Oral insulin using Eligen technology	Emisphere Technologies	T2DM	P 1/2
	rHuPH20 (hyaluronidase/insulin)	Halozyme Therapeutics	DM	P 1
	Technosphere (inhaled insulin)	MannKind	DM	Clinical trials
	VIAject (rapid insulin)	Biodel	T1DM	P 3
	VIAtab (oral/sublingual insulin)	Biodel	T1DM	P 1
	Albulin (albumin/insulin)	Teva Pharmaceuticals USA	T1DM	P 1
Insulin secretogogue	Glinsuna (mitiglinide)	Elixir Pharmaceuticals	T2DM	P 3
(glucose-dependent)	MBX-2982 (GPR-119)	Metabolex	T2DM	P 1
Insulin sensitizer	CRx-401 (benzafibrate + diflunisal)	CombinatoRx	T2DM	P 2
	CVT-3619 (adenosine receptor agonist)	CV Therapeutics	DM	P 1
PPAR agonist	376501	GlaxoSmithKline	T2DM	P 1
	625019	GlaxoSmithKline	T2DM	P 1
	Avandamet XR (extended release)	GlaxoSmithKline	T2DM	P 3
	Avandia (rosiglitazone)	GlaxoSmithKline	T2DM prevention	P 3
	AVE0897 (balanced PPAR agonist)	Sanofi-aventis	T2DM	P 1
	Balaglitazone	Dr. Reddy's Laboratories	T2DM	P 3
	INT-131	InteKrin Therapeutics	T2DM	P 2
	K 111	Kowa Pharmaceuticals	T2DM	P 2
	MBX-102 (non-TZD, metaglidasen)	Johnson & Johnson	T2DM	P 2/3
	MBX-2044	Johnson & Johnson	T2DM	P 2
	MCC-555 (netoglitazone)	Mitsubishi Pharma	T2DM	P 2
	MSDC-0160	Metabolic Solutions	T2DM	P 2

(*continued overleaf*)

Table 102.6 (*continued*).

Mechanism	Drug	Company	Target	Development (phase)
	Netoglitazone	Perlegen Sciences	T2DM	P 1
	ONO-5129	Ono Pharma USA	T2DM	P 2
	PPM-204 (indeglitazar)	Plexxikon	T2DM	P 2
	R1439 (aleglitazar)	Roche	T2DM	P 2
	Rivoglitazone	Daiichi Sankyo	T2DM	P 3
	Sodelglitazar	GlaxoSmithKline	T2DM	P 2
PYY3-36 analogue	PF-4325667	Pfizer	DM	P 1
SGLT2 inhibitor	AVE2268 (SGLT2 inhibitor)	Sanofi-aventis	T2DM	P 2
	BI-10773	Boehringer Ingelheim	T2DM	P 1
	BI-44847	Boehringer Ingelheim	T2DM	P 2
	Dapagliflozin (SGLT2 inhibitor)	AstraZeneca/BMS	DM	P 3
	Dapagliflozin/metformin	AstraZeneca/BMS	T2DM	P 3
	R7201	Roche	T2DM	P 1
	Remogliflozin	GlaxoSmithKline	T2DM	P 2
	SAR7226 (SGLT1/2 inhibitor)	Sanofi-aventis	T2DM	P 1
	TA-7284 (canagliflozin)	Johnson & Johnson	T2DM	P 1
	YM543	Astellas Pharma US	T2DM	P 2
Sirtuin-1 activator	SRT-2104 (resveretrol analogue)	Sirtris Pharmaceuticals	T2DM	P 1
Sweetener	Naturlose (tagatose)	Spherix	T2DM	P 3
Synthetic steroid	HE-3286 (synthetic steroid)	Hollis-Eden Pharma	T2DM	P 2
TGR5 agonist	INT-777	InteKrin Therapeutics	T2DM	P 2
Tyrosine phosphatase inhibitor	ISIS 113715(tyrosine phosphatase inhibitor)	Isis Pharmaceuticals	T2DM (combo Rx)	P 2
	Trodusquemine (MSI-1436)	Genaera	T2DM	P 1
Vanadium	AKP-020 (vanadium compound)	Akesis Pharmaceuticals	T2DM	P 2

glucose lowering. Therefore, the meal excursions of glucose will be lost into the urine, making dietary restrictions of carbohydrate less important. Beyond antiglycaemia, SGLT2 inhibitors also reduce insulin levels and hepatic steatosis and improve β-cell function. In clinical trials, these drugs have shown a low risk of hypoglycaemia, measurable weight loss and reduced blood pressure.[27] On the other hand, an increase in genito-urinary infections has been noted. Future studies should help to resolve potential safety issues, including fluid and electrolyte imbalances and long-term renal function.

Insulin analogues and new delivery approaches: God did not make human insulin to be injected subcutaneously

The direction of insulin development is to be longer, faster and easier. We will not discuss advances in closed-loop patch pump therapies since those are primarily for T1DM. Insulin therapies have not been shown to reduce CVD or slow the progression of T2DM. Perhaps that is because insulin therapy is started very late in the course of the disease. To test whether earlier initiation of insulin therapy will address these problems, the Outcome Reduction with an Initial Glargine Intervention (ORIGIN) trial will start newly diagnosed T2DM and IGT patients on glargine insulin. The results of CVD reduction and T2DM progression are pending.

Basal insulin

SIBA (soluble insulin basal analogue, degludec) is a modified detemir molecule with a very flat, smooth-action profile lasting more than 24 h. It has the potential for thrice weekly dosing. Unlike current basal insulins, degludec can be mixed with a rapid-acting insulin to give basal/bolus therapy in one injection.

Table 102.7 Emerging antiglycaemics and their selected characteristics[a].

Class	Insulin levels	Insulin sensitivity	β-Cell	Glucose	Hypo	BW	RF	Comments
Dual PPAR agonist	↔	↑	↑	0	↔	↑	↓	Some have cardiac or renal toxicity
SGLT2 inhibitors	↔	?	↑	↓	↔	↔	↓	Genitourinary infections
Insulin analogues	↑	↔	?	↓	↑	↑	↔	Earlier insulin Rx may be needed to see benefits
Glucokinase agonists	↑	↔	↑	↓	↑	?	?	Hypos and collateral organ adverse events are of concern
FBPase inhibitors	?	?	?	↓	↔	?	?	Metformin-like with less lactate production
GPR119 agonists	↑	↔	↑	↓	↔	↓	?	Action may be augmented with DPP4I
TGR5 agonists	↑	↔	↑	↓	↔	↓	?	↑energy expenditure in brown fat and muscle
FABR agonists	↑	↔	?	↓	↔	?	?	Concern about lipotoxicity in β-cells
DGAT inhibitors	↔	↑	?	?	?	↓	?	Hepatic steatosis ↓
11BHSD inhibitors	?	?	?	?	?	?	?	Clinical studies have shown little efficacy
Oxyntomodulin analogues	↑	↔	?	↓	↔	↓	?	Combined GLP-1 and glucagon actions
SRBP inhibitor	?	↑	?	↓	?	↓	?	Concern about ↓ hepatic LDL receptor
Bariatric surgery	↑	↔	↑	↓	↔	↓	↓	↓in CVD and mortality demonstrated

[a]β-Cell = β-cell function or mass; Glucose = blood glucose levels; Hypo = hypoglycaemia; BW = body weight; RF = CVD risk factors.

Bolus insulin

VIAject is a formulation of human insulin which has been disassociated into the monomers by the addition of EDTA and citric acid. Pharmacokinetic data demonstrate a faster onset of action than lispro insulin.

New delivery approaches

Buccal, oral and dermal insulins have been under development for some time without much reported success. Nasal and inhaled insulins have been reported to have better absorption rates, but a previously approved inhaled insulin (Exubera) was taken off the market by its manufacturer (Pfizer) owing to poor sales. Before Exubera left the market, however, the FDA required labelling to include a warning for smokers about the risk for lung cancer.

Glucokinase activators: targeting two organs–pancreas and liver – with one pill

Glucokinase activators (GKAs) are a new class of T2DM drugs which target both the pancreas and liver. Glucokinase (GK) is an enzyme that catalyses the phosphorylation of glucose an important step in regulating glucose metabolism. In the β-cell GK activity serves as a glucose sensor for insulin release and in the liver it regulates glycogen production. The activity of this enzyme is regulated endogenously by regulatory proteins. GK activation by these proteins causes the β-cells and hepatocytes to 'sense glucose', thus releasing insulin and taking up glucose to make glycogen, respectively.

Pharmacological GK activation has been an attractive target for T2DM because it addresses two fundamental defects in T2DM: decreased insulin secretion and increased hepatic glucose output. GKA may also decrease β-cell failure, another problem in T2DM.[28]

Several GKAs undergoing clinical testing show efficacy in controlling both FPG and PPG and with other antiglycaemics, including insulin sensitizers and incretin-based therapies. Several concerns need to be resolved, however, including profound hypoglycaemia (the insulin secretion is not glucose dependent), GK activation in other tissues may have untoward effects (e.g. pituitary) and augmented hepatic lipid synthesis (with steatohepatitis). It is also notable that the development of one of most advanced GKAs, Piragliatin, by Hoffman-La Roche was discontinued for undisclosed reasons. Nevertheless, this is a very promising and active area of drug development.

Fructose 1,6-bisphosphatase (FBPase) inhibitors – a metformin mimic

Inhibition of hepatic gluconeogenesis with metformin has proved to be a very successful treatment strategy for T2DM. FBPase is a key enzyme in gluconeogenesis and it has an inhibitory AMP-binding site which is a therapeutic target. AMP mimetics which produce FBPase inhibition should have many of the same efficacy attributes as metformin. One candidate, MB07803 monotherapy, in recent T2DM clinical trials resulted in rapid and pronounced fasting and postprandial glucose lowering. This drug has less effect on lactate metabolism and acid–base balance, which have been problems with earlier compounds.

Antiglycaemic therapies that evolved from G protein-coupled receptor (GPCR) 'orphans'

The discovery of many orphan GPCRs resulted from identifying genes with sequence similarity from large genomic data pools. They were orphans because the ligand for the receptor had not yet been discovered. Some of these orphan GPCRs were involved in glucose and lipid metabolism. Subsequent discovery of their ligands, a strategy called 'deorphanization', has had an impact on drug discovery for T2DM – including a few discussed below: the bile acid-binding receptor TGR5, the fatty acid-binding receptors GPR40 and GPR120 and the glucose-dependent insulinotrophic receptor GPR119.

GPR119 agonists: this orphan has been adopted

GPR119 is a deorphanized GPCR located on β-cells of the pancreas, GLP-1-producing L-cells of the intestine and incretin-producing K-cells of the stomach. Although GPR119's physiological ligand is still uncertain, pharmacological agonists have been found which will produce glucose-dependent insulin secretion both directly and via GLP-1 and other incretins. Animal studies demonstrate glucose lowering, delayed gastric emptying, reduction of body weight, decreased glucagon secretion and preservation of β-cell loss. These effects can be augmented by concomitant DPP4 inhibition.

TGR5 (bile acid receptor) agonists: lower the glucose and raise the heat

Bile acids were once thought of as simple detergents to help with digestion. New evidence, however, points to bile acids as potent hormones helping to regulate body metabolism and glucose homeostasis. Bile acids appear to function as nutrient signalling molecules when they return from the intestines to the liver following a meal. Bile acids bind to several receptors, including the GPCR TGR5, which increases the conversion of the thyroid hormone T4 to its active product T3 and in the gut stimulates GLP-1 secretion. The conversion of T4 to T3 is intracellular in brown fat and muscle and T3 does not enter the circulation, thereby avoiding a state of hyperthyroidism.

The dual antiglycaemic and hypermetabolic actions of TGR5 could complement each other in T2DM therapy. TGR5 agonists have been synthesized with this idea in mind.[29] In animal studies, INT-777, a TGR5 agonist, has been shown to stimulate GLP-1 levels, improve glucose tolerance, protect pancreatic islets and reduce hepatic steatosis and obesity on a high-fat diet. Preliminary data suggest that this class of drugs will be useful in obese T2DM patients.

Fatty acid-binding receptor (FABR) agonists trick the body into thinking you have just been to McDonalds

Fatty acids are part of an important nutrient signalling pathway which modulates the metabolic effects of food intake. FABR agonists use this strategy to 'trick' the body into thinking it has just eaten a fat-laden meal. The FABR responds to this perception of gastronomic gluttony by initiating a cascade of physiological events, including activation of the incretin system and secretion of insulin from the pancreas and leptin from the adipocytes.

Two FABRs are potential therapeutic targets, GPR40 and GPR120.[30] Both are deorphanized GPCRs with medium- and long-chain fatty acids as their ligands. GPR40 is of most interest since it is expressed on pancreatic β-cells and in the presence of glucose will amplify insulin secretion. A number of GPR40 agonists are currently being evaluated for T2DM therapy. One of these compounds, P-1736 (Piramal Life Sciences), is being tested in humans. One unresolved controversy, however, is whether GPR40 may also be responsible for the β-cell lipotoxicity produced by a chronic high-fat diet.

GPR120 is less well studied than GPR40. GPR120 is expressed in enteroendocrine cells which secrete GLP-1 and cholecystokinin. This receptor also has a role in adipogenesis and in inhibiting bone resorption. Further studies will be needed to define its role in T2DM, obesity and bone metabolism.

Anti-obesity therapies for 'diabesity'

The term 'diabesity' is a description for T2DM caused by excessive weight – the condition of having both diabetes and excessive weight. Many of the drugs that target obesity are antiglycaemic and benefit T2DM. We review some of these developing therapies.

Bariatric surgery

Bariatric surgery is unquestionably the most efficacious therapy for T2DM. Results show reductions in CVD, mortality, β-cell failure and glucose levels. In fact, the blood glucose normalizes in the majority of surgery patients for up to 2 years. Interestingly, the type of procedure may make a difference. The Roux-en-Y gives better antiglycaemia results than gastric banding, perhaps because the Roux-en-Y expedites nutrient supply to the distal small intestine. This results in increased incretin secretion. Evidence for a possible incretin mechanism is that many patients become euglycaemic well before the weight loss. Furthermore, some of these patients go on to develop β-cell hyperplasia (nesidioblastosis), resulting in hyperinsulinaemic hypoglycaemia and requiring partial pancreatectomy. Further investigations on the mechanisms of bariatric surgery may lead to new therapeutic opportunities for T2DM.

Diacylglycerol acyltransferase (DGAT) inhibitors

DGAT catalyses the last step in triglyceride synthesis. When this enzyme is inhibited, body weight decreases due to increased energy expenditure, insulin levels decrease and hepatic steatosis is reduced. DGAT1 inhibitor studies have not been reported for T2DM, but the weight loss and increased insulin sensitivity are therapeutically promising.

11β-Hydroxysteroid dehydrogenase-1 (11BHSD) inhibitors

T2DM manifest many of the key features in Cushing syndrome, including adiposity, insulin resistance, dyslipidaemia and hypertension. 11BHSD converts inactive cortisone to cortisol in peripheral tissues and inhibition of this enzyme should reduce cellular cortisol activity. Therefore, 11BHSD inhibitors have been given to T2DM patients to examine the benefits of lowering cellular cortisol activity. To date, the theory has advanced beyond reality. The results so far show only a modest reduction in glucose with no other benefits. Further studies with other inhibitors are needed to evaluate this drug class fully.

Oxyntomodulin analogues with dual GLP-1 and glucagon activity

Oxyntomodulin is produced from the L-cells of the distal small bowel, the same cells that also produce GLP-1. This incretin combines GLP-1's antiglycaemia action and weight loss with glucagon's lipolytic activity and weight loss. GLP-1's glucose-lowering offsets the glucagon's hyperglycaemia and the weight loss benefits are additive. In order to augment oxyntomodulin's activity, pegylated forms have been produced to prolong stability and activity. Combinations of GLP-1 secretogogues and DPP4 inhibition, which promote the release and prolong the activity of oxyntomodulin, may also be pharmacological approaches.

Sterol-regulating element-binding protein inhibitor – fatostatin

Many of the lipogenic enzymes are encoded by genes regulated by sterol regulatory element-binding proteins (SREBPs). An inhibitor of these transcription, fatostatin, produces reductions in body weight, visceral adiposity and blood glucose in animals.

Endocannabinoid receptor (CB1) antagonists – may also prevent the 'marijuana munchies'

Endocannabinoid receptors bind both the psychoactive drug in marijuana (cannabis) and also endogenous ligands to produce a variety of physiological processes involved in memory, mood and appetite. Blocking the receptor suppresses appetite, producing reductions in body weight, lipids, blood pressure and glycaemia. Although one CB1 inhibitor (rimonabant) was initially approved for use in Europe, reports of severe depression led to withdrawal from the market and discontinuation of development. It is unlikely that other drugs in this class will continue development.

Lorcaserin (serotonin agonist) – Redux all over again?

Lorcaserin (APD-356) is a serotonergic weight-loss drug developed by Arena Pharmaceuticals that is pending drug approval by the FDA. A previous serotonergic agonist, dexfenfluramine (Redux), which was considered very efficacious, was taken off the market, however, because of its association with valvular cardiac lesions. Echocardiogram studies of lorcaserin users have not shown similar cardiac problems.

Anti-obesity combos – it takes two to tango

Pramlintide and metreleptin

Amylin and leptin are secreted from the pancreas and adipocytes, respectively, and they function as satiety signals resulting in reduced food intake and weight loss. Pramlintide and metreleptin are synthetic analogues and given in combination produce more weight loss than either given alone.

Contrave (naltrexone and bupropion)

Contrave is a combination of bupropion, a dopamine and noradrenaline reuptake inhibitor, with naltrexone, an opioid antagonist used to treat various addictive disorders. These two agents are reported to synergistically block β-endorphin-mediated inhibition of POMC (pro-opiomelanocortin) neurones, leading to increased hypothalamic anorexigenic neuronal activity. They have each on their own been shown to reduce appetite and body weight and these effects are additive when the two drugs are combined.

Qnexa (phentermine and topiramate)

Qnexa is a combination of low-dose phentermine and the anticonvulsant agent topiramate. Both drugs independently produce weight loss, and the effects are additive when the drugs are combined. In addition to weight loss, lowering of blood pressure in hypertensives and antiglycaemia in T2DM patients have been reported.

Empatic (zonisamide and bupropion)

Empatic is almost like a cross between the two drugs mentioned above, Contrave and Qnexa, combining an anticonvulsant, zonisamide, and a dopamine/noradrenaline reuptake inhibitor, bupropion.

Conclusion

Given the recent explosion of T2DM in the USA, there is an urgent and tremendous need for improved antiglycaemic therapies for T2DM. Current therapies lack the ability to stop the progression of this disease or its macrovascular complications and mortality. Newer therapies will need to do more than just lower glucose. Many of the new and emerging drugs, especially in the incretin class, appear to have positive β-cell and cardiac benefits. Time will tell, however, since in the past other classes of diabetic therapies have promised but failed to deliver.

Key points

- Numerous new drugs for the treatment of diabetes are being developed.
- Anti-obesity drugs have so far been minimally effective.
- Avoidance of hypoglycaemia is a key issue in older persons.

References

1. American Diabetes Association. Standards of medical care in diabetes – 2009. *Diabetes Care* 2009;**32**(Suppl 1):S13–61.
2. Rodbard H, Jellinger PS, Davidson JA *et al.* Statement by an American Association of Clinical Endocrinologists/American College of Endocrinology consensus panel on type 2 diabetes mellitus: an algorithm for glycemic control. *Endocrine Pract* 2009;**15**:541–59.
3. Nathan DM, Buse JB, Davidson MB *et al.* Medical management of hyperglycemia in type 2 diabetes: a consensus algorithm for the initiation and adjustment of therapy: a consensus statement of the American Diabetes Association and the European Association for the Study of Diabetes. *Diabetes Care* 2009;**32**:193–203.
4. Gerstein HC, Miller ME, Byington RP *et al.* Effects of intensive glucose lowering in type 2 diabetes. *N Engl J Med* 2008; **358**:2545–59.
5. Patel A, MacMahon S, Chalmers J *et al.* Intensive blood glucose control and vascular outcomes in patients with type 2 diabetes. *N Engl J Med* 2008;**358**:2560–72.
6. Duckworth W, Abraira C, Moritz T *et al.* Glucose control and vascular complications in veterans with type 2 diabetes. *N Engl J Med* 2009;**360**:129–39.
7. Landman GW, Kleefstra N, van Hateren KJ *et al.* Metformin associated with lower cancer mortality in type 2 diabetes: ZODIAC-16. *Diabetes Care* 2010;**33**:322–6.
8. Gaede P, Lund-Andersen H, Parving HH and Pedersen O. Effect of a multifactorial intervention on mortality in type 2 diabetes. *N Engl J Med* 2008;**358**:580–91.
9. Cushman WC, Evans GW, Byington RP *et al.* Effects of intensive blood-pressure control in type 2 diabetes mellitus. *N Engl J Med* 2010;**362**:1575–85.
10. Ginsberg HN, Elam MB, Lovato LC *et al.* Effects of combination lipid therapy in type 2 diabetes mellitus. *N Engl J Med* 2010;**362**:1563–74.
11. Pignone M, Alberts MJ, Colwell JA *et al.* Aspirin for primary prevention of cardiovascular events in people with diabetes. A Position Statement of the American Diabetes Association, a Scientific Statement of the American Heart Association and an Expert Consensus Document of the American College of Cardiology Foundation. *Circulation* 2010;**121**:2694–701.
12. Khalangot M, Tronko M, Kravchenko V *et al.* Body mass index and the risk of total and cardiovascular mortality among patients with type 2 diabetes: a large prospective study in Ukraine. *Heart* 2009;**95**:454–60.
13. Risérus U, Arnlöv J, Brismar K *et al.* Sagittal abdominal diameter is a strong anthropometric marker of insulin resistance and hyperproinsulinemia in obese men. *Diabetes Care* 2004;**27**:2041–6.
14. Nissen SE and Wolski K. Effect of rosiglitazone on the risk of myocardial infarction and death from cardiovascular causes. *N Engl J Med* 2007;**356**:2457–71.
15. Bolen S, Feldman L, Vassy J *et al.* Systematic review: comparative effectiveness and safety of oral medications for type 2 diabetes mellitus. *Ann Intern Med* 2007;**147**:386–99.
16. Hadden DR. Goat's rue – French lilac – Italian fitch – Spanish sainfoin: *Gallega officinalis* and metformin: the Edinburgh connection. *J R Coll Physicians Edinb* 2005;**35**: 258–60.
17. Chong CR and Chabner BA. Mysterious metformin. *Oncologist* 2009;**14**:1178–81.
18. Holman RR, Haffner SM, McMurray JJ *et al.* Effect of nateglinide on the incidence of diabetes and cardiovascular events. *N Engl J Med* 2010;**362**:1463–76.
19. Zinman B, Harris SB, Neuman J *et al.* Low-dose combination therapy with rosiglitazone and metformin to prevent type 2 diabetes mellitus (CANOE trial): a double-blind randomised controlled study. *Lancet* 2010;**376**:103–11.
20. Fonseca VA, Rosenstock J, Wang AC *et al.* Colesevelam HCl improves glycemic control and reduces LDL cholesterol in patients with inadequately controlled type 2 diabetes on sulfonylurea-based therapy. *Diabetes Care* 2008;**31**:1479–84.
21. Scranton R and Cincotta A. Bromocriptine – unique formulation of a dopamine agonist for the treatment of type 2 diabetes. *Expert Opin Pharmacother* 2010;**11**:269–79.
22. Peters A. Incretin-based therapies: review of current clinical trial data. *Am J Med* 2010;**123**:S28–37.
23. Frederich R, Alexander JH, Fiedorek FT *et al.* A systematic assessment of cardiovascular outcomes in the saxagliptin

drug development program for type 2 diabetes. *Postgrad Med* 2010;**122**(3): 16–27.

24. Brown NJ, Byiers S, Carr D *et al.* Dipeptidyl peptidase-IV inhibitor use associated with increased risk of ACE inhibitor-associated angioedema. *Hypertension* 2009;**54**:516–23.

25. Balakumar P, Rose M, Ganti SS *et al.* PPAR dual agonists: are they opening Pandora's Box? *Pharmacol Res* 2007;**56**:91–8.

26. Goodyear LJ. The exercise pill – too good to be true? *N Engl J Med* 2008;**359**:1842–4.

27. Bakris GL, Fonseca VA, Sharma K and Wright EM. Renal sodium–glucose transport: role in diabetes mellitus and potential clinical implications. *Kidney Int* 2009;**75**:1272–7.

28. Matschinsky FM. Assessing the potential of glucokinase activators in diabetes therapy. *Nat Rev Drug Discov* 2009;**8**: 399–416.

29. Tiwari A and Maiti P. TGR5: an emerging bile acid G-protein-coupled receptor target for the potential treatment of metabolic disorders. *Drug Discov Today* 2009;**14**:523–30.

30. Hara T, Hirasawa A, Sun Q *et al.* Novel selective ligands for free fatty acid receptors, GPR120 and GPR40. *Naunyn Schmiedebergs Arch Pharmacol* 2009;**380**:247–55.

SECTION 11

Urogenital Disorders

CHAPTER 103

Gynaecology and the older patient[1]

Radha Indusekhar, Fidelma O'Mahony and P.M Shaughn O'Brien
University Hospital of North Staffordshire, Stoke-on-Trent, UK

Introduction

The ageing population presents a major challenge for the society and the health services worldwide. It is a reflection of longer life expectancy because of improvements in living standards and healthcare and falling mortality. In the United Kingdom, people aged 60 and above had outnumbered children under 16 (21% compared to 20%). By 2026, nearly 28% of the UK population will be over the age of 60.[2] Women constitute a majority of the elderly population as they outlive males by 5–7 years. Sixty-five years is the accepted starting point of old age, that is, the official retirement age (at time of writing) in the Western world. Female ageing is unique in that it represents a combination of the ageing processes and hormone deficiency. This chapter reviews the problems of the old-age gynaecology patient with reference to the common symptomatology, the menopause, hormone replacement therapy, sexuality and malignancies.

Effect of ageing on the genital tract

Vulva and vagina

The lower genital tract undergoes atrophic changes with loss of connective tissue elasticity and thinning of the mucosa. There is a decline in intracellular glycogen production in the vagina, leading to a decrease in lactobacillae and lactic acid and an increase in the vaginal pH from acid to alkaline. These changes lead to an increase in colonization by pathogenic bacteria and infective vaginitis. Senile or atrophic vaginitis is also common due to loss of vaginal tissue elasticity and shrinkage of the vagina with subsequent loss of lubrication. This can lead to postmenopausal bleeding and dyspareunia.

Cervix and uterus

The cervix becomes atrophic and the ectocervix becomes flush with the vaginal vault. The squamocolumnar junction of the cervix recedes into the endocervical canal and it becomes difficult to obtain an accurate representative cervical smear. The uterus undergoes atrophy of myometrium and the uterine body becomes smaller. The endometrium becomes thinner and the glands become inactive.

Ovary and fallopian tube

In the perimenopausal years, the few remaining primordial follicles become unresponsive to the pituitary gonadotrophins and therefore the estrogen secretion falls. The ovaries become smaller and more wrinkled in appearance. The fallopian tubes become shorter with muscle replaced by fibrous tissue.

Pelvic floor

Pelvic floor muscle weakness is due to the combined effects of estrogen withdrawal and age. This is compounded by the mechanical effects of previous childbirth. The endopelvic fascia surrounding both the genital tract and urinary tract atrophies. The fascial condensations of cardinal and uterosacral ligaments also atrophy, leading to an increased incidence of genital prolapse as age increases. In the elderly, chronic cough, constipation and increased intra-abdominal pressure are other factors contributing to this.

Urethra and bladder

Both the urethra and trigone of the bladder are sensitive to estrogen as they have estrogen receptors and there is deterioration in structure and function as a woman ages.

[1]This chapter is based in part on the chapter 'Gynaecology' by Jarmila Wiener and Joan Andrews, which appeared in *Principles and Practice of Geriatric Medicine*, 3rd Edition.

Principles and Practice of Geriatric Medicine, Fifth Edition. Edited by Alan J. Sinclair, John E. Morley and Bruno Vellas.

The urethral lumen becomes more slit shaped and the folds become coarser. The mucosal lining changes from transitional in the proximal two-thirds to non-keratinizing squamous epithelium.[2] Urethral closure becomes less competent. There is a reduction in detrusor contraction power during voiding and the contractions fade shortly after initiation of voiding. Bladder capacity is also reduced in the elderly. All these features contribute to the greater prevalence of urinary incontinence in elderly women. Estrogen withdrawal may also lead to a high prevalence of urinary tract infection in the elderly, which is aggravated by voiding difficulty and may lead to stress incontinence, urge incontinence, frequency, urgency and nocturia.[3]

Hormonal changes

In premenopausal women, ovarian function is controlled by the two pituitary gonadotrophins, follicle stimulating hormone (FSH) and luteinizing hormone (LH). These are controlled by the pulsastile secretion of gonadotrophin releasing hormone (GnRH) from the hypothalamus. The ovary has the maximum number of oocytes at 20–28weeks of intrauterine life. There is a reduction in these cells from mid-gestation onwards and the oocyte stock becomes exhausted in the perimenopausal age group. The ovary gradually becomes less responsive to gonadotrophins resulting in a gradual increase in FSH and LH levels, and a fall in estradiol concentration. As ovarian unresponsiveness becomes more marked, cycles tend to become anovulatory and complete failure of follicular development occurs. Estradiol production from the granulosa and theca cells of the ovary ceases and there is insufficient estradiol to stimulate the endometrium; amenorrhoea ensues. FSH and LH levels are persistently elevated. FSH level >30 IU l^{-1} is generally considered to be the postmenopausal range

The menopause and HRT (hormone replacement therapy)

Menopause is defined as the permanent cessation of menstruation. The word menopause is derived from the Greek words *menos* (the month) and *pausos* (ending). It is a retrospective diagnosis since a woman is menopausal only after 12 months of amenorrhoea. The average age of menopause is 51 years and the female life expectancy is now over 80 years. Postmenopausal women spend more than 30 years in a profound estrogen-deficient state. The early symptoms of menopause are vasomotor symptoms, principally hot flushes, night sweats and insomnia. The long-term consequences are osteoporosis, urogenital atrophy, cardiovascular disease and connective tissue atrophy.

Vasomotor symptoms

There is good evidence from randomized placebo-controlled studies that estrogen is effective in treating hot flushes and improvement is noted within four weeks.[4] Relief of vasomotor symptoms is the commonest indication for HRT and current recommendations for the duration of use is for up to five years. In general, as old age approaches, the symptoms of the menopause appear to resolve spontaneously, though of course, the risk of osteoporosis increases. However, there are a small proportion of women whose menopausal symptoms (hot flushes in particular) last well into later life. Since non-hormonal treatments for hot flushes are universally ineffective management of this group can be a challenging problem. There is subsequently a small group of women who request HRT well beyond the five years normally recommended.

Osteoporosis

Osteoporosis has been defined by the World Health Organization (WHO) as a 'disease characterized by low bone mass and micro-architectural deterioration of bone tissues, leading to enhanced bone fragility and a consequent increase in fracture risk'. In postmenopausal women, there is accelerated bone loss, so that by the age of 70 years, 50% of bone mass is lost. The risk factors for osteoporosis include family history, low BMI, cigarette smoking, alcohol abuse, early menopause, sedentary lifestyle, corticosteroids. Fractures are the clinical consequences of osteoporosis. The most common sites of osteoporotic fractures are the distal forearm (wrist or Colles fracture), proximal femur and vertebrae. Vertebral fractures lead to loss of height and curvature of the spine with typical dorsal kyphosis ('Dowager's hump'). This affects their overall QOL and may ultimately impair respiratory function. There is evidence from randomized controlled trials that HRT reduces the risk of osteoporotic fractures.[5,6] However, recent advice from regulatory authorities has been that HRT should not be used for osteoporosis prevention as the risks of such treatment outweigh the benefits.[7] After the publication of the Million Women study in 2003, the Committee on Safety of Medicines (CSM) pronounced that HRT was no longer to be considered as first-line therapy for the prevention of osteoporosis. Bisphosphonates may be the best choice for the over 60s, though there is actually less data on long-term safety.

Urogenital symptoms

Symptoms such as vaginal dryness, soreness, superficial dyspareunia and urinary frequency and urgency respond well to local estrogen, in the form of pessaries, rings and tablets. Estradiol tablets (Vagifem® Novo Nordisk) are associated with minimal or no systemic absorption. In light of this it is believed that long-term use of Vagifem is safe in contrast with other vaginal estradiol preparations. However, there is currently no clear evidence to support its long-term safety,

Risks of HRT

Breast cancer

HRT appears to confer a similar degree of risk as that associated with late natural menopause. In absolute terms, the excess risk in the Women's Health Initiative (WHI) study with continuous combined HRT at 50–59 years was 5; 60–69 years, 8; and 70–79 years, 13 cases of breast cancer per 10 000 women per year.[8] The unopposed estrogen-only arm of this study did not show any evidence of an excess increase in breast cancer risk. The Million Women study found an increased risk with all HRT regimens, the greatest degree of risk was with combined HRT.[9] So the addition of progestogen increases breast cancer risk compared with estrogen alone but this has to be balanced against the reduction in risk of endometrial cancer provided by combined therapy.[8,10] Irrespective of the type of HRT prescribed, breast cancer risk falls after cessation of use, risk being no greater than that in women who have never been exposed to HRT by five years.

Endometrial cancer

Unopposed estrogen replacement therapy increases endometrial cancer risk. Most studies have shown that this excess risk is not completely eliminated with monthly sequential progestogen addition especially when continued for more than five years. No increase has been found with continuous combined regimens.[11] Administration of the progestogen by the intrauterine route (Mirena® (levanorgestrol-releasing system)) would seem to have the benefit of maximal endometrial dose with low systemic effects.

Venous thromboembolism

HRT increases risk of venous thromboembolism (VTE) twofold with the highest risk occurring in the first year of use. Advancing age and obesity significantly increase this risk. The absolute rate increase is 1.5 VTE events per 10 000 women in one year. This risk is lower with transdermal estradiol compared to oral due to avoiding the first pass metabolism effect in the hepatic circulation.

Cardiovascular disease (coronary heart disease and stroke)

The role of HRT either in primary or secondary prevention of cardiovascular disease remains uncertain and so it should not be used primarily for this indication. The WHI study showed an early transient increase in coronary events. The excess absolute risk at 50–59 years was 4; 60–69 years, 9; and 70–79 years, 13 cases of stroke per 10 000 women per year. However, the timing, dose, and possibly type of HRT may be crucial in determining cardiovascular effects. In hypertensive patients it is recommended that once the blood pressure is under control estrogen can be given. Therefore, HRT should currently not be prescribed solely for possible prevention of cardiovascular disease. The merits of long-term use of HRT need to be assessed for each woman at regular intervals. It should be targeted to the individual woman's needs.

Alzheimer's disease

While estrogen may delay or reduce the risk of Alzheimer's disease, it does not seem to improve established disease. WHI study found a twofold increased risk of dementia in women receiving the particular combined estrogen and progestogen regimen. However, this risk was only significant in the group of women over 75 years of age. More evidence is required before definitive advice can be given in relation to Alzheimer's disease.

Common symptoms in the elderly

Older women are often reluctant to approach their practitioners due to embarrassment when they suffer from the symptoms as in Table 103.1.

Postmenopausal bleeding (PMB)

Postmenopausal bleeding is defined as bleeding from the genital tract after one year of amenorrhoea. A woman not taking HRT who bleeds after the menopause has a 10% risk of having a genital cancer'.[12] In the vast majority of cases, the cause is benign, mainly atrophic vaginitis. The causes are as in Table 103.2.

Diagnosis

History should include the symptoms, drug history and smear history. Assessment may be difficult in an elderly patient and is frequently complicated by dementia, immobility, obesity and arthritis. A thorough examination including BMI, abdominal examination for masses, pelvic examination including speculum and bimanual examination should be carried out.

Investigation

The principal aim of investigation is to exclude the possibility of cancer. Transvaginal ultrasound measurement

Table 103.1 Common symptoms in the elderly.

Postmenopausal bleeding
Discharge per vagina
Pelvic mass
Prolapse
Urinary incontinence
Vulval soreness or itching
Vulval pain
Vulval swelling

Table 103.2 Causes of postmenopausal bleeding.

Atrophic – Senile vaginitis
  Decubitus ulcer from a prolapse

Neoplasia – Endometrial cancer
  Cervical cancer, vaginal cancer
  Vulval cancer, estrogen-secreting tumours, ovarian tumours
  Fallopian tube cancer, secondary deposits
  Endometrial polyps

Iatrogenic – Bleeding on HRT
  Bleeding on tamoxifen
  Local ulceration due to Ring, shelf pessary

Infection – Vaginal, endometrial
Others – Haematuria, rectal bleeding, trauma, foreign body

of endometrial thickness will help in directing the need for an endometrial biopsy. An endometrial thickness of less than 5 mm is reassuring that the cavity is empty. The myometrium and ovaries can also be visualized for evidence of tumours. Hysteroscopy and endometrial biopsy is now the 'gold standard' investigation for postmenopausal bleeding. Increasingly this procedure is carried out under local anaesthetic in the outpatient setting. In some cases technical difficulties such as cervical stenosis associated with atrophic change may require a general anaesthetic. A full assessment will include cystoscopy and sigmoidoscopy if there is any doubt concerning the source of the bleeding.

Treatment

Treatment depends on the cause of the bleeding. If atrophic vaginitis is diagnosed treatment is by local estrogen therapy. Where ulceration is caused by a pessary, removal of the pessary until the area has healed is the correct course of action. A course of vaginal estrogen is often helpful in preventing further ulceration. In cases of procidenta with decubitus ulceration the woman may have to be admitted to hospital for vaginal estrogen packs and urinary catheterization. Where a malignancy is suspected or diagnosed management is in a multidisciplinary forum in accordance with local and national Cancer Network Guidelines.

Table 103.3 Causes of discharge per vagina.

Atrophic – Postmenopausal vaginitis
Infective – Bacterial vaginosis, trichomoniasis, Chlamydia, gonorrhoea
Tumours – Cervical polyp, intrauterine polyp
  Cervical cancer, endometrial cancer,
  Fallopian tube cancer – rare

Fistulae – Vesicovaginal fistula, rectovaginal fistula
Pyometra – associated with carcinoma of the endometrium
Others – foreign body, pessary

Discharge per vagina

Vaginal discharge is a common gynaecological complaint seen in the elderly. The causes are as in Table 103.3. Owing to the loss of vaginal tissue elasticity and shrinkage of the vagina, atrophic vaginitis is very common. Infective vaginitis is also common due to colonization by pathogenic bacteria when the vaginal pH shifts from acid to alkali. In addition sexually transmitted infections are increasing in prevalence in the older population.

Uterovaginal prolapse

Uterovaginal prolapse is a herniation of the female genital tract. It is extremely common with an estimated 11% of women undergoing at least one operation for this condition. The aetiology is multifactorial but the principle factors responsible for the development of prolapse are damage occurring during pregnancy and childbirth along with weakening of fascia and muscle support following the menopause. Raised intra-abdominal pressure due to obesity, chronic constipation or cough is also a major contributory factor. Finally loss of suspensory support following hysterectomy or a congenital predisposition are other significant causes of prolapse. Due to a shared aetiology uterovaginal prolapse is commonly associated with urinary incontinence.

Classification

1 Anterior vaginal wall prolapse
  i Urethrocele – Urethral descent
  ii Cystocele – Bladder descent
  iii Cystourethrocele – Descent of bladder and urethra
2 Posterior vaginal wall prolapse
  i Rectocele – Rectal descent
  ii Enterocele – Small bowel descent
3 Apical vaginal prolapse
  i Uterovaginal – Uterine descent with inversion of vaginal apex
  ii Vault – Post hysterectomy inversion of vaginal apex

Diagnosis

Most commonly, the presenting symptom is a feeling of a lump coming down the vagina. Women also present with a dragging or bearing down sensation of gradual onset which is worse with activity and settles with rest. A minor prolapse may become symptomatic in the presence of marked atrophic vaginitis. Atrophic ulceration may occur with discharge and bleeding. Urinary symptoms such as frequency, urgency, incontinence, incomplete, or slow emptying result from distortion of the prolapsed bladder and urethra. Digital replacement of the anterior or posterior vaginal wall is sometimes necessary before micturition or defecation respectively.

A detailed obstetric history to identify causative factors and a comprehensive medical history to assess co-morbidities, which may have an aetiological role such as constipation or cough, is essential. A detailed social history to assess QOL must be taken and most importantly a sexual history to assess the desire for future sexual function is central to planning management.

General examination: To assess if surgery is safe, to check BMI, and cardio-respiratory system examination.

Abdominal examination: Looking for pelvic masses.

Pelvic examination: Prolapse may be obvious when examining the patient in the dorsal position if it protrudes beyond the introitus, ulceration and/or atrophy may be apparent. The anterior and posterior vaginal walls and cervical descent should be assessed with the patient in the left lateral position, using a firm Sims speculum. Combined rectal and vaginal digital examination can be an aid to differentiate rectocele from enterocele. Vaginal examination should be performed and pelvic mass excluded. Urine culture and sensitivity, cystometry and cystoscopy to be considered when symptoms include both stress and urge incontinence and especially prior to consideration of surgery.

Management

The management of prolapse depends on the severity of symptoms, the degree of incapacity and the patient's operative fitness. Operative treatment by repair of prolapse with or without vaginal hysterectomy is most effective. Obesity, heavy smoking and constipation require improvement before surgery. Most patients tolerate surgery very well because of improved anaesthetics and minimal post-operative morbidity. When such surgery is undertaken in an older woman, it is important to ascertain the level of sexual activity as this will influence the degree of narrowing achieved by surgery. Age *per se* is not a contraindication to surgery. Medical disorders develop with advanced age and these dictate any reasons for avoiding anaesthesia.

When surgery is contraindicated or declined, conservative methods may be used. A polyvinyl ring pessary will be successful, providing there is adequate perineum to retain the pessary. Some patients, particularly those with large prolapses and very little perineum, may do better with a shelf pessary. Either type needs changing at 4–6 month intervals and the vagina should be inspected to ensure no ulceration has occurred. If ulceration occurs, the pessary should be removed for a few weeks and local estrogen used daily to allow epithelial healing.

Physiotherapy: Pelvic floor exercises are useful for the prevention and improvement of incontinence. But they require good patient motivation. Physiotherapy may improve symptoms from a small prolapse but it is unlikely to help with a greater degree of herniation.

Urinary incontinence

Urinary incontinence is defined as the involuntary loss of urine that is objectively demonstrable and is a social or hygiene problem. The causes are as in Table 103.4. The prevalence increases with age, with approximately 10% of those aged between 45 and 64 years of age being affected, rising to 20% of those greater than 65 years. It is even higher in women who are institutionalized and may affect up to 40% of those in residential nursing homes. This places huge financial demands on health resources, with 2% of the total budget being spent on incontinence services alone. Many women will not seek advice because of embarrassment.

Uninhibited detrusor muscle contractions are usually the cause in geriatric patients owing to age-related changes in the central nervous system. Genuine stress incontinence (GSI) occurs when the bladder pressure exceeds the maximum urethral pressure in the absence of any detrusor contraction and this is common in the early postmenopausal years. In many women, the two conditions exist together.

Assessment

A good history will help to differentiate GSI from detrusor instability to some extent. Examination to rule out any associated prolapse or pelvic mass should be carried out in

Table 103.4 Causes of urinary incontinence.

1. Genuine/urodynamic stress incontinence – Bladder neck hypermobility, urethral sphincter weakness
2. Detrusor instability – Idiopathic, secondary to neurological disease – hyperreflexia
3. Retention with overflow – Motor neurone lesions, drugs, pelvic mass, severe prolapse
4. Fistulae – Ureteric, vesical, urethral
5. Miscellaneous – Urinary infection

these patients. Urodynamic studies are necessary to confirm the diagnosis, especially prior to any surgical treatment.

Management

Simple measures like exclusion of urinary tract infection, restriction of fluid intake, modifying medication like diuretics when possible, play an important role in the management of urinary incontinence.

Genuine stress incontinence (GSI)

Conservative management: The treatment of GSI should be non-operative initially, and the best results for mild/moderate leakage are with pelvic floor exercises. The rationale behind pelvic floor education is the reinforcement of cortical awareness of the levator ani muscle group, hypertrophy of existing fibres and a general increase in muscle tone and strength. Motivation and good compliance are the key factors associated with success. Local estrogen therapy may have a small effect by improving the urethral mucosa in women with estrogen deficiency.

Surgical management – the aims of surgery:

- Restoration of the proximal urethra and bladder neck to the zone of intra-abdominal pressure transmission
- To increase urethral resistance.

The procedures are vaginal tapes (TVT, TOT), periurethral bulking using collagen, macroplastique.

Detrusor instability (DI)

DI can be treated by bladder retraining and biofeedback, all of which tend to increase the interval between voids and inhibit the symptoms of urgency. Drug treatment is mainly by anticholinergics like oxybutynin, tolteridine, regurin combined with local estrogen.

Sexuality and old age

In the past, it was mistakenly assumed that a woman well past the menopause will not be sexually active. In 1953, Kinsey *et al.* described reduced sexual activity in elderly women. In this group of women, orgasm was more likely to be achieved by masturbation than by coitus.[13] In fact, sexual drive is not exhausted with ageing, and as life expectancy increases it is necessary to recognize that continued sexual activity is an important requirement to promote satisfactory relationships, personal well-being and QOL.[14] Many older people grew up in sexually restricted times so that ignorance is widespread. The organization of institutions for elderly people does not recognize their sexuality, so their needs are ignored.[15] It has been proved that sexual activity remains relatively constant within a stable relationship and declines only following death or illness of the partner.[16]

Sexual response and ageing

In the elderly, the changes of vasocongestion, pudendal swelling and vaginal lubrication are reduced and delayed, and resolution occurs more rapidly. Also, vaginal lubrication diminishes and there is less vaginal elasticity leading to shrinkage of the vagina. Coital trauma to the vagina and urethra causes dyspareunia, dysuria and postmenopausal bleeding. Lesions of the vulva like lichen sclerosus (LS) and surgical scarring may make intercourse impossible for some older women.

Health factors that inhibit sexual activity in elderly people

Physical factors

- Stress incontinence
- Diminishing mobility
- Decreasing muscle tone
- Uterine prolapse
- Skin tone and sensitivity
- Diseases like diabetes and cardiovascular problems
- Chronic conditions like arthritis.

Psychological factors

- Sense of unattractiveness
- Facing mortality; depression, bereavement and grief reactions
- Loss of partner or friends
- Lack of contact with others and loneliness.

Effect of chronic illness and surgery on sexuality

Chronic urological and gynaecological conditions causing pain on intercourse, chronic anxiety and stress, neurological disorders, depression and fatigue can result in loss of sexual desire. Disfiguring and mutilating operations, especially of the breasts, genitals and reproductive organs, often have a deleterious effect on a woman's self image and sexuality. Dyspareunia can be a major problem, not only because of lack of arousal or secondary vaginismus after surgery but also because of the amount of scar tissue within the pelvis. Women who have a stoma-like colostomy or ileostomy also experience psychological problems. Patients' greatest fears are loss of control, bad odour, noise, leaking bags and their partner's feelings toward them. Healthy adaptation to a stoma depends on preoperative and postoperative counselling and understanding by stoma nurses.

Management

A detailed sexual history including the problem, the duration, the couple's past life together and emotional relationship should be taken. Early experiences, difficulties with a previous partner and any episode of sexual assault is also important. Examination should aim to look for a physical cause of the sexual problem. Behavioural techniques play an important part in the management of sexual dysfunction. Ignorance about sexuality is common. Changing negative attitudes resulting from past experiences, parental or religious influences will help. Talking to each other about sexual anxieties or needs, and discussion with a therapist increases their mutual understanding and ability to communicate.

Psychological therapy

The psychological approaches include giving accurate information, general counselling, psychosexual therapy, behavioural therapy, sexual and relationship therapy. Before any operation, it is essential to discuss with the woman, preferably with her partner, the full implications of the operation on their sexual life. This helps to minimize sexual dysfunction after the operation.

Pharmacological therapy

There is now evidence from randomized controlled studies that testosterone therapy improves sexual satisfaction and mood in surgically menopausal women treated with concurrent estrogen.[17,18] However, long-term safety data for combined estrogen-testosterone therapy are lacking, and the effects of testosterone-only therapy on such factors as plasma lipids in postmenopausal women are unknown.

The use of appropriate creams to help with vaginal soreness – such as vaginal estrogen, KY Jelly, Sylk or aromatic oils may enable a woman and her partner to enjoy sexual activity much more fully.

Vulval disorders

As the lower genital tract undergoes atrophic changes, the labia majora lose their fat and elastic tissue content and become smaller. The vulval epithelium becomes thin, leading to vulval irritation. Other symptoms are itching and soreness. The conditions affecting the vulva can be a part of a more widespread problem, such as psoriasis or conditions specific to the vulva. Vulval disorders are important because of the chronicity and severity of symptoms and the association with carcinoma. The common benign vulval disorders are as follows:

1 Lichen sclerosus
2 Squamous cell hyperplasia
3 Other dematoses
4 Vulvodynia or chronic vulval pain.

Lichen sclerosus (LS)

LS is a chronic skin condition characterized by the thinning of the epithelium with loss of keratin which frequently extends around the anus. The aetiology is uncertain, but there is an association with genetic and hormonal factors and autoimmune disease.[19] The clinical signs include pale ivory white plaques often with a crinkly atrophic surface, purpura and scarring with gradual destruction of the normal vulval architecture. Complications include narrowing of the introitus and rarely squamous cell carcinoma. Punch biopsies should be taken of any suspicious areas. Squamous cell carcinoma is more likely when there is ulceration, raised lesions or lymph node involvement. The most effective treatment is to use topical steroid ointment clobetasol propionate 0.05% plus a soap substitute.

Squamous cell hyperplasia

The skin is usually reddened with exaggerated folds. In certain areas, after rubbing, lichenification can be seen. The term squamous cell hyperplasia is applied for those women who have histological evidence for the cause.

Other dermatoses

The most common general diseases causing vulval itching or discomfort are diabetes, uraemia and liver failure. Other causes are allergic dermatitis caused by irritants such as perfumed soap, washing powder and so on. General dermatological conditions such as psoriasis, lichen planus and scabies may also affect the vulva.

Vulvodynia (vulval pain)

Vulvodynia is defined as chronic pain, discomfort or burning in the absence of a relevant skin condition. This condition is common in elderly women. The aetiology is uncertain but psychological and physical factors play a role. Depression is also a compounding factor. Treatment initially is empirical using topical steroids, anaesthetic and estrogen cream. The use of antidepressants and antiepileptic therapy should be considered for its analgesic effects. A multidisciplinary approach involving specialists in dermatology, pain relief, psychiatry and gynaecology is essential for intractable cases.

Gynaecological cancer

The most common types of gynaecological malignancies are cervical cancer, ovarian cancer, endometrial cancer and vulval cancer. Occasionally, skin cancers or sarcomas can also be found in the female genitalia.

Cervical cancer

Worldwide, cervical cancer is the most common gynaecological malignancy. The aetiological factors include multiple sexual partners, early age of coitus, human papilloma virus (HPV) 16 and 18 infection. In developed countries, there is an overall decline in incidence and mortality from cervical cancer as a result of the cervical screening programme. There is a defined premalignant stage, namely, cervical intraepithelial neoplasia – CIN1, CIN2 and CIN3. Screening for cervical cancer is by cervical smear. Liquid-based cytology and HPV testing are new developments taking place in this field. Abnormal cytological findings are an indication for further investigation by colposcopy and if necessary, directed biopsies or excision biopsy.

Approximately 500 000 new cases of cervical cancer are diagnosed each year in the world with 80% of these occurring in the less developed world.[20] More than 80% of cervical cancers are squamous cell carcinomas. The presenting symptoms are postcoital bleeding, vaginal discharge, or postmenopausal bleeding. Pain is experienced late and is due to pelvic infiltration or bony metastases. The first sign of this cancer may be obstructive renal failure from hydronephrosis due to advanced disease. On inspection, cancer of the cervix presents as an ulcer, growth, or a friable warty looking mass which bleeds on touch. As the carcinoma progresses, the mobility of the cervix is affected and the cervix eventually becomes fixed. Diagnosis is by biopsy of suspicious areas, preferably under general anaesthesia so that clinical staging can be done. Treatment for clinical invasive carcinoma of the cervix is by surgery, chemo-radiotherapy or a combination of all three. The management of gynaecological cancer patients is now mostly centralized in units staffed by gynaecological oncologists, so that all the treatment modalities can be offered to patients. In early disease confined to the cervix, then either surgery or radiotherapy may be offered since the prognosis is equally good for both. Surgery is by radical hysterectomy and pelvic node dissection, that is, Wertheim's hysterectomy. In the elderly, radiotherapy is usually offered because of the fear of surgical complications. However, a fit patient will tolerate the procedure well and age by itself should be no bar to surgery. If the disease is in a late stage, then chemo-radiotherapy is the treatment of choice. In an unfit patient with advanced disease, palliative care may be the only option.

Endometrial cancer

Carcinoma of the endometrium is considered as the gynaecological cancer with a relatively favourable prognosis because of its early presentation with postmenopausal bleeding. The median age of patients with endometrial cancer is 61 years, with 80% of women being postmenopausal. The risk factors are obesity, diabetes mellitus, hypertension, nulliparity, late menopause, unopposed estrogen therapy and prior history of polycystic ovary syndrome. The presenting symptom in the elderly is almost always postmenopausal bleeding. Late diagnosis includes pain and discharge from a pyometra. The diagnosis is by transvaginal ultrasound determination of endometrial thickness and endometrial biopsy. Outpatient hysteroscopy also may be undertaken, but if there is cervical stenosis, then hysteroscopy should be done under general anaesthesia. Early disease is treated by total abdominal hysterectomy and bilateral salpingo-oophorectomy. In a poorly differentiated tumour or if the myometrium is involved beyond the inner third, postoperative radiotherapy is given. Advanced cancers are treated with radiotherapy. Progestational agents are used for recurrent disease to control vaginal bleeding and to reduce the pain from bony metastases.

Ovarian cancer

Carcinoma of the ovary is common in developed countries. The peak incidence is in the 50–70 year age group. Ovarian cancer remains the most lethal gynaecological malignancy despite trials of many different treatment regimens to try to improve the poor prognosis. Most women present with advanced disease. There is no satisfactory screening method for ovarian neoplasia, but women with a family history of breast or ovarian cancer should be offered regular ultrasonic assessment and measurement of the tumour marker, Ca 125. This test is not sensitive or specific enough to be applied to the general population.

Ninety percent of ovarian carcinomas in older women are epithelial adenocarcinomas, but sex cord and germ cell tumours may also be seen in this age group. Also, metastases may be seen from elsewhere, particularly colon and breast. Granulosa cell tumour is the most common sex cord tumour. This produces estrogen which can cause postmenopausal bleeding due to the resulting endometrial hyperplasia.

The presenting symptoms are often vague including abdominal discomfort, swelling, malaise and weight loss. Later symptoms include abdominal pain and distension, ascites and pleural effusion. Investigations include haematological, biochemical, imaging techniques like ultrasound and CT scan. Solid areas within an ovarian cyst and ascites are strongly suggestive of malignancy. The final diagnosis is by laparotomy.

Management

The mainstay of treatment is by debulking of the tumour with bilateral salpingo-oophorectomy, total hysterectomy and omentectomy. Postoperative chemotherapy is used in all but early stages and indeed many patients will have residual disease after surgery. Radiotherapy is limited to patients with symptomatic recurrence and is used only for palliation.

Vulval cancer

Vulval cancer is a less common cancer and is most frequently seen in the 60–70 year age group. The presenting symptoms are soreness, pruritus, irritation, ulceration, lump, or bleeding. Many women present very late because of embarrassment. Ninety-five percent of vulval carcinomas are squamous cell carcinomas, but basal cell carcinoma, malignant melanoma and adenocarcinoma of the Bartholin's gland may occur rarely. Diagnosis can be confirmed only by vulval biopsy.

Management

Radical vulvectomy with bilateral groin node dissection is the treatment of choice. The common complications are wound breakdown and infection. The primary tumour is resected and separate groin node dissections are performed to improve wound healing and reduce infection. The other complications are deep vein thrombosis, osteitis pubis, secondary haemorrhage and so on. For patients unfit for surgery, wide excision of the lesion may be used as palliation. Pelvic irradiation is available for extensive nodal involvement.

HIV and old age

The majority of those infected and affected by HIV are younger adults. The ability of highly active antiretroviral therapies (HAART) to extend survival means that those infected when younger may reach older age and so an increase in numbers of older individuals living with HIV is expected. There is evidence that older individuals engage in risky sexual behaviours and are drug users, suggesting potential for HIV transmission.[21] For older women after menopause, condom use becomes unimportant, and normal ageing changes such as a decrease in vaginal lubrication and thinning vaginal walls can put them at higher risk during unprotected sexual intercourse.

Key points

Doctors often do not consider the possibility of HIV/AIDS in older patients because they do not perceive them to be at risk or they presume symptoms to be age related. As a result, many older people are diagnosed at a later stage in their infection, and many have an AIDS diagnosis the first time they become aware of their HIV infection. Older people are more likely to be diagnosed with HIV at a generally higher viral load and lower CD4+ cell count, making them more susceptible to opportunistic infections. More aggressive therapy may be required to successfully suppress the virus.

Data from the Centers for Disease Control (CDC) HIV/AIDS surveillance report showed that 11% of all AIDS cases reported in 1999 were among people aged 50 and above.[22] This percentage has remained stable since 1991. However, the CDC notes an alarming trend in that older AIDS patients had a greater increase in opportunistic infections than did younger AIDS patients. The report also says a higher proportion of people aged 50 and above died within one month of AIDS diagnosis. These deaths can be attributed to original misdiagnosis and immune systems that naturally weaken with age. These statistics seem to confirm the idea that older adults are naive about their risk of contracting HIV and their providers are not discussing that risk with them. A 1997 study of Texas doctors found that most physicians rarely or never discussed HIV and risk factors with their older patients.[23] Compounding the problem, AIDS symptoms often are more difficult to diagnose in older people because they mimic some common diseases associated with old age. Because of the stigma, it can be difficult for women to disclose their HIV status to family, friends and their community.

For these reasons, physicians should keep HIV in mind as a possibility, even with their older patients. HIV experts recommend that physicians routinely ask all patients about their sexual behaviour during the annual physical or gynaecological examination. Providers should educate the population over 50 years about possible exposures to HIV and safer sex practices.

Conclusion

Gynaecology for the elderly patient includes the whole spectrum of gynaecological disorders of which cancer, prolapse, urinary incontinence and the problems of late menopause are the most important ones. The advice given for such women changes with each decade. Of particular note is our increasing reluctance to give long-term HRT and our increasing likelihood of undertaking surgery in women who are healthy despite their age. Many women, through fear and embarrassment, avoid telling their problems to general practitioners, geriatricians, or gynaecologists and so present with long-standing disease.

Key points

- The female ageing process is unique in that it represents a combination of the ageing processes and hormone deficiency.

- Managing the menopause should be targeted to individual women's needs. The benefit of hormone replacement often outweighs the risks, provided the appropriate regimen has been instigated in terms of dose, route and combination.
- Age *per se* should not be a contraindication to surgical management for any gynaecological problem.
- There is no age limit for the expression of sexuality. The management of sexual problems should be guided by the same principles irrespective of age and condition of the patient.
- Older women, out of fear and embarrassment, neglect early symptoms of gynaecological diseases, some of which are potentially lethal.

References

1. Dening T, Barapatre C. Mental health and the ageing population. *J Br Menopause Soc* 2004;**10**:49–53.
2. Stanton SL. Gynaecology in the elderly. In: RW Shaw, WP Soutter, SL Stanton (eds), *Gynaecology*, 2nd edn, Churchill Livingstone, Edinburgh, 1997, pp. 915–9.
3. Dantas A, Kasviki-Charvati P, Papanawiotou P, Marketos S. Bacteriuria and survival in old age. *N Engl J Med* 1981;**304**: 939–43.
4. MacLennan A, Lester S, Moore V. Oral oestrogen replacement therapy versus placebo for hot flushes. *Cochrane Database Syst Rev* 2001;**1**: CD002978.
5. Cauley JA, Robbins J, Chen Z *et al*. Women's Health Initiative Investigators. Effects of estrogen plus progestin on risk of fracture and bone mineral density: the Women's Health Initiative randomised trial. *JAMA* 2003;**290**:1729–38.
6. The Women's Health Initiative Steering Committee. Effects of conjugated equine estrogen in postmenopausal women with hysterectomy: the Women's Health Initiative randomised controlled trial. *JAMA* 2004;**291**:1701–12.
7. Managing the Menopause – British Menopause Society Council. *Consensus Statement on Hormone Replacement Therapy*, June 2004.
8. Chlebowski RT, Hendrix SL, Langer RD *et al*. Influence of estrogen plus progestin on breast cancer and mammography in healthy postmenopausal women. The Women's Health Initiative randomised trial. *JAMA* 2003;**289**:3243–53.
9. Million Women Study Collaborators. Breast cancer and hormone replacement therapy in the Million Women Study. *Lancet* 2003;**362**:419–27.
10. Li CI, Malone KE, Porter PL *et al*. Relationship between long durations and different regimens of hormone replacement therapy and risk of breast cancer. *JAMA* 2003;**289**:3254–63.
11. Anderson GL, Judd HL, Kaunitz AM *et al*. Women's Health Initiative Investigators. Effects of estrogen plus progestin on gynaecologic cancer and associated diagnostic procedures: the Women's Health Initiative randomised trial. *JAMA* 2003; **290**:1739–48.
12. Gredmark T, Kvint S, Havel G, Mattsson L-A. Histopathological findings in women with postmenopausal bleeding. *BJOG* 1995;**102**:133–6.
13. Kinsey AC, Pomeroy WB, Martin CE, Gebhard PH. *Sexual Behaviour in the Human Female*, WB Saunders, Philadelphia, 1953.
14. Brown ADG, Cooper TK. Gynaecological disorders. In: *Geriatric Medicine: Women's Health, Section 2*, Churchill Livingstone, 2003, Ch. 90, pp. 1135–44.
15. White CB. Sexual interest, attitudes, knowledge and sexual history in relation to sexual behaviour in the institutionalised aged. *Arch Sex Behav* 1982;**11**:11–22.
16. George L, Weiler SJ. Sexuality in middle and late life. *Arch Gen Psychiatry* 1981;**38**:919–23.
17. Burger HG, Hailes J, Nelson J, Menelaus M. Effect of combined implants of oestradiol and testosterone on libido in postmenopausal women. *Br Med J* 1987;**294**:936–7.
18. Davis S, Rees M, Ribot J, Moufarege A. Efficacy and safety of testosterone patches for the treatment of low sexual desire in surgically menopausal women. *59th Annual Meeting of the American Society for Reproductive Medicine*, San Antonio, 11–15 October 2003.
19. Meyrick TRH, Ridley CM, McGibbon DH *et al*. Lichen sclerosis et atrophicus and autoimmunity; a study of 350 women. *Br J Dermatology* 1988;**118**:41–6.
20. CancerStats. *Cervical cancer – UK*, January 2003, Cancer Research UK, London.
21. Dougan S, Payne LJ, Brown AE *et al*. Past it? HIV and older people in England, Wales and Northern Ireland. *Epidemiol Infect* 2004;**132**:1151–60.
22. Centers for Disease Control. AIDS among persons aged greater than or equal to 50 years – United States, 1991–1996. *Morbidity and Mortality Weekly Report* 1998;**47**:21–7.
23. Skiest DJ, Keiser P. Human immunodeficiency virus infection in patients older than 50 years. A survey of primary care physicians' beliefs, practices, and knowledge. *Arch Fam Med* 1997;**6**:289–94.

CHAPTER 104

The ageing bladder

James M. Cummings and Kimberly C. Berni
University of Missouri, Columbia, MO, USA

Introduction

The increase in human life expectancy unmasked a variety of genitourinary complaints. Most physicians are familiar with lower urinary tract symptoms suffered by the ageing male related to prostatic enlargement. Equally debilitating though are bladder symptoms found in both sexes totally unrelated to obstruction of any kind. Symptoms of frequency, urgency and urge incontinence, commonly lumped together under the term 'overactive bladder' are very prevalent in the ageing patient and confront the physicians who care for them on a daily basis.

A multitude of other influences on the bladder also exist that affect its performance over a lifetime. Certainly injury from infection or surgery can affect vesical function over both long- and short-term horizons. Changes in the bladder outlet via prostatic obstruction in males or overzealous surgery in women can have effects ranging from mild to devastating on detrusor function. Alterations in the neurological milieu of the lower urinary tract can profoundly alter bladder function. These variations, when severe enough, can not only create difficult symptomatology for the patient but also occasionally be detrimental to renal function.

In this chapter, we examine the ageing bladder from a number of angles. The alterations in vesical anatomy both gross and microscopic are important in dysfunctional voiding and incontinence associated with ageing. Neuronal and hormonal changes influence the ageing bladder. Pharmaceutical agents are under intense scrutiny as to their effect in urinary tract as well as their side effects in the elderly patient. Finally, special disease states found mostly in the older population have specific effects on the urinary tract that must be considered in the overall therapy for those diseases.

Anatomy of the ageing bladder

The normal bladder is characterized grossly by its pelvic position in the adult. In the older male, the macroscopic anatomy of the bladder is most commonly affected by the growth of the prostate gland. Although most commonly benign prostate growth occurs in the transition zone surrounding the urethra, occasionally this growth becomes unrestrained in a cephalad manner and pushes the trigone superiorly to give the bladder an elevated appearance radiographically. Gross inspection of the bladder interior often demonstrates a trabeculated appearance. Trabeculations are often thought to be a sign of chronic obstruction but have also been observed in the female bladder as well.[1]

In women, the anatomical position of the bladder is most often altered by defects in the pelvic floor musculature. This leads to the presentation of cystoceles, effectively a herniation of the bladder through the anterior vaginal muscle layers. This defect, as well as rectoceles and enteroceles are commonly noted in parous individuals although the impact of ageing, obesity and possibly neurological dysfunction can be substantial.[2,3] Perucchini has demonstrated localized striated urethral muscle loss with ageing at the bladder neck and dorsal wall of the urethra.[4] Others have shown an increase in paraurethral connective tissue in elderly females with a reduction of blood vessels.[5] Falconer has demonstrated that altered collagen production in women with stress incontinence and poor quality collagen seen in postmenopausal women possibly contribute to disorders related to prolapse in the elderly.[6]

The histologic appearance of the ageing bladder can give clues to its ultimate ability to function as a storage facility for urine. Ultrastructural changes in the ageing bladder include collagen deposition, muscle degeneration and axonal degeneration. The degree of these changes

Principles and Practice of Geriatric Medicine, Fifth Edition. Edited by Alan J. Sinclair, John E. Morley and Bruno Vellas.

may correlate with specific abnormalities in voiding and incontinence such as detrusor overactivity and impaired contractility.[7] Chronic ischaemia of the bladder may play a large causative role in these changes.[8]

Surgical procedures in both sexes can alter vesical anatomy. Certainly in females with pelvic prolapse and/or stress incontinence, operations can successfully reposition the bladder and other pelvic organs towards normalcy. They also can cause difficulties if for example, bladder neck prolapse is overcorrected and obstruction occurs. Certain women will suffer urgency and frequency symptoms even if no obstruction is present.[9] In males, relief of obstruction at the level of the prostate may improve symptoms but changes in bladder configuration may not occur at the same rapid rate seen in symptom reduction. Furthermore, radical prostatectomy in the man with prostate cancer may alter bladder dynamics as well as cause sphincteric incontinence.[10] The anatomical changes of the ageing bladder are summarized in Table 104.1.

Bladder physiology and correlation to anatomy of the ageing bladder

Bladder function involves both the storage of urine and the expulsion of urine at a socially appropriate time. To maintain continence the storage of urine must occur under low pressures and the bladder must empty adequately. Unfortunately, ageing results in changes that occur intrinsically and extrinsically to the bladder that affect continence and emptying. Pathological changes are seen in the bladder due to ageing. In addition, nerve transmission can be altered due to age, disease states, surgical procedures, or drugs. Anatomic obstruction or lack of adequate support of the bladder neck also changes the ability of the bladder to empty and store urine.

The bladder consists of two parts: the body and the base or bladder neck. The smooth muscle fibres of the body are arranged randomly and those of the bladder neck are arranged in an inner longitudinal and outer circular layer. In the male urethra the sphincter consists of both smooth muscles and striated muscles. The external sphincter consists of the periurethral striated muscle and the intramural striated muscle or rhabdosphincter. In the female these muscle are attenuated. DeLancey proposes that female continence is created by a combination of muscular coaptation and passive compression of the urethra by the pubourethral hammock.[11]

Table 104.1 Anatomical changes of the ageing bladder.

Gross anatomical changes
Trabeculations
Cystocele (females)
Muscle loss at bladder neck (females)
Histological changes
Collagen deposition
Muscle degeneration
Axonal degeneration

During urine storage, low-level afferent bladder stimulation signals sympathetic contraction of the bladder neck and relaxation of the detrusor muscle or body of the bladder. This results in storage of urine under low pressure. The voiding reflex is initiated when afferent activity becomes intense. The pontine micturition centre stimulates the parasympathetic pathway and inhibits the sympathetic pathway resulting in relaxation of the bladder outlet and contraction of the detrusor muscle and thus bladder emptying. The striated external sphincter, which has separate innervation from the bladder neck, is also influenced by the pontine micturition and storage centres. The voiding reflex results in inhibition of the external sphincter and the storage reflex results in activation of the pudendal nerve.

The bladder must be able to distend and contract to adequately function. Structural changes in the tissues and abnormalities in bladder shape can alter urinary storage and emptying. Bladder compliance is a measurable value defined as the change in volume divided by the change in intravesical pressure. A normally functioning bladder fills under a low pressure therefore the bladder is compliant. Compliance is greatly affected by tissue composition, innervation and vascular supply.

Histological studies have shown that as collagen levels increase compliance is lost. Landau demonstrated that in bladders with poor compliance the ratio of type III to type I collagen was significantly higher than that of normal bladders.[12] The aged bladder has a higher deposition of collagen; in addition, innervation of the detrusor smooth muscle changes with age. Neurochemical studies of human detrusor strips have shown an increase in purinergic neurotransmission and a decrease in cholinergic neurotransmission with age. It is felt that the shift in neurochemical transmission may change the resting tone of the bladder and contribute to the overactive bladder symptoms in aged bladders.[13]

Bladder wall blood flow is affected by the intramural tension. A bladder with poor compliance has increased intravesical pressure and intramural tension therefore, a greater decrease in bladder blood flow. Ischaemia can result in diminished contractility and can result in patchy denervation. The end result is a bladder that poorly empties and may have detrusor instability.[14] Injured areas of the bladder can become weak and form diverticulum resulting in ineffective bladder emptying.

The complexity of voiding dysfunction in the aged bladder makes if difficult to determine changes in the bladder secondary to the normal ageing process versus changes as the result of bladder outlet obstruction or diseases effecting the nervous system and/or vascular supply. Certainly the lower urinary tract symptoms of obstruction, instability and impaired detrusor function often overlap. The changes seen in bladder function with ageing must certainly overlap as well. A study by Homma found the symptoms of urgency, frequency and nocturia increased with age in both men and women. The cystometric capacity declined with age in both sexes.[15]

Histological changes in the aged bladder have been documented including increased collagen deposition, widened spaces between muscle fibres and ultrastructural changes of the smooth muscle cell membrane.[7] Elbadawi also showed that aged bladders without urodynamic evidence of obstruction had muscle cell membranes with dominant dense bands and depleted caveolae.[7] These finding were reproducible and different from the ultrastructural changes seen with obstruction, overactive or hypocontractile bladders. These findings are felt to represent dedifferentiation of the smooth muscle fibres.

Changes in bladder compliance, nerve transmission and vascularity occur as the bladder ages. Certainly multiple disease processes may worsen these changes. With advanced age expected bladder symptoms might include increasing frequency and urgency with a decreased bladder capacity.

Special disease states

Several disease states especially affect the bladder in the geriatric population. Whether caused by neurological disease, endocrine problems, iatrogenic intervention or the ageing process itself, these problems exact particular mor bidity on the lower genitourinary tract. The following conditions are particularly important.

Parkinson's disease

Parkinson's disease affects 1% of all patients over the age of 60 and is rarely seen in those under 40. In addition to the characteristic tremors and motion deficits, the loss of dopaminergic neurons in the substantia nigra of the basal ganglia affects voiding by reducing the inhibitory effect of the basal ganglia on the micturition reflex as demonstrated in several animal studies.[16]

The voiding symptoms of Parkinson's disease are frequency, urgency and urge incontinence. These irritative symptoms are present in well over half of all patients with the disorder.[17] A significant problem from a diagnostic viewpoint is the presence of these symptoms in elderly males. These irritative voiding symptoms mimic the lower urinary tract symptoms (LUTS) associated with bladder outlet obstruction related to benign prostatic hyperplasia (BPH). Without urodynamic evaluation, the neurogenic component to the symptoms may be overlooked or not quantified well and inappropriate therapy instituted. Furthermore, men with multiple systems atrophy rather than in true Parkinson's disease may actually have mild detrusor-sphincter dyssynergia, which again could mimic the obstructive symptoms of BPH.[18]

The typical urodynamic findings of Parkinson's are detrusor hyperreflexia on filling cystometry. As much as 79% of bladder dysfunction in these patients can be related to hyperreflexia.[19] Other findings are not uncommon though. Hyporeflexia is present in 16% of patients in Araki's study.[19] Obstruction can also be present particularly in the male with prostatic enlargement or stricture disease from previous interventions. Multichannel urodynamics is essential to the evaluation of voiding dysfunction in patients with Parkinson's disease.

Cerebrovascular accident (CVA)

Stroke can be considered a major health problem among elderly patients. Approximately three-quarters of the roughly 400 000 stroke patients per year in the United States are over 65 years old. The impact of this disorder on voiding and continence can range from mild to profound. When occurring in the aged patient, its effects can magnify pre-existing bladder conditions and cause great confusion as to proper therapy. Depending on the location of the ischaemic event, the bladder may range from hyperreflexic to areflexic. One can therefore present with an entire range of symptoms anywhere from nocturia and urgency/urge incontinence to voiding difficulties and urinary retention.[20] The presence of urinary incontinence in the acute phase of a CVA is a powerful predictor of a negative outcome.[21]

The patient presenting with lower urinary tract symptoms following a CVA can be a diagnostic dilemma. In one study, detrusor hyperreflexia was seen in 68% of patients, detrusor-sphincter dyssynergia in 14%, and uninhibited sphincter relaxation in 36%.[20] In that same study, there were patients with retention who were noted to have detrusor areflexia with an unrelaxing sphincter. No correlation was seen between site of lesion and urodynamic findings. In the elderly post-CVA male, neurogenic bladder problems may coexist with obstruction from the prostate gland. Nitti found in a group of men with a mean age of 70 with voiding complaints following a stroke that detrusor hyperreflexia was present in 82% of the group, but pressure-flow characteristics of definite obstruction were present in 63%.[22] Multichannel urodynamics can be an important adjunct in the urological management of these patients.

Nocturia

Nocturia is commonly listed as a symptom by the older patients. In males it is often perceived as related to prostate enlargement. But this symptom is commonly noted in ageing women.[23] Menopausal status may contribute to the presence of nocturia.[24] In all likelihood, nocturia is a manifestation of normal ageing.

Other factors impacting the presence of nocturia in the ageing individual include sleep difficulties and nocturnal polyuria. Sleep disturbances are common in the elderly population and nocturia may be more related to those problems as opposed to a urinary tract dysfunction. Furthermore, the patient with nocturia from whatever cause will have poorer sleep.[25] The problem of nocturnal polyuria in many of the elderly, which is reported as nocturia can be difficult to manage. With lower renal concentrating ability, poorer conservation of sodium, loss of the circadian rhythm of antidiuretic hormone secretion, decreased production of renin-angiotensin-aldosterone, and increased release of atrial natriuretic hormone, there is an age-related alteration in the circadian rhythm of water excretion leading to increased night-time urine production in the older population. Exacerbated by age-related diminution in functional bladder volume and detrusor instability, nocturnal polyuria often leads to a dramatic version of nocturia.[26] Whatever the cause, nocturia is a significant problem both from a QOL standpoint and as a risk factor for falls leading to hip fractures.[27] Essentially, nocturia more than twice per night is significantly associated with the risk of falls and subsequent fractures.

Dementias

The elderly patient with dementia faces the dual difficulties of having to face an ageing bladder with its consequences and in addition, the difficulties caused by an altered perception of his or her internal and external environments. This can lead to urinary incontinence and/or retention based on either bladder factors or due to central neurological misperceptions of urinary activity. The difficulties in management of these patients' other significant conditions often pushes concerns over incontinence aside but the fact is that incontinence issues are the primary cause for institutionalization of the elderly patient.

Evidence of combined cerebral and urinary tract dysfunction comes from perfusion studies in elderly patients. From PET scan studies it has been demonstrated that the pontine micturition centre in the dorsomedial pontine tegmentum, the periaqueductal grey matter and the pre-optic area of the hypothalamus are all active during various phases of micturition.[28] Furthermore, urge incontinence has been associated with underperfusion of the frontal areas of the brain.[29] Clearly, cerebral atrophy due to whatever cause can lead to disinhibition of the bladder and resulting incontinence. Treatment routines combining anticholinergic medications with prompted or timed voiding have been utilized to circumvent the loss of cerebral control over the micturition process in elderly patients afflicted with bladder dysfunction.[30]

Pharmacology as it relates to the ageing bladder

With so many elderly at risk for bladder dysfunction, the use of medications among the elderly for urinary tract problems is rising almost exponentially. The number of prescriptions for overactive bladder drugs number in the millions, many presumably to older sufferers of the condition. Clearly an understanding of how the common drugs for these urinary conditions work is essential to proper prescribing and monitoring. Proper use of pharmaceuticals for urinary conditions can give maximum benefit to the patient's symptoms and pathology without engendering any undue risk in the ageing population.

Receptors

The pharmacology of the bladder is primarily related to either the bladder itself or in the nervous innervation of the organ. At the level of the bladder itself, a number of receptor sites exist to varying degrees. These receptors govern to a great degree the function of the lower urinary tract and become more prominent in the elderly patient as various bladder conditions become more prevalent.

Among the adrenergic receptors, alpha and beta-receptors are found in the bladder although it has been thought that beta-receptors predominate in the bladder body and alpha-receptors in the bladder base and bladder neck region. Urine storage is facilitated by relaxation caused by beta stimulation and tonic contraction in the area enriched by alpha-receptors. More recent work has elucidated (at least in the rabbit) that the division by receptors into bladder base and body may be overly simplistic and that further regionalization of the bladder based on differing mixes of alpha- and beta-receptors might be more appropriate.[31] Alpha-receptors are also well characterized in the prostatic urethra and stroma. Stimulation of these receptors causes contraction and thus possibly obstruction of the bladder neck.[32]

Muscarinic receptors are the other major group of receptors influencing bladder behaviour. These receptors, particularly the M2 and M3 subtypes are responsible for bladder contraction.[33] The pharmacology of these receptors is influenced by their ubiquity. They are also found in gastrointestinal, airway and salivary gland smooth muscle. Table 104.2 gives a summary of receptors located within the bladder and the effects of ageing on these receptors.

Adrenergic stimulation/blockade

Alpha stimulation in the elderly patient is most often a deleterious side effect from a pharmaceutical designed for action elsewhere. With the rich supply of alpha-receptors

Table 104.2 Bladder receptors and ageing.

Receptor	Location	Action	Effect of ageing
Alpha- adrenergic	Prostate	Contraction	Stimulation – causes smooth muscle urinary retention Blockade – improves urine flow
Alpha- adrenergic	Bladder base	Contraction smooth muscle	Shift in subtype may ameliorate bladder symptoms
Beta-adrenergic	Bladder body	Relaxation smooth muscle	Unknown at present
Muscarinic	Detrusor muscle (primarily M3)	Relaxation smooth muscle	Urinary retention Worsening of side effects at other locations

in the prostate, stimulation can cause contraction and thus obstruction and urinary retention.[34] Alpha blockade, although originally designed with hypertension in mind, has become a mainstay in the therapy of lower urinary tract symptoms related to prostatic enlargement.[35]

One effect of ageing is the possible change in the type, sensitivity and number of these receptors. With increasing age, alpha adrenoceptor responsiveness either decreases or remains unchanged.[36] Furthermore, alpha-receptors in the ageing bladder itself show a shift from the alpha-1a subtype to an alpha-1d predominance.[37] If alpha-blockers have an effect in the bladder that aids in relief of lower urinary tract symptoms as well as its effect on obstruction itself, then this change with ageing could have implications for both short-term as well as long-term use in elderly men with prostate disease.

Antimuscarinics

These drugs are utilized primarily in the therapy of symptoms of overactive bladder. Although the M2 subtype is the predominant population, it appears the smaller population M3 subtype is the functionally important group.[38] Although several antimuscarinic agents exist in oral, intravesical and transdermal forms, the lack of bladder M3 selectivity remains a problem.

In the elderly, antimuscarinic can be very effective for symptoms of frequency, urgency and urge incontinence.[39] Changes in the ageing patient may, however, alter the pharmacology of these drugs in an adverse manner. Side effects such as dry mouth and constipation may be of more concern and less well tolerated in the elderly individual. Decreases in force of detrusor contraction in the ageing male with an enlarged obstructing prostate gland may well push the patient into urinary retention. At least one of these agents crosses the blood-brain barrier and thus particularly in the ageing patient could have a higher incidence of confusion as a side effect.[40] These effects could play a role in limiting the usefulness of the antimuscarinics in treating bladder dysfunction.

5-alpha reductase inhibitors

This group of drugs, although having therapeutic activity in the prostate gland, are known for their beneficial effect on the bladder complaints caused by obstruction from the prostate gland. These agents inhibit the conversion of testosterone to dihydrotestosterone in the prostate gland and thus cause reduction in the size of the periurethral prostatic tissue. This leads to improvement in urinary flow and BPH-related symptomatology. In the PLESS study, the main side effects in all age groups are sexual side effects particularly ejaculatory disturbances.[41] This may be more profound in the elderly male with borderline sexual dysfunction although this was not borne out in the PLESS study.

Surgical disease of the ageing bladder

Lower urinary tract surgery in the aged patient is common for two conditions with large impact on the bladder – stress urinary incontinence in women and bladder outlet obstruction from prostatic enlargement in men. The elderly suffer disproportionately from these disorders but have benefited from advances in therapy for these conditions. With proper selection of treatment, this group of patients can enjoy great improvement in their QOL related to their lower urinary tract. Furthermore, minimally invasive techniques for overactive bladder conditions have also evolved and may be useful in the older population.

Female stress urinary incontinence

Stress incontinence occurs when abdominal pressure generated by such actions as coughing, sneezing or other Valsalva manoeuvres causes bladder pressure to exceed urethral pressure without a detrusor contraction and urine is expelled. Stress incontinence is associated with parturition, previous pelvic surgery and ageing. Previously, major abdominal surgery was the only method considered for treatment and older age could be considered a relative contraindication. But with newer therapies, elderly women can be considered excellent candidates for improvement in their condition.

Pelvic floor conditioning

Pelvic floor exercises have become a mainstay of conservative therapy for stress incontinence. They are absolutely safe and can be performed either alone or with biofeedback. Effectiveness as measured both subjectively by patient report as well as objectively with pad weights has been demonstrated in several studies.[42]

Some concern over the effectiveness in the elderly of pelvic floor rehabilitation can be raised. The reduction in estrogen effect on the vaginal tissues may reduce the benefit of these exercises in the elderly woman. Furthermore, the overall reduction of muscle tone with ageing may also make these exercises less efficacious.[43] Patients with significant intrinsic sphincter deficiency may not respond as well to pelvic floor conditioning. These exercises however are essentially risk-free which makes them especially appealing as a first-line effort in the elderly woman.

Pharmacological management

Stress urinary incontinence has been remarkably resistant to drug therapy in the past. Pharmacological agents with alpha-adrenergic properties such as pseudoephedrine were occasionally utilized with moderate success in women with mild incontinence.[44] These medications were effective due to the presence of alpha-receptors in the bladder neck. These agents though have more recently been pulled from use due to adverse events and so are not readily available for use. Estrogen therapy may also play a role in the medical management of stress incontinent in the older, postmenopausal woman[45] but its true benefit is controversial.

Anticholinergic agents, although truly indicated for urgency and urge incontinence, are often prescribed for stress incontinence. These drugs may be helpful in women with mixed incontinence (urge and stress incontinence) by reduction of the urge component and thus improving overall continence. In the patient with pure stress incontinence though, the patient may perceive a worsening of the problem in that the bladder capacity will increase and the patient will leak larger volumes of urine with stress manoeuvres.[46]

Although it is appealing to consider these pharmaceuticals as first-line therapy for stress incontinence in the ageing woman, one must consider certain factors. Alpha-adrenergic agents have been associated with cerebrovascular accidents and increases in blood pressure.[34] Certain anticholinergic medications cross the blood-brain barrier and can cause confusion and drowsiness in the older patient.[40] These adverse effects may outweigh the usually small benefits from these drugs on stress incontinence.

The serotonin-norepinephrine reuptake inhibitors (SNRIs) are being shown to have a therapeutic effect in female stress incontinence. These drugs have been shown to facilitate urine storage and facilitate rhabdosphincter activity. Thus a positive effect on stress incontinence could be expected and trials are underway to study this possibility.[47] Safety in the geriatric population would also need evaluation.

Injection therapy

The concept of injecting substances at the bladder neck to aid in coaptation and thus improve continence dates back to the use of sodium morrhuate by Murless in the 1930s.[48] This led later to the use of Teflon popularized by Politano with good results.[49] Concerns over the safety of Teflon injection led to the use of glutaraldehyde cross-linked bovine collagen and later development of other injectables such as carbon beads. Injection treatments have been shown to have an improvement rate of about 40%[50] with best results occurring in women without low leak point pressures or maximum urethral closure pressures.

This therapy may be a good alternative for the older female. It is minimally invasive with a low rate of complications. The anaesthetic requirements are not significant with some reporting use of local anaesthetic only. The major downside, especially for the geriatric patient is the frequent need for multiple injections to achieve success but newer injection materials may be longer lasting. Still, this is an excellent option for the older woman desiring aggressive treatment but reluctant to undergo major surgical procedures.[51]

Operative therapy

With multiple procedures described for female stress urinary incontinence, it is difficult to discern what the role of surgery might be for the ageing female. Several factors are clear though. Older women are, as a rule, healthier now and thus better able to tolerate surgery. Surgery offers the best chance for successful resolution of stress incontinence. Finally, modifications of many procedures have allowed good results with less morbidity than was seen with older operations.

Sling procedures have evolved from being a procedure designed only for those with severe incontinence to a rational alternative for all women desiring operative therapy.[52] The procedure is commonly done today with alternative materials for the sling such as cadaveric fascia or dermis as opposed to the classic descriptions of harvesting the patient's own fascia. Fixation can be accomplished either at the rectus fascia or at the pubic bone.

The taping procedures for stress incontinence have also shown good results with minimal morbidity and may be ideal alternatives for the elderly female. The tension-free vaginal tape procedure as popularized by Ulmsten[53] and its modifications (suprapubic tapes and transobturator tapes) place a sling-like material at the midurethra and are often done under local anaesthetic with light sedation only.

These procedures have been shown to be safe enough and have good enough results to be a reasonable alternative for the more active older female who requires aggressive treatment but desires minimal morbidity.[54] Newer fixation approaches lend themselves well to a transvaginal approach.

Benign prostatic hyperplasia (BPH) in the older male

Benign enlargement of the prostate gland in the human male is a condition inexorably linked with ageing. When the vesicourethral junction becomes obstructed by the growing tissue, symptoms such as slowing of the urinary stream, hesitancy, straining to void and a sensation of incomplete emptying result. Furthermore, irritative symptoms such as urinary frequency, urgency and nocturia may also become common. It is estimated that the prevalence of symptoms related to BPH may be as high as 50% in a multinational survey.[55]

Medical therapy

Two broad classes of drugs are utilized as therapy for BPH, alpha-receptor blockers and 5-alpha reductase inhibitors. The bladder neck region in males is rich in alpha-receptors and blockade of these causes relaxation of the smooth muscle in the prostatic urethra. This results in a decrease in the tonic luminal pressure in the prostatic fossa and allows for more efficient urine outflow from the bladder.[56]

Early alpha-antagonists were designed primarily for use as antihypertensives and thus a major side effect when used for relief of voiding dysfunction from BPH was orthostasis. Normotensive men complained also of asthenia and fatigue.[57] In older men with hypertension, attempted medical management of BPH along with hypertension became complex. Over the last several years, the introduction of alpha-adrenergic antagonists selective to the prostatic alpha-receptors has broadened the population that can be managed with these agents and includes with safety many elderly men.[35]

The 5-alpha reductase inhibitors block the conversion in the prostate gland of testosterone to dihydrotestosterone, which is the active form stimulating prostate growth. With blockade, the prostate gland involutes and a reduction in prostate volume of up to 30% may be seen. This can result in an improvement in urinary flow and a decrease in symptomatology. The safety profile of these drugs is very good making them a good choice in the older male particularly those with very large prostate glands.[41]

Combination therapy may also be of benefit in the elderly male. The recently completed Medical Therapy of Prostate Symptoms (MTOPS) study demonstrated a 66% decrease in acute urinary retention compared to placebo. Alpha blockade alone and 5 alpha-reductase therapy alone showed 39% and 34% reductions respectively.[58] Acute urinary retention in the elderly is a morbid event with an impact on QOL similar to that of myocardial infarction so prevention via combined therapy may be worthwhile for the older population with lower urinary tract symptoms related to BPH.

Minimally invasive therapy

A plethora of minimally invasive treatments for BPH now exist. Many are safe enough to be office based and thus particularly applicable to the older male population. These therapies involve the delivery of energy to the prostate gland in order to heat the tissues to greater than 60° C which leads to protein denaturation and ultimately destruction of prostatic tissue and relief of obstruction. The differences in the methods lie in the delivery system whether by externally generated microwaves[59] or internally placed systems for radiofrequency energy[60] or laser energy.[61]

Safety makes these procedures particularly appealing for the older male.[62] Most of the complications centre around irritative voiding symptoms. Bleeding essentially does not occur but post-procedure retention can be a problem. Furthermore, it takes several weeks before improvement in symptoms and flow occurs.

Transurethral resection of the prostate gland (TURP)

This procedure is still considered the 'gold standard' of treatment for bladder outlet obstruction from BPH.[63] It works quickly since the obstructing tissue is removed immediately at the time of surgery. Symptom scores drop rapidly and flow rates are instantly improved. Although not without morbidity, improvements in instrumentation and optics have made this procedure much safer for the elderly patient and in those with severe symptoms or retention it is still the best choice for therapy no matter the age of the patient if he can reasonably tolerate anaesthesia.

Minimally invasive therapy of overactive bladder

Since many older patients do not tolerate anticholinergic/ antimuscarinic drugs well, alternatives for urgency/ frequency type symptoms have been sought. The techniques involve modification of the neural pathways leading to muscular contraction in the bladder. Submucosal injection of botulinum toxin under cystoscopic guidance leads to chemodenervation at the motor terminal and increases in bladder capacity and decreases in detrusor pressure.[64]. Sacral nerve stimulation also is an effective mode of treatment for symptoms of urgency and frequency. With this technique, a programmable generator sends electrical impulses along the S3 nerve root thus stimulating the innervation of the pelvic floor. Aboseif demonstrated a large reduction in costs associated with bladder complaints after implantation of this stimulator.[65]

Conclusion

The effects of ageing on lower urinary tract function and dysfunction can be profound. Anatomic variations, both at the macroscopic and ultrastructural levels occur frequently and induce functional changes. Disease states commonly seen in the older patient have significant impact on the bladder, which should be recognized as a major portion of the syndromes. Bladder changes from ageing significantly impact on pharmaceutical effectiveness and alter the ability to manage many conditions. A multimodal approach including surgery to common geriatric disorders of the lower urinary tract can be safe and very effective.

Key points

- Bladder anatomy changes with ageing both macroscopically due to prostate enlargement in men and pelvic prolapse in women as well as microscopically due to collagen deposition.
- Changes in anatomy lead to physiological changes such as loss of compliance and variation in response to neurotransmitters and pharmaceuticals
- Certain extravesical disease processes common in the older patient have a profound effect on the bladder.
- The common lower urinary tract symptom complexes of stress incontinence in women and obstructive voiding in women can be safely treated by a variety of means including surgery.

References

1. Groutz A, Samandarov A, Gold R *et al.* Role of urethrocystoscopy in the evaluation of refractory idiopathic detrusor instability. *Urology* 2001;**58**:544–6.
2. Constantinou CE, Hvistendahl G, Ryhammer A, Nagel LL, Djurhuus JC. Determining the displacement of the pelvic floor and pelvic organs during voluntary contractions using magnetic resonance imaging in younger and older women. *BJU Int* 2002;**90**:408–14.
3. Cummings JM, Rodning CR. Urinary stress incontinence among obese women: review of pathophysiology and therapy. *Int Urogynecol J* 2000;**11**:41–4.
4. Perucchini D, DeLancey JO, Ashton-Miller JA, Galecki A, Schaer GN. Age effects on urethral striated muscle. II. Anatomic location of muscle loss. *Am J Obstet Gynecol* 2002; **186**:356–60.
5. Verelst M, Maltau JM, Orbo A. Computerised morphometric study of the paraurethral tissue in young and elderly women. *Neurourol Urodyn* 2002;**21**:529–33.
6. Falconer C, Ekman-Ordeberg G, Ulmsten U *et al.* Changes in paraurethral connective tissue at menopause are counteracted by estrogen. *Maturitas* 1996;**24**:197–204.
7. Elbadawi A. Pathology and pathophysiology of detrusor in incontinence. *Urol Clin North Am* 1995;**22**:499–512.
8. Azadzoi KM, Tarcan T, Kozlowski R, Krane RJ, Siroky MB. Overactivity and structural changes in the chronically ischemic bladder. *J Urol* 1999;**162**:1768–78.
9. Dunn JS Jr, Bent AE, Ellerkman RM, Nihira MA, Melick CF. Voiding dysfunction after surgery for stress incontinence: literature review and survey results. *Int Urogynecol J Pelvic Floor Dysfunct* 2004;**15**:25–31.
10. Sebesta M, Cespedes RD, Luhman E, Optenberg S, Thompson IM. Questionnaire-based outcomes of urinary incontinence and satisfaction rates after radical prostatectomy in a national study population. *Urology* 2002;**60**:1055–8.
11. DeLancey JO. Anatomy and embryology of the lower urinary tract. *Obstet Gynecol Clin North Am* 1989;**16**:717–31.
12. Landau EH, Jayanthi VR, Churchill BM *et al.* Loss of elasticity in dysfunctional bladders: Urodynamic and histochemical correlation. *J Urol* 1994;**152**:702–5.
13. Yoshida M. Miuamee K. Iwashita H. Otani M. Inadome A. Management of detrusor dysfunction in the elderly: changes in acetylcholine and adenosine triphosphate release during ageing. *Urology* 2004;**63**(3 Suppl 1):117–23.
14. Brading AF. A myogenic basis for the overactive bladder. *Urology* 1997;**50**(Suppl):57–67.
15. Homma Y, Imajo C, Takahashi S, Kaqae K, Aso Y. Urinary symptoms and urodynamics in a normal elderly population. *Scand J Urol Nephrol* 1994;**157**(Suppl):27–30.
16. Yoshimura N, Sasa M, Yoshida O, Takaori S. Dopamine D-1 receptor-mediated inhibition of the micturition reflex by central dopamine from the substantia nigra. *Neurourol Urodyn* 1992;**11**:535–45.
17. Pavlakis AJ, Siroky MB, Goldstein I, Krane RJ. Neurourologic findings in Parkinson's disease. *J Urol* 1983;**129**:80–3.
18. Stocchi F, Carbone A, Inghilleri M *et al.* Urodynamic and neurophysiological evaluation in Parkinson's disease and multiple system atrophy. *J Neurol Neurosurg Psychiatry* 1997; **62**:507–11.
19. Araki I, Kitahara M, Oida T, Kuno S. Voiding dysfunction and Parkinson's disease: urodynamics abnormalities and urinary symptoms. *J Urol* 2003;**164**:1640–3.
20. Sakakibara R, Hattori T, Yasuda K, Yamanishi T. Micturitional disturbance after acute hemispheric stroke: analysis of the lesion site by CT and MRI. *J Neurol Sci* 1996;**137**:47–56.
21. Wade DT, Hewer RL. Outlook after an acute stroke: urinary incontinence and loss of consciousness compared in 532 patients. *Q J Med* 1985;**56**:601–8.
22. Nitti VW, Adler H, Combs AJ. The role of urodynamics in the evaluation of voiding dysfunction in men after cerebrovascular accident. *J Urol* 1996;**155**:263–6.
23. Lose G, Alling-Moller L, Jennum P. Nocturia in women. *Am J Obstet Gynecol* 2001;**185**:514–21.
24. Chen YC, Chen GD, Hu SW, Lin TL, Lin LY. Is the occurrence of storage and voiding dysfunction affected by menopausal transition or associated with the normal ageing process? *Menopause* 2003;**10**:203–8.
25. Middelkoop HA, Smilde-van den Doel DA, Neven AK, Kamphuisen HA, Springer CP. Subjective sleep characteristics of 1485 males and females aged 50–93: effects of sex and

age, and factors related to self-evaluated quality of sleep. *J Gerontol A Biol Sci Med Sci* 1996;**51**: M108–15.

26. Miller M. Nocturnal polyuria in older people: pathophysiology and clinical implications. *J Am Geriatr Soc* 2000;**48**: 1321–9.
27. Temml C, Ponholzer A, Gutjahr G *et al*. Nocturia is an age-independent risk factor for hip-fractures in men. *Neurourol Urodyn* 2009;**28**:949–52.
28. Blok BF, Holstege G. The central nervous system control of micturition in cats and humans. *Behav Brain Res* 1998;**92**: 119–25.
29. Griffiths D. Clinical studies of cerebral and urinary tract function in elderly people with urinary incontinence. *Behav Brain Res* 1998;**92**:151–5.
30. Burgio KL, Locher JL, Goode PS *et al*. Behavioral vs drug treatment for urge urinary incontinence in older women: a randomized controlled trial. *JAMA* 1998;**280**:1995–2000.
31. Chou EC, Capello SA, Levin RM, Longhurst PA. Excitatory alpha1-adrenergic receptors predominate over inhibitory beta-receptors in rabbit dorsal detrusor. *J Urol* 2003;**170**: 2503–7.
32. Caine M. Alpha-adrenergic mechanisms in dynamics of benign prostatic hypertrophy. *Urology* 1988;**32**(Suppl):16–20.
33. Ehlert FJ. Contractile role of M2 and M3 muscarinic receptors in gastrointestinal, airway and urinary bladder smooth muscle. *Life Sci* 2003;**74**:355–66.
34. Beck RA, Mercado DL, Seguin SM, Andrade WP, Cushner HM. Cardiovascular effects of pseudoephedrine in medically controlled hypertensive patients. *Arch Intern Med* 1992; **152**:1242–5.
35. Dunn CJ, Matheson A, Faulds DM. Tamsulosin: a review of its pharmacology and therapeutic efficacy in the management of lower urinary tract symptoms. *Drugs Ageing* 2002;**19**: 135–61.
36. Docherty JR, O'Malley K. Ageing and alpha-adrenoceptors. *Clin Sci (Lond)* 1985;**68** (Suppl 10): 133s–136s.
37. Hampel C, Gillitzer R, Pahernik S, Melchior SW, Thuroff JW. Changes in the receptor profile of the ageing bladder. *Urologe A* 2004;**43**:535–41.
38. Fetscher C, Fleichman M, Schmidt M, Krege S, Michel MC. M(3) muscarinic receptors mediate contraction of human urinary bladder. *Br J Pharmacol* 2002;**136**:641–3.
39. Wein AJ. Diagnosis and treatment of the overactive bladder. *Urology* 2003;**62**(5 Suppl 2):20–7.
40. Todorova A, Vonderheid-Guth B, Dimpfel W. Effects of tolterodine, trospium chloride, and oxybutynin on the central nervous system. *J Clin Pharmacol* 2001;**41**:636–44.
41. Roehrborn CG, Bruskewitz R, Nickel JC *et al*.; Proscar Long-Term Efficacy and Safety Study Group. Sustained decrease in incidence of acute urinary retention and surgery with finasteride for 6 years in men with benign prostatic hyperplasia. *J Urol* 2004;**171**:1194–8.
42. Bo K, Talseth T, Holme I. Single blind, randomised controlled trial of pelvic floor exercises, electrical stimulation, vaginal cones, and no treatment in management of genuine stress incontinence in women. *BMJ* 1999;**318**:487–93.
43. Aukee P, Penttinen J, Airaksinen O. The effect of ageing on the electromyographic activity of pelvic floor muscles. A comparative study among stress incontinent patients and asymptomatic women. *Maturitas* 2003;**44**:253–7.
44. Cummings JM. Current concepts in the management of stress urinary incontinence. *Drugs of Today* 1996;**32**:609–614.
45. Ishiko O, Hirai K, Sumi T, Tatsuta I, Ogita S. Hormone replacement therapy plus pelvic floor muscle exercise for postmenopausal stress incontinence. A randomized, controlled trial. *J Reprod Med* 2001;**46**:213–20.
46. Chutka DS, Takahashi PY. Urinary incontinence in the elderly. Drug treatment options. *Drugs* 1998;**56**:587–95.
47. Thor KB, Donatucci C. Central nervous system control of the lower urinary tract: new pharmacological approaches to stress urinary incontinence in women. *J Urol* 2004;**172**:27–33.
48. Murless BC. The injection treatment of stress incontinence. *J Obstet Gynaecol Br Empire* 1938;**45**:67–73.
49. Lopez AE, Padron OF, Patsias G, Politano VA. Transurethral polytetrafluoroethylene injection in female patients with urinary continence. *J Urol* 1993;**150**:856–8.
50. Groutz A, Blaivas JG, Kesler SS, Weiss JP, Chaikin DC. Outcome results of transurethral collagen injection for female stress incontinence: assessment by urinary incontinence score. *J Urol* 2000;**164**:2006–9.
51. Khullar V, Cardozo LD, Abbott D, Anders K. GAX collagen in the treatment of urinary incontinence in elderly women: a two-year follow-up. *Br J Obstet Gynaecol* 1997;**104**:96–9.
52. Morgan TO Jr, Westney OL, McGuire EJ. Pubovaginal sling: 4-year outcome analysis and quality of life assessment. *J Urol* 2000;**163**:1845–8.
53. Ulmsten U, Falconer C, Johnson P *et al*. A multicenter study of tension-free vaginal tape (TVT) for surgical treatment of stress urinary incontinence. *Int Urogynecol J Pelvic Floor Dysfunct* 1998;**9**:210–3.
54. Walsh K, Generao SE, White MJ, Katz D, Stone AR. The influence of age on quality of life outcome in women following a tension-free vaginal tape procedure. *J Urol* 2004;**171**:1185–8.
55. Rosen R, Altwein J, Boyle P *et al*. Lower urinary tract symptoms and male sexual dysfunction: the multinational survey of the ageing male (MSAM-7). *Eur Urol* 2003;**44**:637–49.
56. Debruyne FM. Alpha blockers: are all created equal? *Urology* 2000;**56**(5 Suppl 1):20–2.
57. Lepor H, Jones K, Williford W. The mechanism of adverse events associated with terazosin: an analysis of the Veterans Affairs cooperative study. *J Urol* 2000;**163**:1134–7.
58. McConnell JD, Roehrborn CG, Bautista OM *et al*.; Medical Therapy of Prostatic Symptoms (MTOPS) Research Group. The long-term effect of doxazosin, finasteride, and combination therapy on the clinical progression of benign prostatic hyperplasia. *N Engl J Med* 2003;**349**:2387–98.
59. Osman Y, Wadie B, El-Diasty T, Larson T. High-energy transurethral microwave thermotherapy: symptomatic vs urodynamic success. *BJU Int* 2003;**91**:365–70.
60. Hill B, Belville W, Bruskewitz R *et al*. Transurethral needle ablation versus transurethral resection of the prostate for the treatment of symptomatic benign prostatic hyperplasia: 5-year results of a prospective, randomized, multicenter clinical trial. *J Urol* 2004;**171**:2336–40.
61. Costello AJ, Agarwal DK, Crowe HR, Lynch WJ. Evaluation of interstitial diode laser therapy for treatment of benign prostatic hyperplasia. *Tech Urol* 1999;**5**:202–6.

62. Berger AP, Niescher M, Spranger R *et al.* Transurethral microwave thermotherapy (TUMT) with the Targis System: a single-centre study on 78 patients with acute urinary retention and poor general health. *Eur Urol* 2003;**43**:176–80.
63. Minardi D, Galosi AB, Yehia M *et al.* Transurethral resection versus minimally invasive treatments of benign prostatic hyperplasia: results of treatments. Our experience. *Arch Ital Urol Androl* 2004;**76**:11–8.
64. Flynn MK, Amundsen CL, Perevich M, Liu F, Webster GD. Outcome of a randomized, double-blind, placebo controlled trial of botulinum A toxin for refractory overactive bladder. *J Urol* 2009;**181**:2608–15.
65. Aboseif SR, Kim DH, Rieder JM *et al.* Sacral neuromodulation: cost considerations and clinical benefits. *Urology* 2007;**70**:1069–73.

CHAPTER 105

Prostate diseases

Clement Gaudin[1], Nicolas Doumerc[1], Loic Mourey[2], Stephane Gerard[1] and Laurent Balardy[1]
[1]Gérontopôle, CHU Toulouse, Toulouse, France
[2]Institut Claudius Regaud, Toulouse, France

Introduction

The prostate is a small gland, surrounding the urethra, located between the penis and the bladder. The prostate is perhaps the most disease-affected organ in the male body. The three main conditions that can affect the prostate are:

- Benign prostatic hyperplasia (BPH), that is, an enlarged prostate that causes urinary problems. It is a common condition that is associated with ageing. About 60% of men who are 60 years of age or over have some degree of prostate enlargement. BPH can be treated with medication, a minimally invasive procedure or, in extreme cases, surgery that removes the prostate.
- Cancer of the prostate is one of most common cancers in men over 65 years old. The risk of developing prostate cancer increases with age. The progression of this cancer is very slow and it can take up to 15 years to develop metastasis (most often in bones), so the specific mortality is weak. The screening of prostate cancer is based on digital rectal examination and prostate-specific antigen (PSA) assay. Prostate cancer can be cured when treated in its early stages. Treatments include removing the prostate, hormone therapy and radiotherapy. All the treatment options carry the risk of significant side effects, including loss libido, sexual dysfunction and urinary incontinence.
- Prostatitis is inflammation of the prostate gland. There are different forms of prostatitis based on causes and chronology (acute or chronic). The inflammation can be due to bacterial infection with an acute or chronic presentation. These forms are treated with antibiotics. Most often (in ~95% of cases) the diagnosis is a chronic non-bacterial prostatitis or male chronic pelvic pain syndrome that is treated with a large variety of modalities.

This chapter reviews these main diagnostic entities and the approach to treatment in the ageing male.

Benign prostatic hyperplasia

BPH is very common and its incidence is correlated with the ageing population. Autopsy data show that nearly 90% of all men aged 80 years and above have anatomical or microscopic evidence of hyperplasia and that pathology is found in half of men in their 50s.[1]

BPH is commonly associated with bothersome lower urinary tract symptoms (LUTS) such as urinary frequency, urgency, nocturia, decreased and intermittent strength of stream and the sensation of incomplete bladder emptying, which can seriously impair quality of life.

The term 'BPH' actually refers to a histological condition, namely the presence of stromal-glandular hyperplasia within the prostate gland.[2] The condition becomes clinically relevant if and when it is associated with bothersome LUTS. However, the relationship between BPH and LUTS is complex, because some men with histological BPH will develop significant LUTS, whereas other men who do not have histological BPH will develop LUTS.[3] Epidemiology, clinical expressions, diagnostic approach and treatment of BPH are discussed is this chapter.

Epidemiology

Mortality

BPH is a common problem among elderly men and leads to substantial disability. However, it is not a frequent cause of death. Mortality from BPH declined dramatically in industrialized countries from the 1950s to the 1990s.[4] Moreover, a cohort study of 4708 men who underwent transurethral resection of the prostate (TURP) between 1976 and 1984 at the Kaiser Permanente Medical Center in Oakland, OR, revealed no greater mortality than age-matched men who did not undergo TURP.[5]

Principles and Practice of Geriatric Medicine, Fifth Edition. Edited by Alan J. Sinclair, John E. Morley and Bruno Vellas.

The decrease in mortality can result either from a reduction in disease prevalence or from improvements in survival. To date, there is no evidence that the decrease in BPH mortality is likely to be related to improvements in medical and surgical treatments provided. Indeed, it could be considered as a health care performance indicator.[6]

Prevalence

BPH is increasingly common with advancing age. About 8% of men aged 31–40 years show histological evidence of BPH. This rate increases sharply to 50, 70 and 90 in men aged 51–60, 61–70 and 81–90 years, respectively.[7] Clinical BPH, defined by moderate-to-severe LUTS, occurs in ~25% of men aged 50–59 years, in 33% of men aged 60–69 years and in 50% of men older than 80 years.[7] Aetiologies of LUTS are multifactorial but BPH is a major contributing factor. Age-elated, detrusor dysfunction, neurogenic disease and diabetes are other major causes of LUTS.[8] The prevalence of LUTS in Europe varies with age, ranging from 14% in the fourth decade to >40% in the sixth decade. Based on an overall prevalence of LUTS of 30%, approximately four million men older than 40 years suffer from LUTS in the UK.[9] Furthermore, with the ageing population, the prevalence of BPH and its impact on medical practice will increase dramatically in the future.[3]

Pathogenesis and risk factors of BPH

BPH initially grows in the periurethral or transitional zone, with a fourfold increase in stromal tissue and a twofold increase in glandular components. However, the pathogenesis of BPH remains vague. Multiple factors contribute to the development of BPH[10] but the two main ones are changes in hormone level with age. Thus, the development of BPH requires both functional Leydig cells and ageing. However, given that testosterone, dihydrotestosterone and estrogen may be involved in BPH development, these hormones are not sufficient to cause BPH. Other factors influence the risk of developing BPH:

- *Age:* Several studies have demonstrated a relationship between age and markers of BPH progression.[11,12]
- *Genetic susceptibility:* Positive family history of BPH increases the risk of having more moderate to severe LUTS.[13] Moreover, twin studies suggest that heredity is a more important determinant of lower urinary tract symptoms than age, transition zone volume or total prostate volume.[14]
- *Race:* Black men are more likely than white men to have more moderate to severe LUTS.[13] In contrast, Asian men are less likely than white and black men to have BPH.[15]
- *Free PSA levels:* Higher free PSA levels increase the risk of BPH.[16]
- *Heart disease:* Heart disease increases the risk of BPH.[16]
- *Physical activity:* Lack of physical exercise increase the risk of BPH.[16]
- *Inflammation:* Epidemiological data show a strong relationship between prostatitis and BPH.[17]
- *Medications:* Use of β-blockers increases the risk of BPH.[16]
- *Other factors:* Conditions such as hyperinsulinaemia, dyslipidaemia, elevated blood pressure and obesity have been identified as risk factors of BPH.[18,19]

Natural history

Lower urinary tract symptoms (LUTS) include increased frequency of urination, nocturia, hesitancy, urgency and weak urinary stream. These symptoms typically appear slowly and progress gradually over years. Untreated BPH can cause acute urinary retention (AUR), recurrent urinary tract infections, hydronephrosis and renal failure.

One of the largest longitudinal studies, the Olmsted County study conducted in the USA, enrolled 2215 men aged 40–79 years. At 92 months' follow-up, 31% of participants reported a ≥3-point increase in AUA Symptom Index (AUA-SI; identical with the seven symptom questions of the IPSS) score and the mean annual increase in AUA-SI was 0.34 points.[20,21] Moreover, in the placebo arm of the Medical Therapy Of Prostatic Symptom (MTOPS) study, the overall clinical progression rate (defined as an increase in AUA-SI of ≥4 points, AUR, urinary incontinence, renal insufficiency or recurrent urinary tract infections) was 17.4% over the 4 year follow-up. About 78% of progression events were worsening symptoms.[22]

Although AUR and surgery are less common than overall symptomatic worsening, they represent important progression events with financial, emotional and health-related consequences for patients. Untreated men with symptomatic BPH have about a 2.5% per year risk of developing AUR.[23,24] Age, LUTS, urinary flow rate and prostate volume are risk factors for AUR in population-based studies, but not in all clinical trials. Moreover, serum PSA seems to be a stronger predictor of prostate growth than age or baseline prostate volume[25] and should be a good risk predictor of AUR.[22]

Diagnostics

Patient evaluation

Urinary symptoms may be evaluated using the American Urologic Association (AUA) symptoms score or the International Prostate Symptoms Score (IPSS) (Table 105.1).

The AUA symptom score should only be used to assess the BPH severity symptoms (not for differential diagnosis). It includes seven questions: frequency, nocturia, urinary stream weakness, straining, intermittency, incomplete emptying and urgency. Each of these items is scored on a scale from 0 (not present) to 5 (almost always present). Symptoms

Table 105.1 AUA Benign Prostatic Hyperplasia Symptom Score (AUA Practice Guidelines Committee, 2003).

	Not at all	Less than 1 time in 5	Less than half the time	About half the time	More than half the time	Almost always
Over the last month how, often have you had a sensation of not emptying your bladder completely after you finish urinating?	0	1	2	3	4	5
During the last month, how often have you had to urinate again less than 2 h after you finished urinating?	0	1	2	3	4	5
During the last month, how often have you stopped and started again several times when you urinate?	0	1	2	3	4	5
During the last month, how often have you found it difficult to postpone urination?	0	1	2	3	4	5
During the last month, how often have you had a weak urinary stream?	0	1	2	3	4	5
During the last month, how often have you had to push or strain to begin urination?	0	1	2	3	4	5
During the last month, how many times did you most typically get up to urinate from the time you went to bed until the time you got up in the morning?	None	1 time	2 times	3 times	4 times	5 or more times

Add the score for each number above and write the total in the space to the right
SYMPTOM SCORE = 1–7 MILD; 8–19 MODERATE; 20–35 SEVERE. TOTAL____

are classified from mild (total score 0–7) to moderate (total score 8–19) or severe (total score 20–35). The AUA symptom score is a useful tool for assessing symptoms over time in a quantitative way. The International Prostate Symptom Score (IPSS) uses the same items and adds a disease-specific quality of life question: 'If you were to spend the rest of your life with your urinary condition the way it is now, how would you feel about that?'.

However, before one concludes that a man's symptoms are related to BPH, other disorders which can cause similar symptoms should be excluded by history, physical examination and several simple tests.

The history may provide important diagnostic information:

- History of type 2 diabetes: nocturia.
- Symptoms of neurological disease: neurogenic bladder.
- Sexual dysfunction related LUTS.
- Gross haematuria or pain in the bladder area: bladder tumour or calculi.
- History of urethral trauma, urethritis or urethral instrumentation: urethral stricture.
- Family history of BPH and prostate cancer.
- Treatment with drugs that can impair bladder function (anticholinergic drugs) or increase outflow resistance (sympathomimetic drugs).

Physical examination should include digital rectal examination (DRE) to assess prostate size and consistency and to detect nodules or induration suggesting a prostate cancer. Rectal sphincter tone should be determined and a neurological examination performed.

A general health and cognitive status evaluation is useful for choosing the best treatment, especially if a surgical procedure is required. Clearly, dementia among many neurological conditions could affect urinary condition.

Laboratory evaluation

Urinalysis should be done to detect urinary infection and haematuria. Urine cytology may be helpful for bladder tumour diagnosis in men with predominantly irritative symptoms (frequency, urgency, nocturia) or haematuria especially with a smoking history.

A high serum creatinine may be due to bladder outlet obstruction or to underlying renal or prerenal disease; it also increases the risk of complications and mortality after prostatic surgery. Serum creatinine used to be recommended, but studies have shown that it is not mandatory without comorbidity.[26] In contrast, the European Association of Urology considers it to be a cost-effective test. Bladder, ureters and kidneys ultrasounds are indicated if the serum creatinine concentration is subnormal.

PSA measurement remains controversial. Serum PSA specificity in men with obstructive symptoms is lower compared with asymptomatic patients. PSA is not cancer specific and could be increased in different prostatic disorders, including BPH. Moreover, 25% of patients with a prostate cancer have a normal PSA (4.0 ng ml^{-1} or less, a widely used cut-off value).

Regarding BPH guidelines,[26] recommendations refer to patients with a life expectancy of >10 years.

Treatment[2]

LUTS of BPH progress slowly, with some patients progressing more rapidly than others. The physician can predict the risk of progression from the patient's clinical profile. Also, increased symptom severity, a poor maximum urinary flow rate and a high post-void residual urine volume are major risk factors for overall clinical progression of LUTS/BPH.[27] Also, therapeutic decision-making should be guided by the severity of the symptoms, the degree of bother, the patient's risk profile for progression and patient preference. Information on the risks and benefits of BPH treatment options should be explained to all patients.

The treatment for LUTS can be separated into four groups: watchful waiting, medical therapy, minimally invasive treatment and invasive surgical therapy.

Watchful waiting

Patients with mild symptoms (IPSS <7) should be counselled about a combination of lifestyle and watchful waiting. They should have periodic physician-monitored visits. Patients with mild symptoms and severe bother should undergo further assessment.

A variety of life style changes may be suggested:

- fluid restriction, particularly prior to bedtime
- avoidance of caffeinated beverages and spicy foods
- avoidance/monitoring of some drugs (e.g. diuretics)
- timed or organized voiding (bladder retraining)
- pelvic floor exercises
- avoidance or treatment of constipation.

Medical treatment

α-Blockers

α-Blockers are an excellent first-line therapeutic option for men with symptomatic bother who desire treatment. Alfuzosin, doxazosin, tamsulosin, terazosin and silodosin are appropriated treatment options for LUTS secondary to BPH. They do not alter the natural progression of the disease. Adverse side effects commonly reported with different alpha-blockers include dizziness, headache, asthenia, postural hypotension, rhinitis and sexual dysfunction, most commonly occurring in ~5–9% of patient populations.

5α-Reductase inhibitors

The 5α-reductase inhibitors (duasteride and finasteride) are appropriate and effective treatments for patients with LUTS associated with demonstrable prostatic enlargement. Because of the mechanism of action, it takes 3–6 months for full clinical effect.

Combination therapy

The combination of an α-adrenergic receptor blocker and a 5α-reductase inhibitor is an appropriate and effective treatment strategy for patients with LUTS associated with prostatic enlargement. The MOST trial demonstrated maximum effect in reducing prostate size and improving symptoms by combining an α-blocker (doxazosin) with an α-reductase inhibitor (finasteride).[22] Combination medical therapy can effectively delay symptomatic disease progression, while combination therapy and/or 5α-reductase monotherapy is associated with decreased risk of urinary retention and/or prostate surgery. Patients successfully treated with combination therapy may be given the option of discontinuing the α-blocker after 6–9 months of therapy. If symptoms recur, the α-blocker should be restarted.

Role of anticholinergic medications

Evidence suggests that for selected patients with bladder outlet obstruction due to BPH and concomitant detrusor overactivity, combination therapy with an α-receptor antagonist and anticholinergic can be helpful.[28]

Caution is recommended, however, when considering these agents in men with an elevated residual urine volume or a history of spontaneous urinary retention. These kinds of medications also increase the risk of delirium in patients with cognitive impairment.

Phytotherapies

Phytotherapies for BPH are becoming increasingly popular and, although many physicians remain sceptical of their value, patients generally seem satisfied with their utility. Two of the more common herbal medications used include *Serenoa repens* (saw palmetto) and *Pygeum africanum* (*Prunus africana*). They have shown some efficacy in several small clinical series but cannot be recommended as the standard treatment of BPH.

Minimally invasive treatment

Transurethral microwave therapy (TUMT)

TUMT is a reasonable treatment consideration for the patient who has moderate symptoms, small to moderate gland size and a desire to avoid more invasive therapy for potentially less effective results.[29] TUMT may be associated with a higher retreatment rate over a 5 year follow-up interval than for men receiving TURP.[29]

Transurethral needle ablation (TUNA)

TUNA is an other minimally invasive therapy recommended as treatment options. The TUNA device is a rigid cystoscope-like instrument passed transurethrally under vision. Utilizing a radiofrequency signal, the tissue is heated to between 46 and 100 °C. TUNA may be a therapeutic option for the relief of symptoms in the younger, active individual in whom sexual function remains an important quality of life issue (less risk of retrograde ejaculation); however, limited data are available on long-term outcomes.[30]

Surgery

Transurethral resection of the prostate (TURP)

A TURP can be performed with a regional block under or general anaesthesia. The procedure takes 60–90 min and generally requires a 24 h observation period in the hospital. A resectoscope loaded with a diathermy loop is introduced into the bladder. Under direct vision, strips of prostatic adenoma are resected one at a time and dropped into the bladder. This is continued until the entire adenoma is resected. At the end of the operation, the prostate chips are evacuated from the bladder and haemostasis achieved with electrocautery. The prostatic fossa is left with a wide open, bound by its capsule. The cavity will be lined by a regenerated epithelial surface in 6–12 weeks. Until the fossa is completely epithelialized, the patient is vulnerable to bleeding; the patient should avoid straining for at least 6 weeks.

TURP remains the gold standard treatment for patients with bothersome moderate or severe LUTS who request active treatment or who either fail or do not want medical therapy. Furthermore, patients should be informed that the procedure may be associated with short- and long term complications.[31] For frail patients, transurethral plasma vaporization of the prostate in saline (TUVis) could be useful. As opposed to the conventional transurethral resection of the prostate, this new procedure does not cut and shave off tissue with a loop but energetically vaporizes the tissue with a small electrode. Bleeds during and after this surgery can be avoided. This surgical technique should be proposed to frail patients especially with blood thinner treatments.

Transurethral incision of the prostate (TUIP)

TUIP is appropriate surgical therapy for men with prostate gland sizes <30 g. These patients should experience symptom improvements similar to TURP with a lower incidence of retrograde ejaculation.[32]

Laser prostatectomy

Several methods for laser prostatectomy have been developed, including ultrasound- and endoscopic-guided approaches.[33] A systematic review evaluated 20 randomized trials involving 1898 patients, including 18 comparing TURP with contact lasers, non-contact lasers and hybrid techniques:[34]

- The pooled percentage improvements for mean urinary symptoms ranged from 59 to 68% with laser treatments and from 63 to 77% with TURP.
- Improvements in mean peak urinary flow ranged from 56 to 119% with laser treatments and from 96 to 127% with TURP.
- Laser-treated subjects were less likely to require transfusions (<1 versus 7%) or develop strictures (4 versus 8%) and their hospitalizations were 1–2 days shorter.
- Surgical reintervention occurred more often after laser procedures than TURP (5 versus 1%).

Data were too limited to draw conclusions about the preferred laser technique or to compare laser treatment with other minimally invasive procedures, but patients treated with non-contact laser prostatectomy were more likely to have dysuria than patients treated with TURP or contact laser prostatectomy. In many centres, laser treatment of BPH has evolved from coagulation to enucleation with the holmium laser (HoLEP: holmium laser enucleation of the prostate). This instrument is not dependent upon prostate size and tissue can be preserved for histology. A meta-analysis of four small randomized trials comparing TURP with HoLEP found significant heterogeneity across studies, but concluded that peak flow rates were similar after either therapy and that TURP required less operating room time but resulted in more blood loss, longer catheterization times and longer hospital stays.[35]

Open prostatectomy

Open prostatectomy accounts for <5% of operations for BPH in the USA,[36] but it is performed more often in other countries. Open prostatectomy remains indicated for men whose prostates, in the view of the treating urologist, are too large for TURP for fear of incomplete resection, significant bleeding or the risk of dilutional hyponatraemia.

Prostate cancer

Epidemiology

Prostate cancer is an extremely frequent malignant disease. It represents the second most common cancer in men after lung cancer and the fifth cause of death by cancer in the world. According to GLOBOCAN statistics, 679 023 new cases of prostate cancer were diagnosed worldwide in 2002 and 2 21 002 men died of this disease during the same year, representing 5.8% of cancer mortality in humans.[37]

The epidemiological impact of prostate cancer varies from one country to another because of health policies or screening, but Western countries such as the USA, Australia and New Zealand and Western Europe are particularly concerned. Given the ageing population and its increasing incidence with age, prostate cancer affects mainly elderly men. In the USA, according to SEER data (Surveillance Epidemiology and End Results) from 2000 to 2005, the median age at diagnosis of prostate cancer was 68 years, with 25.7% of cases diagnosed in men ≥75 years of age.

Over 90% of deaths occurred in men ≥65 years of age and 71.2% in men ≥75 years of age.[38]

Principal individual risks factors of developing a prostate cancer are increasing age and heredity and ethnicity. In the USA, compared with white men, black men have a 40% higher risk of the disease and twice the rate of death.[39] Exogenous factors (food consumption, pattern of sexual behaviour, alcohol consumption and occupational exposure) may have an important impact on this risk. Several ongoing large randomized trials are trying to clarify the role of such risk factors and the potential for successful prostate cancer prevention.[40]

Diagnosis and screening

In the PSA era, procedures for prostate cancer diagnosis have changed considerably. Diagnosis is based clinically, on digital rectal examination (DRE), and biologically, on PSA assay. Diagnosis is confirmed by pathological evaluation of prostate biopsies. Regarding pathology, adenocarcinoma represents 98% of cases and most often arises from the peripheral part of the prostate. Among pathological features, differentiation of tumour tissue given by the Gleason score is particularly important.[39,40]

Based on the preliminary results of large ongoing screening trials, widespread mass screening is not appropriate at present. However, major urological societies recommend early diagnosis in well-informed men.[40] Thus, the French Urological Association (AFU) recommends performing a DRE and PSA test per year from age 55 years (or 45 years if there are risk factors) to 69 years according to the results the results of the European screening study ERSPC. Before 55 and after 69 years, tests should be proposed based on individual criteria.[41]

For elderly patients, in case of symptoms, it is necessary to obtain pathological evidence of prostate cancer to propose specific management. Therapeutic options (hormonal therapy, radiotherapy, analgesics) are usually feasible in this situation.

For asymptomatic patients, it is necessary take into account the individual probability of survival to propose early diagnosis tests. It is important, however, to maintain regular DRE assessment in older men to detect the onset of locally advanced prostate cancer potentially responsible for disabling symptoms. In this situation, even frail elderly patients may benefit from the specific treatment.

Management of localized prostate cancer

The management of localized prostate cancer[40] is based on classifications depending on relapse risk. The most widely used classification is that of D'Amico *et al.*[42] Patients are divided into three groups depending on the probability of biological relapse after local treatment of prostate cancer by surgery, radiotherapy or brachytherapy. This classification is based on DRE, PSA and Gleason score (Table 105.2).

Low-risk patients

- Watchful waiting:

Eligibility criteria
  - DRE T1 or T2a (Table 105.3)
  - PSA <10 ng ml^{-1}
  - Gleason score ≤6, no grade 4
  - ≤2 positive biopsies
  - ≤50% of cancer in each biopsy.
- Radical prostatectomy (bilateral ilio-obturator lymphadenectomy is optional).
- Brachytherapy:

Eligibility criteria
  - ≤cT2b
  - PSA <10 ng ml^{-1}
  - Gleason score ≤6
  - prostatic volume ≤50 cm^3
  - IPSS <12.
- Conformational external beam radiation therapy (prostate volume alone, dose of 70 Gy or more).

Intermediate-risk patients

- Radical prostatectomy with lymphadenectomy.
- Conformational external beam radiation therapy dose ≥74 Gy.
- Conformational external beam radiation therapy with a short course of hormonal therapy with LH–RH agonists (6 months).

High-risk patients

- The standard of care is the association of conformational external beam radiation therapy with hormonal therapy (if life expectancy exceeds 10 years).

Table 105.2 Groups of D'Amico *et al.*[42]

Low risk	Intermediate risk	High risk
Stage <T2b *AND* PSA ≤10 ng ml^{-1} *AND* biopsy Gleason score <7	Stage T2b *OR* 11≤ PSA ≤20 ng ml^{-1} *OR* biopsy Gleason score = 7	Stage ≥T2c *OR* PSA >20 ng ml^{-1} *OR* biopsy Gleason score ≥8

Table 105.3 TNM classification.

T1–T2	*Localized prostate cancer not extending beyond the capsule (no lymph node, absence of metastasis, that is, N0M0)*
T1	*Only histological finding (not visible to imaging and non-palpable)*
T1a	<5% of cancer cells on the samples
T1b	>5%
T2	*Cancer palpable on rectal examination*
T2a	Cancers with <50% of both prostate lobes
T2b	>50%
T2c	Involvement of both lobes
T3: Extension of cancer in the peripheral tissues (crossing of the prostate capsule)	
T3a	Extension beyond capsule
T3b	Involvement of seminal vesicles
T4: extension to adjacent organs: bladder, rectum, pelvic wall	
N0 or N1	Absence or presence of lymph node(s)
M0 or M1	Presence or absence of metastasis(es)

- A long-term adjuvant hormonal therapy (3 years) is beneficial.
- The radiation dose must be at least 70 Gy.
- Irradiation of pelvic lymph nodes is optional; it will be performed according to the risk of lymph node invasion.
- Non-conservative radical prostatectomy with lymphadenectomy is an option for locally advanced tumours with low metastatic risk in patients with long life expectancy and as part of a multimodal treatment.

Treatment modalities for localized prostate cancer in the elderly

Total prostatectomy

Technically, this is associated with bilateral resection of seminal vesicles and may be associated with bilateral pelvic lymph node dissection according to the prognostic group of D'Amico *et al.*[42] Radical retropubic prostatectomy or perineal prostatectomy is performed through open incisions. More recently, laparoscopic and robot-assisted prostatectomy have been developed. Available data are not sufficient to show differences in terms of oncological and functional results between these different techniques.[40]

Although data are limited, no significant differences exist between oncological outcomes and morbidity and mortality of radical prostatectomy done in the elderly compared with younger patients, apart from erectile dysfunction and urinary continence, which is more frequent in men ≥75 years of age. However, patient selection appears to be an important element in ensuring a balance between the expected benefit of surgery and the risks involved. This selection appears clearly from series available in the literature and corresponds perfectly with the 'oncogeriatric approach'.[40,43–47]

Radiotherapy

Technically, the current standard is 3D conformational radiotherapy, which can be further optimized by intensity modulation technology (IMRT).

These technological advances actually allow dose escalation in the volume to be treated to improve local control without increasing acute side effects on critical organs, particularly the bladder and rectum. Available data on the late side effects also appear to be in favour of IMRT.

In the literature, efficacy and tolerability of radiotherapy are not dependent on age. Nevertheless, comorbidities should be taken into account because they have an impact on the incidence of complications, particularly diabetes and vascular disease. Tolerance also depends on the size of irradiation fields. Irradiation of pelvic lymph node will be avoided if the probability of pelvic lymph node involvement is low.

Similarly, the possibility of associating a hormone therapy for 6 months in the intermediate prognosis group, which is a standard for younger patients, should be assessed with caution in elderly patients with moderate to severe comorbidities. The side effects of hormonal treatment could reduce or cancel the benefit in terms of overall survival. On the other hand, it appears that the benefit of hormone therapy in combination with radiotherapy in high-risk forms is found in elderly patients without or with minor comorbidities.[38,40,43,48–52]

Brachytherapy

Brachytherapy is a curative treatment of prostate cancer, most often consisting in the introduction of permanent implants of iodine-125 in the prostate gland. The implantation is performed by the perineal route under ultrasound guidance during general anaesthesia or spinal block.

This technique is used to deliver a very important dose in prostate volume, while sparing relatively periprostatic tissues, the dose falling rapidly at the periphery of the settlement area. Brachytherapy is therefore indicated in tumours with good prognosis: usually Gleason ≤6, initial PSA ≤10 $ng\,ml^{-1}$, absence of capsular damage and low proportion of adenocarcinoma on core biopsies.

This technique should not be applied in case of severe pre-existing urinary dysfunctions, in patients with a history of transurethral resection of prostate or in case of too large a prostate volume (>55 cm^3).

In terms of tolerance, the most frequent complications of brachytherapy arise in the urinary tract or rectum or affect erectile function. They are related to age and comorbidities which are a stronger predictor than age in multivariate analysis.[38,40,43,53]

Active monitoring

Currently, because of the widespread early diagnosis of prostate cancer through PSA testing, more and more prostate cancers are found with size and aggressiveness presumed to be low. Many men with localized prostate cancer will not, in fact, benefit from a definitive treatment. In order to reduce the risk of over-treatment in these patients, conservative management strategies have been proposed.

For elderly patients, a waiting strategy may be proposed in several situations:

- Good prognosis disease according to the classification of D'Amico *et al.*,[42] since in this group, the specific risk of death is almost zero in patients over 70 years old.
- Low individual probability of survival due to a very advanced age or severe comorbidities.
- Patients who wish to avoid or delay the side effects of curative treatments.

The advantages of such a strategy are obvious, since it allows the patient to avoid treatment and side effects. However, it often induces anxiety in the patient and his family. It can also lead to a delayed diagnosis with a risk of more advanced disease.[38,40,43]

High-intensity focused ultrasound (HIFU)

This technique is still under evaluation. The high-intensity focused ultrasound is administered through the rectum, under general or spinal anaesthesia and guided by echography. Transurethral resection of the prostate to prevent postoperative urinary retention is mandatory. When validated, this technique will be useful in patients with small to moderate prostate volume and in patients relapsing after radiotherapy.

Other techniques such as cryotherapy and focal treatments are currently being developed, and will certainly soon strengthen our therapeutic tools.[38,40,43,54,55]

Hormone therapy

Hormone therapy alone is a treatment modality widely used in elderly patients with localized prostate cancer but considered unable to receive curative treatment. Nevertheless, these treatments are associated with a significant number of side effects, with an important impact on quality of life in elderly patients. Moreover, recent studies have shown a clear advantage for combined radiotherapy and hormone therapy in terms of progression-free survival and even overall survival in comparison with hormone therapy alone.

Hormone therapy alone should be considered only in symptomatic patients whose life expectancy is short due to significant competitive comorbidities.[38,40,43,54,56–61]

The management of localized prostate cancer in an elderly man is possible, but is it beneficial for the patient? To answer this question, some authors have tried to model the value of a curative treatment of prostate cancer in elderly men using a Markov model. Alibhai *et al.*[62] compared the probability of survival adjusted for quality of life (QALE) of patients stratified on age and differentiation of prostate cancer, according to their management by active surveillance, surgery or radiotherapy. They concluded that there was no advantage to treat patients >70 years of age with well-differentiated prostate cancer whatever their level of comorbidity. On the other hand, a benefit in terms of survival and QALE was found in patients >70 years of age with moderately to poorly differentiated prostate cancer including patients with intermediate comorbidities.

Advanced and metastatic prostate cancer

Despite earlier diagnosis, we have to take care of many patients with advanced or metastatic prostate cancer. Given the epidemiological and demographic data, this situation is frequently encountered in elderly men. The median overall survival of metastatic prostate cancer patients is 28–53 months, regardless of age, with only 7% of patients alive at 7 years.

Prognostic factors of survival are the initial PSA, Gleason score, volume of metastatic disease and presence of specific symptoms, particularly bone pain.

In metastatic disease, the cornerstone of treatment is androgen deprivation therapy. First-line treatment is surgical castration or medical castration by LH–RH agonists with 'flare-up syndrome' prevention or antagonists of LH–RH.

Hormone treatment should be started early and may be conducted continuously or intermittently. Patients with a normalization of PSA within 6 months are good candidates for intermittent treatment.

with disease progression, modifications of hormonal therapy can be carried out:

- Anti-androgens are used to complete androgen blockade.
- Cessation of anti-androgens since ~30% of patients derive a benefit from the anti-androgen withdrawal approach.[38,40,43]

Castration-refractory prostate cancer

Castration-refractory prostate cancer is defined in the Guidelines of the European Association of Urology:[40]

- Serum castration level of testosterone (testosterone $<50\,\mathrm{ng\,dl^{-1}}$ or $<1.7\,\mathrm{nmol\,l^{-}}$).
- Three consecutive rises of PSA, 1 week apart, resulting in two 50% increases over the nadir, with a PSA $>2\,\mathrm{ng\,ml^{-1}}$.
- Anti-androgen withdrawal for at least 4 weeks.
- PSA progression despite consecutive hormonal manipulations.

The standard treatment of this situation is chemotherapy with docetaxel $75\,\mathrm{mg\,m^{-2}}$ every 3 weeks combined with prednisone following the studies of Tannock *et al.*[63] and Petrylak *et al.*[64] This regimen has shown a significant benefit in overall survival and symptoms compared with chemotherapy using mitoxantrone/prednisone. The weekly administration of docetaxel has not shown the same benefit in survival compared with mitoxantrone while symptomatic gain was found.

The survival benefit obtained with docetaxel is not influenced by patient age, as demonstrated by studies of subgroups (above and below 69 years of age). However, it is difficult to extrapolate these results to daily practice because patients in the trials represent a selected population very different from our daily practice or geriatric oncology 'routine'. In such a situation, the choice of weekly docetaxel therapy may be preferred because of better tolerance, including haematological tolerance.

Docetaxel chemotherapy feasibility, administered every week or every 3 weeks, in a population of unselected patients ≥75 years old was studied in a retrospective French study, involving 175 patients. This study confirmed good results in terms of safety and efficacy (no significant difference in terms of response on the PSA between the 3 weeks docetaxel group and the weekly docetaxel group. Overall survival reached 15 months in the global population without a significant difference between the two groups.[65]

After first-line chemotherapy, there is no standard treatment but therapies can be can be proposed to our patients such as second-line hormonal therapy (e.g. diethylstilbestrol) or second-line chemotherapy, such as docetaxel again and mitoxantrone. Second-line hormone therapy or chemotherapy is an option for symptomatic disease since no survival benefit has yet been established.

Moreover, hormone refractory bone metastasis of prostate cancer is an indication for zoledronic acid. This derives from a study by Saad *et al.* that assessed the effect of 2 years of monthly injections of zoledronic acid in patients with bone metastases from castration-resistant prostate cancer.[66] This treatment significantly increased the time to first skeletal event and reduced the rate of bone complications.

In 2010, several study results were presented and management of patients after chemotherapy with docetaxel will change in the coming months. In particular, a new taxane chemotherapy usingcabazitaxel with prednisone showed an overall survival benefit compared with mitoxantrone after docetaxel. Abiraterone, a novel anti-androgen, has also shown a significant overall survival benefit in this setting compared with placebo.[67,68]

Side effects of androgen suppressive hormones[38,40,43,57,69–71]

The side effects are frequent and many of them are generally well known to doctors and patients, such as hot flashes, lower libido and erectile dysfunction. However, other side effects have to be taken into account in elderly men.

Among them, osteoporosis is important, given the risk of fractures. Bone loss due to physiological ageing is estimated at 1–4.6% per year for men who receive androgen deprivation therapy with the risk of fracture increasing up to 45% over the long term.

Therefore, for these patients it is recommended to seek osteoporosis risk factors (family history, low weight, fracture history, alcohol abuse, smoking, use of glucocorticoids, low blood levels of vitamin D) and prescribe calcium and vitamin D. Bisphosphonates are not recommended routinely but only in cases of established osteoporosis.

In addition, hormone therapy causes an increase in fat mass and sarcopenia, which may have a very important impact in the elderly by promoting loss of autonomy, falls and fractures. Hormone therapy in prostate cancer seems also to be responsible for an increased cardiovascular risk even if the published results are sometimes contradictory. However, androgen suppression is responsible for an altered lipid profile, increase in insulin resistance and diabetes mellitus and an increased prevalence of metabolic syndrome. In some studies, such as the RTOG 92-02 study, an increased cardiovascular risk was demonstrated.

These factors are sufficient, in our view, to push clinicians to consider the cardiovascular risk in the indication of hormone therapy in elderly patients and suggest preventive measures when these treatments are needed. Already mentioned for osteoporosis, modifications of diet and lifestyle (walking, adapted diet and smoking cessation) are needed in order to reduce the metabolic and cardiovascular impact of hormone therapy.

Comprehensive care

Management of metastatic prostate cancer is not limited to the prescription of hormone therapy or chemotherapy. The patient must be accompanied throughout his disease in all dimensions of his existence: psychological and physical symptoms and social issues must be taken into account. To achieve this global care, a multidisciplinary approach is essential, as illustrated by the examples of management listed below:

- psychological and social considerations
- optimization of analgesic treatment
- possible urological intervention such as prostatic drilling
- palliative radiotherapy for bone pain or symptomatic prostate tumour
- use of radiopharmaceuticals, for multiple bone pains
- use of bisphosphonates.

Recommendations for management of elderly patients

In 2010, the International Society of Geriatric Oncology (SIOG) published guidelines for the management of prostate cancer in elderly patients.[38,43] Despite epidemiological data, very little is known about the management of elderly patients. Of course, the evaluation of health status is the cornerstone of these guidelines and experts at SIOG

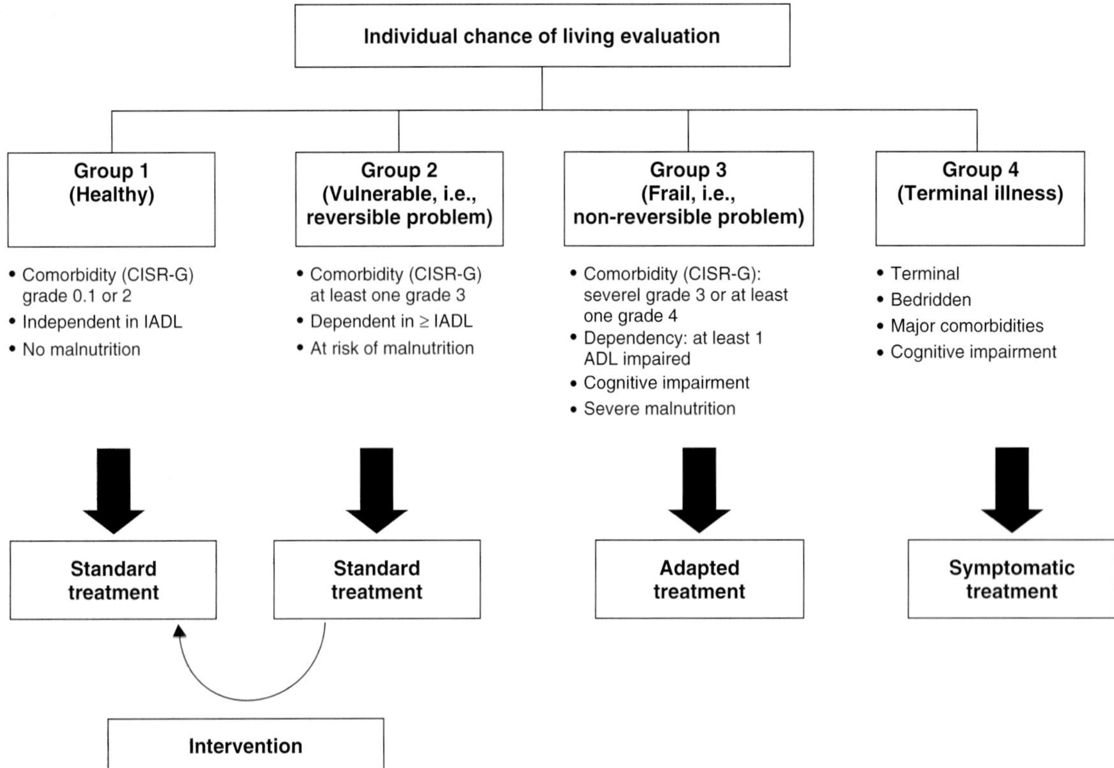

Figure 105.1 General scheme for the treatment decision-making in senior adults with prostate cancer.[38]

recommend treating patients according to their individual health status, mainly driven by their comorbidities and not according to their chronological age. In these recommendations the evaluation of individual health status is based on comprehensive geriatric assessment. This individual evaluation is necessary because of the high heterogeneity of this population. It is designed to estimate the individual probability of survival of each patient, to determine his vulnerability factors that may affect the result or tolerance of the proposed treatment and possibly offer a geriatric intervention.

The SIOG task force proposed a distribution of elderly patients into four groups, according to geriatric evaluation, focusing on comorbidities (Cumulative Illness Rating Scale – Geriatric),[72] cognitive functions (Mini Mental State Examination),[73] dependency (instrumental activities of daily living[74] and activities of daily living[75]) and nutritional status [estimated very simply by the variation (%) of weight during the last 3 months] (Figure 105.1):

- *Group 1 or 'healthy':* are able to receive standard treatment as younger patients.
- *Group 2 or 'vulnerable, i.e. with reversible problems':* may be treated as younger patients (except prostatectomy for localized disease) after geriatric intervention.
- *Group 3 or 'frail, i.e. with non reversible problems'* may receive specific but adapted treatments.
- *Group 4 or 'terminal illness'* should receive only symptomatic treatments.

This evaluation and this classification help physicians to make the best management proposal to the patient according to the medical findings and the patient's preferences

Prostatitis

Definition

The prostate is subject to various inflammatory disorders. Inflammatory or irritative conditions of the prostate were traditionally classified according to the following scheme:

- Acute prostatitis.
- Chronic bacterial prostatitis.
- Non-bacterial prostatitis, which presents with similar symptoms and signs as chronic prostatitis (including pyuria) except that cultures of urine and expressed prostatic secretions are negative.
- Prostatodynia, which also presents with similar symptoms and signs as chronic prostatitis except that the cultures are negative and pyuria is absent.

A classification approach supported by the National Institutes of Health (NIH) to standardize definitions and facilitate research made the following recommendations:[76]

• Adding an entity called asymptomatic inflammatory prostatitis.
• Combining non-bacterial prostatitis and prostatodynia into an entity called chronic prostatitis/pelvic pain syndrome.

The inflammatory subset of this syndrome included patients with significant numbers of inflammatory cells in expressed prostatic secretions, post-prostate massage urine or seminal fluid. The non-inflammatory chronic prostatitis/pelvic pain subset included the remainder of the patients with chronic prostatitis or pelvic pain.

Thus, the newer scheme defined the following categories:

1 acute prostatitis
2 chronic bacterial prostatitis
3 chronic prostatitis/pelvic pain syndrome, inflammatory
4 chronic prostatitis/pelvic pain syndrome, non-inflammatory
5 asymptomatic inflammatory prostatitis.

Manoeuvres performed in the urology office can help refine the categorization of patients. For example, including post-massage urine and seminal fluid for the assessment of inflammatory cells effectively doubles the number of people in the inflammatory subset (as compared with the older distinction using only purulent prostatic secretions).[77]

Acute prostatitis

Entry of microorganisms into the prostate gland almost always occurs via the urethra. In most cases, bacteria migrate from the urethra or bladder through the prostatic ducts, with intraprostatic reflux of urine. As a result, there may be concomitant infection in the bladder or epididymis.

Prostatitis can occur in patients with chronic indwelling bladder catheters and in those with intermittent catheterization.

Microbiology

The flora of acute prostatitis reflects the spectrum of agents causing urinary tract infection (UTI) and deeper genital infection. Gram-negative infections (typically *Escherichia coli* or *Proteus* spp.) are most common.[78] Recurrent infection after completion of therapy is usually caused by the same organism that was found in the original infection.[79]

Clinical presentation

The typical signs and symptoms of acute prostatitis include spiking fever, chills, malaise, myalgia, dysuria, pelvic or perineal pain and cloudy urine. With the exception of fever and chills, these symptoms are similar to those of lower urinary tract infection; it is important to appreciate, however, that isolated acute cystitis does not commonly occur in men, in whom virtually all lower UTIs are due to prostatitis. Men with acute cystitis often have a functional or anatomical abnormality. Swelling of the acutely inflamed prostate can cause obstructive symptoms.

Diagnosis

Clinical symptoms, together with an oedematous and tender prostate on physical examination, should prompt a presumptive diagnosis of acute prostatitis. DRE should be performed gently; vigorous prostate massage should be avoided since it is uncomfortable, allows no additional diagnostics and increases the risk for bacteraemia.

A urine Gram stain and culture should be obtained in all men suspected of having acute prostatitis. Confirmatory laboratory findings include pyuria, peripheral leukocytosis and, occasionally, positive blood cultures.

An elevated serum PSA level is also potentially consistent with a diagnosis of acute prostatitis, although a PSA should not be considered to be a standard diagnostic test for prostatitis. Elective serum PSA for prostate cancer screening should be deferred for 1 month following acute prostatitis.[80]

Treatment

A variety of antimicrobials may be used for the treatment of acute prostatitis. The barrier between the microcirculation and the prostate gland stroma limits drug entry to passive diffusion, which only permits non-protein-bound, lipophilic antimicrobial agents to reach therapeutic levels within the gland. In addition, the low pH of prostatic fluid permits antibiotics with alkaline pK_as (such as quinolones and sulfonamides) to achieve high concentrations in prostatic tissue. However, antibiotic prostatic penetration in the setting of inflammation occurs more readily. Patients with acute bacterial prostatitis may need to be hospitalized for parenteral antibiotic therapy if they cannot tolerate oral medication or if they demonstrate signs of sepsis. In such cases, shock due to Gram-negative bacteraemia may occur abruptly and be life threatening. In general, broad antibiotic coverage should be administered empirically pending the culture results.

Patients with Gram-negative rods should be treated with trimethoprim–sulfamethoxazole or a fluoroquinolone if oral therapy is indicated. Other agents with good to excellent penetration into prostatic fluid and tissue include tetracyclines, macrolides, sulfonamides and nitrofurantoin. For patients who need parenteral therapy, an aminoglycoside may be combined with intravenous fluoroquinolones. The patient should be treated as if infected with Gram-negative rods until additional culture data are available. Gram-positive cocci in chains usually indicate enterococcal infection, which should be treated with amoxicillin. Gram-positive cocci in clusters are most often due to *Staphylococcus aureus* or coagulase-negative staphylococci (e.g. *Staphylococcus epidermidis*). When *S. aureus* is recovered from a urine culture, it is important to perform blood cultures to be certain that the bacteriuria reflects local infection and not seeding of the urine in association with bacteraemia.

Chronic bacterial prostatitis

Chronic prostatitis may present as a complication of acute prostatitis or in the absence of previously recognized initial infection. The diagnosis should be considered in men who have dysuria and frequency in the absence of the signs of acute prostatitis, in those with recurrent UTIs in the absence of bladder catheterization and in the setting of incidental bacteriuria. Gram-negative rods are the most common aetiological agent, with *E. coli* causing ~75–80% of episodes.[81] Other organisms, including enterococci, aerobic Gram-negative rods (other than *E. coli*) and *Chlamydia trachomatis* have also been associated with chronic infection.

Clinical presentation

Chronic prostatitis has more subtle clinical findings than acute prostatitis. Patients may be asymptomatic or have typical complaints of a lower urinary tract infection such as frequency, dysuria, urgency, perineal discomfort and perhaps a low-grade fever. In some cases, the diagnosis may be suspected by the incidental finding of bacteriuria. Sexual dysfunction may accompany chronic prostatitis.[82] Rectal examination may demonstrate prostatic hypertrophy, tenderness and oedema, but is frequently normal.

Diagnosis

The diagnosis of chronic prostatitis can be made by analysing specimens obtained following prostatic massage for leukocytes and bacteria. The periurethral area is cleaned and four samples are taken – the so-called four-glass test.[81] The initial 5–10 ml (VB1) and a midstream specimen (VB2) are obtained for quantitative culture. The patient should stop voiding before the bladder is empty and the prostate should then be massaged. Any prostatic secretions that are expressed (EPS) should be cultured and have a leukocyte count performed, in addition to the first 5–10 ml of subsequently voided urine (VB3). For the test to be interpretable, the colony count in VB2 must be less than 10^3 ml^{-1}, since bladder bacteriuria prevents identification of the frequently small number of organisms from the prostate. Chronic prostatitis is suspected when VB3 has more than 12 leukocytes per high power field; more than 20 leukocytes per high power field is almost diagnostic unless leukocytes were also present in VB2.

Cultures of urine or expressed prostatic secretions are almost always positive in chronic prostatitis. However, negative cultures do not necessarily exclude the possibility of bacterial prostatitis. Although the four-glass test has been described extensively in the literature, it is not clear that it is frequently used in practice. Furthermore, the results of the test apparently did not influence the use of antibiotics, since urologists who used the test routinely did not differ in antibiotic prescribing from others who used it less often. Ultrasonography may also be useful for the evaluation of prostatitis sequelae, including prostatic abscess and prostatic calcification.[83]

Treatment

Selection of agents for and duration of therapy for chronic prostatitis have not been studied using comparative trials. In cases series, there has been a general sense that various fluoroquinolone regimens have a satisfactory outcome in about two-thirds of patients who can tolerate them for >4 weeks. Failures of therapy appear to be related to underlying prostate disease, infecting agent, incomplete adherence or some other less understood component. Courses exceeding 4 weeks should be considered in patients who have previously failed treatment, who have a relatively difficult to treat organism or who cannot tolerate first-line therapy and need other agents. *Chlamydia trachomatis* should be considered in patients with clinical chronic prostatitis and negative results of urine and prostatic secretion cultures. *C. trachomatis* infection can be treated with doxycycline, azithromycin or fluoroquinolone. Chronic bacterial prostatitis often recurs and is usually treated with a second course of antibiotics. A fluoroquinolone is once again the treatment of choice.

Chronic prostatitis/chronic pelvic pain syndrome

Chronic prostatitis/chronic pelvic pain syndrome (CP/CPPS) is a clinically defined syndrome, defined primarily on the basis of urological symptoms and/or pain or discomfort in the pelvic region. Despite the use of the term 'prostatitis', it is unclear to what extent and how often the prostate is the source of symptoms.

Definitions

A number of terms have been used to describe the syndrome now commonly called chronic prostatitis/chronic pelvic pain syndrome (CP/CPPS). These include prostatodynia and abacterial prostatitis. Research guidelines define CP/CPPS as chronic pelvic pain for at least 3 of the preceding 6 months in the absence of other identifiable causes.[84]

The inflammatory subset of CP/CPPS includes patients with inflammatory cells in expressed prostatic secretions, post-prostate massage urine or seminal fluid. The non-inflammatory CP/CPPS subset includes the remainder of the patients with chronic prostatitis or pelvic pain.

Epidemiology

CP/CPPS is common. Most men diagnosed with 'prostatitis' have CP/CPPS rather than acute or chronic bacterial prostatitis. Thus, CP/CPPS is likely responsible for nearly 2 million physician visits annually in the USA.[85] In a large population-based Canadian questionnaire study, over 20% of the men had complaints compatible with chronic prostatitis and 8–10% had moderate to severe symptoms.[77] The men with the most severe symptoms also had poorer general health and recurrent complaints.

Aetiology

The aetiology of CP/CPPS is unknown. As mentioned above, it is uncertain whether the prostate is the culprit in many cases.[86] Although bacterial infection has been suspected, particularly in the inflammatory subset of CP/CPPS, a bacterial aetiology has not been proven. Most experts believe that inflammatory and non-inflammatory CP/CPPS are both non-infectious disorders.[87] Additionally, there appears to be little correlation between histological prostatic inflammation and the presence or absence of CP/CPPS symptoms.[88]

Studies of *Chlamydia*, *Mycoplasma* and *Ureaplasma*, which have all been implicated in chronic prostatitis, have generally concluded that they are not responsible for CP/CPPS.[89–92] Non-infectious aetiologies have been proposed for CP/CPPS, but none has been proven. These include inflammation due to trauma, autoimmunity, reaction to normal prostate flora or some other factor, neurogenic pain, increased prostate tissue pressure and the interplay of somatic and psychological factors. Psychological stress appears to be common in men with symptoms of CP/CPPS.

Clinical manifestations

The clinical presentation of CP/CPPS can be similar to that of chronic bacterial prostatitis (frequency, dysuria, perineal pain). To meet the NIH consensus definition, patients should not have active urethritis, urogenital cancer, urinary tract disease, functionally significant urethral stricture or neurological disease affecting the bladder.[76]

Diagnosis

The symptoms of prostatitis are common and often not recognized by physicians. These symptoms include pain (in the perineum, lower abdomen, testicles and penis and with ejaculation), bladder irritation, bladder outlet obstruction and sometimes blood in the semen. Impotence is occasionally attributed to prostatitis; however, it occurs no more commonly than in men of a similar age without prostatitis. CP/CPPS is a diagnosis of exclusion and the evaluation is designed to rule out identifiable causes of pelvic pain:

- On physical examination, patients should be evaluated for hernias, testicular masses, rectal masses and haemorrhoids. Patients with CP/CPPS are typically afebrile. On rectal examination, the prostate is usually not tender but may sometimes be mildly tender; severe tenderness suggests acute prostatitis.
- A urinalysis should be performed.[93] Patients with haematuria should have an evaluation that includes urine cytology (looking for carcinoma *in situ* of the bladder), cystoscopy and upper tract imaging with intravenous pyelography or computed tomography scan.
- A urine culture is required to rule out UTI.[93] Patients with recurrent UTIs should be evaluated for chronic bacterial prostatitis.
- In patients who report a sensation of incomplete emptying of the bladder, a post-void residual should be checked by catheterization or ultrasound.

The classic four-glass test is no longer routinely performed. A PSA test is not indicated and if PSA is measured and found to be elevated, the elevation should not be ascribed to CP/CPPS.[94]

Imaging studies are appropriate in some patients. Patients with concomitant abdominal pain may require imaging with CT to exclude an intra-abdominal process. Testicular pain should be evaluated with a scrotal ultrasound. Lumbar radiculopathy can produce pelvic pain, so patients with signs and symptoms suggesting this diagnosis (e.g. lower extremity paraesthesias or weakness) may require imaging of the spine with magnetic resonance imaging.

In primary care practice, patients suspected of having acute or chronic bacterial prostatitis will frequently receive an empirical trial of an antibiotic and the diagnosis of CP/CPPS will only be entertained in those patients who relapse or do not respond to such therapy.

Treatment

A number of therapies have been tried for CP/CPPS; however, there is no uniformly effective treatment. One group attempted a meta-analysis to examine diagnostic testing and treatments but found substantial methodological problems with the studies assessed.[95,96] The NIH developed a chronic prostatitis symptoms index that was validated and can be used to evaluate different treatment measures.[97] In addition to the validation set of referral patients to the NIH, this symptom index has also proven useful in the assessment of patients presenting to general medicine and urology clinics. The maximum possible symptom score is 43, where higher numbers indicate more severe symptoms.

Antibiotics

Randomized trials in men with CP/CPPS have not found significant benefits with quinolone antibiotics.[98,99]

α-Blockers

Even in the studies showing benefit with α-blockers, the overall decrease in symptom scores was small and likely of only marginal clinical significance. Given the evidence showing a lack of benefit, we recommend not treating pain attributed to CP/CPPS with α-blockers.[100–104] Since the

NIH–CPSI score focuses mainly on pain, it remains possible that α-blockers could improve urinary symptoms in men with CP/CPPS. A trial of α-blockers in men with CP/CPPS and troublesome urinary symptoms is reasonable.

5α-Reductase inhibitors

Randomized trials of finasteride in men with CP/CPPS have suggested possible small benefits.[101,105] The degree of clinical benefit was not sufficient to warrant the routine use of 5α-reductase inhibitors in men with CP/CPPS who do not have another indication such as benign prostatic hyperplasia.[101]

Anti-inflammatory drugs

Non-steroidal anti-inflammatory drugs (NSAIDs) may be of some benefit in controlling symptoms in men with CP/CPPS. A randomized trial found a trend towards benefit with rofecoxib compared with placebo, particularly at higher doses.[98] Rofecoxib is no longer available, but non-selective NSAIDs can be tried for symptomatic control.

Other

A number of other treatments have been tried for CP/CPPS: pollen extract or saw palmetto does not appear to be effective; a small study suggested that transurethral needle ablation of the prostate is no more effective. Sitz baths may provide some pain relief. Psychotherapy has been recommended if there is sexual dysfunction. Physical therapy aimed at achieving myofascial trigger point release may have benefit in some patients.[106]

Key points

- Benign prostatic hypertrophy (BPH), cancer and prostatitis are the three main conditions affecting the prostate gland in older men.
- BPH is a major contributing factor in the development of LUTS – lower urinary tract symptoms.
- Prostate cancer is an extremely frequent malignant disease. It represents the second most common cancer in men after lung cancer and the fifth cause of death by cancer in the world.
- Clinical symptoms, together with an oedematous and tender prostate on physical examination, should prompt a presumptive diagnosis of acute prostatitis.

References

1. Berry SJ *et al*. The development of human benign prostatic hyperplasia with age. *J Urol* 1984;**132**:474–9.
2. Roehrborn CG. Benign prostatic hyperplasia: an overview. *Rev Urol* 2005;**7**(Suppl 9): S3–14.
3. Emberton M *et al*. Benign prostatic hyperplasia as a progressive disease: a guide to the risk factors and options for medical management. *Int J Clin Pract* 2008;**62**:1076–86.
4. Levi F *et al*. Recent trends in mortality from benign prostatic hyperplasia. *Prostate* 2003;**56**:207–11.
5. Cattolica EV, Sidney S and Sadler MC. The safety of transurethral prostatectomy: a cohort study of mortality in 9,416 men. *J Urol* 1997;**158**:102–4.
6. Duncan ME and Goldacre MJ. Mortality trends for benign prostatic hyperplasia and prostate cancer in English populations 1979–2006. *BJU Int* 2011;**107**:40–5.
7. McVary KT. BPH: epidemiology and comorbidities. *Am J Manag Care* 2006;**12**(5 Suppl): S122–8.
8. Kelly CE *et al*. Clinical evaluation of lower urinary tract symptoms due to benign prostatic hyperplasia, In: PT Scardino and KM Slawin (eds), *Atlas of the Prostate*, Current Medicine, Philadelphia, PA, 2003, pp. 11–23.
9. Speakman MJ *et al*. Guideline for the primary care management of male lower urinary tract symptoms. *BJU Int* 2004;**93**:985–90.
10. Untergasser G, Madersbacher S and Berger P. Benign prostatic hyperplasia: age-related tissue remodeling. *Exp Gerontol* 2005;**40**:121–8.
11. Chute CG *et al*. The prevalence of prostatism: a population-based survey of urinary symptoms. *J Urol* 1993;**150**:85–9.
12. Li MK, Garcia LA and Rosen R. Lower urinary tract symptoms and male sexual dysfunction in Asia: a survey of ageing men from five Asian countries. *BJU Int* 2005;**96**: 1339–54.
13. Roberts RO *et al*. Association between family history of benign prostatic hyperplasia and urinary symptoms: results of a population-based study. *Am J Epidemiol* 1995; **142**:965–73.
14. Meikle AW *et al*. Heritability of the symptoms of benign prostatic hyperplasia and the roles of age and zonal prostate volumes in twins. *Urology* 1999;**53**:701–6.
15. Kang D *et al*. Risk behaviours and benign prostatic hyperplasia. *BJU Int* 2004;**93**:1241–5.
16. Meigs JB *et al*. Risk factors for clinical benign prostatic hyperplasia in a community-based population of healthy aging men. *J Clin Epidemiol* 2001;**54**:935–44.
17. Collins MM *et al*. Prevalence and correlates of prostatitis in the health professionals follow-up study cohort. *J Urol* 2002;**167**:1363–6.
18. Hammarsten J and Hogstedt B. Hyperinsulinaemia: a prospective risk factor for lethal clinical prostate cancer. *Eur J Cancer* 2005;**41**:2887–95.
19. Hammarsten J and Hogstedt B. Clinical, anthropometric, metabolic and insulin profile of men with fast annual growth rates of benign prostatic hyperplasia. *Blood Press* 1999;**8**:29–36.
20. Roberts RO *et al*. Longitudinal changes in peak urinary flow rates in a community based cohort. *J Urol* 2000;**163**:107–13.
21. Jacobsen SJ, Girman CJ, Jacobson DJ *et al*. Long-term (92-month) natural history of changes in lower urinary tract symptom severity. *J Urol* 2000;**163**(Suppl. 4):248–9.

22. McConnell JD *et al.* The long-term effect of doxazosin, finasteride and combination therapy on the clinical progression of benign prostatic hyperplasia. *N Engl J Med* 2003; **349**:2387–98.
23. Barry M and Roehrborn C. Management of benign prostatic hyperplasia. *Annu Rev Med* 1997;**48**:177–89.
24. Marberger MJ *et al.* Prostate volume and serum prostate-specific antigen as predictors of acute urinary retention. Combined experience from three large multinational placebo-controlled trials. *Eur Urol* 2000;**38**:563–8.
25. Roehrborn CG *et al.* Serum prostate specific antigen is a strong predictor of future prostate growth in men with benign prostatic hyperplasia. PROSCAR long-term efficacy and safety study. *J Urol* 2000;**163**:13–20.
26. AUA Practice Guidelines Committee. AUA guideline on management of benign prostatic hyperplasia (2003). Chapter 1. Diagnosis and treatment recommendations. *J Urol* 2003;**170**(2 Pt 1): 530–47.
27. Trachtenberg J. Treatment of lower urinary tract symptoms suggestive of benign prostatic hyperplasia in relation to the patient's risk profile for progression. *BJU Int* 2005;**95**(Suppl 4):6–11.
28. Kaplan SA *et al.* Tolterodine and tamsulosin for treatment of men with lower urinary tract symptoms and overactive bladder: a randomized controlled trial. *JAMA* 2006;**296**:2319–28.
29. de la Rosette JJ *et al.* Transurethral microwave thermotherapy: the gold standard for minimally invasive therapies for patients with benign prostatic hyperplasia? *J Endourol* 2003;**17**:245–51.
30. Bouza C *et al.* Systematic review and meta-analysis of transurethral needle ablation in symptomatic benign prostatic hyperplasia. *BMC Urol* 2006;**6**: 14.
31. Rassweiler J *et al.* Complications of transurethral resection of the prostate (TURP) – incidence, management and prevention. *Eur Urol* 2006;**50**: 969–79; discussion, 980.
32. Yang Q *et al.* Transurethral incision compared with transurethral resection of the prostate for bladder outlet obstruction: a systematic review and meta-analysis of randomized controlled trials. *J Urol* 2001;**165**:1526–32.
33. McAllister WJ *et al.* Does endoscopic laser ablation of the prostate stand the test of time? Five-year results from a multicentre randomized controlled trial of endoscopic laser ablation against transurethral resection of the prostate. *BJU Int* 2000;**85**:437–9.
34. Hoffman RM, MacDonald R and Wilt TJ. Laser prostatectomy for benign prostatic obstruction. *Cochrane Database Syst Rev* 2004;(1): CD001987.
35. Tan A *et al.* Meta-analysis of holmium laser enucleation versus transurethral resection of the prostate for symptomatic prostatic obstruction. *Br J Surg* 2007;**94**:1201–8.
36. Sidney S *et al.* Reoperation and mortality after surgical treatment of benign prostatic hypertrophy in a large prepaid medical care program. *Med Care* 1992;**30**:117–25.
37. Parkin DM *et al.* Global cancer statistics 2002. *CA Cancer J Clin* 2005;**55**:74–108.
38. Droz JP *et al.* Background for the proposal of SIOG guidelines for the management of prostate cancer in senior adults. *Crit Rev Oncol Hematol* 2010;**73**:68–91.
39. Walsh PC, DeWeese TL and Eisenberger MA. Clinical practice. Localized prostate cancer. *N Engl J Med* 2007;**357**: 2696–705.
40. Heidenreich A, Bellmunt J, Bolla M *et al.* EAU Guidelines on Prostate Cancer. Part 1: Screening, Diagnosis and Treatment of Clinically Localised Disease. *Eur Urol* 2011;**59**:61–71
41. Peyromaure M *et al.* The screening of prostate cancer in 2009: overview of the oncology committee of the French Urological Association. *Prog Urol* 2010;**20**(1):17–23 [in French].
42. D'Amico AV *et al.* Biochemical outcome after radical prostatectomy, external beam radiation therapy or interstitial radiation therapy for clinically localized prostate cancer. *JAMA* 1998;**280**:969–74.
43. Droz JP *et al.* Management of prostate cancer in older men: recommendations of a working group of the International Society of Geriatric Oncology. *BJU Int* 2010;**106**(4):462–9.
44. Froehner M *et al.* Comorbidity is poor predictor of survival in patients undergoing radical prostatectomy after 70 years of age. *Urology* 2006;**68**:583–6.
45. Poulakis V *et al.* Laparoscopic radical prostatectomy in men older than 70 years of age with localized prostate cancer: comparison of morbidity, reconvalescence and short-term clinical outcomes between younger and older men. *Eur Urol* 2007;**51**:1341–8; discussion, 1349.
46. Thompson RH *et al.* Radical prostatectomy for octogenarians: how old is too old? *Urology* 2006;**68**:1042–5.
47. Xylinas E, Ploussard G, Paul A *et al.* Laparoscopic radical prostatectomy in the elderly (>75 years old): oncological and functional results. *Prog Urol* 2010;**20**:116–20 [in French].
48. D'Amico AV *et al.* Advanced age at diagnosis is an independent predictor of time to death from prostate carcinoma for patients undergoing external beam radiation therapy for clinically localized prostate carcinoma. *Cancer* 2003;**97**:56–62.
49. D'Amico AV *et al.* Androgen suppression and radiation vs radiation alone for prostate cancer: a randomized trial. *JAMA* 2008;**299**:289–95.
50. Geinitz H *et al.* 3D conformal radiation therapy for prostate cancer in elderly patients. *Radiother Oncol* 2005;**76**:27–34.
51. Nguyen TD, Azria D, Brochon D *et al.* Prostate cancer: what role for curative radiotherapy in elderly? *Cancer Radiother* 2009;**13**:623–7 [in French].
52. Pignon T *et al.* Age is not a limiting factor for radical radiotherapy in pelvic malignancies. *Radiother Oncol* 1997; **42**:107–20.
53. Chen AB *et al.* Patient and treatment factors associated with complications after prostate brachytherapy. *J Clin Oncol* 2006;**24**:5298–304.
54. Blana A *et al.* High-intensity focused ultrasound for the treatment of localized prostate cancer: 5-year experience. *Urology* 2004;**63**:297–300.
55. Thuroff S *et al.* High-intensity focused ultrasound and localized prostate cancer: efficacy results from the European multicentric study. *J Endourol* 2003;**17**:673–7.
56. Isbarn H *et al.* Androgen deprivation therapy for the treatment of prostate cancer: consider both benefits and risks. *Eur Urol* 2009;**55**:62–75.

57. Mohile SG *et al.* Management of complications of androgen deprivation therapy in the older man. *Crit Rev Oncol Hematol* 2009;**70**:235–55.
58. Mottet N, Peneau M, Mazeron J *et al.* Impact of radiotherapy (RT) combined with androgen deprivation (ADT) versus ADT alone for local control in clinically advanced prostate cancer. *J Clin Oncol* 2010;**28**: 343s.
59. Studer UE *et al.* Immediate or deferred androgen deprivation for patients with prostate cancer not suitable for local treatment with curative intent: European Organisation for Research and Treatment of Cancer (EORTC) Trial 30891. *J Clin Oncol* 2006;**24**:1868–76.
60. Studer UE *et al.* Using PSA to guide timing of androgen deprivation in patients with T0–4N0–2M0 prostate cancer not suitable for local curative treatment (EORTC 30891). *Eur Urol* 2008;**53**:941–9.
61. Mason MD, Warde PR, Sydes MR *et al.* Intergroup randomized phase III study of androgen deprivation therapy (ADT) plus radiation therapy (RT) in locally advanced prostate cancer (CaP) (NCIC–CTG, SWOG, MRC-UK and INT: T94-0110; NCT00002633). *J Clin Oncol* 2010;**28**: 343s,
62. Alibhai SM *et al.* Do older men benefit from curative therapy of localized prostate cancer? *J Clin Oncol* 2003;**21**:3318–27.
63. Tannock IF *et al.* Docetaxel plus prednisone or mitoxantrone plus prednisone for advanced prostate cancer. *N Engl J Med* 2004;**351**:1502–12.
64. Petrylak DP *et al.* Docetaxel and estramustine compared with mitoxantrone and prednisone for advanced refractory prostate cancer. *N Engl J Med* 2004;**351**:1513–20.
65. Italiano A *et al.* Docetaxel-based chemotherapy in elderly patients (age 75 and older) with castration-resistant prostate cancer. *Eur Urol* 2009;**55**:1368–75.
66. Saad F *et al.* A randomized, placebo-controlled trial of zoledronic acid in patients with hormone-refractory metastatic prostate carcinoma. *J Natl Cancer Inst* 2002;**94**:1458–68.
67. de Bono JS *et al.* Prednisone plus cabazitaxel or mitoxantrone for metastatic castration-resistant prostate cancer progressing after docetaxel treatment: a randomised open-label trial. *Lancet* **376**:1147–54.
68. De Bono JS, Logothetis CJ, Fizazi K *et al.* Abiraterone acetate (AA) plus low dose prednisone (P) improves overall survival (OS) in patients (pts) with metastatic castration-resistant prostate cancer (mCRPC) who have progressed after doxetaxel-based chemotherapy (chemo): results of COU-AA-031, a randomised double-blind placebo-controled phase II study. *Ann Oncol* 2010;**21**(Suppl 8): viii3.
69. Mitsiades N *et al.* Cognitive effects of hormonal therapy in older adults. *Semin Oncol* 2008;**35**:569–81.
70. Mohile SG, Lachs M and Dale W. Management of prostate cancer in the older man. *Semin Oncol* 2008;**35**:597–617.
71. van Londen GJ, Taxel P and Van Poznak C. Cancer therapy and osteoporosis: approach to evaluation and management. *Semin Oncol* 2008;**35**:643–51.
72. Linn BS, Linn MW and Gurel L. Cumulative illness rating scale. *J Am Geriatr Soc* 1968;**16**:622–6.
73. Folstein MF, Folstein SE and McHugh PR. 'Mini-mental state'. A practical method for grading the cognitive state of patients for the clinician. *J Psychiatr Res* 1975;**12**:189–98.
74. Lawton MP and Brody EM. Assessment of older people: self-maintaining and instrumental activities of daily living. *Gerontologist* 1969;**9**:179–86.
75. Katz S *et al.* Studies of illness in the aged. The Index of Adl: a standardized measure of biological and psychosocial function. *JAMA* 1963;**185**:914–9.
76. Krieger JN, Nyberg L Jr and Nickel JC. NIH consensus definition and classification of prostatitis. *JAMA* 1999;**282**:236–7.
77. Krieger JN, Jacobs RR and Ross SO. Does the chronic prostatitis/pelvic pain syndrome differ from nonbacterial prostatitis and prostatodynia? *J Urol* 2000;**164**:1554–8.
78. Cornia PB, Takahashi TA and Lipsky BA. The microbiology of bacteriuria in men: a 5-year study at a Veterans' Affairs hospital. *Diagn Microbiol Infect Dis* 2006; **56**:25–30.
79. Smith JW *et al.* Recurrent urinary tract infections in men. Characteristics and response to therapy. *Ann Intern Med* 1979;**91**:544–8.
80. Game X *et al.* Total and free serum prostate specific antigen levels during the first month of acute prostatitis. *Eur Urol* 2003;**43**:702–5.
81. Schaeffer AJ. Clinical practice. Chronic prostatitis and the chronic pelvic pain syndrome. *N Engl J Med* 2006;**355**: 1690–8.
82. Muller A. and Mulhall JP. Sexual dysfunction in the patient with prostatitis. *Curr Opin Urol* 2005;**15**:404–9.
83. Shoskes DA *et al.* Incidence and significance of prostatic stones in men with chronic prostatitis/chronic pelvic pain syndrome. *Urology* 2007;**70**:235–8.
84. Nickel JC, Nyberg LM and Hennenfent M. Research guidelines for chronic prostatitis: consensus report from the first National Institutes of Health International Prostatitis Collaborative Network. *Urology* 1999;**54**:229–33.
85. Collins MM *et al.* How common is prostatitis? A national survey of physician visits. *J Urol* 1998;**159**:1224–8.
86. Potts JM. Chronic pelvic pain syndrome: a non-prostatocentric perspective. *World J Urol* 2003;**21**:54–6.
87. Krieger JN and Egan KJ. Comprehensive evaluation and treatment of 75 men referred to chronic prostatitis clinic. *Urology* 1991;**38**:11–9.
88. Nickel JC *et al.* Examination of the relationship between symptoms of prostatitis and histological inflammation: baseline data from the REDUCE chemoprevention trial. *J Urol* 2007;**178**(3Pt 1):896–900; discussion, 900–1.
89. Ohkawa M *et al.* *Ureaplasma urealyticum* in the urogenital tract of patients with chronic prostatitis or related symptomatology. *Br J Urol* 1993;**72**:918–21.
90. Shortliffe LM, Sellers RG and Schachter J. The characterization of nonbacterial prostatitis: search for an etiology. *J Urol* 1992;**148**:1461–6.
91. Berger RE *et al.* Case–control study of men with suspected chronic idiopathic prostatitis. *J Urol* 1989;**141**:328–31.
92. Doble A *et al.* The role of *Chlamydia trachomatis* in chronic abacterial prostatitis: a study using ultrasound guided biopsy. *J Urol* 1989;**141**:332–3.
93. Schaeffer AJ. Etiology and management of chronic pelvic pain syndrome in men. *Urology* 2004;**63**(3 Suppl 1): 75–84.

94. Nickel JC. Clinical evaluation of the man with chronic prostatitis/chronic pelvic pain syndrome. *Urology* 2002;**60**(6 Suppl):20–2; discussion, 22–3.

95. McNaughton Collins M, MacDonald R and Wilt TJ. Diagnosis and treatment of chronic abacterial prostatitis: a systematic review. *Ann Intern Med* 2000;**133**:367–81.

96. McNaughton Collins M, MacDonald R and Wilt TJ. Interventions for chronic abacterial prostatitis. *Cochrane Database Syst Rev* 2001;(1): CD002080.

97. Litwin MS *et al*. The National Institutes of Health chronic prostatitis symptom index: development and validation of a new outcome measure. Chronic Prostatitis Collaborative Research Network. *J Urol* 1999;**162**:369–75.

98. Nickel JC *et al*. Levofloxacin for chronic prostatitis/chronic pelvic pain syndrome in men: a randomized placebo-controlled multicenter trial. *Urology* 2003;**62**:614–7.

99. Alexander RB *et al*. Ciprofloxacin or tamsulosin in men with chronic prostatitis/chronic pelvic pain syndrome: a randomized, double-blind trial. *Ann Intern Med* 2004; **141**:581–9.

100. Mehik A *et al*. Alfuzosin treatment for chronic prostatitis/chronic pelvic pain syndrome: a prospective, randomized, double-blind, placebo-controlled, pilot study. *Urology* 2003;**62**:425–9.

101. Nickel JC *et al*. A randomized placebo-controlled multicentre study to evaluate the safety and efficacy of finasteride for male chronic pelvic pain syndrome (category IIIA chronic nonbacterial prostatitis). *BJU Int* 2004;**93**:991–5.

102. Cheah PY *et al*. Terazosin therapy for chronic prostatitis/chronic pelvic pain syndrome: a randomized, placebo controlled trial. *J Urol* 2003;**169**:592–6.

103. Nickel JC *et al*. Alfuzosin and symptoms of chronic prostatitis-chronic pelvic pain syndrome. *N Engl J Med* 2008; **359**:2663–73.

104. Weidner W. Treating chronic prostatitis: antibiotics no, alpha-blockers maybe. *Ann Intern Med* 2004;**141**:639–40.

105. Leskinen M, Lukkarinen O and Marttila T. Effects of finasteride in patients with inflammatory chronic pelvic pain syndrome: a double-blind, placebo-controlled, pilot study. *Urology* 1999;**53**:502–5.

106. Anderson RU *et al*. Integration of myofascial trigger point release and paradoxical relaxation training treatment of chronic pelvic pain in men. *J Urol* 2005;**174**:155–60.

CHAPTER 106

Urinary incontinence

Ramzi R. Hajjar
American University of Beirut Medical Center, Beirut, Lebanon and St Louis University School of Medicine, St Louis, MO, USA

Introduction

Urinary incontinence (UI) is defined as an involuntary loss of urine in sufficient amounts or frequency as to constitute a medical, hygienic, or psychosocial problem. It is not a single disease, but the clinical manifestation of a diverse set of pathophysiological mechanisms, which must be understood in order to provide optimal management. In its mildest form incontinence may present as an occasional dribbling of small amounts of urine – an inconvenience to which the patient may adapt well. In severe cases it is a potentially devastating condition with serious health consequences. It is associated with significant functional decline and frailty resulting in increased risk of institutionalization and even death. In community-dwelling elderly with progressive debility, UI is cited as a leading factor resulting in nursing home placement.[1]

The prevalence of UI increases with age and frailty. It is up to twice as common in women than in men. Reports of prevalence vary greatly and depend on the definition and degree of incontinence, the method of investigation, and the target population studied. Approximately 1 in 3 women and 1 in 5 men over the age of 65 years have some degree of incontinence, and 5–10% of community-dwelling elderly experience sufficient incontinence as to require modification of lifestyle and/or use daily incontinent pads.[2] By the age of 80 years, 15–40% of community-dwelling elderly have experienced incontinence.[3] In nursing home residents, the prevalence increases to 60–80 %.[4] Despite the high prevalence of UI in the elderly, and its profound impact on quality of life (QOL), UI continues to be under-reported and under-diagnosed. The reluctance of both patients and providers to address the problem is due, in part, to the stigma associated with incontinence and the false belief that it is an unavoidable consequence of ageing.[5,6] Despite great strides that have been made in dissociating social stigma from a variety of diseases (e.g. acquired immune deficiency syndrome and sexually transmitted diseases), UI continues to suffer from a negative stereotypical bias, which hinders a frank discussion of the problem at the primary care level and therefore delays timely intervention (Table 106.1). It is estimated that 50–70% of incontinent persons do not seek help for their problems,[7,8] and in a survey of primary care physicians, the majority enquired about incontinence in 25% or fewer of their patients.[9] For these reasons, it is essential that questions about incontinence be included in the routine assessment of every older patient.

Pathophysiology and types of urinary incontinence

Normal bladder control is a complex process that depends on a functional autonomic and somatic nervous system, sufficient cognitive and physical function, and an adequate environment. Multiple pathological mechanisms exist, both age-related and disease-specific, that result in the various types of incontinence. Age alone, however, is not a necessary factor in the development of urinary incontinence, nor is UI a normal consequence of ageing. Bladder relaxation is a physiologically active process under sympathetic (adrenergic) control. Voiding, which consists of detrusor contraction with relaxation of the internal urethral sphincter, is mediated by the parasympathetic (cholinergic) system. Parasympathetic nerves act directly on the detrusor muscle, as well as by inhibiting sympathetic tone. Normal bladder capacity ranges between 250–600 ml. In most simplified terms, during bladder filling afferent autonomic sensory pathways carry information on bladder volume to the sacral micturition centre. Sympathetic output inhibits parasympathetic activity, relaxes the detrusor muscle, and constricts the internal urethral sphincter, thus allowing the bladder to fill. Normally, intravesicular pressure remains low as the bladder actively distends. Once bladder volume reaches approximately 50% bladder capacity, the first urge to urinate occurs and sensory impulses are sent to the detrusor motor centre in the pons. Frontal lobe neurons exert

Principles and Practice of Geriatric Medicine, Fifth Edition. Edited by Alan J. Sinclair, John E. Morley and Bruno Vellas.

Table 106.1 Reasons for under-reporting and under-management of urinary incontinence.

Patient-related concerns

- Persons with incontinence are ashamed or embarrassed about their condition.
- Persons with incontinence are in denial.
- Persons with incontinence have fear of stigmatization.
- Insidious onset and long trajectory course allows older persons to adapt to incontinence.
- The elderly believe incontinence is an inevitable consequence of ageing.
- Patients believe that nothing can be done for incontinence.
- Patients fear that surgery is necessary to cure incontinence.
- Elderly patients prioritize health conditions, and incontinence is viewed as an inconvenience compared to more serious conditions.
- Lack of appropriate communication and encouragement from healthcare provider.
- Patients with incontinence fear impending institutionalization.

Provider related concerns

- Provider is uncomfortable managing incontinence.
- Absence of routine screening.
- Providers prioritize other complaints due to time constraints.
- Provider views incontinence as sign of other conditions being addressed.

a predominantly inhibitory influence on pontine activity, which allows for suppression or delay of urination. Similarly voluntary contraction of pelvic floor musculature, including the external sphincter, inhibits parasympathetic tone, as occurs when urination is interrupted in mid-stream. Once conditions are appropriate to urinate, conscious disinhibition of parasympathetic outflow is initiated. Disorders of the cerebral cortex such as stroke, dementia, or Parkinson's disease or spinal cord injury can interfere with these pathways and cause incontinence.

In addition to the aforementioned conditions, several age-related changes challenge the lower urinary tract control mechanisms in the elderly. Diminished detrusor compliance effectively decreases bladder capacity, and when combined with impaired bladder contractility, urinary frequency and urgency results. Urethral pathology can further compound the problem. The urethra measures approximately 18–22 cm in men and 4 cm in women. Anatomic urethral obstruction in men due to prostatic enlargement, and urethral incompetence in women due to urethra shortening or sphincter weakness are common age-related problems. Increased nocturnal urine production can occur due to blunting of the circadian rhythm of arginine vasopressin[10] and reabsorption of leg oedema resulting from venous insufficiency, heart failure, or low serum albumin levels. Other common geriatric conditions associated with increased risk if UI are polyuria due to uncontrolled hyperglycaemia, hypercalcaemia, constipation and frailty. Impaired cognitive function and functional decline may precipitate incontinence as a manifestation of global decompensation. Available data suggests that cerebrovascular disease increases the risk of developing UI in older women by as much as twofold.

Based on those mechanisms, urinary incontinence is classified into four groups (Table 106.2).

Urge incontinence

Urinary urgency with or without incontinence affects 1 in 4 adults over the age of 65 years. It is the most common cause of UI in the elderly and accounts for up to 70% of all cases of incontinence. Urge incontinence is characterized by an insuppressible urge to void resulting in loss of urine, sometimes in large amounts (>100 ml). Clinically, patients with urge incontinence will typically have a sudden strong urge to void, fear of leakage, inability to suppress the urge, and not enough time to get to the bathroom. This type of incontinence is often associated with neurological disorders, such as stroke, spinal stenosis, Parkinson's disease, or dementia. The terms 'overactive bladder', 'detrusor hyperreflexia', and 'detrusor instability' have sometimes been used interchangeably. All result in urge incontinence, but strictly, detrusor hyperreflexia is reserved for conditions in which a neurological problem is identified; if no neurological disorder is present, detrusor instability is the proper term. Not all cases of urge incontinence are associated with involuntary detrusor contractions, however. A subtype of urge incontinence is detrusor hyperactivity with impaired contractility, in which incomplete bladder emptying occurs due to involuntary contractions, resulting in high postvoid residuals. This condition can mimic overflow incontinence and the diagnosis may require urodynamic testing. Establishing the proper diagnosis is of critical therapeutic importance, since treating urge incontinence misdiagnosed as overflow can worsen symptoms. Detrusor overactivity with impaired contractility frequently occurs in conjunction in patients with diabetes mellitus, and is sometimes classified under the separate category of *mixed incontinence*.

Stress incontinence

Stress incontinence occurs more often in women than men in all age groups. It is the involuntary loss of urine, usually in small amounts, with increased intra-abdominal pressure such as occurs during coughing, sneezing, lifting, or laughing. Stress incontinence accounts for approximately 25% of all cases of all UI in women. It has multiple anatomic and pathological causes but the underlying common mechanism is incompetence of bladder outlet support tissue. This may include urethral sphincter weakness, atrophy of pelvic

Table 106.2 Clinical presentation in types of incontinence.

Symptom	Urge	Stress	Overflow	Functional
Urgency	yes	no	no	variable
Leakage with straining	no	yes	variable	no
Volume leaked	large	small	small	large
Strength of urine stream	variable	normal	weak	normal
Nocturia	yes	no	variable	yes
Ability to reach toilet in time	reduced	normal	normal	reduced
Bladder distention	no	no	yes	no

floor musculature, hypermobile urethra, or disruption of the angle between bladder neck and urethra. Risk factors include vaginal childbirth, hysterectomy, lack of estrogen and obesity. In advanced cases, large amounts of urine loss may occur with minimal strain, such as during change in posture from sitting to standing, and may render the person housebound.

Overflow incontinence

While urge and stress incontinence primarily involve problems with storing urine, the hallmark of overflow incontinence is a failure to properly empty the bladder. This can be due to increased bladder outflow resistance or a poorly contractile bladder, or both. Common causes include prostatic enlargement, urethral stricture and neuropathic bladder due to diabetes. Less common but potentially treatable causes may include bladder prolapse, spinal injury or stenosis, or pelvic masses such as uterine fibroids. Incontinence occurs when the build up of intra-vesicular pressure in an overdistended bladder finally exceeds that of outlet resistance. Patients with overflow incontinence report trickling of urine, usually in small amounts, in the presence of suprapubic fullness. Additional symptoms include urinary frequency, hesitancy and urgency, as well as a weak urine stream, nocturia and postvoid dribbling. Urine loss with increased intra-abdominal pressure may mimic stress incontinence, except for the differentiating sign of an uncomfortably distended bladder. Medications with strong anticholinergic or α-agonist effects are rarely the sole cause of overflow incontinence, but can exacerbate mild or subclinical cases, and may cause complete obstruction in more advanced stages.

Functional incontinence

Functional incontinence occurs when a patient is unable or unwilling to access toilet facilities in time to void. Factors include musculoskeletal problems, neurological problems, advanced dementia, psychological problems, physical restraints and frailty. Iatrogenic aetiologies include overuse of sedatives or hypnotics, restricting mobility and use of restraints and barriers. Implicit in functional incontinence is that the problem lies outside the lower urinary tract. However, patients with functional incontinence due to any of above factors will almost certainly also have abnormalities affecting the lower urinary tract, and it is sometimes difficult to determine where the predominant problem lies.

Complications and impact of incontinence

Medical complications of urinary incontinence are varied and have been well documented. Aside from the natural progression of the underlying condition causing incontinence, incontinence itself may result in potentially serious complications. In women over the age of 65 years, there is a significant increase in the incidence of traumatic falls associated with incontinence. Up to 40% of women with UI will fall within a year, 10% of which will result in fractures. Acute hospitalization, institutionalization and social isolation have all been associated with UI in older patients. Thirty percent of incontinent women over the age of 65 years are likely to be hospitalized within 12 months.[11] In older men, the risk of hospitalization associated with incontinence is double. Pressure ulcers are more prevalent in frail incontinent patients, as are skin infections, balanitis and cystitis. Not surprisingly, the economic cost of urinary incontinence can be extremely burdensome on affected individuals and long-term care facilities. The cost of care for UI is difficult to determine with accuracy due to the wide-ranging and overlapping nature of this condition. It is estimated that the annual direct cost of managing UI in the US exceeded US$20 billion in 2004.[12] Birnbaum *et al.* estimated the lifetime medical cost of treating an older adult with UI at close to US$60 000,[13] and long-term care facilities shoulder an additional annual financial burden of approximately US$5000 per resident with incontinence. None of this direct cost accounts for reduced work productivity, loss of self-esteem, or caregiver burden and burnout.

The psychosocial impact of UI continues to receive less attention than it commands, despite the inescapable effect on the QOL of affected persons. Great strides have been made in the past 20 years in developing and validating psychosocial assessment tools specifically for incontinence, but UI continues to be viewed by clinicians as a unidimensional medical condition. The impact of a potentially chronic non-life-threatening disease is highly subjective and varies greatly among individuals and even within the same individual over time. It is influenced by cultural, social and psychological factors, as well as the personal concept of self-image, self-worth and health expectations. These human experiences are difficult to measure, but are important nonetheless, because they not only determine the patient's willingness to seek professional help, but also their ability to adapt to the situation and benefit from treatment. A failure to identify the broader consequence of UI is to deny comprehensive management of this complex condition. Even if the underlying condition is incurable, much can be done to alleviate the psychosocial anguish that may accompany UI. Multiple condition-specific and dimension-specific QOL questionnaires have been devised for this purpose and are summarized elsewhere.[14] These tools have also been proven an invaluable component of clinical research, particularly in outcome studies.

Diagnosis and assessment of urinary incontinence

Given the strong intrusion of UI on everyday life, one might assume that incontinent persons would seek help early and often. This is not the case. Although up to 70% of incontinent patients do not freely report the problem, more than 75% will report the condition when asked by their physician.[15] Symptom reporting tends to be marginalized or minimized because of insecurity, fear of hostile distancing, or stigmatization (Table 106.1). In one study, only approximately one third of women with incontinence reported it as bothersome,[16] and 60% of people identified through surveys as being incontinent had not reported their condition to a healthcare provider.[8] When medical attention is sought, it often is after symptoms have been present for a long time, sometimes years, and there is almost complete failure of the underlying physiological regulatory or compensatory mechanisms. The onus lies within providers to screen for UI and identify risk factors in all patients being evaluated.

The objective of the initial evaluation is to identify potentially reversible causes of incontinence (particularly in cases of acute-onset), to classify incontinence in order to devise a treatment plan, and to identify conditions that warrant surgical intervention. In most cases, a detailed history and physical examination suffices to formulate a working diagnosis and guide initial therapy (Table 106.2). The history should cover characteristics of voiding and incontinent episodes, concurrent medical problems of relevance, and an assessment of QOL and caregiver burden. Special attention should focus on quantity of urine loss, duration of the problem, frequency and urgency, as well as strength of the urine stream, dribbling, dysuria, nocturia and leakage during activity. When indicated, inquiry should be made regarding diabetes mellitus, neuromuscular disorders, pelvic surgery, childbirth, cognitive and functional impairment, and alcohol/coffee/fluid intake. Presence of specific risk factors can add support to an uncertain diagnosis, and guide further investigation. A detailed list of prescription and over-the-counter medications should be made, and any temporal association between symptom onset or exacerbation and medication use (or stoppage) should be noted. Many commonly used medications contribute to incontinence (Table 106.3), and surreptitious, casual, or impulsive use of non-prescription medications should be investigated. As with most chronic conditions, the outcome and tolerance of previous treatment attempts can be of immense value in formulating a current treatment plan. An incontinence diary is an important tool when classification of incontinence remains unclear and further information is necessary. Repeat or serial diaries also facilitate assessment of intervention outcome and are often more accurate than the patient's subjective report from memory. A seven-day diary, or longer, may be necessary for infrequent episodes of incontinence, but a shorter 2–3 day voiding diary appears to be comparable in reliability and validity when incontinent episodes are more frequent. Furthermore, patients are more likely to comply with the shorter diary, as they perceive it as being less burdensome and intrusive.[17]

Physical examination of patients with UI should include an abdominal, neurological, rectal and pelvic examination. Abdominal examination does not reliably detect elevated postvoid residuals until urine retention exceeds 500 ml. An overdistended bladder can usually be detected by palpating or percussing the suprapubic area, and will often be uncomfortable to deep palpation. Similarly, prostate size on digital rectal examination does not correlate well with symptoms of bladder outlet obstruction and overflow incontinence. However, valuable information regarding prostate nodules, symmetry and tenderness, as well as rectal tone and reflex tightening of the anal sphincter with coughing renders this examination essential. Pelvic examination in women should include inspection for prolapse, infection and atrophic vaginitis. Clinically significant prolapse of the uterus, bladder, urethra, or intestine warrants prompt referral to specialist for consideration of surgical and non-surgical modalities to relieve the obstruction. During pelvic examination, a cough test should be performed for stress incontinence. Patients with intact perineal sensation and reflexes will exhibit reflex tightening of the anal and urethral sphincter tone during coughing. Persons with stress incontinence may be observed leaking urine while

Table 106.3 Examples of common medications and substances that can worsen incontinence.

Medication class	Possible effect	Type of incontinence most affected
Alcohol	Polyuria, impaired mobility	Overflow, stress, functional
Caffeine	Polyuria, bladder irritant	Stress, urge, overflow
Smoking	Bladder irritant, cough	Urge, stress
Antihistamines	Urine retention, increased urethral tone, decreased bladder contraction	Overflow
Diuretics	Polyuria	Urge, overflow, stress
Alpha-adrenergic blockers	Decreased bladder outlet resistance	Stress
Alpha-adrenergic agonists	Increased bladder outlet resistance Urine retention	Overflow
Opiate analgesics	Sedation, decreased detrusor activity, increased bladder outlet resistance, urine retention	Overflow, functional
Tricyclic antidepressants	Urine retention, increased urethral tone, decreased bladder contraction	Overflow

coughing. Loss of urine during coughing is highly specific for stress incontinence, but can also occur in overflow incontinence, and the absence of a positive test does not rule out stress incontinence. Finally, a comprehensive assessment of UI should include evaluation of cognitive impairment and mobility, and the role each may have in causing or worsening incontinence.

Few diagnostic tests are necessary in the workup of urinary incontinence. In most cases, a urinalysis is performed to look for infections, haematuria and glucosuria. Cytology and imaging tests are only indicated if unexplained haematuria is present. With the exception of infections, urinalysis rarely is expected to assist in the diagnosis or alter the management of incontinence. In fact, guidelines of various agencies, including those of the American Medical Director Association, recommend urinalysis only in cases of suspected infection or with worsening symptoms.[18] It may be prudent, however, to obtain a urinalysis during the initial workup of new incontinence, particularly if symptoms developed acutely or progressed rapidly. Overt urinary tract infections are clearly associated with acute urinary incontinence, but the role of asymptomatic bacteriuria on incontinence is much less clear. In frail elderly patients with chronic stable UI, such as nursing home residents, treatment of asymptomatic bacteriuria is not advised. It is reasonable to initiate a course of antibacterial therapy when clinical symptoms of infection develop, or during initial management of incontinent patients with bacteriuria. Urinary stasis dramatically increases the risk of asymptomatic bacteriuria as well as acute symptomatic cystitis, particularly when bladder catheterization is necessary. In poorly controlled diabetes mellitus, the diuretic effect of hyperglycaemia worsens most types of incontinence. Additionally, autonomic neuropathy of diabetes can worsen urinary urgency and urine retention. Measurement of postvoid residual (PVR) performed by bedside ultrasound bladder scan or by in-and-out catheterization is effective in diagnosing urine stasis and consequently overflow incontinence. Not all patients require PVR assessment. Only patients at high risk for urine retention should have a PVR measurement. Symptoms and physical examination are poor and unreliable predictors of urine retention. Normal postvoid residual volume in older patients is less than 100 ml. A PVR volume of 200 ml or more strongly indicates urinary retention, and is consistent with either outlet obstruction or atonic bladder. Volumes between 100 ml and 200 ml are difficult to interpret but at least suggest inadequate bladder emptying. Portable ultrasound scan is preferred to urethral catheterization for PVR measurement. It is non-invasive and highly reliable when performed by a competent operator. Bladder catheterization carries the risk of infection and urethral trauma, even with a single in-and-out event, but has the therapeutic advantage of draining an overdistended bladder. In severe cases of retention, the catheter may remain in place until a long-term treatment plan is devised.

Most incontinent patients will not require further workup, but when the type of incontinence remains uncertain after the initial assessment, referral for formal urodynamic studies must be considered. Patients that may benefit from urodynamic studies include those with competing pathological mechanisms, history of pelvic surgery or radiation therapy, treatment failure, and those being considered for surgery. Bedside cytometric studies are no longer done mainly due to poor diagnostic accuracy and failure to modify management based on clinical criteria. Furthermore, bedside cytometric studies correlated poorly with formal urodynamic studies.

Management of urinary incontinence

Effective management of persistent incontinence will generally incorporate elements of both non-pharmacological and pharmacological strategies. Traditionally, pharmacological therapy was withheld until non-pharmacological strategies proved ineffective. Some experts, however, have suggested that a parallel approach to therapy may yield better results.[19] Nevertheless, the risk of adverse drug effects and polypharmacy justifies caution in starting medications without fully appreciating other modalities in older patients.

Non-pharmacological modalities

Several non-pharmacological interventions have been used for the management of UI with varying degrees of success. The modality choice and goal of treatment varies with the type of incontinence. Degree of incontinence and comorbid conditions also determine optimal treatment plan. Options include supportive management, including the use of protective undergarments, bedding and topical barrier creams, intended to manage rather than treat incontinence, as well as more involved measures such as behavioural intervention aimed at modifying the progression and impact of the disease. Several studies have shown behavioural modification to be comparable to drug therapy in alleviating symptoms, particularly for stress and urge incontinence. Patient-dependent behavioural therapy is intended to restore continence, and requires the patient to have functional independence, cognitive competence and, above all, motivation. When patients are unable or not willing to participate, caregiver-dependent toileting protocols are more appropriate and are effective in maintaining a hygienic and safe environment, and minimizing incontinent episodes. Neither supportive care, nor behavioural modification address the underlying pathogenic process, except, perhaps, in the case of stress incontinence secondary to bladder outflow incompetence where perineal strengthening exercises may retard the natural progression of the disorder, and in some cases of urge incontinence where biofeedback may actively inhibit bladder contractions.

Rehabilitation exercises of pelvic muscles with biofeedback therapy may prove highly effective in patients with stress or mixed incontinence. Pelvic floor exercises, such as the Kegel exercise, consist of repetitive contraction and relaxation of pelvic floor muscles, a manoeuvre somewhat opposite to that of the Valsalva manoeuvre. The success of pelvic muscle exercises is dependent on a knowledgeable and committed instructor. In addition, biofeedback is helpful in identifying the proper muscle group during initial training, particularly in patients who tend to bear down which is a more natural manoeuvre but may trigger leakage in stress incontinence. It was estimated in one study that only about half the patients who received only verbal instructions on pelvic floor muscle exercises were able to perform the technique properly.[20] Biofeedback can be electronic-based using intra-vaginal pressure transducers and computer feedback, or more simply by manual sensation during the rectal or vaginal examination. Once learned, the frequency and duration of contractions can be increased, and the manoeuvre should be performed several times a day. Highly motivated persons can be trained to perform the contraction with activities that precipitate leakage during their daily routine, such as laughing or sneezing.

In functionally dependent or cognitively impaired patients, *prompted voiding* is likely to be more effective. It is a caregiver-dependent strategy that offers the patient regular opportunities to void by asking about the need to use the restroom and providing assistance and encouragement at routine intervals, usually every two hours during the daytime. Positive reinforcement and social interaction are additional benefits, but clearly a dedicated caregiver is necessary for this approach to succeed. *Habit training* is a variant of prompted voiding, in which the encouragement to void is linked to specific daily activities, such as meals, bathing, or naptime, rather than routine predetermined intervals. The intent is that with continued training, a *habit* to address toileting needs develops with these frequent daily activities. The variability of this approach allows the schedule to be personalized to the patient's daily habits and routine. With more advanced dementia, *timed (or scheduled) toileting* consists of routinely toileting a patient at fixed intervals, whether or not he/she expresses a need to void. This labour-intensive process is dependent on staff or caregiver availability and dedication, and in long-term care facilities may be constrained by the regimented schedule of custodial care. Furthermore some patients with advanced dementia will resist routine toileting, and agitated behaviour may ensue.

Pharmacological management

Detrusor contractility is primarily dependent on activation of the muscarinic acetylcholine receptors. Consequently, anticholinergic agents have been the mainstay of treatment for patients with urge incontinence. This class of drugs can be quite effective. Various studies estimate a 50–70% reduction in the frequency of incontinent episodes in older patients with urge incontinence treated with antimuscarinic agents.[21] Drug selection, however, is based on efficacy as well as tolerability, and this class of medications has been plagued by an unacceptable high frequency of intolerable side effects such as dry mouth, constipation, blurred vision, cognitive dysfunction, delirium and orthostatic hypotension. Five subtypes of muscarinic receptors (M1-M5) have been identified in the central nervous system and peripheral organs. The receptors differ in end-organ targeted, as well as their capacity for activation or inhibition by certain molecules. Systemic effects of anticholinergic drugs are linked to receptor selectivity, and until recently, prohibitive side effects of non-selective drugs rendered them of limited use in older adults. Oxybutinine and tolterodine are the most widely used drugs for the management of urge incontinence in the United States. Oxybutinine, has been shown to reduce incontinent episodes by half in most patients with urge incontinence, but also has a high rate of discontinuation due to side effects. It is an older medication with antagonistic effect on the M1, M2 and M3 acetylcholine receptors, and hence not highly selective in activity or effect. Approximately 75% of patients on oxybutynin will experience bothersome side effects, and 25% will discontinue the medications due to peripheral anticholinergic effects.[22] Tolterodine appears to be comparable to oxybutynin in efficacy. It affects predominantly the M2 and M3 receptor subtypes, and therefore has a more favourable tolerance profile. Sustained release formulations of both drugs are favoured over the immediate release due to simplicity of dosing and better tolerability. More recently, oxybutynin transdermal patch and 10% gel have been approved in the United States for urge or mixed incontinence. Oxybutinine is also the only antimuscarinic available in generic form. The cost benefit is the primary reason for initiating treatment with a trial of this drug.

In 2004, the Food and Drug Administration (FDA) approved solifenacin and darifenacin in the United States for treatment of urge incontinence. These drugs are more selective muscarinic receptor inhibitors (M3), and appear to be at least as effective as tolterodine and equally well tolerated. It is not yet clear, however, whether increased receptor selectivity translates to better tolerability. In a three-month randomized trial of 1200 adults, dry mouth and constipation occurred *more* frequently with solifenacin than with tolterodine (30 vs 24, and 6 vs 3 respectively), thought the difference was not statistically significant.[23] Also in 2004, trospium was approved by the FDA in the United States for the management of OAB. Trospium has been used effectively in Europe for over three decades, and accumulated literature indicate a favourable safety profile. Unlike the M2/M3 selective agents that are lipophilic tertiary amines, trospium exhibits less receptor selectivity but is a hydrophilic quaternary amine. This biochemical property renders it relatively impermeable to the blood-brain barrier and hence limits unwanted central nervous system side effects. Trospium is not metabolized by the cytochrome p450 system and so is less prone to drug interaction. Renal excretion accounts for approximately 70% of drug clearance, and in older patients with renal impairment it must be dosed accordingly. As with other antimuscarinic drugs, the extended release formulation was better tolerated than immediate release in one small study.[24] With current data, there is no compelling evidence that among selective antimuscarinics, any one is vastly superior to another in efficacy or tolerability. In one large study, discontinuation rate for this class of medication was 58–71% at six months.[25]

All patients on antimuscarinic drugs should be monitored for urine retention, particularly older males with potential prostate enlargement. Postvoid residuals should be measured, and when retention is present, dose reduction or discontinuation of drug altogether may be necessary. In older men with bladder outflow obstruction, alpha-adrenergic antagonist treatment prior to starting antimuscarinic agents may reduce the complication of problematic urine retention.

Pharmacological management of stress incontinence has been far less rewarding than urge incontinence. Estrogen has a direct effect on urethral mucosa. Postmenopausal women experience a loss of periurethral tissue, diminished mucosal blood flow, and decreased number and responsiveness of alpha-receptors. On pelvic examination of postmenopausal women, dry, inflamed, friable, or dusky-coloured mucosa with loss of rugae suggests atrophic vaginitis. Hence, intuitive reasoning has driven estrogen to the forefront of treatment options for stress incontinence in older women. In fact, estrogen replacement therapy, both topical and systemic, has been widely used for decades, despite the absence of compelling evidence of efficacy. Vaginal estrogen in the form of creams, tablets, or medicated rings can decrease the frequency of recurrent cystitis and alleviate dyspareunia. Anecdotal evidence suggests improvement in symptoms of stress and mixed incontinence, but a recent large prospective cohort study found that vaginal estrogen cream in women 55–75 years of age was independently associated with incident incontinence during two years of follow-up (OR, 2.0; CI, 1.1–3.7).[26] When effective, several months of therapy is necessary to notice clinical improvement, and patient inconvenience or embarrassment may limit the duration of treatment. Oral conjugated estrogen, with and without progesterone, has been better studied and is no more effective than topical estrogen. In fact, in the Women's Health Initiative (WHI) study of over 23 000 subjects, women who were continent at baseline had an increased risk for all types of incontinence at one and three years follow-up compared to placebo.[27] The greatest increase in risk was for stress incontinence. Women who were incontinent at baseline had worsening incontinence and frequency with treatment. These results have been replicated in other large controlled trials, such as the Heart and Estrogen/Progestin Replacement Study,[28] and Nurses' Health Study,[29] though the latter only included younger subjects. Based on the existing evidence, estrogen is not recommended, or approved, for the treatment of stress incontinence.

Duloxetine is a serotonin and norepinephrine reuptake inhibitor that has been approved in Europe since 2004 for the treatment of stress incontinence. It affects the lower urinary tract function via alpha-adrenergic central nervous system mechanisms. Despite evidence for improvement in QOL and a moderate decrease in frequency of incontinence compared to placebo,[30–32] the Cochrane Collaboration in 2005 and University of Minnesota review in 2008 independently concluded that cure rates with duloxetine were no better than placebo. In addition to the modest transient therapeutic effect, potentially serious side effects have further deterred clinicians from utilizing this drug for incontinence. In the United States, duloxetine is approved for major depressive disorder, but recently failed to gain FDA approval for the treatment of incontinence.

Surgical management

For patients who respond poorly to behavioural and pharmacological interventions surgical procedures may prove effective. Age *per se* is not a contraindication for surgical consideration; however, comorbid conditions, which accrue with age, are. As with any surgery in older persons, patient selection and preparation are paramount. Since mixed incontinence is not uncommon with advancing age, urodynamic studies must be performed in patients being considered for surgery. This procedure delineates the underlying pathological mechanism(s), and allows better prognostication of postsurgical course.

Surgery should be considered in women with urine retention due to pelvic prolapse that has failed conservative measures. Surgery is also a well-accepted treatment choice for stress incontinence. Minimally invasive procedures for bladder outlet incompetence include bladder neck suspension, periurethral collagen injections, and tension-free vaginal tape (TVT). Mid-urethral synthesis slings (TVT) can be used as a first-line treatment in older women with stress incontinence. The TVT sling procedure is a 30-minute outpatient procedure and has a cure rate above 85%. Refractory cases will require the more invasive wide sling procedure rather than a simple bladder neck suspension. The varied procedures are intended to restore the 90° angle between the urethra and bladder neck, and provide bladder support in case of prolapse. Complications include bladder perforation, urine retention, haematoma/thrombosis, and infection. Periurethral bulking injections with collagen and other agents provides mechanical resistance by external compression of the urethra, and is an alternative to traditional surgery when the urethra is immobile.

Electrical stimulation has been used in urge incontinence refractory to medical treatment. External sacral nerve stimulation via cutaneous electrodes in the lower back is safe and can be effective. If significant improvement in symptoms is noted with a trial of external stimulation, a permanent device can be implanted. This 'bladder pacemaker' is placed in the hip or gluteal area, and a lead wire within the sacral canal stimulates the pudendal and sacral nerves. External programming results in the delivery of a painless electrical stimulus, which regulates bladder function. Initial reports have indicated promising long-term results.[33]

Key points

- Urinary incontinence is a very common problem in older persons.
- Mixed incontinence is common, making treatment difficult.
- Lower urinary tract symptomatology occurs in both men and women and is not directly related to prostate size.
- Nocturia is a common problem especially in older males.

References

1. Thom DH, Haan MN, Van Den Eeden SK. Medically recognized urinary incontinence and risk of hospitalization, nursing home admission and mortality. *Age Ageing* 1997;**26**: 367–74.
2. Zunzunegui Pastor MV, Rodriguez-Lasso A, Garcia de Yebenes MJ *et al.* Prevalence of urinary incontinence and linked factors in men and women over 65. *Atencion Primaria* 2003;**32**:337–42.
3. Herzog AR, Diokno AC, Fultz NH. Urinary incontinence: medical and psychosocial aspects. *Ann Rev Gerontol Geriatr* 1989;**9**:74–119.
4. Ouslander JG, Kane RL, Abrass IB. Urinary incontinence in the elderly nursing home patients. *JAMA* 1982;**248**:1194–8.
5. Dugan E, Roberts CP, Cohen SJ *et al.* Why older community-dwelling do not discuss urinary incontinence with their primary care physicians. *J Am Geriatr Soc* 2001;**49**:462–5.
6. Horrocks S, Somerset M, Stoddart H, Peters TJ. What prevents older people from seeking treatment for urinary incontinence? A qualitative exploration of barriers to the use of community continence services. *Family Practice* 2004;**21**: 689–96.
7. Thomas TM, Plymat KR, Blamnin J, Meade TW. Prevalence of urinary incontinence. *BMJ* 1980;**281**:1243–5.
8. Burgio KL, Ives DG, Locher JL, Arena VC, Kuller LH. Treatment seeking for urinary incontinence in older adults. *J Am Geriatr Soc* 1994;**42**:208–12.
9. Branch LG, Walker LA, Stoner D. Prevention survey of physicians for an evaluation of Educational Demonstration of Urinary Continence Assessment and Treatment for the Elderly (EDUCATE). Abt Associates report prepared for the Massachusetts Department of Public Health, Abt Associates Inc., Cambridge, MA, 1993.
10. Morley JE. (2003) Hormones and the aging process. *J Am Geriatr Soc* 2003;**51**(7 Suppl S): S333–S337.
11. Wilson MM. Urinary incontinence: a treatise on gender, sexuality, and culture. *Clin Geriatr Med* 2004;**20**:565–70.

12. Hu TW, Wagner TH, Bentkover JD *et al.* Cost of urinary incontinence and overactive bladder in the United States: a comparative study. *Urology* 2004;**63**:461–5.
13. Birnbaum H, Leong S, Kabra A. Lifetime medical costs for women: cardiovascular disease, diabetes, and stress urinary incontinence. *Women's Health* 2003;**13**:204–13.
14. Hajjar RR. Psychosocial impact of urinary incontinence in the elderly population. *Clin Geriatr Med* 2004;**20**:553–64.
15. Umlauf MG, Goode PS, Burgio KL. Psychosocial issues in geriatric urology: problems in treatment and treatment seeking. *Urol Clin North Am* 1996;**23**:127–36.
16. Hannestad YS, Rortveit G, Sandvik H, Hunskaar S. A community-based epidemiological survey of female urinary incontinence: the Norwegian EPINCOT study. Epidemiology of Incontinence in the County of Nord-Trondelag. *J Clin Epidemiol* 2000;**53**:1150–7.
17. Ku JH, Jeong IG, Lim DJ *et al.* Voiding diary for the evaluation of urinary incontinence and lower urinary tract symptoms: prospective assessment of patient compliance and burden. *Neurourol Urodyn* 2004;**23**:331–5.
18. Resnick B, Quinn C, Baxter S. Testing the feasibility of implementation of clinical practice guidelines in long-term care facilities. *JAMDA* 2004;**5**:1–8.
19. Goode PS. Behavioral and drug therapy for urinary incontinence. *Urology* 2004;**63**(3 Suppl 1):20–5.
20. Bump RC, Hurt WG, Fantl JA, Wyman JF. Assessment of Kegel pelvic muscle exercise performance after brief verbal instruction. *Am J Obstet Gynecol* 1991;165:322–7.
21. Kane, RL, Ouslander JG, Abrass IB, Resnick B. Incontinence. In: RL Kane, JG Ouslander, IB Abrass, B Resnick (eds), *Essentials of Clinical Geriatrics*, 6th edn, McGraw-Hill, New York, 2009, pp. 213–63.
22. Chapple C, Khullar V, Gabriel Z, Dooley JA. The effects of antimuscarinic treatments in overactive bladder: a systemic review and meta-analysis. *Eur Urol* 2005;**48**:5–26.
23. Chapple CR, Matinez-Garcia R, Selvaggi L *et al.* A comparison of the efficacy and tolerability of solifenacin succinate and extended release tolterodine at treating overactive bladder syndrome: results of the STAR trial. *Eur Urol* 2005;**48**:464–70.
24. Dmochowski RR, Sand PK, Zinner NR, Staskin DR. Trospium 60mg one daily (QD) for overactive bladder syndrome: results from a placebo-controlled interventional study. *Urology* 2008;**71**:449–54.
25. Gopal M, Haynes K, Bellamy SL, Araya LA. Discontinuation rates of anticholinergic medications used for treatment of lower urinary tract symptoms. *Obstet Gynecol* 2008; **112**:1311–18.
26. Jackson SL, Scholes D, Boyko EJ, Abraham L, Fihn SD. Predictors of urinary incontinence in a prospective cohort of postmenopausal women. *Obstet Gynecol* 2006;**108**:855–62.
27. Hendrix SL, Cochran BB, Nygaard IE *et al.* Effects of estrogen with and without progestin on urinary incontinence. *JAMA* 2005;**293**:935–48.
28. Grady D, Brown JS, Vittinghoff E *et al.* Postmenopausal hormones and incontinence: The heart and estrogen/progestin replacement study. *Obstet Gynecol* 2001;**97**:116–20.
29. Townsend MK, Curhan GC, Resnick NM, Grodstein F. Postmenopausal hormone therapy and incident urinary incontinence in middle-aged women. *Am J Obstet Gynecol* 2009; **200**:86.e1–5.
30. Dmchowski RR, Miklos JR, Norton PA *et al.* Duloxetine versus placebo for the treatment of North American women with stress urinary incontinence. *J Urol* 2003;**170**:1259–63.
31. Millard RJ, Moore K, Rencken R *et al.* Duloxetine vs placebo in the treatment of stress urinary incontinence: a four-continent randomized clinical trial. *BJU* 2004;**97**:311–18.
32. Van Kerrebroeck PE, Abrams P, Lang R *et al.* Duloxetine versus placebo in the treatment of North American women with stress urinary incontinence. *BJOG* 2004;**111**:249–57.
33. Van Kerrebroeck PE, van Voskuilen AC, Heesakkers JP *et al.* Results of sacral neuromodulation therapy for urinary voiding dysfunction: outcomes of a prospective, worldwide clinical study. *J Urol* 2007;**178**:2029–34.

CHAPTER 107

Geriatric nephrology

Carlos G. Musso[1] and Dimitrios G. Oreopoulos[2]
[1]Hospital Italiano de Buenos Aires, Argentina
[2]University Health Network, Toronto, Canada

Introduction

The border between normal ageing and disease is sometimes blurred because the ageing process consists of a loss of *complexity*, as a result of which the different systems of a senile organism start working without harmony among them, a situation that predisposes to clinical alterations and disease. The kidney also is under this general rule of the ageing process. The discipline of geriatric nephrology includes the normal renal ageing changes, their clinical consequences, and the renal diseases that occur in the elderly population as a result of these changes.[1]

Normal ageing: Glomerular level

Decrease in glomerular filtration (senile glomerulosclerosis)

In senile glomerulosclerosis, the glomeruli are replaced by fibrous tissue (glomerular obsolescence), a process that begins at approximately 30 years of age, and is present in between 1% and 30% of persons aged 50 years or older. The mesangium increases to nearly 12% by age of 70, and microangiographic examination shows the obliteration particularly of the juxtamedullary nephrons that is followed by the formation of a direct channel between afferent and efferent arterioles (*aglomerular circulation*). Presumably, this change contributes to medullary hypotonicity (wash-out) in the aged. These changes with ageing are accompanied by a decrease in the glomerular filtration rate (GFR) and the effective renal plasma flow (ERPF). However, because ERPF decreases proportionally more than GFR – 10% per decade from 600 ml min^{-1} 1.73 m^{-2} in youth to 300 ml min^{-1} 1.73 m^{-2} by the age of 80 years, the filtration fraction (FF), which is the ratio of GFR/ERPF, usually increases in the elderly because the denominator (EFRF) is disproportionately lower than the numerator (GFR).[2–4]

Measurement of the GFR with ^{51}Cr EDTA confirms that the healthy elderly have a lower GFR than the young. At the third decade of life, GFR peaks at approximately 140 ml min^{-1} 1.73 m^{-2}, and from then on, GFR progressively declines at an approximate rate of 8 ml min^{-1} 1.73 m^{-2} per decade. A similar fall in creatinine clearance (Ccr) is accompanied by a concomitant decrease in creatinine production (senile sarcopenia), and consequently serum creatinine does not increase with the progressive decrease in GFR.[5]

However, in approximately one third of old people the GFR does not decrease with age. Since Kimmel *et al.* have demonstrated that old people who were on a high protein diet maintained a normal GFR, it has been hypothesized that 'normal' GFR in the elderly could be the consequence of increased protein intake that is followed by glomerular hyperfiltration.[5]

In clinical practice, Ccr is estimated using the Cockcroft and Gault equation: Ccr = (140-age) × (body weight)/72 × serum creatinine (15% lower in women).[6] Another frequently used equation is the MDRD (modification of diet in renal disease) formula: GFR = 186 × serum $creatinine^{-1.154}$ × age (in years) $^{-0.203}$ × (0.742 if female) × (1.210 if black race). When applied to the elderly each of these formulas has its advantages and disadvantages. Thus, the Cockcroft-Gault formula underestimates GFR in people >80 years, while the MDRD equation has the advantage of not requiring the patient's weight for calculating GFR. There is a poor correlation between GFR obtained by MDRD formula and the measured creatinine clearance with cimetidine, which is a proxy of the GFR gold standard measured by inulin clearance; conversely this study showed a good correlation between the Ccr obtained by Cockcroft-Gault (CG) formula and that measured by creatinine clearance with cimetidine.[6] Keller believes that the easiest formula for estimating GFR in people between

Principles and Practice of Geriatric Medicine, Fifth Edition. Edited by Alan J. Sinclair, John E. Morley and Bruno Vellas.

25 and 100 years old is as follows: GFR = 130-age (in years) ml min^{-1}, but this has not been validated by direct comparison with creatinine clearance with cimetidine.[5–8]

Regarding cystatin-C as a GRF marker, it has been demonstrated that in elderly persons with glomerular filtration lower than 60 ml min^{-1}, it is not superior to that calculated by the CG and MDRD formulae.[5,9]

Consequences of senile hypofiltration

- A serum creatinine concentration of 1 mg dl^{-1} reflects a GFR of 120 ml min^{-1} in a 20-year-old and 60 ml min^{-1} in an 80-year-old.[5,9]
- Senile hypofiltration and diastolic cardiac failure predispose healthy old people to cardiac failure, and to lung congestion after a saline load.[9]
- The dose of prescribed drugs must be adjusted to the estimated GFR in the elderly.[8]
- In old people senile hypofiltration differs from chronic kidney disease because the glomerular filtration value is stable over a period of 6–12 months and there is no haematuria or significant proteinuria (> 0.30 g day^{-1}).[10]

Diseases: At the glomerular level

Glomerulonephritis

Renal biopsy is useful in guiding the prognosis and therapy for renal disorders in this population. In the elderly who underwent a diagnostic renal biopsy, 59% had primary glomerulonephritis, and 20% secondary glomerulonephritis. Even though the aged accounted for only 23% of patients undergoing biopsy, the elderly in the biopsy series were more numerous than the proportion of elderly people in the general population (16%). Primary glomerulonephritis was the most frequent biopsy-proven renal disease in the elderly, even more frequent than primary glomerulonephritis in adults. Although the indications and incidence of complications of renal biopsy are the same for both elderly and adults, when older persons have a complication of renal biopsy, generally such complications are more serious. Crescentic, membranous nephropathy, membranoproliferative glomerulonephritis, minimal change disease, and acute post-streptococcal glomerulonephritis are all more frequent in the elderly than in younger patients. Only focal segmental glomerulosclerosis, IgA and non-IgA mesangioproliferative nephritis were less frequent in elderly patients than in the younger ones.[11–13]

In some elderly patients membranous nephropathy is related to drugs ingestion or an underlying malignancy (20%) (mainly lung or colon adenocarcinoma). Regarding minimal change disease, senile structural renal changes make histological diagnosis difficult; its clinical presentation is usually 'atypical' with hypertension, microhaematuria and/or renal failure; also it may be associated with drugs (NSAIDs) or malignancies (lymphoma). Crescentic glomerulonephritis reaches its greatest incidence between 60–79 years of age, and its typical clinical presentation is an acute renal failure of rapid evolution. Steroids and other immunosuppressive drugs (cyclophosphamide, etc.) can be used in the elderly as in adults, though with special attention to their side effects. Secondary glomerulopathies such as diabetic nephropathy, nephroangiosclerosis secondary to essential hypertension, glomerular vasculitis, and those associated with abnormal plasma-cell proteins (light chain, fibrillary, immunotactoid nephropathy) are frequent in the elderly. Nephrotic syndrome accounts for 50% of renal biopsy indications, its most prevalent causes are: membranous, minimal change, diabetic and amyloidosis nephropathies.[12–14]

Normal ageing: Renovascular level

Senile renal vascular changes

Prearterioles show subendothelial deposition of hyaline and collagen fibres that produce intimal thickening. In the small arteries the intima is thickened due to proliferation of the elastic tissue, and the media shows atrophy. Another characteristic of the ageing kidney is the formation of the above-mentioned *aglomerular circulation*, and dysfunction of the autonomic vascular reflex.[2,3,10,14]

Consequences of the senile vascular changes

- Renovascular atherosclerosis, which can lead to renovascular hypertension, ischaemic nephropathy and chronic kidney disease.[9,14]
- In patients with bilateral renal artery stenosis reversible renal failure may develop after the use of angiotensin-converting enzyme (ACE) inhibitors.[14,15]
- Intrarenal atheroembolism appears when plaque material breaks free from the diseased renal artery and enters the renal circulation. The kidney rarely recovers from this acute insult.[14]
- Renal dysautonomia leads to kidney damage during hypotensive or hypertensive states.[9]

Diseases: Reno-vascular level

Renal vasculitis in the elderly

It has become increasingly clear that renal vasculitis is more common with advancing age and probably this disease is the most common primary cause of renal failure in the elderly. The incidence of Wegener's granulomatosis and microscopic polyangeitis increases with age. Since immunosuppression is the main treatment for these entities, a careful monitoring of therapy can minimize adverse effects in this population.[13,14]

Other diseases: renovascular atherosclerosis and atheroembolic disease.

Normal ageing: Tubular-interstitial level

Senile tubular-interstitial changes

Renal tubules undergo fatty degeneration, and irregular thickening of their basal membrane. Diverticula arise from the distal and convoluted tubules, and it has been suggested that, in the aged, these may serve as reservoirs for recurrent urinary tract infections in the elderly. In addition, the aged kidney also shows increasing zones of tubular atrophy and fibrosis.[2,3]

Consequences of tubular-interstitial changes

The physiological and clinical consequences of these changes in the aged renal tubules can be summarized in three groups: (1) tubular dysfunction, (2) medullary hypotonicity, and (3) tubular frailty.

1 ***Tubular dysfunction:*** Compared to younger individuals tubular handling of many substances is modified in healthy elderly people: [9]

- **Sodium** The 24-hour urinary sodium output and fractional excretion of sodium are significantly greater in old and very old people. The mean half time for the excretion of a sodium load is 17.7 hours in persons under 30 years of age, reaching 30.9 hours in persons over 65. Because GFR declines with age and the amount of filtered sodium is lower than in young subjects, a salt load given to an aged person takes longer to eliminate. However, when sodium is restricted to 50 mmol day^{-1}, the period required to start saving urinary sodium is five days in the young and nine days in the elderly, and therefore the capacity of the ageing kidney to adapt to a low salt intake (50 mmol $24h^{-1}$) is clearly blunted. The proximal nephron behaves similarly in the young, old and very old, whereas in the thick ascending loop of Henle the reabsorption of sodium is reduced in the old and very old people. This phenomenon has two important consequences: first, the amount of sodium loss is increased; and second, the capacity of the medullar interstitium to concentrate is also diminished (medullary hypotonicity). Thus, old subjects exhibit both an increased sodium excretion and an inability to maximally concentrate the urine (water saving). Despite this tendency to an exaggerated natriuresis, total body sodium is not significantly decreased with age. The basal plasma concentrations of renin and aldosterone and the response to their stimuli are diminished in old age, which is another mechanism for the enhanced sodium loss in this population. Finally, elevated serum and urinary natriuretic peptide levels in the elderly may be another cause of the characteristic urinary sodium loss of the aged.[4,16,17]

  Clinical consequences: For therapeutic reasons or due to reduced appetite, salt-restricted elderly can develop hyponatraemia (senile 'sodium leakage' hyponatraemia), volume depletion (hypotension, hypernatraemia) and even acute renal failure (ARF).[4,16,17]

- **Potassium** Total body potassium content is lower in the old than in the young, and the correlation with age is linear. This phenomenon can be explained by the reduced muscle mass (main body potassium stores), and poor potassium intake characteristic of the elderly. On the other hand, the renal excretion of potassium is significantly lower in the aged. A trend to hyperkalaemia in the elderly is explained by the reduced serum aldosterone and reduced tubular response to this hormone. In addition, there is an increase in the activity of the H+K+ATPase pump (potassium reabsorption) in the intercalated cells of the aged collecting ducts (in rats). This mechanism could also explain the trend to hyperkalaemia in old people.[18–20]

  Clinical consequences: Usually serum potassium is normal in the elderly, but when they take diuretics, they develop hypokalaemia more rapidly than do the young. On the other hand elderly persons are predisposed to hyperkalaemia, particularly when they are treated with non-steroidal anti-inflammatory drugs (NSAIDs), angiotensin-converting enzyme inhibitors, beta-blockers and/or potassium-sparing diuretics.[18–20]

- **Urea, creatinine and uric acid** In healthy old and very old people, fractional excretion of urea is increased compared to that in younger persons: 65% and 50% respectively. This phenomenon could be explained by a reduced distal urea reabsorption secondary to the diminished UT1 (urea channels) demonstrated in the collecting tubules in old rats. Regarding the handling of creatinine, it has been shown that healthy older people have a net creatinine tubular reabsorption. Serum uric acid levels and its urinary fractional excretion are similar in the young and the old.[6,21]

  Clinical consequences: The increased urinary loss of urea contributes to osmotic diuresis (nocturia), and medullary hypotonicity that can lead to dehydration in hot weather, febrile syndromes, as well as a characteristic low serum urea level in healthy old. Also creatinine clearance can lead to underestimation of glomerular filtration in the healthy old individuals because this group shows net creatinine reabsorption.[6,21,22]

- **Calcium, phosphate and magnesium** Serum calcium, phosphorus and magnesium levels and their urinary fractional excretion are similar in the healthy young, old and very old. However, since the elderly frequently have a low vitamin D diet, reduced sunlight exposure, decreased vitamin D renal hydroxylation and a low level of serum sexual hormones, they tend to develop calcium metabolism disorders. The latter phenomenon in combination with a poor calcium intestinal absorption leads to the development of senile secondary hyperparathyroidism. When healthy old people undergo a volume overload, renal magnesium excretion is increased to a degree that significantly lowers their serum Mg level. Since, in healthy old people, sodium reabsorption is reduced in the thick ascending loop of Henle and magnesium reabsorption occurs chiefly at this tubular segment, one could hypothesize that a urinary magnesium loss could explain the increased Mg excretion. In addition, it is known that the elderly often need magnesium supplements probably because of a combination of diminished spontaneous intake of magnesium and poor intestinal absorption.[22]

Clinical consequences: Even though renal handling of calcium, phosphate and magnesium are not altered in the elderly, their lower ingestion and intestinal absorption can easily lead to hypocalcaemia, hypomagnesaemia, hypophosphatemia, and secondary hyperparathyroidism.[22]

- **Urinary acidification** Macias *et al.* found no differences in titratable acid, ammonia or net acid excretion in response to an acute acid overload in the elderly compared to young controls. However, following an acid load, the maximal values of ammonia and titratable acid excretion were reached in four hours in the young and between six and eight hours in the old.

Clinical consequences: elderly subjects take longer to reach peak proton (acid) excretion, and experience a greater difficulty in handling states of acidosis.[22]

- **Erythropoietin** Erythropoietin is mainly produced by the peri-tubular interstitial cells near the proximal convoluted tubules. Erythropoietin production is not affected by age and therefore its plasma levels are normal in the healthy old and very old people.

Clinical consequences: Normal ageing process does not explain the presence of anaemia.[23]

2 ***Medulla hypotonicity: water handling:*** Total body water is diminished with age; in the elderly it comprises only 54% of total body weight compared to 65% in the young. As in healthy young people, total body water content is lower in elderly women, than in elderly men. Since the reduction in senile water content takes place in the intracellular compartment, hypovolaemia always represents a pathological state in the elderly. Senescence reduces the capacity of the kidney to concentrate the urine. The maximum urinary concentration capacity remains normal until about the third decade and then it falls by about 30 mOsmol kg^{-1} per decade. This phenomenon can be explained by the *aglomerular circulation*, the defect in sodium reabsorption in the ascending limb of Henle's loop, and the reduced distal urea reabsorption, which in the young kidney induces the development of a hypertonic medulla. Another mechanism for the impairment of the urine concentration ability is the decrease in responsiveness of tubular epithelium of the collecting tubules to antidiuretic hormone. Also this may explain why plasma vasopressin levels are higher in the elderly compared to mature adults. Furthermore, when healthy active elderly volunteers were water-restricted for 24 hours, their threshold for thirst was increased and water intake was reduced compared with a control group of younger subjects. Dryness of the mouth, a decrease of taste, alteration in mental capacity or cortical cerebral dysfunction, and a reduction in the sensitivity of both osmoreceptors and baroreceptors all may contribute to this increased threshold for thirst. Finally, concentration of angiotensin, a powerful generator of thirst, is lower in the elderly. Urinary dilution capability is also decreased. Thus, there is a minimum urine concentration of only 92 mOsmol kg^{-1} in the elderly compared to 52 mOsmol kg^{-1} in the young. Maximum free water clearance also is reduced in the elderly from 16.2 ml min^{-1} to 5.9 ml min^{-1}. Again, the functional impairment of the diluting segment of the thick ascending limb, described above, seems to account for the decrease in the capacity to dilute urine observed in the aged.[4,9,24]

Clinical consequences: Elderly people may develop dehydration (hypernatremia) or volume overload (hyponatremia) under conditions of water restriction or water load respectively.

3 ***Tubular frailty:***Tubular cells are frail in the elderly, and because of this they progress easily to acute tubular necrosis, and also they recover slowly from this histological alteration.[9]

Clinical consequences: Acute kidney injury (AKI) is a frequent complication in the elderly, and if the kidney does not recover after approximately three months it remains as *chronic kidney disease* (CKD).[9]

Diseases: Tubular-interstitial level

Interstitial nephritis

Although acute interstitial nephritis may develop following the use of nearly all NSAIDs or diuretics the number of reported cases is small. Most of these patients are elderly. Usually the associated renal abnormalities improve after the drug is discontinued with or without steroid therapy, but possible complications may include chronic kidney disease or even end-stage renal disease (ESRD). Interstitial nephritis results mainly from a delayed hypersensitivity response to drugs (NSAID, diuretics, etc.). Patients taking NSAIDs for months or years may develop papillary necrosis, chronic interstitial nephritis, or even ESRD.[14]

Urinary tract infection (pyelonephritis)

This is the most common infection in the elderly and is especially frequent in debilitated, institutionalized individuals. Its pathogenesis is strongly related to obstructive uropathy. Moreover, the incidence of bacteriuria increases with advancing age because of several non-obstructive conditions such as vaginal and urethral atrophy, puddling related to bed rest, and bladder catheterization which predispose the aged to urinary infection.[25]

Obstructive uropathy

Prostatic hypertrophy occurs to the same degree in almost all ageing males, but in a proportion of them it provides a slow obstruction to urinary outflow, which gradually decreases kidney function. Often this is not recognized until it is too late, largely because the patient becomes polyuric rather than oliguric. By the time, the urinary obstruction is recognized, the damage may be irreversible, so that even with the relief of obstruction, renal function recovers only partially.[9,26]

Acute kidney injury (AKI)

The most common causes of AKI in the elderly are:

1 Prerenal causes: dehydration (main cause), haemorrhage and shock (cardiogenic and septic).

2 Renal causes: acute tubular necrosis (ATN) due to the persistence of prerenal causes and/or to nephrotoxins (e.g. aminoglycosides), rapidly progressive damage due to primary or secondary glomerular disease, or acute interstitial nephritis.

3 Postrenal (obstructive) causes: stones, tumour, stricture, prostatic hypertrophy.

Prerenal and postrenal causes of AKI are of particular importance because their early identification and treatment may prevent the development or reverse established AKI. The cause of AKI is often multifactorial and its incidence is higher in the elderly than in the young, because of the frequency of systemic illnesses (diabetes mellitus, myeloma, etc.), polypharmacy, and because of the renal ageing process itself. However, age *per se* is not an important determinant of survival in patients with AKI. In the elderly, the urinary indices (urinary sodium and fractional excretion of sodium and urea) for diagnosing AKI may be slightly different from those accepted for younger people since a higher value of these indicators does not rule out a prerenal AKI (due to the senile urinary sodium and urea loss). Sometimes temporary or permanent dialysis may be needed.

Although AKI is treated similarly in the elderly and younger patients, old people are more vulnerable to dialysis-related complications such as haemodynamic instability, bleeding and mild disequilibrium syndrome.

Prevention is of paramount importance: maintenance of an adequate extracellular volume and drug dosage regimens tailored to the patient's GFR are essential.[15]

Chronic kidney disease (CKD)

CKD is a syndrome characterized by progressive and generally irreversible deterioration of renal function due to the reduction of the nephron mass. CKD is predominantly a disease of the elderly, because its incidence rises steadily with age, being at least 10 times more common at 75 and over than at 15–45 years· The causes of end-stage renal disease (ESRD) in the elderly differ substantially from those in younger populations. The most common disorders that lead to renal failure in old age are hypertension, nephrosclerosis, diabetes mellitus and obstructive uropathy, although in as many as one third it proves impossible to identify any specific cause. Two common causes of CKD are: vascular disease of the main renal arteries and prostatic hypertrophy. A further cause worth noting is amyloidosis. Pathogenic mechanisms by which the failing kidney may produce specific clinical features are as follows:

- As sclerosis of the glomeruli advances, the remaining nephrons shift to glomerular hyperfiltration in order to eliminate more waste toxic products per functioning nephron (hyperfiltration). This mechanism appears beneficial at the beginning but the price paid for hyperfiltration is an acceleration of glomerular sclerosis;
- Retention of uremic toxins (polyamines, guanidines, middle molecules and hormonal peptides);
- A high level of parathyroid hormone is currently accepted as one of the major uremic toxins;
- Erythropoietin and 1,25-dihydroxycholecalciferol deficiencies result in anaemia and low serum calcium, respectively;
- Phosphate retention leads to secondary hyperparathyroidism and renal osteodystrophy;
- Derangement of the renin angiotensin aldosterone mechanism results in hypertension. As CKD progresses and creatinine clearance falls to about 25 ml min^{-1}, the full clinical picture of uremia appears. The skin acquires a characteristic yellow-brown pallor and pruritus is frequent. Patients complain of asthenia, anorexia and vomiting. From the cardiorespiratory system, hypertension, heart failure, pulmonary oedema, coronary disease and arrhythmia may be seen. From the nervous system the patient may have polyneuropathy, clonus and even uremic coma in the most advanced stage of the disease. Secondary hyperparathyroidism, and hyperprolactinaemia are frequent endocrinological abnormalities. Impaired cellular immunity, and clotting alterations are also present. In the late phase, all of the above abnormalities increase and, when GFR is lower than 10 ml min^{-1}, it is necessary to start replacement therapy (dialysis or transplantation).[7,10]

Dialysis: Age itself does not constitute a contraindication to dialysis and/or transplantation. Elderly patients can be effectively treated by both haemodialysis (HD) or peritoneal dialysis (PD). Old patients on dialysis are prone to develop more serious forms of bone disease than the young, due to osteopenia, unbalanced diet, reduced physical activity and lack of exposure to sunlight. Frequently malnutrition is present and in order to prevent this state, it is advisable to provide more than 1 g kg^{-1} body weight of protein for patients on HD, and more than 1.2 g for those on PD. The most common practical problems during HD in aged patients are: difficulty in creation of the arteriovenous fistula, permanent catheter/graft infection, gastrointestinal bleeding, intradialytic hypotension, headaches, vomiting, cramps, angina, arrhythmias and cardiovascular instability, while in elderly patients on PD most practical problems are: dialysate leakage, formation of hernias, backache, difficulty in learning, social isolation, family burn-out, and worsening of peripheral vascular disease or malnutrition. PD is better for patients with residual diuresis, severe hypotension, complicated and/or short-lived vascular access, intradialytic arrhythmias, angina or cardiovascular instability. Besides, PD is a satisfactory alternative for geriatric ESRD patients. Most studies confirm that elderly patients on PD and HD have similar survivals. Other forms of peritoneal dialysis include various forms of automated peritoneal dialysis (APD) such as continuous cycling peritoneal dialysis (CCPD) and nightly peritoneal dialysis (NPD); the latter can be an alternative treatment for more vulnerable elderly patients (nursing home).

The predictors of poor outcomes in elderly on dialysis are poor nutritional status, dementia, gait disorders, altered activities of daily living (ADL) and instrumental activities of daily living (IADL), and late referral to the nephrology service. Very elderly patients on haemodialysis have a poor life expectancy: median survival time is 15.6 months from 80–84 years of age, and 11.6 months for those 85–89 (USA). The main causes of death in the oldest dialysis patients are elective withdrawal (38%), cardiovascular events (24%) and infection (22%).[27–29]

Transplantation: Success of transplantation in geriatric ESRD patients requires improved patient selection, the use of new immunosuppressive drugs and lower doses of corticosteroids. One can achieve one-year patient and graft survival rates of 85% and 75%, respectively. For patients older than 60–65 years, the five-year 'functional' graft survival is 55–60%. Although overall results are excellent, the management of transplantation in the elderly requires an understanding of pharmacology, immunology and physiology peculiar to this age group. Although these patients experience fewer rejection episodes than do younger patients, graft loss in the elderly transplant recipient is due mainly to death with a functioning graft.[30]

In addition, transplant stress induces senescence changes in the kidney, while the greatest adverse impact factor in cadaver kidney transplant today is donor age. Most common causes of death in the elderly transplant recipient are cardiovascular disease and infection related to peaks of immunosuppression. Regarding the elderly people as kidney donors, their organs are considered as marginal ones, but these can be useful (single or in pair) in a subgroup of elderly recipients.[30]

Renal pharmacology

Many pharmacokinetic parameters are affected by the ageing process such as: the amount of drug that reaches the systemic circulation and therefore the amount at the site of action (bioavailability), the distribution size of the drug (volume of distribution), its renal excretion (GFR), and the length of time needed to reach steady-state serum concentration or to eliminate the drug (four times the halflife). Due to these pharmacokinetic changes, old people are predisposed to drug toxicity, and treatment should be individualized, using low and slowly increasing doses, and trying to avoid polypharmacy.[8]

Key points

- Numerous physiological changes occur in the kidney during ageing.
- Elderly patients can be effectively treated with either haemodialysis or peritoneal dialysis.
- For persons >60 years of age five-year survival of a renal transplantation graft is 55–60%.

References

1. Musso CG, Macías Nú nez JF. Feedback between geriatric syndromes: general system theory in geriatrics. *Int Urol Nephrol* 2006;**38**:785–6.
2. Silva FG. The ageing kidney: a review – Part I. *Int Urol Nephrol* 2005;**37**:185–205.
3. Silva FG. The ageing kidney: a review – Part II. *Int Urol Nephrol* 2005;**37**:419–32.
4. Alvarez Gregori J, Musso C, Macías Nú nez JF. Renal ageing. In: J Sastre, R Pamolona, J Ramón (eds), *Medical Biogerontology*, Ergon, Madrid, 2009, pp. 111–23.
5. Cockcroft DW, Gault MH. Prediction of creatinine clearance from serum creatinine. *Nephron* 1976:**16**:31–41.
6. Musso CG, Michelángelo H, Vilas M *et al.* Creatinine reabsorption by the aged kidney. *Int Urol Nephrol* 2009;**41**:727–31.
7. Daugirdas J, Blake P, Ing T. *Dialysis Handbook*, Kluwer, Philadelphia, 2008.
8. Bennet W. Geriatric renal pharmacology: practical considerations. In: E Friedman, D Oreopoulos, J Sands (eds), Geriatric Nephrology: An epidemiologic and clinical challenge. Postgraduate Education Course of the American Society of Nephrology, 2008, pp. 205–13.
9. Musso CG. Geriatric nephrology and the 'nephrogeriatric giants'. *Int Urol Nephrol* 2002;**34**:255–6.

10. Musso CG, Macías Nú nez JF, Oreopoulos DG. Physiological similarities and differences between renal aging and chronic renal disease. *J Nephrol* 2007;**20**:586–7.
11. Appel G. Glomerular disease in the elderly – Should we be doing more biopsies? In: E Friedman, D Oreopoulos, J Sands (eds), Geriatric Nephrology: An epidemiologic and clinical challenge. Postgraduate Education Course of the American Society of Nephrology, 2008, pp. 97–100.
12. Vendemia F, Gesualdo L, Schena FP, D'Amico G. Epidemiology of primary glomerulonephritis in the elderly. Report from the Italian registry of renal biopsy. *J Nephrol* 2001;**14**:340–52.
13. Ponticelli C, Glassock R. *Treatment of Primary Glomerulonephritis*, Oxford University Press, Oxford, 2009.
14. Cameron JS. Renal disease in the elderly: particular problems. In: G D'Amico, G Colasanti (eds), *Issues in Nephrosciences*, Wichting, Milano, 1995, pp. 111–17.
15. Musso CG. Acute renal failure in the elderly: pearls for its assessment and treatment. *Electron J Biomed* 2005;**1**:1–93.
16. Fish LC, Murphy DJ, Elahi D, Minaker KL. Renal sodium excretion in normal aging: decreased excretion rates lead to delayed sodium excretion in normal aging. *J Geriatr Nephrol Urol* 1994;**4**:145–51.
17. Musso CG, Fainstein I, Kaplan R, Macías Núñez JF. Tubular renal function in the oldest old. *Rev Esp Geriatr Gerontol* 2004;**39**:314–9.
18. Lye M. Distribution of body potassium in healthy elderly subjects. *Gerontologie* 1981;**27**:286–92.
19. Eiam-Ong S, Sabatini S. Effect of ageing and potassium depletion on renal collecting tubule k-controlling ATPases. *Nephrology* 2002;**7**: 87–91.
20. Andreucci V, Russo D, Cianciaruso B, Andreucci M. Some sodium, potassium and water changes in the elderly and their treatment. *Nephrol Dial Transplant* 1996; **11**(Suppl 9):9–17.
21. Musso CG, Alvarez Gregori JA, Macías Núñez JF. Renal handling of uric acid, magnesium, phosphorus, calcium, and acid-base in the elderly. In: JF Macías Núñez, S Cameron, D Oreopoulos (eds), *The Aging Kidney in Health and Disease*, Springer, New York, 2008, pp. 155–171.
22. Macías JF, Garcia-Iglesias C, Tabernero JM *et al*. Behaviour of the ageing kidney under acute acid overload. *Nefrologia* 1983;**3**:11–16.
23. Musso CG, Musso CAF, Joseph H *et al*. Plasma erythropoietin levels in the oldest old. *Int Urol Nephrol* 2004;**36**:259–62.
24. Sands J. Changes in urine concentrating ability in the aging kidney. In: E Friedman, D Oreopoulos, J Sands (eds), Geriatric Nephrology: An epidemiologic and clinical challenge. Postgraduate Education Course of the American Society of Nephrology, 2008, pp. 85–94.
25. Nicolle L. Urinary infection in the elderly. When does it matter? In: E Friedman, D Oreopoulos, J Sands (eds), Geriatric Nephrology: An epidemiologic and clinical challenge. Postgraduate Education Course of the American Society of Nephrology, 2008, pp. 249–60.
26. Alivizatos G, Skolarikos A. Obstructive uropathy and benign prostatic hyperplasia. In: JF Macías Núñez, S Cameron, D Oreopoulos (eds), *The Aging Kidney in Health and Disease*, Springer, New York, 2008, pp. 257–72.
27. Vandelli L, Medici G, Perrone S, Lusvarghi E. Haemodialysis in the elderly. *Nephrol Dial Transplant* 1996;**11**(Suppl 9):89–94.
28. Grapsa E, Oreopoulos D. Chronic peritoneal dialysis in the elderly. In: R Khanna, R Krediet (eds), *Textbook of Peritoneal Dialysis*, Springer, 2009, pp. 737–55.
29. Oreopoulos D. End stage renal disease in the elderly: Does the type of dialysis make a difference? In: E Friedman, D Oreopoulos, J Sands (eds), Geriatric Nephrology: An epidemiologic and clinical challenge. Postgraduate Education Course of the American Society of Nephrology, 2008, pp. 355–71.
30. Halloran P. Age and somatic cell senescence in nephrology and kidney transplantation. In: E Friedman, D Oreopoulos D, J Sands (eds), Geriatric Nephrology: An epidemiologic and clinical challenge. Postgraduate Education Course of the American Society of Nephrology, 2008, pp. 19–30.

SECTION 12

Cancer

CHAPTER 108

Cancer and ageing

Tanya M. Wildes
Washington University School of Medicine, St Louis, MO, USA

Introduction

The risk of most types of cancer increases with age and with the growth in the aged segment of the population, the burden of cancer in the elderly will continue to grow. In this chapter, the scope of this problem is reviewed, as is the biology of cancer and ageing. A discussion on cancer prevention and treatment in the elderly follows. Finally, supportive care, survivorship issues and the multidisciplinary care of the senior adult cancer patient are reviewed.

Epidemiology and disparities

Cancer is the leading cause of death in men and women aged 60–79 years and the second leading cause of death in persons aged 80 years and older.[1] By 2030, more than one-fifth of the population in the USA will be over the age of 65 years.[2] The probability of developing cancer is one in three in men and one in four women over the age 70 years. The leading causes of cancer incidence and mortality are detailed in Figure 108.1.

Over the past 60 years, cancer-specific death rates have decreased among younger individuals, while increasing in older individuals.[3] Significant disparities in outcomes between younger and older individuals are likely due to a number of factors, including differences in screening, more advanced stage at presentation in older individuals or less aggressive treatment in older patients. Older individuals are more likely to experience delays in diagnosis, incomplete evaluation and undertreatment. Half of older women receive substandard treatment for breast cancer, with significantly worse survival.[4] Similar trends have also been noted among patients with ovarian and rectal cancer and these persist even when studies control for comorbidities and functional status. Under-enrolment of older individuals in clinical trials further compounds the situation by resulting in a paucity of data on appropriate management of cancer in the elderly.

Ageing and tumour development

Hanahan and Weinberg proposed that there are six attributes that must be attained by a cell to be transformed into a malignant cell: self-sufficiency in growth signals, insensitivity to anti-growth signals, evasion of programmed cell death, limitless replicative potential, sustained angiogenesis and tissue invasion/metastasis.[5] Mutations cause cellular changes resulting in these altered characteristics and in malignant transformation.

Theories of biological ageing and carcinogenesis overlap in many ways, potentially explaining the increased incidence of many cancers with age. Over time, DNA damage caused by random events or free radicals can cause either cellular dysfunction/death, resulting in ageing, or may cause mutations in proto-oncogenes or tumour suppressors, yielding carcinogenesis. Further, changes seen in cells with ageing are also observed in early carcinogenesis. The formation of DNA adducts, DNA hypomethylation, chromosomal breakage and translocation are associated with age and increase the susceptibility to late-stage carcinogens.[6]

The immune dysregulation associated with ageing may contribute to the increased incidence of cancer with age. With age, changes in T-cell function result in decreased proliferation, increased proportion of memory cells and a decrease in naive T-cells. B-cell function is intact but dysregulated, with an increase in autoantibody formation and monoclonal protein production. Interleukin-2 levels decrease, whereas interleukin-6 levels rise. A prospective cohort study demonstrated that individuals with better NK cell function had lower rates of cancer 10 years subsequently.[6]

In some ways, however, ageing and cancer biology are at odds: cancer requires limitless replicative potential, while finite replicative potential (replicative senescence) is a hallmark of ageing. Most normal human cell types have the capacity for 60–70 doublings. The cellular 'abacus' is the telomere, which consists of several thousand repeats of a

Principles and Practice of Geriatric Medicine, Fifth Edition. Edited by Alan J. Sinclair, John E. Morley and Bruno Vellas.

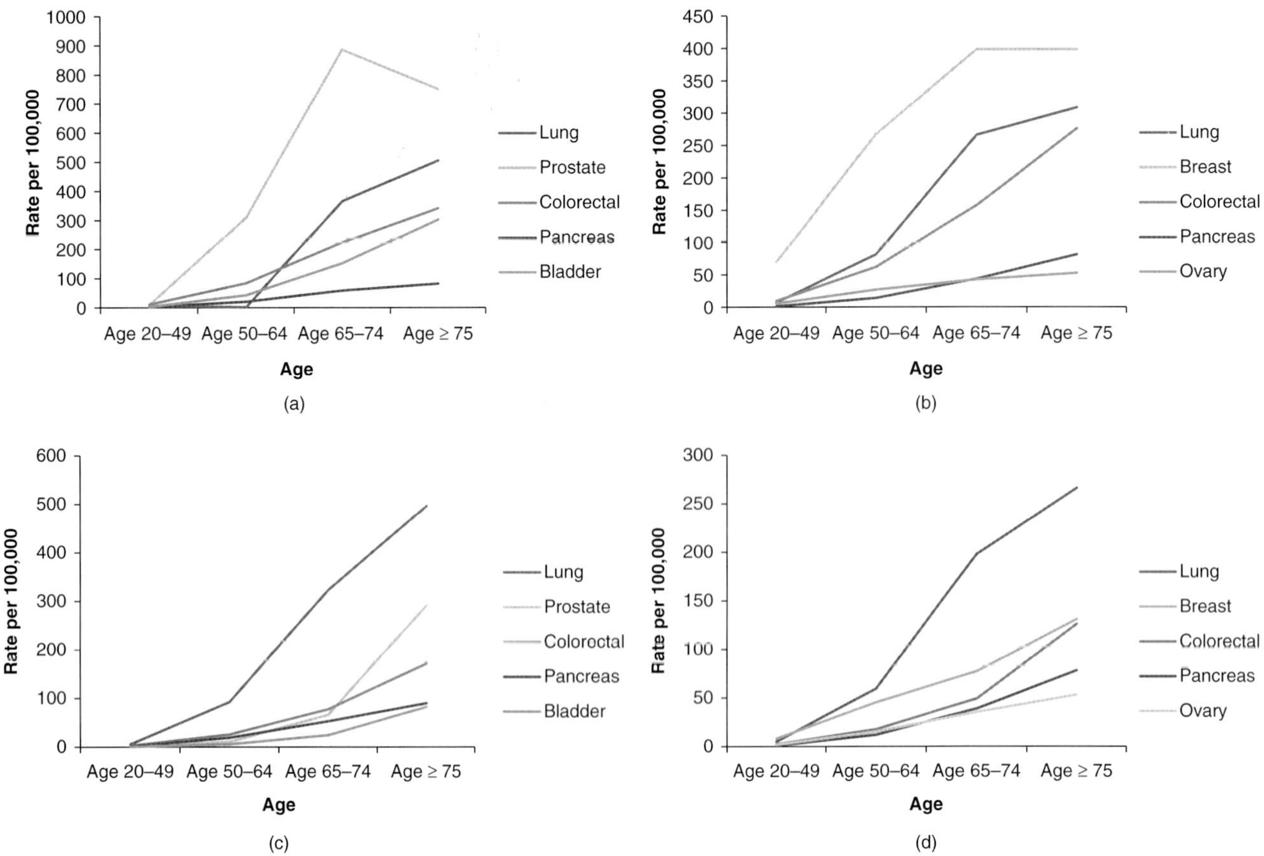

Figure 108.1 (a) Cancer incidence rates in men; (b) cancer incidence rates in women; (c) cancer mortality rates in men; (d) cancer mortality rates in women. All rates age adjusted to 2000 US population. 2006 SEER statistics.

short base pair sequence at the ends of every chromosome. The telomeres protect the chromosomal DNA. With each successive replication, 50–100 base pairs of telomeric DNA are lost from the ends of the chromosomes. Over time, in normal cells, these protective caps are lost; the chromosomal DNA becomes fused end-to-end with other chromosomes, ultimately leading to death of the affected cell. In contrast, in malignant cells, telomeres are maintained through the expression of telomerase, allowing unlimited replication.[7] Another mechanism of senescence, termed 'stress-induced premature senescence', results from cellular events other than telomere shortening. Mutations in an oncogene or double-stranded DNA breaks induced by chemotherapeutic agents can trigger senescence, resulting in a proportion of clonal cells entering senescence. This permanent growth arrest may be as effective as apoptosis as an anti-cancer mechanism.[8]

In some malignancies, there are age-related differences in tumour biology, making the malignancy either more or less aggressive in older patients compared with their younger counterparts. It is a commonly held, though debatable, dogma that solid tumours, including breast, colon, lung and prostate cancer, are more indolent in older patients; however, epidemiological data do not altogether support this observation. It is clear that in some cancers, there are differences in tumour behaviour over the age spectrum. Breast cancers in older women are more likely to be estrogen receptor positive. Acute myeloid leukaemia is more aggressive in elderly patients and more resistant to conventional chemotherapy due to the increased expression of the MDR1 (multidrug resistance) gene.

Cancer prevention

Cancer prevention is an effective way to reduce cancer morbidity and mortality. Cancer prevention strategies include behavioural/lifestyle modification, such as dietary changes, chemoprevention and screening.

Obesity is associated with post-menopausal breast cancer and weight loss lowers circulating estrogen levels. Large cohort studies demonstrate that weight loss is associated with a decreased risk of post-menopausal breast cancer.[9] Further, a randomized trial of a lower fat dietary intervention, which resulted in weight loss in the intervention group, was associated with an 11% reduction (hazard ratio 0.89, 95% confidence interval 0.80–1.00) in estrogen receptor positive (ER+) post-menopausal breast cancer diagnoses in the 8 years of follow-up.[10] Further research is needed into whether it is weight loss *per se* or dietary modification that results in the reduced risk of cancer. In this same trial, however, there was no change in the incidence of colorectal cancer with the dietary intervention.[11]

Epidemiological studies suggest a protective effect of increased calcium and vitamin D intake on the risk of colorectal cancer. Randomized trials have demonstrated a modest but significant decrease in risk of recurrent adenomas. In the Women's Health Initiative randomized trial, supplementation with calcium and vitamin D did not result in a decrease in the risk of colorectal cancer versus placebo.[12] However, this study was criticized for doses of vitamin D_3 (400 IU daily) that are generally inadequate to achieve sufficient serum levels of 25-hydroxyvitamin D.

The inducible enzyme cyclooxygenase 2 (COX-2) is elevated in the majority of colorectal cancers. Aspirin, a non-specific inhibitor of both COX-1 and COX-2, reduces the risk of colorectal cancer by 24% in patients who take at least 300 mg of the medication for at least 5 years and after a latency period of 10 years.[13] However, the benefit of cancer prevention must be weighed against the risk of bleeding complications. The COX-2 inhibitor's more selective mechanism results in lower risk of bleeding. Indeed, the COX-2 inhibitors rofecoxib and celecoxib effectively prevent the formation of precancerous polyps, but are also associated with an increased risk of cardiovascular events.[14] Given the increased risk and no data showing a decreased risk of invasive colorectal cancer, COX-2 inhibitors should not yet be used for colorectal cancer prevention.

The selective estrogen receptor modulators (SERMs) compete with estrogen for binding at the estrogen receptor, inhibiting pathways required for cellular growth and proliferation. A randomized, placebo-controlled trial of tamoxifen for the prevention of breast cancer enrolled over 13 000 women. Tamoxifen reduced the risk of invasive breast cancer by more than 40%. Therapy with tamoxifen was associated with a twofold increased risk of pulmonary embolism and a threefold increased risk of endometrial cancer.[15] Given the serious potential side effects, tamoxifen is recommended only for women at high risk for cancer using risk prediction models such as the Gail model, weighed against the individual risk factors for adverse events.[16]

Another SERM, raloxifene, has been studied with regard to its impact on the incidence of post-menopausal breast cancer. Over the 8 years of follow-up, therapy with raloxifene was associated with a 76% reduction in the incidence of ER+ breast cancers, relative to placebo. Women treated with raloxifene had a twofold increased risk of venous thromboembolic disease.[17] In a head-to-head comparison, postmenopausal women at increased risk for breast cancer were randomized to either raloxifene or tamoxifen. Raloxifene was as effective as tamoxifen at reducing the risk of invasive breast cancer, with a lower risk of venous thromboembolic events.[18]

In summary, several cancer prevention strategies hold promise. However, in an individual patient, the risks and benefits must be considered before recommending chemopreventive strategies.

Cancer screening

Screening as a strategy for prevention is a complicated issue. The goal of screening is to identify a disease during a latent or early symptomatic stage, in order to intervene and alter the natural history of disease. Although there is evidence of benefit of screening for breast, colorectal and cervical cancer in individuals in their 50s and 60s, data for screening older, asymptomatic individuals for these common malignancies is lacking. Complicating the issue are the differences in cancer biology described above, which may result in the detection of more indolent cancers that would not ultimately be life-limiting. The sensitivity and specificity of screening tests may be affected by age-related changes in body composition, such as the change in breast composition with age. The harm due to false-positive screening tests must also be taken into account, including psychological distress and risks of diagnostic procedures. Comorbid medical conditions and functional decline may increase the risk of complications related to screening procedures, such as the sedation required for colonoscopy. Table 108.1 gives a summary of current recommendations regarding screening.

Colorectal cancer screening is effective in selected older patients. In patients aged 70–80 years, randomized trials have shown annual to biennial faecal occult blood testing (FOBT) to be effective at reducing colorectal cancer incidence and mortality, with a lag time of 5 years to mortality benefit. However, the sensitivity and specificity are low. Case–control studies of flexible sigmoidoscopy and colonoscopy in older patients suggest a mortality benefit associated with screening; however, sigmoidoscopy has a lower sensitivity in older individuals given the increase in prevalence of right-sided colon cancers, which sigmoidoscopy does not detect. Colonoscopy is more sensitive and specific than FOBT or sigmoidoscopy, but in a cohort of older patients aged 70–75 years, the rate of major complications of colonoscopy, including perforation, myocardial infarction or stroke, was 0.3%.[19] Computed tomographic (CT) colonography appears to be as effective as colonoscopy in older patients at detecting advanced neoplasias, with a low false-positive rate,[20] but must be followed by traditional colonoscopy to confirm abnormal findings.

Among the randomized trials that established the mortality benefit of mammographic screening for breast

Table 108.1 Recommendations for cancer screening in older adults[a].

Cancer	USPSTF[55]	ACS[56]	AGS
Colorectal cancer	Age 50–75 years: FOBT, sigmoidoscopy or colonoscopy recommended Age 76–85 years: recommends against routine screening, although there may be considerations supporting screening in an individual Age >85 years: recommends against screening	Starting at age 50 years and continuing as long as individual is in good health	Age ≥50 years: screening recommended, unless person is too frail to undergo colonoscopy or life expectancy <5 years[57]
Breast cancer	Age 50–74 years: biennial mammography Age ≥75 years: insufficient evidence to assess risks and benefits of screening mammography	Beginning at age 40 years and continuing as long as the woman is in good health and would be a candidate for breast cancer treatment	Age <75 years: annual or biennial mammography Age ≥75 years: mammography at least every 3 years with no upper age limit for women with an estimated life expectancy of ≥4 years[58]
Cervical cancer	Cessation of screening for women >65 years with adequate prior screening who are not otherwise at high risk for cervical cancer	Cessation of screening for women ≥70 years with ≥3 recent, consecutive negative tests and no abnormal tests in previous 10 years	Age ≤70 years: screening every 1–3 years Age >70 years: little evidence for or against screening women who have been regularly screened in previous years. An older woman of any age should who has never had a pap smear should be screened until two negative pap smears taken 1 year apart[59]
Prostate cancer	Age <75 years: current evidence is insufficient to assess the balance of benefits and harms of prostate cancer screening Age ≥75 years: recommends against screening for prostate cancer	Healthcare provider should discuss risks and benefits of screening with the men at average risk for prostate cancer and with 10 year life expectancy, beginning at age 50 years	No published recommendations

[a]USPSTF, U.S. Preventative Services Task Force: ACS, American Cancer Society; AGS, American Geriatric Society: FOBT, faecal occult blood testing.

cancer, only one included women over the age of 70 years. Although in the overall study mammography decreased the risk of breast cancer death by one-third, there was not a significant reduction in breast cancer mortality in the subgroup of women aged 70–74 years. Interestingly, as the density of breast tissue decreases with age, the sensitivity and specificity of mammography increase. There are several studies demonstrating that among women with multiple comorbidities, detecting early-stage breast cancer does not improve survival. Thus, women with a life expectancy of less than 5 years are unlikely to benefit from breast cancer screening.[19]

There have been no prospective randomized trials of cervical cancer screening in any age group, although multiple observational studies show that screening with Papanicolaou (Pap) smears decreases the incidence and mortality of cervical cancer. With advancing age, the sensitivity of Pap smears decreases due to the migration of the squamo-columnar junction into the cervical canal and specificity declines due to atropic changes causing inflammation. Older women who have been regularly screened are at low risk and those who have significant comorbidity are unlikely to benefit from screening.[19]

Prostate cancer screening is controversial, even in younger populations. Prospective, randomized trials of prostate-specific antigen (PSA) screening are under way, but do not include men over the age of 75 years. Given the indolent nature of most prostate cancers and high prevalence of clinically irrelevant prostate cancers found among octogenarians at autopsy, screening for prostate cancer is generally not recommended in men over the age of 75 years or who have a life expectancy of less than 10 years.[21]

In summary, selected older individuals with longer life expectancy may be appropriate for screening for common cancers.

Cancer treatment

The basic tenets of cancer treatment involve the determination of whether treatment is being undertaken with curative or palliative intent. Radiation therapy and surgery are the modalities of treatment utilized to control the local extent of cancer. Cytotoxic chemotherapy, hormonal therapy, biological therapy or targeted agents are typically administered orally or intravenously for systemic treatment. Treatment may be administered neoadjuvantly, that is, prior to definitive treatment, to limit the chance of systemic spread and to decrease the extent of local treatment. Adjuvant therapy is administered following definitive treatment, to reduce the risk of recurrence in individuals at high risk. Palliative treatment is administered to improve symptoms or prolong life in patients with an incurable malignancy.

Decision-making

Historically, clinical trials of cancer treatment have excluded patients due to advancing age or therapies in older patients. Clinicians have been left to extrapolate from data derived from the treatment of younger individuals. Increasing attention to this problem has yielded both retrospective and prospective studies of the effectiveness of treatment strategies in older adults with cancer, but much work remains to be done. Guidelines for the approach to management of cancer in senior adults have been established (Figure 108.2).

Surgery

Surgery is employed in the treatment of cancer to remove the primary tumour with curative intent. Surgery may also be used to palliate symptoms or prevent serious complications in advanced or metastatic disease, such as colonic diversion for an obstructing colon mass. While some studies have been concerned with increased risk of adverse outcomes in older individuals, often these did not account for comorbidities, advanced cancer stage at presentation, functional impairment and other confounding factors.[22] Appropriate preoperative risk stratification must be employed. A tool developed specifically for use in older cancer patients, the Preoperative Assessment of Cancer in the Elderly (PACE), incorporates measures of cognition, functional status, depression, fatigue, ECOG performance status, American Society for Anesthesiology

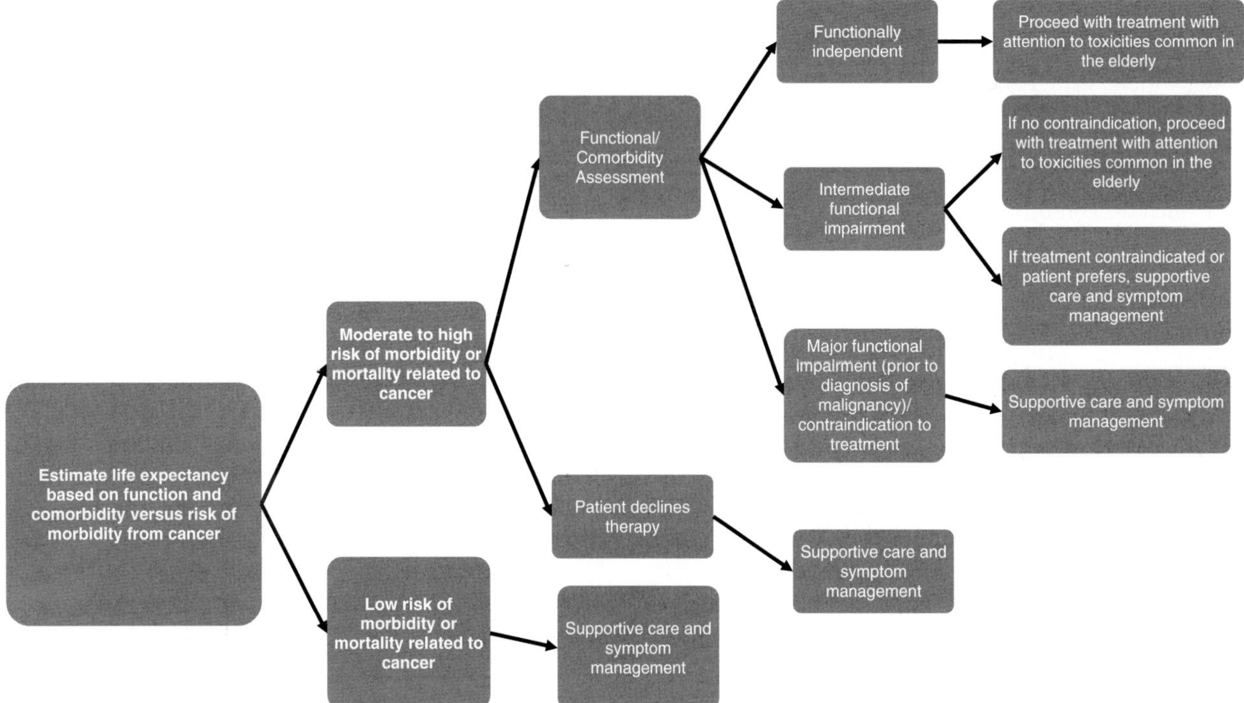

Figure 108.2 Guideline for management of senior adult oncology patients. Adapted with permission from the NCCN 1.2010 Senior Adult Oncology Clinical Practice Guidelines in Oncology. ©National Comprehensive Cancer Network, 2010. The most recent and complete version of the guideline is available at http://www.nccn.org.

scale (ASA) and Satariano's index of comorbidities. In a prospective international study of patient 70 years of age and older undergoing elective cancer surgery for solid tumours under general anaesthesia, 460 patients underwent this oncogeriatric-specific assessment on the day prior to surgery. Any dependencies in instrumental activities of daily living (IADLs), moderate to severe fatigue or abnormal performance status were associated with a 50% increased risk of 30 day morbidity following surgery. Similarly, any dependencies in ADLs or IADLs and abnormal performance status were associated with a longer than expected hospital stay; dependency in ADLs doubled the risk of an extended postoperative hospital stay.[23] Interestingly, in this study, comorbidities did not independently predict postoperative complications. Overall, older adults with cancer should not be excluded from surgery on the basis of age alone, but the decision to proceed should be individualized based on the risks of the procedure, potential benefits, the patient's functional status and goals of care.

Radiation

Radiation therapy can be employed with either curative or palliative intent. Some tumours, such as stage I lung cancers or localized prostate cancer, can be effectively treated with radiation alone. Radiation may also be used in conjunction with surgery to improve local control of cancer, as in post-lumpectomy breast irradiation for breast cancer or preoperative radiation for rectal cancer. Radiation may also provide palliation of symptoms in patients with advanced malignancies. Techniques for the delivery of radiation therapy, utilizing three-dimensional imaging reconstruction, have evolved dramatically recently, allowing improved tolerability with sparing of normal tissues. These include conformal radiation, intensity-modulated radiation and stereotactic radiation therapy. Brachytherapy involves the placement of a radioactive source directly within the site of tumour cells and is used in prostate, breast, cervical and skin cancer. Radiation may be delivered systemically in a few instances. Bone-targeting radioisotopes such as samarium-153 and strontium-89 localize to areas of osteoblastic lesions and are helpful in treating painful osteoblastic bone metastases. Radioimmunotherapy consists of radioactive isotopes conjugated to monoclonal antibodies. Examples of radioimmunotherapy include ibritumomab and tositumomab, which are used in non-Hodgkin lymphomas, target the B-cell marker CD20 and are safe and effective in older patients.

In general, there is no decrement in the benefit of radiation therapy in older compared with younger patients and no increase in toxicity in the elderly. Rectal cancer and malignant gliomas are exceptions to this statement. In older women with high-risk breast cancer, post-lumpectomy radiation improves survival. Elderly prostate cancer patients receiving radiation for localized disease have similar 10 year survival rates and disease-free survival rates compared with younger patients and should not be denied potentially curative therapy based on age alone.[24] Toxicities in the elderly are similar to those in younger patients, although older patients tend to have more functional decline acutely during therapy. In subset analyses of combination chemoradiation for lung cancer, patients over the age of 70 years tended to have more frequent oesophagitis and neutropenia, but still enjoyed a survival benefit without increased long-term complications.[25] Modern radiation techniques can also minimize long-term consequences of therapy, such as sparing the contralateral salivary glands in head and neck radiation to prevent xerostomia.

The toxicity of radiation to the brain in older patients and its effect on cognition warrant specific discussion. *Acute reactions* occur during treatment, are associated with cerebral oedema and can be controlled with corticosteroids. *Early delayed reactions* occur weeks to months after completion of radiotherapy and are characterized by somnolence and lethargy. This is associated with demyelination, endothelial damage, small-vessel thrombosis, accelerated atherosclerosis and long-term memory deficits. *Late delayed injuries* occur months to years after radiation, and are characterized by parenchymal necrosis. Patients may develop papilloedema, visual loss, hemiparesis, speech and language difficulties, seizures or dementia.[26] Despite these potential toxicities, radiation to the brain remains a cornerstone of treatment for central nervous system tumours and may provide the best option for long-term survival. The risk of cognitive changes must be balanced with the potential survival benefits.

In summary, radiation therapy can benefit older patients in both curative and palliative settings and should not be excluded from the management strategy based on the patient's age alone.

Systemic therapy

Systemic therapies include conventional cytotoxic chemotherapy, hormonal therapy, biological agents and targeted agents.

Conventional chemotherapy

Chemotherapy is generally administered intravenously, although in some cases it can be administered orally, intraperitoneally or intrathecally. Age is often considered a risk factor for toxicities and poor tolerance of chemotherapy. Indeed, the physiological changes of ageing may alter the pharmacokinetics of chemotherapeutic drugs. Mucosal changes, altered gastrointestinal motility and reduced intestinal blood flow may reduce the absorption of orally administered agents, such as capecitabine. The age-associated decrease in total body water, reduced plasma protein concentration and lower haemoglobin concentration decrease the volume of distribution of a number of chemotherapeutic agents, increasing the risk of toxicity. Declining renal function may lead to increased toxicity of chemotherapeutic agents that are excreted renally. Changes in hepatic metabolism of chemotherapy with age have not been well studied, but ageing may be associated with increased toxicity due to drugs metabolized by the liver.[27] Polypharmacy is an important consideration, as one-third of hospitalized senior adult cancer patients take at least nine medications,[28] increasing the risk for adverse drug–drug reactions.

Pharmacodynamic effects of chemotherapeutic agents also differ in the elderly, resulting in increased risk of certain toxicities. Older patients are at increased risk of myelosuppression from chemotherapy due to decreased haematopoietic stem cell reserve (see the section below on supportive care). The increased risk of mucositis may also be attributable to a reduced ability to respond to mucosal damage. Older patients receiving anthracyclines are at increased risk for developing cardiomyopathy, which may be mitigated by limiting the total dose of anthracyclines, administering the drug by continuous infusion, using dexrazoxane (which prevents the formation of free radicals) or substituting liposomal doxorubicin. Peripheral neuropathy complicates therapy with a number of classes of chemotherapeutic agents, but is potentially reversible if the clinician monitors for its development (heralded by paraesthesias) and discontinues the offending agent before functional impairment develops.

There is significant interest in utilizing geriatric assessments to predict tolerance of chemotherapy. Preliminary reports suggest that comorbidities, depression, poor performance status and dependence in ADLs predict the development of severe toxicities of chemotherapy. There are currently several ongoing prospective studies utilizing geriatric assessments to predict tolerance of chemotherapy, the development of severe toxicities, hospitalizations and the inability to complete a course of chemotherapy.

Hormonal therapy

A number of cancers prevalent in the elderly, including breast cancer and prostate cancer, are hormonally responsive. Medications aimed at blocking these hormonal pathways can result in prevention of recurrence or prolongation of survival.

The selective estrogen receptor modulator (SERM) tamoxifen reduces the risk of recurrence by 40% and the risk of breast cancer mortality by 31% after primary treatment of estrogen receptor positive (ER+) breast cancer. The same risks of SERMs outlined in the discussion of breast cancer prevention apply, although the potential benefit is greater in the adjuvant setting. One-quarter of women are incompletely adherent to their adjuvant hormonal regimen; older age and increasing numbers of comedications are independent risk factors for non-adherence. Also of importance in the efficacy of adjuvant hormonal therapy is hepatic metabolism and polypharmacy. Tamoxifen is transformed by cytochrome P450 2D6 into the more potent anti-estrogen endoxifen. Women who receive the potent 2D6 inhibitor paroxetine concomitantly with tamoxifen are at increased risk for death from breast cancer; the benefit of tamoxifen is reduced or negated by paroxetine, likely due to reduced metabolism of tamoxifen to the more active form.[29] This interaction is not seen with other selective serotonin reuptake inhibitors.

In post-menopausal women, the aromatase inhibitors letrozole, anastrazole and exemestane are the preferred anti-estrogen therapy. Aromatase inhibitors block the conversion of adrenal androgens to estrogens by the enzyme aromatase. Several studies have shown that aromatase inhibitors either in place of or subsequent to tamoxifen are superior to tamoxifen alone as adjuvant therapy. Both tamoxifen and the aromatase inhibitors are used as first-line therapy in women with ER+ metastatic breast cancer. The aromatase inhibitors cause arthralgias and increase the risk of osteoporosis.

Testosterone fuels prostate cancer growth; thus, androgen deprivation therapy is the cornerstone of first-line therapy for metastatic prostate cancer, although over time, prostate cancer will become insensitive to anti-androgen therapy. Surgical castration was historically utilized, though medical castration is now typically preferred. The gonadotropin-releasing hormone (GnRH) agonists leuprolide and goserelin initially cause the release of FSH and LH with an increase in serum testosterone, with subsequent suppression of gonadotropin secretion. This initial testosterone release may cause increased pain in bone metastases, urinary obstruction or spinal cord compression if already impending. This tumour flare can be prevented by the administration of an androgen receptor antagonist for 2 weeks prior to GnRH agonist initiation. The GnRH antagonist degarelix causes rapid suppression of testosterone levels, but its place in the treatment of prostate cancer remains to be determined. Androgen receptor antagonists (bicalutamide, flutamide or nilutamide) are added after failure of first-line androgen deprivation therapy. Common side effects of androgen deprivation therapy are hot flushes, erectile dysfunction, gynaecomastia and anaemia. Androgen deprivation therapy is associated with an increased risk of osteoporosis.

Biological agents

Biological agents, including interleukin-2 (IL-2) and interferon, have a limited role in selected cancers such as metastatic renal cell carcinoma and melanoma. Their use in the elderly is limited owing to their substantial toxicities. IL-2 is associated with a high likelihood of life-threatening toxicities and is generally reserved for younger patients with excellent functional status and limited comorbidities.

Targeted therapy

Over the past decade, a plethora of cancer therapeutics referred to as 'targeted therapies' have moved rapidly from preclinical development to clinical trial to clinical practice. These drugs, including monoclonal antibodies and small molecule inhibitors of tyrosine kinases, have capitalized on our growing understanding of the molecular mechanisms involved in specific malignancies. Targeting malignant cells holds the promise of less toxic treatments, which is particularly appealing in treating older patients with cancer.

Humanized monoclonal antibodies bind to cell surface receptors on the surface of the malignant cells and induce tumour cell death either by apoptosis, via antibody-dependent cytotoxicity, or through complement-mediated cytotoxicity. Infusion reactions are not uncommon with these agents and require appropriate premedication and observation.

Rituximab is a monoclonal antibody directed against the B-cell antigen CD20. A seminal trial of elderly patients (aged 60–80 years) with diffuse large B cell lymphoma randomized patients to standard combination therapy with cyclophosphamide, doxorubicin, vincristine and prednisone (CHOP) with or without rituximab. The addition of rituximab improved the complete response rate, event-free survival and overall survival with minimal additional toxicity.[30] Rituximab is now widely used in a number of B-cell malignancies, either as monotherapy in some low-grade lymphomas or in combination with chemotherapy.

Bevacizumab is a monoclonal antibody directed against vascular endothelial growth factor (VEGF). It is utilized in combination with chemotherapy in metastatic lung, breast and colorectal cancer. However, there are increasing concerns about toxicity with bevacizumab in older patients with comorbidities. In a randomized trial, patients over the age of 70 years who received bevacizumab in combination with chemotherapy for non-small cell lung cancer had a higher incidence of bleeding, neutropenia and proteinuria compared with both older patients who received chemotherapy alone and patients under the age of 70 years receiving the same therapy, without a significant benefit in response rates or survival.[31] A pooled analysis of randomized trials of patients receiving chemotherapy with or without bevacizumab for metastatic cancer of the breast, lung (non-small cell) or colon/rectum demonstrated a twofold increased risk for arterial thromboembolic events in patients receiving bevacizumab. Risk for arterial thrombotic events was associated with a prior history thromboembolic events and age over 65 years. Aspirin use was associated with an increased risk of bleeding events.[32] Although age alone should not exclude consideration of therapy with bevacizumab, careful attention to the patient's comorbid medical conditions and medications is warranted.

Cetuximab is a monoclonal antibody directed against the epidermal growth factor receptor, utilized in metastatic colorectal cancer and squamous cell carcinoma of the head and neck. Data specific to the elderly are sparse, but in a case series of patients over the age of 70 years with metastatic colorectal cancer, therapy with cetuximab was well tolerated, with toxicities and response to therapy commensurate with those reported in clinical trials.[33]

Trastuzumab is a monoclonal antibody against the HER-2 receptor, present in up to 20% of tumours in older women with breast cancer. In clinical trials, treatment with trastuzumab improved survival in women with HER-2+ breast cancers. A retrospective cohort study of women over the age of 70 years with HER-2 over-expressing tumours who received trastuzumab in combination with chemotherapy showed response rates and survival similar to those in clinical trials, without any increased risk of toxicity compared with clinical trial cohorts.[34] It was noted that 9% of women had a 10–20% decrease in ejection fraction on serial echocardiography. Although this decline did not necessitate discontinuation of therapy, it suggests that close monitoring of cardiac status is warranted in older women receiving trastuzumab.

Imatinib inhibits the tyrosine kinase encoded by the bcr-abl oncogene, and also the receptor tyrosine kinases encoded by the c-kit and platelet-derived growth factor receptor (PDGFR) oncogenes. Imatinib is used in the treatment of chronic myelogenous leukaemia (CML), Philadelphia chromosome-positive acute lymphoblastic leukaemia (Ph+ALL) and gastrointestinal stromal tumours (GISTs). Older patients receiving imatinib for chronic-phase CML are slightly more likely to experience haematological and dermatological toxicities, but are less likely to develop oedema or neurological side effects, in comparison with their younger counterparts. Efficacy is similar, although the time to response is slightly delayed in older individuals.[35] In elderly patients Ph+ALL, imatinib is as effective at inducing remission as conventional chemotherapy, but is markedly less toxic (see Chapter 33, Management of myelodysplastic syndromes and acute leukaemia).

Erlotinib is a small-molecule inhibitor of the epidermal growth factor receptor which is used in patients with non-small cell lung cancer who have progressed after conventional chemotherapy or in whom poor performance status contraindicates chemotherapy. In a phase 3 trial of erlotinib versus placebo, older patients enjoyed a similar benefit to younger patients concerning response and survival. However, this was at the expense of a more frequent severe toxicity, particularly rash, gastrointestinal side effects and fatigue.[36]

The tyrosine kinase inhibitor *sunitinib* is used in the treatment of advanced renal cell carcinoma and GIST. In an expanded access trial of sunitinib in advanced renal cell carcinoma, older patients experienced clinical benefit and survival similar to the entire cohort, with similar frequency of grade III–IV toxicities.[37]

Another multi kinase inhibitor, *sorafenib*, also appears to be safe and effective in older patients. Older patients with advanced renal cell carcinoma had similar response rates and similar rates of toxicities to younger patients and earlier trials.[38]

Lastly, *lapatinib* is an inhibitor of HER-1 and HER-2 indicated for the treatment of metastatic HER-2+ breast cancer. To date, no data on effectiveness or toxicity specifically in the elderly are available.

Supportive care

Senior adults receiving radiation or chemotherapy must receive aggressive supportive care to minimize the toxicities of therapy and adequately address symptoms directly related to their malignancy. Interventions that can decrease the risk of adverse events due to chemotherapy include haematopoietic growth factors, treatment of anaemia and prevention of mucositis.

Neutropenia frequently causes dose delays and dose reductions in older patients, which potentially reduces the chance of cure. Colony-stimulating factors (CSFs) or myelopoietic growth factors, including filgrastim and pegfilgrastim, decrease the incidence and duration of neutropenia and decrease the risk of neutopenic fever and hospitalization. Current recommendations include the use of CSFs for the primary prevention of febrile neutropenia when the risk of febrile neutropenia is greater than 20%. Patients at increased risk for febrile neutropenia due to age >65 years, poor performance status, poor nutritional status or serious comorbidities should receive primary prophylaxis with CSFs, even if the risk of febrile neutropenia is less than 20%.[39]

As several chemotherapeutic drugs are bound to haemoglobin in the circulation, anaemia can result in increased free fraction of cytotoxic drugs. Anaemia may also contribute to fatigue and decreased exercise tolerance. Erythropoiesis-stimulating agents (ESAs), including epoietin alfa and darbopoietin alfa, were initially embraced with enthusiasm to increase haemoglobin levels, reduce need for transfusions and improve fatigue in patients receiving chemotherapy. However, more recent data show that these agents may shorten the time to tumour progression, are associated with a 60% increase in relative risk of venous thromboembolism and are linked to a 10% increased risk of mortality [hazard ratio (HR), 1.10; 95% CI, 1.01–1.20].[40] As such, the US Food and Drug Administration (FDA) has indicated that ESAs should not be used in patients who are undergoing chemotherapy with curative intent. Current guidelines recommend discussion with the individual patient on the risks and benefits of therapy (see www.nccn.org).

In older adults, painful inflammation of the gastrointestinal tract mucosa (mucositis) is a potentially serious complication of chemotherapy. Chemotherapy drugs most commonly associated with oral mucositis include melphalan, cisplatin, 5-FU, methotrexate and cyclophosphamide. Oral mucositis impairs oral intake, causing dehydration and malnutrition. There are few effective interventions for the prevention of oral mucositis. Routine oral hygiene and bland mouth rinses, such as 0.9% saline or bicarbonate solutions, are recommended universally for the prevention and treatment of oral mucositis. Oral cryotherapy (holding ice chips in the mouth) is recommended during infusion for patients receiving stomatotoxic drugs in bolus form; it is hypothesized that vasoconstriction in the oral mucosa prevents delivery of the drug to the oral mucosa, decreasing the risk of oral mucositis.[41] Palifermin, a keratinocyte growth factor, has been approved for prevention of oral mucositis in patients undergoing stem cell transplantation, but it is not used in solid tumours. Amifostine is an organic thiophosphate approved for use in prevention of xerostomia after radiation therapy for head and neck cancer. Whether it prevents oral mucositis is controversial. The infusion can cause hypotension and it is recommended that all anti-hypertensive agents be held for 24 h prior to infusion, which may not be feasible in older adults with comorbidities. The treatment of oral mucositis includes management of xerostomia with sialogogues, management of pain with bland rinses, topical anaesthetics, systemic analgesics and prevention/treatment of superimposed infections, such as thrush.

Diarrhoea also puts patients at increased risk for dehydration; patients and their caregivers must be educated on adequate fluid intake and pre-emptive interventions. Since mucosal injury causes temporary lactase deficiency, milk products should be excluded from the diet for the duration of symptoms. Loperamide and diphenoxylate are both approved for chemotherapy-induced diarrhoea. Octreotide, the long-acting synthetic analogue of somatostatin, is reserved for patients whose diarrhoea does not respond to loperamide.

Remarkably, age over 65 years is *protective* against chemotherapy-induced nausea and vomiting. In addition, new classes of anti-emetics have dramatically reduced the incidence of chemotherapy-induced nausea. Prophylactic anti-emetics are administered with chemotherapeutic regimens having low, moderate or severe emetogenic potential. Routine prophylactic anti-emetics are not required for regimens classified as having minimal emetogenic potential.

The neurokinin (NK1) antagonist aprepitant is used as prophylaxis for highly emetogenic potential; it has no role in the treatment of breakthrough nausea and vomiting. The serotonin-5(HT)$_3$-receptor antagonists, including ondansetron, granisetron, dolasetron and palonosetron, are used in the prevention of acute nausea and vomiting, but have a limited role in the treatment of delayed nausea and vomiting. Drug interactions between these agents and the selective-serotonin reuptake inhibitors have been reported and clinicians should monitor for toxicities. In addition, constipation is a frequent side effect of drugs in this class. Although the mechanism is unknown, corticosteroids play an important role in the prevention of both acute and delayed nausea and vomiting. The dopamine (D)$_2$ receptor antagonists are widely used in both the prevention and treatment of chemotherapy-induced nausea and vomiting.[42] Extrapyramidal side effects are a dose-limiting toxicity of this class and one agent in this class, metoclopramide, has been associated with seizures in older patients with underlying seizure disorder. Benzodiazepines are commonly used for anxiolysis and prevention of anticipatory nausea and vomiting, but should be used with caution in the elderly.

Pain in older patients with cancer is frequently undertreated. Pain may be directly related to the underlying malignancy or may be chronic pain unrelated to the malignancy. Risk factors for failure to receive analgesics for daily pain include age over 75 years, minority race and impaired cognition. Management of pain in cancer patients should follow the World Health Organization Analgesic Ladder.[43] In patients for whom they are indicated, opioids are safe and effective, provided that they are initiated at a low dose and titrated slowly. Opioid-induced constipation should be universally anticipated and treated prophylactically.

The intravenous bisphosphonates pamidronate, zoledronic acid and ibandronate rapidly reduce serum calcium levels when used in treating hypercalcaemia of malignancy. They are also effective at reducing pain and the risk of skeletal-related events in patients with breast cancer metastatic to bone and in multiple myeloma. Caution should be used with the intravenous bisphosphonates when the creatinine clearance is $<30\,\text{ml}\,\text{min}^{-1}$ due to increased risk of nephrotoxicity.[44]

Multidisciplinary care models

Combining the disease-oriented approach of the medical oncologist and the patient-oriented approach of the geriatrician may improve the care of senior adults with cancer.[45] Many models for the delivery of geriatric oncology care exist. In an international panel of clinicians involved in the care of senior cancer patients, 20% reported access to a geriatrician and 34% reported that geriatric oncology was incorporated into general oncology. Among those who reported the presence of a dedicated geriatric oncology programme, 85% were located in oncology departments and 15% were located in geriatric departments. Comprehensive geriatric assessment was much more likely to be performed in institutions with a dedicated geriatric oncology programme than those without. Inpatient multidisciplinary teams usually included a medical oncologist, an advanced practice nurse, a social worker, physical therapists and, in about half of programmes, a geriatrician, nutritionist and pharmacist. Most outpatient multidisciplinary teams also included a surgical oncologist and radiation oncologist.[46]

Survivorship

With advances in cancer treatment, there are increasing numbers of older adult cancer survivors. Cancer survivors may experience long-term morbidity due to effects of the cancer itself or long-term sequelae of their therapy. Older adult cancer survivors are more likely to self-report their health as poor; they more likely to report comorbid medical conditions and functional limitations than their peers without a prior history of cancer.[47,48] In a cohort of older women followed prospectively, the prevalence of functional limitation was highest in women within 2 years of their diagnosis, but improved subsequently. Although the majority of 5-year cancer survivors in this cohort reported no functional limitations, they were more likely to report limitation in activities that required strength and mobility, such as heavy work, walking half a mile or walking up and down stairs, than their peers who had no history of cancer.[49] Studies differ on whether cancer survivors have an increased prevalence of psychological disorders.

Cognitive changes temporally associated with cancer treatment, colloquially known as 'chemobrain', are an area of debate. Early reports of selected younger women following adjuvant chemotherapy for breast cancer revealed an association between chemotherapy and impairments on neuropsychological testing, relative to population norms or controls.[50,51] However, these studies were potentially confounded by a number of factors, including depression and hormonal therapy. Although half of older women reported a subjective decline in their cognitive function 6 months after chemotherapy, prospective longitudinal studies have shown a decline in cognitive testing in only one-quarter of women at 6 months of follow-up.[52,53] Other studies showed no difference in change in neuropsychological testing between patients and controls over time.[54] A large population-based study of people over the age of 65 years showed no difference in the frequency of self-reported memory problems or positive screens for cognitive impairment between long-term cancer survivors and controls.[48] To date, an association between chemotherapy and functional decline due to cognitive impairment in senior adult cancer survivors has not been established. Brain radiotherapy for central nervous system tumours is clearly associated with cognitive decline; older patients are at particularly increased risk for brain atrophy and dementia following brain radiotherapy.[26] Cognitive sequelae of therapy will be an area of continued interest as the number of senior adult cancer survivors increases.

A history of receiving chemotherapy or radiation therapy increases the risk for additional medical problems. Certain chemotherapeutic agents, including the alkylating agents and topoisomerase II inhibitors, are associated with the development of myelodysplastic syndrome and acute myeloid leukaemia. Radiation increases the risk of bone and soft tissue sarcomas within the radiation field. Women who underwent mediastinal radiation for Hodgkin lymphoma are at increased risk for breast cancer. There is also an increased risk of coronary artery disease following mediastinal radiation in early adulthood. Physicians caring for long-term cancer survivor patients must be aware of potential long-term complications of their prior therapy, including second malignancies.

Conclusion

Cancer in the elderly is a growing problem. Older individuals are likely to be diagnosed at a more advanced stage and to receive substandard treatment for their cancer, although there is a growing body of literature showing that older adults may benefit from cancer treatment to the same degree as younger patients.

Biological changes associated with ageing are associated with increased risk of developing cancer. Strategies for prevention of cancer are promising, but most are not widely utilized due to potential risks of treatments. Decisions about screening for common cancers should be individualized, taking into account a patient's wishes, functional status, comorbidities and whether they would be eligible for treatment of a cancer detected during screening.

There is little reason why an older patient should be excluded from treatment of their cancer based on age alone. Again, decisions should be individualized based on a comprehensive assessment of the patient's health status. Geriatric assessments can predict which patients are at increased risk for postoperative morbidity and prolonged hospitalization following cancer surgery. Radiation therapy is well tolerated in elderly patients. Cytotoxic chemotherapy can be tolerated without difficulty in many older patients; results of studies using geriatric assessments to predict which patients are at increased risk for toxicities are eagerly awaited. Targeted therapies are emerging as acceptable, potentially less-toxic options for patients who are not candidates for conventional cytotoxic chemotherapy. Aggressive supportive care with attention to the toxicities most commonly seen in the elderly, such as myelosuppression, will allow older patients to receive treatments with fewer delays or dose reductions, which could otherwise reduce the effectiveness of treatment.

With improvements in survival, there is a burgeoning population of older adult cancer survivors. Some of these patients will have residual functional limitations or cognitive decline following completion of their treatment. Treatments may leave patients at increased risk for secondary malignancies or the development of secondary comorbidities over time.

Multidisciplinary care with the collaboration of geriatricians, medical oncologists, radiation oncologists, surgical oncologists, pharmacists, social workers, nurses and physical and occupational therapists may optimize the treatment of elderly cancer patients.

Key points

- With the growth of the aged segment of the population and the increased incidence of cancer in the elderly, the problem of cancer in the elderly is growing. The historical undertreatment of older adults with cancer must be re-examined, as many older patients with cancer can be safely treated with meaningful prolongation of survival.
- Decisions to pursue cancer screening in the elderly must be individualized based on the patient's life expectancy, functional status, comorbidities and preferences.
- Advanced age is, in general, not a primary consideration for determining surgical risk. Geriatric assessment predicts which older patients are at increased risk for postoperative morbidity. Radiation is well tolerated in older patients and improved techniques further minimize toxicity by sparing normal tissue.
- The decision to utilize systemic cytotoxic chemotherapy depends on the patient's preferences, functional status, comorbidities and goals of therapy. Haematopoietic growth factors decrease the risk of complications associated with neutropenia. Targeted therapies may offer less-toxic treatment options. Polypharmacy must be monitored, as comedications may decrease the efficacy of the anti-cancer treatment, as has been shown with paroxetine and tamoxifen.
- Senior cancer survivors may have unique challenges following therapy and be at increased risk for complications ranging from osteoporosis to dementia to treatment-related acute leukaemia.

References

1. Jemal A, Siegel R, Ward E *et al*. Cancer statistics, 2009. *CA Cancer J Clin* 2009;**59**:225–49.
2. Yancik R and Ries LA. Cancer in older persons: an international issue in an aging world. *Semin Oncol* 2004;**31**:128–36.
3. Wingo PA, Cardinez CJ, Landis SH *et al*. Long-term trends in cancer mortality in the United States, 1930–1998. *Cancer* 2003;**97**(12 Suppl): 3133–275.
4. Bouchardy C, Rapiti E, Fioretta G *et al*. Undertreatment strongly decreases prognosis of breast cancer in elderly women. *J Clin Oncol* 2003;**21**:3580–7.
5. Hanahan D and Weinberg RA. The hallmarks of cancer. *Cell* 2000;**100**:57–70.
6. Denduluri N and Ershler WB. Aging biology and cancer. *Semin Oncol* 2004;**31**:137–48.
7. Irminger-Finger I. Science of cancer and aging. *J Clin Oncol* 2007;**25**:1844–51.
8. Hornsby PJ. Senescence as an anticancer mechanism. *J Clin Oncol* 2007;**25**:1852–7.
9. Eliassen AH, Colditz GA, Rosner B *et al*. Adult weight change and risk of postmenopausal breast cancer. *JAMA* 2006;**296**:193–201.
10. Prentice RL, Caan B, Chlebowski RT *et al*. Low-fat dietary pattern and risk of invasive breast cancer: the Women's Health Initiative Randomized Controlled Dietary Modification Trial. *JAMA* 2006;**295**:629–42.
11. Beresford SA, Johnson KC, Ritenbaugh C *et al*. Low-fat dietary pattern and risk of colorectal cancer: the Women's Health Initiative Randomized Controlled Dietary Modification Trial. *JAMA* 2006;**295**:643–54.
12. Wactawski-Wende J, Kotchen JM, Anderson GL *et al*. Calcium plus vitamin D supplementation and the risk of colorectal cancer. *N Engl J Med* 2006;**354**:684–96.
13. Flossmann E and Rothwell PM. Effect of aspirin on long-term risk of colorectal cancer: consistent evidence from randomised and observational studies. *Lancet* 2007;**369**:1603–13.
14. Half E and Arber N. Colon cancer: preventive agents and the present status of chemoprevention. *Expert Opin Pharmacother* 2009;**10**:211–9.
15. Fisher B, Costantino JP, Wickerham DL *et al*. Tamoxifen for the prevention of breast cancer: current status of the National Surgical Adjuvant Breast and Bowel Project P-1 study. *J Natl Cancer Inst* 2005;**97**:1652–62.
16. Gail MH, Costantino JP, Bryant J *et al*. Weighing the risks and benefits of tamoxifen treatment for preventing breast cancer. *J Natl Cancer Inst* 1999;**91**:1829–46.
17. Martino S, Cauley JA, Barrett-Connor E *et al*. Continuing outcomes relevant to Evista: breast cancer incidence in postmenopausal osteoporotic women in a randomized trial of raloxifene. *J Natl Cancer Inst* 2004;**96**:1751–61.
18. Vogel VG, Costantino JP, Wickerham DL *et al*. Effects of tamoxifen vs raloxifene on the risk of developing invasive breast cancer and other disease outcomes: the NSABP Study of Tamoxifen and Raloxifene (STAR) P-2 trial. *JAMA* 2006;**295**:2727–41.
19. Walter LC, Lewis CL and Barton MB. Screening for colorectal, breast and cervical cancer in the elderly: a review of the evidence. *Am J Med* 2005;**118**:1078–86.
20. Kim DH, Pickhardt PJ, Hanson ME and Hinshaw JL. CT colonography: performance and program outcome measures in an older screening population. *Radiology* 2010; **254**:493–500.
21. Heinzer H and Steuber T. Prostate cancer in the elderly. *Urol Oncol* 2009;**27**:668–72.
22. Audisio RA, Bozzetti F, Gennari R *et al*. The surgical management of elderly cancer patients; recommendations of the SIOG surgical task force. *Eur J Cancer* 2004;**40**:926–38.
23. Audisio RA, Pope D, Ramesh HS *et al*. Shall we operate? Preoperative assessment in elderly cancer patients (PACE) can help. A SIOG surgical task force prospective study. *Crit Rev Oncol Hematol* 2008;**65**:156–63.
24. Horiot JC. Radiation therapy and the geriatric oncology patient. *J Clin Oncol* 2007;**25**:1930–5.
25. Redmond KJ and Song DY. Thoracic irradiation in the elderly. *Thorac Surg Clin* 2009;**19**:391–400.
26. Grau JJ, Verger E, Brandes AA *et al*. Radiotherapy of the brain in elderly patients. *Eur J Cancer* 2000;**36**:443–52.
27. Monfardini S. Prescribing anti-cancer drugs in elderly cancer patients. *Eur J Cancer* 2002;**38**:2341–6.
28. Flood KL, Carroll MB, Le CV and Brown CJ. Polypharmacy in hospitalized older adult cancer patients: experience from a prospective, observational study of an oncology-acute care for elders unit. *Am J Geriatr Pharmacother* 2009;**7**:151–8.
29. Kelly CM, Juurlink DN, Gomes T *et al*. Selective serotonin reuptake inhibitors and breast cancer mortality in women receiving tamoxifen: a population based cohort study. *BMJ* 2010;**340**: c693.
30. Coiffier B, Lepage E, Briere J *et al*. CHOP chemotherapy plus rituximab compared with CHOP alone in elderly patients with diffuse large-B-cell lymphoma. *N Engl J Med* 2002;**346**:235–42.
31. Ramalingam SS, Dahlberg SE, Langer CJ *et al*. Outcomes for elderly, advanced-stage non small-cell lung cancer patients treated with bevacizumab in combination with carboplatin and paclitaxel: analysis of Eastern Cooperative Oncology Group Trial 4599. *J Clin Oncol* 2008;**26**:60–5.
32. Scappaticci FA, Skillings JR, Holden SN *et al*. Arterial thromboembolic events in patients with metastatic carcinoma treated with chemotherapy and bevacizumab. *J Natl Cancer Inst* 2007;**99**:1232–9.
33. Bouchahda M, Macarulla T, Spano JP *et al*. Cetuximab efficacy and safety in a retrospective cohort of elderly patients with heavily pretreated metastatic colorectal cancer. *Crit Rev Oncol Hematol* 2008;**67**:255–62.
34. Brunello A, Monfardini S, Crivellari D *et al*. Multicenter analysis of activity and safety of trastuzumab plus chemotherapy in advanced breast cancer in elderly women (≥70 years). *J Clin Oncol* 2008;**26**(15S): 1096.
35. Pletsch N, Lauseker M, Saussele S *et al*. Therapy with imatinib in elderly CML patients (≥65 years) is well tolerated by cytogenetic and molecular remissions seem to be achieved later compared to younger patients. *Haematologica* 2009;**94**(Suppl.2): 253 abs. 0625.
36. Wheatley-Price P, Ding K, Seymour L *et al*. Erlotinib for advanced non-small-cell lung cancer in the elderly: an analysis of the National Cancer Institute of Canada Clinical Trials Group Study BR.21. *J Clin Oncol* 2008;**26**:2350–7.

37. Gore ME, Szczylik C, Porta C *et al*. Safety and efficacy of sunitinib for metastatic renal-cell carcinoma: an expanded-access trial. *Lancet Oncol* 2009;**10**:757–63.
38. Bukowski RM, Stadler WM, Figlin RA *et al*. Safety and efficacy of sorafenib in elderly patients (pts) ≥65 years: a subset analysis from the Advanced Renal Cell Carcinoma Sorafenib (ARCCS) Expanded Access Program in North America. *J Clin Oncol* 2008;**26**(15S): 5045.
39. Smith TJ, Khatcheressian J, Lyman GH *et al*. 2006 update of recommendations for the use of white blood cell growth factors: an evidence-based clinical practice guideline. *J Clin Oncol* 2006;**24**:3187–205.
40. Bennett CL, Silver SM, Djulbegovic B *et al*. Venous thromboembolism and mortality associated with recombinant erythropoietin and darbepoetin administration for the treatment of cancer-associated anemia. *JAMA* 2008;**299**:914–24.
41. Bensinger W, Schubert M, Ang KK *et al*. NCCN Task Force Report. Prevention and management of mucositis in cancer care. *J Natl Compr Canc Netw* 2008;**6**(Suppl 1): S1–21; quiz S2–4.
42. Jakobsen JN and Herrstedt J. Prevention of chemotherapy-induced nausea and vomiting in elderly cancer patients. *Crit Rev Oncol Hematol* 2009;**71**:214–21.
43. Pergolizzi J, Boger RH, Budd K *et al*. Opioids and the management of chronic severe pain in the elderly: consensus statement of an International Expert Panel with focus on the six clinically most often used World Health Organization Step III opioids (buprenorphine, fentanyl, hydromorphone, methadone, morphine, oxycodone). *Pain Pract* 2008;**8**:287–313.
44. Body JJ, Coleman R, Clezardin P *et al*. International Society of Geriatric Oncology (SIOG) clinical practice recommendations for the use of bisphosphonates in elderly patients. *Eur J Cancer* 2007;**43**:852–8.
45. Terret C, Zulian GB, Naiem A and Albrand G. Multidisciplinary approach to the geriatric oncology patient. *J Clin Oncol* 2007;**25**:1876–81.
46. Monfardini S, Aapro MS, Bennett JM *et al*. Organization of the clinical activity of geriatric oncology: report of a SIOG (International Society of Geriatric Oncology) task force. *Crit Rev Oncol Hematol* 2007;**62**:62–73.
47. Hewitt M, Rowland JH and Yancik R. Cancer survivors in the United States: age, health and disability. *J Gerontol A Biol Sci Med Sci* 2003;**58**:82–91.
48. Keating NL, Norredam M, Landrum MB *et al*. Physical and mental health status of older long-term cancer survivors. *J Am Geriatr Soc* 2005;**53**:2145–52.
49. Sweeney C, Schmitz KH, Lazovich D *et al*. Functional limitations in elderly female cancer survivors. *J Natl Cancer Inst* 2006;**98**:521–9.
50. Wieneke MH and Dienst ER. Neuropsychological assessment of cognitive functioning following chemotherapy for breast cancer. *Psycho-Oncology* 1995;**4**:61–6.
51. van Dam FS, Schagen SB, Muller MJ *et al*. Impairment of cognitive function in women receiving adjuvant treatment for high-risk breast cancer: high-dose versus standard-dose chemotherapy. *J Natl Cancer Inst* 1998;**90**:210–8.
52. Hurria A, Goldfarb S, Rosen C *et al*. Effect of adjuvant breast cancer chemotherapy on cognitive function from the older patient's perspective. *Breast Cancer Res Treat* 2006;**98**:343–8.
53. Hurria A, Rosen C, Hudis C *et al*. Cognitive function of older patients receiving adjuvant chemotherapy for breast cancer: a pilot prospective longitudinal study. *J Am Geriatr Soc* 2006;**54**:925–31.
54. Jenkins V, Shilling V, Deutsch G *et al*. A 3-year prospective study of the effects of adjuvant treatments on cognition in women with early stage breast cancer. *Br J Cancer* 2006;**94**:828–34.
55. U.S. Preventive Services Task Force. *USPSTF Guidelines*, http://www.ahrq.gov/clinic/uspstfix.htm, 2010; last accessed 18 February 2010.
56. Smith RA, Cokkinides V and Brawley OW. Cancer screening in the United States, 2009: a review of current American Cancer Society guidelines and issues in cancer screening. *CA Cancer J Clin* 2009;**59**:27–41.
57. U.S. Preventive Services Task Force. Colon cancer screening (USPSTF recommendation). *J Am Geriatr Soc* 2000;**48**:333–5.
58. American Geriatrics Society Clinical Practice Committee. Breast cancer screening in older women. *J Am Geriatr Soc* 2000;**48**:842–4.
59. American Geriatrics Society. Screening for cervical carcinoma in older women. *J Am Geriatr Soc* 2001;**49**:655–7.

CHAPTER 109

Oncological emergencies

Chantal Bernard-Marty[1], Clement Gaudin[2], Stephane Gerard[2] and Laurent Balardy[2]
[1]Institut Claudius Regaud, Toulouse, France
[2]Gérontopôle, CHU Toulouse, Toulouse, France

Introduction

Most cancer patients experience at least one emergency during the course of the disease. An ageing population is resulting in more people being diagnosed with cancer and an increasing number of treatment options means that many patients live significantly longer with their disease. It is anticipated, therefore, that an increasing number of patients will present to primary and secondary care with acute complications of cancer or the treatment thereof. Physicians should be familiar with oncological emergencies as failure to implement immediate and appropriate treatment may result in significant morbidity or death. This chapter focuses on the common and critical complications of cancer (Table 109.1) in older adults.

Haematological emergencies

Haematological emergencies include febrile neutropenia, thrombocytopenia, intravascular disseminated coagulation and hyperviscosity syndrome.

Febrile neutropenia

Neutropenia is usually defined as an absolute neutrophil count (ANC) of $<500 \times 10^9$ cells l^{-1}. Fever in neutropenic patients is usually defined as a single temperature of >38.3 °C (101 °F) or a sustained temperature >38 °C (100.4 °F) for more than 1 h. However, absence of fever in neutropenic patients does not mean absence of infection, for example,. in the case of corticosteroid use or in elderly patients. A thorough general physical examination should be performed and repeated to identify the infection source: in the absence of neutrophils, signs of inflammation can be extremely subtle, and hypothermia, hypotension or clinical deterioration should be recognized as the initial signs of occult infection. Identified risk factors for occult infection include severe neutropenia, rapid decline in ANC, prolonged duration of neutropenia (>7–10 days), cancer not in remission and comorbid illnesses requiring hospitalization.[1] Approximately 80% of identified infections are believed to arise from patients' own endogenous flora.

Broad-spectrum antibiotics should be given as soon as possible and at full doses (adjusted for renal and/or hepatic function), to avoid the 70% mortality related to the delay of initiation of antibiotics.

Initial antibiotic selection should be guided by the patient's history, allergies, symptoms, signs, recent antibiotic use and culture data and awareness of institutional nosocomial infection pattern. There is no clear optimal choice for empirical antibiotic therapy.[2] Combination therapy and monotherapy (cefepime, ceftazidime) have led to similar outcomes. In critically ill patients, an aminoglycoside should be added for better Gram-negative coverage or a fluoroquinolone or aztreonam when renal function is a cause for concern. (Table 109.2).

In certain circumstances, a drug active against Gram-positive bacteria is recommended. Such circumstances include known colonization with Gram-positive bacteria, suspected infection of a central venous line or device and severe sepsis with or without hypotension. Gram-positive bacteria should also be considered in patients with suspected skin infection or severe mucosal damage and when prophylactic antibiotics against Gram-negative bacteria have been used.[3]

In the case of persistent fever after 5 days without an identifiable source, the following options are valuable:

- Continuing treatment with the initial antibiotic(s) if the patient is clinically stable and the neutropenia is expected to resolve within the ensuing 5 days.
- Changing or adding antibiotic(s) if there is evidence of progressive disease or a new complication (onset of abdominal pain due to enterocolitis, pulmonary infiltrates or drug toxicity).

Principles and Practice of Geriatric Medicine, Fifth Edition. Edited by Alan J. Sinclair, John E. Morley and Bruno Vellas.

Table 109.1 Summary of oncological emergencies.

Emergency	Cause	Clinical findings
Haematological		
Febrile neutropenia	Chemotherapy-associated bacterial or fungal infections	Temperature $>101\,^{\circ}$F ($38.3\,^{\circ}$C), absolute neutrophil count $<500\,\text{mm}^{-3}$ ($0.5 \times 10^{9}\ \text{l}^{-1}$)
Thrombocytopenia	Chemotherapy-induced toxicity, disseminated intravascular coagulation, bone metastasis	Bleeding, platelet count $<150 \times 10^{9}$
Disseminated intravascular coagulation	Metastatic disease	Thrombotic events, Trousseau syndrome, diffuse bleeding
Hyperviscosity syndrome	Waldenström macroglobulinaemia, myeloma, leukaemia	Spontaneous bleeding, retinal haemorrhage, neurological defects, Raynaud syndrome, congestive heart failure, serum viscosity levels >5
Metabolic		
Hypercalcaemia	Lung, breast, prostate and renal cancer, myeloma	Apathy, malaise, weakness, confusion, polyuria–polydipsia, evolving anorexia with nausea plus constipation, renal failure, coma, ECG modifications
Syndrome of inappropriate antidiuretic hormone	Lung cancer	Anorexia, nausea, vomiting, constipation, muscle weakness, myalgia, polyuria-polydipsia, severe neurological symptoms (e.g. seizures, coma)
Tumour lysis syndrome	Haematological malignancies, small-cell lung cancer	Azotaemia, acidosis, hyperphosphataemia, hyperkalaemia, acute renal failure, hypocalcaemia
Neurological		
Spinal cord compression	Breast, lung, renal and prostate cancers and myeloma	New back pain that worsens when lying down, late paraplegia, late incontinence and loss of sensory function
Delirium	Drugs, infection, anaemia, dehydration, surgery, pain	Impairment of consciousness, cognitive impairment of acute onset, disorientation, disturbance of the sleep–wake cycle, illusions, hallucinations
Brain metastases and increased intracranial pressure	Lung cancer, breast cancer, melanoma	Symptoms can be focal or generalized and depend on the location of the lesion within the brain (headaches, seizures, hemiparesis, cognitive disturbance, ataxia)
Cardiologic		
Superior vena cava syndrome	Lung cancer, metastatic mediastinal tumours, lymphoma, indwelling venous catheters	Cough, dyspnoea, dysphagia, head, neck or upper extremity swelling or discoloration, development of collateral venous circulation
Pericardial effusion	Metastatic lung and breast cancer, leukaemia, lymphoma	Dyspnoea, fatigue, distended neck veins, distant heart sounds, tachycardia, orthopnoea, narrow pulse pressure, pulsus paradoxus, water-bottle heart
Structural		
Airway obstruction	All the malignancy from the base of the tongue to the terminal bronchiole	Dyspnoea, stridor (extrathoracic obstruction), wheezing, sudden respiratory distress

Table 109.1 (*continued*).

Emergency	Cause	Clinical findings
Bowel obstruction	Abdominal and gynaecological tumour, mesenteric metastasis	Abdominal pain and distension, vomiting, lack of intestinal emissions
Urinary obstruction	Urinary and gastrointestinal tract cancer, mesenteric metastasis	Flank pain and tenderness, nausea/vomiting, fever, chills, haematuria and oliguria/anuria
Pathological fractures	Breast, lung, prostate, myeloma, thyroid	Bone pain

Table 109.2 Initial antibiotic therapy of neutropenic fever.

Type of therapy	Treatment[a]
Monotherapy	Cefepime Ceftazidime Carbapenem Piperacillin/tazobactam
Combination	Aminoglycoside (or quinolone) + one of the following drugs: Piperacillin Cefepime Ceftazidime Carbapenem

[a]In certain circumstances (e.g. suspected infection of a central venous line or device, skin infection, severe mucosal damage), a drug active against Gram-positive bacteria is recommended. Vancomycin is also the most commonly used drug for suspected infections with Gram-positive bacteria. Reproduced with permission from Halfdanarson *et al.*[3]

- Adding an antifungal drug, with or without changing the antibiotics, if the neutropenia is expected to persist for more than 5–7 days.

If an infectious source of fever is identified, antibiotics should be continued for at least the standard duration (e.g. 14 days for bacteraemia). With no known source, the timing of the discontinuation of antibiotics is usually dependent on resolution of fever and neutropenia. If the ANC increases to $>500 \times 10^9$ cells l^{-1} and the patient becomes afebrile, antibiotics are usually administered for 7 days.

In older patients, primary prophylactic colony-stimulating factor was observed to be effective in reducing the incidence of neutropenia and infection.[4]

Thrombocytopenia

Thrombocytopenia (platelet count $<150 \times 10^9\,l^{-1}$) is mainly a consequence of myelotoxicity induced by chemotherapy[5] or less frequently by radiotherapy, and rarely a sign of disseminated intravascular coagulation. In addition, certain malignant conditions are associated with immune-mediated thrombocytopenia. Multiple causes of thrombocytopenia may coexist in a given patient.

In the case of chemotherapy, neutropenia almost invariably accompanies the low platelet count. If the degree of thrombocytopenia occurs more rapidly or is more severe or more prolonged than anticipated, then a second mechanism should be suspected. The presence of bone marrow metastases should be suspected if anaemia or thrombocytopenia are observed prior to treatment or if chemotherapy induces a sudden or excessive fall in the haemoglobin or platelet count. Immune-mediated destruction of platelets is commonly seen with lymphoid malignancies. As a general rule, patients with autoimmune thrombocytopenia experience less bleeding for a given platelet count compared with patients with chemotherapy-induced thrombocytopenia or other mechanisms of bone marrow failure.

If there is no obvious relationship between platelet count and administration of chemotherapy, a bone marrow aspirate and trephine examination may be indicated. In immune-mediated thrombocytopenia, plentiful megakaryocytes are expected since platelet destruction occurs in the peripheral circulation. If bone marrow metastasis is the primary mechanism of thrombocytopenia, the bone marrow trephine is the most sensitive diagnostic tool.

Patients who have a platelet count of above $10 \times 10^9\,l^{-1}$ with absence of bleeding may be managed conservatively, provided that they have a full daily clinical examination including fundal examination. In the absence of bleeding and of evidence of sepsis or coagulopathy, then observation is adequate.

Platelet counts below $10 \times 10^9\,l^{-1}$ or bleeding need random donor platelets. It should be remembered that the key end point is to arrest the bleeding, and this may occur without a significant platelet rise. However, failure to obtain the expected platelet rise after two consecutive transfusions (platelet refractoriness) may be due to conditions that cause increased platelet consumption (e.g. fever, splenomegaly) or may be related to human leukocyte antigen (HLA) alloimmunization from previous transfusions or pregnancies.

Disseminated intravascular coagulation

Disseminated intravascular coagulation (DIC) is a clinical syndrome characterized by systemic activation of coagulation leading to intravascular deposition of fibrin and thrombosis of small vessels. Depletion of natural anticoagulants such as protein C and antithrombin and suppression of fibrinolysis also add to the prothrombotic state. In addition, there may be consumption of multiple coagulation factors and platelets leading to bleeding. The delicate balance between factors that promote thrombosis and factors that lead to bleeding will determine the clinical presentation of the patient.

Clinical evidence of DIC is seen in 10–15% of patients with metastatic cancer and laboratory markers are found in 50–70% of patients (increased levels of fibrinogen, fibrin degradation products and coagulation factors V, VIII, IX and XI).

There is no single diagnostic test for DIC. The presence of a prolonged prothrombin time (PT) and activated partial thromboplastin time (APTT) with elevated levels of D-dimers and a low or low-normal fibrinogen in a clinical setting known to be associated with DIC will confirm the diagnosis in a bleeding patient. A blood film may show fragmented red blood cells. Patients with thrombosis may have a shortened PT and APTT, a high or high-normal fibrinogen and elevated D-dimers. All features may not be present in every patient. Serial tests are required to monitor progression of the condition and response to therapy and to direct further treatment.

The essence of action is supportive care.[6] Removal of the underlying precipitant is advised. Therefore, the tumour should be treated where possible and concomitant sepsis should be managed aggressively. Random donor platelets should be given until the platelet count is $>20 \times 10^9\,l^{-1}$ or until bleeding has stopped. If bleeding is life-threatening, then the platelet count should be raise to $50 \times 10^9\,l^{-1}$. Fresh frozen plasma (FFP) containing all coagulation factors including fibrinogen and von Willebrand's factor is indicated for bleeding with a prolonged PT and APTT.

Hyperviscosity syndrome

Hyperviscosity is defined as an increased intrinsic resistance of fluid to flow. Marked elevations in paraproteins, marked leukocytosis or erythrocytosis in some cancer patients can result in elevated serum viscosity and the development of significant sludging, decreased perfusion of the microcirculation and vascular stasis with the development of the hyperviscosity syndrome. Common causes of the hyperviscosity syndrome include Waldenstrom macroglobulinaemia, multiple myeloma and leukaemias. Clinical manifestations of the hyperviscosity syndrome, most apparent with a serum viscosity >5 (the relative viscosity of normal serum ranges between 1.4 and 1.8), include a triad of bleeding, visual disturbances and neurological manifestations (Table 109.1). Management of hyperviscosity should aim at urgent reduction of serum viscosity in symptomatic patients by leukopheresis or plasmapheresis. This should be followed by specific chemotherapeutic agents to treat the underlying disease after relief of symptoms. Temporary measures should focus on adequate rehydration and, in patients with coma and established dysproteinaemia, a two-unit phlebotomy with replacement of the patient's red blood cells with physiological saline should be performed.

Metabolic emergencies

Metabolic emergencies include hypercalcaemia, hyponatraemia and tumour lysis syndrome.

Hypercalcaemia

Tumour-induced hypercalcaemia, the most common metabolic emergency in patients with cancer, is due to skeletal metastases or to a paraneoplastic syndrome related to parathyroid hormone-related protein. Hypercalcaemia has been reported in 10–30% of patients with cancer at some time during their disease.[7]

The symptoms of hypercalcaemia are multiple and nonspecific. Classic symptoms include lethargy, confusion, anorexia, nausea, constipation, polyuria and polydipsia (Table 109.1).

Symptoms vary depending on the degree of hypercalcaemia and the rapidity of onset.[8] Changes in mental faculties and strength are more easily recognized in younger individuals, whereas in the elderly such events can be easily blamed on many things, including their poor tolerance of analgesics, anxiolytics, hypnotics and antiemetics.

The definition of hypercalcaemia is an elevation of calcium level above $2.64\,mmol\,l^{-1}$ ($10.6\,mg\,dl^{-1}$) and values above $2.74\,mmol\,l^{-1}$ ($11.0\,mg\,dl^{-1}$) should be considered an indication to initiate treatment. This threshold should be considered (according to the range of normal values from a local laboratory) only in the case of a normal albumin level. If there is any doubt about the validity of the total serum calcium level, measurement of ionized calcium or calculation of the adjusted calcium level to albumin concentrations is essential.

Asymptomatic patients with minimally elevated calcium levels ($<3\,mmol\,l^{-1}$) may be treated as outpatients with encouragement to adopt oral hydration, mobilization and elimination of drugs that contribute to hypercalcaemia (thiazides, lithium). Patients who are symptomatic or have calcium levels $>3\,mmol\,l^{-1}$ should be considered for inpatient management using volume expansion with saline infusion, corticosteroids and bisphosphonates, as follows:

- Rehydration generally has mild and transient effects on calcium levels. The volume of saline infusion depends on the extent of the hypovolaemia and also the patient's cardiac and renal function.

• Bisphosphonates[9] have supplanted all other drugs except calcitonin, still useful in the few cases of severe refractory hypercalcaemia because of its rapid onset of action (2–4 h versus 72 h for bisphosphonates). The recommended dose is 90 mg i.v. over 2–4 h for pamidronate or 4 mg i.v. over 15 min for zoledronate. In patients with pre-existing renal disease, no change in dosage, infusion time or interval is required.
• Glucocorticosteroids can be helpful in the management of hypercalcaemia caused by lymphoma, myeloma and sometimes breast cancer and may be of some value in other malignancies, used at doses of 10–100 mg per day equivalent prednisone.

Hyponatraemia

Serum sodium levels below 135 mmol l^{-1} (135 mequiv l^{-1}), especially with rapid fall, can lead to brain oedema with altered mental status, lethargy, seizures, coma and death. Routine evaluation of serum electrolytes is mandatory in patients with otherwise unexplained alterations of mental status.

Aetiologies are iatrogenic complication[10] (vasopressin, chlorpropamide, carbamazepine, clofibrate, vincristine, ifosfamide and narcotics), water redistribution associated with mannitol infusions, pseudo-hyponatraemia due to hyper-para-proteinaemia or hyperlipidaemia and acute water intoxication, renal sodium loss due to diuretic therapy, extra-renal sodium loss during vomiting/diarrhoea, sudden withdrawal of glucocorticoid therapy and syndrome of inappropriate antidiuretic hormone (SIADH).[11]

SIADH can cause a severe decrease in sodium that may be life-threatening. Diagnostic features include hypo-osmolality of serum, inappropriately high osmolality of urine for the concomitant plasma hypo-osmolality, continued renal excretion of sodium (Table 109.3), associated with clinical normovolaemia, and normal renal, adrenal and thyroid function.

SIADH is a paraneoplastic condition associated with small-cell carcinoma of the lung, central nervous system disease (e.g. metastases, infection and haemorrhage) and pulmonary disorders (e.g., metastases, infection).

Table 109.3 Diagnostic criteria of syndrome of inappropriate antidiuretic hormone (SIADH).

Criterion	Definition
Hyponatraemia	Plasma sodium <135 mequiv l^{-1}
Hypo-osmotic plasma	Plasma osmolality <280 mOsm kg^{-1}
Hyperosmotic urine	Urinary osmolality >500 mOsm kg^{-1}
Hypernatraemic urine	Urinary sodium >20 mequiv l^{-1}

Symptoms depend on the depth and the rate of development. However, elderly patients are more susceptible and may manifest cognitive impairment with less deep hyponatraemia. However, in elderly patients it is difficult to distinguish the hyponatraemia due to SIADH from other causes which are multiple.

The major focus of treatment for SIADH is successful treatment of the underlying disease by chemotherapy and/or radiotherapy. Acute treatment is indicated in patients who have severe hyponatraemia (e.g. plasma sodium <125 mequiv l^{-1}) and who are symptomatic. The goals of therapy are to initiate and maintain rapid diuresis with i.v. furosemide, while restricting the 'free water' intake to 500–1000 ml per day and to replace the sodium and potassium lost in the urine by administering 0.9% saline infusions with added potassium. This rapid correction should not exceed a 20 equiv l^{-1} rise in serum sodium concentration during the first 48 h (1 mequiv l^{-1} h^{-1}) to avoid neurological damage and central pontine myelinolysis.

Tumour lysis syndrome

Tumour lysis syndrome is the set of metabolic abnormalities that results from acute destruction of neoplastic cells and release of their intracellular products into the circulation.[12] The high rate of cell turnover overwhelms the body's normal homeostatic mechanisms for handling potassium, calcium, phosphorus and uric acid, leading to hyperuricaemia, hyperkalaemia, hyperphosphataemia, hypocalcaemia and uraemia. These may be seen alone or in combination with one another.

Also, the release of intracellular purines from fragmented tumour nuclei increases serum uric acid. Uric acid, with a pH of 5.4, exists in a soluble form at physiological pH. However, in the acidic environment of the kidney collecting ducts, uric acid may crystallize in the collecting ducts and ureters. This may lead to an obstructive nephropathy and subsequent renal failure. In addition, purine precursors including adenosine triphosphate, adenosine diphosphate and adenosine regulate vascular tone. With elevation of angiotensin II, adenosine may lead to preglomerular vasoconstriction and postglomerular vasodilatation with a resultant reduction in filtration and renal failure. The risk of renal failure may be increased in the setting of renal parenchymal tumour infiltration or ureteral or venous obstruction from tumour compression. Hyperkalaemia associated with tumour lysis syndrome may be accentuated by associated renal insufficiency and may cause electrocardiographic alterations and potentially fatal cardiac arrhythmia. The major manifestation of hyperphosphataemia is secondary hypocalcaemia caused by precipitation of calcium phosphate in the soft tissues, which may present as renal failure, pruritic or gangrenous changes in the skin or inflammation of the eyes or joints. Signs and symptoms of hypocalcaemia include anorexia, vomiting, cramps, carpopedal spasms, tetany, seizures, alterations in consciousness, cardiac dysrhythmia and occasionally cardiac arrest.

The syndrome is commonly iatrogenic, caused by administration of therapy during the rapid growth phase of aggressive malignancies (high-grade lymphomas, leukaemia patients with high leukocyte counts, less frequently solid tumours).

Patients at risk are men with advanced disease, markedly elevated lactate dehydrogenase level with predisposing factors including volume depletion, concentrated acidic urine pH and excessive urinary uric acid excretion rates.

The diagnosis is based on the development of increased levels of serum uric acid, phosphorus and potassium, decreased levels of serum calcium and oliguric renal failure following chemotherapy.

The incidence of tumour lysis syndrome is rare, due to the use of prophylactic measures in patients at risk: adequate hydration, urine alkalinization, use of allopurinol started 24–48 h before initiation of cytotoxic treatment, monitoring of serum electrolytes, uric acid, phosphorus, calcium and creatinine levels.

Treatment of established tumour lysis syndrome is directed at vigorous correction of electrolytic abnormalities, hydration and haemodialysis (as appropriate in patients with renal failure).

Cardiovascular emergencies

Cardiovascular emergencies include superior vena cava syndrome, cardiac tamponade, venous thromboembolic complication and volume depletion.

Superior vena cava syndrome

Large space-occupying lesions in the upper mediastinal space may compress the superior vena cava (SVC), obstructing the return of blood to the heart. SVC syndrome is seen mainly with (small-cell) lung cancer, lymphoma and mediastinal metastasis of solid tumours or with thrombosis, commonly related to intravascular device complication.

Typically, SVC syndrome produces cough, dyspnoea and dysphagia combined with swelling and discoloration of the neck, face or upper extremities. Depending on the site of the disease, both vocal cord paralysis and Horner syndrome can occur. Clinical findings are greater in complete obstruction than in mildly obstructive disease or in gradual obstruction. Others symptoms may include hoarseness, dysphagia, headaches, dizziness, syncope, lethargy and chest pain. They may be worsened by positional changes, particularly bending forward, stooping or lying down. Physical findings include oedema of the face (periorbital, laryngeal, glossal oedema), neck or arms, dilatation of the veins of the upper body, plethora or cyanosis of the face and mental status changes.

Treatment of tumour-related SVC syndrome includes radiotherapy, chemotherapy or expandable wire stents.[13] For patients known to have small-cell carcinoma of the lung or lymphoma, chemotherapy is the treatment of choice. Life-threatening symptoms, such as respiratory distress, are indications for urgent radiotherapy. The usefulness of anticoagulation must be weighed against the risk of haemorrhage in a venous system under increased pressure. Placement of an expandable wire stent across a stenotic portion of the vena cava is an appropriate therapy when possible. Diuretics and steroids may provide transient symptomatic relief of oedema and respiratory compromise, although no controlled trials support their use.

Catheter-associated SCV thrombosis is best treated by immediate thrombolytic therapy, administered when possibly directly to the thrombus to minimize systemic fibrinolysis. An alternative is anticoagulation and catheter removal.

Cardiac tamponade

Tamponade occurs when fluids accumulate faster than the pericardium can stretch. Compression of all four chambers ensues, with tachycardia and diminishing cardiac output. Dyspnoea is the most common symptom, often with cough or retrosternal chest pain (Table 109.1). There are often distant heart sounds, pulsus paradoxus and pericardial friction rub. With cardiac tamponade, progressive heart failure occurs, with increased shortness of breath, confusion and hypotension.

Asymptomatic, small effusions may be managed with careful follow-up and treatment directed against the underlying malignancy.[14] Cardiac tamponade requires an immediate removal of pericardial fluid as an emergency, under echocardiographic guidance, to ensure symptom relief and cytological diagnosis. In patients with symptomatic, moderate to large effusions who do not present as an emergency, therapy should be aimed at relieving symptoms and preventing recurrence of tamponade. After pericardiocentesis alone, effusion usually recurs rapidly. Percutaneous tube drainage can be performed in addition to pericardial windows or resection, based on the underlying condition of the patient.

Venous thromboembolic complications

Cancer increases the risk of venous thromboembolism (VTE) 4–6-fold. The aetiology of deep venous thrombosis (DVT) and pulmonary embolism (PE) in cancer patients may be attributable to several factors: hypercoagulable states due to abnormalities of blood composition (increased plasma levels of clotting factors, cancer procoagulant A, tissue factors and cytokines) and increased release of plasminogen activator, and indwelling central venous catheter. Chemotherapy agents also increase endothelial cell reactivity to platelets, a phenomenon which may underlie thrombotic thrombocytopenic purpura and haemolytic uraemic syndrome.

Initial treatment[15] of acute VTE starts with heparin, either unfractionated heparin (UFH) or low molecular weight heparin (LMWH), followed by a coumarin derivative (e.g. warfarin). UFH is administered as a bolus followed by a continuous drip, titrated to approximately partial thromboplastin time (PTT) 1.5–2 times control. Oral anticoagulants are usually started on day 1 or 2 of treatment, are monitored by PTT and dosages are adjusted to maintain an international normalized ratio (INR) between 2.0 and 3.0. Patients are maintained on UFH for 4–5 days while the oral anticoagulant is titrated to therapeutic levels. The use of LMWH is easier and does not need laboratory monitoring, except for individuals with renal insufficiency or those with <50 kg body weight or with obesity (plasma anti-factor Xa concentration). LMWH is the treatment of choice in patients receiving chemotherapy since many drugs may alter the anticoagulant response to oral anticoagulants.

Catheter-related thrombosis is treated with fibrinolytic agents (tissue-type plasminogen activator, streptokinase or urokinase). Pre-existing clotting defects, bleeding source, central nervous system metastatsis, recent major surgery and a history of gastrointestinal bleeding or uncontrolled hypertension are contraindications to thrombolytic treatment. Patients who develop recurrent thrombosis while on therapeutic doses of anticoagulation should be considered for inferior vena cava filter placement.

Age alone is not a contraindication to appropriate thrombolytic therapy or anticoagulation, although it may complicate management (e.g. risk of fall, gastrointestinal bleeding and variable appetite and diet).

Volume depletion

Often overlooked, dehydration is very common in cancer patients and volume depletion may lead to hypovolaemic shock more rapidly in elderly than in younger individuals due to a limited reserve of body water and a blunted response of capacitance vessels to sympathetic stimulation. Many studies have reported greater severe 5-fluorouracil-induced toxicity related to advanced age.[16,17] The mechanism does not result from decreased clearance of chemotherapy but from age-related impairment of compensatory mechanisms including a cascade of secondary effects related to poor physiological reserves. Mucositis, leading to dysphagia and diarrhoea, is highlighted among the causes of volume depletion in the elderly. Unfortunately, the presentation of volume depletion may be delayed, including poor appreciation of the initial symptoms of mucositis, inadequate fluid replacement due to swallowing disorders and inadequate access to transportation.

The mainstay of the management of fluid depletion includes timely fluid resuscitation. Early management may prevent both death and complications such as functional dependence.

Neurological emergencies

Neurological emergencies include brain metastases, increased intracranial pressure, spinal cord compression and delirium.

Brain metastases and increased intracranial pressure

Intracranial metastases occur in up to one-quarter of patients dying of cancer.[18] Brain metastases arise from haematologenous spread of the tumour and the distribution within the brain is in accordance with the regional blood flow. Approximately 90% of brain metastases are found in the supratentorial region. The metastases are commonly located at the junction of the grey and white matter and in the so-called watershed areas of the brain. Brain oedema and tumour expansion commonly result in increased intracranial pressure.

In patients with intracranial-occupying lesions (brain tumours, metastases, oedema), the intracranial pressure may rise to 25–30 mmHg, leading to hypoperfusion and to death. Clinical findings (Table 109.1) depend on the rate of the rise in intracranial pressure and signs depend on the lesion's topography. Conservative treatment is aimed reducing vasogenic oedema and maintaining cerebral perfusion thanks to patient position, control of arterial blood pressure, hypertonic infusions (mannitol 20%, 1 g kg^{-1} in 15–30 min twice per day for 3 days) and corticosteroids (dexamethasone 4 mg four times per day).

Spinal cord compression

Spinal cord compression, due to extradural tumour mass, usually resulting from involvement of the vertebral column, is not immediately life-threatening unless it involves level C3 or above, but it may lead to profound, permanent morbidity. Paraplegia or loss of sphincter control or both not only diminishes a patient's quality of life but also predisposes to further complications such as venous thrombosis, decubitus ulcers and urinary obstruction. It often presents insidiously with back pain radiating in a belt-like fashion and may progress rapidly to overt neurological dysfunction (weakness and sensory loss), leading to irreversible paralysis.

Treatment outcome correlates with the degree and duration of neurological impairment prior to therapy. The choice of treatment[19] depends on the clinical presentation, rapidity of the clinical course, type of malignancy, site of spinal involvement and previous treatment. Corticosteroids (dexamethasone 10 mg intravenously followed by an oral dose of 16 mg daily) are used until efficacy of definitive treatment, radiotherapy (30 Gy in 10 fractions over 2 weeks) or surgical decompression (laminectomy or vertebral body resection) in selected patients.

Delirium

Delirium remains the most common and distressing neuropsychiatric complication in patients with advanced cancer. Delirium is defined as an acute, transient, fluctuant and usually reversible cause of cerebral dysfunction and manifests clinically with a wide range of psychiatric abnormalities. The cause of hospitalization for 10–22% of elderly patients, delirium has been found in 14–56% of elderly medical inpatients[20] and even more in intensive care units (41–87% of patients).[21]

Delirium is associated with an increased risk of mortality not only during the stay but also[22] during the months following discharge.[23] The consequences of delirium include not only increased mortality but also lengthened hospital stays and the need for increased services after hospital discharge.

Unfortunately, delirium is often unrecognized by the patients' physicians and nurses,[24,25] because of its fluctuating nature, its overlap with dementia, lack of formal cognitive assessment and under appreciation of its clinical consequences.

The clinical features of delirium are numerous and encompass a variety of neuropsychiatric symptoms common to other psychiatric disorders. Delirium or acute confusional state is characterized by impairment of consciousness and global cognitive impairment of acute onset. Other key features include disorientation and disturbance of the sleep–wake cycle. Psychomotor behaviour may be altered. Patients may be hypoactive or hyperactive; in the latter case patients can be agitated and even physically combative. Perception can be altered with patients experiencing illusions (misinterpretations of external stimuli, for example, believing that patterns in the bed sheets are insects) or hallucinations (perceptions in the absence of stimuli). Frank paranoid ideas or delusions may occur. The syndrome is frequently worse at night and periods of relative lucidity can occur.

Several delirium assessment and rating scales have been designed to aid clinicians in the diagnosis of delirium, such as the Confusion Assessment Method (CAM).[26]

The pathophysiology of delirium remains poorly understood, but perturbations of neurotransmitters (cholinergic balance) may play a role.[27,28] Given the clinical heterogeneity and multifactorial nature of delirium, it is likely that multiple pathogenic mechanisms contribute to its development, with a complex interrelationship between vulnerability (patient with predisposing factors) and exposure to precipitating factors or noxious insults: in vulnerable patients (e.g. those with dementia and multiple coexisting conditions), delirium may develop as a result of relatively benign insults, such as one dose of a sleeping medication. Conversely, delirium may develop in patients who are not vulnerable after exposure to multiple noxious insults, such as general anaesthesia, major surgery and psychoactive medications (Table 109.4).

In a recent series of 100 cancer patients, the aetiology of delirium was multifactorial (two or more in 40% of patients) and the 1 week reversibility increased when the number of insults decreased.[29] Furthermore, in elderly cancer patients, the most frequent and reversible aetiology is drug-induced delirium resulting from opioids and other psychoactive medications.[30]

Treatment of any physical cause underlying the delirium should be started promptly. General principles include

Table 109.4 Main predisposing and precipitating factors of delirium.

Predisposing factors	Precipitating factors
Demographic characteristics	*Drugs*
Age 65 years or older	Sedative hypnotics
Male gender	Narcotics
	Anticholinergic drugs
Cognitive status	Polypharmacy
Dementia	Alcohol or drug withdrawal
Cognitive impairment	
History of delirium	*Primary neurological diseases*
Depression	Stroke
	Intracranial bleeding
Functional status	Meningitis or encephalitis
Functional dependence	
Immobility	*Intercurrent illnesses*
Low level of activity	Infections
	Iatrogenic complications
History of falls	Severe acute illness (hypoxia, fever, anaemia, dehydration)
Sensory impairment	
Visual impairment	*Surgery*
Hearing impairment	
Decreased oral intake	*Environmental*
Dehydration	Hospitalization
Malnutrition	Use of physical restraints
	Use of urinary catheter
Drugs	Use of multiple procedures
Treatment with multiple psychoactive drugs	Pain
	Emotional stress
Polypharmacy	
Alcohol abuse	

Adapted from Inouye.[27]

nursing in bright conditions with familiar staff members. If wandering is problematic, 'one-to-one' nursing management may have to be implemented for the patient's safety. The most effective supportive treatment is haloperidol with an initial dose of 0.5 mg twice daily.[31] Short-term use of antipsychotic agents is advised as these agents have been associated with a higher risk of mortality and possibly stroke when used in patients with dementia.[32] Benzodiazepines have a more rapid onset of action than the psychotics, but they can worsen confusion and sedation.

Structural emergencies

Structural emergencies include airway, bowel and urinary obstructions and pathological fractures.

Airway obstruction

Airway obstruction in elderly cancer patients may have different causes, from swallowing disorders to tumours involving the upper (hypopharynx, larynx and trachea to carina) or lower airway.

Clinical differentiation between upper and lower airway obstructions can be difficult because both can cause cough, wheezing, dyspnoea, infection, respiratory failure and death.

A rapid evaluation must ensure that no foreign body is inhaled. In the case of an upper airway tumour mass, emergency visualization of the larynx by an otolaryngologist or anaesthesiologist must be performed in order to pass an endotracheal tube, based mainly on the condition and life expectancy of the patient. Treatment associates low tracheotomy with placement of a long tracheostomy tube, adjunctive therapy such as corticosteroids (to reduce oedema), humidified oxygen and bronchodilators and definitive therapy, based on underlying disease (chemotherapy for sensitive cancers, radiotherapy, surgery, endoscopic laser and stenting for the others). Similarly, endobronchial obstruction is treated with radiation therapy, surgical or endoscopic procedures.

Bowel obstruction

Lack of intestinal emission is frequent in the elderly and a clinical distinction must be made between constipation and intestinal occlusion. Faecal impaction must be kept in mind, especially in bedridden patients. Cancer-related obstruction may have mechanical and/or functional causes. Within the lumen, obstruction can occur owing to annular or polypoïd lesions. Externally, malignant or surgical adhesions, radiotherapy-related fibrosis and omental or mesenteric tumours may result in obstruction. Finally, tumour infiltration to the bowel muscle or mesentery may cause motility disorders (pseudo-obstruction).

Intestinal colic, abdominal pain and vomiting are associated with anorexia, intermittent borborygmi and abdominal distension. Significant sequelae of bowel obstruction include potential life-threatening perforation, intravascular volume depletion and sepsis.

Based on a threshold of 75 years, preoperative complication and emergency surgery rates are more common in elderly patients. Whereas postoperative surgical morbidity rates are similar to those observed in younger patients, postoperative non-surgical morbidity is higher in the elderly group, which influences postoperative mortality.[33] When a surgical procedure is contraindicated, alternative therapy includes the use of a nasogastric tube, analgesics, centrally acting antiemetics (haloperidol, prochlorperazine), antisecretory agents (octreotide rather than anticholinergic agents) and corticosteroids (tapered to the minimum effective dose that controls symptoms).

Urinary obstruction

Obstruction of the upper urinary tract, primarily the ureters, is common in a variety of cancers. When compression is bilateral either simultaneously or sequentially, early intervention may prevent life-threatening complications such as anuria and renal failure. This may be caused by obstruction to bladder outflow or to one or both ureters and occurs commonly in genitourinary malignancy. Ureteric obstruction may be produced by intraluminal, intramural or extramural tumours. Retroperitoneal fibrosis and stricture caused by radiotherapy, chemotherapy or surgery may also lead to progressive upper tract obstruction.

Patients commonly present with the insidious onset of uraemia and reduced urine output. Pain is rarely a feature, unless there is acute obstruction of a ureter. If there is concomitant infection, then urosepsis may intervene unless prompt drainage is performed using percutaneous nephrostomy or retrograde stenting of the ureter. Procedure choice depends on life expectancy, comorbidity and patient preference.

Pathological fractures

Fractures of weight-bearing bones are common in the elderly due to osteopenia. This tendency is enhanced in patients with cancer due to local metastasis or to tumour-enhanced osteopenia. Bone pain is the most common presenting feature of either pathological fracture or of impending pathological fracture, but it is not absolutely essential for the diagnosis. Around 50% of events are due to metastasis from breast cancer and the commonest site for pathological fracture is the femur.

Whether fractures are displaced, non-displaced, impending in weight-bearing bones or in non-weight-bearing bones are all important factors for management decisions. These tumour-related factors, along with patient-related factors, such as performance status, comorbidity, previous mobility and geriatric evaluation, need to be assessed. For example, surgical intervention for fractures in non-weight-bearing bones may be considered worthwhile when survival is expected to be at least 3 months, whereas for fractures in weight-bearing bones it should be considered even with a life expectancy limited to 1 month. Pain relief may be an objective as important as stability or mobility. Radiation therapy is a highly effective modality for treating painful bones metastases. Where a fracture has occurred, surgical intervention should always be considered in the first instance, unless it involves regions not amenable to orthopaedic intervention such as ribs, scapula or pelvis. In these cases, radiotherapy can provide pain relief in up to 80% of patients, while promoting bone healing. For long bone fractures, rigid immobilization with internal fixation should be performed prior to irradiation, in order to give the lesion the best chance of healing.

Acute pain emergencies

Acute cancer pain in the elderly population is an increasingly common clinical situation. Previous studies indicate a high prevalence rate (between 25 and 40% of elderly patients with cancer experience daily pain)[34] and poor management of cancer pain in the elderly. Pain is often considered as an expected concomitant of ageing and older patients are considered more sensitive to opioids. Furthermore, no physiological changes in pain perception in the elderly have been demonstrated. In fact, the elderly may be less likely to complain of pain than younger people.[35] However, the assessment of pain in elderly individuals with cancer may pose significant and specific challenges, notably in emergency. The presence of multiple concurrent medical problems, the increased likelihood of cognitive and sensory impairment and the presence of depression may all contribute to underestimation of pain.

In practice, because of the many variables in pain, it is essential to have a standard approach to assessment, notably in elderly cancer patients. This includes

- taking an accurate pain history
- using an assessment tool
- standard clinical examination
- appropriate laboratory and radiological investigation.

Pain assessment tools help in understanding the patient's pain and facilitate monitoring of the effects of analgesics and other interventions. Furthermore, not all tools for pain assessment are equally reliable in the elderly. Numerical rating scales, pictorial pain scales and verbal descriptor scales are more reliable than visual analogue scales.[36]

The most important is to use the same scale during follow-up evaluation, ensuring reproducibility and easy comparison. Moreover, the key to performing pain assessment in the cognitively impaired patient is to assess pain frequently (because of poor recall) and recognize changes. Behavioural cues, such as a change in cognitive level or appearance, increased agitation or change in respiratory status, may indicate pain.[37]

Subsequently, physical examination should be aimed at identifying causes of pain, for example, tenderness from bone metastases, evidence of bowel obstruction and neurological dysfunction as a pointer to neuropathic pain or patterns suggestive of cancer pain syndromes. Investigation may be necessary to confirm areas of suspected disease.

Finally, the general principles in managing acute cancer pain in the elderly are similar to those in the general population, but with a greater degree of caution. Effective pain management may be achieved by any one of the following modalities: delay tumour progression (chemotherapy, radiotherapy, ...), palliative surgery (spinal cord decompression, ...) and analgesics and adjuvant analgesic drugs. Frequently a combination is necessary.

However, analgesic pain management in elderly patients requires taking into consideration the physiological and pharmacokinetic changes that occur in the geriatric population, the phenomenon of poly-pharmacy, which is common in the elderly, and the treatment goals. Elderly patients are potentially more likely to be affected by opioid toxicity because of the physiological changes associated with ageing. Nevertheless, appropriate dosage and administration may limit these risks. Cancer patients with acute pain not responding to increased opioid doses because they develop adverse effects before achieving acceptable analgesia may be switched to alternative opioids. Adjuvant analgesics, including antidepressants, antiepileptics, corticosteroids and bisphosphonates, may help in the treatment of certain types of pain. On the other hand, the elderly are at increased risk of developing toxicity from non-steroidal anti-inflammatory drugs (NSAIDs) and the overall safety of these drugs in frail elderly patients should be considered.

Finally, with an appropriate and careful approach, it should be possible to soothe acute cancer pain in most elderly patients. Then, the goal of optimal pain management is to maximize quality of life and independence.[38]

The role of geriatric evaluation in the prediction of oncological emergencies

The prevalence of cancers increases with age, half of them being diagnosed after 70 years of age, which implies new healthcare management challenges.[39,40] Both the US National Comprehensive Cancer Network (NCCN) and the International Society of Geriatric Oncology (SIOG)[41] recommend some form of pretreatment geriatric assessment to identify older adults fit enough to undergo standard treatment and those who need adjusted treatment.[42,43]

However, a geriatric assessment is time consuming and the benefits have not yet been demonstrated,[44] and traditional geriatric assessment may not be a sensitive tool to predict treatment toxicity in well-functioning and autonomous older adults. A more sensitive way to characterize health and functional status is to use the concept of frailty.[45] Frailty represents a state of reduced homeostasis and resistance to stress that leads, in turn, to increased vulnerability and risk of adverse outcome. Measures of frailty proposed by Fried *et al.* include weakness, poor endurance, reduced physical activity, slow walking speed and unintentional weight loss during the preceding year.[46] The concept of frailty is intended to identify older persons at risk of adverse outcome, with the aim of preventing or delaying the occurrence of adverse outcome. In a prospective pilot study, low grip strength and poor cognitive functioning were associated with treatment-related toxicity in unadjusted analyses.[45] Furthermore, the only frailty marker to be a statistically significant predictor of severe toxicity in the adjusted analyses was low grip strength, shown to predict disability in the elderly and mortality. Bohannon suggested that grip strength should be considered as a vital sign for older person.[47]

Moreover, among newly diagnosed older cancer patients, suspicion of cognitive impairment is associated with emergency department visits.[48] According to Kurtz *et al.*, lower physical functioning increases the risk of emergency department visits during the active treatment and the follow-up period.[49,50] However, many patients were included after the start of cancer treatment, hence it is unclear whether the low physical functioning was treatment induced or due to the pre-existing comorbid conditions.

Finally, in older patients, cancer treatments, especially chemotherapy, are considered strong stressors that reveal patients with sufficient functional reserve to regain stable homeostasis. Frailty markers may add important information to that obtained using traditional geriatric tools such as instrumental activities of daily living and basic activities of daily living in detecting potential vulnerability. However, further longitudinal studies are needed to investigate the usefulness of frailty markers in predicting the risk of oncological emergencies.

Conclusion

Cancer is predominantly a disease of the elderly. More than 60% of all incident cases of cancer and more than 70% of all deaths from malignant tumours occur in older individuals. Elderly patients with malignancies are subject to developing a unique set of complications that require urgent evaluation and treatment. Geriatricians must be able to recognize these conditions and to institute appropriate therapy. With timely intervention, many of these elderly cancer patients can return to their previous level of function and independence. Therefore, it is important that geriatric physician have a sound knowledge of the most common oncological emergencies.

Key points

- The majority of deaths in those with malignant tumours occur in older patients.
- Physicians should be familiar with oncological emergencies, as failure to implement immediate and appropriate treatment may result in significant morbidity or death.
- Common problems include haematological emergencies, infections, neurological and metabolic derangements and tumour lysis syndrome.

References

1. Hosmer W, Malin J and Wong M. Development and validation of a prediction model for the risk of developing febrile neutropenia in the first cycle of chemotherapy among elderly patients with breast, lung, colorectal and prostate cancer. *Support Care Cancer* 2011;**19**:333–41.
2. Serefhanoglu K, Ersoy Y, Serefhanoglu S *et al.* Clinical experience with three combination regimens for the treatment of high-risk febrile neutropenia. *Ann Acad Med Singapore* 2006;**35**:11–6.
3. Halfdanarson TR, Hogan WJ and Moynihan TJ. Oncologic emergencies: diagnosis and treatment. *Mayo Clin Proc* 2006;**81**:835–48.
4. Gruschkus SK, Lairson D, Dunn JK *et al.* Comparative effectiveness of white blood cell growth factors on neutropenia, infection and survival in older people with non-Hodgkin's lymphoma treated with chemotherapy. *J Am Geriatr Soc* 2010;**58**:1885–95.
5. Elting LS, Rubenstein EB, Martin CG *et al.* Incidence, cost and outcomes of bleeding and chemotherapy dose modification among solid tumor patients with chemotherapy-induced thrombocytopenia. *J Clin Oncol* 2001;**19**:1137–46.
6. Levi M, Toh CH, Thachil J *et al.* Guidelines for the diagnosis and management of disseminated intravascular coagulation. British Committee for Standards in Haematology. *Br J Haematol* 2009;**145**:24–33.
7. Stewart AF. Clinical practice. Hypercalcemia associated with cancer. *N Engl J Med* 2005;**352**:373–9.
8. Bushinsky DA and Monk RD. Electrolyte quintet: calcium. *Lancet* 1998;**352**:306–11.
9. Body JJ, Coleman R, Clezardin P *et al.* International Society of Geriatric Oncology (SIOG) clinical practice recommendations for the use of bisphosphonates in elderly patients. *Eur J Cancer* 2007;**43**:852–8.
10. Ishikawa S, Fujita N, Fujisawa G *et al.* Involvement of arginine vasopressin and renal sodium handling in pathogenesis of hyponatremia in elderly patients. *Endocr J* 1996;**43**:101–8.

11. Flombaum CD. Metabolic emergencies in the cancer patient. *Semin Oncol* 2000;**27**:322–34.
12. Pumo V, Sciacca D and Malaguarnera M. Tumor lysis syndrome in elderly. *Crit Rev Oncol Hematol* 2007;**64**:31–42.
13. Lonardi F, Gioga G, Agus G *et al.* Double-flash, large-fraction radiation therapy as palliative treatment of malignant superior vena cava syndrome in the elderly. *Support Care Cancer* 2002;**10**:56–60.
14. Soler-Soler J, Sagrista-Sauleda J and Permanyer-Miralda G. Management of pericardial effusion. *Heart* 2001;**86**:235–40.
15. Di Nisio M, Squizzato A, Klerk CP *et al.* Antithrombotic therapy and cancer. *Curr Opin Hematol* 2004;**11**:187–91.
16. Stein BN, Petrelli NJ, Douglass HO *et al.* Age and sex are independent predictors of 5-fluorouracil toxicity. Analysis of a large scale phase III trial. *Cancer* 1995;**75**:11–7.
17. Tsalic M, Bar-Sela G, Beny A *et al.* Severe toxicity related to the 5-fluorouracil/leucovorin combination (the Mayo Clinic regimen): a prospective study in colorectal cancer patients. *Am J Clin Oncol* 2003;**26**:103–6.
18. Posner JB and Chernik NL. Intracranial metastases from systemic cancer. *Adv Neurol* 1978;**19**:579–92.
19. Rades D, Hoskin PJ, Karstens JH *et al.* Radiotherapy of metastatic spinal cord compression in very elderly patients. *Int J Radiat Oncol Biol Phys* 2007;**67**:256–63.
20. Fick DM, Agostini JV and Inouye SK. Delirium superimposed on dementia: a systematic review. *J Am Geriatr Soc* 2002;**50**:1723–32.
21. Ely EW, Margolin R, Francis J *et al.* Evaluation of delirium in critically ill patients: validation of the Confusion Assessment Method for the Intensive Care Unit (CAM-ICU). *Crit Care Med* 2001;**29**:1370–9.
22. O'Keeffe S and Lavan J. The prognostic significance of delirium in older hospital patients. *J Am Geriatr Soc* 1997;**45**:174–8.
23. Curyto KJ, Johnson J, TenHave T *et al.* Survival of hospitalized elderly patients with delirium: a prospective study. *Am J Geriatr Psychiatry* 2001;**9**:141–7.
24. Cole MG. Delirium in elderly patients. *Am J Geriatr Psychiatry* 2004;**12**:7–21.
25. Inouye SK, Foreman MD, Mion LC *et al.* Nurses' recognition of delirium and its symptoms: comparison of nurse and researcher ratings. *Arch Intern Med* 2001;**161**:2467–73.
26. Inouye SK, van Dyck CH, Alessi CA *et al.* Clarifying confusion: the confusion assessment method. A new method for detection of delirium. *Ann Intern Med* 1990;**113**:941–8.
27. Inouye SK. Delirium in older persons. *N Engl J Med* 2006;**354**:1157–65.
28. Trzepacz P and van der Mast R. The neuropathophysiology of delirium. In: J Lindesay, K Rockwood and A Macdonald (eds), *Delirium in Old Age*, Oxford University Press, Oxford, 2002, pp. 51–90.
29. Sagawa R, Akechi T, Okuyama T *et al.* Etiologies of delirium and their relationship to reversibility and motor subtype in cancer patients. *Jpn J Clin Oncol* 2009;**39**:175–82.
30. Bush SH and Bruera E. The assessment and management of delirium in cancer patients. *Oncologist* 2009;**14**:1039–49.
31. Olofsson SM, Weitzner MA, Valentine AD *et al.* A retrospective study of the psychiatric management and outcome of delirium in the cancer patient. *Support Care Cancer* 1996;**4**:351–7.
32. Schneider LS, Dagerman KS and Insel P. Risk of death with atypical antipsychotic drug treatment for dementia: meta-analysis of randomized placebo-controlled trials. *JAMA* 2005;**294**:1934–43.
33. Latkauskas T, Rudinskaite G, Kurtinaitis J *et al.* The impact of age on post-operative outcomes of colorectal cancer patients undergoing surgical treatment. *BMC Cancer* 2005;**5**: 153.
34. Bernabei R, Gambassi G, Lapane K *et al.* Management of pain in elderly patients with cancer. SAGE Study Group. Systematic Assessment of Geriatric Drug Use via Epidemiology. *JAMA* 1998;**279**:1877–82.
35. Melding PS. Is there such a thing as geriatric pain? *Pain* 1991;**46**:119–21.
36. Herr KA and Garand L. Assessment and measurement of pain in older adults. *Clin Geriatr Med* 2001;**17**:457–78.
37. Maxwell T. Cancer pain management in the elderly. *Geriatr Nurs* 2000;**21**:158–63.
38. Mercadante S and Arcuri E. Pharmacological management of cancer pain in the elderly. *Drugs Aging* 2007;**24**:761–76.
39. Yancik R and Ries LA. Cancer in older persons: an international issue in an aging world. *Semin Oncol* 2004;**31**:128–36.
40. Yancik R. Population aging and cancer: a cross-national concern. *Cancer J* 2005;**11**:437–41.
41. Smith BD, Smith GL, Hurria A *et al.* Future of cancer incidence in the United States: burdens upon an aging, changing nation. *J Clin Oncol* 2009;**27**:2758–65.
42. Carreca I, Balducci L and Extermann M. Cancer in the older person. *Cancer Treat Rev* 2005;**31**:380–402.
43. Fentiman IS, Tirelli U, Monfardini S *et al.* Cancer in the elderly: why so badly treated? *Lancet* 1990;**335**:1020–2.
44. Hurria A, Zuckerman E *et al.* A prospective, longitudinal study of the functional status and quality of life of older patients with breast cancer receiving adjuvant chemotherapy. *J Am Geriatr Soc* 2006;**54**:1119–24.
45. Puts MT, Monette J, Girre V *et al.* Are frailty markers useful for predicting treatment toxicity and mortality in older newly diagnosed cancer patients? Results from a prospective pilot study. *Crit Rev Oncol Hematol* 2011;**78**:138–49.
46. Fried LP, Tangen CM, Walston J *et al.* Frailty in older adults: evidence for a phenotype. *J Gerontol A Biol Sci Med Sci* 2001;**56**: M146–56.
47. Bohannon RW. Hand-grip dynamometry predicts future outcomes in aging adults. *J Geriatr Phys Ther* 2008;**31**:3–10.
48. Puts MT, Monette J, Girre V *et al.* Does frailty predict hospitalization, emergency department visits and visits to the general practitioner in older newly-diagnosed cancer patients? Results of a prospective pilot study. *Crit Rev Oncol Hematol* 2010;**76**:142–51.
49. Kurtz ME, Kurtz JC, Given CW and Given BA. Utilization of services among elderly cancer patients – relationship to age, symptoms, physical functioning, comorbidity and survival status. *Ethn Dis* 2005;**15**: S17–22.
50. Kurtz ME, Kurtz JC, Given CW and Given BA. Predictors of use of health care services among elderly lung cancer patients: the first year after diagnosis. *Support Care Cancer* 2006;**14**:243–50.

CHAPTER 110

Breast cancer

Robert E. Mansel and Bedanta P. Baruah
Cardiff University, Cardiff, Wales, UK

The presentation

Diagnosis of breast cancer in the elderly is made by the discovery of a lump in 60–80% women. Since screening is applied less rigorously to elderly patients, the majority of women present with a palpable lump. Several studies have revealed that the stage at presentation is more advanced in elderly women.[1,2] A patient care evaluation survey was conducted by the Commission on Cancer of the American College of Surgeons for 1983 and 1990.[3] They surveyed all States of USA, including Puerto Rico, and Canada and studied 17 029 women in 1983 and 24 004 women in 1990. Some 20% women in 1983 and 23% in 1990 were 75 years of age or older. The survey included 2000 hospitals (25 patients from each). The percentage of cancers detected by physicians' examination decreased in the younger group from 27% in 1983 to 21% in 1990, whereas in the elderly the corresponding figures were 41 and 34%, respectively.

Veronesi's group in Milan reported various features of presentation and choice of therapy in the elderly.[4] They studied 2999 postmenopausal patients referred for surgery at the European Institute of Oncology, Milan, from 1997 to 2002. The patients were grouped according to age: young postmenopausal (YPM, age 50–64 years, $n = 2052$), older postmenopausal (OPM, age 65–74 years, $n = 801$) and elderly postmenopausal (EPM, age $\geq$75 years, $n = 146$). EPM patients had larger tumours compared with YPM patients (pT4: 6.7 versus 2.4%) and more nodal involvement (lymph node positivity: 62.5 versus 51.3%). EPM patients showed a higher degree of estrogen and progesterone receptor expression, less peritumoral vascular invasion and less human epidermal growth factor receptor-2 (HER-2)/*neu* expression than YPM patients. Although comorbidities were more often recorded for elderly patients (72% EPM versus 45% YPM), this did not influence surgical choices, which were similar across groups (breast conservation: 73.9, 76.9 and 72.9%, respectively). No systemic therapy was recommended for 19.1% of the EPM group compared with 5.4 and 4.7% of the two other groups. A recent epidemiological study in The Netherlands[5] of 127 805 adult female patients with their first primary breast cancer diagnosed between 1995 and 2005 showed that elderly breast cancer patients were diagnosed with a higher stage of disease. Elderly patients underwent less surgery (99.2 versus 41.2%), received hormonal treatment as monotherapy more frequently (0.8 versus 47.3%) and less adjuvant systemic treatment (79 versus 53%).

In women over 70 years of age, estrogen receptor-positive tumours are more common, range 69–95%, compared with all tumours, range 53–72%.[3]

Pathologically infiltrating ductal carcinoma accounts for 77–85% of all tumours in elderly women compared with 68% in younger women. There is an increase in the proportion of papillary and mucinous carcinoma with advancing age. Whereas the number of lobular carcinoma *in situ*, comedo, medullary and inflammatory carcinoma decreases with advancing age, the prevalence of ductal carcinoma *in situ* (DCIS) increases until 75 years, after which it declines.[6,7]

In summary, elderly women generally present with large palpable estrogen receptor-positive, infiltrating ductal carcinoma with a positive lymph node.[5,7]

Stage of presentation

There is generally a delay in the diagnosis of breast cancer in elderly women. In a study by Berg and Robbins,[8] the diagnosis was delayed by more than 6 months in 28% of women under 70 years of age compared with 42% in women above the age of 70 years. Similarly, Devitt[9] observed a delay of more than 6 months in diagnosis in 35% of women above the age of 70 years compared to 28% below that age. The tumour is generally advanced in the elderly group, as shown in Table 110.1.

Principles and Practice of Geriatric Medicine, Fifth Edition. Edited by Alan J. Sinclair, John E. Morley and Bruno Vellas.

Table 110.1 TNM stage (%) with age at presentation.

Age (years)	Stage				Ref.
	I	II	III	IV	
>80	52	18	6	24	10
>80	25	49	15	10	11
>73	33	22	12	13	12

Variation in care and undertreatment in the elderly

There is growing evidence that there is significant variation in standard care of breast cancer in the elderly and that elderly patients often receive suboptimal treatment. Monica Morrow, in a review on treatment in the elderly, noted that screening by physical examination and mammography is underutilized for the older women.[13] Since mastectomy offers excellent local control and has only less than 1% operative mortality in women above 65 years of age, it should be offered to more (suitable) patients. She further pointed out that failure to use adjuvant therapy when indicated is one of the most frequent problems in management of elderly.[13]

Pattern of care of elderly women is different from that offered to younger patients. In the study by the Commission on Cancer of the American College of Surgeons for 1983 and 1990,[3] in 1983, 23% of older women received total or partial mastectomy without axillary dissection compared with 8% of younger females. In 1990, the rate of total or partial mastectomy without nodal dissection was 20.6% in older women and 10% in younger women. The use of reconstruction was limited in the older women. The percentage of elderly females receiving reconstruction was 1.2% in 1983 and 1.3% in 1990. The operative mortality rates were higher in the older age-group (2.9% in 1983 and 1.5% in 1990). Radiotherapy was used less frequently in the older group in both study years.

In an editorial in the *Journal of Clinical Oncology*, Rebecca Silliman chided clinicians for not offering definitive treatment to elderly women with breast cancer.[14] Although breast cancer-specific mortality has declined among women younger than 70 years, it is either stable in those aged 70–79 years or increased in women above 65 years of age. This proportion is likely to grow, as older age is the most important risk factor for breast cancer and gains in life expectancy will result in more women being at risk for longer periods. Currently, the average life expectancy of a 75-year-old woman is 12 years (17 years if she is healthy) and that of an 85-year-old is 6 years (9 years if she is healthy). Owing to paucity of good evidence-based data, there is considerable controversy about what constitutes appropriate care for older women. More than one-quarter (27%) of breast cancer deaths in 2001 in the USA were in the age group of 80 years and older. Although the patient's health status, patient and family preferences and support and patient–physician interactions explain in part age-related treatment variations, age alone remains an independent risk factor for less than definitive breast cancer care.

In a cohort of 407 octogenarian women in Canton of Geneva, Switzerland, Bouchardy *et al.*[15] addressed the relationship between undertreatment and breast cancer mortality. They used tumour registry data, including sociodemographic data, comorbidity, tumour and treatment characteristics and the cause of death. The main problem that they noted in analysing these data was the issue of missing information – 20% for comorbidity, 49% for tumour grade and 74% for estrogen receptor (ER) status. Because of loss of data on these important prognostic factors, there was a problem in multivariate analysis and incomplete control of confounding, decreasing the statistical power and precision. Both mastectomy plus adjuvant therapy and breast-conserving surgery plus adjuvant therapy appear to protect against death from causes other than breast cancer, suggesting residual confounding either because comorbidity was not well measured or because undertreatment of breast cancer is associated with undertreatment of other medical conditions. This cohort of Swiss women differed from women presenting elsewhere. The average tumour size in this group was 30 mm, only 22% presented in Stage I, 22% received no therapy and 32% received tamoxifen alone. Despite the limitations of this study, it highlights the link between undertreatment and high rates of breast cancer recurrence and mortality.

A recent retrospective cohort study involving case-note review based on the North Western Cancer Registry database of women aged ≥65 years resident in Greater Manchester with invasive breast cancer registered over a 1 year period ($n = 480$) showed that even after adjusting for tumour characteristics associated with age by logistic regression analyses, older women were less likely to receive standard management than younger women for all indicators investigated.[16] Compared with women aged 65–69 years, women aged ≥80 years with operable (Stage I–IIIa) breast cancer have increased odds of not receiving triple assessment [odds ratio (OR) = 5.5, 95% confidence interval (CI), 2.1–14.5], not receiving primary surgery (OR = 43.0; 95% CI, 9.7–191.3), not undergoing axillary node surgery (OR = 27.6; 95% CI, 5.6–135.9) and not undergoing tests for steroid receptors (OR = 3.0; 95% CI, 1.7–5.5). Women aged 75–79 years have increased odds of not receiving radiotherapy (RT) following breast-conserving surgery compared to women aged 65–69 years (OR = 11.0; 95% CI, 2.0–61.6). These results demonstrate that older women in the UK are less likely to receive standard management for breast cancer compared with younger women and this disparity cannot be explained by differences in tumour characteristics.

In a recent German clinical cohort study, 1922 women aged >50 years with histologically confirmed invasive breast cancer treated at the University of Ulm from 1992 to 2005 were enrolled.[17] Adherence to guidelines and effects on overall survival (OAS) and disease-free survival (DFS) for women aged >70 years were compared with those for younger women (aged 50–69 years). The study found that women aged >70 years less often received recommended breast-conserving therapy (70–79 years, 74–83%; >79 years, 54%) than women aged <69 years (93%). Non-adherence to the guidelines on RT (<70 years, 9%; 70–79 years, 14–27%; >79 years, 60%) and chemotherapy (<70 years, 33%; 70–79 years, 54–77%; >79 years, 98%) increased with age. Omission of RT significantly decreased OAS [<69 years, hazard ratio (HR) = 3.29; $p < 0.0001$; >70 years, HR = 1.89; $p = 0.0005$] and DFS (<69 years, HR = 3.45; $p<0.0001$; >70 years, HR = 2.14; $p< 0.0001$). OAS and DFS did not differ significantly for adherence to surgery, chemotherapy or endocrine therapy. This study showed that substandard treatment increases considerably with age and omission of RT had the greatest impact on OAS and DFS in the elderly population.

Women suffering from heart disease, obstructive airway disease, stroke or other major incapacitating illnesses receive inadequate diagnostic and therapeutic attention. One study found that the main cause of under treatment in the over-65 age group patients was cited as prohibitive associated medical conditions.[18]

Nicolucci *et al.*[19] analysed the data on 1724 women treated in 63 general hospitals in Italy. A comorbidity index was computed from individual disease value (IDV) and functional status (FS). IDV summates the severity and presence of specific complications for each disease suffered on a scale of 0–3, with 0 = full recovery and 3 = life-threatening disease. FS from signs and symptoms of 12 system categories evaluated the impact of all conditions, whether diagnosed or not, on patients' health status. The study showed higher proportions of inadequate diagnosis and therapy in the elderly group. The quality of care was assessed by a score based on observed degree of compliance with standard care. The median value of overall diagnostic and staging score was 60%. About one-third of surgical operations were inappropriate; 24% of cases with Stage I–II disease had unnecessary Halsted mastectomy and breast conservation in smaller tumours of ≤2 cm was underutilized. The presence of one or more coexisting diseases was associated with failure to undergo axillary dissection and lower utilization of conservative surgery.

Alvan Feinstein, a famous clinical epidemiologist from Yale, has said that the failure to classify and analyse comorbid disease has led to many difficulties in medical statistics.[20] There are four reasons for measuring comorbidity correctly: (1) to be able to correct for confounding, thus improving the internal validity of the study, (2) to be able to identify effect modification, (3) the desire to use comorbidity as a predictor of outcome and (4) to construct a comprehensive single comorbid scale that is valid, to improve the statistical efficiency. de Groot *et al.*[21] reviewed various comorbidity indices. The following indices have been applied for patients with breast cancer. The Charlson index is the most extensively studied method and includes 19 diseases which are weighted on the basis of strength of association with mortality. The disease count index simply counts the coexisting diseases but lacks a consistent definition and weighting for different diseases. The Kaplan index uses the type and severity of comorbid condition, for example, types are classified vascular (hypertension, cardiac disease, peripheral vascular disease) and non-vascular (lung, liver, bone and renal disease). It has good predictive validity for mortality. It may be worthwhile for all the agencies involved in breast cancer research to adopt one of the above indices and record it prospectively.

Screening in the elderly

Currently, all women in the UK between ages 50 and 70 years are offered breast cancer screening, which is saving ~1400 lives every year (2009 NHSBSP Annual Review). Although previously women between 65 and 70 years of age were eligible, they were not offered screening routinely. Extended age pilot schemes are now under way in which the age of inclusion includes women between 47 and 73 years of age. In 2007–08, 16 449 new cancers were detected under this programme. In England, in 2008–09 just under 1.8 million women (aged 45 years and over) were screened within the programme, an increase of 3.5% over 2007–08. The previous 10 years saw the programme grow by 43.9% from 1.2 million in 1998–99. There were 14 166 cases of cancer diagnosed in women screened aged 45 years and over, similar to the previous year (14 110) and nearly double the number in 1998–99 (7561). Of all cancers diagnosed, 11 212 (79.1%) were invasive and of these 5850 (52.2%) were 15 mm or less in size, which could not have been detected by clinical examination alone.

It has been observed that with increasing age the number of screening-detected cancers detected increases (Table 110.2).

In order to enhance the rate of breast examination by doctors of women above 65 years of age and to increase compliance with mammography, Herman *et al.*[22] conducted a randomized clinical trial (RCT) at the Metro Health Medical Center, Cleveland, OH. All house staff in Internal Medicine were asked to complete a questionnaire about their attitude towards prevention of breast cancer in elderly people after providing some basic information (monograph and a lecture). In one arm (controls), no specific interventions were offered. In the next group (education),

Table 110.2 Result of UK breast cancer screening – 2004 review NHS Breast Cancer Screening Programme in the UK, 2005.

Age (years)	Cancer detected per 1000 women screened
50–64	7.6
65–69	20.6

Table 110.3 Rates of examination and mammography by intervention.

Group	Breast examination (%)	Mammography (%)
Control (n = 192)	18	18
Education (n = 183)	22	31
Prevention (n = 165)	32	36

nurses provided educational leaflets to patients attending the clinics. In the third group (prevention), nurses filled the request forms and facilitated women to undergo mammography. The results are given in Table 110.3. The study suggested that encouragement and education of older women by motivated doctors and nurses improves compliance.

Chen *et al.*[23] reported the mortality rate of women aged 65–74 years screened in the Swedish two-county trial – 77 080 women were randomized to undergo screening every 33 months and 55 985 women served as controls. Of the screened group, 21 925 were in the age group 65–74. In the control arm, 15 344 women belonged to the age group 65–74 years. The relative breast cancer mortality in the screened group was 0.68, demonstrating a survival advantage in the elderly population.

Risk factors in the elderly

With advancing age, the risk of developing breast cancer rises. In a cohort of National Surgical Adjuvant Breast and Bowel Project's breast cancer prevention trial in the USA, the presence of non-proliferative lower category benign breast disease (LCBBD) was found to increase the risk of invasive breast cancer. The overall relative risk (RR) of breast cancer was 1.6 for LCBBD compared with women without any LCBBD. This risk increased to 1.95 (95% CI, 1.29–2.93) among women aged 50 years and over.[24]

Hormone replacement therapy (HRT) has been identified as a risk factor for breast cancer. The impact of HRT on the incidence and death due to breast cancer in the UK was assessed through a study of over 1 million women.[25] In this prospective cohort of 1 084 110 women aged 50–64, current users of HRT were found to have a higher risk of developing breast cancer than non-users (RR = 1.66; 95% CI, 1.58–1.75). The risk was highest for combined estrogen + progestogen (RR = 2; 95% CI, 1.88–2.12) than for estrogen alone (RR = 1.3; 95% CI, 1.2–1.4) and for tibolone (RR = 1.45; 95% CI, 1.25–1.68) compared with those who never used this treatment. There was a dose–response relationship of increasing risk of cancer with increasing duration of HRT usage, the highest being with combined estrogen + progestogen used for 10 years or more (RR = 2.31; 95% CI, 2.08–2.56).

The Danish Nurses Cohort study[26] provided data on 10 874 nurses (aged 45 years and above). Of these, 244 women developed breast cancer. After adjusting for confounding, increased risk was found with current use of estrogens (RR = 1.96; 95% CI, 1.16–3.35), for combined use of estrogen + progesterone (RR = 2.7; 95% CI, 1.96–3.73), for current use of tibolone (RR = 4.27; 95% CI, 1.74–10.51), compared with never used HRT. In current users of combined HRT with progestins, continuous combined use has a higher risk (RR = 4.16; 95% CI, 2.56–6.75) than cyclical combined use (RR = 1.94; 95% CI, 1.26–3).

Natural history of breast cancer in the elderly

It has long been thought that breast cancer in the elderly is rather indolent and a biologically less aggressive disease. Singh *et al.*[27] studied the metastatic proclivity as indicated by the virulence (defined as the rate of appearance of distant metastasis) and metastagenecity (defined as the ultimate likelihood of developing distant metastasis). They examined 2136 women who underwent mastectomy without systemic adjuvant therapy at the University of Chicago Hospitals between 1927 and 1987. The median follow-up period was 12 years. Distant disease-free survival (DDFS) was determined and virulence (V) and metastagenecity (M) were obtained from log-linear plots of DDFS. No significant difference was observed between size of primary tumour in the age groups <40, 40–70 and >70 years. Significantly, fewer women above 70 years of age presented with positive nodes. In women with negative nodes, the DDFS was higher among those aged 40–70 years, compared with those aged >70 years. However, no significant difference was observed in the DDFS in the node-positive group in any of the age categories. The 10 year DDFS for age 40–70 years was 33% and for women aged >70 years it was 38%. Among the node-negative women, V was 3% per year for age 40–70 years and also for age >70 years and M was 0.2 for age 40–70 years and 0.35 for age >70 years. In women with positive nodes, both V (11 versus 10% per year) and M (0.7 versus 0.65) were similar in both age groups. It was concluded that there was no evidence that breast cancer was more indolent in the elderly. Therefore, similar diagnostic and therapeutic efforts should be made in elderly as in younger women, the only modification being made on the basis of comorbidity.

Treatment of operable disease

The optimum treatment of breast cancer in the elderly is not yet well established. It is reasonable to apply the principles of therapy largely learned from studies in younger cohorts of women, namely breast conservation therapy (BCT) and sentinel lymph node biopsy (SLNB)/axillary clearance for smaller lesions, mastectomy for larger tumours, tamoxifen or aromatase inhibitors for ER-positive lesions and chemotherapy for node-positive or >1 cm tumours and RT for locally advanced lesions. SLNB is now the operative technique of choice for intraoperative staging of the axilla as established by major RCTs. Axillary clearance should now only be reserved for patients who are found to have biopsy- or fine-needle cytology-proven node-positive disease preoperatively or proven sentinel node metastases following an SLNB.

Unlike the treatment of younger women, which is based on sound high-level evidence from meta-analyses of large RCTs, the therapy for the elderly is not evidence based, as there is a paucity of large RCTs. Women over 65 years of age have been excluded from many trials. In order to fill this lacuna in knowledge, two European Organization for Research and Treatment of Cancer (EORTC) trials were set up. In the UK, a CRC trial and a trial at Nottingham were conducted to answer the question of what would be the best therapy for the elderly. Moreover, a decision analysis has also been performed by Punglia *et al.*[28] Truong *et al.*[29] reported an overview of the literature on BCT in elderly women with early breast cancer. They found a paucity of prospective data and numerous retrospective series of diverse treatments with conflicting results. Their observation supports BCT + postoperative RT as the standard of care for the elderly.

As mentioned previously, treatment of elderly patients with breast cancer is limited by the lack of evidence-based medicine due to the exclusion of elderly patients from clinical studies and the difficulty of decision-making in an elderly population comprising subjects with heterogeneous health backgrounds. Among cooperative group clinical trials sponsored by the National Cancer Institute for early-stage breast cancer, women aged 65 years and above constitute only 18% of participants, although they constitute 49% of the eligible pool of all newly diagnosed cases. Physicians have been incriminated as the key barrier to enrolling older women in trials.[30] The difficulty of recruitment into clinical trials aimed at elderly patients is also a major issue. A recent trial looking at the efficacy of anastrozole with or without surgery for older women with breast cancer (ESTEeM) in the UK was suspended after failing to recruit suitable patients.

Crowe *et al.*[31] reported the outcome of modified radical mastectomy (MRM) in a group of 1353 women (age range 22–75 years). The HR for death was similar in all the three age-groups (<45, 46–65 and >65 years), demonstrating that older women achieve similar results to younger ones, provided that they are treated adequately.

The Cancer Research UK Breast Cancer Trial Group[32] conducted an RCT for women over 70 years of age with operable breast cancer. Of 455 patients, from 27 hospitals in the UK, 225 were randomized to surgery + tamoxifen and 230 to receive tamoxifen alone. The analysis was based on a median follow-up of 12 years. The local control was better achieved when surgery was combined with tamoxifen. Fifty-seven patients randomized to surgery and 141 to tamoxifen alone progressed. The HR for local progression for tamoxifen compared with mastectomy was 17.24 (95% CI, 6.4–47.6) and for tamoxifen compared with BCT it was 5.99 (95% CI, 4.12–8.7). The risk of local progression was greater in the BCT arm compared with mastectomy (HR = 2.98; 95% CI, 1.06–8.39). The 5 year risk of local progression was 8% after mastectomy, 18% after breast conservation and 64% in women who had tamoxifen alone. The 10 year survival was 37.7% for surgery + tamoxifen and 28.8% for tamoxifen alone. Primary tamoxifen therapy is inferior to mastectomy and breast-conserving surgery in achieving local control. Among patients randomized to surgery + tamoxifen, the risk of local progression was greater in those who had breast conservation than in those who had a mastectomy.[32]

A Cochrane review noted that data based on an estimated 869 deaths in 1571 women were unable to show a statistically significant difference in favour of either surgery or primary endocrine therapy in respect of overall survival.[33] However, there was a statistically significant difference in terms of progression-free survival, which favoured surgery with or without endocrine therapy. The HRs for overall survival were 0.98 (95% CI, 0.74–1.30; $p = 0.9$) for surgery alone versus primary endocrine therapy and 0.86 (95% CI, 0.73–1.00; $p = 0.06$) for surgery plus endocrine therapy versus primary endocrine therapy. The HRs for progression-free survival were 0.55 (95% CI, 0.39–0.77; $p = 0.0006$) for surgery alone versus primary endocrine therapy and 0.65 (95% CI, 0.53–0.81; $p = 0.0001$) for surgery plus endocrine therapy versus primary endocrine therapy (each comparison based on only one trial). It was concluded that primary endocrine therapy should only be offered to women with ER-positive tumours who are unfit for or who refuse surgery. In a cohort of women with significant comorbid disease and ER-positive tumours, it is possible that primary endocrine therapy may be a superior option to surgery. Trials are needed to evaluate the clinical effectiveness of aromatase inhibitors as primary therapy for an infirm older population with ER-positive tumours.

Role of radiotherapy

In a study by the University of Pennsylvania of 558 women aged ≥50 years who had been treated with breast conservation and RT for Stage I and II breast cancer, there were 173 women who were aged ≥65 years. Treatment included complete gross excision of tumour, pathological axillary lymph node staging and breast irradiation. Women aged ≥65 years and those between 50 and 64 years were found to have large T2 lesions (43 versus 34%; $p = 0.05$) and ER negativity (9 versus 16%; $p = 0.13$). The proportions of axillary node positivity (24%) and also the mortality rates due to breast cancer at 10 years (13%) were similar in elderly patients and those in the 50–64 year age group. The overall survival at 10 years (77 versus 85%; $p = 0.14$), local failure (13 versus 12%; $p = 0.6$) and freedom from distant metastasis (83 versus 78%; $p = 0.45$) were similar. The study revealed that breast cancer in the elderly is not an indolent disease and has many aggressive prognostic factors. Moreover, breast-conserving surgery and RT achieves good local control and a survival comparable to that in women aged <65 years.[34]

It is thought by some that in a selected group of elderly women, RT could be avoided. Gruenberger *et al.*[35] at the University of Vienna evaluated the need for RT in a retrospective review of 356 women aged >60 years, treated by quadrantectomy + axillary dissection followed or not followed by adjuvant radiation. Among node-negative, ER-positive cases, there was no benefit of RT as the locoregional recurrence (LR) rate was 3% with or without radiation. In this subgroup (ER-positive, node-negative women), adjuvant tamoxifen reduced the LR rate to 2% with or without radiation. The authors suggested that elderly women aged ≥60 years with a T1, ER-positive, node-negative tumour may be spared the toxicity of RT when treated by conservation surgery, axillary dissection and tamoxifen.

The instigator of the Milan trials of breast conservation, Professor Umberto Veronesi of the Milan Institute has been a great proponent of breast conservation. He initially developed the technique of quadrantectomy plus radiotherapy (QUART) and later reduced the extent of resection to only lumpectomy. The results of the Milan trials were published in a meta-analysis of data from 1973 patients treated in three consecutive randomized trials by four different radiosurgical procedures: Halsted mastectomy, QUART, lumpectomy plus RT and quadrantectomy without RT).[36] The median follow-up for all patients was 82 months. The annual rates of local recurrence were 0.2 for patients treated with Halsted mastectomy, 0.46 for QUART, 2.45 for lumpectomy plus RT and 3.28 for quadrantectomy without RT. The local recurrences were much higher in women under 45 years of age than those over 55 years of age. The overall survival was identical in the four groups of patients. This study indicated that in elderly patients, lumpectomy plus RT is a satisfactory option. RT should be considered as standard treatment in fit patients, but there is some evidence that it can be omitted in certain selected cases.

Adjuvant endocrine therapy

Since the majority of tumours in postmenopausal women are ER positive, hormonal manipulation by anti-estrogen molecules or aromatase inhibitors is used with advantage in over 60% of cases. Tamoxifen has been the standard adjuvant endocrine therapy in women with breast cancer for more than 25 years. However, aromatase inhibitors including anastrazole and letrozole should now be considered as first-line therapy for all ER-positive breast cancers in postmenopausal women. Tamoxifen should only be used if an aromatase inhibitor is not tolerated or contraindicated. The recent NICE guideline (February 2009) for the management of early breast cancer also recommends the above strategy based on the results of large RCTs.

The Arimidex, Tamoxifen, Alone or in Combination (ATAC) trial was designed to compare the efficacy and safety of anastrozole (1 mg) with tamoxifen (20 mg), both given orally every day for 5 years, as adjuvant treatment for postmenopausal women with early-stage breast cancer. A proportional hazards model was used to assess the primary endpoint of disease-free survival and the secondary endpoints of time to recurrence, time to distant recurrence, incidence of new contralateral breast cancer, overall survival and death with or without recurrence in all randomized patients (anastrozole $n = 3125$, tamoxifen $n = 3116$) and hormone receptor-positive patients (anastrozole $n = 2618$, tamoxifen $n = 2598$). After completion of treatment, data on fractures and serious adverse events in a masked fashion (safety population: anastrozole $n = 3092$, tamoxifen $n = 3094$) continued to be collected. Patients were followed up for a median of 120 months (range 0–145); there were 24 522 woman-years of follow-up in the anastrozole group and 23 950 woman-years in the tamoxifen group. The study found that in the full study population, there were significant improvements in the anastrozole group compared with the tamoxifen group for disease-free survival (HR 0.91; 95% CI, 0.83–0.99; $p = 0.04$), time to recurrence (HR 0.84; 95% CI, 0.75–0.93; $p = 0.001$) and time to distant recurrence (HR 0.87; 95% CI, 0.77–0.99; $p = 0.03$). For hormone-receptor-positive patients, the results were also significantly in favour of the anastrozole group for disease-free survival (HR 0.86; 95% CI, 0.78–0.95; $p = 0.003$), time to recurrence (HR 0.79; 95% CI, 0.70–0.89; $p = 0.0002$) and time to distant recurrence (HR 0.85; 95% CI, 0.73–0.98; $p = 0.02$). In hormone receptor-positive patients, absolute differences in time to recurrence between anastrozole and tamoxifen increased over time (2.7% at 5 years and 4.3% at 10 years) and recurrence rates remained significantly lower on anastrozole than tamoxifen after completion of treatment (HR 0.81; 95% CI, 0.67–0.98; $p = 0.03$), although the carryover benefit was smaller after 8 years. There was weak evidence of fewer deaths after recurrence with anastrozole compared with tamoxifen treatment in the hormone receptor-positive subgroup (HR 0.87; 95% CI, 0.74–1.02; $p = 0.09$), but there was little difference in overall mortality (HR 0.95; 95% CI, 0.84–1.06; $p = 0.4$). Fractures were more frequent during active treatment in patients receiving anastrozole than those receiving tamoxifen (451 versus 351; OR 1.33; 95% CI, 1.15–1.55; $p < 0.0001$), but were similar in the post-treatment follow-up period (110 versus 112; OR 0.98; 95% CI, 0.74–1.30; $p = 0.9$). Treatment-related serious adverse events were less common in the anastrozole group than the tamoxifen group (223 anastrozole versus 369 tamoxifen; OR 0.57; 95% CI, 0.48–0.69; $p<0.0001$), but were similar after completion of treatment (66 versus 78; OR 0.84; 95% CI, 0.60–1.19; $p = 0.3$). No differences in non-breast cancer causes of death were apparent and the incidence of other cancers was similar between groups (425 versus 431) and continue to be higher with anastrozole for colorectal (66 versus 44) and lung cancer (51 versus 34) and lower for endometrial cancer (6 versus 24), melanoma (8 versus 19) and ovarian cancer (17 versus 28). No new safety concerns were reported. These data confirm the long-term superior efficacy and safety of anastrozole over tamoxifen as initial adjuvant therapy for postmenopausal women with hormone-sensitive early breast cancer.[37]

The Breast International Group (BIG) 1–98 study was a randomized, Phase III, double-blind trial that compared 5 years of treatment with various adjuvant endocrine therapy regimens in postmenopausal women with hormone receptor-positive breast cancer: letrozole, letrozole followed by tamoxifen, tamoxifen and tamoxifen followed by letrozole. The aromatase inhibitor letrozole is a more effective treatment for metastatic breast cancer and more effective in the neoadjuvant setting than tamoxifen. In this study, letrozole was compared with tamoxifen as adjuvant treatment for steroid hormone receptor-positive breast cancer in postmenopausal women. A total of 8010 women with data that could be assessed were enrolled, 4003 in the letrozole group and 4007 in the tamoxifen group. After a median follow-up of 25.8 months, 351 events had occurred in the letrozole group and 428 events in the tamoxifen group, with 5 year disease-free survival estimates of 84.0 and 81.4%, respectively. Compared with tamoxifen, letrozole significantly reduced the risk of an event ending a period of disease-free survival (HR 0.81; 95% CI, 0.70–0.93; $p = 0.003$), especially the risk of distant recurrence (HR 0.73; 95% CI, 0.60–0.88; $p = 0.001$). Thromboembolism, endometrial cancer and vaginal bleeding were more common in the tamoxifen group. Women given letrozole had a higher incidence of skeletal and cardiac events and of hypercholesterolaemia. The study group concluded that in postmenopausal women with endocrine-responsive breast cancer, adjuvant treatment with letrozole, as compared with tamoxifen, reduced the risk of recurrent disease, especially at distant sites.[38]

Chemotherapy

Owing to concerns about excessive toxicity, there is a negative attitude towards chemotherapy in the elderly. Hence women above 65 years of age are not included in chemotherapy trials. In the National Institute of Health (NIH) consensus, chemotherapy is recommended only for women below 70 years of age.

Allocation to about 6 months of anthracycline-based polychemotherapy [e.g. with 5-fluorouracil, adiamycin and cytoxan (FAC) or 5-fluorouracil, epirubicin and cyclophosphamide (FEC)] reduces the annual breast cancer death rate by about 38% (SE 5) for women younger than 50 years of age when diagnosed and by about 20% (SE 4) for those aged 50–69 years when diagnosed, largely irrespective of the use of tamoxifen and of ER status, nodal status or other tumour characteristics. Such regimens are significantly ($2p = 0.0001$ for recurrence, $2p < 0.00001$ for breast cancer mortality) more effective than cyclophosphamide, methotrexate and 5-fluorouracil (CMF) chemotherapy. Few women of age $\geq$70 years entered these chemotherapy trials.[39]

Recently, taxanes have been tried in older women with good tolerance. Taxanes are considered a very effective drug in breast cancer and have been tried on weekly regimens. The toxicity of weekly therapy is much lower than that of 3 weekly courses. Since there is decreased clearance of both paclitaxel and docetaxel in the elderly, it seems safer to use lower doses of weekly regimens. A dose of paclitaxel of 80 mg m^{-2} per week and docetaxel 36 mg m^{-2} per week is usually well tolerated, with impressive response. Severe neutropenia, the dose-limiting toxicity of the 3 weekly regimen, is rare in weekly therapy.[40] In a Phase II study of weekly docetaxel 36 mg m^{-2} among 47 frail or elderly patients with metastatic breast cancer, a response rate of 30% with low toxicity was achieved.[41]

A recent review on the use of cytotoxic therapy noted that even in the in the fit elderly breast cancer patient, the use of chemotherapy has been tempered with concerns regarding age, physical function and comorbid illness.[42] In the appropriate patient with biologically aggressive disease, such as receptor-poor breast cancer, it is reasonable to consider combination chemotherapy as part of an adjuvant programme. If this approach is to be employed, the physician must also consider the patient's comorbid conditions and status of function in society as potential indicators of toxicity or lack of benefit. In this case, a formal geriatric assessment is of value. A Cancer and Leukemia Group B (CALGB) trial of monotherapy versus combination cytotoxic therapy as adjuvant treatment for localized breast cancer patients over 65 years of age determined that the combination approach is superior to single-agent therapy.

In an unplanned analysis of receptor-rich and receptor-poor tumours, the patients with receptor-poor tumours seemed to achieve the greatest benefit from combination cytotoxic therapy. Adjuvant chemotherapy can also be considered for patients with high-risk receptor-rich breast cancers. However, the use of chemotherapy in the elderly patient with breast cancer is largely based upon data emerging from trials in younger patients. Studies specifically for patients over 65 years of age are urgently needed in this population to provide evidence-based proof of the current approach.

Nowadays, trastuzumab (Herceptin) can be considered along with chemotherapy for patients with HER2+ breast cancer. There is currently no evidence of efficacy of adjuvant trastuzumab without concurrent use of chemotherapy. There is evidence to suggest that capecitabine, an oral chemotherapeutic drug, is safe and effective in elderly breast cancer patients.[43]

Treatment of advanced disease

Patients with locally advanced disease need evaluation by a combined breast care team and should be offered good local control by limited surgery and radiation followed by aromatase inhibitors and chemotherapy (preferably taxanes). Women presenting with a fungating or bleeding ulcer should not be denied the benefit of limited surgical ablation and coverage of the defect with a myocutaneous flap. Palliative haemostatic fractions of radiation may help arrest bleeding. Women with dissemination of cancer need systemic chemoendocrine administration until the level of tolerance and, later, tender loving care for the debility.

Prognostic factors in elderly breast cancer

Ian Fentiman, in an editorial in the *British Journal of Surgery*,[44] pointed out that 60% of deaths from breast cancer occurred in women of age 65 years and above because of late diagnosis and treatment.

The outcome for elderly patients and the post-treatment quality of life (QOL) has been studied by a number of groups. Age has been considered an important determinant of the type of treatment and hence the outcome. In the CRUK trial, age and tumour size were found to predict mortality independently.[32]

Data from six regional National Cancer Institute Surveillance Epidemiology End Result Cancer registries evaluated a population-based random sample of 1800 patients in the age group ≥55 years. About 73% of the women presented with Stage I and II breast cancer, 10% with Stage III and IV and 17% did not have stage assignment. Of the 1017 cases with Stage I and II node-negative disease, 95% of women received therapy in agreement with NIH consensus. Patients in older age groups were less likely to receive therapy according to the consensus statement. Women aged ≥70 years were significantly less likely to receive axillary lymph node dissection. Diabetes, renal failure, stroke, liver disease and history of smoking were significant predictors of early mortality in a statistical logistic regression model that included age and disease stage. The authors concluded that patient care decision making occurs in the context of age and other comorbid conditions. Comorbidity in older patients results in smaller number of axillary dissections. As a result, information on axillary nodes is not available in many elderly patients. Breast cancer was the underlying cause of death in 51% and heart disease in 17%. The number of women receiving breast conservation therapy is also reduced and comorbidity also increases the risk of death from breast cancer.[45]

Quality of life issues

The impact of the diagnosis of breast cancer and the effect of different therapeutic modalities has been addressed by a number of authors. Kroenke *et al.*[46] of the Harvard School of Medicine and Harvard School of Public Health reported changes in physical and psychological functions before and after breast cancer by age at diagnosis. Of 122 969 women from the Nurses' Health Study (NHS) and NHS2 of age 29–71 years who responded to a pre- and postfunctional status assessment who were included, 1082 women were diagnosed with breast cancer between 1992 and 1997. Functional status was assessed using Short-Form SF-36. Mean changes in health-related quality of life (HRQOL) scores was computed. Compared with women ≤40 years of age without breast cancer, women with breast cancer experienced a functional decline. Young women who developed breast cancer experienced the largest decline in HRQOL as compared with older women in multiple domains such as physical roles, bodily pain, social functioning and mental health. Much of the decline in HRQOL was age related (age ≥65 years).

A telephone survey was conducted from a random cross-sectional sample of 1812 Medicare beneficiaries aged ≥67 years treated for breast cancer 3–5 years earlier. The QOL and satisfaction with treatment were evaluated. The use of axillary dissection was the only surgical treatment that affected outcome, increasing the risk of arm problems fourfold (95% CI, 1.56–10.51). Having arm problems exerted a negative independent effect on all outcomes. Processes of care were also associated with QOL and satisfaction. Women who perceived high levels of ageism or felt that they had no choice of treatment reported more bodily pain, lower mental health scores and less general satisfaction. These same factors and also high perceived racism were significantly associated with diminished satisfaction with the medical care system. The authors concluded that with the exception of axillary dissection, the processes of care and not the therapy itself are the most important determinants of long-term QOL in older women.[47]

Conclusion

Breast cancer in the elderly is inadequately diagnosed, with a significant delay. Many women are improperly treated, as there is a lack of practice guidelines for women above 65 years of age. Screening and prevention strategies need to be applied more rigorously to older women. The same therapeutic principles and selection criteria should be utilized as established for younger women. Breast care providers need to be cognizant of the associated illnesses and tailor therapy to suit the tolerance of the individual case.

Guidelines for therapy

The present knowledge base supports the following general guideline for the elderly:

- <4 cm tumour, ER+ → BCT + SLNB/ANC + RT + aromatase inhibitor.
- <4 cm tumour, ER− → BCT + SLNB/ANC + RT + chemotherapy; consider Herceptin.
- <4 cm tumour, ER+ → MRM + RT + aromatase inhibitor.
- <4 cm tumour, ER- → MRM + RT + chemotherapy; consider Herceptin.

Consider Herceptin in all HER+ cases who are eligible for chemotherapy. Consider downstaging for large tumours by neoadjuvant anastrozole/tamoxifen with or without chemotherapy prior to surgery. More elderly patients should be recruited in trials to expand the evidence base not confounded by ageist bias. Oncologists ought to explore newer modes of delivering less toxic chemotherapy, intraoperative radiotherapy and biological response modifiers. Interventions to address the physical and emotional needs of older women with breast cancer should be developed.

Key points

- Improve awareness among geriatric care providers for early diagnosis.
- Apply screening and prevention strategies similar to those applied to younger women to reduce the burden of disease and morbidity of therapy.
- Apply the same therapeutic principles as in younger women.
- Recruit more elderly women in therapeutic trials and develop practice guidelines.
- Be cognizant of comorbidity and tailor therapy accordingly.

References

1. Goodwin JS, Samet JM, Key CR *et al.* Stage at diagnosis of cancer varies with the age of the patient. *J Am Geriatr Soc* 1986;**34**:20–6.
2. Homes FF and Hearne E. Cancer stage-to-age relationship: implication for cancer screening in the elderly. *J Am Geriatr Soc* 1981;**29**:55–7.
3. Busch E, Kemeny M, Fremgen A *et al.* Patterns of breast cancer care in the elderly. *Cancer* 1996;**78**:101–11.
4. Gennari R, Curigliano G, Rotmensz N *et al.* Breast carcinoma in elderly women: features of disease presentation, choice of local and systemic treatments compared with younger postmenopausal patients. *Cancer* 2004;**101**:1302–10.
5. Bastiaannet E, Liefers GJ, de Craen AJ *et al.* Breast cancer in elderly compared to younger patients in The Netherlands: stage at diagnosis, treatment and survival in 127,805 unselected patients. *Breast Cancer Res Treat* 2010;**124**:801–7.
6. Rosen P, Lesser M and Linne D. Breast carcinoma at the extremes of age: a comparison of patients younger than 35 years and older than 75 years. *J Surg Oncol* 1985;**28**:90–6.
7. Law TM, Hesketh PJ, Porter KA *et al.* Breast cancer in elderly women. *Surg Clin North Am* 1996;**76**:289–308.
8. Berg JW and Robbins GF. Modified mastectomy for older, poor risk patients. *Surg Gynecol Obstet* 1961;**113**:631–4.
9. Devitt JE. The influence of age on the behaviour of carcinoma of the breast. *Can Med Assoc J* 1970;**103**:923–6.
10. Robin RE and Lee D. Carcinoma of the breast in women 80 years of age and older: still a lethal disease. *Am J Surg* 1985;**140**:606–9.
11. Davis SJ, Karrer FW, Moose BJ *et al.* Characteristics of breast cancer in women over 80 years of age. *Am J Surg* 1985;**150**:655–8.
12. Host H. Age as a prognostic factor in breast cancer. *Cancer* 1986;**57**:2217–21.
13. Morrow M. Breast disease in elderly women. *Surg Clin North Am* 1994;**74**:145–61.
14. Silliman RA. What constitutes optimal care for older women with breast cancer? *J Clin Oncol* 2003;**21**:3554–6.
15. Bouchardy C, Rapiti E, Fioretta G *et al.* Undertreatment strongly decreases prognosis of breast cancer in elderly women. *J Clin Oncol* 2003;**21**:3580–7.
16. Lavelle K, Todd C, Moran A *et al.* Non-standard management of breast cancer increases with age in the UK: a population based cohort of women > or = 65 years. *Br J Cancer* 2007;**96**:1197–203.
17. Hancke K, Denkinger MD, König J *et al.* Standard treatment of female patients with breast cancer decreases substantially for women aged 70 years and older: a German clinical cohort study. *Ann Oncol* 2009;**21**:748–53.

18. Velanovich V, Gabel M, Walker EM *et al.* Causes for the undertreatment of elderly breast cancer patients: tailoring treatments to individual patients. *J Am Coll Surg* 2002;**194**:8–13.
19. Nicolucci A, Mainini F, Penna A *et al.* The influence of patient characteristics on the appropriateness of surgical treatment for breast cancer patients. *Ann Oncol* 1993;**4**:133–40.
20. Feinstein AR. The pre-therapeutic classification of co-morbidity in chronic disease. *J Chron Dis* 1970;**23**:455–68.
21. de Groot V, Beckerman H, Lankhorst GJ and Bouter LM. How to measure comorbidity: a critical review of available methods. *J Clin Epidemiol* 2003;**56**:221–9.
22. Herman CJ, Speroff T and Cebul RD. Improving compliance with breast cancer screening in older women. *Arch Intern Med* 1995;**155**:717–22.
23. Chen H-H, Tabar L, Faggerberg G and Duffy SW. Effect of breast screening after age 65. *J Med Screen* 1995;**2**:10–4.
24. Wang J, Costanino JP, Tan-Chiu E *et al.* Lower-category benign breast disease and the risk of invasive breast cancer. *J Natl Cancer Inst* 2004;**96**:616–20.
25. Million Women Study Collaborators. Breast cancer and hormone replacement therapy in the million women study. *Lancet* 2003;**362**:419–27.
26. Stahlberg C, Pedersen AT, Lynge E *et al.* Increased risk of breast cancer following different regimens of hormone replacement therapy frequently used in Europe. *Int J Cancer* 2004;**109**:721–7.
27. Singh R, Hellman S and Heimann R. The natural history of breast carcinoma in the elderly, implications for screening and treatment. *Cancer* 2004;**100**:1807–13.
28. Punglia RS, Kuntz KM, Lee JH and Recht A. Radiation therapy plus tamoxifen versus tamoxifen alone after breast-conserving surgery in postmenopausal women with stage I breast cancer: a decision analysis. *J Clin Oncol* 2003;**21**:2260–7.
29. Truong PT, Wong E, Bernstein V *et al.* Adjuvant radiation therapy after breast-conserving surgery in elderly women with early-stage breast cancer: controversy or consensus? *Clin Breast Cancer* 2004;**4**:407–14.
30. Kemeny MM, Peterson BL, Kornblith AB *et al.* Barriers to clinical trial participation by older women with breast cancer. *J Clin Oncol* 2003;**21**:2268–75.
31. Crowe JP, Gordon NH, Shenk RR *et al.* Age does not predict breast cancer outcome. *Arch Surg* 1994;**129**:483–8.
32. Fennessy M, Bates T, MacRae K *et al.* Late follow-up of a randomized trial of surgery plus tamoxifen versus tamoxifen alone in women aged over 70 years with operable breast cancer. *Br J Surg* 2004;**91**:699–704.
33. Hind D, Wyld L, Beverley C *et al.* Surgery versus primary endocrine therapy for operable primary breast cancer in elderly women (70 years plus). *Cochrane Database Syst Rev* 2006;(1): CD004272.
34. Solin LJ, Schultz DJ and Fowble BL. Ten year results of the treatment of early stage breast carcinoma in elderly women using breast-conserving surgery and definitive breast irradiation. *Int J Radiat Oncol Biol Phys* 1995;**33**:45–51.
35. Gruenberger T, Gorlitzer M, Soliman T *et al.* It is possible to omit postoperative irradiation in a highly selected group of elderly breast cancer patients. *Breast Cancer Res Treat* 1998;**50**:37–46.
36. Veronesi U, Salvadori B, Luini A *et al.* Breast conservation is a safe method in patients with small cancer of the breast. Long-term results of three randomised trials on 1,973 patients. *Eur J Cancer* 1995;**31A**:1574–9.
37. Cuzick J, Sestak I, Baum M *et al.* Effect of anastrozole and tamoxifen as adjuvant treatment for early-stage breast cancer: 10-year analysis of the ATAC trial. *Lancet Oncol* 2010;**11**:1135–41.
38. Thürlimann B, Keshaviah A, Coates AS *et al.* A comparison of letrozole and tamoxifen in postmenopausal women with early breast cancer. *N Engl J Med* 2005;**353**:2747–57.
39. Early Breast Cancer Trialists' Collaborative Group (EBCTCG). Effects of chemotherapy and hormonal therapy for early breast cancer on recurrence and 15-year survival: an overview of the randomised trials. *Lancet* 2005;**365**:1687–717.
40. Wildiers H and Paridaens R. Taxanes in elderly breast cancer patients. *Cancer Treat Rev* 2004;**30**:333–42.
41. D'hondt R, Paridaens R, Wildiers H *et al.* Safety and efficacy of weekly docetaxel in frail and/or elderly patients with metastatic breast cancer: a phase II study. *Anticancer Drugs* 2004;**15**:341–6.
42. Leung M, Shapira I, Bradley T *et al.* Adjuvant chemotherapy for early breast cancer in the elderly. *Curr Treat Options Oncol* 2009;**10**:144–58.
43. Bajetta E, Procopio G, Celio L *et al.* Safety and efficacy of two different doses of capecitabine in the treatment of advanced breast cancer in older women. *J Clin Oncol* 2005;**23**:2155–61.
44. Fentiman IS. Improving the outcome for older women with breast cancer. *Br J Surg* 2004;**91**:655–6.
45. Yancik R, Wesley MN, Ries LAG *et al.* Effect of age and comorbidity in postmenopausal breast cancer patients aged 55 years and older. *JAMA* 2001;**285**:885–92.
46. Kroenke CH, Rosner B, Chen WY *et al.* Functional impact of breast cancer by age at diagnosis. *J Clin Oncol* 2004;**22**: 1849–56.
47. Mandelblatt JS, Edge SB, Meropol NJ *et al.* Predictor of long-term outcomes in older breast cancer survivors: perceptions versus patterns of care. *J Clin Oncol* 2003;**21**:855–63.

CHAPTER 111

Maintaining functional status

Miriam B. Rodin
Saint Louis University Medical Center, St Louis, MO, USA

Introduction

Cancers are largely diseases of ageing. The most recent SEER (Surveillance, Epidemiology and End Results) summaries through 2006 show that 61% of all cancers occur in people over age 65 years, an important fact for Medicare in the USA and similar health insurance programmes elsewhere. Age-specific rates continue to rise well into the ninth decade of life. Even though cancer mortality in the elderly is also higher and 71% of all cancer deaths occur in people of Medicare age, there are nonetheless 6.5 million cancer survivors over age 65 years, of whom 4.4 million are long-term, that is, >5 year, survivors. Therefore population studies of cancer and cancer survivorship are studies of ageing.[1,2]

Cancer is the leading cause of death for men and women aged 60–79 years, followed by heart disease. This is reversed among those aged 80 years and over, with heart disease causing more deaths than cancer.[3] Table 111.1 shows that cancer as a cause of death declines in importance relative to cardiovascular diseases in advanced old age.[3] As shown in Table 111.2, among the 10 most common cancers affecting adults, by a wide margin breast, prostate, lung and colon cancer occur mostly among the elderly.

In Table 111.3, it can be seen that the common cancers have good prospects for prolonged survival. All except lung cancer, if detected at an early stage, have better than a 50% 5 year survival.[3] Therefore, the goal of optimizing physical and mental function for elderly cancer patients and survivors affects hundreds of thousands of people. Treatment protocols tested in clinical trials have included few if any elderly participants over age 70 years, so individualizing cancer treatment for elderly patients requires individualizing functional assessments also.[4]

A role for geriatricians in cancer care

There is a strong referral bias for more fit elderly people in cancer clinical samples.[5] Clinical decision-making in cancer is further complicated by marked under-representation of elderly persons in cancer clinical trials.[6] Analyses of population treatment data through the linked SEER–Medicare database suggest that frail elderly people are unlikely to be referred to cancer specialists in community practice. Hurria *et al.*[7] performed standard geriatric functional screening on elderly CALGB trial enrollees and found that functional impairment defined as any ADL (activity of daily living), IADL (instrumental activity of daily living) or cognitive deficit was rare. For example, Gupta and Lamont[8] showed that the proportion of elderly with a diagnosis of dementia was lower among Medicare beneficiaries treated for colon cancer than in the general population. More recently, Lamont *et al.* used the SEER–Medicare database to compare treatment outcomes in community practice with those of trial participants and found that poorer results in the community treatment cohorts were not entirely explained by comorbidities.[9] Either trial participants were fitter regardless of comorbidity or receiving treatment through a trials centre conferred better clinical management.

Balducci adapted the consensus frailty phenotype as defined by Fried and co-workers'[10,11] to making decisions about cancer therapy.[12] He included ADL and IADL disability, non-cancer severe comorbidity and presence of 'geriatric syndromes' including cognitive impairment, falls and delirium as probably excluding an older cancer patient from receiving full dose or any chemotherapy.[12] Further, he effectively explained in terms of cancer-related life expectancy why frail elderly patients may be harmed with highly toxic therapy. There appears to be a tacit agreement in community practice not to subject obviously frail and otherwise incapacitated elderly people to toxic therapy.

The role of geriatrics in these decisions is to identify vulnerabilities that are not evident in apparently well elderly subjects, to prescribe and provide supportive interventions for patients with good prognosis cancers, to participate in the transition from disease control to symptom palliation and to communicate clearly with patients and families when the trajectory of disease is approaching end-of-life.

Principles and Practice of Geriatric Medicine, Fifth Edition. Edited by Alan J. Sinclair, John E. Morley and Bruno Vellas.

Table 111.1 Five leading causes of death: US men and women aged 60 years and older, 2009.

Age 60–79 years		Age 80 years and older	
Men	Women	Men	Women
Cancer	Cancer	Heart disease	Heart disease
Heart disease	Heart disease	Cancer	Cancer
COPD	COPD	Stroke	Stroke
Stroke	Stroke	COPD	Alzheimer's disease
Diabetes	Diabetes	Alzheimer's disease	COPD

Table 111.2 Five most common sites of cancer mortality: US adults, 2009.

Age 60–79 years		Age 80 years and older	
Men	Women	Men	Women
Lung	Lung	Lung	Lung
Colon	Breast	Prostate	Colon
Prostate	Colon	Colon	Breast
Pancreas	Pancreas	Urinary bladder	Pancreas
Oesophagus	Ovary	Pancreas	Non-Hodgkin's lymphoma

Table 111.3 Percentage 5+ year survival by cancer site, 1996–2004.

Cancer site	Survival rate (%)
All cancers	66
Prostate	99
Breast	89
Urinary bladder	81
Rectal	67
Colon	65
Non-Hodgkin's lymphoma	65
Ovarian	46
Oesophagus	17
Lung and bronchus	16
Multiple myeloma	16
Pancreas	5

Additionally, geriatricians inevitably care for long-term cancer survivors. Survivorship care entails awareness of cancer-specific sequelae. Survivors experience continuing adverse health for years after the event compared with those who never had a malignancy.[13,14] Ganz and Hahn[15] and others[16,17] therefore proposed specific survivorship care plans that go beyond mere surveillance for recurrences.

Functional status as used by geriatricians refers to activities of daily living (ADL), the ability to care for oneself at home, and instrumental ADL (IADL), the ability to live alone and manage one's own household affairs. This is different from oncologists' construct of performance status, which has more to do with exercise tolerance, grading activity levels from fully physically active outside the home to bedbound. Using a summary Karnofsky Performance Score (KPS)[17] or Eastern Cooperative Oncology Group Performance Score (ECOG-PS), oncologists make very accurate predictions about survival and ability to tolerate toxic therapies. Summary KPS or ECOG scores, however, are relatively insensitive to risk for functional decline and fail to identify the so-called vulnerable elderly. The summary scores do not identify specific functional disabilities that might be reversible, nor do they suggest how that might be done.[18] A short functionally based screening such as the ACOVE VES-13 has been proposed as a quick way to select apparently fit elderly cancer patients for further evaluation.[19,20] A more extensive battery of screening tools has been shown to be feasible to perform in the outpatient oncology setting.[7] Several studies have suggested that abbreviated geriatric measures of function provide actionable data.[21] For example, Extermann *et al.* addressed fall risk reduction for breast cancer patients.[22] Bylow *et al.* established a high prevalence of previously under-reported falls among prostate cancer patients on hormonal deprivation therapy.[23]

There have yet to be any randomized trials to test whether routine geriatric assessment could improve patient tolerance of cancer therapy. Cohen *et al.* reported a randomized clinical trial of continuity of care for geriatric veterans who received inpatient geriatric assessment and intervention with follow-up in outpatient GEM (geriatric evaluation and management) and home-based care.[24] *Post hoc* subgroup analysis revealed that older veterans with a cancer diagnosis benefited the most from geriatric continuum of care. Although they did not live longer, quality of life measures were statistically significantly improved.[25]

Staging the ageing of the elderly cancer patient

Cancer treatment often involves sequencing multimodal interventions including surgery, chemotherapy and radiation. There are several key aspects of geriatric assessment that are particularly salient for patients and physicians planning surgical cancer treatment. In addition to standard preoperative risk stratification, preoperative assessments should be able to anticipate whether subacute care[26,27] at home or at a long-term care facility (LTCF) will be needed. The goal is to prevent SNF placement but if it becomes necessary, selecting a LTCF or SNF (skilled nursing facility) on the day of discharge is disconcerting for families and patients. Since it is usually predictable, shopping for acceptable facilities should begin early. If surgery will involve the head and neck or a long intubation, facilities' capacity to provide specialized oral care and speech and swallow therapies should be considered carefully, not just their ability to provide tracheostomy care. Nutritional support and evaluation are required to re-establish oral feeding.[28] Furthermore, early feeding when possible with use of protein–calorie supplements have been shown to improve surgical outcomes in elderly surgical patients.[29] Cancer surgery outcomes for the elderly are improved by early mobilization and early nutritional support.[26,27]

Use structured methods to establish decisional capacity prior to treatment

If chemotherapy is contemplated, geriatric assessments should be performed proactively to determine the patient's decisional capacity, that is, whether the patient is cognizant of the risks and benefits of the alternative courses. If there is any doubt, formal evaluation of decisional capacity is mandatory.[30] If decisional capacity is impaired, this should be factored into treatment decisions since at all stages of disease, cognitively impaired patients fare substantially worse.[8,31] Unrecognized cognitive impairment[32] and delirium[33] are common in elderly cancer patients. The complexity of the decision to be made needs to be titrated to the patient's cognitive capacity. There are four established legal standards for determining capacity: the patient is aware of the treatment options and expresses a treatment preference clearly and consistently; the patient can give a conventionally understandable reason that is consistent with their past behaviour; the patient retains and reproduces the information given as the context for the decision; the patient understands what their decision means for their own state of health.[30]

Figure 111.1 shows a schematic diagram of the decisional standard required to consent to each level of therapy offered. Physically robust, cognitively intact older patients have been shown to derive equal benefit from equal treatment in clinical trials and should not therefore be excluded from standard therapy and clinical trials on age alone.[6,34–36] Therefore, staging the ageing is as important as staging the cancer.

The diagonal axis in Figure 111.1 describes the ratio of risk to benefit for the course of treatment. The hierarchy of legal standards used to determine decisional capacity is arrayed on the y-axis. Usual care and clinical trials are marked on the diagonal suggesting the standard required for consent. Cancer care options are inclusive from least to most risky.

The short term impact of chemotherapy on functional capacity should be assessed proactively. Is the patient at risk for delirium? This bears directly on the patient's

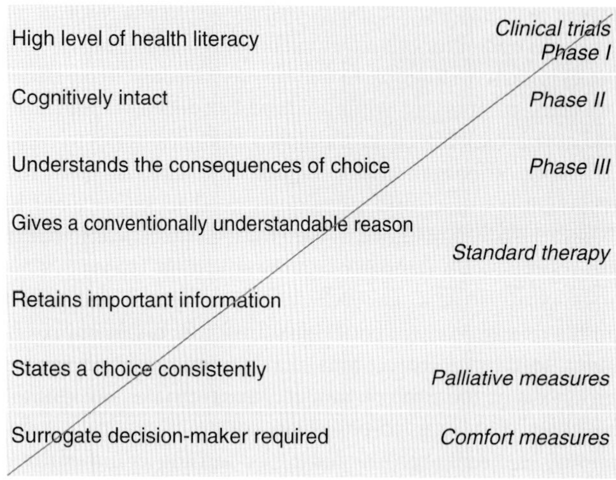

Figure 111.1 Matching the complexity of clinical decision-making to the decisional capacity of the patient.

ability to self-manage chemotherapy-associated toxicities, medications and nutrition. What is the patient's home support system? An elderly person living alone who manages fairly well in their usual state of health is judged fit for chemotherapy by having an ECOG-PS of 2 or less. They are likely to do well in the infusion suite but may develop problems with delayed toxicities. It is critical that spousal, family or pre-emptive home care supports be put in place to prevent unplanned hospitalizations due to falls, delirium, malnutrition and volume depletion. The National Cancer Care Network (NCCN), which represents the largest number of community-based cancer treatment centres, has adopted these recommendations as part of its body of treatment guidelines for specific cancer sites in the elderly. An extensive summary statement of the evidence for these guidelines has been prepared by the International Society for Geriatric Oncology (SIOG) based in Geneva.[18]

Although numerous studies have reported that fit elderly patients tolerate cancer therapy without undue acute toxicities, elderly cancer patients have several specific chemotherapeutic risk factors. Dosing must be adjusted for reduced renal and hepatic function. Still, it has been well described that elderly patients experience more severe and more prolonged neutropenia from cytotoxic agents. Although studies are not entirely consistent, the NCCN has also recommends prophylactic use of granulocyte colony-stimulating factors to prevent neutropenia in elderly patients based on a high incidence of severe bone marrow toxicity observed in the elderly in clinical trials and increased risk for sepsis.[37,38] With the high risk for delirium, the use of 'prn' ('when necessary') advice to an elderly patient living alone, even with 'drop-ins', is simply not adequate. Outpatient management must prevent hospitalizations for toxicities which can spiral into loss of functional capacity and nursing home placement. Elderly cancer patients should be vigilantly screened for risk of delirium and clinical suspicion should be high.[32]

Giving chemotherapy to a long-stay resident in an LTCF presents an array of complex medical decisions and ethical concerns. However, short-stay SNF residents may be receiving outpatient chemotherapy and radiation and the responsible nurses and physicians need to know what to expect. Hence transitions of care for elderly cancer patients are fraught with danger of communication lapses.[39] This is especially true since SNF care assumes, indeed based on the reimbursement codes, requires, functional improvement. Without a correct and clearly communicated cancer prognosis at the time of transfer, appropriate care cannot be given. Physician-to-physician communication by telephone, electronic record-sharing or writing is imperative. Prognostic errors go both ways, unrealistically optimistic and pessimistic, on both sides. The idea that an elderly patient with any malignancy is hospice appropriate can be as mistaken as the idea that a patient with an untreatable advanced malignancy can be functionally upgraded.

It often falls to the long-term care physician to state what was not clearly understood at hospital discharge. Over 65% of oncologists report that they do not routinely discuss prognosis, advance directives or end-of-life until the patient is within days to weeks of death. This contrasts with younger oncology physicians who report having these discussions before the need.[40] There is an interesting correspondence with patient preference in this study. A similar >60% of cancer patients preferred not to have these discussions with their oncologists; rather, they expressed no unwillingness to discuss advance directives and end-of-life with hospital doctors, which means typically hospitalists and house staff.[40]

Supportive management during cancer treatment is just good geriatric care

Supportive oncology is the branch of palliative medicine that addresses the management of symptoms due to cancer and to the debilitating effects of cancer treatment with the goal of maintaining patients' quality of life. All major cancer centres have invested in supportive care because it offers the best chance for patients to be able to complete treatment. When treatments fail and cancer progresses, supportive oncology manages the transition to hospice.

Four randomized clinical trials have compared palliative care delivered with cancer treatment to usual care with optional palliative referral as determined by the treating physician. Patients with advanced cancer in rural Vermont, $N = 322$, mean age about 65 years, were randomized to psychoeducational intervention with monthly telephone follow-up by advanced practice nurses. At the end of the study, quality of life and mood scores were higher in the intervention group, but there was no difference in symptom intensity or hospital days.[41] Two additional trials also showed improvements in self-reported quality of life among patients randomized to palliative care along with usual cancer care, but the differences were not statistically significant.[42,43] Similarly, a Norwegian trial was suggestive but inconclusive.[44] A more recent study reported that 151 advanced-stage lung cancer outpatients were randomized to concurrent palliative care or usual care. The mean age was again about 65 years. Mean change scores on symptom scales and quality of life scales favoured the experimental group, but the differences were not statistically significant. The experimental group survived on average 2.7 months (30%) longer and used fewer hospital days at the end-of-life.[45] One reason for the more definitive findings of this study is that participants were more homogeneous in terms of type and stage of disease and therefore had less variance in clinical course. Previous studies mixed different cancers and stages and lacked statistical power due to small numbers.

As with randomized controlled trials (RCTs) of geriatric interventions, it may not be possible to identify which interventions explain the results. That is, both GEM and palliative care involve multiple disciplines individualizing care, doing different things for each patient. This is a profoundly unsettling model of care for physicians trained to use drug trials of single agents, multidrug protocols in the case of oncology, to decide what works. It is unsettling to rely on questionnaire responses as endpoints over so-called 'hard' end-points such as disease progression, hospitalization and death. If similarly designed studies reproduce the finding of less hospitalization and longer survival, it shows that it is feasible to develop 'harder' evidence.

In the supporting oncology literature, it is clear that the burden of symptoms and also the stage of disease drive functional status. Targeting the most troublesome symptoms should improve functional status. The caveat in this literature is that the outcome measures, the portfolio of standardized symptom scales, are different from the functional geriatric measures, they are subjective, the numbers are small, patients are not particularly old and a variety of tumour types and stages are reported. The construct 'quality of life' includes functional status and a number of other things such as satisfaction, mood and energy. One review enumerated over 100 different definitions of quality of life.[46] It is easier to focus on studies of specific symptoms to sort out how treating that symptom affects quality of life, however it is defined. For example, a recently reported RCT of preventive treatment for chemotherapy-associated mucositis showed a significant drop in unplanned hospitalizations in the experimental group who reported less pain and better nutrition.[47]

In keeping with the purpose of this chapter, to focus on maintaining function and not on end-of-life, the next section addresses specific symptoms that occur during cancer treatment, including pain, fatigue, nausea and vomiting and anorexia. Successful management of these symptoms can make the difference between loss of functional independence due to treatment and obtaining the benefit of treatment. The reader is referred to an excellent summary by Rao and Cohen.[48] Geriatricians immediately recognize the fatigue–anorexia symptom complex as age-related frailty. Supportive modalities include pharmacological agents, mind–body alternatives, rehabilitation and cognitive behavioural strategies. The following section looks at randomized trials of pharmacological agents. This is not intended to dismiss non-pharmacological, alternative and mind–body interventions. The level of evidence for these is weak but improving, reflecting the difficulty in designing and conducting trials of complex interventions. Readers are by no means dissuaded from trying them with willing patients.

Follow AGS guidelines to treat pain in the elderly cancer patient

There is not much more to be said about treating pain. People, patients, everyone functions better when the pain is treated. There is no plausible rationale for not treating pain, only that there may be different ways to treat pain and patients may differ in how aggressively they wish to be treated for pain. Cancer pain is complex. It is both nociceptive and neuropathic. There may be components of anxiety and depression. There are specific pain syndromes associated with surgeries, with radiation and tumour invasion plexopathies, bone pain and visceral pain, post-chemotherapeutic neuropathies and oral pain from mucositis. To the specialist, each has an appropriate treatment. Patients with specific surgical pain syndromes should be referred to specialist care, including head-and-neck centres, interventional pain clinics and postoperative rehabilitation centres.

The mainstay of cancer pain management has been the WHO approach to titrating non-opiate and opiate therapy.[49] The AGS pain management guidelines focus on how to assess pain in frail or cognitively impaired elderly and on caregiver education to recognize and treat pain.[50] Most moderate to severe cancer pain will respond to opiates. In the elderly, the conventional wisdom is to expect a higher peak effect due to a lower number of neural receptor sites (saturation) and a longer duration of action due to slower elimination. An advantage of opiates is the lower likelihood of gastrointestinal (GI) bleeding or renal failure compared with non-steroidal anti-inflammatory drugs (NSAIDS), but NSAIDS are particularly useful for bone pain. There is a higher risk for delirium, falls, nausea and constipation with opiates. In general, opiates with complex metabolism and active metabolites should be avoided, including meperidine, propoxyphene, fentanyl patches and methadone.[50] The geriatric practice of choosing the least number of agents by the least invasive route at the lowest dose is good advice with opiates. In general, short-acting agents are to be preferred, such as immediate-release morphine, oxycodone and hydromorphone, titrated under close scrutiny, especially for patients with impaired executive and short-term memory function. Opiates should always be accompanied by a bowel regimen to prevent constipation. Sennosides with stool softeners and osmotic agents together are preferred. Severe opiate bowel may precipitate hospitalizations. Methylnaltrexone is an injectable which blocks mu-opiate receptors in the bowel that does not cross the blood–brain barrier. It can be used for bowel rescue when oral agents fail.

Once the best level of pain relief versus sedation has been achieved, short-acting agents can be converted to a long-acting agent with breakthrough coverage using one of many available conversion tables or calculators. Adjuvants for neuropathic pain should be selected for lowest anticholinergic burden and evidence-based supporting literature. Consideration should be given to topicals, such as lidocaine gels and sports creams. Therapeutic massages, heat, cold, oral rinses and focused physical therapy all have a role. For example, moderate weight lifting proved superior to usual protective advice in reducing post-mastectomy lymphoedema pain in middle-aged women without affecting the actual volume of fluid retained.[51]

Treat fatigue in elderly cancer patients to limit functional decline

Considerable research has gone into understanding the non-pain symptoms of cancer and cancer therapy. Whether fatigue is the cause or the effect, elderly cancer patients who report extreme fatigue also report poor nutritional intake, poor sleep, immobility and loss of functional capacity.[52,53] Extreme fatigue is often a reason given for terminating cancer treatment. There are no specific diagnostic features to distinguish the fatigue of cancer from the fatigue of primary frailty. Both are characterized by unregulated cytokine production.[54] However, cancer fatigue generally dates to the clinical onset of cancer or to cancer treatment. Students of fatigue describe a multicomponent disturbance of neuroendocrine regulation, cytokine peripheral and central effects including depression and diurnal cycle dysregulation.[53] The association between cancer fatigue and anaemia is not as strong as initially thought, although severe anaemia certainly exacerbates fatigue. It has also been difficult to show a simple association between stage of disease and severity of fatigue or between specific treatment modalities and fatigue.[53] A follow-up study of clinical trial participants found that fatigue persisted years after the completion of presumably successful cancer treatment.[55] There is no consistent association between cancer fatigue and age.[52,53]

Fatigue outranks pain as a symptom for cancer patients.[52,55,56] It is a common complaint among frail elderly people who do not have cancer. Fatigue has been hard to define and hard to treat as it is embedded in a complex cluster of symptoms and disease-related perturbations. It has to be evaluated in the context of the disease trajectory and untangled from cancer-related anaemia, cancer treatment-related anaemia, radiation sickness and radiation-induced hypothyroidism, depression, disturbed sleep and undernutrition. Nonetheless, clinicians believe that it is a distinct cytokine-related syndrome. Studies have tried to define it and measure it so that it may be quantified. NCCN adopted a narrative definition: 'a persistent, subjective sense of physical, emotional and/or cognitive tiredness or exhaustion (related to cancer or cancer treatment) that is not proportional to recent activity and *that significantly interferes with usual functioning*'.[57,58] Provisional ICD-10 criteria for the E&M code include six of the following complaints: weakness, heaviness in the limbs, subjective problems with concentration and short-term memory, no motivation to participate in activities, a subjective sense of having to struggle to get moving, not getting the usual daily tasks done, feeling bad rather than pleasantly tired for several hours after exercise, sleeping too much or not enough and never feeling refreshed after sleep.[59] Minton *et al.* reviewed available standardized, validated fatigue screening and severity scales.[60–62]

Fatigue is worsened by depression. Depression is underdiagnosed among cancer patients.[61] Mor *et al.* have shown that elderly breast cancer patients are less likely to suffer from new onset depression than younger breast cancer patients.[62] However, in evaluating an elderly patient with fatigue, depression should be addressed routinely and explicitly.[18]

Symptomatic anaemia is treatable and should be treated in elderly patients, particularly those with underlying coronary artery disease (CAD), congestive heart failure (CHF), chronic obstructive pulmonary disease (COPD) or increasing exertional dyspnoea. In one study, correction of anaemia with erythropoietin improved FACT-Fatigue scores but only if FACT-Anemia was also positive.[63] Recent clinical studies have dimmed hopes that erythropoietin supplementation for cancer-associated anaemias would solve the fatigue problem and have additional functional and survival benefits.[64] Transfusion or correction above 9–10 g dl^{-1} offered no further symptomatic improvement and increased the risk for thromboembolic and cardiac events.[65]

Research on the treatment of fatigue has focused on psychostimulants. The best studied is methylphenidate. A double-blinded placebo-controlled randomized trial of short-acting methylphenidate in cancer patients demonstrated improvement and maximum effect within 8 days and a sustained effect over the 4 weeks of the trial that was durable for up to 6 months on drug as measured by the Brief Fatigue Inventory (BFI). However, there was no statistically significant difference between the treated arm and the placebo arm except among patients with BFI-rated >6, severe fatigue.[66] Sustained-release methylphenidate showed benefit equivalent to short-acting methylphenidate in a trial enrolling patients undergoing cancer treatment and was also not different from placebo except among the subgroup of patients with BFI >6, severe fatigue.[67] A head-to-head comparison of methylphenidate and modafinil favoured methylphenidate.[68] Two trials have been reported that tested whether donepezil effectively addresses the cognitive component of cancer-related fatigue. Patients treated with donepezil reported 56% improvement of fatigue symptoms, not different from placebo.[69] A randomized trial of placebo versus 'no-cebo' reported 56% improvement of fatigue symptoms on placebo versus 36% on 'no-cebo'.[70] In summary, if there are no contraindications, methylphenidate appears to be safe for a trial of treatment for severe cancer-related or cancer treatment-related fatigue in elderly patients.

Anticipate anorexia, recognize cachexia and support nutrition

Anorexia means loss of appetite. Loss of appetite and distortions of taste commonly occur in cancer patients and it is critical to determine whether the symptoms are due to the cancer or to cancer treatment. If anorexia causes failure to eat and weight loss, and the patient is not at end-of-life due to the cancer, it is reasonable to try to stimulate appetite and nutritional intake.[29,71] The key differential diagnosis is to recognize cancer cachexia, a cytokine-mediated hypercatabolic state in which both fat and muscle are degraded. Cytokines have central effects on appetite and peripheral effects on metabolism.[72–74] Cancer cachexia, unlike protein–calorie starvation, is not reversible solely with nutritional interventions.[75] Some cancers induce cachexia early in their course and treating the cancer may induce a brief period of remission with improved appetite and possible modest weight gain. Pancreatic cancer is highly inflammatory and is one such example. Among the common solid tumours including non-small-cell lung, prostate, breast and colon, rapid weight loss occurs late in advanced disease and signals impending death. Haematological malignancies in general do not precipitate cachexia, although immunotherapies may.

In starvation, resting energy expenditure declines and metabolism slows to divert available calories to high-priority end-users such as the brain and heart. Patients with very poor intake can sometimes maintain a remarkable level of physical activity. Hence it is crucial to differentiate weight loss due to cachexia from just poor nutritional intake with or without anorexia. In cancer patients, there may be physical causes for not eating even if hungry. Mucositis, radiation oesophagitis, diarrhoea and nausea, surgical interruption of the GI tract, pain, sedation and drug effects affect eating. Families are often more anxious about disturbances of appetite than the patient in the author's experience. Treating proximal symptoms can improve intake. High caloric density snacks and liquid protein–calorie supplements are easy to consume and not over-filling.

Anorexia has been the subject of a number of randomized clinical trials. There are four basic classes of orexigenics. Corticosteroids, dexamethasone 4 mg 1–4 times per day or prednisone 5–10 mg per day initially induces a mild euphoria, suppresses nausea and may increase appetite. The risks include further immune suppression, Cushingoid changes with long use, myopathies, HPA (hypothalamic–pituitary–adrenal) axis suppression and hyperglycaemia.[76] There is no convincing evidence that they cause weight gain with short-term use and the weight gained with prolonged use is largely fat and water. The progestationals are the best studied orexigenics. These include megestrol acetate 400–800 mg per day or medroxyprogesterone 500 mg twice daily.[76] As shown by Yeh *et al.* in an RCT that did not include cancer patients, frail veterans did gain weight and the maximum effect was seen by 12 weeks of treatment. After 1 year there was no difference in the weight of the experimental and control groups.[77] On treatment, participants had lowered cytokine levels.[78] There is an increased risk of venous thromboembolism with progestationals and potential for HPA suppression, so they should be tapered once the treatment goal has been reached or stopped if no response is obtained after 12 weeks.

Cannabinoids include medical marijuana, which is not usually considered for elderly patients regardless of diagnosis, and dronabinol 2.5–20 mg twice daily. One widely cited study of advanced HIV patients showed improved appetite but no weight gain after 1 year.[79] A head-to-head comparison of megestrol acetate (MA) and dronabinol in 469 cancer patients was reported. The 73% of patients randomized to MA reported better appetite and 13% gained >10% of their starting weight compared with 47% and 3%, respectively, in the dronabinol group. There was no added benefit to combining the drugs and the older patients did not tolerate the dronabinol.[80] Recent reports suggest a role for the novel GI peptide ghrelin in managing cancer-related anorexia.[81,82] A number of novel agents, including SARMs (selective androgen receptor modulators) and anti-TNF (tumour necrosis factor) antibodies, have been studied in small numbers of subjects and second-look studies of atypical antipsychotics, thalidomide and anabolic steroids including oxandrolone are under way, but so far definitive evidence is lacking.[83]

Anticipate and prevent nausea and vomiting

Nausea and vomiting are a normal part of the host defence system among omnivores and carnivores that is not shared by ungulates. It is designed to rid the body of toxic ingested substances. The physiology of nausea is shown in Figure 111.2. The area postrema at the base of the fourth ventricle where the blood–brain barrier is permeable provides early central sensing of toxins in the bloodstream. Stimuli are forwarded to the vomiting centre in the medulla to coordinate the vomiting reflex with feedback to the upper GI tract. Central causes of nausea and vomiting include increased intracranial pressure, vestibular toxicity, motion sickness, acid–base disorders, electrolyte disturbances, chemotherapy and anxiety, so-called anticipatory nausea and vomiting. Elderly patients have been described as less likely to suffer from anticipatory nausea and vomiting than younger patients.[84] Many anticancer drugs cause nausea and vomiting.[85] Opiates are also highly likely to cause nausea and vomiting, particularly in the opiate-naïve patient and when doses are rapidly escalated.

Chemotherapeutic agents are ranked as minimally to highly emetogenic and infusion therapists generally incorporate premedication into the protocol to prevent acute chemotherapy-induced nausea and vomiting (CINV).[85] Perhaps because of less anxiety or because of the selection of less toxic chemotherapeutic agents, elderly cancer patients appear to suffer less with acute CINV. Delayed CINV is also well described and it is a more serious problem for elderly cancer patients. Around 4–10 days after chemotherapy, it is caused by a combination of central and peripheral disturbances and by direct GI tract toxicity. Specific toxicities include oral and pharyngeal pain, digestive endothelial mucosal injury due to cytotoxins and antimetabolites, radiation, increased vagal tone, autonomic failure, hiccups associated with phrenic nerve and diaphragmatic irritation. Gastritis, gastric reflux and gastroparesis cause nausea. These problems are often accompanied by severe diarrhoea and a high risk for volume depletion, falls, delirium and injury.

Elderly patients undergoing chemotherapy should not be left alone or treated with prn measures during this vulnerable period. When the acute infusions go well it may be assumed that there is no further problem. An able caregiver should be present at all times and preventive treatment of side effects should involve scheduled dosing, not as needed. Non-pharmacological treatment has limited efficacy. Small, frequent snacks of preferred foods and liquids may be all that is tolerated. The choice of drugs should be identified as closely as possible to the presumed aetiology with the understanding that there is a large placebo effect.[76,86]

Six classes of agents are available for control of central and upper GI-induced nausea and vomiting. Benzodiazepines are useful for anticipatory CINV and to induce sleep. Opiate-related nausea should be treated if possible with dose reduction or rotation of drugs. Central nausea is helped by a variety of agents as shown in Figure 111.2. There are currently three serotonin 5-HT3 antagonists

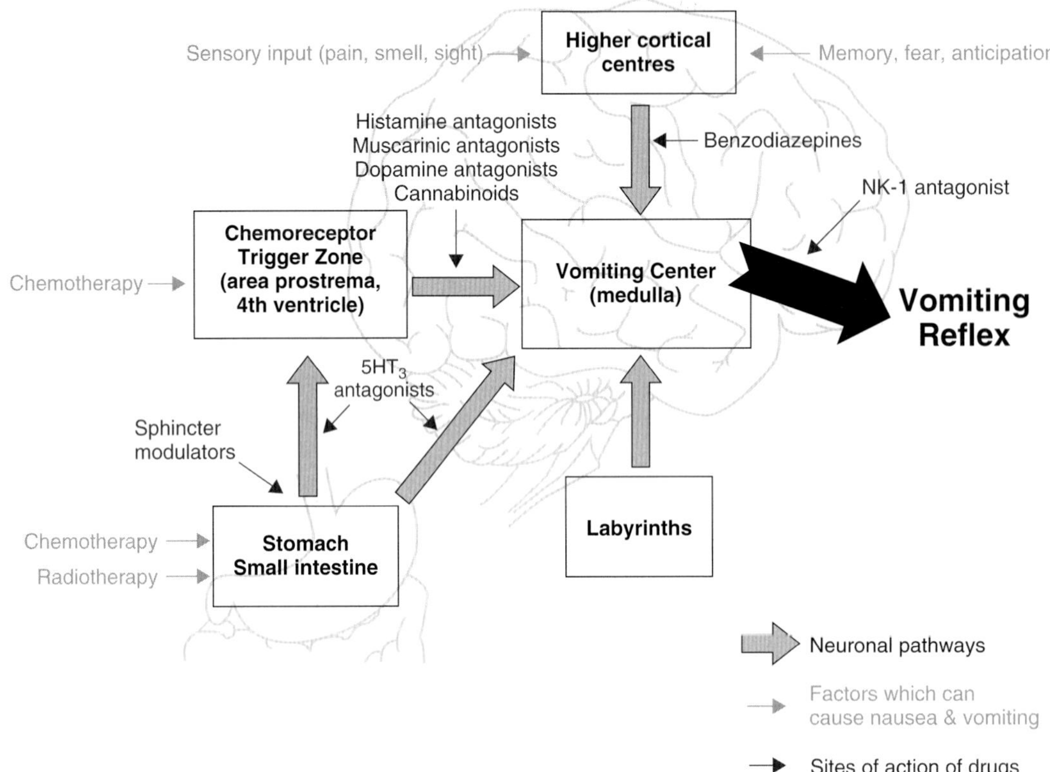

Figure 111.2 Nausea and vomiting pathways.

available, ondansetron, granisetron and dolasetron. They are favoured for effectiveness and lack of side effects. Generics are becoming available. A newer agent, the NK-1 receptor agonist aprepitant, blocks substance P in the medulla to the vomiting centre. Antihistamines include H1 blockers such as diphenhydramine and meclizine. Several D2 blockers, including prochlorperazine, chlorpromazine, metaclopramide and haloperidol, are used for their antihistaminic effects and also sedation. Anti-M1 muscarinic agents include atropine and scopolamine and act on the pathways between the chemoreceptor zones and the medulla. Anticholinergic side effects should be expected. The mechanisms by which corticosteroids manage CINV are not known. Dexamethasone 4 mg four times per day and 8 mg twice daily or prednisone 10 mg daily for 3–4 days have been used prophylactically to cover acute CINV. This treatment is usually combined with metaclopramide and a 5-HT3 antagonist.[76,86]

Delayed CINV is treated with 5-HT3 antagonists. Cannabinoids have fallen out of favour for this indication among medical oncologists. There is considerable popular support, however, for legalizing medical cannabis. Gastroparesis can be treated with promotility agents such as metaclopramide.[86] Physicians need to review carefully all the medications that the patient is taking in order to minimize polypharmacy, especially non-cancer drugs that may aggravate GI symptoms such incretin analogues for diabetes, calcium channel blockers, iron supplements, other anticholinergics and antihyperglycaemics that can cause severe hypoglycaemia when the patient stops eating.

Exercise

Exercise maintains function. How good is it for elderly cancer patients and survivors?

The impact of exercise on functional status and disease management has been reported to be beneficial for the management of frail elderly patients[87] and many of the common chronic illnesses. Cancer is a somewhat different proposition. First, it is not one disease. The functional impact of cancer depends on both the type and the stage. Furthermore, cancer treatments vary considerably in how debilitating they are to the patient. Whether to treat the cancer or only the symptoms may depend as much on a patient's performance status as it does on the effectiveness of the cancer treatment. The value of exercise in cancer treatment is of great interest and some complexity. In summarizing this literature, it will be noted that virtually no studies have explicitly addressed exercise for elderly cancer patients despite the fact that they are the majority of patients and the majority of survivors. It is therefore, like chemotherapy trials, a problem in extrapolation. We can see what kind of cancer patients were exercised and we can estimate the extent to which elderly people with cancer fit this profile.

How cancer affects exercise tolerance

A sedentary lifestyle is associated with low cardiorespiratory fitness. If inactivity due to pain, cytokine-induced fatigue, nausea, anorexia, treatment-induced fatigue, joint pain,[88–90] mucositis, neuropathy and diarrhoea is superimposed on pre-existing disuse atrophy and inactivity, tolerance is further affected.[57] One survey of cancer survivors confirmed that 70% are sedentary.[91] Observational studies also confirmed that activity levels drop during cancer treatment, generally after the second or third cycle of chemotherapy, and are unlikely to return to pretreatment baselines.[92,93] A second survey of cancer patients during and after treatment reported that 70% of respondents engaged in exercise over this period, but this survey has limited generalizability since 66% of the respondents were white, married women under 60 years of age and 88% were rated as 90% or better KPS by their physicians.[94]

The combined effects of pre-existing organ dysfunction, tumour cachexia and drug toxicity need to be disaggregated in order to understand the role of exercise in cancer. For example, the oxygen consumption of middle-aged post-pneumonectomy patients was shown to compensate out of proportion to the volume of lung resected.[95] It is unclear whether this would be replicated in aged patients with age-related loss of lung compliance. Two small pilot studies by the same group reported fewer perioperative complications among patients with a mean age over 65 years and resectable lung cancer who were given preoperative conditioning exercise.[96,97] Although the idea of neoadjuvant physical training prior to cancer surgery, as in elective joint replacement surgery, is intriguing, no studies of other tumour types have been reported.

In a follow-up study to a preoperative lung resection study, the investigators found no change in pre- and post-exercise inflammatory markers.[98] Similarly, 10 young patients with acute leukaemia were exercised during induction therapy with self-reported improved mood and endurance, but no change in cytokine levels was observed.[99] Little can be generalized from these small studies. Results may be affected by limited variability in measures of cytokine activity, small numbers and the brief intervention. The fact that observations were concurrent with pro-inflammatory treatment may also mask an effect.[75] In patients who already have advanced chronic disease such CHF and COPD or primary frailty, background inflammation may well have preceded cancer effects. As had been shown, cytokine levels are also associated with non-cancer frailty.[54,100]

Choosing appropriate exercise along the trajectory of disease

The onset of rapid wasting, exhaustion, anorexia and weakness is a sign of advanced cancer and portends imminent death.[101] In this setting, physical therapy and exercise need to be evaluated for whether they provide pain relief or other comfort. It is not credible, at least to the author, that functional improvement or strengthening is an appropriate goal for dying patients. A cancer diagnosis, especially a verified diagnosis of metastatic cancer, is a hospice-qualifying diagnosis, but as the diagnosis and actual survival are poorly correlated, the rapid decline in performance status is a better prognostic indicator for cancer survival. A dying patient cannot benefit from rehabilitation. However, a patient with a cancer may not imminently be dying. Typically, hospice companies will not pay for restorative therapy to return a patient to a previous level of function on the presumption that a terminal diagnosis means irreversible decline. Conversely, eligible patients who are not offered hospice care or refuse hospice admission may have no way to afford long-term care and so their Medicare Part A benefits are used for 'subacute' even when death is near. A skilled clinician ought to be able to make a reasonably accurate diagnosis of early death. As shown in Figure 111.3, functional decline due to advanced cancer is usually irreversible. This contrasts with the up-and-down course of other end-stage diseases such as CHF and COPD in which some functional recovery after exacerbations is the rule.[101] It is reasonable to provide gentle mobilization therapies, therapeutic massage and mind–body interventions to patients with advanced malignancy who want them and who are able to participate. However, it is also appropriate to withhold restorative therapies for patients with advanced malignancy who are dying, the last stage of a predictable course of disease.

Figure 111.3 tracks the functional status over 1 year of two geriatric outpatients that the author cared for. One was a 76-year-old woman with mild dementia and colon

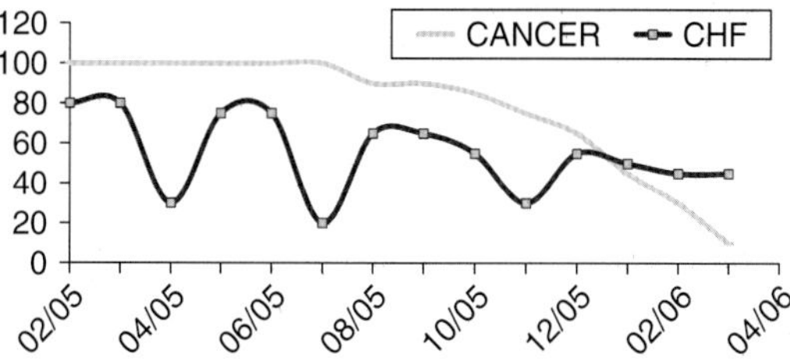

Figure 111.3 Comparing the course of chronic disease to cancer. The y-axis is the Karnofsky Performance Score and the x-axis is the time course over 12 months.

cancer receiving single-agent maintenance for what had been stable Stage IV disease. The other patient was an 85-year-old man with CHF, NYHA Stage II–III, and recurrent hospitalizations. It illustrates the observations of Teno *et al.*[101] that with many chronic diseases, the course of the final year of life is often difficult to predict but cancer is quite predictable.

There are few data on the benefit of rehabilitation in patients with advanced malignancy. Jones *et al.* reported accrual data for their study of exercise for inoperable lung cancer patients. Of the 20% who were fit enough for exercise screening, 40% consented. Hence only 8% of non-operative stage lung cancer patients were willing and able to exercise.[102] In another study, less than half of 25 highly selected patients with advanced lung cancer enrolled in a feasibility study were able to complete an 8 week fitness programme.[103] At the very end of life, complementary therapies might be more helpful. Stretching, yoga, massage and relaxation therapies are likely appropriate physical modalities for end-of-life cancer patients.[104] Long-term care facilities are often enough given the job of recognizing an imminently terminal prognosis when patients are sent from hospitals with inadequate records and no clear understanding of life expectancy.[39] In this situation, adequate consultation for prognostication is an important part of care planning.

Exercise and radiation toxicity

Radiotherapy is a rapidly evolving field. Radiation oncologists undertake a variety of dose modulation, shielding and pharmacological measures to limit healthy tissue damage. However, they also recognize that there are long-term delayed pulmonary and cardiac toxicities experienced by lung, lymphoma and breast cancer patients treated for loco-regional disease.[105] No study has actually evaluated the effect of pulmonary rehabilitation on post-radiotherapy pulmonary function. Some degree of permanent scarring is inevitable.[106] Patients with poor cardiopulmonary function measured by the 6 min walk distance (6MWD) sustained greater tissue damage after palliative radiation for inoperable lung cancer than did fitter subjects.[107,108] One small trial reported generally positive but essentially marginal performance benefit to patients with mixed tumour types who exercised at home during outpatient radiation therapy.[109]

Exercise and chemotherapy toxicity

Several chemotherapeutic agents have toxic effects on cardiopulmonary fitness. Specifically, the anthracyclines, which are among the most effective agents for lung and breast cancer, ovarian cancer and lymphomas, have direct cardiac myocyte toxicity.[110–112] Oncologists now will generally avoid using anthracyclines in elderly and heart patients if there is an acceptable alternative. However, the current cohort of long-term survivors did receive these agents when they were younger and the debt is coming due. Primary care physicians may not have access to chemotherapy records from the past.

New biological agents such as bevacizumab, an anti-VEGF monoclonal antibody, show effectiveness in treating a number of cancers by blocking their ability to grow an arterial supply. However, early on in trials with breast cancer patients, excess cardiovascular mortality was seen in older women and it is not recommended for older patients.[12] Trustazumab was very effective in Her2+ breast cancers, but the benefit was deemed marginal in elderly women, even those with appropriate histology.[113] The '–abs' are one class of targeted agents, the tyrosine kinase inhibitors (TKIs), that are not directly cytotoxic to cancer cells but rather modulate their ability to sustain oxidative metabolism and to migrate. Nearly all in common use have been shown to have cardiotoxic potential.[114] They are relatively new agents that early on showed excess toxicity in elderly patients, but long-term effects for survivors are not yet known.

The effect of exercise on TKI toxicity has been examined in only one study. Middle-aged women with Her2+ breast cancer were provided with supervised aerobic exercise during 4 months of adjuvant trustazumab therapy; 17 women experienced statistically significant LV dilation and reduced ejection fraction despite training.[115] These findings do not support the speculation that exercise during chemotherapy with TKIs is cardioprotective, but there was no control group so it is possible that cardiotoxicity was lessened by the intervention. Further empirical studies are needed.[116] Since aerobic and resistance exercise promote angiogenesis in muscle, there is a theoretical reason to think that exercise could also promote tumour angiogenesis.[95]

IGF-1 is another growth factor implicated in tumour growth. Several solid tumour cell lines express IGF receptors that present targets for new blocking agents. Observational studies have noted an association between fasting insulin levels in non-diabetic women and time to progression in breast cancer patients[117] and in colon cancer patients.[118] Exercise increases insulin receptor sensitivity and decreases insulin secretion. Strength and endurance training lowered insulin levels in breast cancer survivors in two randomized trials but the effect on late recurrence is unknown.[119,120] Limitations of these studies were small numbers, brief follow-up and relatively younger participants. Furthermore, the interventions were intense, requiring supervision in exercise physiology laboratories. Whether similar results can be obtained in community settings with elderly patients is the subject of current research.

Breast and prostate cancer survivors experience accelerated ageing

Support for the general efficacy of exercise interventions would require showing that elderly representatives of community-living elderly would adhere to an intervention that is rigorous enough to achieve endpoints such as modifying cardiovascular risk factors, markers of inflammation and measures of fitness and body composition. Such trials have been reported. Project LEAD randomized 182 recently diagnosed older breast and prostate cancer survivors to a home-based diet and exercise intervention.[121] A follow-up study randomized 641 >5 year survivors of breast, prostate and colon cancer aged 65–91 years to a home-based programme. Their self-reported SF-36 physical function sub-scale scores declined less in the intervention group. The intervention group increased their exercise time on average by about 15 min per week and on average the intervention group lost about 1.1 kg more weight.[122] Nearly all of the self-reported comparisons were favourable and statistically significant for the intervention group, but no physiological measures were taken and actual clinical improvement is to be inferred. A trial of supervised exercise in 177 middle-aged women showed marginal increases in 6MWD after a 12 week intervention that was maintained for 6 months.[123]

Main-line therapy for oestrogen/progesterone receptor-positive breast cancer is now daily oral aromatase inhibitors to deprive residual tumour of trophic oestrogen. The anticancer effectiveness of these agents appears to result in exaggerated adverse changes associated with endocrine ageing, including worsening of cardiovascular risk factors and accelerated bone loss.[124] Standard of care for postmenopausal women on aromatase inhibitors includes measuring their bone mineral density (BMD), supplemental vitamin D and bisphosphonate therapy.[15] The aromatase inhibitors and bisphosphonates have both been associated with bone and joint pain.[88,125] Because these women experience adverse changes in cardiovascular and bone health risk factors, they are an important target for exercise interventions aimed not at the cancer but at the adverse risk factor profiles induced by cancer therapy. One systematic review focused on trials of endurance and resistance training immediately after initial treatment of breast cancer (54% of all subjects in all trials), prostate cancer or all other cancers. They concluded that there was support for improved oxygen consumption and one-repetition arm or leg strength, but no effect on body composition or other physiological measures.[126] Most studies were of small size and short duration and suffered other methodological weaknesses such that fitness measures ought to be regarded as intermediate measures for a potential risk reduction that has yet to be shown. The studies were also not explicit as to whether the risk reduction of interest was for cancer recurrence or for cardiac outcomes.

Early studies documented the basis for women's complains of weight gain during breast cancer treatment.[127] Small studies showed that this adverse effect was blunted by vigorous exercise.[128] The small studies were positive and likely reflect a publication bias. Larger studies later confirmed the benefit of multimodal fitness training for overall wellbeing, strength, curbing weight gain and improved activity levels, except among women who received anthracycline treatment.[129] Two systematic reviews that included many of the same studies confirmed a generally beneficial effect for measures of performance, but were unable to draw conclusions about metabolic outcomes due to inconsistent reporting of biochemical markers of cardiovascular risk.[130,131] Most recently, Friedenreich and colleagues reported on a large RCT of 320 sedentary post-menopausal breast cancer survivors who engaged in supervised aerobic activity for 45 min per day for 5 days per week for 1 year. After adjusting for weight loss from baseline, the treatment group had statistically significantly lower estrogen levels than the observational control. Androgen levels in these women did not change.[132] The investigators did not report on changes in lipids, inflammatory markers, fitness outcomes or the radiodensity of mammograms, but they did demonstrate that sedentary women can be engaged in vigorous exercise.

Observational studies appear to support the interventional studies. The Nurses Study followed nearly 3000 women after the diagnosis of breast cancer and found about a 6% lower mortality from hormone-sensitive breast cancer between the lowest quintile <3 MET (metabolic units) per week and the upper half >9 MET per week activity levels. The highest quintile experienced no additional benefit.[133] A similar reduction in cancer-specific and total mortality was observed among 668 male physicians followed after treatment for localized colon cancer. The median exercise level was 18 MET per week. Men who exercised >27 MET per week had a relative risk reduction (RRR) of about 50% compared with sedentary men on <3 MET per week.[134] The usual caveats apply to these observational data since there may be numbers of unmeasured covariates. For example, the burden of progressive disease may have been much lower among the active survivors, explaining their higher activity levels. This bias is attenuated but not entirely removed by statistical adjustment for stage of disease.

Androgen ablation is the cornerstone of prostate cancer management. Achieving castrate levels of endogenous testosterone deprives prostate cancers and satellite metastases of hormonally mediated growth factors. Prostate cancers remain hormonally susceptible for a median of 6 years before they develop hormone independence. Because of this, many urogenital oncologists are less eager to treat biochemical recurrences in the absence of evaluable disease.[135] Five year survival after a diagnosis of prostate cancer, for example, is well over 90%.[3] However, increasing evidence for long-term adverse effects of androgen deprivation on cardiac risk and physical performance are accumulating.[32,90,135–140] Androgen ablation affects men in many serious ways. Hot flashes, fatigue, loss of libido and depression are subjective toxicities. Loss of muscle mass and increased body fat are recognized side effects.[139] The adverse change in body composition also contributes to the observation of increased incidence of type 2 diabetes and cardiovascular disease.[136,141,142] Our consecutive series of elderly men attending prostate cancer clinic reported an unexpectedly high rate of falls.[23] Combined with hypogonadal bone loss, the risk for fractures is increased.[137,140,143]. Epidemiological associations with physical activity[144] provide part of the rationale for trials of extreme lifestyle interventions for men with prostate cancer.[145,146] Severely restricted diets, especially those with low protein content, are potentially dangerous for elderly men experiencing accelerated muscle ageing due to hormonal manipulation.

Given the well-understood toxicities of androgen ablation in elderly men, it is surprising that so few exercise intervention trials have been reported.[147] The standard of care has acknowledged these. Loss of muscle is measurable before 1 year of therapy is completed.[138] Hence current guidelines include using pulsed androgen ablation to limit toxicity, measuring BMD and giving prophylactic bisphosphonates.[135] Into this gap one group has reported a well-designed trial aimed at metabolic risk factor modification. The RADAR trial plans to enrol 370 men undergoing androgen ablative therapy from multiple sites in Australia. They were randomized to 6 months of supervised resistance and aerobic exercise versus standard public health recommendations for exercise for cardiovascular health.[148] Their report of preliminary findings with the first 60 subjects at 12 weeks is encouraging. There were statistically significant increases in muscle mass, strength and gait speed over short distances and significantly improved rapid clinical balance test (backward gait speed). The authors caution about ceiling effects due to selection bias. C-reactive protein levels dropped significantly in the intervention group, but there was no change in body composition, lipid total or fraction levels, insulin, homocysteine or blood glucose. The authors attribute this disappointing aspect of the trial to the short duration of exercise participation and to the less than 250 min per week of aerobic exercise in the protocol.[149]

Exercise and subjective quality of life

Physical exercise is the most widely studied intervention to treat cancer fatigue. Several systematic reviews have evaluated exercise interventions to relieve cancer fatigue.[93,150,151] Part of the difficulty in performing these analyses is the overall poor quality of studies. Some were restricted to one tumour type, others were mixed. Some involved variations on circuit training with resistance and aerobic conditioning components. Others examined mild activities such as walking or walking and stretching. Relatively few were randomized and controlled and all but a handful were crippled by small numbers. The most common endpoint was subjectively rated fatigue. Several studies measured fitness outcomes including gait speed, muscle strength and aerobic performance. The association between physical training effects and subjective fatigue was not as direct or as simple as expected. In other words, fit and fatigued was as common as fit or fatigued.

Of the main group of studies, subjects over the age of 65 years were routinely excluded. In a systematic review, 19 of 34 studies enrolled participants over the age of 65 years.[152] Four of 19 studies enrolled only subjects over 65 years old.[153]. One meta-analysis concluded that the benefit was probably real but small. Calculated effect sizes were less than 0.5 SDs in nearly all comparisons.[130] The most recent meta-analysis found 28 of 54 published studies to be adequate for analysis.[150] While adjusting for heterogeneity, the analysis did not attempt sensitivity analysis to control for publication bias. The analysis found consistent positive findings for exercise compared with no exercise controls. The largest effect sizes (ES) were reported for the breast cancer subgroup of 18 studies ($N = 977$), ES–0.36 (95% CI,–0.49 to–0.23). and for 11 studies ($N = 491$) comparing exercise with no exercise among long-term survivors, ES–0.37 (95% CI,–0.55 to–0.18).[154] Another group of investigators reported that elderly women aged over 75 years adhered poorly to their exercise protocols and were therefore pessimistic about this intervention.[155] It is possible that their protocol was not 'gero-friendly' and that age-tailored interventions would obtain better adherence.

Although the best clinical trial evidence in cancer patients is graded as only moderate in quality and weakly supportive of structured exercise interventions, for the elderly in general the evidence of benefit of increased physical activity is broadly supported. Table 111.4 presents an heuristic algorithm with no empirical evidence that attempts to summarize the results of published research as a prescriptive model for exercise in elderly cancer patients and cancer survivors. It should be validated empirically. As a 'thought experiment', scores <4 suggest that exercise is unlikely to be beneficial or accepted. Scores of 4–5 suggest that symptomatic relief of fatigue and stiffness through low- to moderate-intensity exercise would be beneficial. Scores of 6 or more suggest moderate-intensity training, such as structured walking programmes and resistance training, would be beneficial for long-term survivors. Baseline performance can be estimated from any validated, available activity questionnaire or standardized observational fitness

Table 111.4 A proposed algorithm for exercise prescription for elderly cancer patients.

Item	Points
1. Current exercise capacity[a]	
Immobile (PS 3–4)	0
Sedentary but mobile (PS 2)	0
Low-intensity exercise (PS 1)	1
Moderate-intensity exercise (PS 0)	2
2. Estimated remaining life expectancy with cancer	
<6 months	0
1–2 years	1
3–5 years	1
>5 years or cure	2
3. Duration and toxicity of current cancer therapy[74,85]	
Intense high-toxic therapy, e.g. bone marrow transplantation	0
Episodic high-toxicity therapy with no therapy while in remission	1
Continuous low-toxicity cytotoxic therapy depending on continued response	1
Continuous hormonal or pulse deprivation[b]	2
Long-term survivor on no anticancer therapy[b]	2
4. Patient exercise goal	
Comfort	0
Symptom management	1
Health improvement	2

[a]Reverse scoring of ECOG-PS: 0–1 = 2, 2 = 1, 3–4 = 0.
[b]May require cardiac risk stratification.

evaluation. Estimating remaining life expectancy eliminates the need for an age-based scoring requirement.

For example, an 80-year-old man on androgen deprivation therapy maintains a moderately active lifestyle. He walks every evening with his wife. He accrues one point for life style, two points for therapy and one point for estimated life expectancy. His choice of symptom management only for hot flashes and fatigue vs choosing health improvement for maintenance of strength and muscle mass adds one point to total five with a recommendation to continue moderate exercise.

In another example, a 75-year-old woman is diagnosed with estrogen receptor-positive breast cancer. She chooses not to undergo lymph node sampling, fearing postoperative lymphoedema. She is treated with simple mastectomy and an aromatase inhibitor. She has multiple comorbidities, including arthritis, NYHA Stage II congestive heart failure, diabetes and Stage II chronic renal insufficiency. She is able to do light housekeeping and drive a car, but she engages in no regular exercise. She accrues no points for lifestyle, one point for survival based on her comorbidities, two points for rigour of cancer therapy and she prefers symptom management. Her points total is four and a prescription for light weight-bearing exercise such as walking to maintain mobility and for bone preservation would be appropriate.

Conclusion

Elderly patients with a new diagnosis of cancer are heterogeneous and the specific cancer diagnosis introduces another layer of complexity to clinical decision-making. Decisions about treatment must take into account the patient's functional status and remaining life expectancy. Clinicians must be able to distinguish with some certainty whether impairments in functional status are attributable to age-related frailty, non-cancer comorbidities or the malignancy. Geriatric assessment screening tools have been proposed as a way of stratifying geriatric risk for cancer treatment toxicity. Several expert bodies now recommend routinely assessing for ADL and IADL dependency, and screening for falls, delirium and depression, for cognitive impairment and nutritional deficits. In some cases, directly observed performance measures are helpful in determining danger of falls and functional decline during treatment. Determining whether there is adequate caregiver and social support is also crucial as a safety net if disease or treatment effects cause falls, delirium, malnutrition and unplanned hospitalizations leading to functional decline. Highly selected fit elderly patients in clinical trials appear to derive equal benefit from equal treatment. Specifically, cognitively impaired patients fare poorly in cancer treatment, with excess mortality and questionable benefit.[31] Both physical frailty and decisional incapacity will preclude aggressive cancer treatment.

Limited clinical trial evidence suggests that elderly cancer patients benefit from geriatric interventions during and after treatment. Clinical trial evidence suggests that formal and continuous palliative interventions in addition to usual cancer care may improve quality of life measures and possibly survival. For the elderly cancer patient, proactive management of treatment toxicity is critical to maintaining function and preventing hospitalizations for treatment-related toxicity that lead to further functional decline and loss of independence. Important acute toxicities include mucositis and poor oral intake due to radiation and cytotoxic chemotherapy, volume depletion from poor intake, vomiting and diarrhoea. Elderly patients appear to suffer less acute and more delayed nausea and vomiting, hence treatment should be preventive rather than reactive. Anorexia with weight loss must be distinguished from cancer cachexia. Proactive pharmacological symptom management and nutritional support are necessary during treatment. An important component of pharmacological management is smart polypharmacy, which means stopping unnecessary drugs to minimize drug interactions. Using scheduled drugs rather than prns makes it easier for caregivers to supervise, especially if delirium occurs. In the absence of a 24/7 family caregiver, preventive home care should be considered for monitoring.

Among the most problematic symptoms is fatigue. Fatigue clusters with depression, weakness, anaemia and sleep disturbances. Fatigue, after pain, is the most troubling symptom for elderly cancer patients. There is some evidence that treatment with methylphenidate is helpful once anaemia is corrected and sleep is addressed. Use of erythropoietin for cancer-related anaemia has been only modestly useful for addressing fatigue and carries its own risks if not used according to current guidelines. Compared with middle-aged patients, elderly cancer patients are less likely to suffer with depression and anxiety but more likely to suffer extreme fatigue. Pain management should be addressed following the American Geriatrics Society pain management guidelines. Delirium is markedly underdiagnosed by oncologists, perhaps because it is so common.[33] However, the risk for elderly outpatients is significant if delirium is missed and caregivers and providers need to be vigilant

The numbers of long-term cancer survivors are increasing and the majority, over 4 million in the USA, are of Medicare age. These survivors may be at risk for second cancers or late recurrences. In addition, they may experience late effects of surgery and chemo- and radiation therapy. Several analyses of large databases indicate that elderly cancer survivors continue to have moderately decreased quality of life compared with non-cancer survivors. Late effects include radiation proctitis and cystitis from treatment of prostate and anorectal cancers and sclerosis of the soft tissues of the neck and oral cavity. Lymphoedema can be painful and even with improved surgical techniques continues to impair upper extremity function for breast cancer survivors. Specialized therapies are often necessary. Cognitive impairment due to cancer chemotherapy has been difficult to characterize, most likely because it is multifactorial.[156] However, studies which obtained pretreatment measures indicate that unrecognized cognitive impairment is not uncommon among elderly cancer patients[32] and survivors.[157] Further research is needed to determine whether there are specific phenotypes at greater risk for developing chemotherapy-related cognitive impairment.[158] Patients on hormonal ablation therapies for breast and prostate cancer suffer accelerated ageing, including subtle cognitive impairment, osteoporosis, fractures, falls and adverse changes in cardiac risk factors. Patients who received chest radiation or any of several cardiotoxic chemotherapy agents develop late cardiomyopathies and coronary artery disease. Neuropathies causing pain, denervation and balance problems may persist. For these reasons, it is recommended that cancer survivors have specific care plans so that their primary care physicians can manage their symptoms and risk factors appropriately. The role of exercise interventions, especially among cancer survivors, is under active investigation in several centres. For the elderly cancer survivor, exercise prescriptions should be appropriate to the patient's goals and abilities. On-line resources for medical care of elderly cancer survivors are becoming available. In sum, the best way to maintain function in elderly cancer patients and cancer survivors is to provide good, evidence-based geriatric care.

Key points

- Function is important in planning the management of oncology patients.
- Palliative management improves outcomes.
- Fatigue is an important area to be addressed during chemotherapy.
- Exercise therapy may improve quality of life in cancer patients.

References

1. Smith BD, Smith GL, Hurria A *et al.* Future of cancer incidence in the United States: burdens upon an aging, changing nation. *J Clin Oncol* 2009;**27**:2758–65.
2. Yancik R. Population aging and cancer. *Cancer* 2005;**11**:437–41.
3. Jemal A, Siegel R, Ward E *et al.* Cancer statistics 2009. *CA Cancer J Clin* 2009;**59**:1–25.
4. Aapro M, Claus-Henning SK, Cohen HJ and Extermann M. Never too old? Age should not be a barrier to enrollment in cancer clinical trials. *Oncologist* 2005;**10**:198–204.
5. Repetto L, Fratino L, Audisio R *et al.* Comprehensive geriatric assessment adds information to Eastern Cooperative Group performance status in elderly cancer patients: an Italian Group for Geriatric Oncology Study. *J Clin Oncol* 2002;**20**:494–502.
6. Holmes CE and Muss HB. Diagnosis and treatment of breast cancer in the elderly. *CA Cancer J Clin* 2003;**53**:227–44.
7. Hurria A, Hurria E, Zuckerman E *et al.* A prospective, longitudinal study of the functional status and quality of life of older patients with breast cancer receiving adjuvant chemotherapy. *J Am Geriatr Soc* 2006;**54**:1119–24.
8. Gupta SK and Lamont EB. Patterns of presentation, diagnosis and treatment in older patients with colon cancer and comorbid dementia. *J Am Geriatr Soc* 2004;**52**:1681–7.
9. Lamont EB, Landrum MB, Keating NL *et al.* Differences in clinical trial patient attributes and outcomes according to enrollment setting. *J Clin Oncol* 2010;**28**:215–221.

10. Fried LP, Tangen CM, Walston J *et al*. Frailty in older adults: evidence for a phenotype. *J Gerontol A Biol Sci Med Sci* 2001;**56**: M146–56.
11. Walston J, Hadley EC, Ferrucci L *et al*. Research agenda for frailty in older adults: toward a better understanding of physiology and etiology: summary from the American Geriatrics Society/National Institute on Aging Research Conference on Frailty in Older Adults. *J Am Geriatr Soc* 2006;**54**:991–1001.
12. Balducci L. Aging, frailty and chemotherapy. *Cancer Control* 2007;**14**:7–12.
13. Alfano CM, Day JM, Katz ML *et al*. Exercise and dietary change after diagnosis and cancer-related symptoms in long term survivors of breast cancer: CALGB 79804. *Psycho-oncology* 2009;**18**:128–33.
14. Seo P, Pieper C and Cohen HJ. Effects of cancer history and comorbid conditions on mortality and health care use among older cancer survivors. *Cancer* 2004;**101**:2276–84.
15. Ganz P and Hahn E. Implementing a survivorship care plan for patients with breast cancer. *J Clin Oncol* 2008;**26**:759–67.
16. OncoLink. *LIVESTRONG Care Plan*, 2011, www.livestrong careplan.org. OncoLink, Abramson Cancer Center of the University of Pennsylvania (last accessed 7 September 2011).
17. Karnofsky DA. Determining the extent of the cancer and clinical planning for cure. *Cancer* 1968;**22**:730–4.
18. Extermann M, Aapro M, Bernabei R *et al*. Use of comprehensive geriatric assessment in older cancer patients: recommendations from the task force on CGA of the International Society of Geriatric Oncology (SIOG). *Crit Rev Oncol Hematol* 2005;**55**:241–52.
19. Saliba D, Elliott M, Rubenstein LZ *et al*. The Vulnerable Elders Survey: a tool for identifying vulnerable older people in the community. *J Am Geriatr Soc* 2001;**49**:1691–9.
20. Mohile SG, Bylow K, Dale W *et al*. A pilot study of the vulnerable elders survey-13 compared with the comprehensive geriatric assessment for identifying disability in older patients with prostate cancer who receive androgen ablation. *Cancer* 2007;**109**:802–10.
21. Overcash JA, Beckstead J, Moody L *et al*. The abbreviated comprehensive geriatric assessment (aCGA) for use in the older cancer patient as a prescreen: scoring and interpretation. *Crit Rev Oncol Hematol* 2006;**59**:205–10.
22. Extermann M, Meyer J, McGinnis M *et al*. A comprehensive geriatric intervention detects multiple problems in older breast cancer patients. *Crit Rev Oncol Hematol* 2004;**49**:69–75.
23. Bylow K, Dale W, Mustian K *et al*. Falls and physical performance deficits in older patients with prostate cancer undergoing androgen deprivation therapy. *Urology* 2008;**72**:422–7.
24. Cohen HJ, Fuessner JR, Weinberger M *et al*. A controlled trial of inpatient and outpatient geriatric evaluation and management. *N Engl J Med* 2002;**346**:905–12.
25. Rao AV, Hsieh F, Fuessner JR and Cohen HJ. Geriatric evaluation and management units in the care of the frail elderly cancer patient. *J Gerontol A Biol Sci Med Sci* 2005;**60**:798–803.
26. Kristjansson SK, Farinella E, Gaskell S and Audisio RA. Surgical risk and post-operative complications in older unfit cancer patients. *Cancer Treat Rev* 2009;**35**:499–502.
27. Pope D, Ramesh H, Gennari R *et al*. Pre-operative assessment of cancer in the elderly (PACE): a comprehensive assessment of underlying characteristics of elderly cancer patients prior to elective surgery. *Surg Oncol* 2007;**15**:189–97.
28. Guigoz Y, Lauque S and Vellas B. Identifying the elderly at risk for malnutrition. *Clin Geriatr Med* 2002;**18**:737–57.
29. Bozzetti F. Nutritional issues in the care of the elderly patient. *Crit Rev Oncol Hematol* 2003;**48**:113–21.
30. Rodin MB and Mohile SG. Assessing decisional capacity in the elderly. *Semin Oncol* 2008;**35**:625–32.
31. Robb C, Boulware D, Overcash J and Extermann M. Patterns of care and survival in cancer patients with cognitive impairment. *Crit Rev Oncol Hematol* 2010;**74**:218–24.
32. Mohile SG, Lacy M, Rodin MB *et al*. Cognitive effects of androgen deprivation therapy in an older cohort of men with prostate cancer. *Crit Rev Oncol Hematol* 2010;**75**:152–9.
33. Bial AK, Schilsky RL and Sachs GA. Evaluation of cognition in cancer patients: special focus on the elderly. *Crit Rev Oncol Hematol* 2006;**60**:242–55.
34. Balducci L. The geriatric cancer patient: equal benefit from equal treatment. *Cancer Control* 2001;**8**(2 Suppl):1–25; quiz 27-8.
35. Habermann TM, Weller EA, Morrison VA *et al*. Rituxamab plus CHOP vs CHOP alone or with maintenance rituxamab in older patients with diffuse large B cell lymphoma. *J Clin Oncol* 2006;**24**:3121–7.
36. Gridell C. The ELVIS Trial: a phase III study of single agent vinorelbine as first line therapy in elderly patients with advanced non-small cell lung cancer: Elderly Lung Cancer Vinorelbine Italian Study. *Oncologist* 2001;**6**(Suppl 1):4–7.
37. Gruschkus SK, Lairson D, Dunn JK *et al*. Comparative effectiveness of white blood cell growth factors on neutropenia, infection and survival in older people with non-Hodgkin's lymphoma treated with chemotherapy. *J Am Geriatr Soc* 2010;**58**:1885–95.
38. Shayne M, Culakova E, Poniewierski MS *et al*. Dose intensity and hematologic toxicity in older cancer patients receiving systemic chemotherapy. *Cancer* 2007;**110**:1611–20.
39. Rodin M. Cancer patients in nursing homes: what do we know ? *J Am Med Dir Assoc* 2008;**9**:149–56.
40. Dow LA, Matsuyama RK, Ramakrishnan V *et al*. Paradoxes in advance care planning: the complex relationship of oncology patients, their physicians and advance medical directives. *J Clin Oncol* 2010;**28**:299–304.
41. Bakitas M, Lyons KD, Hegel MT *et al*. Effects of a palliative care intervention on clinical outcomes in patients with advanced cancer: the Project ENABLE II randomized controlled trial. *JAMA* 2009;**302**:741–9.
42. Rabow M, Dibble SL, Pantilat SZ and McPhee SJ. The comprehensive care team: a controlled trial of outpatient palliative medicien consultation. *Arch Intern Med* 2004;**164**:83–91.
43. Rummans T, Clark MM, Sloan JA *et al*. Impacting quality of life for patients with advanced cancer with a structured multidisciplinary intervention: a randomized controlled trial. *J Clin Oncol* 2006;**24**:635–42.
44. Jordhoy MS, Fayers P, Loge JH *et al*. Quality of life in palliative cancer care: results from a clustered randomized trial. *J Clin Oncol* 2001;**19**:3884–94.

45. Temel, JS, Greer JA, Musikansky A *et al.* Early palliative care for patients with metastatic non-small cell lung cancer. *N Engl J Med* 2010;**363**:733–42.
46. Gill T and Feinstein A. A critical appraisal of the quality of quality-of-life measurements. *JAMA* 1994;**272**:619–26.
47. Vadhan-Raj S, Trent J, Patel S *et al.* Single-dose palifermin prevents severe oral mucositis during multicycle chemotherapy in patients with cancer: a randomized trial. *Ann Intern Med* 2010;**153**:358–67.
48. Rao A. and Cohen HJ. Symptom management in the elderly cancer patient: fatigue, pain and depression. *J Natl Cancer Inst Monogr* 2004;**32**:150–7.
49. World Health Organization. *Cancer Pain Relief and Palliative Care. Report of a WHO Expert Committee.* World Health Organization Technical Report Series, No. 804. WHO, Geneva, 1990, pp. 1–75.
50. American Geriatrics Society. *AGS Clinical Practice Guideline: Pharmacological Management of Persistent Pain in Older Persons (2009).* http://www.americangeriatrics.org/health_care_professionals/clinical_practice/clinical_guidelines_recommendations/2009/ (last accessed 7 September 2011).
51. Schmitz KH, Ahmed RL, Troxel A *et al.* Weight-lifting in women with breast-cancer-related lymphedema. *N Engl J Med* 2010;**361**:664–73.
52. Miaskowski C, Dodd M and Lee K. Symptom clusters: the new frontier in symptom management research. *J Natl Cancer Inst Monogr* 2004;**32**:7–21.
53. Rao AV and Cohen HJ. Fatigue in older cancer patients: etiology, assessment and treatment. *Semin Oncol* 2008;**35**:633–42.
54. Cesari M, Pennix BW, Pahor M *et al.* Inflammatory markers and physical performance in older persons: the InChianti study. *J Gerontol A Biol Sci Med Sci* 2004;**59**: M242–8.
55. Curt GA, Breitbart W, Cella D *et al.* Impact of cancer-related fatigue on the lives of patients: new findings from the Fatigue Coalition. *Oncologist* 2000;**5**:353–60.
56. Vogelzang NJ, Breitbart W, Cella D *et al.* Patient, caregiver and oncologist perceptions of cancer-related fatigue: results of a tri-part assessment survey. *Semin Oncol* 1997;**34**:4–12.
57. Luciani A, Jacobsen PB, Extermann M *et al.* Fatigue and functional dependence in older cancer patients. *Am J Clin Oncol* 2008;**31**:424–30.
58. National Comprehensive Cancer Network. *NCCN Guidelines. Cancer-Related Fatigue.* http://www.nccn.org/professionals/physician_gls/PDF/fatigue.pdf (last accessed 23 November 2010).
59. Cella D, Davis K, Breitbart W *et al.* Cancer-related fatigue: prevalence of proposed diagnostic criteria in a United States sample of cancer survivors. *J Clin Oncol* 2001;**19**:3385–91.
60. Minton O, Richardson A, Sharpe M *et al.* Drug therapy for the management of cancer-related fatigue. *Cochrane Database Syst Rev* 2008;(1): CD006704.
61. Pirl WF, Muriel A, Hwang V *et al.* Screening for psychosocial distress: a national survey of oncologists. *J Support Oncol* 2007;**5**:499–504.
62. Mor V, Allen S and Malin M. The psychosocial impact of cancer on older vs younger patients. *Cancer* 1994;**72**:2118–27.
63. Littlewood TJ, Kallich JD, San Miguel J *et al.* Efficacy of darbepoetin alfa in alleviating fatigue and the effect of fatigue on quality of life in anemic patients with lymphoproliferative malignancies. *J Pain Symptom Manage* 2006;**31**:317–25.
64. Aapro MS, Cella D and Zagari M. Age, anemia and fatigue. *Semin Oncol* 2002;**29**(Suppl 8):55–9.
65. Lappin T, Maxwell A and Johnston P. Warning flags for erythropoiesis-stimulating agents and cancer-associated anemia. *Oncologist* 2007;**12**:362–65.
66. Bruera E, Valero V, Driver L *et al.* Patient-controlled methylphenidate for cancer fatigue: a double-blind, randomized, placebo-controlled trial. *J Clin Oncol.* 2006;**24**: 2073–8.
67. Moraska AR, Sood A, Dakhil SR *et al.* Phase III, randomized, double-blind, placebo-controlled study of long-acting methylphenidate for cancer-related fatigue: North Central Cancer Treatment Group NCCTG-N05C7 trial. *J Clin Oncol* 2010;**28**:3673–9.
68. Breitbart W and Alici Y. Psychostimulants for cancer-related fatigue. *J Natl Compr Cancer Netw* 2010;**8**:933–42.
69. Bruera E, El Osta B and Valero V. Donepezil for cancer fatigue: a double-blind, randomized, placebo-controlled trial. *J Clin Oncol* 2007;**25**:3475–81.
70. de la Cruz M, Hui D, Parsons HA and Bruera E. Placebo and nocebo effects in randomized double-blind clinical trials of agents for the therapy for fatigue in patients with advanced cancer. *Cancer* 2010;**116**:766–74.
71. Baldwin C, McGough C, Norman AR *et al.* Failure of dietetic referral in patients with gastrointestinal cancer and weight loss. *Eur J Cancer* 2006;**42**:2504–9.
72. Yeh SS, Blackwood K and Schuster MW. The cytokine basis of cachexia and its treatment: are they ready for prime time? *J Am Med Dir Assoc* 2008;**9**:219–36.
73. Puccio M and Nathanson L. The cancer cachexia syndrome. *Semin Oncol* 1997;**24**:277–87.
74. Yeh SS and Schuster MW. Geriatric cachexia: the role of cytokines. *Am J Clin Nutr* 1999;**70**:183–97.
75. Argiles J, Lopez-Soriano F and Busquets S. Mechanisms to explain wasting of muscle and fat in cancer cachexia. *Curr Opin Support Palliat Care* 2007;**1**:293–8.
76. American Society of Clinical Oncology. *ASCO Curriculum: Cancer Care in the Older Population.* American Society of Clinical Oncology, Alexandria, VA, 2003, Section 8, pp. 15–33.
77. Yeh SS, Wu SY, Lee TP *et al.* Improvement in quality-of-life measures and stimulation of weight gain after treatment with megestrol acetate oral suspension in geriatric cachexia: results of a double-blind, placebo-controlled study. *J Am Geriatr Soc* 2000;**48**:485–92.
78. Yeh SS, Wu SY, Levine DM *et al.* The correlation of cytokine levels with body weight after megestrol acetate treatment in geriatric patients. *J Gerontol A Biol Sci Med Sci* 2001;**56**: M48–54.
79. Abrams DI, Hilton JF, Leiser RJ *et al.* Short-term effects of cannabinoids in patients with HIV-1 infection: a randomized, placebo-controlled clinical trial. *Ann Intern Med* 2003;**139**:258–66.

80. Jatoi A, Windshitl HE, Loprinzi CL *et al*. Dronabinol versus megestrol acetate versus combination therapy for cancer-associated anorexia: a North Central Cancer Treatment Group study. *J Clin Oncol* 2002;**20**:567–73.
81. Lundholm K, Gunnebo L, Korner U *et al*. Effects by daily long term provision of ghrelin to unselected weight-losing cancer patients: a randomized double-blind study. Cancer 2010;**116**:2044–52.
82. Neary NM, Small CJ, Wren AM *et al*. Ghrelin increases energy intake in cancer patients with impaired appetite: acute, randomized, placebo-controlled trial. *J Clin Endocrinol Metab* 2004;**89**:2832–6.
83. Madeddu C and Mantovani G. An update on promising agents for the treatment of cancer cachexia. *Curr Opin Support Palliat Care* 2009;**3**:258–62.
84. Balducci L and Extermann M. Management of cancer in the older person. *Oncologist* 2000;**5**:224–37.
85. Oken MM, Creech RH, Tomney DC *et al*. Toxicity and response criteria of the Eastern Cooperative Oncology Group. *Am J Clin Oncol* 1982;**5**:649–55.
86. Mercadante S. Nausea/vomiting. In: E Bruera *et al*. (eds), *Textbook of Palliative Medicine*, Hodder Arnold, London, 2006, pp. 546–53.
87. Seyennes O, Fiatarone-Singh MA, Hue O *et al*. Physiologic and functional responses to low-moderate vs high intensity progressive resistance training in frail elderly. *J Gerontol A Biol Sci Med Sci* 2004;**59**:503–9.
88. Crew KD, Greenlee H, Capodice J *et al*. Prevalence of joint symptoms in postmenopausal women taking aromatase inhibitors for early-stage breast cancer. *J Clin Oncol* 2007;**25**:3877–83.
89. Clough-Gorr KM, Stuck AE, Thwin SS *et al*. Older breast cancer survivors: geriatric assessment domains are associated with poor tolerance of treatment adverse effects and predict mortality over 7 years of follow-up. *J Clin Oncol* 2010;**28**:380–6.
90. Bylow K, Mohile SG, Stadler WM and Dale W. Does androgen-deprivation therapy accelerate the development of frailty in older men with prostate cancer?: a conceptual review. *Cancer* 2007;**110**:2604–13.
91. Blanchard CM, Courneya KS and Stein K. Cancer survivors' adherence to lifestyle behavior recommendations and associations with health-related quality of life: results from the ACS SCS-II. *J Clin Oncol* 2008;**26**:198–204.
92. Kasymjanova G, Correa JA, Kreisman H *et al*. Prognostic value of the six-minute walk in advanced non-small cell lung cancer. *J Thorac Oncol* 2009;**4**:602–7.
93. Luctkar-Flude M, Groll D, Woodend K and Tranmer J. Fatigue and physical activity in older patients with cancer: a six-month follow-up study. *Oncol Nurs Forum* 2009;**36**:194–202.
94. Mustian, KM, Griggs JJ, Morrow GR *et al*. Exercise and side effects among 749 patients during and after treatment for cancer: a University of Rochester Cancer Center Community Clinical Oncology Program study. *Support Care Cancer* 2006;**14**:732–41.
95. Jones LW, Eves ND, Haykowsky M *et al*. Exercise intolerance in cancer and the role of exercise therapy to reverse dysfunction. *Lancet Oncol* 2009;**4**:602–7.
96. Jones LW, Peddle CJ, Eves ND *et al*. Effects of presurgical exercise training on cardiorespiratory fitness among patients undergoing thoracic surgery for malignant lung lesions. *Cancer* 2007;**110**:590–8.
97. Bobbio A, Chetta A, Ampollini L *et al*. Preoperative pulmonary rehabilitation in patients undergoing lung resection for non-small cell cancer. *Eur J Cardiothorac Surg* 2008;**33**:95–8.
98. Jones LW, Eves ND, Peddle CJ *et al*. Effects of presurgical exercise training on systemic inflammatory markers among patients with malignant lung lesions. *Appl Physiol Nutr Metab* 2009;**34**:197–202.
99. Battaglini CL, Hackney AC, Garcia R *et al*. The effects of an exercise program in leukemia patients. *Integr Cancer Ther* 2009;**8**:130–8.
100. Taaffe DR, Harris TB, Ferrucci L *et al*. Cross-sectional and prospective relationships of interleukin-6 and C-reactive protein with physical performance in elderly persons: MacArthur Studies of successful aging. *J Geron A Biol Sci Med Sci* 2000;**55**: M709–15.
101. Teno JM, Weitzen S, Fennell ML and Mor V. Dying trajectory in the last year of life: does the cancer trajectory fit other diseases ? *J Palliat Med* 2001;**4**:457–64.
102. Jones LW, Eves ND, Mackey JR *et al*. Safety and feasibility of cardiopulmonary exercise testing in patients with advanced lung cancer. *Lung Cancer* 2007;55:225–32.
103. Temel, JS, Greer JA, Goldberg S *et al*. A structured exercise program for patients with advanced non-small cell lung cancer. *J Thorac Oncol* 2009;**4**:595–601.
104. Cassileth BR, Deng GE, Gomez JE *et al*. Complementary therapies and integrative oncology in lung cancer. ACCP evidence-based clinical practice guidelines (2nd ed.). *Chest* 2007;**132**(Suppl): 340S–54S.
105. Bentzen S. Preventing or reducing late side effects of radiation therapy: radiobiology meets molecular pathology. *Nat Rev Cancer* 2006;**6**:702–13.
106. Jones LW, Eves ND, Waner E and Joy AA. Exercise therapy across the lung cancer continuum. *Curr Oncol Rep* 2009;**11**:255–62.
107. Miller KL, Kozak Z, Kahn D *et al*. Preliminary report of the 6-minute walk test as a predictor of radiation induced pulmonary toxicity. *Int J Radiat Oncol Biol Phys* 2005;**62**:1009–13.
108. American Thoracic Society. ATS Statement. Guidelines for the six-minute walk test. Official statement of the American Thoracic Society. *Am J Respir Crit Care Med* 2002;**166**:111–7.
109. Mustian KM, Peppone L, Darling TV *et al*. A 4-week home-based aerobic and resistance exercise program during radiation therapy: a pilot randomized clinical trial. *J Support Oncol* 2009;**7**:158–67.
110. Swain SM, Whaley FS and Ewer MS. Congestive heart failure in patients treated with doxorubicin: a retrospective analysis of three trials. *Cancer* 2003;**97**:2869–79.
111. Swain SM, Whaley FS, Ewer MS and Lippmann SM. Type II chemotherapy-related cardiac dysfunction: time to recognize a new entity. *J Clin Oncol* 2005;**23**:2900–2.
112. Jones LW, Haykowsky M, Pituskin EN *et al*. Cardiovascular reserve and risk profile of postmenopausal women after chemoendocrine therapy for hormone receptor positive operable breast cancer. *Oncologist* 2007;**12**:1156–64.

113. Hurria A, Wong L, Pal S *et al.* Perspectives and attitudes on the use of adjuvant chemotherapy and trustazumab in older adults with HER-2+ breast cancer: a survey of oncologists. *Oncologist* 2009;**14**:883–90.

114. Verheul H and Pinedo H. Possible molecular mechanisms involved in the toxicity of angiogenesis inhibition. *Nat Rev Cancer* 2007;**7**:475–85.

115. Haykowsky MJ, Mackey JR, Thompson RB *et al.* Adjuvant trustazumab induces ventricular remodeling despite aerobic exercise training. *Clin Cancer Res* 2009;**15**:4963–7.

116. Wonder K and Reigle B. Trustazumab and doxorubicin-related cardiotoxicity and the cardioprotective role of exercise. *Integr Cancer Ther* 2009;**8**:17–21.

117. Goodwin PJ, Ennis M, Pritchard KI *et al.* Fasting insulin and outcome in early stage breast cancer: results of a prospective cohort study. *J Clin Oncol* 2002;**20**:42–51.

118. Haydon AM, MacInnis RJ, English DR *et al.* Physical activity, insulin-like growth factor binding protein and survival from colon cancer. Gut 2006;**55**:689–94.

119. Fairy AS, Courneya KS, Field CJ *et al.* Effects of exercise training on fasting insulin, insulin resistance, insulin-like growth factors and insulin-like growth factor binding proteins in postmenopausal breast cancer survivors: a randomized controlled trial. *Cancer Epidemiol Biomarkers Prev* 2003;**12**:721–7.

120. Ligibel, JA, Campbell N, Partridge A *et al.* Impact of a mixed strength and endurance exercise intervention on insulin levels in breast cancer survivors. *J Clin Oncol* 2008;**26**:907–12.

121. Demark-Wahnefried, W, Clipp ED, Morey MC *et al.* Lifestyle intervention development study to improve physical function in older adults with cancer: outcomes from project LEAD. *J Clin Oncol* 2006;**24**:3465–73.

122. Morey MC, Snyder DC, Sloan R *et al.* Effects of home-based diet and exercise on functional outcomes among older, overweight long-term cancer survivors. RENEW: a randomized controlled trial. *JAMA* 2009;**301**:1883–91.

123. Murtrie N, Campbell AM, Whyte F *et al.* Benefits of supervised group exercise programmme for women being treated for early stage breast cancer: a pragmatic randomized controlled trial. *BMJ* 2007;**334**: 517.

124. Mouridsen H, Keshaviah H, Coates AS *et al.* Cardiovascular adverse events during adjuvant endocrine therapy for early breast cancer using letrazole or tamoxifen: safety analysis of BIG 1-98 Trial. *J Clin Oncol* 2007;**25**:5715–22.

125. Henry NL, Giles JT, Ang D *et al.* Prospective characterization of musculoskeletal sympotms in early stage breast cancer patients treated with aromatase inhibitors. *Breast Cancer Res Treat* 2008;**111**:365–72.

126. DeBacker IC, Schep G, Backx FJ *et al.* Resistance training in cancer survivors: a systematic review. *Int J Sports Med* 2009;**30**:703–12.

127. Demark-Wahnefried W, Hars V, Conaway MR *et al.* Reduced rates of metabolism and decreased physical activity in breast cancer patients receiving adjuvant chemotherapy. *Am J Clin Nutr* 1997;**65**:1495–501.

128. MacVicar M, Winningham M and Nickel J. Effects of aerobic interval training on cancer patients' functional capacity. *Nurs Res* 1989;**38**:348–51.

129. Courneya KS, Segal RJ, Mackey JR *et al.* Effects of aerobic and resistance exercise in breast cancer patients receiving adjuvant chemotherapy: a multicenter randomized controlled trial. *J Clin Oncol* 2007;**25**:4396–404.

130. Schmitz KH, Holtzman J, Courneya KS *et al.* Controlled physical activity trials in cancer survivors: a systematic review and meta-analysis. *Cancer Epidemiol Biomarkers Prev* 2005;**14**:1588–95.

131. McNeeley MI, Campbell KL, Rowe BH *et al.* Effects of exercise on breast cancer patients and survivors: a systematic review and meta-analysis. CMAJ 2006;**175**:34–41.

132. Friedenreich, CM, Woolcott CG, McTiernan A *et al.* Alberta physical activity and breast cancer prevention trial: sex hormone changes in a year-long exercise intervention among postmenopausal women. *J Clin Oncol* 2010;**28**:1458–66.

133. Holmes, MD, Chen WY, Feskanich D *et al.* Physical activity and survival after breast cancer diagnosis. *JAMA* 2005;**293**:2479–86.

134. Meyerhardt JA, Giovannucci EL, Ogino S *et al.* Physical activity and male colorectal cancer survival. *Arch Int Med* 2009;**169**:2102–8.

135. Droz JP, Balducci L, Bolla M *et al.* Background for the proposal of SIOG guidelines for the management of prostate cancer in senior adults. *Crit Rev Oncol Hematol* 2010;**73**:68–91.

136. Alibhai SMH, Minh DM, Sutradhar M *et al.* Impact of androgen deprivation therapy on cardiovascular disease and diabetes. *J Clin Oncol* 2009;**27**:3452–8.

137. Daniell HW, Dunn SR, Ferguson DW *et al.* Progressive osteoporosis during androgen deprivation therapy for prostate cancer. *J Urol* 2000;**163**:181–6.

138. Galvao DA, Spry NA, Taafe DR *et al.* Changes in muscle, fat and bone mass after 36 weeks of maximal androgen blockade for prostate cancer. *BJU Int* 2008;**102**:44–7.

139. Galvao DA, Taafe DR, Spry NA *et al.* Reduced muscle strength and functional performance in men with prostate cancer undergoing androgen suppression: a comprehensive cross-sectional investigation. *Prostate Cancer Prostat Dis* 2009;**12**:198–203.

140. Ross R and Small E. Osteoporosis in men treated with androgen deprivation therapy for prostate cancer. *J Urol* 2002;**167**:152–6.

141. Keating N, O'Malley A and Smith M. Diabetes and cardiovascular disease during androgen deprivation therapy for prostate cancer. *J Clin Oncol* 2006;**24**:4448–56.

142. Tsai HK, D'Amico AV, Sadetsky N *et al.* Androgen deprivation therapy for localized prostate cancer and the risk of cardiovascular disease. *J Natl Cancer Inst* 2007;**99**:1516–24.

143. Shahinian VB, Kuo YF, Freeman JL *et al.* Risk of fracture after androgen deprivation for prostate cancer. *N Engl J Med* 2005;**352**:154–64.

144. Giovannucci EL, Liu Y, Leitzman MF *et al.* A prospective study of physical activity and incident and fatal prostate cancer. *Arch Int Med* 2005;**165**:1005–10.

145. Ornish D, Weidner G, Fair WR *et al.* Intensive life-style changes may affect the progression of prostate cancer. *J Urol* 2005;**174**:1065–9.

146. Tymchuk CN, Barnard RJ, Heber D and Aronson WJ. Evidence of an inhibitory effect of diet and exercise on prostate cancer cell growth. *J Urol* 2001;**166**:1185–9.

147. Galvao D and Newton R. Review of exercise intervention studies in cancer patients. *J Clin Oncol*. 2005;**23**:899–909.

148. Galvao DA, Spry N, Taafe DR *et al*. A randomized controlled trial of an exercise intervention targeting cardiovascular and metabolic risk factors for prostate cancer patients from the RADAR trial. *BMC Cancer* 2009;**9**: 419.

149. Galvao DA, Taafe DR, Spry N *et al*. Combined resistance and aerobic exercise program reverses muscle loss in men undergoing androgen suppression therapy for prostate cancer without bone metastases: a randomized controlled clinical trial. *J Clin Oncol* 2010;**28**:340–7.

150. Cramp F and Daniel J. Exercise for the management of cancer-related fatigue in adults. *Cochrane Database Syst Rev* 2008;(2): CD006145–.

151. Kuchinski A, Reading M and Lash A. Treatment-related fatigue and exercise in patients with cancer: a systematic review. *Medsurg Nurs* 2009;**18**:174–80.

152. Knols R, Aaronson NK, Uebelhart D *et al*. Physical exercise in cancer patients during and after medical treatment: a systematic review of randomized and controlled clinical trials. *J Clin Oncol* 2005;**23**:3830–42.

153. Luctkar-Flude MF, Groll DI, Tranmer J and Woodend K. Fatigue and physical activity in older adults with cancer. A systematic review of the literature. *Cancer Nurs* 2007;**30**:35–45.

154. Mustian KM, Sprod LK, Palesh OG *et al*. Exercise for the management of side effects and quality of life among cancer survivors. *Curr Sports Med Rep* 2009;**8**:326–30.

155. Courneya KS, Vallence JKH, McNeeley ML *et al*. Exercise issues in older cancer survivors. *Crit Rev Oncol Hematol* 2004;**51**:249–61.

156. Ahles TA, Saykin AJ, McDonald BC *et al*. Longitudinal assessment of cognitive changes associated with adjuvant treatment for breast cancer: impact of age and cognitive reserve. *J Clin Oncol* 2010;**28**:4434–40.

157. Ahles TA, Saykin AJ, McDonald BC *et al*. Cognitive function in breast cancer patients prior to adjuvant treatment. *Breast Cancer Res Treat* 2008;**110**:143–52.

158. Sloan CD, Shen L, West JD *et al*. Genetic pathway-based hierarchical clustering analysis of older adults with cognitive complaints and amnestic mild cognitive impairment using clinical and neuroimaging phenotypes. *Am J Med Genet B Neuropsychiatr Genet* 2010;**153B**:1060–9.

SECTION 13

Functional Disorders and Rehabilitation

CHAPTER 112

Multidimensional geriatric assessment

Laurence Z. Rubenstein[1] and Andreas E. Stuck[2]

[1]University of Oklahoma College of Medicine, Oklahoma City, OK, USA
[2]Geriatrics Inselspital University Hospital, Bern, Switzerland

Introduction

The essence of good geriatric practice is the expert management of the medical, psychological and social needs of elderly patients and their family caregivers. For this to be accomplished, the members of the interdisciplinary geriatric team – whether based in a hospital geriatric unit, an outpatient clinic, a nursing home, or a home-care programme – must work closely together to assess carefully the patient's risks and problems and translate this knowledge into care plans that will have far-reaching effects on both the patient's and caregiver's lives.

Such multidimensional assessment implies the detailed investigation of the elderly individual's total situation in terms of physical and mental state, functional status, formal and informal social support and network, and physical environment. This requires the clinician to become involved in collecting, interpreting, synthesizing and weighing a formidable amount of patient-specific information. Much of this differs in kind from the physical symptoms and signs, laboratory values, radiology results and other data that are traditionally combined to reach a medical diagnosis.

Definition

Multidimensional geriatric assessment (MGA) (often called comprehensive geriatric assessment or CGA) is a diagnostic process, usually interdisciplinary, intended to determine an older person's medical, psychosocial, functional and environmental resources, and problems with the objective of developing an overall plan for treatment and long-term follow-up. It differs from the standard medical evaluation in its concentration on older people with their often complex problems, its emphasis on functional status and quality of life (QOL), and its frequent use of interdisciplinary teams and quantitative assessment scales.

As described in this chapter, multidimensional geriatric assessment can vary in its the level of detail, its purpose, and other aspects depending on the clinical circumstances. Therefore, multidimensional assessment denotes both the relatively brief multidimensional screening assessment for preventive purpose in a patient's home as well as the interdisciplinary work-up of a newly hospitalized patient. Despite this broad definition, the term must meet the primary criteria above. For example, a multidimensional evaluation of an older person without link to the overall plan for treatment and follow-up does not meet these criteria. Similarly, a home visit emphasizing psychosocial and environmental factors, but not including a medical evaluation of the older person, is not a multidimensional assessment, since one of the key components of the multidimensionality is not included.

Rationale

While the principles of geriatric assessment may be valid in the treatment of younger persons as well, since bio-psycho-social factors play an important role in medicine for patients of all age groups, there is additional justification for using this multidimensional approach in older persons for various reasons:

– Multi-morbidity and complexity: Many older persons suffer from multiple conditions, and multidimensional assessment helps to deal with these complex situations through its systematic approaches and its setting of priorities.

– Unrecognized problems: Many older persons suffer from problems that have not been reported to the physician or may not even be known to the older person. One of the reasons problems may go undetected is that they may be falsely considered non-modifiable consequences of ageing. Multidimensional geriatric assessment is a method for identifying previously unknown problems.

– Chronic conditions: Many older persons suffer from chronic conditions. Diagnostic information without

Principles and Practice of Geriatric Medicine, Fifth Edition. Edited by Alan J. Sinclair, John E. Morley and Bruno Vellas.

information on functional relevance of the underlying condition is often of limited value for therapeutic decisions or for monitoring follow-up.

– Interaction with social and environmental factors: Once functional impairments or dependencies arise, the older person's condition is strongly influenced by his or her social and physical environment. For example, the arrangement of the older person's in-home environment and the availability of his or her social network might determine whether a person can continue to live in his or her home.

– Functional status: One of the main objectives of medicine for older persons is to prevent or delay the onset of functional status decline. Epidemiological research has shown that functional status decline is related to medical, functional, psychological, social and environmental risk factors. Therefore, both for rehabilitation as well as for prevention the approach of multidimensional assessment helps to take into account potentially modifiable factors in all relevant domains.

– Intervention studies: Multiple intervention studies that compared the effects of programmes based on the concept of multidimensional geriatric assessment with usual care did show benefits of geriatric assessment, including better patient outcomes and more efficient healthcare use.

Brief history of geriatric assessment

The basic concepts of geriatric assessment have evolved over the past 70 years by combining elements of the traditional medical history and physical examination, the social worker assessment, functional evaluation and treatment methods derived from rehabilitation medicine, and psychometric methods derived from the social sciences.

The first published reports of geriatric assessment programmes came from the British geriatrician Marjorie Warren, who initiated the concept of specialized geriatric assessment units during the late 1930s while in charge of a large London infirmary. This infirmary was filled primarily with chronically ill, bedfast and largely neglected elderly patients who had not received proper medical diagnosis or rehabilitation and who were thought to be in need of lifelong institutionalization. Good nursing care kept the patients alive, but the lack of diagnostic assessment and rehabilitation kept them disabled. Through evaluation, mobilization and rehabilitation, Warren was able to get most of the long bedfast patients out of bed and often discharged home. As a result of her experiences, Warren advocated that every elderly patient receive comprehensive assessment and an attempt at rehabilitation before being admitted to a long-term care hospital or nursing home.[1]

Since Warren's work, geriatric assessment has evolved. As geriatric care systems have been developed throughout the world, geriatric assessment programmes have been assigned central roles, usually as focal points for entry into the care systems. Geared to differing local needs and populations, geriatric assessment programmes vary in intensity, structure and function. They can be located in different settings, including acute hospital inpatient units and consultation teams, chronic and rehabilitation hospital units, outpatient and office-based programmes, and home visit outreach programmes. Despite diversity, they share many characteristics. Virtually all programmes provide multidimensional assessment, utilizing specific measurement instruments to quantify functional, psychological and social parameters. Most use interdisciplinary teams to pool expertise and enthusiasm in working toward common goals. Additionally, most programmes attempt to couple their assessments with an intervention, such as rehabilitation, counseling, or placement.

Today, geriatric assessment continues to evolve in response to increased pressures for cost-containment, avoidance of institutional stays, and consumer demands for better care. Geriatric assessment can help achieve improved quality of care and plan cost-effective care. This has generally meant more emphasis on non-institutional programmes and shorter hospital stays. Geriatric assessment teams are well positioned to deliver effective care for elderly persons with limited resources. Geriatricians have long emphasized judicious use of technology, systematic preventive medicine activities, and less institutionalization and hospitalization.

Components of geriatric assessment

A typical geriatric assessment begins with a functional status 'review of systems' that inventories the major domains of functioning.[2–6] The major elements of this review of systems are captured in two commonly used functional status measures – basic activities of daily living (ADL) and instrumental activities of daily living (IADL). Several reliable and valid versions of these measures have been developed, perhaps the most widely used being those by Katz,[7] Lawton[8] and Barthel.[9] These scales are used by clinicians to detect whether the patient has problems performing activities that people must be able to accomplish to survive without help in the community. Basic ADL include self-care activities such as eating, dressing, bathing, transferring and toileting. Patients unable to perform these activities will generally require 12- to 24-hour support by caregivers. Instrumental activities of daily living include heavier housework, going on errands, managing finances and telephoning – activities that are required if the individual is to remain independent in a house or apartment.

To interpret the results of impairments in ADL and IADL, physicians will usually need additional information about the patient's environment and social situation. For example, the amount and type of caregiver support available, the strength of the patient's social network, and the level of social activities in which the patient participates will all influence the clinical approach taken in managing deficits detected. This information could be obtained by an experienced nurse or social worker. A screen for mobility and fall risk is also extremely helpful in quantifying function and disability, and several observational scales are available.[10,11] An assessment of nutritional status and risk for undernutrition is also important in understanding the extent of impairment and for planning care.[3] Likewise, a screening assessment of vision and hearing will often detect crucial deficits that need to be treated or compensated for.

Two other key pieces of information must always be gathered in the face of functional disability in an elderly person. These are a screen for mental status (cognitive) impairment and a screen for depression.[2,3,6] Of the several validated screening tests for cognitive function, the Folstein Mini-mental State is one of the best because it efficiently tests the major aspects of cognitive functioning.[3,12] Of the various screening tests for geriatric depression, the Yesavage Geriatric Depression Scale,[13] and the Zung Self-Rating Depression Scale[3] are in wide use, and even shorter screening versions are available without significant loss of accuracy.[14]

The major measurable dimensions of geriatric assessment, together with examples of commonly used health status screening scales, are listed in Table 112.1.[2–16] The instruments listed are short, have been carefully tested for reliability and validity, and can be easily administered by virtually any staff person involved with the assessment process. Both observational instruments (e.g. physical examination) and self-report (completed by patient or proxy) are available. Components of them – such as watching a patient walk, turn around and sit down – are routine parts of the geriatric physical examination. Many other kinds of assessment measures exist and can be useful in certain situations. For example, there are several disease-specific measures for stages and levels of dysfunction for patients with specific diseases such as arthritis, dementia and parkinsonism. There are also several brief global assessment instruments that attempt to quantify all dimensions of the assessment in a single form.[17,18] These latter instruments can be useful in community surveys and some research settings but are not detailed enough to be useful in most clinical settings. More comprehensive lists of available instruments can be found by consulting published reviews of health status assessment.[2–6]

Settings of geriatric assessment

A number of factors must be taken into account in deciding where an assessment should take place – whether it is done in the hospital, in an outpatient setting, or in the patient's home. Mental and physical impairment make it difficult for patients to comply with recommendations and to navigate multiple appointments in multiple locations. Functionally impaired elders must depend on families and friends, who risk losing their jobs because of chronic and relentless demands on time and energy and in their roles as caregivers, and who may be elderly themselves. Each separate medical appointment or intervention has a high

Table 112.1 Measurable dimensions of geriatric assessment with examples of specific measures

Dimension	Basic context	Specific examples
Basic ADL	Strengths and limitations in self-care,basic mobility and incontinence	Katz (ADL),[7] Lawton Personal Self-Maintenance Scale,[8] Barthel Index [9]
IADL	Strengths and limitations in shopping cooking, household activities, finances	Lawton (IADL)[8] OARS, IADL Section [3,4]
Social Activities and Supports	Strengths and limitations in social network and community activities	Lubben Social Network Scale[16] OARS, Social Resources Section [3,4]
Mental Health Affective	Degree of anxiety, depression, happiness	Geriatric Depression Scale [12,14] Zung Depression Scale [3]
Mental Health Cognitive	Degree of alertness, orientation concentration, mental task capacity	Folstein Mini-mental State[12] Kahn Mental Status Questionnaire [3,4]
Mobility Gait and Balance	Quantification of gait, balance and risk of falls	Tinetti Mobility Assessment [10] Get up and go test [11]
Nutritional Adequacy	Current nutritional status and risk of malnutrition	Nutritional Screening Checklist [3] Mini-nutritional Assessement [15]
Special Senses	Hearing and vision impairments	Whispered Voice Test or Hearing Handicap Inventory [3–6] Snellen chart or Vision Function Questionnaire [3–6]
Oral Health	Impairments of oral health	Geriatric Oral Health Assessment Index [5,6]

ADL, activities of daily living; IADL, instrumental activities of daily living time-cost to these caregivers. Patient fatigue during periods of increased illness may require the availability of a bed during the assessment process. Finally, enough physician time and expertise must be available to complete the assessment within the constraints of the setting.

Most geriatric assessments do not require the full range of technology nor the intense monitoring found in the acute care inpatient setting. Yet hospitalization becomes unavoidable if no outpatient setting provides sufficient resources to accomplish the assessment fast enough. A specialized geriatric setting outside an acute hospital ward, such as a day hospital or subacute inpatient geriatric evaluation unit, will provide the easy availability of an interdisciplinary team with the time and expertise to provide needed services efficiently, an adequate level of monitoring, and beds for patients unable to sit or stand for prolonged periods. Inpatient and day hospital assessment programmes have the advantages of intensity, rapidity and ability to care for particularly frail or acutely ill patients. Outpatient programmes are generally cheaper and avoid the necessity of an inpatient stay.

Assessment in the office practice setting

A streamlined approach is usually necessary in the office setting. An important first step is setting priorities among problems for initial evaluation and treatment. The 'best' problem to work on first might be the problem that most bothers a patient or, alternatively, the problem upon which resolution of other problems depends (alcoholism or depression often fall into this category).

The second step in performing a geriatric assessment is to understand the exact nature of the disability through performing a task or symptom analysis. In a non-specialized setting, or when the disability is mild or clear-cut, this may involve only taking a careful history. When the disability is more severe, more detailed assessments by a multidisciplinary or interdisciplinary team may be necessary. For example, a patient may present with difficulty dressing. There are multiple tasks associated with dressing, any one of which might be the stumbling block (e.g. buying clothes, choosing appropriate clothes to put on, remembering to complete the task, buttoning, stretching to put on shirts, or reaching downward to put on shoes). By identifying the exact areas of difficulty, further evaluation can be targeted toward solving the problem.

Once the history has revealed the nature of the disability, a systematic physical examination and ancillary laboratory tests are needed to clarify the cause of the problem. For example, difficulty dressing could be caused by mental status impairment, poor finger mobility, or dysfunction of shoulders, back, or hips. Evaluation by a physical or occupational therapist may be necessary to pinpoint the problem adequately, and evaluation by a social worker may be required to determine the extent of family dysfunction engendered by or contributing to the dependency. Radiological and other laboratory testing may be necessary.

Each abnormality that could cause difficulty dressing suggests different treatments. By understanding the abnormalities that contribute most to the functional disability, the best treatment strategy can be undertaken. Often one disability leads to another – impaired gait may lead to depression or decreased social functioning; and immobility of any cause, even after the cause has been removed, can lead to secondary impairments in performance of daily activities due to deconditioning and loss of musculoskeletal flexibility.

Almost any acute or chronic disease can reduce functioning. Common but easily overlooked causes of dysfunction in elderly people include impaired cognition, impaired special senses (vision, hearing, balance), unstable gait and mobility, poor health habits (alcohol, smoking, lack of exercise), poor nutrition, polypharmacy, incontinence, psychosocial stress and depression. To identify contributing causes of the disability, the physician must thus look for worsening of the patient's chronic diseases, occurrence of a new acute disease, or appearance of one of the common occult diseases listed above. The physician does this through a refocused history guided by the functional disabilities detected and their differential diagnoses, and a focused physical examination. The physical examination always includes, in addition to usual evaluations of the heart, lungs, extremities and neurological function, postural blood pressure, vision and hearing screening, and careful observation of the patient's gait. The mini-mental state examination, already recommended as part of the initial functional status screen, may also determine what parts of the physical examination require particular attention as part of the evaluation of dementia or acute confusion. Finally, basic laboratory testing including a complete blood count and a blood chemistry panel, as well as tests indicated on the basis of specific findings from the history and physical examination, will generally be necessary.

Once the disability and its causes are understood, the best treatments or management strategies for it are often clear. When a reversible cause for the impairment is found, a simple treatment may eliminate or ameliorate the functional disability. When the disability is complex, the physician may need the support of a variety of community or hospital-based resources. In most cases, a strategy for long-term follow-up and often, formal case management should be developed to ensure that needs and services are appropriately matched up and followed through.

Preventive home visits

Preventive home visitation programmes in elderly people are part of national policy in several countries. The rationale is to delay or prevent functional impairment and subsequent nursing home admissions by primary prevention (e.g. immunization and exercise), secondary prevention (e.g. detection of untreated problems), and tertiary prevention (e.g. improvement of medication use).

This is a typical description of a preventive home visitation programme:[19] 'The assessment included a medical history-taking, a physical examination, haematocrit and glucose measurements in blood samples obtained by finger stick, a dipstick urinalysis and a mail-in faecal occult-blood test. The subjects were also evaluated for functional status, oral health, mental status (presence or absence of depression and cognitive status), gait and balance, medications, percentage of ideal body weight, vision, hearing, extensiveness of social network, quality of social support and safety in the home, and ease of access to the external environment. The nurse practitioners discussed each case with the project geriatricians, developed rank-ordered recommendations, and conducted in-home follow-up visits every three months to monitor the implementation of the recommendations, make additional recommendations if new problems were detected, and facilitate compliance. If additional contact was considered necessary, the nurse practitioner telephoned the participant or was available by telephone. All the participants were encouraged to take an active role in their care and to improve their ability to discuss problems with their physicians. Only in complex situations did the nurse practitioners or study physicians contact the patients' physicians directly.'

Various studies have shown the advantage of the home environment in conducting a multidimensional assessment. The yield of a home visit does not seem to be limited to the preventive application, home visits can also play an important role as part of outpatient or inpatient programmes.

Inpatient geriatric assessment

If referral to a specialized geriatric setting has been chosen, the process of assessment will probably be similar to that described above, except that the greater intensity of resources and the special training of all members of the multidisciplinary team in dealing with geriatric patients and their problems will facilitate carrying out the proposed assessment and plan more quickly, and in greater breadth and detail. In the usual geriatric assessment setting, key disciplines involved include, at a minimum, physicians, social workers, nurses and physical and occupational therapists, and optimally may include other disciplines such as dieticians, pharmacists, ethicists and home-care specialists. Special geriatric expertise among the interdisciplinary team members is crucial.

Geriatric assessment and management programmes were developed for both the acute care and the post-acute care settings. A typical example of an acute care programme is the 'acute care for elderly (ACE) unit', specifically designed for the the special needs of unselected acutely ill elderly inpatients, combining a structured geriatric assessment approach with other adaptations of the process of patient care, such as early discharge planning or interdisciplinary care in the acute care setting for co-existing conditions (e.g. for immobility, confusion, malnutrition).[20] In addition, these units contain specific structural characteristics, for example related to personnel staffing (e.g. additional physical therapists) and environmental adaptations (e.g. rails for the prevention of falls or calendars for better orientation). On the other hand, programmes for the post-acute care setting are focused to in-hospital care of selected older patients who had initial acute care treatment. These programmes admit patients with ongoing need for postacute and rehabilitative care. Typically, these programmes contain a rehabilitation component with an interdisciplinary team assigning patients to specific therapies based on individual geriatric assessment of each patient.[21]

The interdisciplinary team conference, which takes place after most team members have completed their individual assessments, is critical. Most successful trials of geriatric assessment have included such a team conference. By bringing the perspectives of all disciplines together, the team conference generates new ideas, sets priorities, disseminates the full results of the assessment to all those involved in treating the patient, and avoids duplication or incongruity. Development of fully effective teams requires commitment, skill and time as the interdisciplinary team evolves through the 'forming, storming and norming' phases to reach the fully developed 'performing' stage. Involvement of the patient (and carer if appropriate) at some stage is important in maintaining the principle of choice.[22]

Hospital-home assessment programmes

A number of additional published reports have described another multidimensional assessement model in which hospitalized older patients in need of comprehensive assessment are referred to an in-home assessment programme that occurs in their homes following the hospital discharge. The advantages of this approach include shortening the hospital stay, providing the assessment in the home environment that allows evaluation of the home itself and how the patient functions therein, and allowing careful targeting of the in-home assessment to individuals who can derive maximal benefit.

A special approach has been tested in older patients with cardiac risk. In these patients, geriatric assessment in the hospital was combined with a systematic ambulatory follow-up. Early detection of heart failure and optimizing patient adherence with medication prescriptions were key ingredients of these programmes.[23] Several studies have confirmed that geriatric assessment also reduces unnecessary or inappropriate medications use.

Geriatric assessment in the care of older cancer patients

The International Society of Geriatric Oncology (SIOG) created a task force to review the evidence on the use of a comprehensive geriatric assessment in older cancer patients.[24] Based on a systematic review of the evidence strong evidence was found that a comprehensive geriatric assessment detects many problems missed by a regular assessment in general geriatric and in cancer patients. However, there was corroborative evidence only from a few studies conducted in cancer patients. A recent study confirmed that geriatric assessment conducted in breast cancer survivors is associated with treatment side effects, and long-term survival.[25] Screening tools exist and were successfully used in settings such as the emergency room, but globally were poorly tested. Based on these findings, it was concluded that a comprehensive geriatric assessment, with or without screening, and with follow-up, should be used in older cancer patients, in order to detect unaddressed problems, improve their functional status, and possibly their survival. The task force could not recommend any specific tool or approach above others at this point and general geriatric experience should be used.

Geriatric assessment in the care of nursing home patients

Geriatric assessment is also an important component in the care of older patients in the nursing home. One of the most widely disseminated systems of assessment is the Resident Assessment Instrument.

Effectiveness of geriatric assessment programmes

The pioneering studies of geriatric assessment

A large and still growing literature supports the effectiveness of geriatric assessment programmes (GAPs) in a variety of settings. Early descriptive studies indicated a number of benefits from GAPs such as improved diagnostic accuracy, reduced discharges to nursing homes, increased functional status, and more appropriate medication prescribing. Because they were descriptive studies, without concurrent control patients, they were not able to distinguish the effects of the programmes from simple improvement over time. Nor did these studies look at long-term, or many short-term, outcome benefits. Nonetheless, many of these early studies provided promising results.[2,3,26]

Improved diagnostic accuracy was the most widely described effect of geriatric assessment, most often indicated by substantial numbers of important problems uncovered. Frequencies of new diagnoses found ranged from almost one to more than four per patient. Factors contributing to the improvement of diagnosis in GAPs include the validity of the assessment itself (the capability of a structured search for 'geriatric problems' to find them), the extra measure of time and care taken in the evaluation of the patient (independent of the formal elements of 'the assessment'), and a probable lack of diagnostic attention on the part of referring professionals.

Improved living location on discharge from healthcare setting was demonstrated in several early studies, beginning with TF Williams' classic descriptive pre–post study of an outpatient assessment programme in New York.[27] Of patients referred for nursing home placement in the county, the assessment programme found that only 38% actually needed skilled nursing care, while 23% could return home, and 39% were appropriate for board and care or retirement facilities. Numerous subsequent studies have shown similar improvements in living location.[2,3] Several studies that examined mental or physical functional status of patients before and after comprehensive geriatric assessment coupled with treatment and rehabilitation showed patient improvement on measures of function.[2,3]

Evidence from controlled studies

Beginning in the 1980s, controlled studies appeared that corroborated some of the earlier studies and documented additional benefits such as improved survival, reduced hospital and nursing home utilization, and in some cases, reduced costs.[2,3,28–33] These studies were by no means uniform in their results. Some showed a whole series of dramatic positive effects on function, survival, living location, and costs, while others showed relatively few if any benefits. However, the GAPs being studied were also very different from each other in terms of process of care offered and patient populations accepted. To this day, controlled trials of GAPs continue, and as results accumulate, we are able to understand which aspects contribute to their effectiveness and which do not.

One striking effect confirmed for many GAPs has been a positive impact on survival. Several controlled studies of different basic GAP models demonstrated significantly increased survival, reported in different ways and with varying periods of follow-up. Mortality was reduced for Sepulveda geriatric evaluation unit patients by 50% at one year, and the survival curves of the experimental and control groups still significantly favoured the assessed group at two years.[3,28] Survival was improved by 21% at one year in a Scottish trial of geriatric rehabilitation consultation. Two Canadian consultation trials demonstrated significantly improved six-month survival. Two Danish community-based trials of in-home geriatric assessment and follow-up demonstrated reduction in mortality, and two Welsh studies of in-home GAPs had beneficial survival effects among patients assessed at home and followed for two years. On the other hand, several other studies of geriatric assessment found no statistically significant survival benefits.[3,31,33]

Multiple studies followed patients longitudinally after the initial assessment and thus were able to examine the longer-term utilization and cost impacts of assessment and treatment. Some studies found an overall reduction in nursing home days. Hospital utilization was examined in several reports. For hospital-based GAPs, the length of hospitalization was obviously affected by the length of the assessment itself. Thus, some programmes appear to prolong initial length of stay while others reduce initial stay. However, studies following patients for at least one year have usually shown reduction in use of acute-care hospital services, even in those programmes with initially prolonged hospital stays.[3,31,33]

Compensatory increases in use of community-based services or home-care agencies might be expected with declines in nursing home placements and use of other institutional services. These increases have been detected in several studies but not in others. Although increased use of formal community services may not always be indicated, it usually is a desirable goal. The fact that several studies did not detect increases in use of home and community services probably reflects the unavailability of community service or referral networks rather than that more of such services were not needed.[3,31,33]

The effects of these programmes on costs and utilization parameters have only seldom been examined comprehensively, due to methodological difficulties in gathering comprehensive utilization and cost data, as well as statistical limitations in comparing highly skewed distributions. The Sepulveda study found that total first-year direct healthcare costs had been reduced due to overall reductions in nursing home and rehospitalization days, despite significantly longer initial hospital stays on the geriatric unit.[28] These savings continued through three years of follow-up. Hendriksen's in-home programme reduced the costs of medical care, apparently through successful early case-finding and referral for preventive intervention.[3,31,33] Williams' outpatient GAP detected reductions in medical care costs due primarily to reductions in hospitalization.[3,31,33] Although it would be reasonable to worry that prolonged survival of frail patients would lead to increased service use and charges, or, of perhaps greater concern, to worry about the quality of the prolonged life, these concerns may be without substance. Indeed, the Sepulveda study demonstrated that a GAP could improve not only survival but prolong high-function survival,[3,28,31,33] while at the same time reducing use of institutional services and costs.

Meta-analytic data

A 1993 meta-analysis attempted to resolve some of the discrepancies between study results, and to try to identify whether particular programme elements were associated with particular benefits.[3,31] This meta-analysis included published data from the 28 controlled trials completed as of that date, involving nearly 10 000 patients, and was also able to include substantial amounts of unpublished data systematically retrieved from many of the studies. The meta-analysis identified five GAP types: hospital units (six studies), hospital consultation teams (eight studies), in-home assessment services (seven studies), outpatient assessment services (four studies), and hospital-home assessment programmes (three studies). The meta-analysis confirmed many of the major reported benefits for many of the individual programme types. These statistically and clinically significant benefits included reduced risk of mortality (by 22 for hospital-based programmes at 12 months, and by 14% for all programmes combined at 12 months), improved likelihood of living at home (by 47% for hospital-based programmes and by 26% for all programmes combined at 12 months), reduced risk of hospital (re)admissions (by 12% for all programmes at study end), greater chance of cognitive improvement (by 47% for all programmes at study end), and greater chance of physical function improvement for patients on hospital units (by 72% for hospital units).

Clearly not all studies showed equivalent effects, and the meta-analysis was able to indicate a number of variables at both the programme and patient levels that tended to distinguish trials with large effects from ones with more limited ones. When examined on the programme level, hospital units and home-visit assessment teams produced the most dramatic benefits, while no major significant benefits in office-based programmes could be confirmed. Programmes that provided hands-on clinical care and/or long-term follow-up were generally able to produce greater positive effects than purely consultative programmes or ones that lacked follow-up. Another factor associated with greater demonstrated benefits, at least in hospital-based programmes, was patient targeting; programmes that selected patients who were at high risk for deterioration yet still had 'rehabilitation potential' generally had stronger results than less selective programmes.

The 1993 meta-analysis confirmed the importance of targeting criteria in producing beneficial outcomes. In particular, when use of explicit targeting criteria for patient selection was included as a covariate, increases in some programme benefits were often found. For example, among the hospital-based GAPs studies, positive effects on physical function and likelihood of living at home at 12 months were associated with studies that excluded patients who were relatively 'too healthy'. A similar effect on physical function was seen in the institutional studies that excluded persons with relatively poor prognoses. The reason for this effect of targeting on effect size no doubt lies in the ability of careful targeting to concentrate the intervention on patients who can benefit, without diluting the effect with persons too ill or too well to show a measurable improvement.

Since 1993 many new controlled studies on the effects of geriatric assessment programmes have been conducted. However, with principles of geriatric medicine and geriatric asssessment becoming more diffused into usual care, particularly at places where controlled trials are being undertaken, differences between geriatric assessment programmes and control groups seem to be narrowing. Given discrepancies in results between individual trials, several additional meta-analyses and systematic analyses have been conducted over the past few years.[31,33–38]

Assessment in the office practice setting: effects of outpatient geriatric assessment programmes have been less impressive, with a recent meta-analysis showing no favourable effects on mortality outcome.[35] For cost reasons, growth of inpatient units has been slow, despite their proven effectiveness, while outpatient programmes have increased, despite their less impressive effect size in controlled trials. However, some newer trials of outpatient programmes have shown significant benefits in areas not found in earlier outpatient studies, such as functional status, psychological parameters and well-being, which may indicate improvement in the outpatient care models being tested.[3,31,33]

Inpatient geriatric assessment programmes: several meta-analyses on inpatient geriatric assessment studies confirm favourable effects of these programmes on multiple outcomes (e.g. reduction of nursing home admissions and re-admissions to acute care hospital, improvement of functional status outcome), but continue to identify an important heterogeneity in findings and research methodology among published trials. A 2005 meta-analysis confirmed that inpatient comprehensive assessment programmes for older hospital patients may reduce mortality, increase the chances of living at home at one year and improve physical and cognitive function.[34] Two recent meta-analyses conducted separate meta-analyses on inpatient geriatric assessment units, one as part of acute care[36] and one on inpatient geriatric rehabilitation.[21] These two studies, and one additional meta-analysis[37] confirm favourable outcomes, and a large heterogeneity of care processes among these programmes.

Most recently, a 2011 Cochrane meta-analysis concluded that inpatient GAPs increase patients' likelihood of being alive and in their own homes at follow-up, and result in a potential cost reduction compared to general medical care.[38]

Hospital-home assessment programmes: Individual randomized controlled trials evaluated more refined models of hospital-home assessment programmes. For example, Rich *et al.*[23] developed and evaluated the effects of a programme specifically designed for older patients at high risk for recurrent heart failure after hospital discharge. Geriatric assessment was combined with follow-up in the hospital and at home after hospital discharge, and included monitoring of follow-up and compliance adherence. This programme resulted in a reduction of hospital re-admissions, improvement of QOL on participating patients, and in net cost savings.

Preventive home visitation programmes: There is an ongoing debate on the effects of community-based programmes geared towards the prevention of functional status decline and reduction of nursing home admissions among older persons. Meta-analysis of preventive home visits revealed that home visitation programmes are effective if based on multidimensional geriatric assessments with extended follow-up, and if offered to older persons with relatively good function at baseline.[33] Based on a large number of trials, the findings from this meta-analysis indicate that preventive home visitation programmes are effective only if interventions are based on multidimensional geriatric assessment, include multiple follow-up home visits and target persons with relatively good function at baseline. The number needed to visit (NNV) to prevent one admission in programmes with frequent follow-up visits is around 40.

These results have important policy implications. In countries with existing national programmes of preventive home visits, the process and organization of these visits should be reconsidered based on the criteria identified in this meta-analysis. In the United States, a system for functional impairment risk identification and appropriate intervention to prevent or delay functional impairment seems promising. There are a variety of chronic disease management programmes specifically addressing the care needs of the elderly. Engrafting the key concepts of home-based preventive care programmes into these programmes should be feasible, as they continue to evolve, and cost-effective. Identifying risks and dealing with them as an essential component of the care of older persons is central to reducing the emerging burden of disability and improving the QOL in elders.

Conclusion

Published studies of multidimensional geriatric assessment have confirmed its efficacy in many settings. A continuing challenge has been obtaining adequate financing to support adding geriatric assessment services to existing medical care. Despite GAPs' many proven benefits, and their ability to reduce costs documented in controlled trials, healthcare financers have been reluctant to fund geriatric assessment programmes – presumably out of concern that the programmes might be expanded too fast and that costs for extra diagnostic and therapeutic services might increase out of control. Many practitioners have found ways to 'unbundle' the geriatric assessement process into component services and receive adequate support to fund the entire process. In this continuing time of fiscal restraint, geriatric practitioners must remain constantly creative in order to reach the goal of optimal patient care.

While there is no single optimal blueprint for geriatric assessment, the participation of the multidisciplinary team and the focus on functional status and QOL as major clinical goals are common to all settings. Although the greatest benefits have been found in programmes targeted to the frail subgroup of older persons, a strong case can be made for a continuum of GAPs – screening assessments performed periodically for all older persons and comprehensive assessment targeted to frail and high-risk patients. Clinicians interested in developing these services will do well to heed the experiences of the programmes reviewed here in adapting the principles of geriatric assessment to local resources. Future research is still needed to determine the most effective and efficient methods for performing geriatric assessment and on developing strategies for best matching needs with services.

Key points

- Multidimensional geriatric assessment is an efficient and effective way for evaluating complex elderly patients and planning improved care.
- The process of multidimensional geriatric assessment usually involves the systematic evaluation of function, medical conditions, psychological parameters and social networks through use of an interdisciplinary team and validated assessment measures.
- Multidimensional geriatric assessment has been shown to improve function and survival while reducing healthcare utilization and costs.

References

1. Matthews DA. Dr. Marjory Warren and the origin of British geriatrics. *J Am Geriatr Soc* 1984;**32**:253–8.
2. Rubenstein LZ, Campbell LJ, Kane RL. *Geriatric Assessment*, WB Saunders, Philadelphia, 1987.
3. Rubenstein LZ, Wieland D, Bernabei R. *Geriatric Assessment Technology: The State of the Art*, Kurtis Publishers, Milan, 1995.
4. Kane RL, Kane RA. *Assessing Older Persons*, Oxford University Press, New York, 2004.
5. Osterweil D, Brummel-Smith K, Beck JC. *Comprehensive Geriatric Assessment*, McGraw-Hill, New York, 2000.
6. Gallo JJ, Fulmer T, Paveza GJ, Reichel W. *Handbook of Geriatric Assessment*, 3rd edn, Aspen Publishers, Rockville, MD, 2000.
7. Katz S, Ford AB, Moskowitz RW *et al*. Studies of illness in the aged. The index of ADL: a standardized measure of biological psychosocial function. *JAMA* 1963;**185**:914–19.
8. Lawton MP, Brody EM. Assessment of older people: self-maintaining and instrumental activities of daily living. *Gerontologist* 1969;**9**:179–86.
9. Wade DT, Colin C. The Barthel ADL Index – a standard measure of physical disability. *Int Disabil Studies* 1988;**10**:64–7.
10. Tinetti ME. Performance oriented assessment of mobility problems in elderly patients. *J Am Geriatr Soc* 1986;**34**:119–26.
11. Mathias S, Nayak USL, Isaacs B. Balance in elderly patients: the 'get up and go' test. *Arch Phys Med Rehab* 1986;**67**:387–9.
12. Folstein M, Folstein S, McHugh P. Mini-mental state: a practical method for grading the cognitive state of patients for the clinician. *J Psychiatr Res* 1975;**12**:189–98.
13. Yesavage J, Brink T, Rose T *et al*. Development and validation of a geriatric screening scale: a preliminary report. *J Psychiatr Res* 1983;**17**:37–49.
14. Hoyl T, Alessi CA, Harker JO *et al*. Development and testing of a 5-item version of the geriatric depression scale. *J Am Geriatr Soc* 1999;**47**:873–8.
15. Rubenstein LZ, Harker JO, Salva A, Guigoz Y, Vellas B. Screening for undernutrition in geriatric practice: developing the short-form Mini-nutritional Assessment (MNA-SF). J *Gerotol Med Sci* 2001;**56A**: M366–M372.
16. Lubben JE. Assessing social networks among elderly populations. *Family and Community Health* 1988;**8**:42–52.
17. Stewart AL, Hays RD, Ware JE. Communication: the MOS short-form general health survey: reliability and validity in a patient population. *Med Care* 1988;**26**:724–35.
18. Jette AM, Davies AR, Calkins DR *et al*. The functional status questionnaire: reliability and validity when used in primary care. *J Gen Intern Med* 1986;**1**: 143–.
19. Stuck AE, Aronow HU, Steiner A *et al*. A trial of annual comprehensive geriatric assessments for elderly people living in the community. *N Engl J Med* 1995;**333**:1184–9.
20. Landefeld CS, Palmer RM, Kresevic DM *et al*. Randomied trial of care in a hospital medical unit designed for older patients. *N Engl J Med* 1995;**332**:1338–44.
21. Bachmann S, Finger C, Huss A, Egger M, Stuck AE, Clough-Gorr KM. Post-acute impatient rehabilitation specifically designed for geriatric patients: a systematic review and a meta-analysis of randomised controlled trials. *BMJ* 2010;**340**: c1718. doi: 10.1136.
22. Wieland D, Kramer BJ, Waite MS, Rubenstein LZ. The interdisciplinary team in geriatric care. *Am Behav Sci* 1996;**39**:655–64.
23. Gwadry-Sridhar FH, Flintoft V, Lee DS, Lee H, Guyatt GH. A systematic review and meta- analysis of studies comparing readmission rates and mortality rates in patients with heart failure. *Arch Intern Med*. 2004;**164**:2315–20.
24. Extermann M, Aapro M, Bernabei R *et al*.; Task Force on CGA of the International Society of Geriatric Oncology. Use of comprehensive geriatric assessment in older cancer patients: recommendations from the task force on CGA of the International Society of Geriatric Oncology. *Crit Rev Oncol Hematol* 2005;**55**:241–52.

25. Clough-Gorr KM, Stuck AE, Thwin SS, Silliman RA. Older breast cancer survivors: Geriatric assessment domains are associated with poor tolerance of treatment side-effects and predict mortality over seven-years of follow-up. *J Clin Oncol* 2010;**28**:380–6.
26. William J, Stokoe IH, Gray S *et al*. Old people at home: their unreported needs. *Lancet* 1964;**i**:1117–20.
27. Williams TF, Hill JH, Fairbank ME, Knox KG. Appropriate placement of the chronically ill and aged: a successful approach by evaluation. *JAMA* 1973;**266**:1332–5.
28. Rubenstein LZ, Josephson KR, Wieland GD *et al*. Effectiveness of a geriatric evaluation unit: a randomized clinical trial. *N Engl J Med* 1984;**311**:1664–70.
29. Hendriksen C, Lund E, Stromgard E. Consequences of assessment and intervention among elderly people: three-year randomized controlled trial. *BMJ* 1984;**289**:1522–4.
30. Pathy MSJ, Bayer A, Harding K, Dibble A. Randomized trial of casefinding and surveillance of elderly people at home. *Lancet* 1992;**340**:890–3.
31. Stuck AE, Siu AL, Wieland GD *et al*. Comprehensive geriatric assessment: a meta-analysis of controlled trials. *Lancet* 1993;**342**:1032–6.
32. Stuck AE, Minder CE, Peter-Wuest I *et al*. A randomized trial of in-home visits for disability prevention in community-dwelling older people at low and high risk for nursing home admission. *Arch Intern Med* 2000;**160**:977–86.
33. Stuck AE, Egger M, Hammer A, Minder CE, Beck JC. Home visits to prevent nursing home admission and functional decline in the elderly: Systematic review and meta-regression analysis. *JAMA* 2002;**287**:1022–8.
34. Ellis G, Langhorne P. Comprehensive geriatric assessment for older hospital patients. *Br Med Bull* 2005;**71**:43–57.
35. Kuo HK, Scandrett KG, Dave J, Mitchell SL. The influence of outpatient comprehensive geriatric assessment on survival: a meta-analysis. *Arch Gerontol Geriatr* 2004;**39**:245–54.
36. Baztan JJ, Suarez-Garcia FM, Lopez-Arrieta J, Rodriguez-Manas L, Rodriguez-Artalejo F. Effectiveness of acute geriatric units on functional decline, living at home, and case fatality among older patients admitted to hospital for acute medical disorders: meta-analysis. *BMJ* 2009;**338**:b50.
37. Van Craen K, Braes T, Wellens N *et al*. The effectiveness of inpatient geriatric evaluation and management units: a systematic review and meta-analysis. *J Am Geriatr Soc* 2010; **58**:83–92.
38. Ellis G, Whitehead MA, Robinson D *et al*. Comprehensive geriatric assessment for older adults admitted to hospital: meta-analysis of randomised controlled trials. *BMJ* 2011;**343**:d6553.

CHAPTER 113

Frailty

John E. Morley
Saint Louis University School of Medicine and St Louis Veterans' Affairs Medical Center, St Louis, MO, USA

Introduction

Frailty can be defined as that condition when a person loses the ability to carry out important, practiced social activities of daily living when exposed to either psychological or stressful conditions.[1] It should be distinguished from disability. Frailty represents a form of predisability.

Frailty has been objectively defined by Linda Fried and colleagues (Table 113.1).[2,3] Their definition includes weight loss, exhaustion, weakness, walking speed and low physical activity. By this definition, ~6.9% of the older population are frail. Females are more often classified as frail than are males of the same age. Two other similar definitions of frailty that are easier to use in the clinic have been validated[4,5] (Table 113.1). Rockwood *et al.*[6] defined frailty as an increasing number of disabilities. Frailty is the beginning of a cascade that leads to functional deterioration, hospitalization, institutionalization and death (Figure 113.1). Over our lifetime, there is a peak in vitality between 20 and 30 years of age, after which there is a gradual physiological decline in performance (Figure 113.2). This decline can be delayed by positive behaviours such as exercise or accelerated by negative factors such as disease. However, eventually all individuals, if they live long enough, will cross the frailty threshold. This chapter discusses the factors involved in the acceleration of the life slope towards the frailty threshold.

Pathophysiology of frailty

The causes of frailty are multifactorial. The backdrop for the development of frailty is the physiological changes of ageing. The interaction of normal physiology with genes, lifestyle, environment and disease determines which individuals will become frail. In most individuals, frailty is caused by the failure to generate adequate muscle power and/or the failure to have sufficient executive function to utilize the available executive function appropriately. The major causes of frailty are illustrated in Figure 113.3.

Disease

Numerous disease processes can directly or indirectly result in frailty. Many diseases produce an excess of cytokines that can lead to a decrease in muscle mass, food intake and cognitive function. Diseases also lead to a decline in levels of the anabolic hormone testosterone.

Congestive heart failure (CHF) is a condition that is classically associated with frailty. Persons with CHF have a marked decline in their $VO_{2\,max}$, leading to an inability to perform endurance or resistance tasks. Left-sided heart failure leads to intestinal wall oedema. This results in bacterial translocation into the lymphatic and systemic circulation. The bacterial endotoxins (lipopolysaccharides) result in the activation of the immune system and release of cytokines, such as TNF-α. This results in anorexia, loss of muscle mass, weight loss, hypoalbuminaemia and hypocholesterolaemia (Figure 113.4). In CHF, the best predictors of poor outcome are weight loss and hypocholesterolaemia.[7] Activation of the angiotensin II system that leads to cleavage of actomyosin and subsequent clearance of muscle protein by the ubiquitin–proteasome system may also play a role. Angiotensin-converting enzyme inhibitors reverse weight loss and frailty in some persons with CHF.

Persons with chronic obstructive pulmonary disease have a decrease in endurance, weight loss due to poor food intake and increased resting metabolic rate and thermic energy of eating. They lose muscle because of low testosterone levels and increased circulating cytokine levels.

Diabetes mellitus is classically associated with an increase in frailty, injurious falls, disability and premature death (Figure 113.5). Again, the causes are multifactorial and include low testosterone, increased angiotensin II, increased cytokines, peripheral neuropathy, reduced executive function and accelerated atherosclerosis.

Persons with anaemia have reduced endurance, decreased muscle strength, orthostasis, increased falls, increased frailty, decreased mobility, increased disability and increased mortality (Figure 113.6). Both erythropoietin

Principles and Practice of Geriatric Medicine, Fifth Edition. Edited by Alan J. Sinclair, John E. Morley and Bruno Vellas.

Table 113.1 Comparison of three frailty scales.

Cardiovascular Health Study	Study of Osteoporotic Fractures	International Association of Nutrition and Aging
• Weight loss (10 lb in year) • Exhaustion (self-report) • Weakness (grip strength, lowest 20%) • Walking speed (15 ft, slowest 20%) • Low physical activity (kcal per week, lowest 20%)	• Weight loss • Inability to rise from chair five times without using arms • Reduced energy level	• Fatigue • Resistance (climb one flight of stairs) • Aerobic (walk one block) • Illnesses (>5) • Loss of weight (5%)

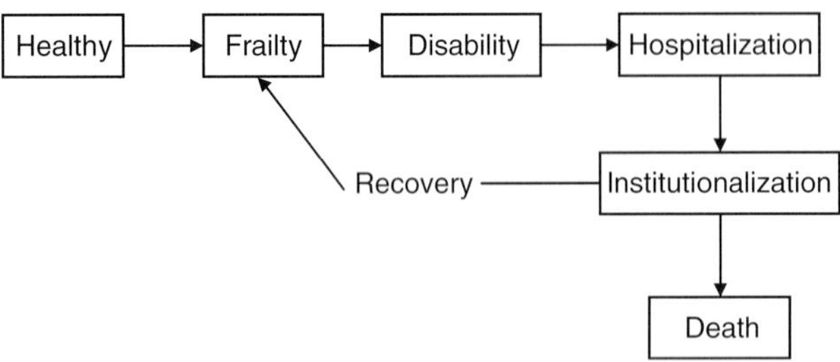

Figure 113.1 The pathway from frailty to death

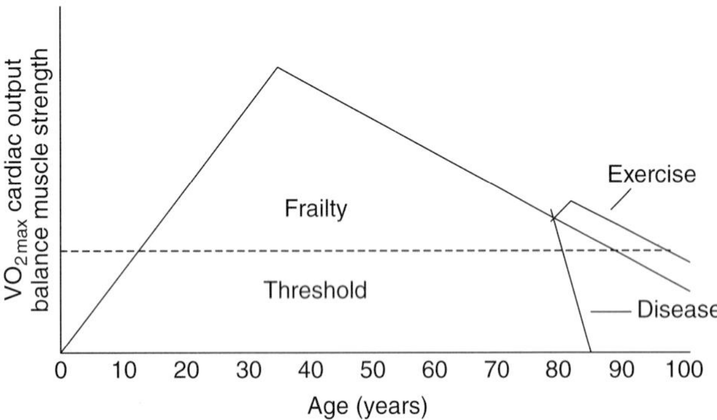

Figure 113.2 The frailty threshold

and darbepoetin-α can reverse the anaemia and many of these changes.[8] The use of these agents has led to a marked increase in the quality of life of patients with chronic kidney failure, anaemia of chronic disease and myelofibrosis.

Polymyalgia rheumatica results in painful muscles with proximal myopathy. The diagnosis is confirmed by finding an elevated erythrocyte sedimentation rate. Treatment of this condition with corticosteroids reverses the frailty that it produces. Unfortunately, this totally reversible condition is often misdiagnosed by clinicians.

Endocrine disorders, such as hyperthyroidism, hypothyroidism and hypoadrenalism, can have insidious onset. Joint pain, that is, the arthritides, is classically associated with immobility. Immobility, over time, leads to loss of muscle mass and power and to a decline in endurance, the hallmarks of frailty. Pain can further induce frailty secondarily to increasing depression in older persons.

Decreased food intake

Older persons develop a physiological anorexia of ageing that is associated with a loss of weight. The causes of the anorexia of ageing are multifactorial.[9] Social causes, such as isolation and dysphoria, and the decline in smell and increase in taste threshold are obvious causes. Recently, there have been a number of studies that demonstrated that decreased compliance and adaptive relaxation of the stomach result in a more rapid antral filling and early satiety. Excess production of cholecystokinin from the duodenum in response to a fatty meal is another cause of anorexia in older persons. High circulating cytokine levels in older persons have been associated with anorexia. Males have a greater decrease in both absolute and relative amounts of food intake over the lifespan. This appears to be due to the fall in testosterone, which results in an increase in leptin levels and, therefore, greater anorexia.

In addition to the physiological anorexia of ageing, many reversible causes of anorexia occur in older persons. These are easily remembered by the mnemonic MEALS-ON-WHEELS (Table 113.2).

Sarcopenia

Sarcopenia is the excessive loss of muscle mass that occurs in older persons.[10–12] It is usually defined as a greater than two standard deviations amount of lean tissue compared with that of younger persons. It occurs in 13–24% of persons aged 60–70 years and in about 50% aged over 80 years. The best measure of sarcopenia is based on the appendicular skeletal mass as measured by dual-energy X-ray absorptiometry (DEXA), divided by the height in metres squared. It can also be calculated using magnetic resonance imaging (MRI), computed tomography (CT) or bioelectrical impedance. DEXA and MRI measures are highly correlated. Ultrasound is proving to be an excellent

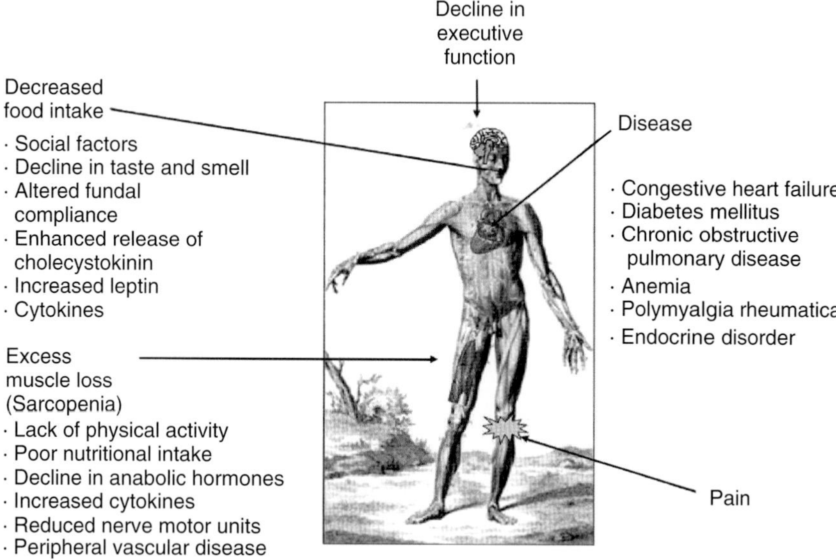

Figure 113.3 The major causes of frailty

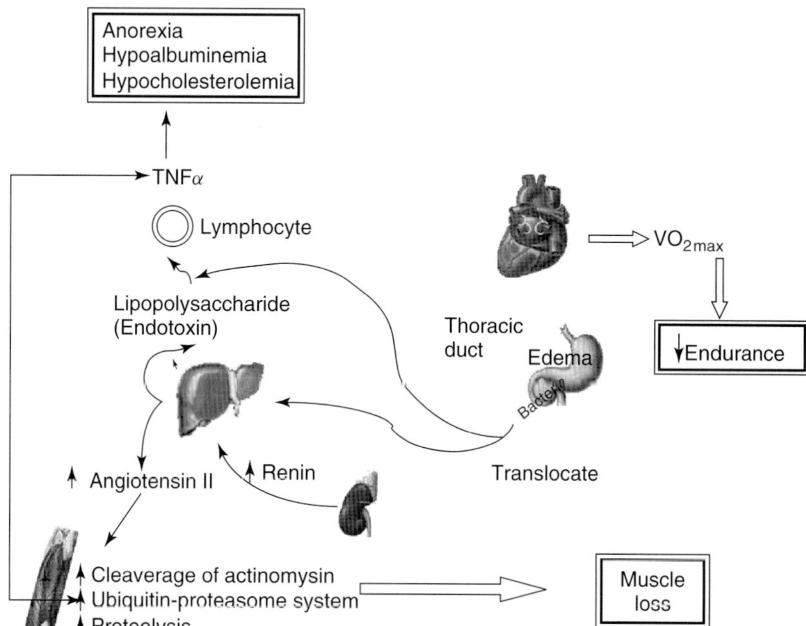

Figure 113.4 The pathogenesis of frailty in congestive heart failure

measure of muscle mass loss in older persons.[13] Sarcopenia is strongly correlated with disability. Most sarcopenic individuals have also lost fat. However, a subset of individuals remain fat while losing muscle mass. These individuals have been characterized as the 'sarcopenic obese' or the 'fat frail'. Longitudinally, those with obese sarcopenia have been found to be the most likely to develop future disability and mortality.[14] Myosteatosis – the infiltration of fat into muscle – appears to be a separate condition related to insulin resistance. Mitochondrial failure or elevated circulating triglycerides lead to the accumulation of triglycerides within the cell. This alters the function of the insulin receptor substrate and, therefore, the GLUT transporter, leading to insulin resistance.

The development of sarcopenia and its effect on frailty have been characterized in the worm *Caenorhabditis elegans*. In *C. elegans*, muscle deterioration (sarcopenia) with ageing leads to a decline in body movement. The muscle deterioration also correlates with behaviour deficits (a frailty equivalent). These changes rarely correlated with a decreased lifespan. Mutations in daf-2 (the worm's IGF-1) delay these changes.

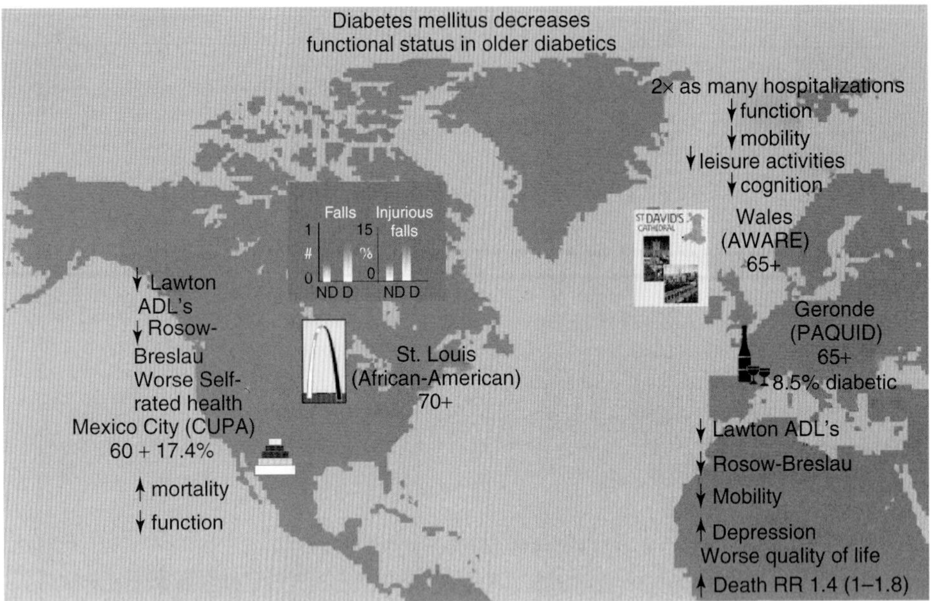

Figure 113.5 Frailty and diabetes mellitus

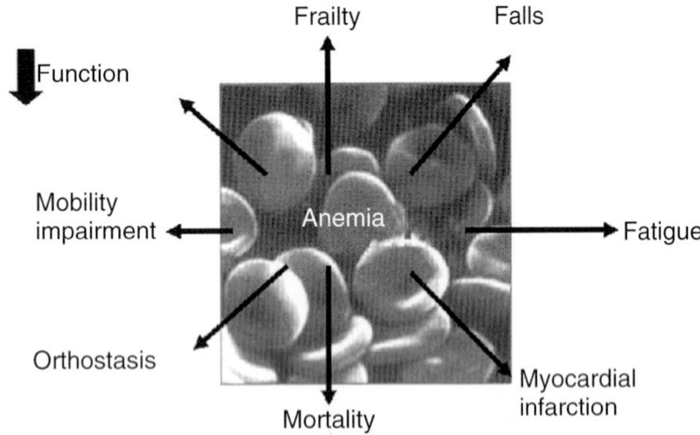

Figure 113.6 Frailty and anaemia

There is evidence that sarcopenia originates at birth. In the Hertfordshire cohort study, it was shown that grip strength correlates with birth weight. Genetic studies have shown that persons with a single I or double I allele for angiotensin-converting enzyme appear to be able to generate more power when exercising regularly than those with D allele. Epidemiological studies have suggested that the best predictors of muscle mass and strength in older persons are age, energy intake, physical activity, IGF-1, testosterone and cytokines.[15] Hypovitamin D is also associated with decreased muscle strength and falls.[16]

Testosterone levels decline at the rate of 1% per year from the age of 30 years in men and rapidly between 20 and 40 years in women.[17,18] Testosterone inhibits the movement of pluripotential stem cells into the fat cell lineage and stimulates the muscle cell lineage to result in the production of satellite cells. Satellite cells are essential for the repair of skeletal muscle.[19] Testosterone also stimulates muscle protein synthesis and inhibits the ubiquitin–proteasome pathway, resulting in a decrease in muscle protein turnover. Testosterone replacement, even in non-hypogonadal males, increases muscle mass.[20] Pharmacological doses of testosterone or testosterone replacement in hypogonadal males lead to an increase in muscle strength and muscle power.[21] These changes have now been shown to lead to functional improvement. However, there is a small amount of evidence that testosterone has similar effects in older women.

Table 113.2 MEALS-ON-WHEELS mnemonic for treatable causes of weight loss.

Medications (e.g. digoxin, theophylline, cimetidine)
Emotional (e.g. depression)
Alcoholism, elder abuse, anorexia tardive
Late-life paranoia
Swallowing problems
Oral factors
Nosocomial infections (e.g. tuberculosis)
Wandering and other dementia-related factors
Hyperthyroidism, hypercalcaemia, hypoadrenalism
Enteral problems (e.g. gluten enteropathy)
Eating problems
Low salt, low cholesterol and other therapeutic diets
Stones (cholecystitis)

Reproduced from Jette AM *et al.* *J Gerontol A Biol Sci Med Sci* 2002;**57**:M209–16, by permission of The Gerontological Society of America.

Three studies in older persons with frailty have shown some functional improvement.[22–24] An important side effect is oedema. More persons died in the placebo arms of these studies than in the testosterone treatment arms. Similarly, testosterone treatment has improved function in older persons with heart failure.[25]

A number of selective androgen receptor molecules (SARMs) are being developed, in an attempt to find androgenic compounds that have a specific effect on muscle but are less likely to produce side effects (Table 113.3). Ostarine is a SARM that increases muscle mass and power performance in older persons. Dehydroepiandrosterone (DHEA), a weak androgen, failed to produce an effect on muscle strength or muscle mass when given at 50 mg daily for 1 year to 288 men and women.

Another anabolic hormone, growth hormone, increases muscle mass but not strength in older persons.[26] The effect of growth hormone is predominantly on type II muscle fibres. Ghrelin, a growth hormone secretagogue produced in the fundus of the stomach, also appears to increase muscle mass.

Table 113.3 Selective androgen receptor molecules.

Steroids
Nandrolone
Oxymethalone
Oxandrolone
Non-steroidal
2-Quinoline
Coumarin
Phthalimide
Bicalutamide
Acetothiolutamide

Insulin growth factor (IGF) is produced in three alternative forms in muscle. One of these forms, a mechanogrowth factor (MGF), is produced in response to mechanical overload.[27] The ability of MGF to be produced in response to mechanical overload declines with ageing. Resistance exercise increases MGF in human quadriceps and this increase is greater when growth hormone is also given. IGF enhances satellite cell production. Localized

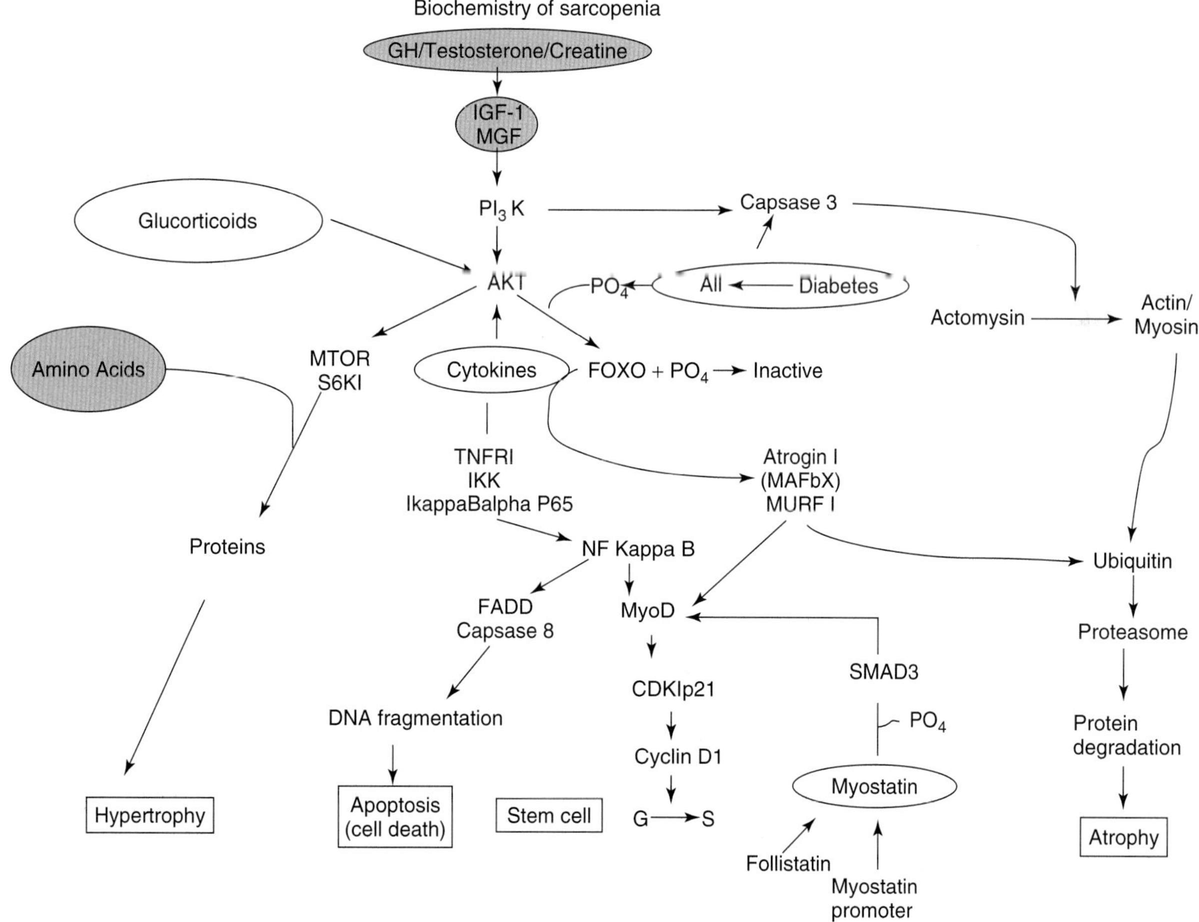

Figure 113.7 Schematic view of the biochemistry of sarcopenia

IGF transgene expression sustains hypertrophy and regeneration of senescent skeletal muscle.[28]

Myostatin D inhibits muscle growth. A double deletion of myostatin D in mice leads to muscle hypertrophy, a veritable 'mighty mouse'. Double deletions of myostatin D in cows, whippets and in a single human result in marked muscle hypertrophy.[29] Myostatin produces its effect through the activin II receptors. A soluble circulating the activin IIb receptor can scavenge activan and lead to muscle and bone hypertrophy in rodents, monkeys and humans.[30]

Motor unit functioning is essential for the maintenance of muscle function. The motor unit firing rate is significantly decreased in the old-old, that is, those over 80 years of age. Ciliary neurotrophic factor (CNTF) levels decline with age and this decline correlates with the decrease in muscle strength with ageing. Administration of CNTF leads to a twofold increase in soleus muscle size.

Cytokines are soluble peptide messengers that are synthesized by white cells, neuronal cells and adipocytes. Excess of TNF-α and interleukin-6 leads to loss of muscle strength. High levels of C-reactive protein and interleukin-6 are associated with a decrease in handgrip strength and in physical performance.[31]

Elevated homocysteine levels and peripheral vascular disease lead to poor blood flow to muscles, with muscle atrophy and decreased function. Creatine is an essential amino acid for muscle. Creatine, together with exercise, may improve muscle performance in older persons.[32]

In the end, the development of sarcopenia depends on an imbalance of the normal everyday renewal cycle of muscle. There is either an excess of atrophy and apoptosis or a diminution of hypertrophy and satellite cell production. Figure 113.7 provides a schematic view of the biochemistry of sarcopenia.

Conclusion

Frailty is a predisability state. It is been defined objectively. The causes of frailty are multifactorial. Frailty can have a single cause, such as anaemia. Reversal of the anaemia with iron, folate, vitamin B_{12} or erythropoietin will, in this case, reverse frailty. In other cases, frailty is due to the interplay of hormones and cytokines with disease processes and poor-quality nutritional intake. In these cases, the management of frailty requires a careful assessment of the causative factors and a multifaceted treatment regimen. One approach to the preventive strategies necessary to slow the onset of frailty is given in Table 113.4.

Table 113.4 Preventive strategies to slow the onset of frailty.

Food intake maintenance
Resistance exercises
Atherosclerosis prevention
Isolation avoidance (i.e. depression)
Limit pain
Tai Chi and other balance exercises
Yearly check for testosterone deficiency

Key points

- Frailty is predisability and has been objectively defined.
- Frail persons are precipitated into disability by experiencing a stressful event.
- Causes of frailty include chronic diseases, pain, poor-quality nutritional intake, impaired executive function and sarcopenia.
- The interplay of hormones and cytokines is an important determinant of frailty.

References

1. Morley JE. Developing novel therapeutic approaches to frailty. *Curr Pharm Des* 2009;**15**:3384–95.
2. Fried LP, Tangen CM, Walston J *et al.* Frailty in older adults: evidence for a phenotype. *J Gerontol A Biol Sci Med Sci* 2001;**56**: M146–56.
3. Fried LP, Ferrucci L, Darer J *et al.* Untangling the concepts of disability, frailty, and comorbidity: implications for improved targeting and care. *J Gerontol A Biol Sci Med Sci* 2004;**59**:255–63.
4. Abellan van Kan G, Rolland Y, Bergman H *et al.* The I.A.N.A. Task Force on frailty assessment of older people in clinical practice. *J Nutr Health Aging* 2008;**12**:29–37.
5. Ensrud KE, Ewing SK, Taylor BC *et al.* Comparison of 2 frailty indexes for prediction of falls, disability, fractures, and death in older women. *Arch Intern Med* 2008;**168**:382–9.
6. Rockwood K, Abeysundera MJ and Mitnitski A. How should we grade frailty in nursing home patients ? *J Am Med Dir Assoc* 2007;**8**:595–603.
7. Von Haehling S, Jankowska EA and Anker SD. Tumour necrosis factor-alpha and the failing heart-pathophysiology and therapeutic implications. *Basic Res Cardiol* 2004;**99**:18–28.
8. Cesari M, Penninx BW, Lauretani F *et al.* Hemoglobin levels and skeletal muscle: results from the InCHIANTI study. *J Gerontol A Biol Sci Med Sci* 2004;**59**:249–54.
9. Morley JE. Weight loss in older persons: new therapeutic approaches. *Curr Pharm Des* 2007;**13**:3637–47.
10. Morley JE, Baumgartner RN, Roubenoff R *et al.* Sarcopenia. *J Lab Clin Med* 2001;**137**:231–43.
11. Roubenoff R. Sarcopenia: effects on body composition and function. *J Gerontol A Biol Sci Med Sci* 2003;**58**:1012–7.
12. Rolland Y, Czerwinski S, Abellan van Kan G *et al.* Sarcopenia: its assessment, etiology, pathogenesis, consequences and future perspectives. *J Nutr Health Aging* 2008;**12**:433–50.

13. Narici MV, Maganaris CN, Reeves ND *et al*. Effect of aging on human muscle architecture. *J Appl Physiol* 2003;**95**:2229–34.
14. Baumgartner RN, Wayne SJ, Waters DL *et al*. Sarcopenic obesity predicts instrumental activities of daily living disability in the elderly. *Obes Res* 2004;**12**:1995–2004.
15. Baumgartner RN, Waters DL, Gallagher D *et al*. Predictors of skeletal muscle mass in elderly men and women. *Mech Ageing Dev* 1999;**48**:378–84.
16. Scott D, Blizzard L, Fell J *et al*. A prospective study of the associations between 25-hydroxyvitamin D, sarcopenia progression and physical activity in older adults. *Clin Endocrinol* 2011;**73**:581–7.
17. Morley JE. Anorexia of aging-physiologic and pathologic. *Am J Clin Nutr* 1997;**66**:760–73.
18. Harman SM, Metter JE, Tobin JD *et al*. Longitudinal effects of aging on serum total and free testosterone levels in healthy men. *J Clin Endocrinol Metab* 2001;**86**:724–31.
19. Bhasin S. Testosterone supplementation for aging-associated sarcopenia. *J Gerontol A Biol Sci Med Sci* 2003;**58**:1002–8.
20. Wittert GA, Chapman IM, Haren MT *et al*. Oral testosterone supplementation increases muscle and decreases fat mass in healthy elderly males with low-normal gonadal status. *J Gerontol A Biol Sci Med Sci* 2003;**58**:618–25.
21. Matsumoto AM. Andropause: clinical implications of the decline in serum testosterone levels with aging in men. *J Gerontol A Biol Sci Med Sci* 2002;**57**: M76–99.
22. Kenney AM, Kleppinger A, Annis K *et al*. Effects of transdermal testosterone on bone and muscle in older men with low bioavailable testosterone levels, low bone mass, and physical frailty. *J Am Geriatr Soc* 2010;**58**:1134–43.
23. Srinivas-Shankar U, Roberts SA, Connolly MJ *et al*. Effects of testosterone on muscle strength, physical function, body composition, and quality of life in intermediate-frail and frail elderly men: a randomized, double-blind, placebo-controlled study. *J Clin Endocrinol Metab* 2010;**95**:639–50.
24. Basaria S, Coviello AD, Travison TG *et al*. Adverse events associated with testosterone administration. *N Engl J Med* 2010;**363**:109–22.
25. Iellamo F, Rosano G and Volterrani M. Testosterone deficiency and exercise intolerance in heart failure: treatment implications. *Curr Heart Fail Rep* 2010;**7**:59–65.
26. Harman SM and Blackman MR. Use of growth hormone for prevention or treatment of effects of aging. *J Gerontol A Biol Sci Med Sci* 2004;**59**:652–8.
27. McKoy G, Ashley W, Mander J *et al*. Expression of insulin growth factor-1 splice variants and structural genes in rabbit skeletal muscle induced by stretch and stimulation. *J Physiol* 1999;**516**:583–92.
28. Musaro A, McCullagh K, Paul A *et al*. Localized IGF-1 transgene expression sustains hypertrophy and regeneration in senescent skeletal muscle. *Nat Genet* 2001;**27**:195–200.
29. Schuelke M, Wagner KR, Stolz LE *et al*. Brief report-myostatin mutation associated with gross muscle hypertrophy in a child. *N Engl J Med* 2004;**350**:2682–8.
30. Zhou X, Wang JL, Lu J *et al*. Reversal of cancer cachexia and muscle wasting by ActRIIB antagonism leads to prolonged survival. *Cell* 2010;**142**:531–43.
31. Cesari M, Penninx BWJH, Pahor M *et al*. Inflammatory markers and physical performance in older persons: the InCHIANTI study. *J Gerontol A Biol Sci Med Sci* 2004;**59**:242–8.
32. Morley JE, Argiles JM, Evans WJ *et al*. Nutritional recommendations for the management of sarcopenia. *J Am Med Dir Assoc* 2010;**11**:391–6.

CHAPTER 114

Rehabilitation

Michael Watts and Paul Finucane
Graduate-Entry Medical School, University of Limerick, Limerick, Ireland

Introduction

The human and economic consequences of avoidable dependency in older people are considerable. This reality was first stated by Marjorie Warren over 60 years ago when she emphasized the need to help sick elderly people to regain their functional independence, the primary elements of which are mobility and independent self-care.[1]

Older people who typically benefit from rehabilitation will have had a disabling event of recent onset. This is commonly an age-related event such as a stroke, hip fracture, other fall-related injury or deconditioning following a major illness. Many elderly people will have ongoing limitations from other diseases such as osteoarthritis or Parkinson's disease.

Though there are many reasons why rehabilitation in the old differs from that in the young, perhaps the greatest is the lack of physiological reserve with which to combat a disabling insult. As a consequence, recovery is typically prolonged and the pre-morbid functional state is never fully regained. The specific diseases to which elderly people are susceptible are described throughout this text. This chapter focuses on the process of optimizing recovery from the major disabling diseases of old age and on strategies for adaptation to their long-term sequelae.

Terminology and classifications

For many years, the World Health Organization (WHO) has sought to classify aspects of health and disease, most notably through its International Classification of Disease, now in its tenth revision (ICD-10).[2] Such systems provide a standard language and framework for the description of health and health-related states across geographical boundaries, disciplines and sciences.

To complement the ICD, in 1980 the WHO introduced its International Classification of Impairments, Disabilities and Handicaps (ICIDH).[3] This stated that any illness could be considered at three levels: impairment, disability and handicap. In simple terms, *impairment* refers to the pathological process affecting the person, *disability* to the resulting loss of function, and *handicap* to any consequent reduction in that individual's role in society.

The ICIDH had significant limitations, including the use of pejorative terms that emphasized the negative consequences of ill health and played down its social and societal dimensions. Consequently, in 2001, WHO produced a revised classification, the International Classification of Functioning, Disability and Health (ICF), which challenged traditional views on health and disability and allowed positive experiences to be described. In particular, the ICF focuses on the impact of the social and physical environment on a person's functioning.

The ICF contains two *parts*, each with two *components*:

Part 1 Functioning and Disability
- (a) Body Functions and Structures
- (b) Activities and Participation

Part 2 Contextual Factors
- (c) Environmental Factors
- (d) Personal Factors

Under this classification, each component is further divided into various *domains* and each domain into a number of *categories*, which form the units of classification.

The ICF has the following definitions:

Impairment: problems in body function or structure such as a significant deviation or loss.

Activity: the execution of a task or action by an individual.

Activity limitations: difficulties an individual might have in executing activities.

Participation: involvement in a life situation.

Participation restrictions: problems an individual may experience in involvement in life situations.

Environmental factors: the physical, social and attitudinal environment in which people live and conduct their lives.

Components of the ICF can be expressed in both positive and negative terms. Thus, *functioning* is an umbrella term for all body functions, activities and participation while

Principles and Practice of Geriatric Medicine, Fifth Edition. Edited by Alan J. Sinclair, John E. Morley and Bruno Vellas.

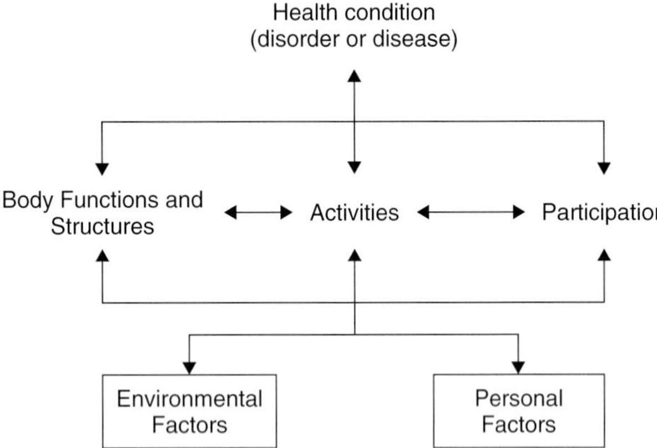

Figure 114.1 The complex interaction between health status, activity and participation.

disability is a collective term for impairments, activity limitations or participation restrictions.

As illustrated by Figure 114.1, an individual's functioning is a result of a complex interaction between the health condition and contextual factors (i.e. environmental and personal factors). Their interaction is highly dynamic such that any intervention in one area might impact on the other, perhaps in unpredictable ways.

Consider, for example, an individual with Parkinson's disease, whose impairment (problems in body function or structure) is described elsewhere in this text. As a consequence, the person may have some activity limitations such as difficulty with personal care and mobility. In turn, the person cannot pursue former hobbies and interests (participation restriction), restrictions that might be exacerbated if widowed and living alone in a first floor apartment. Now suppose that she falls and fractures her hip. This new impairment causes her to lose confidence. Further restrictions in activity and participation ensue and she becomes even more isolated, withdrawn and depressed. The feedback loops shown in Figure 114.1 indicate how vicious cycles can develop with the person's level of activity and participation spiralling downwards.

Simply stated, rehabilitation is a process that seeks to minimize activity and participation restrictions resulting from impairment. Many and more comprehensive definitions exist; perhaps the most widely accepted is the UN definition:[5]

> Rehabilitation means a goal-orientated and time-limited process aimed at enabling an impaired person to reach an optimum mental, physical and/or social functional level, thus providing him or her with the tools to change his or her own life. It can involve measures intended to compensate for a loss of function or a functional limitation (for example the use of technical aids) and other measures intended to facilitate social adjustment or readjustment.

Figure 114.1 also illustrates how rehabilitation programmes can impact at various points in the impairment-activity-participation cycle. Not only can they prevent the progression of impairment to activity restriction and of activity restriction to participation restriction, they can also prevent further impairments and the development of vicious cycles.

Determinants of activity and participation restrictions

As summarized in Table 114.1, many factors determine the activity and participation restrictions that result from a given impairment. The type of impairment is of paramount importance, with some diseases being inherently more likely to cause restrictions than others. The site of a pathological lesion is also important as is well illustrated by stroke disease, where large lesions in some parts of the brain may be asymptomatic while smaller lesions in strategic areas may cause major problems.

Older patients often have pre-existing impairments contributing to activity and participation restrictions and rehabilitation programmes can be influenced as much by these as by any new impairments.

Regarding reduced physiological reserve, the ageing process is characterized by a gradual functional decline in most bodily systems – a phenomenon which tends to be unimportant when organs and physiological systems are 'at rest' but is often critical when they are placed under stress by a disabling illness or event. However, it must be emphasized that even very old people can recover from major illness

Table 114.1 Determinants of activity and participation restrictions.

Determinants of activity restriction
Type of impairment (nature and severity of the disease process)
Presence of associated impairments
Degree of physiological reserve
Level of physical fitness
Determinants of participation restriction
Intrinsic factors
Attitude
Personality
Ability to adjust
Cultural issues
Extrinsic factors
Financial resources
Housing
Other resources
Social supports (spouse, family, neighbours, friends, pets)

and failure to make progress at rehabilitation can seldom be attributed to reduced physiological reserve alone. Of far greater importance is the lack of activity and physical fitness that typifies elderly people in modern societies.[6] Many of today's older people grew up in an era when exercise was not encouraged and sports and recreation facilities were relatively inaccessible. An age-related decline in muscle mass (sarcopenia) and strength is aggravated by physical inactivity[7] and numerous studies have shown an association between sarcopenia and activity restriction.[8]

Such age-associated phenomena are reversible. For example, weight training increases muscle strength in older people and improves functional capacity[9] and older people who participate in lifelong aerobic or strength training have comparable muscle strength to sedentary middle-aged individuals.[10] Although there is little data on the relationship between prior physical fitness and recovery from impairment, it is probable that those who are physically unfit have worse outcomes.

The degree of participation restriction resulting from activity restriction is influenced by several intrinsic and extrinsic factors (Table 114.1). Intrinsic factors include the person's attitude in adjusting to activity restriction. Somebody who suffers a functional loss typically experiences a grief-like reaction. Some demonstrate better coping strategies than others; they are more positive in their approach, assume greater control of their situation and find solutions to their problems. These issues are discussed in more detail later.

Extrinsic factors that impact on participation include the available resources and supports in dealing with activity restriction. In societies where health and welfare systems are poorly developed, personal finance is required for the many components of a rehabilitation programme. These include the provision of physical therapy, prosthetic devices, home modification and ongoing care. Of even greater importance are the social supports on which the person can rely at all stages of the rehabilitation programme, and particularly upon returning to their former environment. In this regard elderly females are particular disadvantaged, often being widowed and living alone. In Australia, for example, 20% of people aged 65 years and over and 27% of elderly people with activity restriction live alone.[11] In recent decades, other demographic trends, such as the loss of the nuclear family and the recruitment of informal carers into paid employment have further reduced the supports available to elderly people.

Psychological aspects of rehabilitation

The onset of impairment, particularly if unexpected or catastrophic, is generally associated with some emotional disturbance. Expected feelings include a sense of loss with regard to one's physical or mental faculties, to relationships with others or to inanimate objects such as one's home or other possessions. A typical grief reaction involves phases of denial, anger and depression leading to enough acceptance to allow a relatively normal life to be resumed. However, adjustment to impairment is sometimes abnormal. For example, over 40% of older people become depressed following a myocardial infarction and this worsens the prognosis.[12] High levels of depression have also been found following stroke,[13,14] despite participation in a rehabilitation programme.[15]

Some are inherently more adaptable and optimistic than others when faced with an impairment and this greatly influences the development of activity and participation restriction. At one end of the spectrum of responses are 'highly motivated' people who set ambitious goals and work hard to achieve them. At the other end are those who submit to their impairment, disengage, surrender power and autonomy and adopt the 'sick role'.

There are psychological theories to explain such different responses, such as that proposed by Kemp,[16] who contends that motivation is a dynamic process driven by four elements: the individual's wants, beliefs, the rewards to achievement, and the cost to the patient. The first three elements drive motivation in one direction and this is counteracted by the cost in terms of pain and effort. Thus, if a person really wants something, believes it to be attainable and potentially rewarding, he will strive to achieve it, provided the cost is acceptable. The converse also holds. Using this framework, the rehabilitation specialist can help individuals by setting goals, challenging incorrect beliefs, establishing rewards and minimizing the physical and mental cost of the rehabilitation process (cf. section on Psychosocial Support).

Principles of rehabilitation

The principles of rehabilitation are broadly similar irrespective of the underlying problem and of the working environment. *Early intervention* is crucial, as avoidable activity and participation restriction can occur soon after the onset of impairment. Problems should be anticipated and avoided as once established, they may prove irremediable. For example, a person with a flaccid hemiplegia is at risk of shoulder subluxation and its long-term sequelae. Proper handling and limb positioning in the immediate post-stroke period will minimize this risk.

A *team approach* is also essential. A properly resourced team will have input from medical and nursing staff, physiotherapists, occupational therapists, speech pathologists, clinical psychologists, dieticians and social workers. Doctors are primarily concerned with the assessment and management of impairment while remedial therapists are skilled in managing activity restriction and social workers in managing participation restriction. Nursing staff have an holistic brief with areas of expertise capable of influencing both activity and participation restriction.

To function effectively, team members need to communicate with each another. When they are co-located (e.g. in a designated rehabilitation unit), exchange of information occurs regularly and informally. Most teams also have regular formal meetings to discuss the progress of patients, to revise goals, plan discharge and organize follow-up in the community.

The rehabilitation process

The steps in any rehabilitation process are summarized in Table 114.2. Though presented in chronological order, in practice there is considerable overlap between the elements, many of which occur simultaneously and some of which must be regularly revisited. For example, while the assessment of a patient's impairment, activity and participation restriction is an important initial step, this needs to be repeated frequently (at least weekly) as the rehabilitation programme proceeds.

Assessment

It is essential that patients be assessed before entry into a rehabilitation programme to ensure that their problems are remediable and to determine their optimal management. The selection of patients for rehabilitation can be difficult as it is unfair to subject a person who cannot benefit to a demanding programme and in the process to raise false expectations and waste resources. On the other hand, those who can benefit even to a limited extent should not be denied access.

Assessment should focus on both the problem in the individual and the individual with the problem. The nature and severity of all impairments, whether new or longstanding, should be determined. It is essential to obtain a baseline measure of functional status, so that progress can be monitored and the efficacy of rehabilitation reviewed. A variety of assessment tools are available, ranging from simple subjective measures to the more complex and time consuming. The best choice of tool depends on the clinical context. Busy clinicians can often estimate the extent of activity and participation restriction by asking a few simple questions and by making some equally simple observations. Detailed assessment of activity and participation restrictions using standardized scales is generally left to remedial therapists and social workers.

Table 114.2 Steps in the rehabilitation process.

1 Assessment
2 Setting goals
3 Therapy
4 Aids and adaptations
5 Education
6 Psychological support
7 Evaluation
8 Follow-up

Assessment of activity and activity restriction

Assessment begins with the clinical history. For the person with a recent impairment, it is important to determine the premorbid as well as the current functional status. A common approach is to focus on activities of daily living (ADLs). These are classified as items of personal care (e.g. washing, grooming, dressing, using toilet, eating, etc.) and those involving the use of 'instruments' – hence known as instrumental ADLs (IADLs). The latter include such tasks as preparing meals, using the telephone, doing laundry and other housework, gardening, shopping and using public transport. If any difficulties are reported, it is important to determine how the person manages. Are these tasks neglected or do others provide help?

More formal, objective and standardized assessment of activity restriction is generally required when patients are entering a rehabilitation programme. Several assessment scales exist and their strengths and weaknesses have been analysed.[17] As yet, there is no consensus on the best assessment scales and a lack of uniformity inhibits comparative research.

The education literature provides a model drawn to explain the difficulty in reaching such a consensus.[18] This contends that the utility (U) of any assessment tool is governed by the formula:

$$U = \frac{V \times R \times A}{C}$$

where V = validity; R = reliability; A = acceptability and C = cost. While the ideal tool will score highly in the first three areas and be low on cost, in practice, assessment tools with high validity and reliability are invariably costly (i.e. resource intensive) and/or have low acceptability (e.g. are intrusive). The converse is equally true; tools that are easy and cheap to administer often have poor validity and reliability. The multiplication factor in the equation is important, because if any one element of the equation is close to zero, then the overall utility of the assessment tool will also be close to zero. In practice, the utility of any assessment tool is a trade-off between these elements.

Despite these considerations, the UK's Royal College of Physicians and British Geriatrics Society jointly endorse a number of standardized functional assessment scales for elderly patients, all of which have stood the test of time (Table 114.3). Collectively, they assess competence with activities of daily living, vision, hearing, communication, cognitive function and memory, depression and quality of life.[27]

Table 114.3 Standardized functional assessment scales for elderly patients.

Domain assessed	Recommended scale	Comments
Basic activities of daily living (ADL)	Barthel Index[19,20]	Observation of what the patient *does*. Ceiling effect in ambulatory patients.
Vision, Hearing, Communication	Lambeth Disability Screening Questionnaire[21]	Postal questionnaire
Memory and Cognitive Function	Abbreviated Mental Test (AMT)[22,23]	10 questions from longer Roth-Hopkins test
Depression	Geriatric Depression Scale[24]	Screening test with 30 questions; 15 questions in short form[25]
Subjective morale	Philadelphia Geriatric Center Morale Scale[26]	Distinct from depression, although some overlap

Reproduced from Royal College of Physicians and British Geriatrics Society Joint Workshops (1992), [27] with permission.

Such standardized scales facilitate the exchange of information across acute, rehabilitation and community-based healthcare settings. They allow the effectiveness of rehabilitation to be measured and foster comparisons of different approaches to treatment. Standardized assessments can also minimize the repeated gathering of identical information by the various members of multidisciplinary rehabilitation teams.

Other assessment scales deserve special consideration. Neurodegenerative disorders are common in older patients and Wade has provided a valuable reference for commonly used assessment measures in neurological rehabilitation.[28] A drive towards output-driven health funding in many countries has stimulated the development of specific outcome measures in rehabilitation. The Functional Independence Measure (FIM) scores patient progress in 18 common functions concerning self-care, sphincter control, mobility, locomotion, communication and social cognition.[29] Attempts have been made to use the FIM to identify the most effective and efficient aspects of rehabilitation programmes.[30,31]

Assessment of participation and participation restriction

As individuals uniquely interact with their environment, so any reduced role in society (participation restriction) resulting from activity restriction will be unique to the individual. Furthermore, it is possible for somebody to develop major participation restriction in one area and have little or no restriction in another. Thus, the person who loses mobility following a lower limb amputation may no longer be able to play golf but can continue to drive a car. As explained earlier, the level of participation restriction is mainly determined by one's ability to adapt. While some fail in this regard, for others the onset of activity restriction prompts a redefinition rather than a loss of social role. Potential losses in one area can be offset by gains elsewhere, thus minimizing participation restriction. The authors occasionally encounter people who consider their lives to have been enriched through developing an impairment and associated activity restriction.

It follows that an assessment of participation restriction can only be obtained through gaining an in-depth understanding of the individual and the manner in which he or she has come to terms with activity restriction. Such measurements are always subjective. They are also unstable over time and can be influenced by psycho-behavioural variables such as mood. For these reasons the assessment of participation restriction is largely neglected in both clinical and research settings.

Goal setting

Assessment should culminate in the setting of rehabilitation goals. To avoid frustration and disappointment for all concerned, goals should be realistic and take account of the individual's impairment and pre-morbid functional status. It is sometimes appropriate to set modest goals, such as helping an amputee patient to become wheelchair-independent rather than to walk. It is essential that all multidisciplinary team members, and particularly the patient, are involved in setting goals and that there is general agreement on the validity of the set targets.[32] A programme can be seriously compromised if key people differ on what each is trying to achieve. Patients with ambitious goals seem to make greater progress than those with more modest targets;[33] a pragmatic approach is to set ambitious but achievable goals.

Short-term (intermediate) as well as long-term (final) goals should be identified; by achieving a succession of intermediate goals, the patient arrives at the final goal. It is important to set realistic time frames for the achievement of goals, bearing in mind that the rate of progress can be difficult to predict, particularly at the outset. Goals and time frames should therefore be flexible, be regularly reviewed and modified when necessary.

Therapy

A detailed description of the role of the various multidisciplinary rehabilitation team members is outside the scope of this chapter. In brief, doctors focus on the identification and management of the presenting problem and coexisting impairments. Underlying risk factors are identified and minimized; potential complications are anticipated and prevented. Thus, in an arteriopath who has had an embolic stroke, the doctor monitors anticoagulation, controls hypertension and manages coexisting angina pectoris and diabetes mellitus. Occupational therapists (OTs) assess and enhance competence with activities of daily living. Physiotherapists provide therapies that target specific problems and enhance cardiorespiratory, neuromuscular and locomotor function. Speech and Language Therapists deal with communication issues and swallowing disorders. In specific situation, input from other health professionals (e.g. clinical psychologists, podiatrists, dieticians) may be invaluable.

Aids and adaptations

The use of aids has the potential to reduce activity and participation restriction for many impaired people. Devices range from the simple and inexpensive to the technologically advanced. They help people in diverse ways, from carrying out activities of daily living to the maintenance of mobility and the promotion of continence. The most commonly used aids have been critiqued by Mulley.[34] The provision of an aid is not always the best option for an impaired person as it can foster dependence rather than independence. However, those in real need often do not avail of even basic and aids and appliances.[35]

Advice on the suitability of aids is best left to OTs or others with particular expertise. Physiotherapists can advise on mobility aids, speech therapists on communication aids, audiologists on hearing aids and continence advisors on continence aids. Such people can also provide follow-up and ensure that aids are properly used and maintained and continue to serve their purpose.

The design, construction and fitting of prostheses (devices which replace body parts) and orthoses (devices applied to the external surface of the body to provide support, improve function, or restrict or promote movement) require particular skill and technological expertise. Well-resourced rehabilitation centres have access to prosthetists and orthotists as part of the multidisciplinary team.

Adapting the home environment also promotes activity and participation. This might include the installation of simple handrails or ramps, or improving access to shower and toilet areas. Early input from an OT, often including a home visit, ensures that modifications will be appropriate and timed to facilitate hospital discharge.

Education and secondary prevention

Education is a vital part of rehabilitation, as it empowers the patient to minimize the activity and participation restrictions that result from impairment. The unique educational needs (in terms of knowledge, skills and attitudes) of the individual must first be determined and the patient has a central role in setting the agenda. A compromise must be reached when there is a discrepancy between the person's perceived needs and actual needs (as determined by health professionals).

Generally, patients need to learn about their impairment, its aetiology, underlying risk factors, management and prognosis. This fosters compliance with treatment and impacts on attitudes. The skills required will be highly specific and can range from cognitive skills to the more practical manual skills. Patients who are empowered through education are more likely to assume responsibility for their health and to institute life changes to maintain it.

Education should be integrated into all stages of the rehabilitation programme through informal daily contact with team members. Formal educational activities can complement the more informal. These can occur on an individual basis or in group settings. The format can vary from the distribution of educational literature to didactic presentations and small group discussions. Discussion groups allow patients to learn from one another and provide mutual support and encouragement.

Psychosocial support

Rehabilitation team members should have at least a basic understanding of those common psychological issues which impact on the rehabilitation process. These include the physiology of grief and loss and the psychology of motivation. They need practical skills in helping patients to mentally and physically adjust to their loss. To this end, they need to get to know and understand the patient, and especially his or her beliefs, goals and fears. This calls for good communication skills and particularly good listening skills. People tend to fear the unknown; an explanation of their condition and the rehabilitation process helps to reduce anxiety. Some will be as concerned about potential future problems (e.g. the risk of a further stroke) as about the immediate one. If such concerns do not surface spontaneously, they should be sought and discussed.

Regular reassurance and positive feedback are simple and effective forms of psychological support. Team members need to maintain a consistently positive approach both to patients and to their progress at rehabilitation; there is much anecdotal evidence for the way in which a careless negative remark can profoundly demoralize a patient. Demonstrating respect for a patient as an individual fosters feelings of self-worth and enhances motivation. However, attempts to providing positive feedback should never lead to dishonesty or insincerity and care must be taken not to generate false expectations.

The need for the psychological support of spouses, partners and other relatives should not be forgotten. In hospital-based rehabilitation settings, patients can offer one other support and encouragement – the so-called 'therapeutic community'. Self-help groups are particularly useful in providing ongoing psychological and practical support following discharged from the rehabilitation programme.

Discharge planning and follow-up

Discharge from hospital should signal a transition in the rehabilitation process rather than its conclusion. Many patients benefit from continuing outpatient therapy aimed at achieving further gains or preventing the loss of what has been achieved. Follow-up arrangements will depend on the needs of the individual and the availability of services. Some follow-up is essential so that any exacerbation of activity or participation restriction can be evaluated and, if possible, remedied.

Evaluation

Rehabilitation programmes are resource intensive and must therefore demonstrate their effectiveness. At a minimum, data should be collected to allow comparison of people on entry and at discharge. Data collection is becoming increasingly standardized; this facilitates comparison between facilities and between different treatment strategies. Such research is now coming of age and holds promise that we will not only be able to prove the overall efficacy of rehabilitation programmes, but also to identify the key elements that contribute to success.[30]

The rehabilitation setting

Rehabilitation can be provided in various settings, including stand-alone rehabilitation hospitals, designated rehabilitation units in general hospitals, undifferentiated hospital wards, nursing homes and residential care centres, day hospitals, community day centres, outpatient rehabilitation centres, and the patient's own home. Each of these has specific advantages and disadvantages, detailed discussion of which is outside the scope of this chapter. Ideally, a range of options should be available to meet the needs of individual patients at a given time.

In larger hospitals, it is usual to co-locate patients with similar rehabilitation needs. Thus, for example, stroke units and ortho-geriatric units have long been in fashion. Such units foster staff expertise and facilitate research, education and training. Though stroke units have been shown to improve survival and functional outcomes,[36] evidence for the efficacy of ortho-geriatric units is less convincing.[37]

Community-based rehabilitation has recently come of age as a compliment to hospital-based rehabilitation. In practice, it only suits patients from the least disabled end of the spectrum and who are otherwise well supported in the community. 'Intermediate care' is a term to describe intensive, short-term, community or home-based rehabilitation that aims to prevent hospitalization, to facilitate early discharge from hospital and/or to maximize independent living.[38]

Emerging technologies and rehabilitation

New technologies have enormous potential in both the assessment and management of the older person in the rehabilitation setting. Many of the existing scoring systems used to quantify disability and document progress (see Table 114.3) are subjective and prone to inter- and intra-observer variability or bias. They are also time-consuming and divert therapists from providing more direct patient care. Remote measuring devices or sensors can objectively record quantitative data and measure an individual's progress in rehabilitation. They can indicate when full rehabilitation potential has been reached or demonstrate ongoing improvement and the need for ongoing therapy.

Technology also has research potential and can provide more accurate evidence of efficacy of interventions (including pharmacological intervention) in clinical trials. For example, a simple accelerometer might be better than a traditional scoring system[39] in demonstrating subtle but important gains in mobility with new drug treatment in a patient with Parkinson's disease.

Technology can also help to tailor a rehabilitation programme to the unique requirements of the individual patient. For example, it can be used to accurately assess a maladaptive gait pattern in a person with osteoarthritis and thus indicate the most appropriate orthotic device to prescribe.[40]

The development of advanced robotic devices to assist in rehabilitation programmes in select patients is equally becoming a reality. The Honda Motor Company is researching a walking assist device which has the potential to not only augment recovery in patients with neuromuscular deficits, but to provide ongoing assistance with activities of daily living including stair walking (Figure 114.2).

Development of devices

Until recently, the clinical use of remote sensor devices was limited by their bulk, weight and battery life. They were often difficulty to attach and there were problems with data storage and transmission. Recent advances in miniaturization, ergonomic design and the availability of wireless transmission have generated patient-friendly devices that

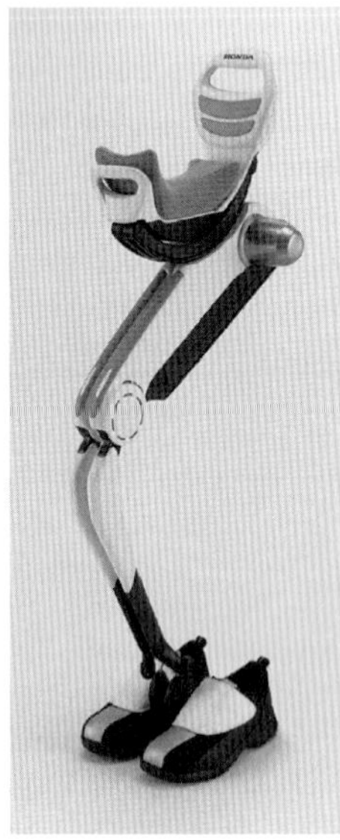

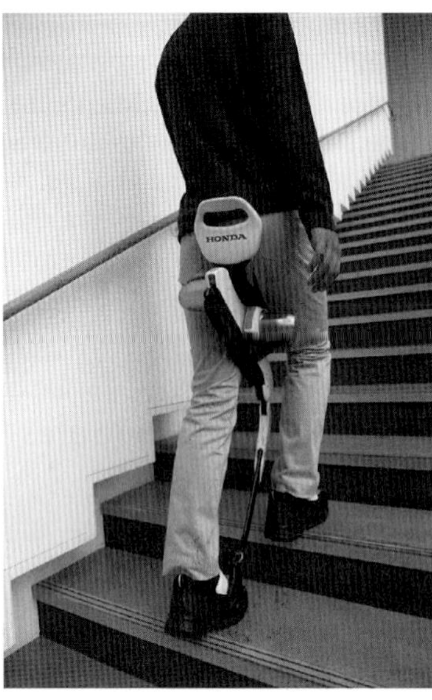

Figure 114.2 Honda's experimental Walking Assist Device with Body Weight Support System. Reproduced by permission of Honda Motor Co., Ltd.

can transmit massive amounts of data for analysis. While devices including accelerometers are now widely used in the gaming industry, their scientific validation in the rehabilitation of older patients is limited.

'Virtual reality' (VR) platforms can provide safe and novel treatment for the older patient with rehabilitation needs. They can provide visual, auditory and tactile sensory input and when used in conjunction with robotic devices, they can also assist with motor skills. For example, a 'robotic glove', when combined with a virtual reality platform can optimize motor function following a hemiparetic stroke. The device can then be attached to an arm orthosis which can be adjusted to overcome gravity by passively counterbalancing arm weight, and providing sensory feedback through virtual environments.[41]

'Video capture' technology combined with remote sensor technology provides an added dimension. Specifically, head-mounted devices designed to track head movements have been used to enhance the virtual environments of patients recovering from stroke.

There have been attempts to use VR platforms to counter impaired postural control and thus reduce falls and injury.[42] In maintaining balance, we know that the CNS integrates visual, vestibular, proprioceptive and somatosensory stimuli. As the intensity and integration of these stimuli decline with advancing age, adaptive mechanisms cause older adults to rely more on visual stimuli and to initiate fewer head movements.[43] By altering sensory inputs and enhancing appropriate corrective strategies, VR can augment such adaptive mechanisms, thus promoting postural stability. VR also provides a safe virtual environment where rehabilitation activities can be risk free and promote patient confidence.

Current barriers to the wider use of sensory-based technological systems include their cost, lack of technical support and a strong evidence base for their efficacy. 'Video capture' technology is, however, much cheaper and is widely available. The gaming industry has been instrumental in developing such systems as the Nintendo Wii, with its built-in accelerometers and infrared camera to track movement. Thus, the potential to develop game-like activities to support rehabilitation already exists. Features designed to enhance motivation, to improve motor function, to reach and to grasp can all be incorporated into specific games. Video games that focus on upper limb function following stroke are being developed. Such games should be meaningful (i.e. provide feedback), should avoid conveying a sense of failure and should try to match the level of challenge to the capability of the player.[41]

Rehabilitation at home

Remote sensors, wireless data transfer (perhaps in combination with global positioning systems – GPS – technology) robotics and mobile computer systems also facilitate early transfer from hospital-based to home-based rehabilitation programmes. Cost savings, reduced hospital-acquired infections and return to familiar environments are just some of the advantages. Such technology can then continue to be used to maintain independence, reduce caregiver burden and prevent institutionalization.

Specific rehabilitation problems

Cardiac rehabilitation

Cardiac rehabilitation is defined as:

> The process by which patients with cardiac disease, in partnership with a multidisciplinary team of health professionals, are encouraged and supported to achieve and maintain optimal physical and psychological health.[44]

It has evolved over the past 60 years, since early mobilization following myocardial infarction was first recommended.[45] Initial programmes were exercise-based and successfully reduced post-infarct morbidity and mortality, with a 27% reduction in all cause mortality being reported.[46] More recently, it has been shown that three months of exercise training in older patients following acute myocardial infarction, improves exercise capacity and a range of biochemical and physiological markers of cardiac performance.[47]

The scope of cardiac rehabilitation has now expanded to include other conditions (e.g. ischaemic heart disease, cardiac failure, coronary revascularization, valve replacement surgery). Modern interventions include education, psychological support, lifestyle advice, risk factor reduction and drug therapy.[48] Home-based programmes complement those that are hospital-based and these particularly suit some elderly people. Outcomes increasingly focus on improved exercise tolerance and quality of life in addition to reduced mortality.[49]

Guidelines on cardiac rehabilitation devised by the Scottish Intercollegiate Guidelines Network (SIGN) have been endorsed by the British Association for Cardiac Rehabilitation and identify four phases of rehabilitation as outlined in Table 114.4.

In Phase 1, early mobilization reduces the risk of thromboembolic disease and other complications of immobility. Low-level self-care activities can begin shortly after the acute event and then gradually increase. Thus, people with an uncomplicated infarct might feed themselves from the outset, sit out of bed within 24 hours and walk to the toilet within 48 hours. Spouses, partners and other family members are ideally involved from this initial stage and should also be offered reassurance and information.

The early post-discharge period (Phase 2) is often a time when patients and families are apprehensive and need support. This can be provided by written information and a telephone 'help line'. Though Phase 3 revolves around a structured and tailored exercise programme, this is just one of its elements (Table 114.4). This phase is increasingly offered in the community rather than in hospital. Physical activity and lifestyle changes need to be maintained (Phase 4) if the gains of rehabilitation are to be sustained. Many people benefit from involvement in a local cardiac support group and participation in group activities.

A detailed description of the exercise programmes suitable for people with cardiac disease is available elsewhere.[44] An initial assessment is essential to identify high-risk patients who either need a modified exercise programme and/or who need to be carefully monitored. Ideally, this will include a simple test of functional capacity such as a shuttle walking test [50] or a six-minute walking test.[51] High-risk patients need careful evaluation, perhaps including an exercise stress test.

Table 114.4 The four phases of cardiac rehabilitation.

1 The inpatient stage, following an acute cardiac event includes medical evaluation, reassurance, education and correction of misconceptions, risk factor assessment, mobilization and discharge planning.
2 Following hospital discharge, when patients may need physical and psychological support.
3 Structured exercise training, together with continuing educational and psychological support and advice on risk factor reduction.
4 Long-term maintenance of physical activity and lifestyle change.

Aerobic, low to moderate intensity exercise is appropriate for the majority of elderly patients in a cardiac rehabilitation programme. This is generally undertaken in a group setting and at least twice weekly for a minimum of eight weeks. However, weekly hospital-based group exercise, together with a home-based exercise programme can be just as effective.

The intensity of exercise can be monitored by perceived exertion or by heart rate, as measured with a pulse monitor. With the former, the aim is to achieve 'comfortable breathlessness'. The target heart rate is derived from the maximal heart rate (estimated at 220-age in years). A training effect is best seen at 65–80% of maximal heart rate.[52]

Patients with unstable angina, valve stenosis or cardiac failure, or with a history of cardiac arrhythmia, are most at risk of an exercise-induced cardiac event. Such patients require a particularly careful evaluation before starting rehabilitation and close medical supervision thereafter. Warm-up and cool-down exercises minimize the risk of musculoskeletal injury and cardiac arrhythmia. Extremes of temperature and over-exertion should be avoided and exercise should cease immediately if the person feels unwell. All symptoms should be reported and medically assessed.

Access to a formal cardiac rehabilitation programme is not always possible and is inappropriate for elderly people with coincidental respiratory, neurological or musculoskeletal disorders. However, even chair-bound elderly people benefit from low-intensity exercise following a cardiac event.

As psychosocial factors predispose to heart disease,[53] it is not surprising that they are particularly prevalent following an acute cardiac event. Thus, over 40% of elderly patients have some depressive symptoms following acute myocardial infarction.[12] Psychological distress in the early post-infarction period predicts a subsequently reduced QOL.[54,55] Though psychological rehabilitation aims to reduce distress, evidence of its efficacy is conflicting.[56,57] The key components are relaxation, stress management and counselling for individuals or groups.

Patient education is the final element of cardiac rehabilitation and should span the entire programme. Activities can range from the highly structured and formal to the informal and opportunistic. Patients need to understand their disease, its implications and the prospect of recovery. They also need to know about underlying risk factors and the scope for secondary prevention. Lifestyle modification should be recommended for those who smoke, are obese, hypertensive, or with lipid abnormalities. Ideally, spouses, partners and other family members should be involved in educational activities.

Pulmonary rehabilitation

Pulmonary rehabilitation is defined as:

> An art of medical practice wherein an individually tailored, multidisciplinary programme is formulated which through accurate diagnosis, therapy, emotional support and education, stabilizes or reverses both the physio- and psycho-pathology of pulmonary disease and attempts to return the patient to the highest possible functional capacity allowed by his pulmonary handicap and overall life situation.[58]

For people with chronic obstructive pulmonary disease (COPD), pulmonary rehabilitation reduces dyspnoea and fatigue, enhances patient control of the disease and increases exercise capacity.[59] It also improves QOL[58] and may prevent hospitalizations.[60] Similar levels of benefit are seen in all adults, including the 'old old'.[61,62] Indeed, the greatest benefits from pulmonary rehabilitation are found in the most impaired patients.[63] People with other significant chronic lung diseases (e.g. asthma, interstitial/restrictive lung disease) also benefit from rehabilitation.[64]

The key elements of pulmonary rehabilitation are summarized in Table 114.5. An initial assessment allows the programme to be tailored to the individual. While clinical and laboratory tests (e.g. radiology, pulmonary function tests) help to define the nature and severity of lung disease, these are unlikely to improve with rehabilitation. Formal exercise testing, together with blood gas analysis (or oximetry) and cardiac monitoring, should be performed at this stage to determine exercise tolerance, the tendency to hypoxia and the risk of cardiac dysrhythmia. For those who are hypoxic at rest or who desaturate with exertion, a modified exercise programme with supplementary oxygen and appropriate monitoring might still be feasible.[65]

Table 114.5 Elements of pulmonary rehabilitation.

Assessment
Define the nature and severity of lung disease
Identify continuing risk factors
Identify comorbidities
Assess nutritional status
Check immunization status (especially against *Pneumococcus* and influenza)
Assess lifestyle factors contributing to activity and participation restriction
Exercise test ± blood gas analysis/oximetry ± ECG monitoring
Intervention
Optimize medical management
Exercise programme
Breathing exercises
Patient education
Lifestyle and dietary modification
Psychosocial support
Follow-up
Establish benefits of rehabilitation
Assess need for continued rehabilitation

Exercise training is the cornerstone of the rehabilitation process and both upper and lower limb exercises improve limb strength and exercise tolerance.[58] Ventilatory muscle training only benefits a minority of patients with COPD. Ideally, exercise should be undertaken three times weekly, should last a minimum of 20 minutes, should induce a heart rate of not less than two-thirds of the maximum expected in the absence of lung disease, and should last at least 6 weeks and preferably 3 months.[66]

In most centres, group exercise programmes are conducted in outpatient settings. Based on the initial assessment, a programme of graded exercises is provided for each individual, leading to a gradual increase in exercise capacity and tolerance. Exercise protocols for people with mild, moderate and severe chest disease are available.[67]

Education aims to enable patients to develop a greater understanding of their disease and the factors contributing to its progression and retardation.[67] Lifestyle and dietary modifications may be required and people may need practical help to achieve these. For example, those who smoke not only need to understand the consequences and the advisability of stopping, but may also need access to smoking cessation programmes. Psychosocial support involves techniques to reduce anxiety and depression; however, there is no clear evidence of their efficacy.[57]

The gains achieved through pulmonary rehabilitation are often lost over time without specific strategies to maintain them.[68] While some form of follow-up is always required, a continuous maintenance programme is ideal. In this regard, self-help groups who encourage and support one another are particularly valuable.

Musculoskeletal disorders

This is a collective term for many heterogeneous conditions that differ in their duration (i.e. acute, sub-acute or chronic), aetiology (e.g. traumatic, inflammatory, degenerative) and the tissues involved (e.g. bone, joint, muscle). They are the commonest cause of disability in old people, such that in the United States, almost 60% of people aged 65 years and over report arthritis or chronic joint symptoms.[69] Such problems will affect over 41 million older Americans by 2030.[70]

Despite their heterogeneity, musculoskeletal disorders tend to result in similar restrictions in activity and participation. Pain, reduced mobility and other functional losses are prominent and these are inter-linked and tend to reinforce one another. For example, people with arthritis may avoid those activities that exacerbate joint pain. As a result, muscles are weakened and joints become unstable and easily injured. This leads to more pain and further avoidance of exercise. Cardio-respiratory fitness may then become critically reduced, particularly in the very old in whom activities of daily living require oxygen uptakes close to the age-associated maximum. The net result is an unfit, inactive, arthritic person whose independence is compromised.

Detailed discussion of the non-pharmacological and pharmacological management of musculoskeletal pain is dealt with elsewhere in this text (see Section 9). However, it should be emphasized that accurate diagnosis is a prerequisite for rational drug prescribing. If analgesics are required, the timing of their use is important. For example, as pain in osteoarthritis is often exacerbated by exercise, it is best to medicate beforehand. Non-pharmacological approaches to pain management should also be considered. For example, moulded splints can protect arthritic hand joints and allow pain-free function with minimal loss of dexterity. A cane held in the contralateral hand limits pain by reducing weight on an arthritic hip. For knee pain, the patient should experiment with holding a cane in either hand. Cane length is important to avoid secondary problems with other joints. Length should equal the distance from the wrist crease to the floor. Stick rubbers should be regularly checked and replaced when worn, to reduce the risk of falls. Resistant pain is best managed by a multidisciplinary approach and nowadays most large centres have access to a pain management team and with it the expertise of anaesthetists, psychiatrists and others.

Daily range-of-motion exercises are particularly important in attempting to restore function in arthritic joints. However, compliance with such measures is low for people of all ages. Joining others in group activities adds a social component and increases compliance. Footwear must be appropriate. Patients with painful knees will benefit from wearing soft-soled shoes with cushioned heels (e.g. jogging shoes). A rocker bottom shoe (Figure 114.3) can reduce pain from rigid toes by assisting in weight transfer from posterior to anterior. This reduces the force needed to propel the body over the metatarsophalangeal (MTP) joints. Metatarsalgia can be reduced by an internal pad placed proximal to the MTP joints. When the hind foot is involved through medial arch collapse, an orthosis which supports the medial arch often helps. Heat, including baths and spas, has been traditionally used for arthritic joints. There is no evidence that hydrotherapy causes measurable functional improvement in arthritic joints, although it does promote self-confidence.[71]

With regard to loss of function, a home-based assessment by an OT is often invaluable. Simple ergonomic measures and aids (e.g. tap turners, zipper pulls, sock pulls, stretch laces, long-handled shoe-horns and Velcro fasteners) can notably reduce joint strain and consequent pain.

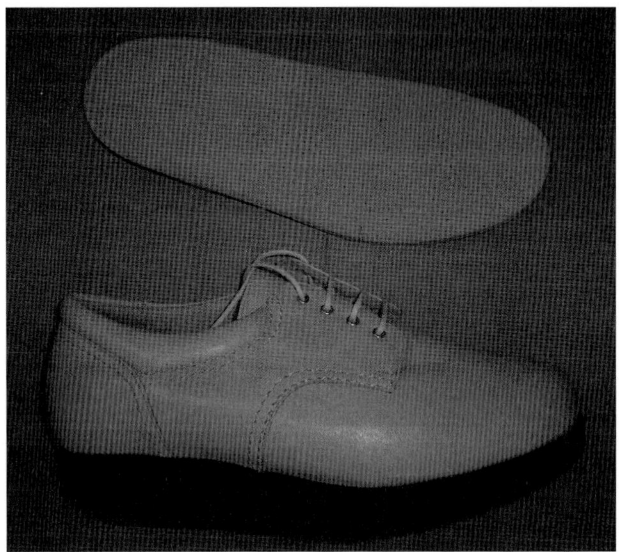

Figure 114.3 Rockerbottom shoe with an insole.

Pathological changes occur against a backdrop of age-related changes in joints and soft tissues, which themselves limit flexibility. However, these age-related changes are reversible and exercise will increase joint flexibility[72] and improve the strength, size and resilience of cartilage, ligaments and muscles. The arthritic patient should be encouraged to develop physical fitness and set realistic goals.

In the context of musculoskeletal disorders, there is little evidence for the efficacy of structured rehabilitation programmes perhaps because research of sufficient rigor has yet to be undertaken. Multidisciplinary rehabilitation, based on time-limited and goal-directed interventions, is only of proven benefit in the management of chronic back pain, other types of chronic pain and following hip fracture in frail elderly people.[73] The prevalence and impact of musculoskeletal disorders on elderly people, means that further research to identify the effective elements of rehabilitation should become an even greater priority.

The elderly amputee patient

Most lower limb amputations in elderly patients are a consequence of peripheral vascular disease.[74] While limb-threatening ischaemia is occasionally due to a sudden embolic event, most patients have a long period of worsening ischaemia prior to amputation. Many people are diabetic and have coexisting cardiac and other vascular disease, while others have smoking-induced chronic lung disease. Despite this, rehabilitation has much to offer the older amputee[75] and many rise to the challenge of walking even with bilateral below-knee prostheses.

That stated, elderly people who require a lower limb amputation are a high-risk group. Perioperative mortality is in the range of 10–30%, two-year survival is 40–50% and five-year survival is 30–40%. These rates have not changed significantly in the past 50 years, even with better anaesthetic and surgical techniques.[76]

When faced with an ischaemic limb that cannot be salvaged by vascular reconstruction, the surgeon often has to choose between a transfemoral (i.e. above-knee) or transtibial (i.e. below-knee) amputation. Preservation of the knee is critical in maintaining proprioceptive and neuromuscular control and particularly in minimizing energy expenditure. It takes 40% more energy to walk with an above-knee than with a below-knee prosthesis.[77] However, injudicious efforts to salvage a knee joint can result in an ischaemic stump which fails to heal and later necessitates a more proximal amputation. The need for a second surgical procedure is potentially disastrous as it increases the anaesthetic risk, prolongs the period of immobility, increases the risk of deconditioning and delays entry into rehabilitation.

Following limb amputation, stump management involves the use of rigid removable dressings to reduce oedema, promote healing and protect against incidental trauma. It is important that early physical therapy be directed at strengthening the arms, the abdominal muscles, the lower back and the remaining leg. Irrespective of age, prescription of a lower limb prosthesis is almost always indicated, even in the presence of other major medical problems. However, it has been shown that older amputees are less likely than their younger counterparts to receive a prosthesis, even when potential confounding factors such as comorbidities and functional status are considered.[78]

The prosthesis facilitates transfers, standing and walking and has cosmetic value. It used to be argued that an older amputee should have crutch-walking capacity before being offered a prosthesis. However, as walking without bearing weight on the amputated side has a higher energy cost than walking on the prosthesis, this criterion is invalid. While some refuse a prosthesis and accept wheelchair mobility, most elderly people and particularly those with few comorbidities, are happy with their prosthesis and use it well.[79] As with any other medical intervention, a prosthesis should never be prescribed without considering the unique needs and wishes of each patient. The demands of using a prosthesis should be fully explained. For a below-knee amputee, the full range of knee extension should be maintained. It is therefore important to avoid prolonged periods of sitting without corrective exercises and a minimum of 20–30 minutes of prone lying should occur twice daily to promote full extension. The skin coming into contact with the prosthesis needs to be durable and toughened; this is best achieved by graded use of the prosthesis. Massaging the stump improves circulation and prevents adhesions during the healing process and patients should be encouraged to do this.

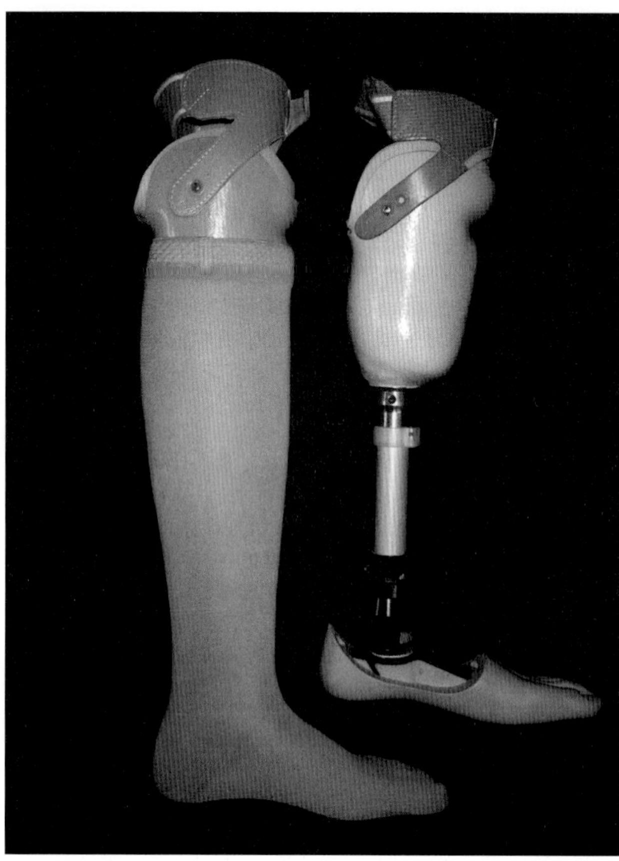

Figure 114.4 Two types of lower limb prostheses are shown with a solid ankle-cushion heel (SACH) foot on the left and an articulated flexible ankle mechanism fitted on the right prosthesis, which additionally shows the central pylon before final covering.

Modern trans-tibial prostheses consist of a socket, a shank and an ankle and foot mechanism (Figure 114.4). The socket is the major determinant of the comfort and stability of the prosthesis. In general, it is designed to transfer most of the weight onto the patellar tendon and a good fit is critical. The stump will be oedematous in the early post-operative period and then shrinks over time. Temporary sockets are therefore required until this process is complete and a permanent socket is cast. Plastic laminate is the most commonly used socket material. The socket may incorporate a suction device to suspend the limb. When a non-suction socket is used, an interface material (stump socks or other plastic resilient material) is needed. Stump socks should be washed daily with mild soap and warm water, rinsed thoroughly and allowed to dry flat. The inner surface of the socket should be cleaned each evening with a warm soapy cloth.

Shanks have traditionally had an 'exoskeletal' design, using willow or lightweight balsa wood covered with laminated plastic. A more modern 'endoskeletal' limb (Figure 114.4) has a central pillar, made of carbon-fibre or lightweight metal to support the body weight, and is surrounded by a soft cover approximating the feel of a normal limb.

A prosthetic foot may be rigid or have an ankle that allows movement in one or more planes. Prescription is dependent on the level of client activity and on the condition of the stump. There is no evidence that any one design is inherently superior.[80] The advantages of a rigid ankle are lightness, low initial and maintenance cost, easy fitting and good appearance. The solid ankle-cushion heel (SACH) foot has a rigid ankle, a compressible heel and a light foot. It is particularly suited to the frail, less active patient who does not take long steps. SACH feet provide long service and are now almost always used for below-knee limbs.

Once a comfortable, stable and functional limb has been provided, the next stage of training is to help the patient to walk on it properly. Gait retraining and the provision of additional mobility aids are complex subjects, discussion of which is outside the scope of this chapter.

When peripheral vascular disease leads to limb amputation, the remaining limb is often significantly ischaemic such that 15–20% of people undergo a contralateral amputation within two years and some 40% within four years.[81] The viability of the remaining leg can often be enhanced by surgery and by minimizing risk factors for vascular disease (e.g. poor diabetic control, cigarette smoking, etc.). Foot hygiene should be promoted and trauma to the leg should be avoided, particularly by wearing appropriate footwear.

Comprehensive rehabilitation of the elderly amputee involves more than the provision of a prosthesis. Comorbidity, prosthetic component selection and resettlement with tenuous or absent social supports all present formidable challenges. A more comprehensive review of this area, including the care of the bilateral amputee, is available.[82]

The non-painful sensation of a phantom limb is normal after amputation. Initially, this can be so deceptive that a patient inadvertently attempts to walk or to scratch the missing limb. Over time, patients sense the limb retracting or 'telescoping' into the stump. Phantom pain is a separate though perhaps related phenomenon, which affects some 50–80% of people following a limb amputation.[83]

The pathophysiology of phantom pain is poorly understood, though central and peripheral nervous system factors together with psychological factors are implicated.[79] It can usually be differentiated from stump pain, as it is localized in the phantom and is variously described as burning, crushing or lancinating. Phantom pains may be continuous or intermittent and the limb may be perceived as twisted or deformed. Management includes explaining the nature of the phenomenon to the patient. While patients with chronic pain before amputation have a higher incidence of phantom pain, attempts to control pain before and during surgery do not consistently reduce the subsequent development of phantom pain.

The management of phantom pain is challenging, particularly on the rare occasion when it is very debilitating. There is little evidence from randomized controlled trials to guide clinicians and when reported, improvement rates are little better than with placebo.[84] Anaesthetic and surgical techniques (e.g. local anaesthesia, sympathectomy, cordotomy) are as disappointing as pharmacological approaches. Tricyclic antidepressants and sodium-channel blocks are often used because of their efficacy in neuropathic pain, but are of no proven benefit. Transcutaneous electrical nerve stimulation (TENS) provides modest relief at best[85] and patients need ongoing psychological help to develop coping strategies.[86]

Neurological rehabilitation

The pathological processes that involve the brain and other parts of the nervous system tend to divide into those that are acute and non-progressive (e.g. stroke, acquired brain injury, spinal cord injury) and those that are chronic and progressive (e.g. Parkinson's disease, motor neurone disease). Collectively, they present an array of rehabilitation challenges, particularly relating to mobility, balance and stability, communication and swallowing, and cognition. The management of chronic pain in older people can be a particular challenge.[87]

This brief section deals only with the rehabilitation of some common chronic progressive neurological disorders of old age. The complex area of rehabilitation following stroke is addressed elsewhere in this text (Chapter 58), while acquired brain injury and spinal cord injury are so uncommon in elderly people as to not warrant discussion here.

A key matter to consider is the rationale for rehabilitation in people with progressive neurological disorders as it can be argued that their relentless nature makes resource-intensive approaches to rehabilitation inappropriate. This raises complex ethical and practical issues regarding the overlap between rehabilitation and palliative care. In the context of a progressive dementing illness, particular challenges arise when, for example, patients lack both the intellectual capacity to fully engage in rehabilitation and to provide informed consent to participate. However, the loss of intellectual capacity cannot justify a decision to deny a person access to potentially beneficial therapy.

With progressive neurological disorders such as Parkinson's disease, rehabilitation has tended to focus on gait and speech problems.[88] While these are often the most distressing aspects of the disease, they are also the most difficult to modify with remedial therapy.[89,90]

Dementia is by far the commonest progressive neurological disorder in older people. Here, two particular considerations arise: the impact of rehabilitation on the dementing process *per se* and the impact of a coincidental dementia on rehabilitation for another disorder (e.g. hip fracture or stroke). With regard to the former, most research to date has focused on the potential benefits of exercise; a meta-analysis of 30 trials involving over 2000 patients concluded that exercise training increases fitness, physical function, cognitive function and positive behaviour in people with dementia.[91] There is also evidence that those with mild to moderate dementia benefit from rehabilitation for such problems as hip fracture.[92]

Future challenges

While the principles and practice of rehabilitation have evolved considerably in recent decades, progress has been slow in at least two areas. The first concerns access to rehabilitation for elderly people even in countries with well-developed health services. For example, it is estimated that only 2% of Canadians who might benefit access pulmonary rehabilitation and only 1% of those in need access musculoskeletal rehabilitation.[93,94] The mis-match between resources and demand is even greater in developing countries.

The second area of slow progress is in identifying the most cost-effective elements of rehabilitation in different clinical situations. Further research in this area is essential for resources to be optimally targeted, for funding to be secured and for geriatric rehabilitation to advance as a discipline. Many healthcare systems are struggling with demographic change and a consequent increased demand for hospital resources at a time when acute hospital beds are being reduced. As acute hospital care and long-term residential care tend to be separately funded and poorly coordinated, pressures to reduce lengths of acute hospital stay tend to erode rehabilitation services in the acute hospital. Community-based rehabilitation services are not expanding to fill the gap and are anyway unsuited to many elderly people who lack the live-in support of a carer.

A lack of investment in rehabilitation is a false economy as it leads to avoidable and costly institutional care.[95] Sixty years ago, Marjorie Warren highlighted the social injustice of failing to optimally meet the rehabilitation needs of elderly people and their families. Such concerns are still relevant today.

Key points

- In 2001, the WHO introduced its International Classification of Functioning, Disability and Health (ICF). This challenges traditional views on health and disability, while providing a mechanism to document the impact of the social and physical environment on a person's functioning.
- Rehabilitation is a step-wise process where the various stages often overlap, may occur concurrently and may need to be regularly revisited.
- Education is a vital component of rehabilitation as through it the patient acquires the knowledge, skills and attitudes to minimize the activity and participation restrictions that can result from impairment.
- A failure to optimally meet the rehabilitation needs of older people and their families is socially unjust, just as a lack of investment in rehabilitation is a false economy, leading to avoidable and costly institutional care.

References

1. Warren M. Care of the chronic aged sick. *Lancet* 1946;**i**:841–3.
2. World Health Organization (WHO). International Statistical Classification of Diseases and Related Health Problems, Tenth Revision, Vols 1–3, WHO, Geneva, 1992–1994.
3. World Health Organization. International Classification of Impairments, Disabilities and Handicaps, WHO, Geneva, 1980.
4. World Health Organization. International Classification of Functioning, Disability and Health, WHO, Geneva, 2001.
5. United Nations (UN). World Programme of Action Concerning Disabled Persons. Division for Social Policy Development, 2003. http://www.un.org/esa/socdev/enable/diswpa01.htm (last accessed 6 December 2011).
6. Finucane P, Giles L, Withers RT *et al.* Exercise profile and subsequent mortality in an elderly Australian population. *Aust NZ J Publ Health* 1997;**21**:155–8.
7. Castille EM, Goodman-Gruen D, Kritz-Silverstein D *et al.* Sarcopenia in elderly men and women. The Rancho Bernardo study. *Am J Prevent Med* 2003;**25**:226–31.
8. Janssen I, Heymsfield SB, Ross R. Low relative skeletal muscle mass (sarcopenia) in older people is associated with functional impairment and physical disability. *J Am Geriatr Soc* 2002;**50**:889–96.
9. Lathan N, Anderson C, Bennett D, Stretton C. Progressive resistance strength training for physical disability in older people (Cochrane Review). In: *The Cochrane Library*, Issue 3, John Wiley & Sons, Ltd, Chichester, UK, 2004.
10. Booth FW, Zwetsloot KA. Basic concepts about genes, inactivity and ageing. *Scand J Med Sci Sports* 2010;**20**:1–4.
11. Australian Bureau of Statistics. *Disability, Ageing and Carers Australia*, ABS Catalogue No. 4430.0, Belconnen, ACT, Australia, 1998.
12. Shiotani I, Sato H, Kinjo K *et al.* Depressive symptoms predict 12-month prognosis in elderly patients with acute myocardial infarction. *J Cardiovasc Risk* 2002;**9**:153–60.
13. Whyte, EM, Mulsant, BH. Depression after stroke: A prospective epidemiological study. *J Am Geriatr Soc* 2004;**52**:774–8.

14. Mast BT, MacNeill SE, Lichtenberg PA. Post-stroke and clinically defined vascular depression in geriatric rehabilitation patients. *Am J Psychiatr* 2004;**12**:84–92.
15. Young JB, Forster A. The Bradford community stroke trial: results at six months. *Br Med J* 1992;**304**:1085–9.
16. Kemp BJ. Motivation, rehabilitation and aging: a conceptual model. *Topics Geriatr Rehabil* 1988;**3**:41–51.
17. Barer D. Assessment in rehabilitation. *Rev Clin Gerontol* 1993; **3**:169–86.
18. van der Vluten CPM. The assessment of professional competence: developments, research and practical implications. *Adv Health Sci Educ* 1996;**1**:41–67.
19. Mahoney FJ, Barthel DW. Functional evaluation: the Barthel Index. *Maryland State Med J* 1965;**14**:61–5.
20. Collin C, Wade DT, Davies S, Horne V. The Barthel ADL Index: a reliability study. *Int Disabil Stud* 1988;**10**:61–3.
21. Peach H, Green S, Locker D *et al.* Evaluation of a postal screening questionnaire to identify the disabled. *Int Rehabil Med* 1980;**2**:189–93.
22. Hodkinson HM. Evaluation of a mental test score for assessment of mental impairment in the elderly. *Age Ageing* 1972;**1**: 233–8.
23. Jitapunkul S, Pillay I, Ebrahim SB. The abbreviated mental test: its use and validity. *Age Ageing* 1991;**20**:332–6.
24. Yesavage JA, Brink TL, Rose TL *et al.* Development and validation of a geriatric depression screening scale – a preliminary report. *J Psychiatr Res* 1983;**17**:37–49.
25. Yesavage JA. Geriatric Depression Scale. *Psychopharmacol Bull* 1988;**24**:709–11.
26. Davies B, Challis D. *Matching Resources to Needs in Community Care*, Personal Social Services Research Unit, University of Kent, Canterbury, 1986.
27. Royal College of Physicians and British Geriatrics Society Joint Workshops. *Standardised Assessment Scales for Elderly People*, The Royal College of Physicians of London and the British Geriatrics Society, London, 1992.
28. Wade DT. *Measurements in Neurological Rehabilitation*, Oxford University Press, Oxford, 1992.
29. Keith RA, Granger CV, Hamilton BB, Sherwin FS. The functional independence measure: a new tool for rehabilitation. *Adv Clin Rehabil* 1987;**1**:6–18.
30. Johnston MV, Wood KD, Fiedler R. Characteristics of effective and efficient rehabilitation programmes. *Arch Phys Med Rehabil* 2003;**84**:410–18.
31. Wilkerson DL, Johnston MV. Outcomes research and clinical programme monitoring systems: current capability and future directions. In: M Fuhrer (ed.), *Medical Rehabilitation Outcomes Research*, PH Brookes, Baltimore, 1997.
32. Wade DT. Evidence relating to goal planning in rehabilitation. *Clin Rehab* 1998;**12**, 273–5.
33. Guthrie S, Harvey A. Motivation and its influence on outcome in rehabilitation. *Rev Clin Gerontol* 1994;**4**:235–43.
34. Mulley GP. *Everyday Aids and Appliances*, BMJ Publishing, London, 1989.
35. Edwards NI, Jones DA. Ownership and use of assistive devices among older people in the community. *Age Ageing* 1998;**27**:463–8.
36. Stroke Unit Trialists. Organised inpatient (stroke unit) care for stroke. *Cochrane Database Syst Rev* 2001;**3**: CD000197.
37. Cameron ID, Handoll HHG, Finnegan TP *et al.* Co-ordinated multidisciplinary approaches for inpatient rehabilitation of older persons with proximal femur fractures. *Cochrane Database Syst Rev* 2001;**3**: CD000106.
38. Stevenson J, Spencer L. *Developing Intermediate Care: A Guide for Health and Social Service Professionals*, The King's Fund, London, 2002.
39. Fahn S, Elton RL. Unified Parkinson's disease rating scale. In: S Fahn, CD Marsden, M Goldstein, DB Clane (eds.) *Recent Developments in Parkinson's Disease*, Vol. 2, Macmillan Healthcare Information, Florham Park, NJ, 1987, pp. 153–63.
40. Crevier LM. Wearable technology provides readymade monitoring for musculoskeletal rehabilitation. *J Musculoskeletal Med* 2009;**26**:178–81.
41. Crosbie JH, McNeill MDJ, Burke J, McDonough S. Utilising technology for rehabilitation of the upper limb following stroke: the Ulster experience. *Physical Ther Rev* 2009;**14**:366–7.
42. Virk S, Valter McConville KM. *Virtual reality applications improving postural control and minimizing falls*. Proceedings of the 28th IEEE EMBS annual international conference, New York, USA, 2006.
43. Zettel J, Holbeche A, McIlory W, Maki B. Redirection of gaze and switching of attention during rapid stepping reactions evoked by unpredictable postural perturbation. *Exp Brain Res* 2005;**165**:392–401.
44. Scottish Intercollegiate Guidelines Network. *Cardiac Rehabilitation: A national clinical guideline*, SIGN (SIGN publication No. 57), Edinburgh, 2002.
45. Levine SA, Lown B. Armchair treatment of acute coronary thrombosis. *JAMA* 1952;**148**:1365–9.
46. Jolliffe JA, Rees K, Taylor RS *et al.* Exercise-based rehabilitation for coronary heart disease. *Cochrane Database Syst Rev* 2001;**1**: CD001800.
47. Dalal H, Evans PH, Campbell JL. Recent developments in secondary prevention and cardiac rehabilitation after acute myocardial infarction. *BMJ* 2004;**328**:693–7.
48. Marchionni N, Fattirolli F, Fumagalli S *et al.* Improved exercise tolerance and quality of life with cardiac rehabilitation of older patients after myocardial infarction. *Circulation* 2003;**107**:2201–6.
49. Giallauria F, Lucci R, De Lorenzo A *et al.* Favourable effects on exercise training on N-terminal pro-brain naturetic peptide plasma levels in elderly patients after acute myocardial infarction. *Age Ageing* 2006;**35**:601–7.
50. Tobin D, Thow MK. The 10m shuttle walk test with Holter monitoring: an objective outcome measure for cardiac rehabilitation. *Coronary Health Care* 1999;**3**:3–17.
51. Demers C, McKelvie RS, Negassa A, Yusuf S. Reliability, validity, and responsiveness of the six-minute walk test in patients with heart failure. *Am Heart J* 2001;**142**:698–703.
52. Kavanagh T. The role of exercise training in cardiac rehabilitation. In: D Jones, R West (eds), *Cardiac Rehabilitation*, BMJ Publishing, London, 1995, pp. 54–82.
53. Hemingway H, Marmont M. Psychological factors in the aetiology and prognosis of coronary heart disease: systematic review of prospective cohort studies. *Br Med J* 1999;**318**: 1460–7.

54. Mayou RA, Gill D, Thompson DR *et al.* Depression and anxiety as predictors of outcome after myocardial infarction. *Psychosom Med* 2000;**62**:212–19.
55. Yohannes AM, Doherty P, Yalfani A, Bundy C. Predictors of quality of life in patients with chronic heart disease. *Age Ageing* 2008;**37**(Suppl 1):i1.
56. Jones DA, West RR. Psychological rehabilitation after myocardial infarction: multicentre randomised controlled trail. *BMJ* 1996;**313**:1517–21.
57. Milani RV, Lavie CJ. Prevalence and effects of cardiac rehabilitation on depression in the elderly with coronary heart disease. *Am J Cardiol* 1998;**81**:1233–6.
58. American College of Chest Physicians and American Association of Cardiovascular and Pulmonary Rehabilitation guidelines panel. Pulmonary rehabilitation: joint AACP/AACVPR evidence-based guidelines. *Chest* 1997;**112**: 1363–96.
59. Lacasse Y, Brosseau L, Milne S *et al.* Pulmonary rehabilitation for chronic obstructive pulmonary disease. *Cochrane Database Syst Rev* 2002;**4**: CD003793.
60. Calverley PMA, Walker P. Chronic obstructive pulmonary disease. *Lancet* 2003;**362**:1053–61.
61. Katsura H, Kanemaru A, Yamada K *et al.* Long-term effectiveness of an inpatient pulmonary rehabilitation programme for elderly COPD patients: comparison between young-elderly and old-elderly groups. *Respirology* 2004;**9**: 230–6.
62. Couser JI, Guthmann R, Hamadeh MA, Kane CS. Pulmonary rehabilitation improves exercise capacity in older elderly patients with COPD. *Chest* 1995;**107**:730–4.
63. Di Meo F, Pedone C, Lubich S *et al.* Age does not hamper the response to pulmonary rehabilitation of COPD patients. *Age Ageing* 2008;**37**:530–5.
64. Foster S, Thomas HM. Pulmonary rehabilitation in lung disease other than chronic obstructive pulmonary disease. *Am Rev Resp Dis* 1990;**141**:601–4.
65. Roig RL, Worsowicz GM, Stewart DG, Cifu DX. Geriatric rehabilitation. 3. Physical medicine and rehabilitation interventions for common disabling disorders. *Arch Phys Med Rehabil* 2004;**85**: S12–S17.
66. Clark CJ. Setting up a pulmonary rehabilitation programme. *Thorax* 1994;**49**:270–278.
67. American Association of Cardiovascular and Pulmonary Rehabilitation. *Guidelines for Pulmonary Rehabilitation Programmes*, 3rd edn, AACVPR, 2004.
68. Spruit MA, Troosters T, Trappenburg JCA, Decramer M, Gosselink R. Exercise training during rehabilitation of patients with COPD: a current perspective. *Patient Educ Counseling* 2004;**52**:243–8.
69. Centers for Disease Control. Prevalence of self-reported arthritis or chronic joint symptoms among adults – United States, 2001. *MMWR* 2002;**51**:948–50.
70. Centers for Disease Control. Projected prevalence of self-reported arthritis or chronic joint symptoms among persons aged ≥65 years – United States, 2005–2030. *MMWR* 2003; **52**:489–91.
71. Ahern M, Nicholls E, Siminiato E *et al.* Clinical and psychological effects of hydrotherapy in rheumatic diseases. *Clin Rehabil* 1995;**9**:204–12.
72. Raab DM, Agre JC, McAdam M, Smith EL. Light resistance and stretching exercise in elderly women: effect on flexibility. *Arch Phys Med Rehabil* 1988;**69**:268–72.
73. Cameron ID. How to manage musculoskeletal conditions: when is 'Rehabilitation' appropriate? *Best Practice Res Clin Rheumatol* 2004;**18**:573–86.
74. Ephraim PL, Dillingham TR, Sector M, Pezzin LE, Mackenzie EJ. Epidemiology of limb loss and congenital limb deficiency: a review of the literature. *Arch Phys Med Rehabil* 2003;**84**: 747–61.
75. Esquenazi A. Geriatric amputee rehabilitation. *Clin Geriatr Med* 1993;**9**:731–43.
76. Cutson TM, Bongiorni DR. Rehabilitation of the older lower limb amputee: a brief review. *J Am Geriatr Soc* 1996; **4**:1388–93.
77. James U. Oxygen uptake and heart rate during prosthetic walking in the healthy male unilateral above-knee ampotee. *Scand J Rehabil Med* 1973;**5**:71–80.
78. Kurichi JE, Kwong PL, Reker DM *et al.* Clinical factors associated with prescription of a prosthetic limb in elderly veterans. *J Am Geriatr Soc* 2007;**55**:900–6.
79. Pezzin LE, Dillingham TR, MacKenzie EJ, Ephraim P, Rossbach P. Use and satisfaction with prosthetic limb devices and related services. *Arch Phys Med Rehabil* 2004;**85**:723–9.
80. Hofstad C, Van der Linde H, Van Limbeek J, Postema K. Prescription of prosthetic ankle-foot mechanisms after lower limb amputation. *Cochrane Database Syst Rev* 2002;**4**: CD003978.
81. Weiss GN, Gorton TA, Read RC, Neal LA. Outcomes of lower extremity amputations. *J Am Geriatr Soc* 1990;**38**:877–83.
82. Esquenazi A. Geriatric amputee rehabilitation. *Clin Geriatr Med* 1993;**9**:731–43.
83. Flor H. Phantom-limb pain: characteristics, causes, and treatment. *Lancet Neurology* 2002;**1**:182–9.
84. Halbert J, Crotty M, Cameron ID. Evidence for the optimal management of acute and chronic phantom pain: a systematic review. *Clin J Pain* 2002;**18**:84–92.
85. Katz J, Melzack RA. Auricular transcutaneous electrical nerve stimulation (TENS) reduces phantom limb pain. *J Pain Symptom Manage* 1991;**6**:77–83.
86. Hill A, Niven CA, Knussen C. The role of coping in adjustment to phantom limb pain. *Pain* 1995;**62**:79–86.
87. Helme RD. Chronic pain management in older people. *Eur J Pain* 2001;**5**:31–6.
88. Montgomery EB. Rehabilitative approaches to Parkinson's disease. *Parkinsonism and Related Disorders* 2004;**10**: S43–S47.
89. Deane KHO, Jones D, Ellis-Hill C *et al.* Physiotherapy for Parkinson's disease. Cochrane Movement Disorders Group. *Cochrane Database Syst Rev* 2003;**3**.
90. Deane KOH, Ellis-Hill C, Playford ED, Ben-Shlomo Y, Clarke CE. Occupational therapy for Parkinson's disease. Cochrane Movement Disorders Group. *Cochrane Database Syst Rev* 2003;**3**.
91. Heyn P, Abreu BC, Ottenbacher KJ. The effects of exercise training on elderly persons with cognitive impairment and dementia: a meta-analysis. *Arch Phys Med Rehabil* 2004;**85**:1694–1704.

92. Huusko TM, Karppi P, Avikainen V, Kautiainen H, Sulkava R. Randomized, clinically controlled trial of intensive geriatric rehabilitation in patients with hip fracture: subgroup analysis of patients with dementia. *BMJ* 2000;**321**:1107–11.
93. Brooks D, Lacasse Y, Goldstein RS. Pulmonary rehabilitation programmes in Canada: national survey. *Can Resp J* 1999; **6**:55–63.
94. Arthritis Foundation, Association of State and Territorial Health Officers, CDC. *National Arthritis Plan: a public health strategy*, Arthritis Foundation, Atlanta, GA, 1999.
95. Young J, Robinson J, Dickinson E. Rehabilitation for older persons. *BMJ* 1998;**316**:1109–10.

SECTION 14

Iatrogenic Infections

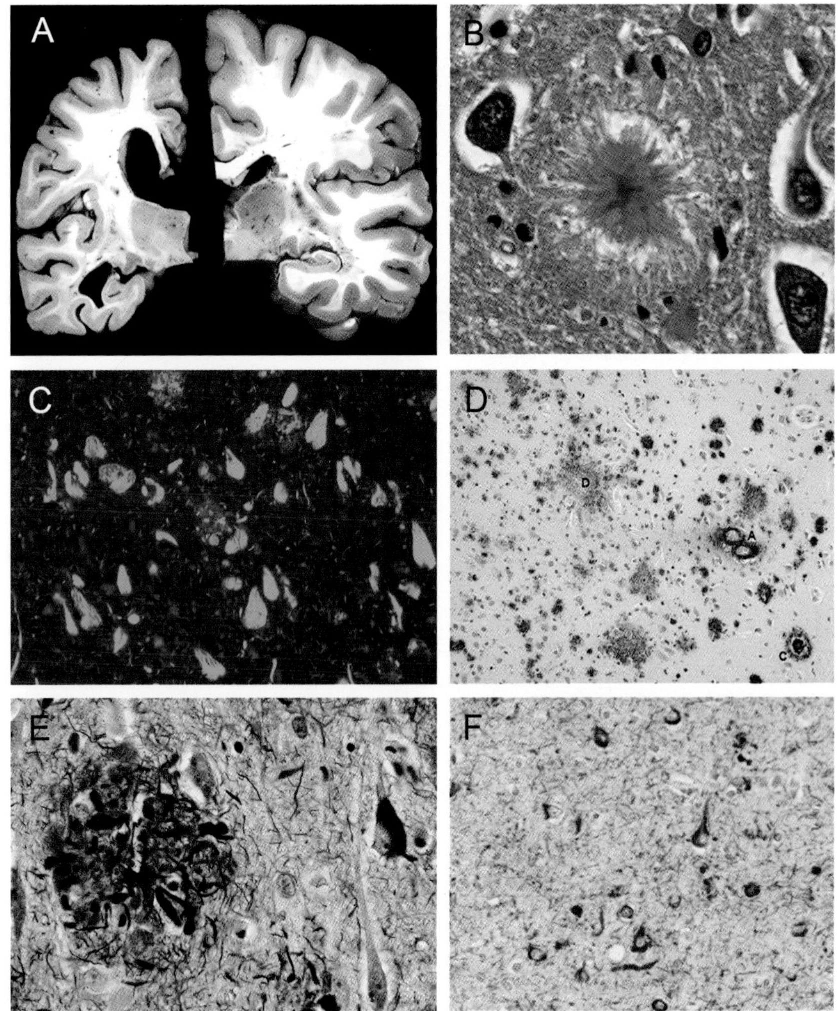

Plate 73.1 The neuropathology of AD. (a) Coronal sections of brain at the level of the hippocampus. On the left is a patient with AD, and on the right is an age-matched individual without cognitive impairment. Note the cortical atrophy and dilatation of the ventricles in the AD patient. (b) Extracellular Aβ senile plaques visualized with haematoxylin and eosin stain. (c) Thioflavin S fluorescent staining of amyloid plaques and neurofibrillary tangles. (d) Immunohistochemistry using Aβ antibodies demonstrating extracellular diffuse and fibrillar amyloid plaques and amyloid deposition in cerebral vessels. (e) Silver impregnation demonstrating fibrillar amyloid with dystrophic neurites and neurofibrillary tangles. (f) Immunohistochemistry using tau antibodies demonstrating neurofibrillary tangles and dystrophic neurites.

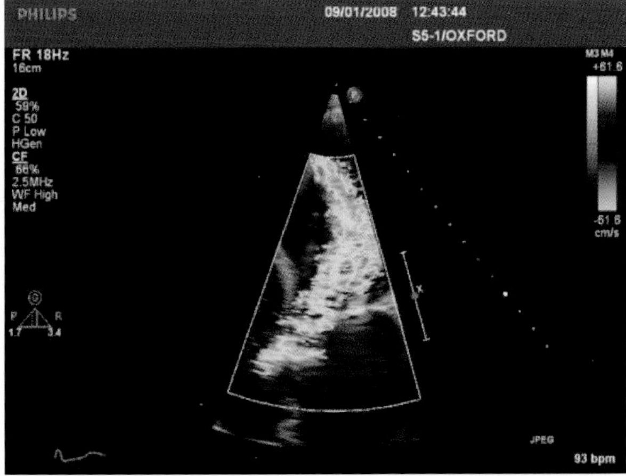

Plate 116.9 Apical five-chamber TTE view demonstrating a wide jet of severe aortic regurgitation in the left ventricular outflow tract extending to the left ventricular apex.

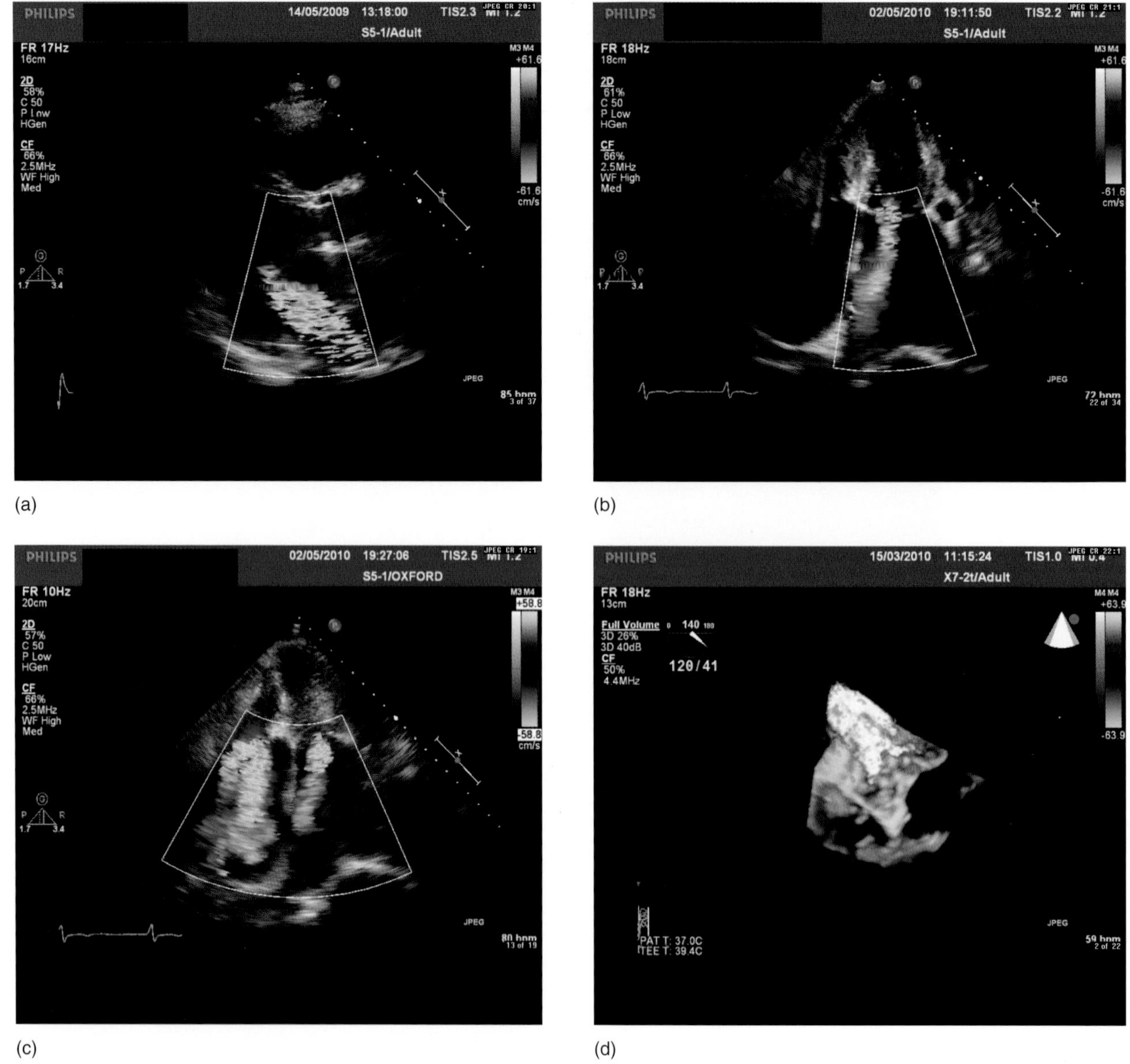

Plate 116.11 (a) TTE parasternal long-axis view with a broad colour jet across the mitral valve demonstrating severe mitral regurgitation. (b) TTE apical view demonstrating severe mitral regurgitation; the broad colour jet occupies over one-third of the left atrium. (c) TTE apical view demonstrating torrential tricuspid regurgitation and concurrent severe mitral regurgitation, causing biatrial dilatation. (d) 3D TOE demonstrating severe mitral regurgitation.

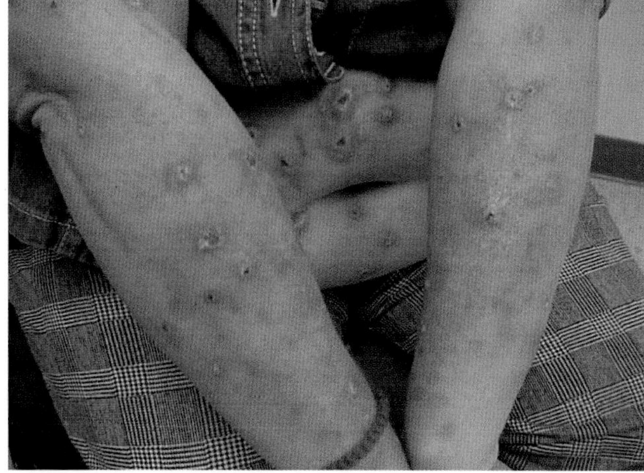

Plate 125.1 Neurotic excoriations of the arms and upper body.

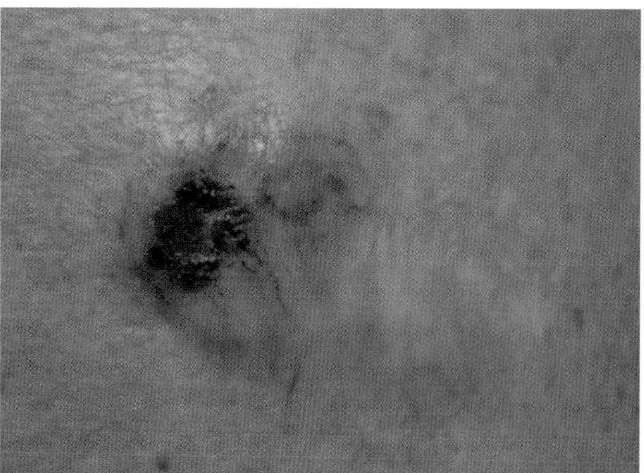

Plate 125.2 Basal cell carcinoma.

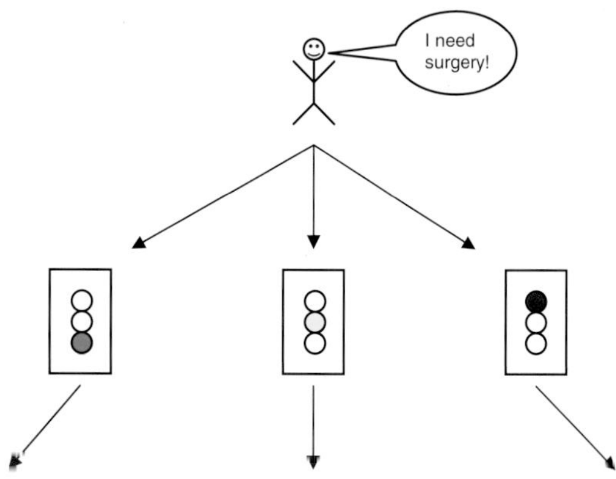

Proceed with surgery without further cardiac testing: ●
1. Emergency surgery
2. No active cardiac condition AND
   - low–risk surgery*
   - functional capacity ≥4 METS†
   - functional capacity <4 METS and no cardiac risk factors+

Consider non-invasive cardiac testing if: ○
1. Intermediate** or high*** risk surgery AND
   - functional capacity <4 METS
   - 1 or 2 cardiac risk factors present
2. Intermediate risk surgery AND
   - functional capacity <4 METS
   - presence of ≥3 cardiac risk factors

Delay surgery for non-invasive cardiac testing if:
● • High risk surgery
AND
- Functional capacity <4 METS

AND
- Presence of ≥3 cardiac risk factors

* Low risk surgery = endoscopic procedures, superficial procedures and cataract, breast and ambulatory surgeries carry <1% risk of sustaining a perioperative cardiac event
** Intermediate risk surgery = all surgeries that do not fall into low or high risk categories carry 1–5% risk of sustaining a perioperative cardiac event
*** High risk surgery = vascular surgery (aortic or other major vascular procedure and peripheral vascular surgery) carry >5% risk of sustaining a perioperative cardiac event)

† 4 METS of activity = light housework or ability to climb a flight of stairs or walk up a hill
+ Cardiac risk factors are defined by the Revised Goldman Cardiac Risk Index

Plate 127.2 Decision tree for evaluation of cardiac risk prior to surgery.

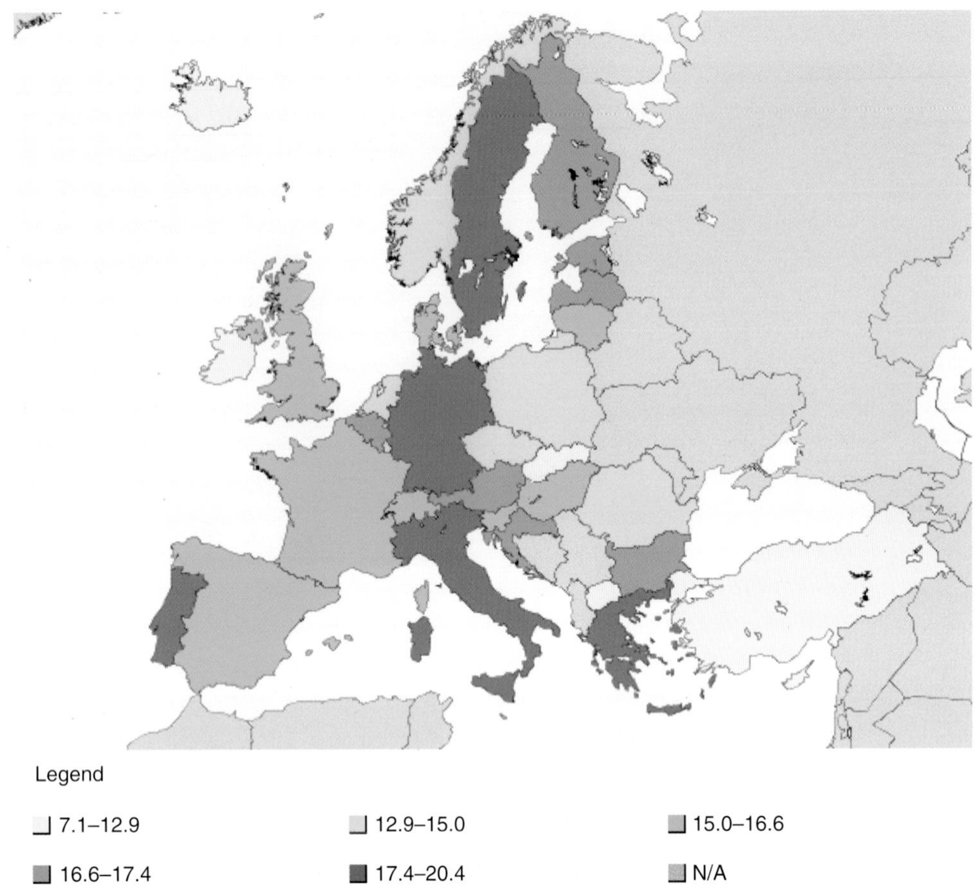

Plate 148.1 Proportion of population aged 65 and over (% of total population).

CHAPTER 115

Tuberculosis

Shobita Rajagopalan[1] and Thomas T. Yoshikawa[2]
[1]Los Angeles County Department of Public Health, Los Angeles, CA, USA
[2]UCLA School of Medicine and VA Greater Los Angeles Healthcare System, Los Angeles, CA, USA

Introduction

In 2008, the World Health Organization (WHO) estimated 8.9–9.9 million incident cases of tuberculosis (TB), 9.6–13.3 million prevalent cases of TB, 1.1–1.7 million deaths from TB among HIV-negative people and an additional 0.45–0.62 million TB deaths among HIV-positive people.[1]

In the USA, during the past three decades, the excess in morbidity reflected a changing epidemiological pattern. HIV infection, poverty, homelessness, substance abuse and immigration from countries with a high prevalence of TB have all contributed to TB morbidity. Overburdened public health TB services were not only unable to manage the resurgence in the 1980s but were also unprepared to cope with emerging multidrug resistance. From the mid-1990s to the present, aggressive TB control, implementation and enhanced resources have resulted in a substantial decline in the overall incidence of TB.

The geriatric population across all racial and ethnic groups and both genders is at substantial risk for *Mycobacterium tuberculosis* (*Mtb*) infection, perhaps because of both biological (compromised nutrition and immune status, underlying disease, medications and possible racial predisposition) and socioeconomic factors (poverty, living conditions and access to healthcare). Frail elderly residents of nursing homes and other long-term care facilities are the most vulnerable group. Because of the highly communicable potential of *Mtb*, the inevitable endemic transmission between residents and from resident to staff has been demonstrated in such facilities. (For the purpose of clarity, TB infection, or latent TB, refers to contained and asymptomatic primary infection with a positive tuberculin skin test reaction, whereas TB disease indicates overt clinical manifestations of TB.)

The Institute of Medicine report *Ending Neglect: the Elimination of TB in the United States*, which was undertaken through sponsorship from the Centers for Disease Control and Prevention (CDC) in 2000, reviews the lessons learned from the neglect of TB between the late 1960s and the early 1990s and reaffirms commitment to a more realistic goal of elimination of TB in the USA.[2] The WHO report *Global Tuberculosis Control: a Short Update to the 2009 Report* includes the latest (2008) estimates of the global burden of TB (incidence, prevalence and mortality).[1] It also includes an assessment of progress in implementing the Stop TB Strategy and the Global Plan to Stop TB to achieve the 2015 global targets for TB control. These targets are that incidence should be falling by 2015 (Millennium Development Goal Target 6.c) and that prevalence and mortality rates should be halved by 2015 compared with their level in 1990.

This chapter reviews the current global epidemiology, pathogenesis, clinical characteristics, diagnosis, management and prevention of *Mtb* infection in community-dwelling and institutionalized ageing adults.

Epidemiology

More than 2 billion people (about one-third of the world population) are estimated to be infected with tuberculosis.[1] The global incidence of TB peaked around 2003 and now appears to be declining slowly. In 2006, the WHO estimated the prevalence of active infection to be 14.4 million and the incidence of new cases 9.2 million; 12 of the 15 countries with the highest estimated TB incidence were reported to be in Africa.

Developed nations including the USA and parts of Southeast Asia report an estimated 380 million persons infected with *Mtb*; about 80% of infected persons in Europe are 50 years of age or older.[3]

In the USA, TB prevails among the foreign-born and minorities. From 1985 to 1992, TB incidence increased among all ethnic groups except non-Hispanic whites and Native Americans/Alaskan Natives. From 1992 to the present, the overall incidence of TB in the USA declined by

Principles and Practice of Geriatric Medicine, Fifth Edition. Edited by Alan J. Sinclair, John E. Morley and Bruno Vellas.

over 45%, largely because of improved funding resources channelled into TB control programmes, which allowed for the implementation of directly observed therapy (DOT). However, the percentage of cases among foreign-born persons increased disproportionately from 27% in 1992 to 46% in 2000.[4] In 2009, the CDC reported 11 540 TB cases; the TB rate was 3.8 cases per 100 000 population, a decrease of 11.4% from the rate of 4.2 per 100 000 reported for 2008.[5] The 2009 rate demonstrated the greatest single-year decrease ever recorded and was the lowest recorded rate since national TB surveillance began in 1953. TB case counts and rates decreased substantially among both foreign-born and US-born persons, although foreign-born persons and racial/ethnic minorities continued to have TB disease disproportionate to their respective populations, and nearly 11 times higher than in US-born persons. The rates among Hispanics and blacks were approximately eight times higher than among non-Hispanic whites and rates among Asians were nearly 26 times higher. The large decrease in reported cases during 2009 might represent a decrease in TB disease resulting from changes in population demographics or improved TB control.

TB also occurs with disproportionate frequency among the elderly.[6,7] Elders living in communal settings such as nursing homes or other long-term care facilities have a TB incidence rate approximately four times greater than the general population.[8] The aggregate TB incidence rate for nursing home residents is 1.8 times higher than the rate seen in community-dwelling elderly.[9] The enhanced efficiency of TB transmissibility within congregate settings such as prisons, nursing facilities (nursing homes), chronic disease facilities and homeless shelters has raised concerns about TB infection and disease in the institutionalized elderly.[10,11] Positive tuberculin reactivity associated with prolonged stay among residents of long-term care facilities for the elderly has been demonstrated, implying an increasing risk of TB infection.

Pathogenesis

The pathogenesis of TB infection and disease begins in most cases with the inhalation of the tubercle bacilli.[12] The usual inoculum is no more than 1–3 organisms, which are taken up by alveolar macrophages and carried to regional lymph nodes. Spread may occur via the lymphohaematogenous route with dissemination to multiple organs. From 2 to 8 weeks after infection, cell-mediated immunity (CMI) and delayed-type hypersensitivity (DTH) responses develop, leading to the characteristic reactive tuberculin test and to the containment of infection. Chemoattractants cause monocytes to enter the area and become transformed into histiocytes forming granulomas. Although the bacilli may persist within macrophages, additional multiplication and spread is curtailed. Healing usually follows with calcification of the infected focus. Caseous necrosis may result secondary to the immune response. Erosion into a bronchiole causes cavity formation where bacilli can multiply and spread. Solid necrosis can result from production of hydrolases from inflammatory cells causing tissue liquefaction and creating a prime medium for microbial replication, generating up to 10 billion bacilli per millilitre. Individuals who develop active disease either fail to contain the primary infection or develop reactivation as a result of relative or absolute immune suppression at a point remote from primary infection. This is most likely to occur in immunocompetent adults within the first 3 years after exposure. Factors related to progression of disease reflect a weakened immune status and include physiological states, for example, normal ageing; associated intercurrent disease – particularly diabetes mellitus, malignancies causing primary immunosuppression or requiring toxic chemotherapy or corticosteroid-dependent diseases such as asthma or collagen vascular disease; poor nutritional status particularly related to alcohol and drug abuse; smoking and HIV infection. Although it is likely that the increased frequency of TB in the elderly could partly be due to CMI that is impaired by senescence (shown in murine models), other concomitant age-related diseases (diabetes mellitus, malignancy), chronic kidney disease and renal insufficiency, poor nutrition and immunosuppressive drugs may also contribute to this increase.[13] In the elderly, approximately 90% of TB disease cases are due to reactivation of primary infection. Persistent infection without disease may occur in 30–50% of individuals. Some elderly persons previously infected with *Mtb* may eventually eliminate the viable tubercle bacilli and revert to a negative tuberculin reactor state. These individuals are therefore at risk of new infection (reinfection) with *Mtb*. There are therefore three subgroups of older persons potentially at risk for TB: one subgroup never exposed to TB that may develop primary TB disease, a second subgroup with persistent and latent primary infection that may reactivate and a third subgroup that is no longer infected and consequently at risk for reinfection.

Clinical characteristics

Clinicians must be aware that frail older persons with TB disease may not demonstrate the overt and characteristic clinical features of TB such as fever, night sweats or haemoptysis. They may exhibit atypical and subtle clinical manifestations of 'failure to thrive' with loss of appetite, functional decline and low-grade fever or weight loss.[13] Although several published works have attempted to delineate clear differences between younger and older TB patients, such studies have provided variable findings. In a meta-analysis of published studies, comparing pulmonary TB in older and younger patients, evaluating the differences in the clinical, radiological and laboratory features of pulmonary TB, no differences were found in the prevalence of cough, sputum production, weight loss, fatigue/malaise, radiographic upper lobe lesions, positive acid-fast bacilli (AFB) in sputum, anaemia or haemoglobin level and serum aminotransferases.[14] A lower prevalence of fever, sweating, haemoptysis, cavitary disease and positive purified protein derivative (PPD), and also lower levels of serum albumin and blood leukocytes, were noticed among older patients. In addition, the older population had a greater prevalence of dyspnoea and some underlying comorbid conditions, such as cardiovascular disorders, chronic obstructive pulmonary disease, diabetes mellitus, gastrectomy history and malignancies. This meta-analytical review identified some subtle differences in clinical presentations of older TB patients compared with their younger TB counterparts. However, most of these differences can be explained by the already known physiological changes that occur during ageing. The majority of older TB patients (75%) with *Mtb* disease manifest active disease in their lungs.[14] Extrapulmonary TB in the elderly is similar to that in younger persons and may involve the meninges, bone and joint and genitourinary systems or disseminate in a miliary pattern.[15–19] Infection of lymph nodes, pleura, pericardium, peritoneum, gall bladder, small and large bowel, the middle ear and carpal tunnel have been described in the literature. Because TB can involve virtually any organ in the body, this infection must be kept in the differential diagnosis of unusual presentations of diseases, especially in the elderly. Thus, TB has been aptly described as 'the great masquerader' of many diseases.

Diagnosis

Clinicians caring for the elderly must maintain a high index of suspicion for TB when possible, in order to recognize and treat infected individuals promptly.

Tuberculin skin testing

The Mantoux method of tuberculin skin testing using the Tween-stabilized purified protein derivative (PPD) antigen is one of the diagnostic modalities readily available to screen for TB infection, despite its potential for false-negative results.[20] In the elderly, because of the increase in anergy to cutaneous antigens, the two-step tuberculin test is suggested as part of the initial geriatric assessment to avoid overlooking potentially false-negative reaction.[21] The American Geriatrics Society routinely recommends two-step tuberculin testing as part of the baseline information for all institutionalized elderly.[22] The two-step tuberculin skin test involves initial intradermal placement of five tuberculin units of PPD and the results are read at 48–72 h. Patients are retested within 2 weeks after a negative response (induration of less than 10 mm). A positive 'booster effect', and therefore a positive tuberculin skin test reaction, is a skin test of 10 mm or more and an increase of 6 mm or more over the first skin test reaction. It is important to distinguish the booster phenomenon from a true tuberculin conversion. The booster effect occurs in a person previously infected with *Mtb* but who has a false-negative skin test; repeat skin test elicits a truly positive test. Conversion (not to be confused with the booster phenomenon) occurs in persons previously uninfected with *Mtb* and who have had a true negative tuberculin skin test, but who become infected within 2 years as demonstrated by a repeat skin test induration that is a positive 10 mm or more during this period. Several factors influence the results and interpretation of the PPD skin test. Decreased skin test reactivity is associated with waning DTH with time, disseminated TB, corticosteroids and other drugs and other diseases in addition to the elimination of TB infection. False-positive PPD results occur with cross-reactions with non-tuberculous mycobacteria and in persons receiving the Bacillus Calmette–Guérin (BCG) vaccine, the latter having been administered to some foreign-born elderly persons, which has an unpredictable effect on the PPD skin test reactivity and is presumed to wane after 10 years. The use of anergy testing has been debated because of lack of a standardized protocol for selection of the number and type of antigens to be used, the criteria for defining positive and negative reactions and administration and interpretation techniques.[23]

Interferon-gamma release assays

In 2005, the CDC published guidelines for using an interferon gamma release assay (IGRA) known as the QuantiFERON-TB Gold test (QFT-G) (Cellestis, Carnegie, Victoria, Australia).[24] Subsequently, two new IGRAs were approved by the US Food and Drug Administration (FDA) as aids in diagnosing both TB infection and disease. These tests are the QuantiFERON-TB Gold In-Tube test (QFT-GIT) (Cellestis) and the T-SPOT.TB test (T-Spot) (Oxford Immunotec, Abingdon, UK). The antigens, methods and interpretation criteria for these assays differ from those for IGRAs approved previously by the FDA. This *in vitro* test measures by an enzyme-linked immunosorbent assay (ELISA) the concentration of interferon-gamma (IFN-γ) released from tuberculin PPD sensitized lymphocytes in heparinized whole blood incubated for 16–24 h. Interpretation of QFT results is stratified by estimated risk for *Mtb* infection in a manner similar to the tuberculin skin test using different induration cut-off values.

Although data on the accuracy of IGRAs and their ability to predict subsequent active TB are limited, to date no major deficiencies have been reported in studies involving various populations.

The role for QFT in targeted testing has not yet been clearly defined and may be a useful alternative to tuberculin skin testing in the future for all infected individuals including the elderly.

Chest radiography

Chest radiography is indicated in all individuals with suspected TB infection, regardless of the primary site of infection. In the elderly, 75% of all TB disease occurs in the respiratory tract and largely represents reactivation disease; 10–20% of cases may be as a result of primary infection.[25] Although reactivation TB disease characteristically involves the apical and posterior segments of the upper lobes of the lungs, several studies have shown that many elderly patients manifest their pulmonary infection in either the middle or lower lobes or the pleura, and also present with interstitial, patchy or cavitary infiltrates that may be bilateral. Primary TB can involve any lung segment, but more often tends to involve the middle or lower lobes in addition to mediastinal or hilar lymph nodes. Therefore, caution must be exercised in dismissing the radiographic diagnosis of pulmonary TB in the elderly because of the atypical location of the infection in the lung fields.

Laboratory diagnosis

Sputum samples must be collected from all patients, regardless of age, with pulmonary symptoms or chest radiographic changes compatible with TB disease and who have not been previously treated with antituberculous agents. In elderly patients unable to expectorate sputum, other diagnostic techniques such as sputum induction or bronchoscopy should be considered. Flexible bronchoscopy to obtain bronchial washings and to perform bronchial biopsies has been shown to be of diagnostic value for TB disease in the elderly; however, in frail and very old patients, the risk of such a procedure must be carefully balanced against the benefits of potentially making a definite diagnosis of TB.[26] In the case of pulmonary and genitourinary TB, three consecutive early-morning sputum or urine specimens, respectively, are recommended for routine mycobacteriological studies. Sputum samples are examined initially by smear before and after concentration and then cultured for *Mtb*. Because routine mycobacterial culture methods may require up to 6 weeks for growth of *Mtb*, many laboratories now use radiometric procedures for the isolation and susceptibility testing of this organism; this method may identify the organisms as early as after 8 days. Sterile body fluids and tissues can be inoculated into liquid media, which also allow the growth and detection of *Mtb* 7–10 days earlier than in the solid media techniques. Histological examination of tissue from various sites such as the liver, lymph nodes, bone marrow, pleura or synovium may show the characteristic tissue reaction (caseous necrosis with granuloma formation) with or without AFB, which would also strongly support the diagnosis of TB disease. Other diagnostic methods for TB that have been clinically evaluated include serology and nucleic acid amplification (NAA) tests such as polymerase chain reaction (PCR) and other methods for amplifying DNA and RNA.[27] The latter may facilitate rapid detection of *Mtb* from respiratory specimens; the interpretation and use of the NAA test results has been updated by the CDC. Similar techniques using DNA probes can be used to track the spread of the organism in epidemiological studies and may be used to predict drug resistance prior to the availability of standard results; such methods are currently being used in some laboratories. The rapid diagnosis of TB is especially important in elderly patients, in addition to HIV-infected persons and patients with multidrug-resistant (MDR) TB.

Treatment

Treatment of TB disease

The recommended treatment regimens are for the most part based on evidence from clinical trials and are rated on the basis of a system developed by the United States Public Health Service (USPHS) and the Infectious Diseases Society of America (IDSA).[28] There are four recommended regimens for treating patients with TB caused by drug-susceptible organisms. Although these regimens are broadly applicable, there are modifications that should be made under specified circumstances, which are described subsequently. Each regimen has an initial phase of 2 months followed by a choice of several options for the continuation phase of either 4 or 7 months. The recommended treatment algorithm and regimens are shown in Figure 115.1 and Table 115.1, respectively.[28] Because of the relatively high proportion of adult patients with TB caused by organisms that are resistant to isoniazid (INH), four drugs are necessary in the initial phase for the 6 month regimen to be maximally effective. Thus, in most circumstances, the treatment regimen for all adults including the elderly with previously untreated TB should consist of a 2 month initial phase of INH, rifampin (RIF), pyrazinamide (PZA) and ethambutol (EMB). If (when) drug susceptibility test results are known and the organisms are fully susceptible, EMB need not be included. If PZA cannot be included in the initial phase of treatment or if the isolate is resistant to PZA alone (an unusual circumstance), the initial phase should consist of INH, RIF and EMB given daily for 2 months. However, since most TB in the elderly is due to reactivation (from infection acquired prior to 1950), the organism will generally be sensitive to INH and other antituberculous drugs.

Treatment of MDR-TB is complex and often needs to be individualized, requiring the addition of a minimum

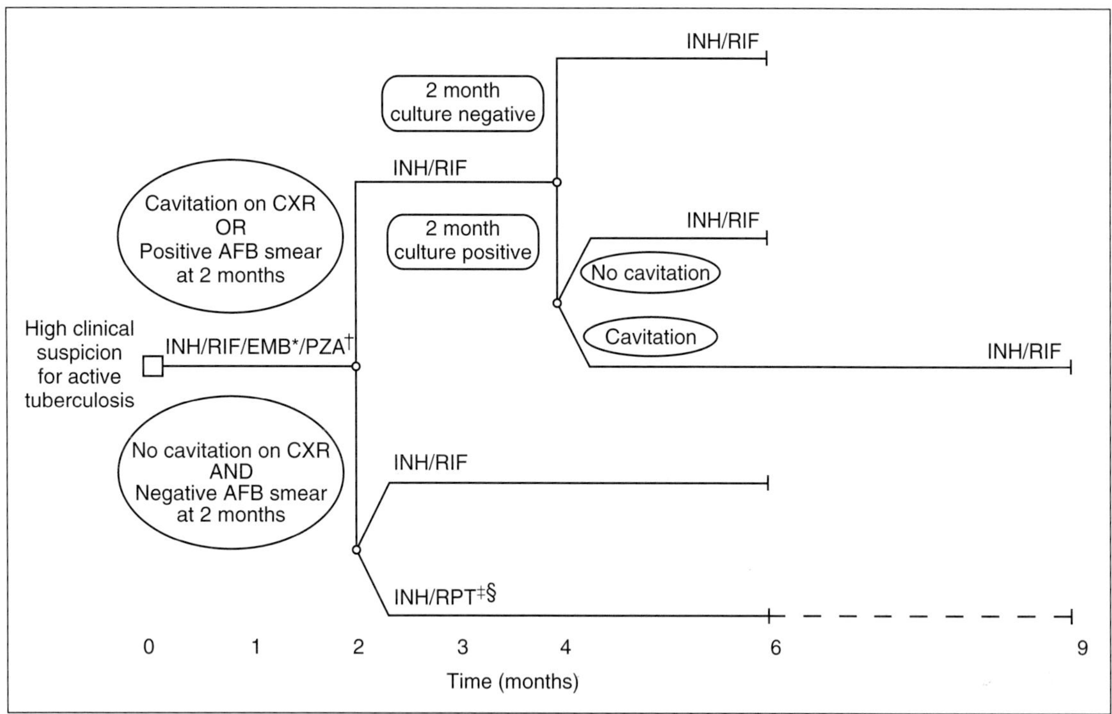

Figure 115.1 Treatment algorithm for tuberculosis. Patients in whom tuberculosis is proved or strongly suspected should have treatment initiated with isoniazid, rifampin, pyrazinamide and ethambutol for the initial 2 months. A repeat smear and culture should be performed when 2 months of treatment has been completed. If cavities were seen on the initial chest radiograph or the acid-fast smear is positive at completion of 2 months of treatment, the continuation phase of treatment should consist of isoniazid and rifampin daily or twice weekly for 4 months to complete a total of 6 months of treatment. If cavitation was present on the initial chest radiograph and the culture at the time of completion of 2 months of therapy is positive, the continuation phase should be lenghened to 7 months (total of 9 months of treatment). If the patient has HIV infection and the $CD4^+$ cell count is <100 per μl, the continuation phase should consist of daily or three times weekly isoniazid and rifampin. In HIV-uninfected patients having no cavitation on chest radiograph and negative acid-fast smears at completion of 2 months of treatment, the continuation phase may consist of either once weekly isonizaid and rifapertine, or daily or twice weekly isoniazid and rifampin, to complete a total of 6 months (bottom). Patients receiving isoniazid and rifapentine and whose 2 month cultures are positive, should have treatment extended by an additional 3 months (total of 9 months). EMB may be discontinued when results of drug susceptibility testing indicate no drug resistance. PZA may be discontinued after it has been taken for 2 months (56 doses). RPT should not be used in HIV-infected patients with tuberculosis or in patients with extrapulmonary tuberculosis. Therapy should be extended to 9 months if 2-month cultures is positive. CXR, chest radiiograph; EMP, ethambutol; INH, isoniazid; PZA, pyrazinamide; RIF, rifampin; RPT, rifapentine. (Source: Centers for Disease Control and Prevention, American Thoracic Society and Infectious Disease Society of America.[28])

of two additional antituberculous agents to which the organism is presumably susceptible, preferably in consultation with a TB expert who is familiar with *Mtb* drug resistance. Alternative drugs such as capreomycin, kanamycin, amikacin, ethionamide and cycloserine, and also the newer quinolones, may have to be used for treatment in such cases.

Monitoring of response to drug therapy

Patients with active pulmonary TB should be monitored on a monthly basis with sputum examination until conversion to negative by culture is achieved; this usually occurs within 3 months in 90% of cases. Continued positive sputum cultures for *Mtb* beyond 3 months of initiation of therapy should raise the suspicion for drug resistance or non-compliance (if not on DOT); such patients should have sputum culture and susceptibility repeated and started on DOT pending results of these data. Follow-up chest radiography is indicated 2–3 months after initiation of drug therapy. Older patients are at greater risk for hepatic toxicity from INH. Although INH therapy poses a small but significant risk for hepatitis, the hepatitis is relatively low in frequency and mild in severity. Therefore, presumably with careful monitoring of the older patient, antituberculous chemotherapy is a relatively safe intervention in this population. It is recommended that clinical assessments and also baseline liver function tests be performed before the administration of INH and RIF (and PZA) in older patients.

Table 115.1 Tuberculosis disease treatment regimens.[28]

Initial phase			Continuation phase				Rating[d] (evidence)[e]	
Regimen	Drugs[a]	Interval and doses[b] (minimal duration)	Regimen	Drugs[a]	Interval and doses[b,c] (minimal duration)	Range of total closes (minimal duration)	HIV⁻	HIV⁺
1	INH RIF PZA EMB	7 days per week for 56 doses (8 wk) or 5 days per week for 40 doses (8 wk)[f]	1a	INH/RIF	7 days per week for 126 doses (18 wk) or 5 days per week for 90 doses (18 wk)[f]	182–130 (26 wk)	A(I)	A(II)
			1b	INH/RIF	Twice weekly for 36 doses (18 wk)	92–76 (26 wk)	A(I)	A(II)[h]
			1c[g]	INH/RPT	Once weekly for 18 doses (18 wk)	74–58 (26 wk)	B(I)	E(I)
2	INH RIF PZA EMB	7 days per week for 14 doses (2 wk),[f] then twice weekly for 12 doses (6 wk) or 5 d/wk for 10 doses (2 wk),[f] then twice weekly for 12 doses (6 wk)	2a	INH/RIF	Twice weekly for 36 doses (18 wk)	62–58 (26 wk)	A(II)	B(II)[h]
			2b[g]	INH/RPT	Once weekly for 18 doses (18 wk)	44–40 (26 wk)	B(I)	E(I)
3	INH RIF PZA EMB	3 times weekly for 24 doses (8 wk)	3a	INH/RIF	3 times weekly for 54 doses (18 wk)	78 (26 wk)	B(I)	B(II)
4	INH RIF EMB	7 days per week for 56 doses (8 wk) or 5 d/wk for 40 doses (8 wk)[f]	4a	INH/RIF	7 days per week for 217 doses (31 wk) or 5 days per week for 155 doses (31 wk)[f]	273–195 (39 wk)	C(I)	C(II)
			4b	INH/RIF	Twice weekly for 62 doses (31 wk)	118–102 (39 wk)	C(I)	C(II)

[a]EMB, Bhambutol; INH, isoniazide; PZA, pyrazinnarnidel; RIF, rifampin; RPT, rifapentine.

[b]When DOT is used, drugs may be given 5 days per week and the necessary number of doses adjusted accordingly. Although there are no studies that compare five with seven daily doses, extensive experience indicates this would be and effective practice.

[c]Patients with cavitation on initial chest radiograph and positive cultures at completion of 2 months of therapy should receive a 7-month [31 week; either 217 doses (daily) or 62 doses (twice weekly)] continuation phase.

[d]Definitions of evidence ratings: A = preferred; B = acceptable alternative; C = offer when A and B cannot be give; E = should never be given.

[e]Definitions of evidence ratings: I = randomized clinical trial; II = data from clinical trials that were not randomized or were conducted in other populations; III = expert opinion.

[f]Five-day-a-week administration is always given by DOT. Rating for 5 days per week regimens is A III.

[g]Not recommended for HIV-infected patients with CD4 + cell counts <100 cells per μl.

[h]Options 1c and 2b should be used only in HIV-negative patients who have negative sputurn smears at the time of completion of 2 months of therapy and who do not have cavitation on initial chest radiograpah (see text). For patients started on this regiment and found to have a positive culture from the 2-month specimen, treatment should be extended and extra 3 months.

Monthly clinical evaluations and periodic measurements of the serum aminotransferase (SGOT) level should be performed in the elderly. If the SGOT rises to five times above normal or if the patient exhibits symptoms or signs of hepatitis, INH (and also other hepatotoxic drugs) should be discontinued. After clinical symptoms improve or the SGOT level normalizes, or both, INH may be resumed at a lower dose (e.g. 50 mg kg^{-1} per day) and gradually increased to a full dose if symptoms and the SGOT level remain stable. In case of relapse of the hepatitis with the INH challenge, the drug should be replaced with an alternative regimen. There is some disagreement among clinicians regarding the monitoring of liver function tests in older patients on INH. Because frail, elderly patients may often be asymptomatic in the presence of worsening hepatitis and may not be able to communicate symptoms, laboratory monitoring seems prudent. The frequency of such monitoring (e.g. monthly or every 2–3 months) remains less clear. RIF, in addition to hepatitis, is also associated with orange discoloration of body fluids.

EMB may cause loss of colour discrimination, diminished visual acuity and central scotomata; older patients receiving this drug should have frequent evaluation of visual acuity and colour discrimination. Streptomycin is associated with irreversible auditory and vestibular damage and generally should not be prescribed in the elderly. Adverse effects of PZA include hyperuricaemia, hepatitis and flushing. Dose adjustment of antituberculous drugs is necessary with streptomycin, when used in the presence of renal impairment; however, no adjustment is needed for INH, RIF or PZA in most elderly patients.

Treatment of latent TB infection

Table 115.2 outlines the revised criteria for positive tuberculin skin test reactivity by size of induration requiring drug treatment.[29] Drug therapy for latent TB (based on tuberculin skin test reactivity) considerably decreases the risk of progression of TB infection to TB disease. Since the LTBI treatment recommendations address adults in general, targeted skin testing and treatment of high-risk populations can be applied to the elderly. The INH daily regimen for 9 months has recently replaced the previously recommended 6 month schedule for treatment of LTBI. Randomized, prospective trials in HIV-negative persons have indicated that a 12 month regimen is more effective than 6 months of treatment; subgroup analyses of several trials indicate that the maximum beneficial effect of INH is likely.

In a community-based study conducted in Bethel, Alaska, persons who took <25% of the prescribed annual dose had a threefold higher risk for TB than those who took more than 50% of the annual dose. In addition, the efficacy decreased significantly if INH was taken for less than 9 months. In instances of known exposure to drug-resistant organisms, alternative preventive therapy regimens may be recommended.

Although these recommendations do not specifically address ageing adults, the concept of targeted skin testing and revised LTBI treatment guidelines for high-risk populations to include the elderly can be applied. Elderly persons receiving isoniazid should continue to be monitored for hepatitis and peripheral neuropathy induced by the drug.

Table 115.2 Skin test criteria for positive tuberculin reaction (mm induration).[29]

≥5 mm

1 HIV-positive persons
2 Recent contacts of person(s) with infectious tuberculosis
3 Persons with chest radiographs consistent with tuberculosis (e.g. fibrotic changes)
4 Patients with organ transplants and other immunosuppressed hosts receiving the equivalent of >15 mg per day of prednisone for >1 month

≥10 mm

1 Recent arrivals (<5 years) from high-prevalence countries
2 Injection-drug users
3 Residents and employees of high-risk congregate settings: prisons, jails, nursing homes, other healthcare facilities, residential facilities for AIDS patients and homeless shelters
4 Mycobacteriology laboratory personnel
5 High-risk clinical conditions: silicosis; gastrectomy; jejunoileal bypass; ≥10% below ideal body weight; chronic renal failure; diabetes mellitus; haematological malignancies (e.g. lymphomas, leukaemias); other specific malignancies (carcinoma of the head or neck and lung) (alcoholics are also considered high risk)

≥15 mm

1 Persons with no risk factors for TB

Infection control issues

The primary goal of an infection control programme is to detect TB disease early and to isolate and treat persons with infectious TB promptly. Prevention of transmission of TB in any healthcare environment is of the utmost importance, for both patients and healthcare workers. Enhanced awareness of drug-resistant TB has prompted public health agencies to institute strict TB identification, isolation, treatment and prevention guidelines. The TB infection control programme in most acute care and long-term care facilities should consist of three types of control measures: administrative actions (i.e. prompt detection of suspected cases, isolation of infectious patients and rapid institution of appropriate treatment), engineering control [negative-pressure ventilation rooms, high-efficiency particulate air (HEPA) filtration and ultraviolet germicidal irradiation (UVGI)] and personal respiratory protection requirements (masks). The Advisory Committee for the Elimination of Tuberculosis of the CDC has established recommendations for surveillance, containment, assessment and reporting of TB infection and disease in long-term care facilities; healthcare professionals, administrators and staff of such extended care programmes should be made aware of these recommendations.[30]

Key points

- Tuberculosis (TB) remains one of the world's most lethal infectious diseases.
- Preventive and control strategies among other high-risk groups such as the elderly remain a challenge.
- Clinical features of TB in older adults may be atypical and confused with age-related diseases.
- Underlying diseases, malnutrition and biological changes with ageing can contribute to age-associated decline in cellular immune responses to infecting agents such as *Mycobacterium tuberculosis*.
- Diagnosis and management of TB in the elderly may be difficult; treatment can be associated with adverse drug reactions.
- The institutionalized elderly are at high risk both for reactivation of latent TB and to new TB infection.

References

1. World Health Organization. *Global Tuberculosis Control: a Short Update to the 2009 Report*, 2009, http://whqlibdoc.who.int/publications/2009/9789241598866_eng.pdf (last accessed 14 October 2010).
2. Institute of Medicine; Geiter L (ed.). *Ending Neglect: the Elimination of Tuberculosis in the United States*, National Academies Press, Washington, DC, 2000.
3. Rajagopalan S. Tuberculosis and aging: a global health problem. *Clin Infect Dis* 2001;**33**:1034–9.
4. Centers for Disease Control and Prevention. Progress toward tuberculosis elimination in low-incidence areas of the United States: recommendations of the Advisory Council for the Elimination of Tuberculosis. *MMWR Morb Mortal Wkly Rep* 2002;**51**:1–16.
5. Centers for Disease Control and Prevention. Decrease in reported tuberculosis cases – United States, 2009. *MMWR Morb Mortal Wkly Rep* 2010;**59**:289–94.
6. Reichman LB and O'Day R. Tuberculosis infection in a large urban population. *Am Rev Respir Dis* 1978;**117**:705–12.
7. Narain J, Lofgren J, Warren E *et al*. Epidemic tuberculosis in a nursing home: a retrospective cohort study. *J Am Geriatr Soc* 1985;**33**:258–63.
8. Schultz M, Hernandez JM, Hernandez NE *et al*. Onset to tuberculosis disease: new converters in long-term care settings. *Am J Alzheimers Dis Other Demen* 2001;**16**:313–8.
9. Hutton MD, Cauthen GM and Bloch AB. Results of a 29-state survey of tuberculosis in nursing homes and correctional facilities. *Public Health Rep* 1993;**108**:305–14.
10. Ijaz K, Dillara JA, Yang Z *et al*. Unrecognized tuberculosis in a nursing home causing death with spread of tuberculosis to the community. *J Am Geriatr Soc* 2002;**50**:1213–7.
11. Rajagopalan S and Yoshikawa TT. Tuberculosis in long-term care facilities. *Infect Control Hosp Epidemiol* 2000;**21**:611–5.
12. Adler JJ and Rose DM. Transmission and pathogenesis of tuberculosis. In: WN Rom and SM Garay (eds), *Tuberculosis*, 1st edn, Little, Brown, New York, 1996.
13. Perez-Guzman C, Vargas MH, Torres-Cruz A *et al*. Does aging modify pulmonary tuberculosis? A meta-analytical review. *Chest* 1999;**116**:961–7.
14. Yoshikawa TT Tuberculosis in aging adults. *J Am Geriatr Soc* 1992;**40**: 178.
15. Mert A, Bilir M and Tabak F. Miliary tuberculosis: clinical manifestations, diagnosis and outcome in 38 adults. *Respirology* 2001;**6**:217–24.
16. Kalita J and Misra UK. Tuberculous meningitis with pulmonary miliary tuberculosis:a clinicoradiological study. *Neurol India* 2004;**52**:194–6.
17. Shah AH, Joshi SV and Dhar HL. Tuberculosis of bones and joints. *Antiseptic* 2001;**98**:385–7.
18. Malaviya A. Arthritis associated with tuberculosis. *Best Pract Res Clin Rheumatol* 2003;**17**:319–43.
19. Lenk S and Schroeder J Genitourinary tuberculosis. *Curr Opin Urol* 2001;**11**:93–8.
20. Markowitz N, Hansen NI, Wilcosky TC *et al*. Tuberculin and anergy testing in HIV-seropositive and HIV-seronegative persons. *Ann Intern Med* 1993;**119**:185–93.
21. Tort J, Pina JM, Martin-Ramos A *et al*. Booster effect in elderly patients living in geriatric institutions. *Med Clin (Barcelona)* 1995;**105**:41–4.
22. American Geriatrics Society. *Two-Step PPD Testing for Nursing Home Patients on Admission*, 1993, www.info.amger@americangeriatrics.org.
23. Slovis BS, Plitman JD and Haas DW. The case against anergy testing as a routine adjunct to tuberculin skin testing. *JAMA* 2000;**283**:2003–7.

24. Mazurek GH, Jereb J, Vernon A *et al.*; IGRA Expert Committee, Centers for Disease Control and Prevention. Updated guidelines for using interferon gamma release assays to detect *Mycobacterium tuberculosis* infection – United States, 2010. *MMWR Recomm Rep* 2010;**54**(RR-15): 49–55.

25. Woodring JH, Vandiviere HM, Fried AM *et al.* Update: the radiographic features of pulmonary tuberculosis. *AJR Am J Roentgenol* 1986;**146**:497–506.

26. Patel YR, Mehta JB, Harvill L and Gatekey K. Flexible bronchoscopy as a diagnostic tool in the evaluation of pulmonary tuberculosis in an elderly population. *J Am Geriatr Soc* 1993;**41**:629–32.

27. Centers for Disease Control and Prevention. Nucleic acid amplification tests for tuberculosis. *MMWR Morb Mortal Wkly Rep* 2000;**49**:593–4.

28. Centers for Disease Control and Prevention, American Thoracic Society and Infectious Disease Society of America. Treatment of tuberculosis. *MMWR Recomm Rep Report;* 2003;**52**(RR-11): 1–77.

29. American Thoracic Society. Targeted skin testing and treatment of latent tuberculosis infection. *Am J Respir Crit Care Med* 2000;**161**: S221–47.

30. Centers for Disease Control and Prevention. Control of tuberculosis in facilities providing long-term care to the elderly: recommendations of the Advisory Committee for the Elimination of Tuberculosis. *MMWR Recomm Rep* 1990;**39**(RR-10): 7–20.

CHAPTER 116

Valvular heart disease and infective endocarditis

Aneil Malhotra*, Sam Dawkins* and Bernard D. Prendergast
John Radcliffe Hospital, Oxford, UK
*Joint first authors

Introduction

Valvular heart disease (VHD) is an increasingly common and important problem despite the decline of rheumatic fever. One of the principal reasons is the relative and absolute ongoing increase in the elderly population, such that the increased requirements for care of degenerative valve disease now outweigh the decreasing burden of rheumatic heart disease.

The widespread availability of echocardiography has revolutionized investigation by providing accurate and non-invasive assessment of severity and a means of monitoring disease progression, while also allowing progress in the application of interventional techniques and reconstructive valve surgery. The indications for valve replacement surgery have been broadened by improvements in prosthetic valve design and reduced perioperative mortality while the advent of transcatheter aortic valve implantation (TAVI) and percutaneous mitral valve repair offer a less invasive alternative for elderly patients whose frailty and comorbidity may preclude conventional surgery.

Epidemiology and pathophysiology

VHD was historically caused by rheumatic fever and this remains a major burden in developing countries. However, industrialized countries face a different type of problem: as rheumatic disease has fallen substantially due to improved living conditions and the introduction of penicillin for streptococcal pharyngitis in the 1940s, degenerative VHD is increasingly common.

With an ever-increasing elderly population over the past half century and the increasing availability of diagnostic tools such as echocardiography, the requirements for care of degenerative valve disease now outweigh the decreasing burden of rheumatic heart disease.

Prevalence of valvular heart disease in an ageing population

The prevalence data for VHD in the elderly are derived mainly from European and North American studies. In 2006, Nkomo *et al.*[1] collated the results of several large population-based studies (total >28 000 adults) to assess the overall prevalence of VHD and its effect on overall survival in the general population of the USA. The prevalence of VHD increased with age, rising from 0.7% in those aged 18–44 years to 13% in those over 75 years of age (Figure 116.1). The most common valve lesion was mitral regurgitation, followed closely by aortic stenosis, whilst mitral stenosis was very uncommon in this population. There was equal gender preponderance. The presence of VHD also had a statistically significant impact on survival, emphasizing its significance as a healthcare issue.

There is also a demonstrable association between the prevalence of VHD and increasing age. In the developed world, low birth rates and increasing life expectancy have inverted the age pyramid. All adult age groups below 65 years will begin to diminish in size throughout most of Europe beyond 2030. In contrast, those aged over 65 years are expected to grow to 107 million by 2025 and 133 million by 2050, with a 180% (19 million to 51 million) increase in those over 80 years of age between 2005 and 2050. Based on a prevalence of VHD of 13% in the over-75 age group, this will result in over 6.5 million new cases of moderate to severe VHD in Europe by 2050.

In the UK, approximately 1 million individuals over 65 years of age are thought to be affected by VHD. This will inevitably increase rapidly as the UK population aged >75 years is projected to rise by ~50% by 2025. In turn, the impact on healthcare resources is likely to grow substantially.

Principles and Practice of Geriatric Medicine, Fifth Edition. Edited by Alan J. Sinclair, John E. Morley and Bruno Vellas.

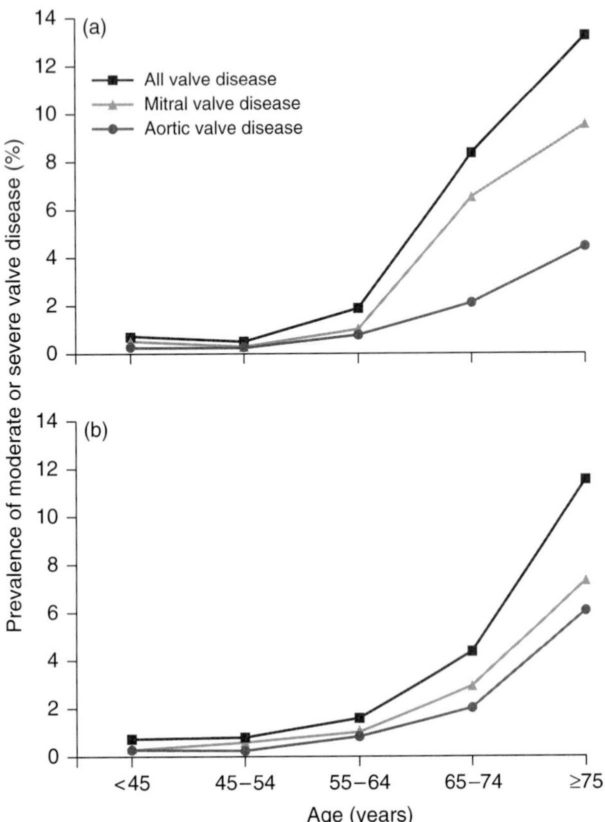

Figure 116.1 The rising prevalence of valvular heart disease according to age. Frequency in (a) population-based studies and (a) the Olmsted County community.[1]

Aetiology of valvular heart disease

The aetiology and management of VHD were assessed across Europe in 2001 in the European Society of Cardiology Euro Heart Survey on Valvular Heart Disease. Prospective data were collected on 5000 patients with significant primary VHD (according to specific criteria) or infective endocarditis, in both in- and outpatient settings across cardiology and cardiothoracic departments in Europe.

In this hospital setting, the most common native left-sided valve lesion was aortic stenosis (43%), followed by mitral regurgitation (32%), aortic regurgitation (13%) and mitral stenosis (12%). The dominant aetiology of aortic stenosis, aortic regurgitation and mitral regurgitation was degenerative, while mitral stenosis resulted from rheumatic disease in 85%. Valvular regurgitation was caused by a wider range of aetiologies than stenosis, with endocarditis and congenital abnormalities featuring prominently in aortic regurgitation and ischaemia an important cause of mitral regurgitation.

Aortic stenosis

Detection of aortic stenosis in the elderly has increased with improved diagnostic tools. Echocardiography has revealed mild calcification of the aortic valve in up to 40% of those aged 60 years or over and 75% of those aged over 85 years. The overall prevalence of clinically significant aortic stenosis in those older than 70 years has become more frequent and is ~1–3%. Recent evidence suggests variation in the left ventricular response to aortic stenosis according to gender: whereas elderly males tend to undergo ventricular dilatation with systolic impairment, females have small, hypertrophied ventricles with preserved contractile function.

Overall, the most common cause of aortic stenosis is a congenitally bicuspid aortic valve, accounting for over 40% of UK cases (Figure 116.2a). Rheumatic aortic stenosis is now much rarer. Bicuspid valves occur in 0.5–2.5% of the general population and are more common in males. Significant stenosis, caused by progressive calcification (Figure 116.2b and 116.2c), develops in up to one-third of affected individuals, often before the age of 70 years.

Aortic sclerosis (thickening of the aortic valve without obstruction) is present in 25% of patients over 65 years of age and is associated with age, hypertension, smoking, male gender, low-density lipoprotein levels and diabetes mellitus. Nearly 9% of these patients progress to aortic stenosis over a 5 year period.

Senile degeneration of an anatomically normal aortic valve is increasingly important in the ageing population. The degeneration is related to repeated minor trauma to the valve cusps leading to fibrosis and deposition of calcium, with consequent immobility and stenosis. These changes are unusual before the age of 70 years but the incidence increases rapidly thereafter.

Aortic stenosis is the result of impaired mobility of the valve cusps, leading to reduced systolic excursion and open valve area (normally 3–4 cm^2). The consequence is an increase in left ventricular systolic pressure and a pressure gradient across the valve between the ventricle and aorta. The ventricle subsequently attempts to accommodate this pressure increase through hypertrophy that in turn leads to falling compliance of the left ventricle. Symptoms of exertional breathlessness, angina and syncope eventually result. Most patients develop these symptoms before a reduction in ejection fraction, but some present with poor ventricular function and overt heart failure.

Aortic regurgitation

Aortic regurgitation is less common than aortic stenosis with a prevalence of <1% in the elderly population. The

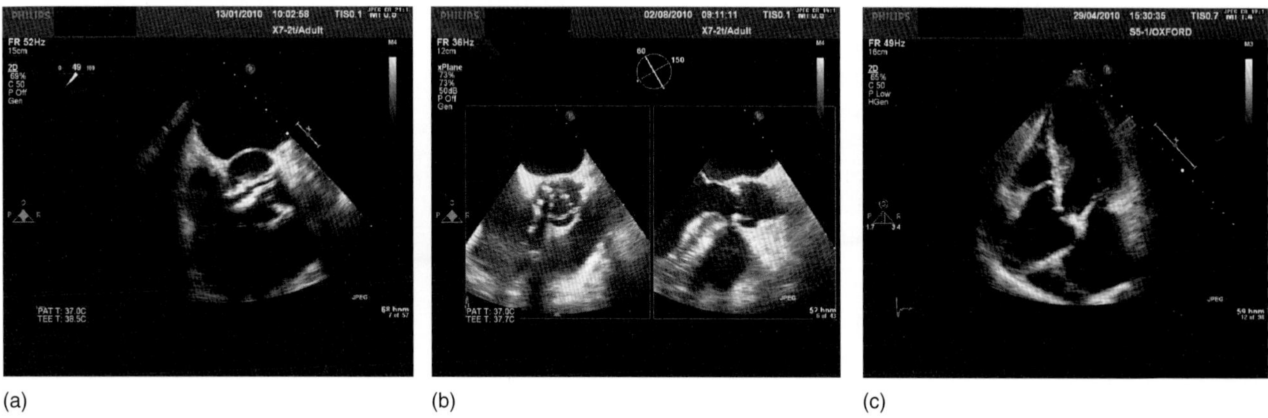

(a) (b) (c)

Figure 116.2 (a) Transoesophageal echocardiogram (TOE) demonstrating severe aortic stenosis in a bicuspid valve with left ventricular dilatation. (b, c) TOE demonstrating a severely calcified tricuspid aortic valve.

usual aetiology is aortic root dilatation, which appears to occur as part of normal ageing and is more frequent in hypertensive patients. Of the valvular causes, bileaflet valves comprise ~60% of cases, infective endocarditis 20% and rheumatic heart disease <10%. Rarer causes include inflammatory aortitis (associated with rheumatoid arthritis, ankylosing spondylitis, giant-cell arteritis and syphilis), aortic root aneurysm and 'silent' chronic dissection. Acute aortic regurgitation is less common and is usually due to infective endocarditis, but may occasionally arise as a result of aortic dissection, dehiscence of a valve prosthesis or trauma.

Aortic regurgitation is caused by inability of the valve cusps to coapt during the diastolic phase of the cardiac cycle. This may be due to an abnormality of the aortic root or a problem with the valve itself that disrupts valve closure. As a result, a proportion of left ventricular stroke volume (>50% in severe cases) leaks back through the aortic valve in diastole, inducing a compensatory response of ventricular hypertrophy to maintain efficient ventricular function. This compensatory response eventually becomes inadequate, resulting in progressive ventricular dilatation and the onset of exertional breathlessness.

Mitral stenosis

The falling incidence of mitral stenosis parallels that of acute rheumatic fever. Rheumatic scarring and inflammation of the valve and subvalvular tissues eventually lead to progressive fibrosis, calcification and stenosis, which usually becomes haemodynamically significant in the fourth and fifth decades.

The major cause of mitral stenosis worldwide is rheumatic fever, usually developing within a few years of acquiring the disease. In contrast, congenital abnormalities of the valve make up a larger proportion of cases in industrialized nations. The stenotic valve is the result of fusion, thickening and reduced mobility of the mitral leaflets and chordae tendinae. Valve area decreases from the normal of around 4 cm^2 to less than 1 cm^2, producing a diastolic gradient between the left atrium and left ventricle, raised left atrial pressure (and consequent enlargement), secondary pulmonary hypertension and right heart failure. The primary symptom is breathlessness on exertion.

Mitral regurgitation

The most common cause of mitral regurgitation in the elderly UK population is myxomatous degeneration. The prevalence appears to be ~2% with a 5:1 male preponderance and an even age distribution. It mainly affects the posterior mitral valve leaflet to cause chordal stretching (and ultimately rupture).

Mitral regurgitation is also a common accompaniment to ischaemic heart disease as a result of ventricular dilatation and papillary muscle dysfunction; ~50% of patients have some degree of mitral regurgitation 1 month after suffering a myocardial infarction. Acute papillary muscle rupture may complicate myocardial infarction to cause acute mitral regurgitation, which may also result from infective endocarditis or dehiscence of a prosthetic valve.

Mitral annular calcification is a common echocardiographic finding which occurs more often in women and affects 8.5–10% of the population above the age of 50 years (although affected individuals are usually much older). In one-third there is associated mitral regurgitation, but this is usually mild and asymptomatic; accompanying mitral stenosis is rare. Other complications are unusual, although there is an associated t2–3-fold increase in the incidence of embolic stroke. Mitral valve prolapse is also frequently detected by echocardiography, although diagnostic criteria vary. Its clinical relevance is often uncertain although in some cases it may be the antecedent of a 'floppy valve' where the chordae are grossly elongated, the valve voluminous and mitral regurgitation more significant.

Pulmonary/tricuspid valve disease

The elderly population rarely presents with primary disease of these valves and there are no meaningful epidemiological data available. Pulmonary hypertension associated with mitral valve disease can cause regurgitation of either or both right heart valves. Tricuspid stenosis may be associated with rheumatic mitral and aortic valve disease and is occasionally seen as a feature of carcinoid syndrome.

History and clinical assessment

Despite technological advances in the investigation and management of cardiovascular disease, an accurate history and careful clinical assessment remain the most important part of diagnosis and management in the elderly. Questioning may be more difficult and it is often necessary to enlist the help of a relative or other carer. This history should seek a background or rheumatic fever, ischaemic heart disease or hypertension and incorporate specific enquiry for symptoms of dyspnoea (either on exertion or at rest, particularly when lying flat) and exertional angina or syncope. However, symptoms in the elderly are often vague and difficult to interpret, particularly if there is concomitant pulmonary or cerebral disease.

The principles of examination are the same as those for any other age group and the weight of the patient and a dental inspection should be routinely included. However, in elderly patients many of the classical manifestations of VHD may be attenuated by the effects of ageing on the cardiovascular system, namely atherosclerosis, hypertension and valve calcification. Thus, for example, a pulse of normal character or the presence of systemic hypertension do not exclude significant aortic stenosis in the elderly. Conversely, a wide pulse pressure is not necessarily indicative of aortic regurgitation. Inspection of the jugular venous pressure is of particular importance as dependent oedema secondary to chronic venous insufficiency is common and may erroneously suggest circulatory overload. Systolic murmurs are common in the elderly and have been reported in up to 60% of normal subjects. They are frequently due to increasing rigidity and calcification of the aortic cusps without significant obstruction or mild mitral regurgitation through a floppy valve. Diastolic murmurs are always abnormal and usually indicate aortic regurgitation or mitral stenosis, although the customary accompanying opening snap in mitral stenosis may be absent in the elderly due to valve calcification.

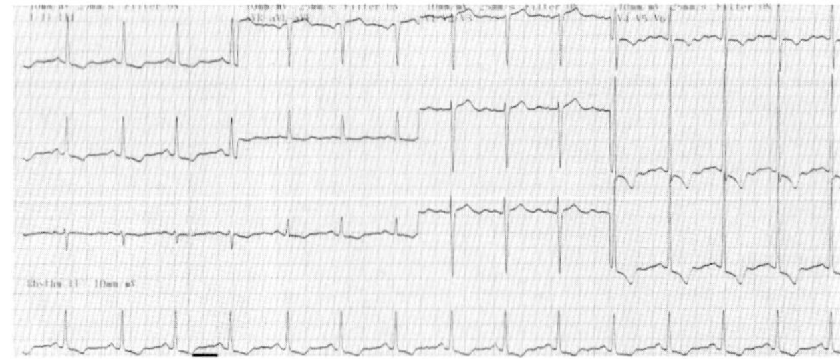

Figure 116.3 ECG demonstrating left ventricular hypertrophy: increased amplitude of the QRS complex, ST-segment depression and T-wave inversion in the lateral and inferior leads.

Investigations

Electrocardiogram (ECG)

This provides important information regarding heart rate and rhythm. The ECG has low sensitivity for the detection of atrial or ventricular hypertrophy and therefore assessment of the severity of valve lesions from the ECG should be cautious (Figure 116.3). Similarly, ST/T wave changes may result from left ventricular hypertrophy or the use of digoxin and do not necessarily indicate the presence of coexisting coronary artery disease.

Chest X-ray

A chest X-ray is useful for the assessment of heart size, the identification of specific chamber enlargement (particularly the left atrium) or aortic dilatation and for detection of pulmonary vascular changes or oedema (Figure 116.4). It can also assist in localizing valve calcification and prosthetic valves, particularly if a lateral radiograph is requested. Finally, the detection of coincident pulmonary disease may be of considerable clinical importance in some cases, especially if invasive investigation is being considered. The cardiothoracic ratio may increase to 60% as part of normal ageing, particularly beyond 75 years, caused by a small increase in cardiac diameter and a larger fall in chest diameter. Hence the use of absolute dimensions may be more appropriate in this age group: a transverse cardiac diameter >15 cm usually indicates significant enlargement.

Echocardiography

This is now the technique of choice for the diagnosis and evaluation of VHD and has negated the need for routine cardiac catheterization in many patients. It provides information regarding valve anatomy and physiology in addition to the effect of valve abnormality on cardiac function and allows serial observation of the patient over time.

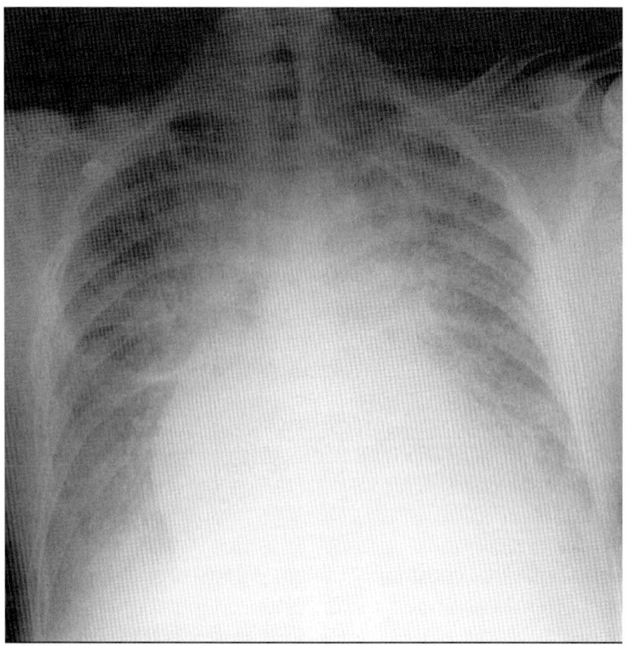

Figure 116.4 Chest X-ray demonstrating pulmonary oedema: cardiomegaly, alveolar shadowing, upper lobe diversion and blunting of the costophrenic angles.

Interpretation can be difficult and requires experience, particularly in the Doppler assessment of valve stenosis when poor signal alignment may lead to underestimation of the peak velocity. Furthermore, it is a sensitive tool and 'physiological' regurgitation is often detected in normal subjects.

There are three principal modalities: M (or motion)-mode, two-dimensional (or cross-sectional) and Doppler echocardiography. M-mode employs a single stationary beam of ultrasound to produce a recording of motion along a single line through the heart and provides a large amount of accurate information allowing the determination of cavity dimensions and wall thickness and physiological measurements of wall motion. Two-dimensional echocardiography images a plane through the heart by sweeping a beam of ultrasound though the sector of interest and is the modality of choice for displaying anatomy (Figure 116.5). Standardized precordial views are employed and a further subcostal view may be invaluable in elderly patients, in whom obesity, lung disease, chest wall deformities or kyphoscoliosis may preclude conventional imaging. Doppler echocardiography permits accurate assessment of the position, direction and velocity of the blood flow within the heart. This information can be anatomically correlated by superimposing a colour flow Doppler map onto the two-dimensional image. Three-dimensional imaging is under development and allows reconstruction of cardiac anatomy, which may be of particular value when percutaneous intervention or surgery is being considered.

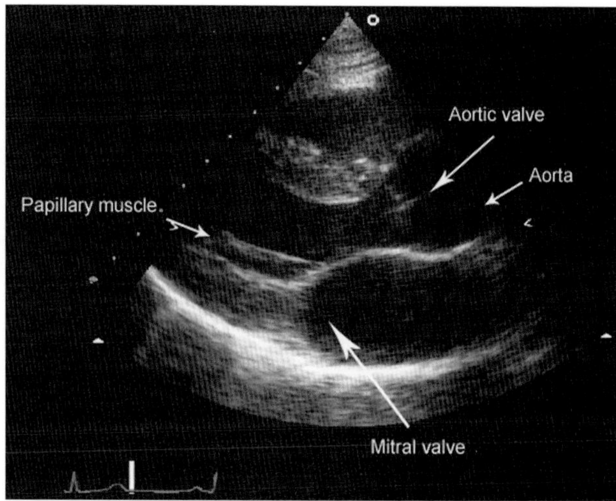

Figure 116.5 Parasternal long-axis TTE demonstrating the left ventricular cavity and mitral and aortic valves.

Transoesophageal echocardiography is a specialized technique which provides excellent image quality in almost every patient. The procedure is tolerated well by the elderly and may be performed on an outpatient basis, usually under light sedation. It has specific indications in the assessment and management of VHD and is highly sensitive in the detection of thrombus, vegetations and abscesses which may not be apparent on precordial imaging.

Cardiac catheterization

The increasing sophistication of echocardiography means that invasive investigations are unnecessary in many patients. Nevertheless, specific questions may remain, most commonly the presence or absence of coronary artery disease in patients being considered for valve surgery. The mortality of the procedure is 0.1–0.2% and other complications (cardiac or vascular trauma, embolism, arrhythmias or contrast reactions) occur in ~1% of cases. Patients at higher risk include the elderly and those with poor left ventricular function, severe aortic stenosis, pulmonary hypertension or peripheral vascular disease. As much information as possible should be obtained using non-invasive techniques to ensure that any invasive investigation is not unnecessarily prolonged. Furthermore, in the emergency setting, coronary angiography should not delay a potentially life-saving operation, such as emergency aortic valve replacement. In these situations, the investigations required should be decided by consultation between the physician and the surgeon and, if necessary, performed on the way to the operating theatre.

Cardiac magnetic resonance

Cardiac magnetic resonance (CMR) is becoming more frequently used in the assessment of VHD. It provides

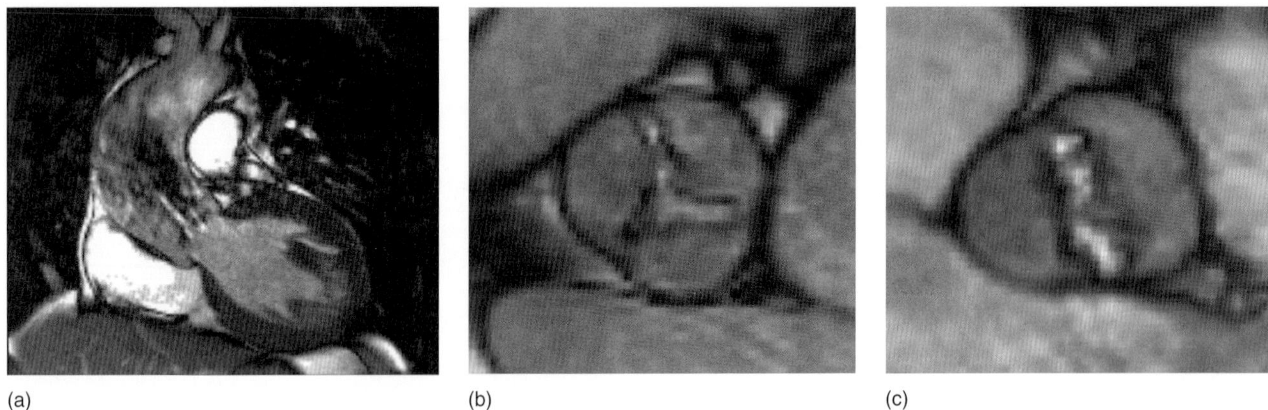

Figure 116.6 Cardiac magnetic resonance imaging in aortic stenosis. (a) A narrow high-velocity jet in the left ventricular outflow tract; (b) 'en-face' view of a stenosed trileaflet aortic valve; (c) 'en-face' view of a stenosed bicuspid aortic valve.

quantitative and reproducible measures of both stenosis and regurgitation, and also accurate measurement of the volume and function of both ventricles (Figure 116.6). A unique feature of CMR is the ability to measure flow through an image slice, with good agreement between invasive measurements and *in vitro* testing, allowing the quantification of regurgitation rather than a qualitative assessment of severity. The aortic root and ascending aorta are also accurately assessed and are important aspects in aortic valve disease. CMR can thus provide a comprehensive and accurate evaluation of the severity of VHD and the consequences for the ventricles. Detailed information on valve leaflet anatomy is less well assessed, however, and transoesophageal echocardiography provides higher resolution imaging.

Measurement of forward and reverse flow across the aortic or pulmonary valves allows the quantification of aortic/pulmonary regurgitation, providing both regurgitant volume and fraction. The high mobility of the mitral and tricuspid valves and turbulent flow across them makes direct flow measurement difficult. In valve stenosis, valve area can be assessed by direct planimetry rather than by calculation and usually provides a better assessment of severity with CMR than velocity across the valve – velocity measurements lack the spatial and temporal resolution of Doppler echocardiography and may underestimate valve severity. Left ventricular mass can also be measured accurately, in addition to volumes and function.

At present, the limited availability of CMR restricts its use in VHD and it has a relatively high cost compared with echocardiography. Acquisition and analysis times are also longer, making it less attractive for outpatient use, although developments in scanners and software technology are likely. Arrhythmias (e.g. atrial fibrillation) may impair image quality and affect the accuracy of flow measurements, although newer imaging sequences can cope with this common problem. Claustrophobic patients can often be scanned by experienced personnel, though about 1–2% of patients may find this too difficult. CMR remains mostly contraindicated in the presence of certain ferromagnetic implants, including cerebral aneurysm clips and cardiac pacemakers/defibrillators. However, prosthetic (including metallic) valves and coronary stents are almost never a problem.

Cardiac computed tomography

Although cardiac computed tomography (CT) is increasingly used in the context of coronary artery disease, its use in VHD is limited. It can provide morphological information on the valves and their associated structures (particularly calcification) and also volume and mass measurements. However, it does not provide haemodynamic information, is sensitive to arrhythmias and requires a slow heart rate (often necessitating beta-blockade or other rate-slowing medication). CT also involves ionizing radiation, although newer scanners utilize techniques to reduce the dose significantly. A major future advantage of CT may be the non-invasive exclusion of coronary artery disease prior to valve surgery.

Aortic stenosis

Symptoms and signs

The normal aortic valve area is 3–4 cm^2 and symptoms of haemodynamic origin, namely syncope, angina and dyspnoea, usually develop when this falls to 1–1.5 cm^2. The onset of symptoms heralds a poor prognosis (Figure 116.7) with a 1 year mortality of 43%. In the elderly, coexisting cerebral or coronary artery disease may make interpretation difficult. Furthermore, many patients with severe aortic stenosis may be asymptomatic and the diagnosis is easily overlooked.

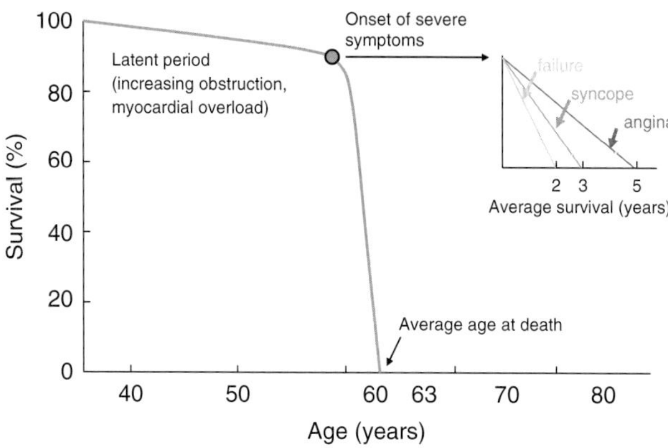

Figure 116.7 The natural history of aortic stenosis demonstrating a long asymptomatic preclinical phase followed by rapid decline associated with poor prognosis following the onset of symptoms.

Syncope, usually associated with exercise, becomes increasingly likely as disease progresses and is associated with an increased incidence of sudden death. The underlying mechanism is probably related to inappropriate vasodilatation secondary to abnormal baroreceptor sensitivity stimulated by elevated left ventricular pressure. In the presence of outflow obstruction, the compensatory increase in cardiac output is limited and cerebral hypoperfusion results.

Angina occurs in two-thirds of patients with aortic stenosis. Contributing factors include myocardial hypertrophy, prolonged systole and high left ventricular pressure, and these are compounded if there is coexisting coronary artery disease. The incidence of associated coronary artery disease increases with age and the need for concomitant coronary artery bypass grafting at the time of aortic valve replacement rises from 20% at 70 years to more than 60% at ages >80 years.

The onset of dyspnoea indicates significant left ventricular impairment. This is associated with a very poor prognosis and is an indication for urgent surgical intervention.

The classical peripheral manifestations of aortic stenosis (a plateau pulse and narrow pulse pressure) are often absent in elderly patients because the pulse waveform is distorted by stiff, atherosclerotic vessels. A normal or elevated blood pressure does not exclude the diagnosis. In many cases, the only physical sign is the presence of a mid systolic murmur which is usually squeaking or musical in character, loudest at the base of the heart, and typically radiates into the neck. In practice, the intensity of the murmur is a poor guide to the severity of the stenosis and in elderly patients its position is often atypical (frequently maximal at the apex). There may be an accompanying thrill and the apex beat is forceful and sustained. The first heart sound is usually normal and an ejection click (associated with a mobile valve) is uncommon in older patients. The aortic component of the second sound may be diminished (or absent) and delayed because of reduced valve mobility and the prolonged ejection time.

The finding of a systolic murmur in conjunction with any of the above symptoms should not be dismissed without further assessment. Given the high prevalence of aortic valve disease in the elderly, the poor prognosis of symptomatic aortic stenosis, the benefits of valve replacement and the difficulty of making precise clinical diagnosis, such patients require echocardiography.

Investigations

The ECG and chest X-ray

A normal ECG and chest X-ray do not exclude the diagnosis. The ECG usually shows left ventricular hypertrophy with repolarization changes; anteroseptal Q waves, occurring most often when there is left-axis deviation, are not unusual and may be mistakenly ascribed to a previous myocardial infarction. Occasionally, conducting tissue calcification can cause atrioventricular or bundle branch block. In the elderly, calcification of the stenosed aortic valve is invariably present on the chest X-ray, particularly in the lateral view. There may be post-stenotic aortic dilatation and cardiac enlargement and pulmonary oedema develop in the late stages.

Echocardiography

Two-dimensional and Doppler echocardiography are the techniques of choice for the assessment of suspected aortic stenosis. Aortic valve thickening and calcification are common in the elderly and associated restriction of cusp mobility is required to confirm the diagnosis. In practice, heavy calcification often obscures visualization of the valve structure and disease severity can only be determined by continuous-wave Doppler echocardiography. Echocardiography also provides the most convenient assessment of ventricular hypertrophy, size and function.

The velocity (V) of blood flow across the valve can be measured by continuous-wave Doppler echocardiography and, using the modified Bernoulli equation, the *peak instantaneous* pressure gradient can be derived (gradient $= 4V^2$). Generally, there is an excellent correlation between the gradients measured using invasive and non-invasive techniques although the *peak-to-peak instantaneous* gradient is usually higher than the *peak-to-peak* gradient measured at cardiac catheterization. A Doppler gradient >70–80 mmHg (equivalent to a catheter gradient of 50 mmHg) indicates significant aortic stenosis (Figure 116.8).

However, the gradient produced by any degree of valve obstruction is smaller if cardiac output falls due to declining left ventricular function. Conversely, the severity of aortic stenosis will be overestimated in the presence of any

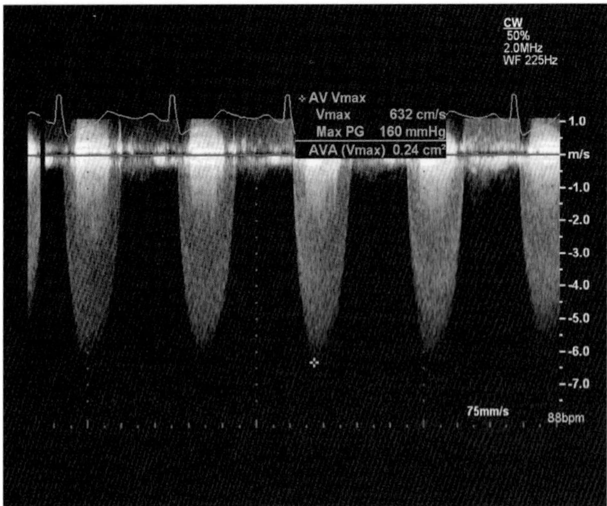

Figure 116.8 Continuous-wave Doppler echocardiography in severe aortic stenosis – the peak velocity is nearly 6 m s^{-1} (equivalent to a trans-valve pressure gradient of ~140 mmHg).

associated aortic regurgitation when the peak velocity is elevated by the large forward stroke volume. Hence clinical assessment is particularly important in these patients.

Cardiac catheterization

As outlined, invasive assessment of the aortic valve by cardiac catheterization is no longer necessary for most patients. In complicated cases, where echocardiography is equivocal or inconsistent, catheterization may be needed to resolve diagnostic doubt, particularly if cardiac output is low. The stenotic valve may be crossed retrogradely or the left ventricle entered trans-septally from the left atrium and aortic and left ventricular pressures measured simultaneously. In most patients, the major purpose of catheterization is to detect concomitant coronary artery disease (present in 50% of cases) prior to aortic valve replacement.

Aortic regurgitation

Symptoms and signs

In chronic aortic regurgitation, the left ventricle dilates and becomes hypertrophied – even when severe, the effective forward stroke volume remains normal. The end-diastolic volume increases but end-systolic volume is initially maintained. Eventually, the end-diastolic pressure rises, systolic function declines and only then does exercise tolerance fall. Thus, symptoms of exertional dyspnoea, orthopnoea and paroxysmal nocturnal dyspnoea usually follow a long asymptomatic period. Angina is less frequent than in aortic stenosis and its presence is strongly suggestive of coexisting coronary artery disease. Syncope is rare. In acute regurgitation, adaptive processes do not come into play and circulatory failure rapidly results.

The pulse pressure is wide with increased systolic and low diastolic pressure, although these signs may be obscured in the elderly by concomitant hypertension and a rigid circulation. During blood pressure measurement, the Korotkoff sounds can often be heard right down to zero although diastolic pressure is usually no lower than 30 mmHg. The apex is displaced laterally and inferiorly and is hyperdynamic. A high-pitched decrescendo early diastolic murmur is typically heard maximally in the third or fourth left intercostal space. In general, the duration of the murmur is a better guide to the severity of regurgitation than its intensity. Finally, there may be a loud ejection murmur secondary to increased forward flow during systole (not necessarily indicative of associated aortic stenosis) and a low-pitched mid-diastolic (Austin Flint) murmur due to fluttering and partial closure of the anterior mitral valve leaflet caused by the regurgitant jet. Clinical signs may be less obvious in acute aortic regurgitation – there is usually a prominent gallop rhythm and the typical murmur may be inaudible.

Investigations

The ECG and chest X-ray

The ECG characteristically shows left ventricular hypertrophy or, less often, left bundle branch block. Cardiomegaly on the chest X-ray is due to left ventricular enlargement. Ascending aortic dilatation is common and often extensive, particularly if there is additional aortic stenosis or if regurgitation is secondary to aortic wall disease.

Echocardiography

Although sensitive in detection, echocardiography is of only moderate value in quantitating valvular regurgitation. The appearances of the aortic valve and root may provide clues to the aetiology and serial measurements of left ventricular dimensions guide clinical decisions in conjunction with the patient's symptoms.

High-frequency fluttering of the anterior mitral valve leaflet in diastole is pathognomonic of aortic regurgitation and is best seen with M-mode imaging. Colour flow Doppler echocardiography is the more sensitive method of detection and clinically insignificant regurgitation may be found in a sizeable proportion of elderly patients. The extent to which the regurgitant jet extends from the aortic cusps into the left ventricle and its width in the left ventricular outflow tract are both useful measures of severity (Figure 116.9). Poor prognostic signs in acute severe aortic regurgitation are premature mitral valve closure (caused by free regurgitation into a non-compliant ventricle) and

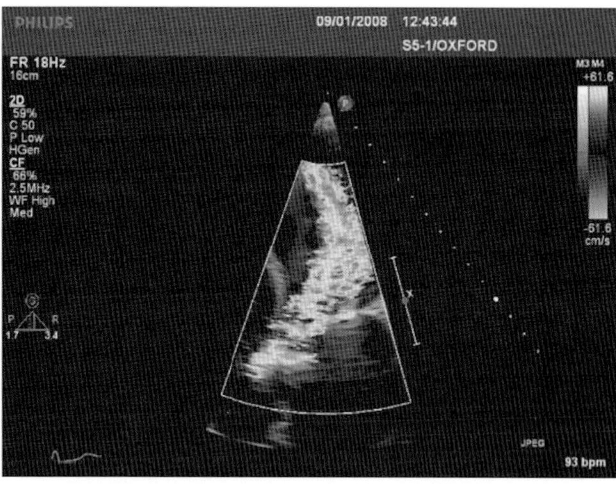

Figure 116.9 Apical five-chamber TTE view demonstrating a wide jet of severe aortic regurgitation in the left ventricular outflow tract extending to the left ventricular apex. See plate section for a colour version of this image.

premature aortic valve opening, caused by the rapid rise in left ventricular diastolic pressure.

Transoesophageal echocardiography provides useful supplementary information regarding the aetiology of aortic regurgitation and is invaluable in the assessment of aortic dissection.

Cardiac catheterization

The diagnosis and severity of aortic regurgitation are usually evident from clinical and echocardiographic assessment, although aortography may provide extra information if root replacement is being considered. As in aortic stenosis, coronary angiography is the main purpose of invasive investigation.

Cardiac magnetic resonance

This is the best technique for the assessment of pathology in the aortic root and arch and is therefore used increasingly in patients with aortic dilatation or dissection, particularly if surgery is planned. If unavailable, then CT is a useful substitute.

Prognosis and treatment

Chronic aortic regurgitation, even if severe, is associated with a good prognosis: with medical treatment alone, 75% of patients survive 5 years and 50% 10 years after diagnosis. The onset of symptoms heralds rapid deterioration and heart failure is usually associated with death within 2 years. Therefore, the early detection of left ventricular dysfunction is of paramount importance.

The progression of disease and need for surgery may be delayed by vasodilators (e.g. nifedipine) in asymptomatic patients with normal left ventricular contraction. Intervention on prognostic grounds alone does not improve outcome in the elderly and surgery for the symptom-free patient is not currently recommended. Unless there are specific contraindications, vasodilator therapy should be given to all elderly patients with aortic regurgitation. This treatment is usually all that is required in the very elderly and those unsuitable for surgery. Otherwise, patients should be monitored frequently (approximately 6 monthly) and serial echocardiographic assessment of left ventricular size and function undertaken. The onset of symptoms associated with evidence of progressive left ventricular dilatation (end-systolic dimension >5.5 cm) or reduced ejection fraction (<50%) indicates the need for surgery. Aortic valve replacement is nearly always necessary in the elderly, although occasionally the native valve can be resuspended, for example, in aortic dissection. Some patients with coexisting aneurysmal dilatation of the ascending aorta (>5.5 cm) may require aortic root replacement.

In patients with severe, long-standing left ventricular impairment, the prognosis is poor and the choice between medical and surgical management is extremely difficult. Left ventricular function may improve following aortic valve replacement, particularly if symptoms are mild and the duration of left ventricular dysfunction is short. However, the operative risk is high (>10%) and in many patients there is no postoperative improvement. Therefore, patients in this category, particularly with other risk factors for surgery, are probably best managed with vigorous medical therapy.

Acute aortic regurgitation requires emergency surgery and interim reduction of afterload using intravenous vasodilators.

Mitral stenosis

Symptoms and signs

The normal mitral valve orifice is 4 cm^2. In severe mitral stenosis this may be reduced to less than 1 cm^2, associated with pulmonary hypertension and raised pulmonary vascular resistance. In mild–moderate disease the cardiac output may remain normal but is unable to increase with exercise, leading to exertional dyspnoea. With more severe degrees of stenosis, cardiac output becomes subnormal, even at rest. Symptoms may also be precipitated during tachycardia (when abbreviation of diastole is associated with impaired left ventricular filling) and by the onset of atrial fibrillation when cardiac output may fall by 20–25% due to loss of atrial transport.

Older patients with mitral stenosis tend to fall into two categories: those with restenosis after a previously successful surgical mitral valvotomy and those with more slowly progressive rheumatic disease which has only become symptomatic in later life. Only 40–65% of patients give a history of rheumatic fever. The symptoms are a combination of exertional dyspnoea, orthopnoea, paroxysmal nocturnal dyspnoea, cough, palpitations and fatigue. These usually arise in the fourth or fifth decade and may remain mild for many years before gradual, often unnoticed, deterioration. Indeed, the diagnosis may not be made until echocardiography is performed to investigate unexplained breathlessness. Occult mitral stenosis is also an important cause of embolic stroke.

The classical signs of mitral stenosis are often absent in the elderly. A malar flush is uncommon and the signs associated with a pliable valve (tapping apex beat, loud first heart sound and opening snap) are unusual because the valve has calcified and become immobile. Auscultation reveals an apical rumbling mid-diastolic murmur; presystolic accentuation is rare as most are in atrial fibrillation. In general, the length of the murmur is proportional to the severity of the lesion, although it is often difficult to hear in its entirety. In advanced disease, signs of pulmonary hypertension may be present: raised venous pressure, right ventricular heave, loud pulmonary second sound, murmurs of pulmonary and tricuspid regurgitation and dependent oedema.

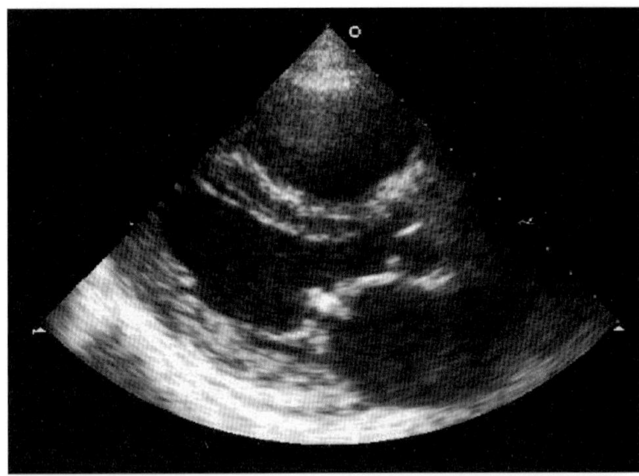

(a)

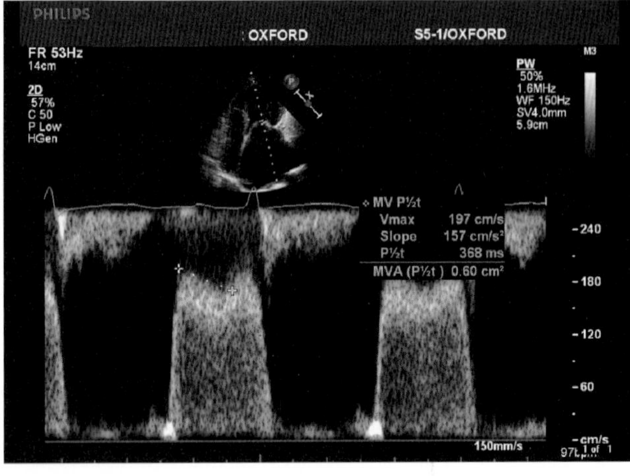

(b)

Figure 116.10 (a) TTE parasternal long-axis view in diastole demonstrating thickened and calcified mitral valve leaflets. (b) The pressure half-time may be estimated by tracing the mitral inflow deceleration slope at 368 ms (severe >220 ms).

Investigations

The ECG and chest X-ray

In sinus rhythm, a broad, notched P wave illustrates left atrial enlargement, although atrial fibrillation is more usual. The development of right ventricular hypertrophy is associated with right-axis deviation and may ultimately cause a prominent R wave in lead V1.

The chest X-ray reveals enlargement of the left atrium and its appendage, causing a double right heart border and widening of the tracheal bifurcation (best seen on a penetrated film). Gross left atrial dilatation usually indicates additional mitral regurgitation. Calcification of the valve, best appreciated on a lateral view, is common and usually indicates long-standing disease. Ultimately, signs of pulmonary venous and arterial hypertension develop and pulmonary oedema may be present.

Echocardiography

In rheumatic mitral stenosis, the valve leaflets are thickened and usually calcified with commissural fusion (Figure 116.10a). Cusp mobility is reduced and bowing of the leaflets occurs in diastole. Associated features such as left atrial enlargement and/or thrombus, pulmonary hypertension and mitral regurgitation may also be apparent. The valve area can be calculated from the two-dimensional image using planimetry, although this is subject to error. A more accurate assessment is obtained by measuring the velocity of flow across the valve using continuous-wave Doppler echocardiography. By this means, a pressure half-time (the time interval for the velocity to fall from its peak value to the peak value divided by the square root of 2, normal <100 ms) can be derived (Figure 116.10b) and the valve area calculated with the following equation:

$$\text{mitral valve area (cm}^2\text{)} = 220/\text{pressure half-time (ms)} \quad (116.1)$$

Tricuspid regurgitation is usually present to some extent and measurement of the velocity of the jet allows estimation of the pulmonary artery pressure.

Transoesophageal imaging may have an additive role in examining the anatomy of the valve and subvalvar apparatus and in excluding the presence of left atrial thrombus. This is important prior to balloon mitral valvuloplasty or DC cardioversion and in the investigation of systemic embolism.

Cardiac catheterization

Although echocardiographic imaging has removed the need for diagnostic catheterization in most cases, right and left heart studies may still be indicated when there is persistent uncertainly in determining disease severity or in patients with multiple valve lesions and/or coexisting pulmonary disease. Assessment of the coronary arteries is indicated in those being considered for interventional treatment.

Prognosis and treatment

Patients may remain asymptomatic for decades. Progression is variable after the onset of symptoms but generally occurs over a 5–10-year period with a 20% 5-year and 40% 10-year mortality for those treated medically. Systemic thromboemboli (most frequently to the cerebral circulation) occur in 20% of patients. Infective endocarditis is relatively unusual.

Most elderly patients with mitral stenosis are in atrial fibrillation and can be improved by good control of the ventricular response. The treatment of choice is digoxin and verapamil is a useful adjunctive therapy. Amiodarone is almost always effective but has many side effects and should be reserved for resistant cases. Beta-blockers also serve a useful role, even in helping to maintain sinus rhythm, and are under-utilized. In cases where atrial fibrillation is of short duration and the left atrium is not significantly enlarged (<4.5 cm on echocardiography), cardioversion should be considered, although this is contraindicated when there is evidence of left atrial thrombus.

Diuretics may be necessary for the control of breathlessness, but high doses may cause volume depletion and should be avoided. Anticoagulation is recommended for all patients with mitral stenosis, especially if there is left atrial enlargement, and is mandatory in those with atrial fibrillation (unless there are obvious contraindications). It reduces the risk of stroke by 60%, although the risk of bleeding is increased, especially in patients over 80 years of age.

All patients who remain symptomatic despite medical treatment should be considered for percutaneous balloon mitral valvuloplasty; the surgical alternatives are open mitral commissurotomy or mitral valve replacement.

Mitral regurgitation

Symptoms and signs

In chronic mitral regurgitation, the impedance to flow from the left ventricle into the left atrium is low and therefore the ventricle is relatively spared from the effects of chronic volume overload. Initially, left ventricular end-diastolic volume is normal, but as time passes the ventricle dilates, develops hypertrophy and ultimately fails. Symptoms can therefore be delayed for years and may only develop after deterioration in left ventricular function has already occurred. In contrast, those with acute regurgitation become unwell suddenly and may deteriorate rapidly.

The main complaints are of chronic fatigue, lethargy and progressive dyspnoea. Some may present with pulmonary oedema and fluid retention. The signs of mitral regurgitation are relatively unaffected by age. The pulse volume is normal and may have a sharp character and the apex beat is heaving and displaced laterally. The murmur is pansystolic, often with a marked crescendo towards the second heart sound, and is heard loudest at the apex radiating to the axilla (although radiation to the base of the heart or carotid arteries frequently accompanies posterior leaflet prolapse). A third heart sound is common. In acute mitral regurgitation, a sinus tachycardia and systemic hypotension are invariable. The apex beat is hyperdynamic but undisplaced unless there has been preceding chronic mitral regurgitation. The apical systolic murmur is harsh and there is often an accompanying thrill. A gallop rhythm may be palpable and signs of pulmonary oedema are usually present.

Investigations

The ECG and chest X-ray

The ECG shows left atrial enlargement or atrial fibrillation. Left ventricular hypertrophy occurs in ~50% of patients. In chronic mitral regurgitation, the chest X-ray shows left ventricular and left atrial dilatation. Calcification of the mitral annulus is best seen in the lateral projection. In acute mitral regurgitation, the heart size is normal and there is usually gross pulmonary oedema.

Echocardiography

Echocardiography demonstrates the enlarged left atrium, the anatomy of the sub-valvar apparatus and may indicate the aetiology of mitral regurgitation (Figure 116.11). Pulsed Doppler and colour flow mapping can detect the most trivial degree of regurgitation and demonstrate its direction. They also provide semiquantitative indices of severity although interpretation is highly subjective and notoriously unreliable. Therefore, assessment may be difficult. Left ventricular dimensions and wall motion are useful clues: in severe regurgitation there is dilatation and vigorous contraction characteristic of volume overload. Quantitative assessment is possible but remains a relatively specialized tool. In practice, it remains common to grade regurgitation as mild, moderate or severe according to the width of the regurgitant colour jet as it enters the left atrium and to base management decisions on left ventricular size and function in conjunction with the patient's symptoms.

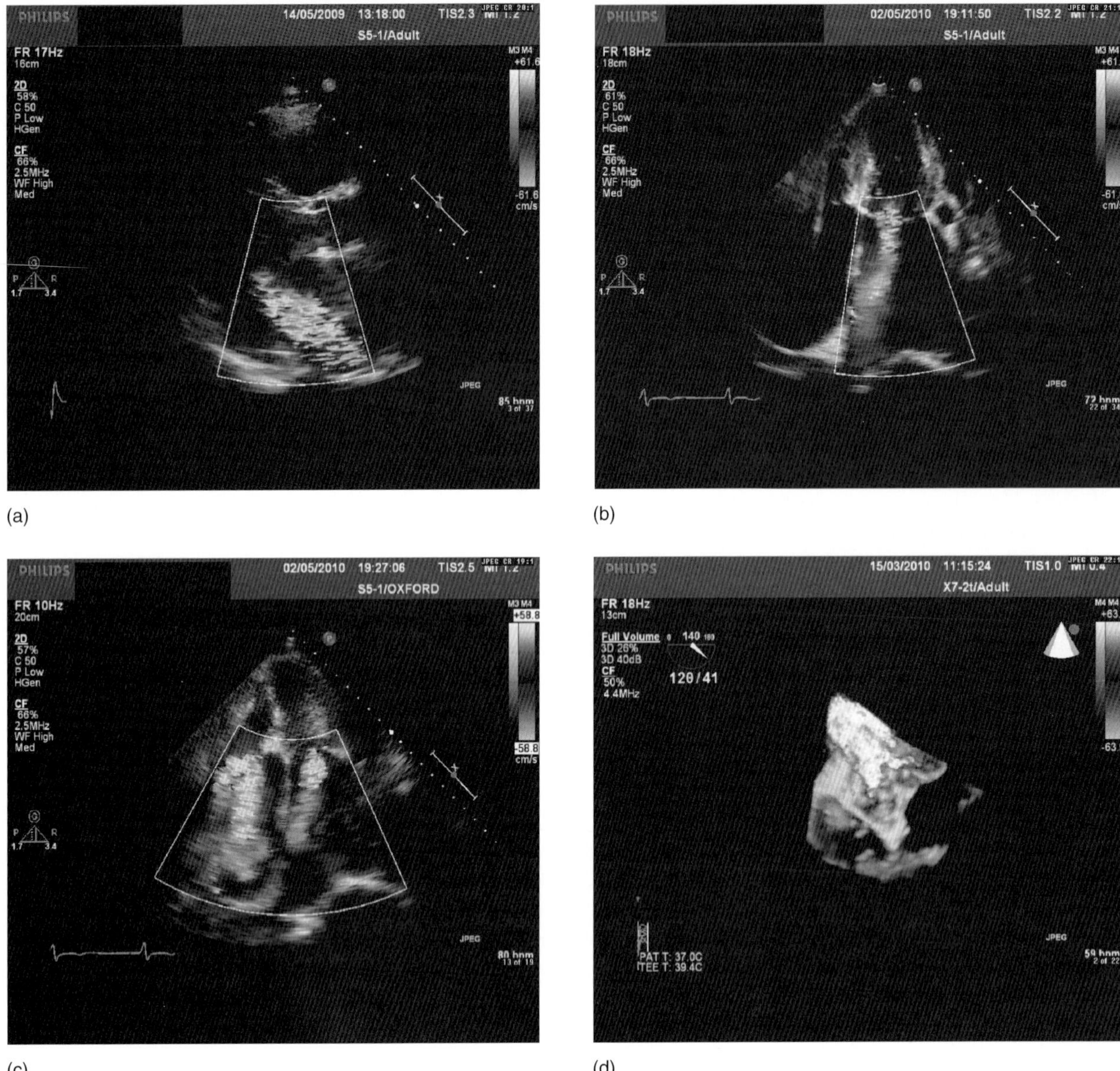

Figure 116.11 (a) TTE parasternal long-axis view with a broad colour jet across the mitral valve demonstrating severe mitral regurgitation. (b) TTE apical view demonstrating severe mitral regurgitation; the broad colour jet occupies over one-third of the left atrium. (c) TTE apical view demonstrating torrential tricuspid regurgitation and concurrent severe mitral regurgitation, causing biatrial dilatation. (d) 3D TOE demonstrating severe mitral regurgitation. See plate section for a colour version of this image.

Transoesophageal echocardiography provides more information regarding valvular morphology and the mechanism of regurgitation. These are of particular importance preoperatively, especially when valve repair rather than replacement is being considered.

Cardiac catheterization

Catheterization is rarely needed for diagnostic purposes but coronary angiography is mandatory in those patients being considered for surgery. Left ventricular angiography can be used to assess left ventricular function and end-diastolic pressure and right heart catheterization may confirm the presence of associated pulmonary hypertension.

Prognosis and treatment

Mitral regurgitation may remain indolent for many years and therefore the timing of invasive investigations is difficult in the elderly. Asymptomatic patients have a 5-year survival rate of >80%, but when symptoms develop this falls to 45%. In chronic regurgitation these may be initially controlled by vasodilators (particularly angiotensin-converting enzyme inhibitors), diuretics and digoxin, but such medical therapy should not be used as a tool to defer surgery in suitable candidates. Those with left atrial enlargement and atrial fibrillation should be anticoagulated; in sinus rhythm the risk of thromboembolism is relatively small and treatment with aspirin alone may be adequate.

Surgical treatment improves survival in symptomatic mitral regurgitation and outcome is related to ventricular function; thus, the combination of symptoms and echocardiographic evidence of progressively increasing left ventricular size (end-systolic dimension >5.5 cm) suggests the need for mitral valve replacement or repair. Age *per se* is not a contraindication to surgery, but advanced left ventricular dysfunction in patients who present late may make the risks unacceptably high.

In acute mitral regurgitation, the outlook with medical therapy alone is bleak. Even in elderly patients, intra-aortic balloon counter pulsation should be considered in addition to standard measures (oxygen, intravenous diuretics, vasodilators and inotropes) in order to improve the haemodynamic situation while patients undergo emergency cardiac catheterization followed by mitral valve surgery and revascularization if appropriate. The operative mortality is high (>50%).

Mixed valve disease

Assessment and treatment comprise a summation of the factors for each individual valve lesion. Some combinations bear a poor prognosis, for example, mitral stenosis and aortic regurgitation, and such patients require careful monitoring. The risk of combined aortic and mitral valve replacement is significantly higher than for single valve replacement, with reported mortality rates of 15–30% in the elderly. Clearly, this may influence the decision to proceed. Occasionally, the need for surgery can be avoided by a 'palliative' balloon procedure, particularly if pure mitral stenosis is the major component, although this decision should only be made after specialist assessment and multidisciplinary team discussion.

Interventional treatment in the elderly

The age of patients undergoing valvular heart surgery in the UK continues to rise and there has been an increase in the number of procedures in which coronary artery bypass grafting and valve surgery are combined (Figure 116.12). More than 20% of patients currently treated by cardiac surgery are over the age of 75 years and 5% are over 80 years old. Overall perioperative mortality in this age group is falling, from 5% in 2004 to 3.4% in 2008. Not only has the risk of surgery diminished, but medium-term survival rates are also remarkably good; for a patient aged 75 years, the 5-year survival following isolated valve surgery is 70%.

General considerations

Risk assessment

When surgical intervention is being considered, it is important to optimize medical therapy, which may warrant specialist referral. For some patients this will improve symptoms sufficiently to avoid the need for intervention and its associated risk.

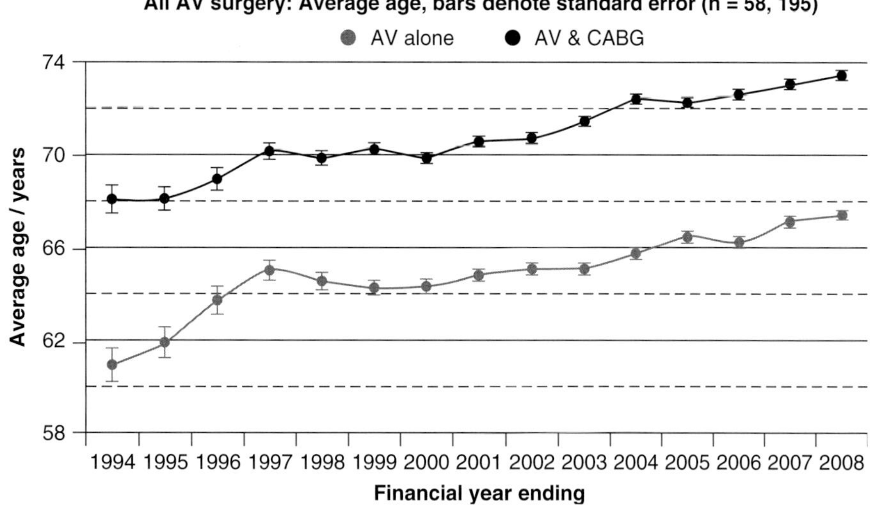

Figure 116.12 The rising age of patients undergoing aortic valve (AV) surgery in the UK. CABG = concomitant coronary artery bypass grafting. Data reproduced from the Sixth National Adult Cardiac Surgical Database Report, Society for Cardiothoracic Surgery in Great Britain and Ireland.

Operative mortality is higher in the elderly and also greater following valve surgery than with coronary artery bypass grafting alone. Nevertheless, with judicious patient selection, early referral and optimization of preoperative status, the results of valve replacement in the elderly can approach those in younger patients. Factors influencing outcome include concomitant coronary artery disease, poor left ventricular function, associated tricuspid valve disease (often associated with pulmonary hypertension), cerebrovascular or peripheral vascular disease, impaired respiratory or renal function, osteoporosis and general frailty, patient motivation, nutritional status and previous or coexisting malignant disease. Of particular concern are pre-existing cardiac, respiratory or renal impairment and neurological status, as these systems are most susceptible to the detrimental effects of cardiopulmonary bypass. There are several risk stratification models that can be used to estimate overall perioperative risk, the best known being the EuroSCORE and the Society of Thoracic Surgeons risk score.

The failure to deal with significant associated coronary disease is now recognized as a frequent cause of early and late mortality following otherwise successful valve replacement and preoperative coronary angiography is an important investigation in the elderly prior to consideration of valve surgery. However, the principle of a simple, quick procedure in the elderly patient is important; additional bypass grafting should only be undertaken for severe coronary artery disease. Urgent or emergency surgery has a higher mortality (often >30%) and the risk is also magnified if second-time surgery (for example, aortic valve replacement following coronary artery bypass grafting some years previously) is being considered.

Complications

The incidence of perioperative myocardial infarction after open heart surgery is usually estimated at around 2–4%. Atrial fibrillation is common preoperatively in patients with VHD but frequently develops *de novo* between the second and fourth postoperative day, especially in the elderly. Treatment with digoxin or amiodarone is usually successful and cardioversion may be required for the small proportion of patients who are haemodynamically compromised.

Major focal neurological abnormalities occur in around 1% of patients undergoing valve replacement and the risk is increased in the elderly (4% in patients over the age of 85 years). Neuropsychological abnormalities can be identified in 30–50% of patients following cardiopulmonary bypass but the majority are subtle and resolve within a few months of surgery. Cardiac surgery results in some degree of respiratory impairment in virtually all patients, but particularly in the elderly patient whose respiratory reserve is already diminished. The overall incidence of acute renal failure requiring dialysis is around 5%, although some degree of reversible renal dysfunction occurs in up to one-third of patients.

Aortic valve disease

Elective surgical valve replacement is the treatment of choice for the management of severe aortic valve disease. In the elderly the procedure can be undertaken with a mortality rate of 2–10%. Long-term outcome is good with late survival rates similar to age- and gender-matched control populations. In general, valve replacement for aortic regurgitation has a less favourable outcome than for aortic stenosis since patients tend to present at a later stage when irreversible left ventricular damage has occurred. Preoperative left ventricular impairment is not a definite contraindication to surgery (particularly in aortic stenosis) but an ejection fraction of <45% is associated with considerably increased operative risk. This risk also rises with increasing age and if valve replacement is combined with coronary artery bypass grafting.

Balloon aortic valvuloplasty (BAV) is a percutaneous technique using a large balloon catheter to dilate a stenosed aortic valve and has been shown to increase aortic valve area, reduce the trans-valve gradient and improve symptoms. However, BAV does not alter the natural history of severe aortic stenosis; symptoms usually recur within a few months and the procedure does not reduce overall mortality or increase long-term survival. Despite this, there are some clearly defined situations where the technique can be considered:

- Bridge to definitive treatment [either open aortic valve replacement or TAVI (Figure 116.13)].
- Bridge to new technology, for example, for those patients whose aortic annulus is too large for the currently available TAVI devices.
- Adjunct to pre-TAVI percutaneous coronary intervention (PCI) (which is often complex and high risk in the setting of severe aortic stenosis).
- Therapeutic trial – particularly in breathless patients with a combination of severe aortic stenosis, significant coronary artery disease and severe airways disease.
- Palliative – although this is more controversial, some feel that offering 3–6 months of symptomatic benefit to very elderly patients (even when recurrence of symptoms is likely) is worthwhile in some clinical scenarios.
- In patients requiring urgent non-cardiac surgery (e.g. for malignancy).

Recently, percutaneous TAVI has become available as another treatment option for patients who are unsuitable or considered too high risk for conventional surgery. In this procedure, which avoids the need for sternotomy or cardiopulmonary bypass, a stent-mounted bioprosthetic aortic valve is deployed within the diseased native aortic valve after predilatation with a valvuloplasty balloon, via the

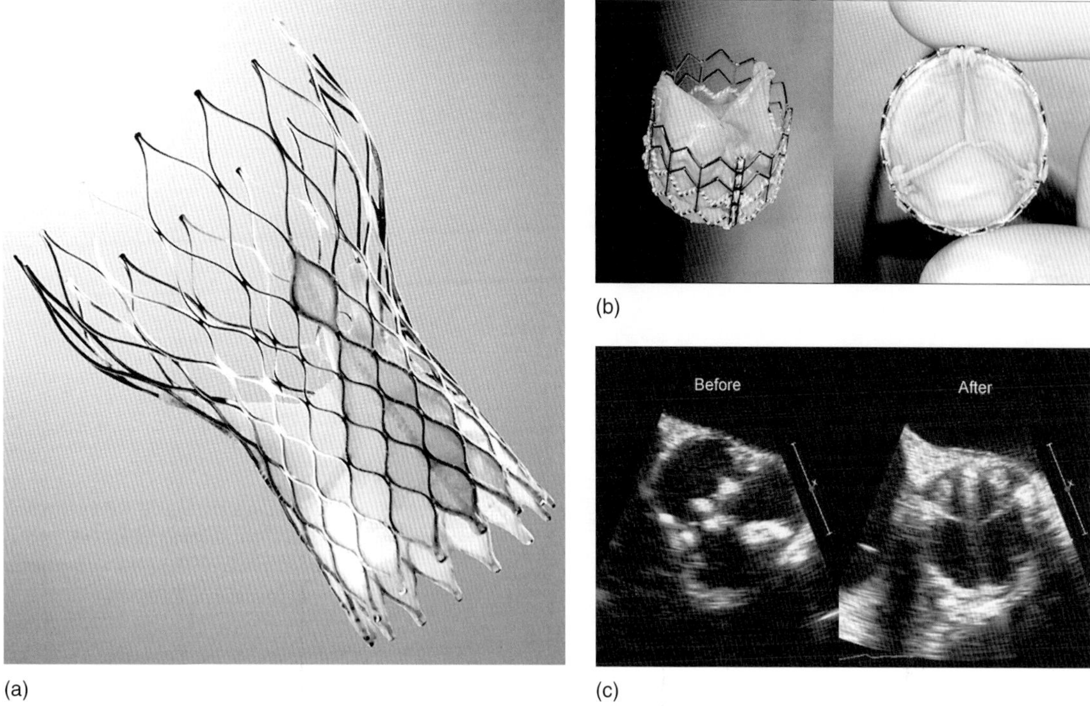

Figure 116.13 Contemporary transcatheter aortic valve implantation devices: (a) Medtronic Corevalve; (b) Sapien–Edwards. (c) TOE images before and after deployment of the Sapien–Edwards TAVI prosthesis.

femoral, subclavian or apical route. In high-risk patients, TAVI has been shown to be superior to standard medical management (including BAV). Although 30 day mortality in patients undergoing TAVI is higher, 1-year cardiovascular mortality is 20% for TAVI patients compared with 42% for standard medical management alone or in conjunction with BAV.

Mitral valve disease

The most common indication for mitral valve intervention in the elderly is mitral regurgitation, whether caused by degenerative or functional mitral valve disease. Patients undergoing mitral valve replacement have a higher perioperative and long-term mortality than those undergoing aortic valve replacement, probably as a consequence of associated left ventricular impairment and pulmonary hypertension. Mortality for elective mitral valve replacement in the elderly is ~15% and this risk is increased if there is associated coronary artery disease or significant left ventricular impairment.

In patients with mitral regurgitation, there is now accumulating evidence of the benefits of mitral valve repair rather than replacement. Valve repair results in better preservation of left ventricular function and may obviate the need for anticoagulation. Compared with valve replacement, mitral repair is associated with lower mortality (5.5 versus 15.6% in one series), reduced risk of stroke and shorter duration of intensive care stay. The procedure is well established in elderly patients and earlier intervention may be favoured if repair is thought to be technically feasible, particularly if mitral regurgitation is due to ischaemic annulo-papillary dysfunction or non-rheumatic disease. Transoesophageal echocardiography is essential for pre- and perioperative assessment and can predict the probability of a successful repair procedure. The role of conservative surgery in rheumatic mitral regurgitation is limited due to poor long-term event-free survival.

Percutaneous balloon mitral valvuloplasty for rheumatic mitral stenosis was originally described by Inoue *et al.*[2] in 1984 and is well established as a less invasive replacement for surgical valvotomy (Figure 116.14). In this procedure, a cylindrical balloon is positioned across the mitral valve and inflated to split the fused commissures. The balloon is waisted to minimize movement during balloon inflation. Mitral valve area and gradient can then be measured and a further inflation carried out in a stepwise approach if required. Although ideally suited to those with pliable, non-calcified valves, there is now increasing evidence that it can be performed safely in the elderly with less suitable valve morphology and in those who have undergone surgical valvotomy in the past. The procedure usually results in a moderate but significant improvement in valve function associated with a clinically useful symptomatic result. The

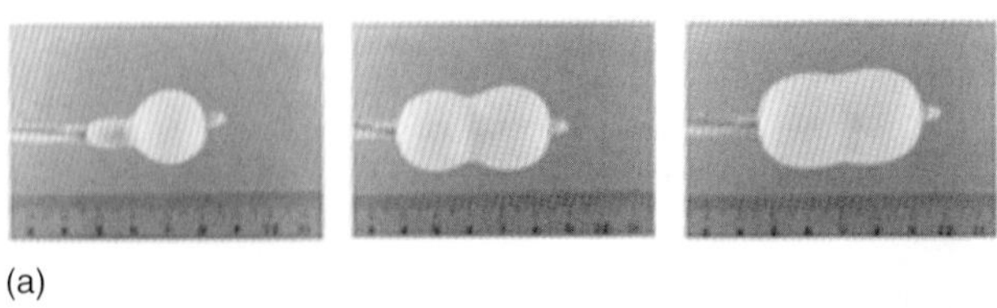

(a)

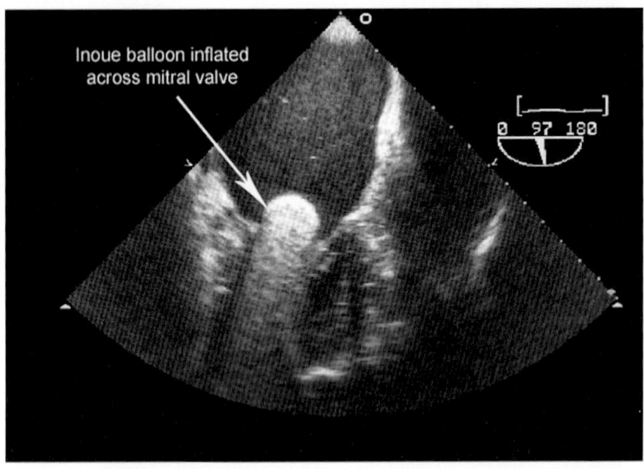

(b)

Figure 116.14 (a) The Inoue balloon used during percutaneous balloon mitral valvuloplasty. (b) TOE demonstrating balloon inflation across the stenosed mitral valve.

procedural mortality of 3% in the elderly is considerably less than with mitral valve replacement. Contraindications include the presence of left atrial thrombus, severe subvalvar involvement or valve calcification and significant mitral regurgitation. These can be detected by preprocedural evaluation with transoesophageal echocardiography which is mandatory. The procedure usually increases mitral valve area by ~1.0 cm^2 associated with an improvement in functional class. Complications include severe mitral regurgitation requiring emergency surgery (<1% of cases), cardiac perforation and restenosis (which is considerably slower and less frequent than after BAV).

Percutaneous options for the treatment of mitral regurgitation are now emerging and two approaches are currently under investigation. One technique for the surgical repair of mitral regurgitation is to suture the central portions of the two leaflets of the mitral valve together (the Alfieri stitch) to create a double orifice of smaller area than the original valve defect. The Mitraclip system has been developed to recreate this procedure using a percutaneous approach and initial results suggest that this may be a useful minimally invasive method for mitral repair (Figure 116.15). Percutaneous mitral valve annuloplasty is an alternative technique for the management of functional mitral regurgitation where an annuloplasty ring is deployed via the coronary sinus, thereby reducing mitral annular size and the degree of mitral regurgitation.

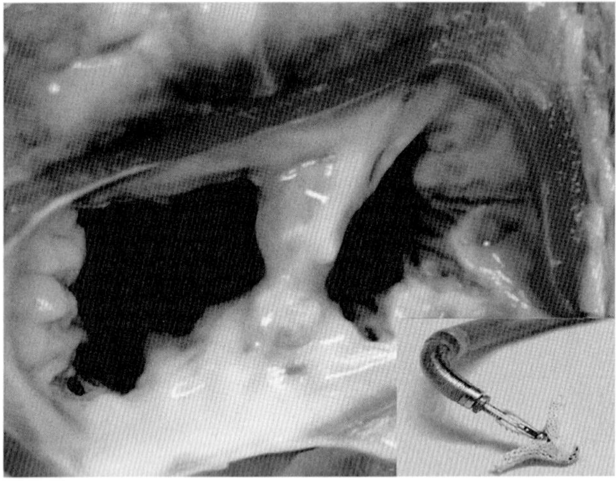

Figure 116.15 The percutaneous Evalve Mitraclip device (inset) provides a central tether for the opposing mitral valve leaflets thereby creating a double orifice and reducing the regurgitant area, as demonstrated in this *ex vivo* porcine model.

Prosthetic valves in the elderly

Choice of prosthesis

There are two broad categories of valve prosthesis that can be used for surgical valve replacement: mechanical valves and bioprostheses (xenograft). In rare cases (usually related to infective endocarditis affecting the aortic valve), alternatives include a human homograft or pulmonary autograft (transplanting the native pulmonary valve to the aortic position and implanting a homograft in the pulmonary position; the Ross procedure).

Mechanical prostheses offer durability and longevity. Despite the problems associated with anticoagulation and small risks of thrombosis *in situ* (usually engendered by a period of under-anticoagulation) and infective endocarditis, they remain the first choice for patients whose life expectancy significantly exceeds 10 years. Patients with significant mitral valve disease usually have another indication for anticoagulation (e.g. atrial fibrillation and/or left atrial enlargement) and mechanical prostheses are therefore most commonly used when mitral repair is not an option.

Bioprostheses avoid the need for obligatory oral anticoagulation and are most commonly used for aortic valve replacement in the elderly (70% in isolated AVR, 82% in patients undergoing AVR and coronary artery bypass graft). Valve lifespan is often quoted as 10 years, although modern stentless bioprostheses may last for considerably longer. Bioprosthetic valve degeneration occurs more slowly in the elderly and affects around 10% of patients over the age of 70 years at 15-year follow-up.

Table 116.1 Target international normalized ratio (INR) for mechanical prostheses.[3]

Prosthesis thrombogenicity[a]	Patient-related risk factors[b]	
	No risk factor	≥1 risk factor
Low	2.5	3.0
Medium	3.0	3.5
High	3.5	4.0

[a]Prosthesis thrombogenicity: low, Carbomedics (aortic position), Medtronic Hall, St Jude Medical (without Silzone); medium, Bjork–Shiley, other bileaflet valves; high, Lillehei–Kaster, Omniscience, Starr–Edwards.
[b]Patient-related risk factors: mitral, tricuspid or pulmonary valve replacement; previous thromboembolism; atrial fibrillation; left atrial diameter >5 cm; dense left atrial spontaneous echo contrast; mitral stenosis of any degree; left ventricular ejection fraction <35%; hypercoagulable state.

Anticoagulation

Comprehensive guidelines for the prevention of thromboembolic events in VHD have been produced by the European Society of Cardiology. The indications for anticoagulation and recommended international normalized ratio (INR) for patients with prosthetic valves or native valve disease are summarized in Table 116.1. The recommended target INR for patients with mechanical prosthetic valves is 2.5–4.0, the intensity of anticoagulation varying according to the type of valve, its position and the patient's innate thrombotic risk.

The main difficulty with anticoagulation, particularly in the elderly, is the small risk of serious haemorrhage, which can be reduced by careful monitoring (with assistance from the family if necessary). Common causes of fluctuating levels are intercurrent illness, dehydration, dietary alterations (particularly excess alcohol consumption) and drug interactions – often no reason can be found. Excessive departures from the desired range (i.e. INR >7.0 or <1.5) may require hospital admission. High-dose intravenous vitamin K can complicate the reintroduction of warfarin and should be avoided unless there is evidence of active bleeding – haematological advice is recommended.

Complications

The symptoms of prosthetic valve dysfunction are often subtle and the clinician should have a low threshold for arranging further investigation or referral to a specialist centre. Prosthetic valve endocarditis is a dangerous condition and the diagnosis should be considered in any patient with a prosthetic valve who becomes unwell; symptoms of infection may be atypical or absent in the elderly. Specialist investigation and treatment are virtually always necessary.

Echocardiography is the investigation of choice for the routine follow-up of elderly patients with prosthetic valves and an integral part of the assessment of suspected malfunction. In many situations transthoracic imaging is inconclusive, particularly in patients with metallic valves, and in these circumstances a transoesophageal study should be performed.

The risk of thromboembolism in patients with prosthetic valves is ~1–3% per year. The rate is higher for mitral than aortic valves and lower in those with bioprostheses. Obstruction of a prosthetic valve is nearly always thrombotic and occurs more frequently with mechanical valves (Figure 116.16). The mortality associated with emergency presentation approaches 50% and early recognition and immediate intervention are essential. Revision surgery is the preferred treatment strategy although thrombolysis may be a preferred option in high-risk elderly patients.

Many elderly patients with bioprosthetic valves are now in their second decade following surgery. Bioprosthetic stenosis or regurgitation may eventually develop secondary to progressive calcification, degeneration and/or rupture of the valve cusps. Aortic regurgitation in this setting has been successfully treated by TAVI within the original prosthesis (the so-called 'valve-in-valve' procedure). Other mechanical complications include suture dehiscence (which may occur in the early postoperative period or as a complication of infective endocarditis), strut fracture or haemolysis.

All patients with a prosthetic valve are at risk of infective endocarditis and should receive antibiotic prophylaxis when appropriate. There is considerable variability between the various national and international bodies as to when antibiotic prophylaxis should be used, but there is agreement that patients with prosthetic valves are at higher

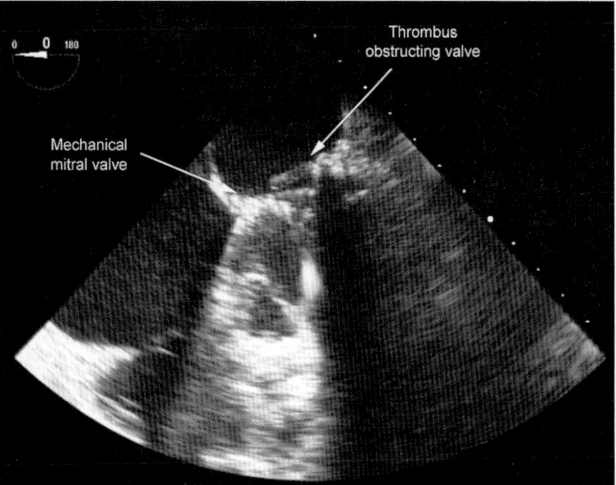

Figure 116.16 TOE demonstrating laminated thrombus (arrowed) obstructing a prosthetic mitral valve.

Table 116.2 UK and European guidelines for antibiotic prophylaxis against infective endocarditis.

	UK guidelines	European guidelines
Patients at higher risk of developing infective endocarditis	Acquired valvular heart disease with stenosis or regurgitation Valve replacement Structural congenital heart disease, including surgically corrected or palliated structural conditions, but excluding isolated atrial septal defect, fully repaired ventricular septal defect or fully repaired patent ductus arteriosus and closure devices that are judged to be endothelialized Hypertrophic cardiomyopathy Previous infective endocarditis	Patients with prosthetic valves Previous infective endocarditis Congenital heart disease: Cyanotic congenital heart disease (either not repaired or repaired with a residual defect) Repaired congenital heart disease (for 6 months post-procedure) Where a residual defect persists at the site of implantation of prosthetic material or a device
Procedures requiring antibiotic prophylaxis in high-risk patients	Gastrointestinal and genitourinary procedures at a site where there is suspected pre-existing infection	*Dental:* recommended for any procedure requiring manipulation of the gingival or periapical region of the teeth or perforation of the oral mucosa *Respiratory tract:* not recommended *GI or urogenital (including TOE)*: not recommended *Skin and soft tissue:* not recommended

risk. Current UK and European guidelines are summarized in Table 116.2.

Infective endocarditis

Introduction

In recent years, the number of elderly patients presenting with infective endocarditis has risen and staphylococcal and prosthetic valve endocarditis are increasingly prevalent in this group. Echocardiography is the principal investigative tool and the wide availability of transoesophageal imaging has greatly increased diagnostic sensitivity and specificity, in addition to providing invaluable preoperative anatomical information when cardiac surgery is necessary. These advances have been reflected by new diagnostic criteria which incorporate echocardiographic data to increase accuracy. Recent European guidelines for prompt diagnosis, specialist assessment, appropriate antibiotic therapy and timely surgery have potential for a significant impact on morbidity and mortality.

Epidemiology

The elderly form an increasing proportion of patients presenting with infective endocarditis and their mortality is higher than in younger patients. Although the absolute incidence in elderly subjects is unknown, the overall annual incidence in Western populations is approximately 2 per 100 000 population, one-third of whom are aged over 65 years. Streptococci and staphylococci are the most common causative organisms in all age groups, the latter being the predominant organism in prosthetic valve endocarditis.

Diagnosis

The classical history and typical physical signs of infective endocarditis may be absent in the elderly and diagnosis is often difficult. Therefore, a high index of suspicion is important. Patients with prosthetic valves represent a particularly high-risk group and the diagnosis of infective endocarditis should be actively sought in those who present with non-specific symptoms, prosthetic obstruction or regurgitation or systemic embolism. Minimum investigations include a full blood count, biochemical screen, inflammatory indices (erythrocyte sedimentation rate and/or C-reactive protein) and at least three sets of blood cultures from two separate sites before starting antibiotic therapy. The first two sets of blood cultures are positive in 90% of cases of infective endocarditis.

Echocardiography is invaluable, allowing the detection of vegetations, assessment of valvular incompetence and investigation of complications, such as cusp perforation or abscess formation (Figure 116.17). Vegetations appear as echogenic masses attached to valve leaflets or occasionally other intracardiac structures, although only those larger than 1–2 mm in size will be detected. Therefore, although transthoracic echocardiography should be performed, a negative study does not exclude the diagnosis. More definitive information may be obtained from a transoesophageal examination, which should be considered in all patients with proven or suspected infective endocarditis. The procedure has a high negative predictive value and is particularly sensitive in the detection of vegetations or abscesses. The old von Reyn diagnostic criteria have now been superseded by the new 'Duke' criteria, which

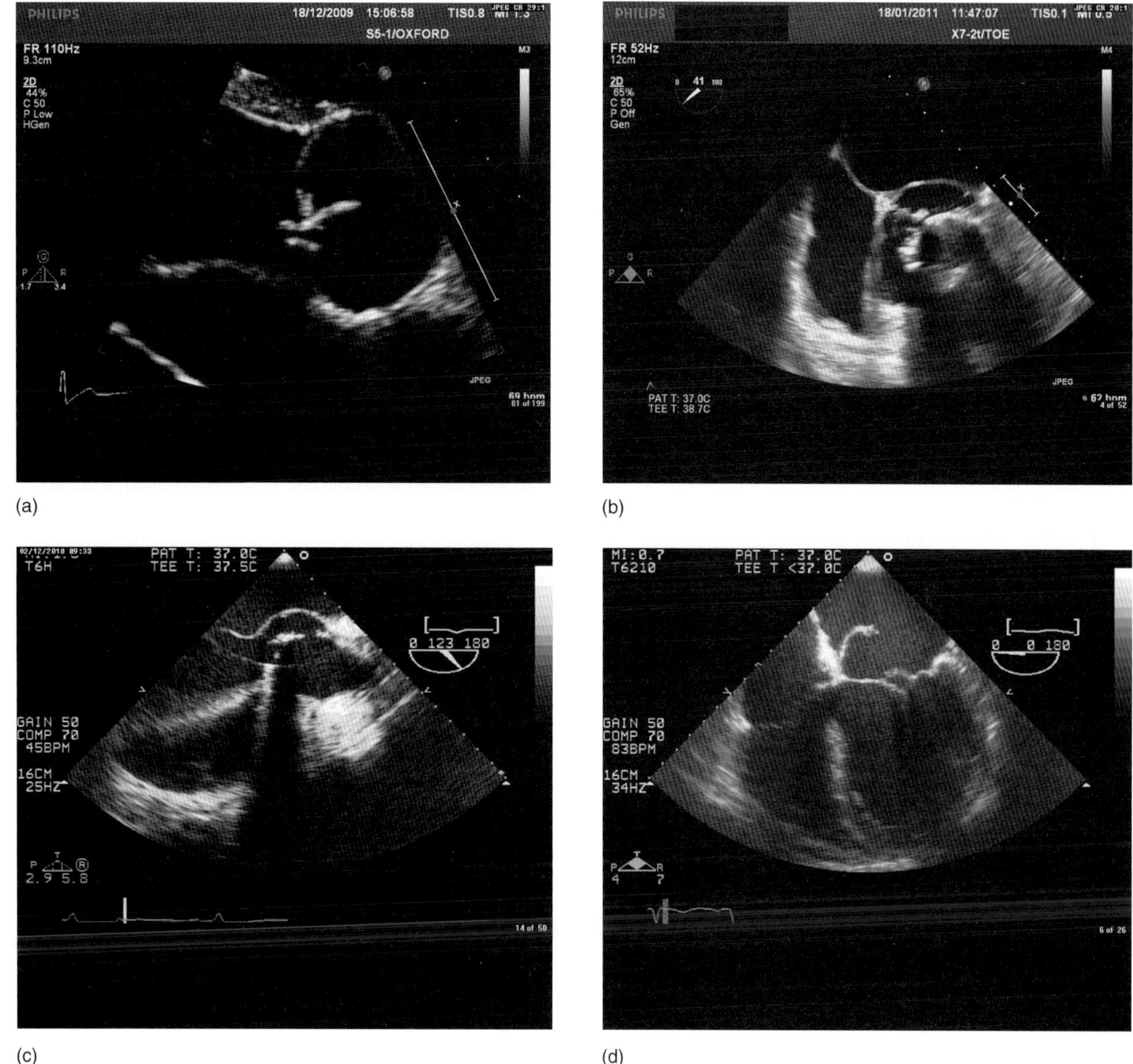

Figure 116.17 (a) Perforation of a bicuspid aortic valve secondary to infective endocarditis causing severe aortic regurgitation. (b) TOE demonstrating a large abscess cavity surrounding a prosthetic aortic valve secondary to infective endocarditis. (c) Large abscess cavity secondary to infective endocarditis with resulting prosthetic valve dehiscence. (d) TOE demonstrating a highly mobile vegetation on the anterior mitral valve leaflet prolapsing into the left atrium during ventricular systole.

include echocardiographic features and provide superior sensitivity and specificity.

Cardiac catheterization should be avoided in infective endocarditis because of the risk of dislodging vegetations or injecting friable tissues.

Treatment

Any febrile illness of doubtful or uncertain origin occurring in a patient with VHD should be considered as infective endocarditis until proven otherwise and referred to hospital urgently prior to *any* antibiotic administration. Optimal management requires close liaison between the cardiologist, cardiac surgeon and microbiologist. Antibiotic therapy should be started promptly after blood cultures have been taken and subsequent treatment is guided by the clinical and microbiological features. Indications for surgery include heart failure secondary to valvular regurgitation, abscess formation, failure to respond to medical therapy, recurrent systemic embolism and an unstable infected prosthetic valve. Urgent surgery should not be delayed to allow an arbitrary period of preoperative antibiotic therapy.

Prosthetic valve endocarditis

The cumulative risk of infective endocarditis is 1–4% during the lifetime of a prosthesis. Antibiotic prophylaxis should be strongly considered in this group of patients, who should also receive careful education regarding the need for rigorous dental and skin hygiene – intravenous cannulae, urinary catheters and indwelling lines should be avoided whenever possible. Prosthetic valve endocarditis is a dangerous disease with a mortality of ~50% and further surgery is usually required, often as an emergency. Therefore, it should always be managed in a cardiothoracic surgical centre unless close communication can be maintained and rapid transfer is possible if needed. Transthoracic echocardiography is inadequate in this situation and prosthetic valve patients with unexplained pyrexia should be referred for transoesophageal imaging.

Conclusion

Valvular heart disease and infective endocarditis are increasingly common in the elderly population. Rheumatic heart disease is now uncommon in industrialized nations but still a major burden in the developing world. Most valvular pathology is now degenerative, particularly in those aged above 75 years. Mitral regurgitation and aortic stenosis are the most common lesions. Symptomatic VHD will continue to rise in the elderly with consequent huge implications for medical resources.

Diagnosis can be difficult and is often complicated by the presence of coincident medical conditions and the physiological effects of ageing. Transthoracic echocardiography is the investigation of choice supplemented by transoesophageal imaging when appropriate. Cardiac catheterization is only necessary if there is diagnostic doubt and for the preoperative detection of coronary artery disease if surgery is required. The risks of valve surgery are relatively low in elderly subjects provided that patients are carefully selected with optimization of their preoperative status: the risks rise significantly in the presence of left ventricular impairment, renal insufficiency and cerebrovascular or coronary artery disease. Balloon mitral valvuloplasty provides an alternative to surgery for suitable elderly patients with mitral stenosis and new percutaneous techniques of TAVI and mitral valve repair have an exciting future. Thus, although medical therapy is useful in specific situations, interventional treatment should not be denied on the grounds of age alone and early referral for expert assessment is recommended.

Key points

- The widespread availability of echocardiography has revolutionized the investigation of valvular heart disease (VHD) by providing accurate and non-invasive assessment of severity and a means of monitoring disease progression.
- In elderly patients, many of the classical manifestations of VHD may be attenuated by the effects of ageing on the cardiovascular system, namely atherosclerosis, hypertension and valve calcification.
- Progression of VHD is variable after the onset of symptoms but generally occurs over a 5–10 year period with a 20% 5 year and a 40% 10 year mortality for those treated medically.
- Echocardiography is the principal investigative tool for infective endocarditis and the wide availability of transoesophageal imaging has greatly increased diagnostic sensitivity and specificity, in addition to providing invaluable preoperative anatomical information when cardiac surgery is necessary.
- Indications for surgery for infective endocarditis include heart failure secondary to valvular regurgitation, abscess formation, failure to respond to medical therapy, recurrent systemic embolism and an unstable infected prosthetic valve.

Key references

1. Nkomo VT, Gardin JM, Skelton TN *et al.* Burden of valvular heart diseases: a population-based study. *Lancet* 2006;**368**:1005–11.
2. Inoue K, Owaki T, Nakamura T *et al.* Clinical application of transvenous mitral commissurotomy by a new balloon catheter. *J Thorac Cardiovasc Surg* 1984;**87**:394–402.
3. NICE. *Antimicrobial Prophylaxis Against Infective Endocarditis: Full Guideline,* National Institute for Health and Clinical Excellence, London, 2008.

Further reading

ACC/AHA. 2006 guidelines for the management of valvular heart disease. *J Am Coll Cardiol* 2006;**48**:e1–48.

Ailawadi G, Swenson BR, Girotti ME *et al.* Is mitral valve repair superior to replacement in elderly patients? *Ann Thorac Surg* 2008;**86**:77–85.

Bertrand OF, Philippon F, St Pierre A *et al.* Percutaneous mitral valve annuloplasty for functional mitral regurgitation: acute results of the first patient treated with the Viacor permanent device and future perspectives. *Cardiovasc Revasc Med* 2010;**11**:265 e1–8.

Bridgewater B, Keigh B, Kinsman R and Walton P. *Sixth National Adult Cardiac Surgical Database Report 2008*. Society for Cardiothoracic Surgery in Great Britain and Ireland, London, 2008.

Bursi F, Enriquez-Sarano M, Nkomo VT *et al*. Heart failure and death after myocardial infarction in the community; the emerging role of mitral regurgitation. *Circulation* 2005;**111**:295–301.

Feldman T, Kar S, Rinaldi M *et al*. Percutaneous mitral repair with the MitraClip system: safety and midterm durability in the initial EVEREST (Endovascular Valve Edge-to-Edge REpair Study) cohort. *J Am Coll Cardiol* 2009;**54**:686–94.

Gogbashian A, Sepic J, Soltesz EG *et al*. Operative and long-term survival of elderly is significantly improved by mitral valve repair. *Am Heart J* 2006;**151**:1325–33.

Government Statistical Service. *UK National Statistics*, www.statistics.gov.uk (last accessed 12 October 2011).

Habib G, Hoen B, Tornos P *et al*. Guidelines on the prevention, diagnosis and treatment of infective endocarditis (new version 2009): the Task Force on the Prevention, Diagnosis and Treatment of Infective Endocarditis of the European Society of Cardiology (ESC). Endorsed by the European Society of Clinical Microbiology and Infectious Diseases (ESCMID) and the International Society of Chemotherapy (ISC) for Infection and Cancer. *Eur Heart J* 2009;**30**:2369–413.

Iung B, Baron G, Butchart EG *et al*. A prospective survey of patients with valvular heart disease in Europe: the Euro Heart Survey on Valvular Heart Disease. *Eur Heart J* 2003;**24**:1231–43.

Lee JL, Naguwa SM, Cheema GS and Gershwin ME. Acute rheumatic fever and its consequences: a persistent threat to developing nations in the 21st century. *Autoimmun Rev* 2009;**9**:117–23.

Leon MB, Smith CR, Mack M *et al*. Transcatheter aortic-valve implantation for aortic stenosis in patients who cannot undergo surgery. *N Engl J Med* 2010;**363**:1597–607.

Marijon E, Celermajer DS, Tafflet M *et al*. Rheumatic heart disease screening by echocardiography: the inadequacy of World Health Organization criteria for optimising the diagnosis of subclinical disease. *Circulation* 2009;**120**:663–8.

Nashef SA, Roques F, Michel P *et al*. European system for cardiac operative risk evaluation (EuroSCORE). *Eur J Cardiothorac Surg* 1999;**16**:9–13.

Novaro CM, Katz R, Gottdiener JS *et al*. Clinical factors but not C reactive protein predict progression of calcific aortic valve disease: The Cardiovascular Health Study. *J Am Coll Cardiol* 2007;**50**:1992–8.

O'Brien SM, Shahian DM, Filardo G *et al*. The Society of Thoracic Surgeons 2008 cardiac surgery risk models: part 2 – isolated valve surgery. *Ann Thorac Surg* 2009;**88**:S23–42.

Roberts WC and Ko JM. Frequency by decades of unicuspid, bicuspid and tricuspid aortic valves in adults having isolated aortic valve replacement for aortic stenosis with or without associated aortic regurgitation. *Circulation* 2005;**111**:920–5.

Stewart BF, Siscovick D, Lind BK *et al*. Clinical factors associated with calcific aortic valve disease: Cardiovascular Health Study. *J Am Coll Cardiol* 1997;**29**:630–4.

Tuzcu EM, Block PC, Griffin BP *et al*. Immediate and long-term outcome of percutaneous mitral valvotomy in patients 65 years and older. *Circulation* 1992;**85**:963–71.

Vahanian A, Baumgartner H, Bax J *et al*. Guidelines on the management of valvular heart disease: the Task Force on the Management of Valvular Heart Disease of the European Society of Cardiology. *Eur Heart J* 2007;**28**:230–68.

CHAPTER 117

Infections of the central nervous system

Michael Blank[1] and Allan R. Tunkel[2]

[1]Firelands Regional Medical Center, Sandusky, OH, USA

[2]Drexel University College of Medicine, Philadelphia, PA and Monmouth Medical Center, Long Branch, NJ, USA

Meningitis

Viral meningitis

Epidemiology and aetiology

Viruses are the major causes of the aseptic meningitis syndrome, which has been defined as any meningitis (infectious or non-infectious) for which a cause is not apparent after initial evaluation and routine stains and cultures of cerebrospinal fluid (CSF). The most common aetiological agents of the aseptic meningitis syndrome in adults are the non-polio enteroviruses (specifically Coxsackie and echoviruses), which account for 85–95% of cases in which a pathogen is identified.[1] These viruses are worldwide in distribution. In temperate climates, infections occur with a peak incidence in the summer and early autumn. Other viral causes of the aseptic meningitis syndrome include arboviruses (e.g. St Louis encephalitis virus, the California encephalitis group of viruses, West Nile virus and the agent of Colorado tick fever), mumps virus, human immunodeficiency virus (HIV) and the herpes viruses [herpes simplex viruses (HSVs) types 1 and 2 and varicella zoster virus (VZV)]. The DNA of HSV (mostly HSV type 2) has been detected in the CSF of patients with recurrent benign lymphocytic meningitis (formerly known as Mollaret's meningitis).[2]

Clinical presentation

Patients with viral meningitis often present with typical symptoms and signs of meningitis, including headache, meningismus, fever and photophobia.[1,3] Symptoms associated with the causative virus may also be present, such as vomiting and diarrhoea with the enteroviruses, vesicular rash with HSV and a mononucleosis-like syndrome with primary HIV infection. The duration of illness in enteroviral meningitis is usually less than 1 week, with many patients reporting improvement after lumbar puncture, probably as a result of a reduction in intracranial pressure.

Diagnosis

In enteroviral meningitis, lumbar puncture usually reveals a lymphocytic pleocytosis (100–1000 cells mm^{-3}), although there may be a predominance of neutrophils early in the course of infection; however, this quickly gives way to a lymphocytic predominance over the first 6–48 h.[1,3,4] CSF protein is elevated, whereas glucose may be normal or low, although these abnormalities, if present, are usually mild. Similar CSF abnormalities are usually observed in other causes of viral meningitis. Viral cultures are rarely helpful in the aetiological diagnosis of the aseptic meningitis syndrome; in one study of viral cultures on 22 394 CSF samples, virus was recovered from only 5.7% of samples, most of which were enteroviruses (98.4%).[5] Acute and convalescent serum titres may be obtained to identify specific aetiological agents but are not helpful in acute diagnosis and management.

The polymerase chain reaction (PCR) has been shown to be useful in the diagnosis of meningitis due to HSV types 1 and 2 and VZV[3] and may be helpful in the identification of HIV in the CSF or plasma of patients with meningitis following primary infection. Reverse transcription-polymerase chain reaction (RT-PCR) has also been utilized for detecting enteroviral RNA, with sensitivity ranging from 86 to 100% and specificity from 92 to 100% in the diagnosis of enteroviral meningitis.[1,3,4]

Therapy

Viral meningitis is usually a self-limited illness and in the majority of cases only supportive therapy is indicated.[1,3] Pleconaril, a novel compound that integrates into the hydrophobic pocket of picornaviruses, has been shown to have beneficial effects on the clinical, virological, laboratory and radiological parameters in patients with severe enterovirus infections. In one randomized, multi-centre, double-blind, placebo-controlled trial of 607 patients with enteroviral meningitis, pleconaril shortened the course of

Principles and Practice of Geriatric Medicine, Fifth Edition. Edited by Alan J. Sinclair, John E. Morley and Bruno Vellas.

illness especially early in the disease course.[6] Pleconaril, however, has not achieved approval by the US Food and Drug Administration (FDA) because it induces CYP3A enzyme activity and has the potential for drug interactions; therefore, the sponsor has not sought approval. In cases associated with HSV infection (most often an initial infection with HSV type 2), treatment of the genital infection with antiviral therapy (e.g. acyclovir) often results in resolution of the meningitis.

Bacterial meningitis

Epidemiology and aetiology

Although numerous bacterial pathogens have been reported to cause meningitis in the elderly, certain agents are isolated more frequently.[3] *Streptococcus pneumoniae* is the most common cause of bacterial meningitis in the elderly. A contiguous (e.g. sinusitis, otitis media or mastoiditis) or distant (e.g. endocarditis or pneumonia) site of infection is often identified. More serious pneumococcal infections occur in elderly patients and in those with underlying conditions such as asplenia, multiple myeloma, alcoholism, malnutrition, diabetes mellitus and hepatic or renal disease. *S. pneumoniae* is also the most common aetiological agent of meningitis in patients with basilar skull fracture and CSF leak. In the USA, the overall mortality rates for pneumococcal meningitis have ranged from 19 to 26%. In one study of 352 episodes of community-acquired pneumococcal meningitis in adults, 70% of cases were associated with an underlying disorder and the overall in-hospital mortality rate was 30%;[7] in patients aged 60 years or older, death was more likely secondary to systemic complications. For this reason, the 23-valent pneumococcal vaccine is recommended for all patients over the age of 64 years and for those in groups at high risk for serious pneumococcal infection.

Persons at risk for infection (including meningitis) with *Listeria monocytogenes* are the elderly (≥50 years of age), those with underlying malignancy, alcoholics, those receiving corticosteroids, immunosuppressed adults (e.g. transplant recipients) and patients with diabetes mellitus and iron overload disorders.[3] Cases have also been reported in patients receiving treatment with anti-tumour necrosis factor alpha agents. Although *L. monocytogenes* is an unusual cause of bacterial meningitis in the USA, it is associated with high mortality rates (15–29%). Outbreaks of *Listeria* infection have been associated with the consumption of contaminated coleslaw, raw vegetables and milk, with sporadic cases traced to contaminated cheese, turkey franks, alfalfa tablets and processed meats; this points to the intestinal tract as the usual portal of entry. However, the incidence has been decreasing, likely as a result of a decrease in the prevalence of *Listeria* in ready-to-eat foods.

Bacterial meningitis caused by aerobic Gram-negative bacilli (e.g. *Klebsiella* species, *Escherichia coli, Serratia marcescens, Salmonella* and *Pseudomonas aeruginosa*) is found in the elderly, occurring after head trauma or neurosurgical procedures and in patients with Gram-negative bacteraemia.[3,8] Some cases have been associated with disseminated strongyloidiasis in the hyperinfection syndrome, in which meningitis caused by enteric bacteria occurs secondary to seeding of the meninges during persistent or recurrent bacteraemias associated with migration of infective larvae; alternatively, the larvae may carry enteric organisms on their surfaces or within their own gastrointestinal tracts as they exit the intestine and subsequently invade the meninges.

Other bacterial species are less common causes of bacterial meningitis in the elderly.[3] *Neisseria meningitidis* may cause meningitis during epidemics (caused by serogroups A and C) or in sporadic outbreaks (serogroup B), although meningitis caused by this microorganism is more common in children and adults. There is an increased incidence of neisserial infections, including that caused by *N. meningitidis*, in persons with deficiencies of the terminal complement components (C5, C6, C7, C8 and perhaps C9), although the case fatality rates in these patients are lower than in those with an intact complement system. *Hemophilus influenzae* meningitis in elderly adults is associated with concurrent infections such as sinusitis, otitis media and pneumonia and underlying conditions such as chronic obstructive pulmonary disease, asplenia, diabetes mellitus, immunosuppression and head trauma with CSF leak. Meningitis caused by *Staphylococcus aureus* is usually found in the early postneurosurgical period or after head trauma or in patients with CSF shunts; other underlying conditions include diabetes mellitus, alcoholism, chronic renal failure requiring haemodialysis, injection drug use and malignancies. *Staphylococcus epidermidis* is the most common cause of meningitis in patients with CSF shunts. The group B streptococcus (*Streptococcus agalactiae*) may cause meningitis in adults; risk factors include age greater than 60 years, diabetes mellitus, cardiac disease, collagen vascular disorders, malignancy, alcoholism, hepatic failure, renal failure, previous stroke, neurogenic bladder, decubitus ulcers and corticosteroid therapy.

Clinical presentation

The classic symptoms and signs in patients with bacterial meningitis include headache, fever and meningismus; these are seen in more than 85% of patients.[3] In a review of community-acquired meningitis in adults, the classic triad of fever, nuchal rigidity and change in mental status was found in only two-thirds of patients. Other findings include cranial nerve palsies (~10–20%), seizures (~30%) and Kernig's and/or Brudzinski's signs. However, in a prospective study that examined the diagnostic accuracy of meningeal signs in adults with suspected meningitis, the sensitivity of Kernig's sign was 5%, Brudzinski's sign 5% and nuchal rigidity 30%, indicating that the presence of these signs did not accurately distinguish patients with meningitis from those without meningitis. In another review of 696 episodes of community-acquired bacterial meningitis, the triad of fever, neck stiffness and altered mental status was found in only 44% of patients,[9] although 95% presented with at least two of four symptoms (fever, headache, stiff neck, altered mental status).

However, elderly patients with bacterial meningitis, especially those with underlying conditions (e.g. diabetes mellitus or cardiopulmonary disease), may present insidiously with lethargy, confusion, anorexia, no fever and variable signs of meningeal inflammation.[3] In one review, confusion was very common in elderly patients on initial examination and occurred in 92 and 78% of those with pneumococcal and Gram-negative bacillary meningitis, respectively. There may be a history of an antecedent or concurrent illness such as sinusitis, otitis media or pneumonia. In the elderly patient, an altered or changed mental status should not be ascribed to other causes until bacterial meningitis has been excluded by CSF examination.

Diagnosis

The diagnosis of bacterial meningitis rests with CSF examination following lumbar puncture.[3] CSF characteristics of bacterial meningitis include an elevated opening pressure in virtually all patients. The white blood cell count is elevated in untreated bacterial meningitis (usually 1000–5000 cells mm^{-3}) with a neutrophilic predominance, although lymphocytes may predominate in *L. monocytogenes* meningitis (~30% of cases). Elevated protein (100–500 mg dl^{-1}) and decreased glucose (<40 mg dl^{-1}) levels are also typically observed; a CSF: serum glucose level of ≤ 0.4 mg dl^{-1} is found in the majority of patients with acute bacterial meningitis.

The CSF Gram stain provides rapid and accurate identification of the causative organism in 60–90% of patients with bacterial meningitis, with a specificity of almost 100%. Bacteria are observed in 90% of cases of meningitis caused by *S. pneumoniae*, but in only about one-third of patients with *L. monocytogenes* meningitis.[3] CSF cultures are positive in 70–85% of patients overall. The probability of identifying the organism in CSF cultures may decrease in patients who have received prior antimicrobial therapy.

Several rapid diagnostic tests are available to aid in the aetiological diagnosis of bacterial meningitis.[3] Latex agglutination tests detect the antigens of *H. influenzae* type b, *S. pneumoniae, N. meningitidis, E. coli* K1 and *S. agalactiae*. The overall sensitivity ranges from 50 to 100% (somewhat lower for *N. meningitidis* because of the limited immunogenicity of the group B meningococcal polysaccharide), although these tests are highly specific. However, the routine use of latex agglutination for the aetiological diagnosis of bacterial meningitis has recently been questioned and is no longer routinely recommended, because the results do not appear to modify the decision to administer appropriate antimicrobial therapy and false-positive tests have been reported.[10] Latex agglutination may be most useful for the patient who has been pretreated with antimicrobial therapy and whose CSF Gram stain and cultures are negative, although it must be emphasized that a negative test does not rule out infection by a specific meningeal pathogen. An immunochromatographic test for the detection of *S. pneumoniae* in CSF has been found to have an overall sensitivity of 95–100% in the diagnosis of pneumococcal meningitis,[11] but more studies are needed to assess the usefulness of this test.

Nucleic acid amplification tests (e.g. PCR) have been used to amplify DNA from patients with bacterial meningitis caused by several pathogens. In one study, broad-based PCR demonstrated a sensitivity of 100%, a specificity of 98.2%, a positive predictive value of 98.2% and a negative predictive value of 100%.[3] The sensitivity and specificity of PCR in CSF for the diagnosis of pneumococcal meningitis are 92–100% and 100%, respectively.[11] There are some problems with false-positive results, but further refinements in PCR may demonstrate its usefulness in the diagnosis of bacterial meningitis in patients who have already received antibiotics and when the CSF Gram stain, bacterial antigen tests and cultures are negative.

Antimicrobial therapy

In patients suspected of having bacterial meningitis, blood cultures should be obtained and a lumbar puncture done immediately. If purulent meningitis is present, targeted antimicrobial therapy should be initiated on the basis of results of Gram staining (i.e. vancomycin and a third-generation cephalosporin if Gram-positive diplococci are seen). However, if no aetiological agent can be identified or if there is a delay in the performance of the lumbar puncture, empirical antimicrobial therapy should be initiated on the basis of the patient's age and the underlying disease status.[3,10] In patients who are immunosuppressed and have a history of central nervous system (CNS) disease, focal neurological deficits or seizures or if papilloedema is found on funduscopic examination, a computed tomographic (CT) scan is recommended prior to lumbar puncture, with empirical antimicrobial therapy initiated before scanning. Empirical therapy for elderly patients with suspected community-acquired bacterial meningitis should include vancomycin, ampicillin and a third-generation cephalosporin (see the following text for specific recommendations). Once the meningeal pathogen has been identified, antimicrobial therapy can be modified for optimal treatment (Table 117.1); recommended dosages for CNS infections are shown in Table 117.2.

For the treatment of bacterial meningitis in elderly persons, choices of antimicrobial therapy should be based on prevalent trends in antimicrobial susceptibility. For meningitis caused by *S. pneumoniae*, therapy in recent years has been significantly altered by changes in pneumococcal susceptibility patterns.[3,10] Numerous reports from around the world have documented strains of pneumococci that are of intermediate susceptibility [minimal inhibitory concentration (MIC) range $0.1–1.0\,\mu g\,ml^{-1}$] and highly (MIC $\geq 2.0\,\mu g\,ml^{-1}$) resistant to penicillin G; susceptible strains have MICs $\leq 0.06\,\mu g\,ml^{-1}$. On the basis of these trends and because achievable CSF concentrations of penicillin are inadequate to treat these resistant isolates, penicillin can never be recommended as empirical therapy for patients with suspected or proven pneumococcal meningitis, pending results of susceptibility testing. As an empirical regimen, we recommend the combination of vancomycin plus a third-generation cephalosporin (either cefotaxime or ceftriaxone). If the isolate is susceptible to penicillin, high-dose intravenous penicillin G or ampicillin is adequate. If the isolate is of intermediate susceptibility to penicillin, only the third-generation cephalosporin need be continued. However, if the pneumococcal isolate is highly resistant to penicillin, the combination of vancomycin and the third-generation cephalosporin should be continued, because vancomycin therapy alone may not be optimal therapy for patients with pneumococcal meningitis. Any patient who is not improving as expected or has a pneumococcal isolate for which the cefotaxime/ceftriaxone MIC is $\geq 2.0\,\mu g\,ml^{-1}$ should undergo a repeat lumbar puncture to document sterility of CSF after 36–48 h of therapy;[10] this may be especially important for patients who are also receiving adjunctive dexamethasone therapy (see the following text). Some experts have also recommended the addition of rifampin for these highly resistant strains, although clinical data are lacking. In patients not responding, administration of vancomycin by the intraventricular or intrathecal route is a reasonable adjunct. Newer fluoroquinolones (e.g. moxifloxacin) that have *in vitro* activity against *S. pneumoniae* may have utility in the treatment of pneumococcal meningitis;[3,10] the newer fluoroquinolones (specifically moxifloxacin), combined with either a third-generation cephalosporin or vancomycin, may emerge as an option in the treatment of bacterial meningitis.

Adjunctive therapy

Despite the availability of effective antimicrobial therapy, the mortality and morbidity from bacterial meningitis have not changed significantly over the past 30 years. A major factor contributing to increased morbidity and mortality is the generation of a subarachnoid space inflammatory response following antimicrobial-induced bacterial lysis;[3] therefore, several clinical trials were performed to examine the effectiveness of adjunctive dexamethasone in attenuating this inflammatory response in patients with bacterial meningitis. Most of these studies were conducted in infants and children with predominantly *H. influenzae* type b meningitis and supported the routine use of adjunctive dexamethasone in this patient population.[3,10] In a prospective, randomized, double-blind trial in 301 adults with bacterial meningitis, adjunctive dexamethasone was associated with a reduction in the proportion of patients who had unfavourable outcomes and in the proportion of patients who died; the benefits were most striking in the subgroup of patients with pneumococcal meningitis and in those with moderate-to severe disease as assessed by the admission Glasgow Coma Scale score. Despite these results, the use of adjunctive dexamethasone in the treatment of bacterial meningitis in the developing world has been more controversial. In one randomized, double-blind, placebo-controlled trial in adolescents and adults in Vietnam with confirmed bacterial meningitis (most often caused by *Streptococcus suis*), adjunctive dexamethasone was associated with reduction in the risk of death or disability.[12] In contrast, in another randomized, double-blind, placebo-controlled trial in Malawi, there were no significant differences in mortality;[13] however, in this trial, almost 90% of patients were infected with HIV and most had advanced disease. These data suggest that adjunctive dexamethasone is not beneficial in patients in resource-poor countries when a substantial number of patients are infected with HIV.

On the basis of these data and the apparent absence of serious adverse outcomes in the patients who received dexamethasone, the routine use of adjunctive dexamethasone ($0.15\,mg\,kg^{-1}$ every 6 h for 4 days, given concomitantly with or just prior to the first dose of an antimicrobial agent for maximum attenuation of the subarachnoid space inflammatory response) is warranted in adults with suspected or proven pneumococcal meningitis.[10] Adjunctive dexamethasone should not be used in patients who have already received antimicrobial therapy; if the meningitis is subsequently found not to be caused by *S. pneumoniae*, dexamethasone should be discontinued, although some experts recommend the use of adjunctive dexamethasone regardless of the microbial aetiology. However, the use of adjunctive dexamethasone is of particular concern in patients with pneumococcal meningitis caused by highly penicillin-resistant strains, since a diminished inflammatory response may significantly impair CSF vancomycin penetration. In an experimental model of *S. pneumoniae* meningitis in rabbits, the concurrent use of dexamethasone with vancomycin decreased the penetration of vancomycin into the CSF and also decreased the rate of bactericidal activity of vancomycin. However, appropriate CSF concentrations of vancomycin may be achieved when

Table 117.1 Specific antimicrobial therapy for meningitis.

Microorganism	Standard therapy	Alternative therapies
Bacteria		
Streptococcus pneumoniae		
Penicillin MIC $<0.1\,\mu g\,ml^{-1}$	Penicillin G or ampicillin	Third-generation cephalosporin[a]; vancomycin
Penicillin MIC $0.1{-}1.0\,\mu g\,ml^{-1}$	Third-generation cephalosporin[a]	Meropenem; vancomycin
Penicillin MIC $\geq 2.0\,\mu g\,ml^{-1}$	Vancomycin plus a third-generation cephalosporin[a,b]	Third-generation cephalosporin[a] + moxifloxacin
Enterobacteriaceae	Third-generation cephalosporin[a]	Aztreonam; fluoroquinolone; trimethoprim–sulfamethoxazole; meropenem
Pseudomonas aeruginosa	Ceftazidime[c] or cefepime[c]	Aztreonam[c]; fluoroquinolone[c]; meropenem[c]
Listeria monocytogenes	Ampicillin[c] or penicillin G[c]	Trimethoprim–sulfamethoxazole
Hemophilus influenzae		
β-Lactamase-negative	Ampicillin	Third-generation cephalosporin[a]; cefepime; chloramphenicol; aztreonam
β- Lactamase-positive	Third-generation cephalosporin[a]	Cefepime, chloramphenicol; aztreonam; fluoroquinolone
Neisseria meningitidis		
Penicillin MIC $<0.1\,\mu g\,ml^{-1}$	Penicillin G or ampicillin	Third-generation cephalosporin[a]; chloramphenicol; fluoroquinolone
Penicillin MIC $0.1{-}1.0\,\mu g\,ml^{-1}$	Third-generation cephalosporin[a]	Chloramphenicol; fluoroquinolone; meropenem
Streptococcus agalactiae	Ampicillin[c] or penicillin G[c]	Third-generation cephalosporin[a]; vancomycin
Staphylococcus aureus		
Methicillin-sensitive	Nafcillin or oxacillin	Vancomycin; meropenem; linezolid; daptomycin
Methicillin-resistant	Vancomycin	Trimethoprim–sulfamethoxazole; linezolid; daptomycin
Staphylococcus epidermidis	Vancomycin[b]	Linezolid
Myobacteria		
Mycobacterium tuberculosis	Isoniazid + rifampin + pyrazinamide + ethambutol	Ethionamide; streptomycin; fluoroquinolone
Spirochetes		
Treponema pallidum	Penicillin G	Doxycycline[d]; ceftriaxone[d]
Borrelia burgdorferi	Third-generation cephalosporin[a]	Penicillin; doxycycline
Fungi		
Cryptococcus neoformans	Amphotericin B deoxycholate[f] + 5-flucytosine	Fluconazole
Candida species	Amphotericin B deoxycholate ± 5-flucytosine	Fluconazole[d]
Coccidioides immitis	Fluconazole	Amphotericin B[e]; itraconazole; voriconazole

[a]Cefotaxime or ceftriaxone.
[b]Addition of rifampin should be considered; see text for details.
[c]Addition of an aminoglycoside should be considered.
[d]The value of these antimicrobial agents has not been established.
[e]Intravenous and intraventricular administration.
[f]See text for indications of utilizing a lipid formulation of amphotericin B.

Table 117.2 Recommended dosages of selected antimicrobial agents for central nervous system infections in adults with normal renal and hepatic function.

Antimicrobial agent	Total daily dose	Dosing interval (h)
Acyclovir	30 mg kg^{-1}	8
Amikacin[a]	15 mg kg^{-1} ←	8
Amphotericin B deoxycholate[b]	0.6–1.0 mg kg^{-1}	24
Amphotericin B lipid formulation	5 mg kg^{-1}	24
Ampicillin	12 g	4
Aztreonam	6–8 g	6–8
Cefepime	6 g	8
Cefotaxime	8–12 g	4–6
Ceftazidime	6 g	8
Ceftriaxone	4 g	12–24
Chloramphenicol[c]	4–6 g	6
Ciprofloxacin	800–1200 mg	8–12
Fluconazole	400–800 mg	24
Flucytosine[d,e]	100 mg kg^{-1}	6
Gentamicin[a]	5 mg kg^{-1}	8
Imipenem	2 g	6
Liposomal amphotericin B (AmBisome)	5 mg kg^{-1}	24
Meropenem	6 g	8
Metronidazole	30 mg kg^{-1}	6
Nafcillin	9–12 g	4
Oxacillin	9–12 g	4
Penicillin G	24 million units	4
Rifampicin (rifampin)	600 mg	24
Tobramycin[a]	5 mg kg^{-1}	8
Trimethoprim–sulfamethoxazole[f]	10–20 mg kg^{-1}	6–12
Vancomycin[g]	30–60 mg kg^{-1}	8–12
Voriconazole[h]	8 mg kg^{-1}	12

[a]Need to monitor peak and trough serum concentrations.
[b]Can increase dosage to 1.5 mg kg^{-1} per day in severely ill patients.
[c]Higher dose recommended for pneumococcal meningitis.
[d]Oral administration.
[e]Maintain serum concentrations from 50 to 100 µg ml^{-1}.
[f]Dosage based on trimethoprim component.
[g]May need to monitor cerebrospinal fluid concentrations in severely ill patients.
[h]Load with 6 mg kg^{-1} i.v. every 12 h for two doses.

patients are receiving adequate dosing of vancomycin; in one study of 14 patients with pneumococcal meningitis, administration of vancomycin at a continuous infusion of 60 mg kg^{-1} per day, after a 15 mg kg^{-1} loading dose, led to a mean CSF concentration of 7.2 µg ml^{-1}.[14] In patients with pneumococcal meningitis caused by strains that are highly resistant to penicillin or cephalosporins, careful observation and follow-up are critical to determine whether the use of adjunctive dexamethasone is associated with adverse clinical outcome in these patients.

Tuberculous meningitis

Epidemiology and aetiology

Almost all cases of tuberculous meningitis are caused by *Mycobacterium tuberculosis*. Risk factors for the development of tuberculous meningitis include a history of prior tuberculous disease, advanced age, homelessness, alcoholism, gastrectomy, diabetes mellitus and immunosuppression.[15] HIV infection has influenced the epidemiology of tuberculosis, in which extrapulmonary disease occurs in more than 70% of patients with AIDS, but in only 24–45% of patients with tuberculosis and less advanced HIV infection.

Clinical presentation

Tuberculous meningitis often has a subacute, indolent presentation with a prodrome characterized by malaise, low-grade fever, headache and personality changes;[15,16] this is followed by a meningitic phase with worsening headache, meningismus, nausea, vomiting and waxing-and-waning mental status. A history of prior clinical tuberculosis is obtained in fewer than 20% of cases. Up to 30% of patients have focal neurological signs on presentation, usually consisting of unilateral or, less commonly, bilateral cranial nerve palsies [cranial nerve (CN) VI is the most frequently affected]. Hemiparesis may result from ischaemic infarction, most commonly in the distribution of the territory of the middle cerebral artery. In one study of 122 patients with tuberculous meningitis, stroke was found in 45% and manifested anywhere from the time of initial presentation to months after the start of therapy.[17]

Diagnosis

CSF examination in patients with tuberculous meningitis often reveals a lymphocytic pleocytosis (5–500 cells mm^{-3}), although early in the course of disease there may be a mix of both lymphocytes and neutrophils.[15,16] Following treatment with antituberculous drugs, a so called 'therapeutic paradox' may develop with a change in the white blood cell differential from a lymphocytic to a neutrophilic predominance. There is usually an elevated CSF protein (median of 150–200 mg dl^{-1}) and often a very low glucose (<20 mg dl^{-1}, although the median value is 40 mg dl^{-1}). Because of the small number of organisms present in the CSF, acid-fast bacilli (AFB) smears are often negative (fewer than 25% of smears are positive).

On the basis of these poor results, several rapid diagnostic tests are under development to aid in the diagnosis of tuberculous meningitis. Although PCR testing, which can detect *M. tuberculosis* DNA in CSF specimens, is promising; the lack of standardization makes interpretation difficult[16,18] and older assays had varying sensitivities (33–90%) and specificities (80–100%). Newer PCR assays have improved sensitivity for the diagnosis of tuberculous meningitis. Although largely experimental, detection of specific CSF antigens and antibodies is another way in which tuberculous meningitis may be diagnosed.

CT and magnetic resonance (MR) scanning may be useful to support the diagnosis of tuberculous meningitis.[15,16] Hydrocephalus is frequently present at diagnosis or develops during the course of infection. The presence of basal cistern enhancement is also supportive evidence for the diagnosis. MR may be superior to CT in the identification of basilar meningeal inflammation and small tuberculoma formation.

Antimicrobial therapy

Therapy for tuberculous meningitis is often initiated on the basis of the patient's clinical presentation, as cultures may take weeks to become positive and may remain negative in up to 20% of patients. Therapy with isoniazid, rifampin, ethambutol and pyrazinamide for 2 months, followed by isoniazid and rifampin for 7–10 months, should be adequate for patients with drug-sensitive tuberculous meningitis.[16,18] In HIV-infected patients, therapy is continued for at least 12 months. However, therapy for tuberculous meningitis may need to be individualized, with longer durations in patients with a higher severity of illness. For patients with suspected tuberculous meningitis caused by multidrug-resistant strains, at least five drugs should be used pending susceptibility testing. The fluoroquinolones (e.g. moxifloxacin) penetrate well into CSF and have good *in vitro* activity against *M. tuberculosis*. Most authorities recommend continuing therapy for a total of 18–24 months in patients with multidrug-resistant tuberculous meningitis.

Adjunctive Therapy

Corticosteroids have been shown to be of value as adjunctive therapy in tuberculous meningitis with resolution of fevers, improved mental status and, most importantly, the ability to treat or avert the development of spinal block.[15,16,18] Despite some controversy, most authorities recommend the use of corticosteroids in patients with tuberculous meningitis. Recommended therapy is prednisone $1\,mg\,kg^{-1}$ per day slowly tapered over 1 month, although varying doses of dexamethasone or hydrocortisone have also been used. In a randomized, double-blind, placebo-controlled trial in Vietnam in patients with tuberculous meningitis, adjunctive dexamethasone improved survival in patients over 14 years of age,[19] although it probably did not prevent severe disability. A systematic review of published studies has noted a decreased risk of death or disabling residual neurological deficits in patients with tuberculous meningitis who received adjunctive dexamethasone therapy.[20]

Spirochetal meningitis

Epidemiology and aetiology

Treponema pallidum (the aetiological agent of syphilis) disseminates to the CNS early during infection, with CSF abnormalities detected in 5–9% of patients with seronegative primary syphilis.[21] The overall incidence of neurosyphilis has increased in association with HIV infection; in one report, 44% of all patients with neurosyphilis had AIDS and 1.5% of AIDS patients were found to have neurosyphilis at some point during the course of their illness.

Approximately 10–15% of patients with Lyme disease will develop signs and symptoms of meningitis, usually early in the course of infection.[22] Infection with *Borrelia burgdorferi* should be suspected in a patient with meningitis in association with other symptoms of Lyme disease, such as erythema migrans, malaise, myalgias and arthralgias. Meningitis usually follows erythema migrans by 2–10 weeks, although only about 40% (range 10–90%) of cases of Lyme meningitis are preceded by this characteristic rash.

Clinical presentation

There are four categories of CNS involvement with *T. pallidum*.[21] Syphilitic meningitis occurs within the first 2 years of infection, with symptoms of headache, nausea, vomiting and less frequently fevers, meningismus and mental status changes. Meningovascular syphilis (found in 10–12% of individuals with CNS involvement), occurring months to years after infection, results in focal neurological findings as a result of focal syphilitic arteritis, which almost always occurs in association with meningeal inflammation; focal deficits may progress to a stroke syndrome with attendant irreversible neurological deficits. Parenchymatous neurosyphilis (10–20 years after infection) manifests as general paresis and tabes dorsalis. Gummatous disease is very rare and generally occurs more than 30 years following initial infection. Coinfection with HIV may alter the clinical course of syphilis, in which patients may be more likely to progress to neurosyphilis and show accelerated disease courses.

Symptoms of CNS infection with *B. burgdorferi* include headache, fever, meningismus, nausea and vomiting.[22] Up to 50% of patients will develop cranial nerve palsies, most commonly involving CN VII; facial nerve palsy is bilateral in 30–70% of patients, although the two sides are affected asynchronously in most cases. In untreated patients the duration of symptoms is 1–9 months and patients typically experience recurrent attacks of meningeal symptoms lasting several weeks, alternating with similar periods of milder symptoms. About half of the patients with Lyme meningitis have mild cerebral symptoms, consisting of somnolence, emotional lability, depression, impaired memory and concentration and behavioural symptoms.

Diagnosis

CSF findings in patients with CNS syphilis are non-specific, revealing a mononuclear pleocytosis (>10 cells mm^{-3} in most patients), elevated protein and a normal or slightly decreased glucose.[21] A reactive VDRL (venereal disease research laboratory) slide test in the CSF has a sensitivity of only 30–70% for the diagnosis of neurosyphilis (although the specificity is high). The treatment for neurosyphilis is indicated in the presence of any of the above abnormalities in association with the appropriate clinical setting. The fluorescent treponemal antibody absorption test (FTA-ABS) in the CSF has been examined as a possible diagnostic test for neurosyphilis; a non-reactive test effectively rules out the likelihood of neurosyphilis, although a positive test may result from leakage of small amounts of antibody absorption from the serum into CSF, making it less specific than the CSF VDRL.

The best currently available laboratory test for the diagnosis of Lyme disease is the demonstration of specific serum antibody to *B. burgdorferi*, in which a positive test in a patient with a compatible neurological abnormality is strong evidence for the diagnosis.[22] It is currently recommended that when the pretest probability of Lyme disease is 0.20–0.80, sequential testing with enzyme-linked immunosorbent assay (ELISA) and Western blot is the most accurate method for ruling in or out the possibility of Lyme disease. The sensitivity and specificity of two-tier testing in one study of patients with later manifestations of Lyme disease were 100% and 99%, respectively.[23] A lymphocytic pleocytosis (usually <500 cells mm^{-3}) is observed in the CSF, along with elevated protein and normal glucose in patients with Lyme meningitis. Antibodies and antigens to *B. burgdorferi* may be detected in the CSF by ELISA or Western blot, respectively, although antibody tests are not standardized with marked variability between laboratories. One study of 123 patients with anti-*Borrelia* antibody in CSF found that determination of the antibody index had a sensitivity of 75% and a specificity of 97% for diagnosis, although another aetiology was responsible for symptoms in 60% of patients.[24] PCR may be a useful tool for the detection of *B. burgdorferi* DNA in CSF, although PCR must still be considered experimental in the diagnosis of CNS Lyme disease.

Antimicrobial therapy

Treatment for neurosyphilis is intravenous penicillin G 18–24 million units per day in divided doses every 4 h for 10–14 days.[21] No large studies have been performed to evaluate alternative antimicrobial agents for the therapy of neurosyphilis; the tetracyclines, chloramphenicol and ceftriaxone may have potential clinical utility based on case reports, clinical experience and extrapolations from experimental animal studies. Although follow-up lumbar puncture every 6 months until the CSF changes have normalized is recommended, one recent study demonstrated that in most patients treated for neurosyphilis, normalization of the serum RPR (rapid plasma reagin) correctly predicted the success of therapy and normalization of CSF parameters after treatment.[25]

Treatment of Lyme meningitis is intravenous ceftriaxone 2 g per day for 14 days (range 10–28 days);[26] the literature contains no agreement on the duration of therapy or on the minimum adequate dose of the antimicrobial. At present, there is no evidence to support treatment durations longer than 4 weeks.

Fungal meningitis

Epidemiology and aetiology

Cryptococcus neoformans is the most common fungal cause of clinically recognized meningitis, with most cases seen in immunocompromised patients, including those with AIDS, transplant recipients and those receiving chronic corticosteroids.[27] Other underlying conditions with an increased risk for cryptococcal disease include sarcoidosis, collagen vascular disorders (e.g. systemic lupus erythematosus), chronic renal and hepatic failure and diabetes mellitus; *C. neoformans* meningitis has also been documented in apparently healthy individuals.

Meningitis due to *Candida* species is relatively rare and is often associated with disseminated disease. Risk factors include malignancy, neutropenia, chronic granulomatous disease, the presence of central venous catheters, diabetes mellitus, hyperalimentation and corticosteroid therapy.[27]

Coccidioides immitis is a fungus endemic to the semi-arid regions and the desert areas of southwestern USA. Extrapulmonary disease develops in 1–5% of symptomatic patients, although, of those, one-third to one-half have meningeal involvement. Dissemination is associated with extremes of age, male gender, non-white race and immunosuppression (e.g. corticosteroid therapy, organ transplantation, HIV infection and treatment with inhibitors of tumour necrosis factor alpha).[27–29]

Clinical presentation

Clinical presentation of cryptococcal meningitis can vary. Most patients present with signs and symptoms of subacute meningitis or meningoencephalitis, such as headache, fever, cranial nerve palsies, lethargy, coma or memory loss over several weeks.[27] HIV-infected patients with cryptococcal meningitis exhibit few differences at presentation from those without HIV. However, several clinical aspects may be more prominent in patients with AIDS given that the burden of yeast in this population is generally higher. However, AIDS patients may present with very minimal symptoms in which the only clinical findings may be fever, headache and lethargy; cranial nerve palsies are often absent. Ocular abnormalities (e.g. cranial nerve palsies and papilloedema) occur in about 45% of patients.

Patients with *Candida* meningitis may present either abruptly or insidiously.[27] Symptoms include fever, headache and meningismus; patients may also have depressed mental status, confusion, cranial nerve palsies and focal neurological signs. The presentation is often similar to that observed with bacterial meningitis.

Meningeal infection with *C. immitis* most often follows a subacute or chronic course.[27–29] Previously healthy people with meningitis may present with the indolent onset of headache that is present for weeks or months at time of diagnosis. The patient may recall the initial infection as a period of fever and cough occurring 2–4 weeks following exposure. Other symptoms include nausea, photophobia, neck pain and stiffness, confusion, declines in cognition or memory, emotional lability and hearing or visual changes. Immunosuppressed patients, including those with AIDS, are more likely to present with a systemic illness, including fever, headache, profound malaise and lesions in the bone or skin.

Diagnosis

In most non-AIDS patients with cryptococcal meningitis, examination of the CSF reveals an elevated opening pressure, lymphocytic pleocytosis (range 20–500 cells mm^{-3}), elevated protein and normal or decreased glucose.[27] AIDS patients with cryptococcal meningitis may have very low or even normal CSF white blood cell counts; 65% of patients have fewer than 5 cells mm^{-3} in CSF. India ink examination is positive in up to 50–75% of patients with cryptococcal meningitis and the rate of positivity is even higher (~88%) in AIDS patients. As the India ink examination is difficult to perform and rates of positivity are dependent upon the experience of the laboratory, the latex agglutination test for cryptococcal polysaccharide antigen in the CSF should be performed and is both sensitive and specific for the diagnosis of cryptococcal meningitis. A presumptive diagnosis is indicated by a titre of ≥1:8. The presence of cryptococcal antigen in the serum is also supportive evidence for the diagnosis and may be detected in severely immunocompromised patients (i.e. those with AIDS); however, the value of the serum cryptococcal polysaccharide antigen for screening patients suspected of having meningeal disease has not been established. Routine fungal cultures of the CSF are often positive.

Examination of the CSF in patients with *Candida* meningitis typically shows a mixture of neutrophils and lymphocytes, elevated protein and decreased glucose. Yeast cells are seen on smear in ~40% of patients, with fungal cultures positive in most cases.

CSF examination in coccidioidal meningitis reveals a pleocytosis, occasionally showing a prominent eosinophilia.[27–29] Unfortunately, only about 15% of patients have positive CSF cultures. Enzyme immunoassay and immunodiffusion methods are commonly used for the detection of both IgM and IgG antibody groups; although positive serological results are helpful in diagnosis, negative results cannot be used to rule out disease. Elevated serum concentrations of complement-fixing antibodies (titres in excess of 1:32–1:64) suggest dissemination. CSF complement-fixing antibodies are present in at least 70% of patients with early meningitis and from virtually all patients as disease progresses, although antibodies may fail to develop in the serum or CSF of patients with immunodeficiencies. When present, the antibody titres appear to parallel the course of meningeal disease.

Antimicrobial therapy

The treatment for cryptococcal meningitis in non-AIDS patients is amphotericin B deoxycholate with 5-flucytosine for at least 4 weeks of induction therapy;[30] the 4 week combination regimen can be used in the subset of patients who, at presentation, have no neurological complications and CSF yeast culture results that are negative after 2 weeks of treatment. In patients experiencing toxicity to amphotericin B deoxycholate, a lipid formulation of amphotericin B may be substituted in the second 2 weeks. In patients with neurological complications, consideration should be given to extending induction therapy for a total of 6 weeks and a lipid formulation of amphotericin B can be given for the last 4 weeks. This is followed by consolidation therapy with fluconazole for 8 weeks and then maintenance therapy of 200 mg daily for 6–12 months.

In AIDS patients with cryptococcal meningitis, amphotericin B deoxycholate with 5-flucytosine for at least 2 weeks of induction therapy is recommended, followed by fluconazole consolidation therapy for a minimum period of 8 weeks.[30] A lipid formulation of amphotericin B can be substituted for amphotericin B deoxycholate among patients with or predisposed to renal dysfunction. Chronic suppressive therapy with fluconazole (200 mg daily) is then continued indefinitely in patients with AIDS to prevent relapse, although discontinuation of suppressive therapy can be considered in patients on antiretroviral therapy with CD4 cell counts >100 mm^{-3} and an undetectable or very low HIV RNA level sustained for ≥3 months (minimum of 12 months of antifungal therapy).

Treatment for meningitis caused by *Candida* species is amphotericin B, with or without 5-flucytosine.[27] Although there have been no studies comparing the efficacy of single versus combination therapy, some investigators recommend combination therapy based on more rapid CSF sterilization and possible reduction of long-term neurological sequelae.

In the management of coccidioidal meningitis, most patients are now treated initially with fluconazole; in one study the response rate was 79%, although 24% of patients exhibited a persistent CSF pleocytosis despite the relative absence of symptoms.[29] On the basis of these results, fluconazole (800–1200 mg daily) is recommended as first-line therapy for coccidioidal meningitis;[28,29,31] itraconazole and voriconazole can be considered as alternative agents, although few data are available. Therapy may need to be continued indefinitely. In patients who fail azole therapy, amphotericin B deoxycholate may be administered both intravenously and intrathecally. Intrathecal administration may be via the lumbar, cisternal or ventricular route (i.e. through an Ommaya reservoir). The usual dosage is 0.5 mg three times weekly for 3 months, although 1.0–1.5 mg combined with hydrocortisone can be used. Antifungal therapy is discontinued once the CSF has been normal for at least 1 year on an intrathecal regimen of once every 6 weeks.

Adjunctive therapy

Increased intracranial pressure and hydrocephalus have been noted in AIDS patients with cryptococcal meningitis. In patients with symptoms of increased intracranial pressure and CSF pressure $\geq$25 cmH_2O during induction therapy, relief of CSF pressure by lumbar puncture is recommended; persistent elevations may require repeat lumbar puncture daily or consideration of temporary placement of a percutaneous lumbar drain or ventriculostomy.[30] Permanent ventriculoperitoneal shunting should be utilized only if the patient has received appropriate antifungal therapy and if more conservative measures to control elevated intracranial pressure have failed.

Focal central nervous system infections

Brain abscess

Epidemiology and aetiology

Bacterial brain abscesses may be due to a single organism or may be polymicrobial in origin.[32] Clues to the likely aetiological agents may be found in the patient's history. Streptococci (aerobic, anaerobic and microaerophilic) are identified in up to 70% of patients. They are normal inhabitants of the oral cavity, gastrointestinal tract and female genital tract. Although streptococcal brain abscesses are seen most often in patients with otopharyngeal infections or infective endocarditis, they are isolated after neurosurgical or other medical procedures. Staphylococci are found in 10–20% of patients, usually those with a history of trauma or injection drug use. *Bacteroides* and *Prevotella* species are identified in 20–40% of patients, often in mixed cultures. Enteric Gram-negative bacilli are isolated in 23–33% of patients with brain abscess, often in patients with otitic foci of infection, septicaemia, following neurosurgical procedures or in those who are immunocompromised. Other bacteria (*S. pneumoniae, H. influenzae* and *L. monocytogenes*) are seen much less frequently (<1% of cases). Patients with defects in cell-mediated immunity (e.g. patients with AIDS, transplant recipients and those receiving corticosteroids) have an increased incidence of brain abscess caused by *Nocardia* species. *Mycobacterium tuberculosis* and non-tuberculous mycobacteria have been increasingly observed to cause focal CNS lesions, with several cases reported in patients with HIV infection.

Brain abscesses caused by *Aspergillus* species are seen in patients with haematological malignancies and those with prolonged neutropenia; other risk groups include patients with Cushing syndrome, diabetes mellitus and hepatic disease.[32,33] Risk factors for development of cerebral mucormycosis include patients with diabetes mellitus (especially in association with diabetic ketoacidosis), haematological malignancies, transplant recipients and corticosteroid or deferoxamine use. Infection caused by either agent may result from direct extension of rhinocerebral disease or from haematogenous spread from a distant focus of infection.

Clinical presentation

Symptoms in patients with bacterial brain abscess result from the presence of a space-occupying lesion and include headache (~70% of cases), nausea, vomiting and seizures.[32] Many patients also experience a change in mental status, ranging from lethargy to coma. Fever is found in only 45–50% of patients. Sudden worsening of the headache, accompanied by a new onset of meningismus, may signify rupture of the abscess into the ventricular space. The clinical presentation also depends upon the location of the abscess. Frontal lobe involvement may result in headache, drowsiness, inattention, hemiparesis, and/or motor disorders. Ataxia, nystagmus and vomiting indicate a cerebellar lesion, while an abscess of the temporal lobe produces headache, aphasia and visual field defects. Involvement of the brainstem may result in cranial nerve palsies, headache, fever and vomiting.

Fungal brain abscesses often present with symptoms similar to those of bacterial brain abscess (see the preceding text).[32,33] However, some differences do exist. *Aspergillus* species have a tendency to invade blood vessels and patients may present with signs and symptoms of cerebral infarction. In patients with rhinocerebral mucormycosis, symptoms may be referable to the eyes and sinuses in which patients present with headache, diplopia and nasal discharge. Physical examination may show nasal ulcers or discharge, proptosis, and/or external ophthalmoplegia. Approximately 60% of patients will have orbital involvement and there is an increased incidence of development of cavernous sinus thrombosis.

Diagnosis

Radiological techniques, such as CT and MR, have revolutionized the diagnosis of brain abscess.[32] CT characteristically reveals a hypodense lesion with peripheral ring enhancement; there may also be a surrounding area of decreased attenuation due to cerebral oedema. MR offers significant advantages over CT in the diagnosis of brain abscess, including early detection of cerebritis, detection of cerebral oedema with greater contrast between oedema and the brain, more conspicuous spread of inflammation into the ventricles and subarachnoid space and the earlier detection of satellite lesions. Contrast enhancement with the paramagnetic agent gadolinium diethylenetriaminepentaacetic acid provides the added advantage of clearly differentiating the central abscess, surrounding enhancing rim and cerebral oedema surrounding the abscess.

In abscesses caused by *Aspergillus* species, radiographic studies (CT or MR) may show evidence of infarction with surrounding abscess formation. In mucormycosis, there may be bony erosion, sinus opacification and evidence of cavernous sinus thrombosis.

CT has also been useful to permit stereotactic guided aspiration of brain abscesses to obtain tissue for microbiological diagnosis.[32] Samples should be sent for Gram stain, aerobic and anaerobic culture and smears and cultures for AFB and fungi. If there is a clinical suspicion of *Nocardia* infection, a modified AFB stain should also be done. Recently, the use of multiple 16S ribosomal DNA sequences was found to increase dramatically the number of infectious agents identified in cerebral abscesses,[34] although confirmation of this study is needed to determine whether these agents are true pathogens in patients with brain abscess. Tissue should also be sent for histopathological examination. Definitive diagnosis in fungal brain abscess is based on biopsy or resection of the lesion, with a characteristic appearance of the causative organism in microbiological and histopathological specimens.

Therapy

Empirical antimicrobial therapy for bacterial brain abscess should include agents active against streptococci, anaerobes, the Enterobacteriaceae and staphylococci, although therapy can usually be chosen on the basis of the likely pathogenic mechanism of brain abscess formation (Table 117.3).[32] Optimal therapy of brain abscesses includes surgical intervention with either stereotactic CT-guided aspiration or craniotomy with resection or debridement; all lesions >2.5 cm in diameter should be excised or stereotactically aspirated. Certain patients may be treated with medical therapy alone and these criteria include the presence of multiple abscesses, location in a surgically inaccessible area, clinical improvement with medical therapy alone and abscess size $\leq$ 2.5 cm. Once culture results are available, antimicrobial therapy may be adjusted for optimal therapy (Table 117.4). Intravenous therapy for 6–8 weeks is recommended for treatment of bacterial brain abscess, often followed by 2–3 months of oral therapy (although the efficacy and necessity of this approach have not been established). Brain abscess caused by *Nocardia* species should be treated for up to 12 months, in conjunction with surgical resection.

The optimal therapy of fungal brain abscess requires a combined medical and surgical approach.[32,33] High-dose amphotericin B deoxycholate (0.8–1.25 mg kg^{-1} per day, with doses up to 1.5 mg kg^{-1} per day depending on the clinical response) was previously recommended for treatment of *Aspergillus* brain abscess. Voriconazole is now the drug of choice, with response rates of ~35%.[35] Mucormycosis should be treated with amphotericin B deoxycholate or one of its lipid formulations, along with correction of underlying metabolic derangements and aggressive surgical debridement.

Table 117.3 Empirical antimicrobial therapy of bacterial brain abscess.

Predisposing condition	Usual bacterial isolates	Antimicrobial regimen
Otitis media or mastoiditis	Streptococci (anaerobic or aerobic), *Bacteroides* and *Prevotella* species, Enterobacteriaceae	Metronidazole + a third-generation cephalosporin[a]
Sinusitis (frontoethmoidal or sphenoidal)	Streptococci, *Bacteroides* species, Enterobacteriaceae, *Staphylococcus aureus, Hemophilus* species	Metronidazole + a third-generation cephalosporin[a,b]
Dental sepsis	Mixed *Fusobacterium* and *Bacteroides* species, streptococci	Penicillin + metronidazole
Penetrating trauma or postneurosurgical	*Staphylococcus aureus*, streptococci, Enterobacteriaceae, *Clostridium*	Vancomycin + a third-generation cephalosporin[a]
Lung abscess, empyema, bronchiectasis	*Fusobacterium, Actinomyces, Bacteroides* species, streptococci, *Nocardia asteroides*	Penicillin + metronidazole + a sulfonamide[c]
Bacterial endocarditis	*Staphylococcus aureus*, streptococci	Vancomycin + gentamicin

[a]Cefotaxime or ceftriaxone; ceftazidime or cefepime is used if *Pseudomonas aeruginosa* is suspected.
[b]Add vancomycin if infection caused by methicillin-resistant *Staphylococcus aureus* is suspected.
[c]Sulfadiazine or trimethoprim–sulfamethoxazole; include if *Nocardia asteroides* is suspected.

Table 117.4 Antimicrobial therapy of brain abscess.[a]

Organism	Standard therapy	Alternative therapies
Actinomyces species	Penicillin G	Clindamycin
Aspergillus species	Voriconazole	Amphotericin B lipid complex; liposomal amphotericin B; amphotericin B deoxycholate
Bacteroides fragilis	Metronidazole	Clindamycin
Candida species	Amphotericin B deoxycholate + 5-flucytosine	Fluconazole
Enterobacteriaceae	Third-generation cephalosporin[b]	Aztreonam; trimethoprim–sulfamethoxazole; fluoroquinolone; meropenem
Fusobacterium species	Penicillin G	Metronidazole
Mucormycosis	Amphotericin B deoxycholate	Liposomal amphotericin B; amphotericin B lipid complex; posaconazole
Nocardia asteroides	Trimethoprim–sulfamethoxazole or sulfadiazine	Minocycline; imipenem; meropenem; third-generation cephalosporoin[b]; amikacin
Pseudomonas aeruginosa	Ceftazidime[c]or cefepime[c]	Aztreonam[c]; fluoroquinolone[c]; meropenem[c]
Staphylococcus aureus		
Methicillin-sensitive	Nafcillin or oxacillin	Vancomycin
Methicillin-resistant	Vancomycin	Trimethoprim–sulfamethoxazole
Streptococcus milleri, other streptococci	Penicillin	Third-generation cephalosporin[b]; vancomycin

[a]Depending upon the pathogenesis of bacterial brain abscess, these bacteria may be part of a mixed infection and treatment for other suspected bacteria should be given.
[b]Cefotaxime or ceftriaxone.
[c]Addition of an aminoglycoside should be considered.

Subdural empyema

Epidemiology and aetiology

The most common predisposing conditions to cranial subdural empyema are otorhinological infections; 50–80% of cases begin in the paranasal sinuses.[36] Other predisposing conditions include skull trauma, neurosurgical procedures and infection of a pre-existing subdural empyema; haematogenous dissemination occurs in only about 5% of cases. The bacterial species isolated from cranial subdural empyema include streptococci (~25–45%), staphylococci (~10–15%) and aerobic Gram-negative bacilli (~3–10%); anaerobes (e.g. anaerobic and microaerophilic streptococci *Bacteroides fragilis*) have been recovered in up to 100% of cases. Polymicrobial infections are common.

Clinical presentation

Subdural empyema can present as a rapidly progressive, life-threatening infection with symptoms and signs related to the presence of increased intracranial pressure, meningeal irritation, and/or focal cortical inflammation.[36] A prominent complaint is headache, which is initially localized to the infected sinus or ear but becomes generalized as the infection progresses. Other clinical findings include vomiting, altered mental status (with progression to obtundation if treatment is not initiated), fever and focal neurological signs (usually within 24–48 h with rapid progression). About 80% of patients have meningeal irritation and seizures occur in more than half of cases. Without treatment, there is a rapid neurological deterioration with signs of increased intracranial pressure and cerebral herniation. However, this fulminant presentation may not be seen in patients with cranial subdural empyema following cranial surgery or trauma, in patients who have received prior antimicrobial therapy, in patients with infected subdural haematomas or in patients with infections metastatic to the subdural space.

Diagnosis

The diagnostic procedure of choice for cranial subdural empyema is either CT with contrast enhancement or MR imaging.[36] CT typically reveals a crescentic or elliptically shaped area of hypodensity below the cranial vault or adjacent to the falx cerebri; with extensive disease, there is often associated mass effect. Following the administration of contrast material, there is a fine, intense line of enhancement that can be seen between the subdural collection and cerebral cortex. Extensive mass effect, manifested as ventricular compression, sulcal effacement and midline shift, is invariably present. MR provides greater clarity of morphological detail than CT and is particularly valuable in detecting subdural empyemas located as the base of the brain, along the falx cerebri or in the posterior fossa. MR can also differentiate empyema from most sterile effusions and chronic haematomas, making it the diagnostic modality of choice for subdural empyema.

Therapy

The therapy of subdural empyema requires a combined medical and surgical approach because antimicrobial agents alone do not reliably sterilize these lesions and surgical decompression is needed to control increased intracranial pressure.[36] Drainage via burr hole placement may be considered in the early stages of subdural empyema when the pus is liquid, although it may not be adequate in 10–20% of patients. For patients requiring craniotomy, a wide exposure should be afforded to allow adequate exploration of all areas of suspected infection. In one report,[37] craniotomy appeared to be superior to burr hole and craniectomy drainage, as patients undergoing burr hole or craniectomy drainage not only required more frequent operations to drain recurrent or remaining pus, but also exhibited higher mortality rates and poorer outcomes.

Following the aspiration of purulent material, antimicrobial therapy is based on the results of Gram stain and predisposing condition. If the primary infection is paranasal sinusitis, otitis media or mastoiditis, therapy with vancomycin, metronidazole and a third-generation cephalosporin (cefotaxime or ceftriaxone; or ceftazidime, cefepime or meropenem if *P. aeruginosa* is suspected) is recommended pending organism identification. Parenteral therapy should be continued for 3–4 weeks and perhaps longer if an associated osteomyelitis is present,[36] although there are no firm data to support a specific duration of antimicrobial therapy in patients with subdural empyema.

Epidural abscess

Epidemiology and aetiology

Epidural abscess refers to a collection between the dura mater and the overlying skull or vertebral column.[36,38] The aetiologies of cranial subdural abscess are usually the same as for subdural empyema (see the preceding text), whereas spinal epidural abscess usually follows haematogenous dissemination from foci elsewhere to the epidural space (25–50% of cases) or by extension from a vertebral osteomyelitis, local trauma or infection (e.g. from penetrating trauma, decubitus ulcers, paraspinal abscess, back surgery, lumbar puncture or epidural anaesthesia). The likely infecting organisms in spinal epidural abscess are staphylococci (50–90%), streptococci (8–17%) and aerobic Gram-negative bacilli (12–17%).

Clinical presentation

Symptoms in patients with cranial epidural abscess are usually insidious, with the presentation overshadowed by the primary focus of infection (e.g. sinusitis or otitis media).[36,38] Cranial epidural abscesses usually enlarge too slowly to produce sudden major neurological deficits unless there is deeper intracranial extension. The typical complaints are fever and headache, focal neurological signs, seizures and papilloedema and other signs of increased intracranial pressure may eventually develop without appropriate therapy.

In contrast, spinal epidural abscess may develop rapidly within hours (following haematogenous dissemination) or pursue a chronic course over months (associated with vertebral osteomyelitis).[36,38] Initially, patients complain of focal vertebral pain (the most consistent symptom seen in 70–90% of patients), followed by root pain, defects of motor, sensory or sphincter function and finally paralysis. These symptoms and signs indicate the need for emergency evaluation, diagnosis and treatment.

Diagnosis

MR imaging is the diagnostic procedure of choice for both cranial and spinal epidural abscess.[36] In cases of spinal epidural abscess, MR is recommended because it can visualize the spinal cord and epidural space in both the sagittal and transverse sections and can also identify accompanying osteomyelitis, intramedullary spinal cord lesions and joint space infection.

Therapy

Recommendations for antimicrobial therapy for cranial epidural abscess are the same as for subdural empyema (see the preceding text). Presumptive therapy for spinal epidural abscess must include an antistaphylococcal agent (i.e. vancomycin); coverage for Gram-negative bacilli (e.g. ceftazidime, cefepime or meropenem) must be included for patients with a history of a spinal procedure or injection drug use.[36,38]

Antimicrobial therapy for an uncomplicated spinal epidural abscess should be continued for 4–6 weeks and for 6–8 weeks if osteomyelitis is present. Surgical therapy for epidural abscess is aimed at drainage of the collection and for patients with neurological changes to minimize the likelihood of permanent neurological sequelae. Some patients with spinal epidural abscess have been treated with antimicrobial therapy alone (i.e. those with an unacceptably high surgical risk or those without neurological deficits), although these patients must be carefully followed for clinical deterioration and for progression by radiological studies.[36,38] Surgical decompression should be performed in patients with increasing neurological deficit, persistent severe pain, increasing temperature or peripheral white blood cell count. Surgery is not likely to be a viable therapeutic option in patients who have experienced complete paralysis for more than 24–36 h, although some would perform surgical therapy in patients with duration of complete paralysis of less than 72 h.

Encephalitis

Encephalitis is characterized by symptoms similar to those seen with acute meningitis, but patients with encephalitis are more likely to experience mental status changes and seizures. Numerous infectious and non-infectious aetiologies may produce encephalitis.[39] Most common are the herpes viruses that are also the most treatable. West Nile encephalitis has been reported in endemic areas and is discussed below.

Herpes simplex virus

Epidemiology and aetiology

Herpes simplex virus accounts for ~10–20% of viral encephalitides and occurs sporadically throughout the year, affecting all age groups;[40] most cases in adults are caused by HSV type 1. The disease is associated with significant morbidity and mortality (as high as 70% if untreated).

Clinical presentation

Patients with HSV encephalitis often present with diminished levels of consciousness and focal neurological signs, such as dysphasia, weakness and paraesthesias.[40] Personality changes and fever are uniformly present and approximately two-thirds of patients develop seizures, often involving the temporal lobes. The clinical course may be slow or progress with alarming rapidity, with progressive loss of consciousness leading to coma.

Diagnosis

CSF examination in HSV encephalitis reveals a lymphocytic pleocytosis in 97% of cases with biopsy-proven disease and an elevated protein.[40] The presence of CSF red blood cells suggests the diagnosis but is not always present. Generally, CSF culture is of limited value.[5] Detection of HSV DNA in the CSF using PCR is both sensitive (96–98%) and specific (95–99%) and is now the optimal method for the diagnosis of HSV encephalitis.[39,40] However, an initially negative CSF PCR result for HSV may become positive if the test is repeated 1–3 days after initiation of treatment, such that in undiagnosed cases in which patients have clinical features of HSV encephalitis or temporal lobe lesions on neuroimaging, consideration should be given to repeating the PCR for HSV 3–7 days later on a second CSF specimen.[39] Several non-invasive tests may also support the diagnosis of HSV encephalitis. The electroencephalogram (EEG) may show a characteristic spike-and-slow wave activity with periodic lateralizing epileptiform discharges over the temporal and frontotemporal regions. MR is more sensitive than CT, revealing temporal lobe abnormalities in more than 90% of PCR-proven HSV encephalitis, and is considered by many experts to be the most important and specific imaging technique.

Antimicrobial therapy

On the basis of its ease of administration and good safety profile, treatment with intravenous acyclovir 30 mg kg^{-1} per day (in patients with normal renal function) in three divided doses for 14–21 days is recommended for patients with suspected HSV encephalitis.[39,40]

Varicella zoster virus

Epidemiology and aetiology

Herpes zoster is a consequence of reactivation of latent VZV and a direct correlation exists between cutaneous dissemination and visceral involvement (including meningoencephalitis).[27] CNS complications associated with recurrent zoster infection result in significantly higher morbidity and mortality than primary varicella infection. This may be due to the advanced age and underlying illnesses of most patients with herpes zoster.

Clinical presentation

Symptoms associated with CNS infection with VZV include headache, fever, vomiting, seizures, altered sensorium and focal neurological deficits.[27] Encephalitis is the most common abnormality associated with herpes zoster, seen most commonly in patients of advanced age, following immunosuppression and in those with disseminated cutaneous zoster. Some patients with ophthalmic zoster present with the distinctive CNS process of contralateral hemiplegia that usually occurs several weeks or more after zoster ophthalmicus; this finding is seen in up to one-third of CNS abnormalities in herpes zoster.

Diagnosis

CSF analysis in patients with herpes zoster encephalitis shows a lymphocytic pleocytosis and elevated protein, although these findings may be seen in up to 40% of zoster patients without CNS involvement.[27] Viral cultures are rarely helpful diagnostically. PCR detection of VZV DNA has a specificity of >95% but the sensitivity is 80–95%.[39] In patients with zoster ophthalmicus with contralateral hemiplegia, a unilateral arteritis or thrombosis of involved vessels may be seen on cerebral angiography and cerebral infarction may be seen on CT or MR imaging.

Antimicrobial therapy

Although no clinical trials have established the efficacy of antiviral therapy in herpes zoster encephalitis, we believe that intravenous acyclovir should be used in this setting.[39]

West Nile virus

Epidemiology and aetiology

West Nile encephalitis is an infection of the brain caused by West Nile virus (WNV), a flavivirus that is commonly found in Africa, West Asia and the Middle East. The virus first appeared in the USA in 1999 with an outbreak of meningoencephalitis reported in New York City.[41] Mosquitos are the primary vectors of WNV and anyone bitten by an infected mosquito can get the disease. It has been estimated that the risk to a person of becoming infected with WNV from the bite of an infected mosquito is about 1%. Transmission can also occur via transplanted organs and infected blood products. Most human infections with WNV are asymptomatic, but, in recent outbreaks, one in five infected persons developed West Nile fever and one in 150 developed CNS disease;[42] the elderly are much more likely to develop serious diseases. Although the risk of infection with WNV may be small, the disease can be fairly serious; mortality from WNV neuroinvasive disease is ~12%.

Clinical presentation

Patients with WNV encephalitis present with fever, headache, mental status changes, nausea and vomiting.[42] Severe generalized muscle weakness was a common feature in cases during the New York City outbreak, and also in other outbreaks in the USA. Seizures are uncommon. Depressed deep tendon reflexes, diffuse muscle weakness, flaccid paralysis and respiratory failure may also occur. The disease progresses to coma in about 15% of patients.

Diagnosis

CSF examination in patients with WNV encephalitis typically reveals a moderate lymphocytic pleocytosis (although no cells or neutrophils may be seen), elevated protein and normal glucose. Laboratories can perform an IgM antibody capture enzyme-linked immunosorbent assay (MAC-ELISA). Using this assay, virus-specific IgM can be detected in nearly all CSF and serum specimens received from WNV-infected patients at the time of their clinical presentation.[39,42] However, the serum IgM antibody may persist for more than 1 year and physicians must determine whether the detection of antibody is the result of a WNV infection in the previous year and unrelated to the current clinical presentation. The IgM in the CSF is specific for CNS infection, with almost all patients having detectable antibody by the first week of presentation.

Treatment

There is no specific treatment for West Nile encephalitis.[39] In more severe cases, intensive supportive therapy is indicated, often involving hospitalization, intravenous fluids, airway management, respiratory support, prevention of secondary infections (e.g. pneumonia, urinary tract infection) and good nursing care.

Postpolio syndrome

Epidemiology

Any discussion of CNS infections in the elderly should include the postpolio syndrome. This syndrome does not appear to be because of persistent poliovirus infection, but rather is likely due to an age-related loss of surviving motor neurons and their inability to innervate the enlarged motor neuron units seen in poliomyelitis patients.[43] In a study of the prevalence and risk factors for postpolio syndrome in a cohort of 551 former poliomyelitis patients in Allegheny County, PA, 137 (~25%) developed symptoms of the postpolio syndrome between 32 and 39 years after the acute illness. Risk factors for the development of the postpolio syndrome were female gender, bulbar disease and the degree of post-recovery residual impairment. Despite the relatively high prevalence of this disorder, the majority of patients (80% in this study) did not require the use of new assisted devices to accomplish their activities of daily living, despite a subjective decline in their functional status.

Clinical presentation

The postpolio syndrome is characterized by muscle weakness, muscle and/or joint pain, fatigue and a decline in functional status occurring 30–40 years after acute poliomyelitis.[43] Some patients have progressive weakness and wasting in muscles that were not necessarily weak at the onset of poliomyelitis.

Diagnosis

Conventional electromyography (EMG) demonstrates chronic denervation; occasionally there may also be new or ongoing denervation manifested as fasciculations, fibrillations and positive sharp waves.[43] Enlarged motor units consistent with highly increased fibre density can be demonstrated in 90% of patients on single-fibre EMG. However, the primary role of EMG is to exclude other causes of the patient's presentation.

Therapy

There is no definitive treatment for the postpolio syndrome, but symptomatic improvement may be obtained with analgesics such as paracetamol (acetaminophen) or non-steroidal anti-inflammatory drugs (NSAIDs), local heat application to affected muscles and joints and a low-impact, non-fatiguing exercise programme to prevent the development of muscle atrophy.[43] Patients may also benefit from rest periods, increased sleep time and other energy conservation methods to overcome fatigue.

Creutzfeldt–Jakob disease

Epidemiology

The most common human prion disease is sporadic, or classic, Creutzfeldt–Jakob disease (CJD), with a worldwide incidence of approximately one case per million population;[44] however, among individuals aged 60–74 years, the incidence is five cases per million population. Symptoms generally begin by age 60–70 years, with a mean age of onset of 60 years.

Clinical presentation

Sporadic CJD is characterized by a rapidly progressive multifocal neurological dysfunction, myoclonus and a terminal state of global severe cognitive impairment.[44] About 40% of patients with sporadic CJD present with rapidly progressive cognitive impairment, 40% with cerebellar dysfunction and the remaining 20% with a combination of both findings. The clinical picture rapidly expands to include behavioural abnormalities, higher cortical dysfunction, cortical visual abnormalities, cerebellar dysfunction and both pyramidal and extrapyramidal signs. Almost all patients with sporadic CJD develop myoclonus that involves either the entire body or a limb; myoclonus may be absent at disease onset, but appears with increasing severity as the disease progresses. After a rapidly progressive illness of 3–9 months, death usually occurs with the patient in an akinetic and mute state.

Diagnosis

The clinical presentation, progressive nature and failure to find any other diagnoses are the hallmarks of sporadic CJD. There are no available, completely reliable diagnostic tests for use before the onset of clinical symptoms in patients with sporadic CJD. During the course of disease, most patients develop a characteristic picture on EEG with periodic paroxysms of sharp waves or spikes on a slow background.[44] These periodic complexes have a diagnostic sensitivity and specificity of 67% and 87%, respectively, on a single EEG; if repeated recordings are obtained, more than 90% of patients show periodic EEG abnormalities. The triad of myoclonus, dementia and EEG periodic sharp waves is a characteristic presentation of sporadic CJD.

Therapy

There is no treatment that can cure or control CJD. About 90% of patients die within 1 year.[44] Current treatment is aimed at alleviating symptoms and making the patient as comfortable as possible. Opiate drugs can help relieve pain; clonazepam and sodium valproate may help relieve involuntary myoclonus. Quinidine has been tested in an uncontrolled and unblinded study of patients with sporadic CJD; despite transient improvement in some patients, they reverted to their previous states and died of progressive disease.

Key points

- Central nervous system infections are frequently devastating and can lead to significant morbidity and mortality.
- Although the brain possesses several defence mechanisms to prevent infection, once microorganisms reach the central nervous system, host defence mechanisms are inadequate to control the infection.
- Antimicrobial therapy is limited by the poor penetration of many agents into the central nervous system.
- Recent developments in diagnosis and therapy of meningitis, brain abscess, subdural empyema, epidural abscess, encephalitis, postpolio syndrome and Creutzfeldt–Jakob disease are reviewed.
- The use of adjunctive treatment strategies is discussed.

References

1. Sawyer MH and Rotbart HA. Viral meningitis and aseptic meningitis syndrome. In: WM Scheld, RJ Whitley and CM Marra (eds), *Infections of the Central Nervous System*, 3rd edn, Lippincott Williams and Wilkins, Philadelphia, 2004, pp. 75–93.
2. Shalaby M and Whitley RJ. Recurrent benign lymphocytic meningitis. *Clin Infect Dis* 2006;**43**:1194–7.
3. Tunkel AR and Scheld WM. Acute meningitis. In: GL Mandell, JE Bennett and R Dolin (eds), *Principles and Practice of Infectious Diseases*, 7th edn, Churchill Livingstone Elsevier, Philadelphia, 2010, pp. 1189–229.
4. Romero JR. Diagnosis and management of enteroviral infections of the central nervous system. *Curr Infect Dis Rep* 2002; **4**:309–16.
5. Polage CR and Petti CA. Assessment of the utility of viral culture of cerebrospinal fluid. *Clin Infect Dis* 2006;**43**:1578–9.
6. Desmond RA, Accortt NA, Talley L *et al*. Enteroviral meningitis: natural history and outcome with pleconaril therapy. *Antimicrob Agents Chemother* 2006;**50**:2409–14.
7. Weisfeldt M, van de Beek D, Spanjaard L *et al*. Clinical features, complications and outcome in adults with pneumococcal meningitis: a prospective case series. *Lancet Neurol* 2006;**5**:123–9.
8. van de Beek D, Drake JM and Tunkel AR. Nosocomial bacterial meningitis. *N Engl J Med* 2010;**362**:146–54.
9. van de Beek D, de Gans J, Spanjaard L *et al*. Clinical features and prognostic factors in adults with bacterial meningitis. *N Engl J Med* 2004;**351**:1849–59.
10. Tunkel AR, Hartman BJ, Kaplan SL *et al*. Practice guidelines for the management of bacterial meningitis. *Clin Infect Dis* 2004;**39**:1267–84.
11. Werno AM and Murdoch DR. Laboratory diagnosis of invasive pneumococcal disease. *Clin Infect Dis* 2008;**46**:926–32.

12. Mai NTH, Chau TTH, Thwaites G *et al.* Dexamethasone in Vietnamese adolescents and adults with bacterial meningitis. *N Engl J Med* 2007;**357**:2431–40.

13. Scarborough M, Gordon SB, Whitty CJM *et al.* Corticosteroids for bacterial meningitis for adults in sub-Saharan Africa. *N Engl J Med* 2007;**357**:2441–50.

14. Ricard JD, Wolff M, Lacherade JC *et al.* Levels of vancomycin in cerebrospinal fluid of adult patients receiving adjunctive corticosteroids to treat pneumococcal meningitis: a prospective multicenter observational study. *Clin Infect Dis* 2007;**44**:250–5.

15. Leonard JM and Des Prez RM. Tuberculous meningitis. *Infect Dis Clin North Am* 1990;**4**:769–87.

16. Zugar A. Tuberculosis. In: WM Scheld, RJ Whitley and CM Marra (eds), *Infections of the Central Nervous System*, 3rd edn, Lippincott Williams and Wilkins, Philadelphia, 2004, pp. 441–59.

17. Kalita J, Misra UK and Nair PP. Predictors of stroke and its significance in the outcome of tuberculous meningitis. *J Stroke Cerebrovasc Dis* 2009;**18**:251–8.

18. Sinner SW. Approach to the diagnosis and management of tuberculous meningitis. *Curr Infect Dis Rep* 2010;**12**:291–8.

19. Thwaites GE, Bang ND, Duang NH *et al.* Dexamethasone for the treatment of tuberculous meningitis in adolescents and adults. *N Engl J Med* 2004;**351**:1741–51.

20. Prasad K and Singh MB. Corticosteroids for managing tuberculous meningitis. *Cochrane Database Syst Rev* 2008;(1): CD002244.

21. Marra CM. Neurosyphilis. In: WM Scheld, RJ Whitley and CM Marra (eds), *Infections of the Central Nervous System*, 3rd edn, Lippincott Williams and Wilkins, Philadelphia, 2004, pp. 649–57.

22. Cadavid D. Lyme disease and relapsing fever. In: WM Scheld, RJ Whitley and CM Marra (eds), *Infections of the Central Nervous System*, 3rd edn, Lippincott Williams and Wilkins, Philadelphia, 2004, pp. 659–90.

23. Steere AC, McHugh G, Damle N *et al.* Prospective study of serologic tests for Lyme disease. *Clin Infect Dis* 2008; **47**:188–95.

24. Blanc FB, Jaulhac M, Fleury J *et al.* Relevance of the antibody index to diagnose Lyme neuroborreliosis among seropositive patients. *Neurology* 2007;**69**:953–8.

25. Marra CM, Maxwell CL, Tantalo LC *et al.* Normalization of serum rapid plasma regain titer predicts normalization of cerebrospinal fluid and clinical abnormalities after treatment of neurosyphilis. *Clin Infect Dis* 2008;**47**:893–9.

26. Wormser GP, Dattwyler RJ, Shapiro ED *et al.* The clinical assessment, treatment and prevention of Lyme disease, human granulocytic anaplasmosis and babesiosis: clinical practice guidelines by the Infectious Diseases Society of America. *Clin Infect Dis* 2006;**43**:1089–134.

27. Tunkel AR and Scheld WM. Central nervous system infection in the compromised host. In RH Rubin and LS Young (eds), *Clinical Approach to Infection in the Compromised Host*, 4th edn, Kluwer Academic/Plenum Publishers, New York, 2002, pp. 163–214.

28. Blair JE. Coccidioidal meningitis: update on epidemiology, clinical features, diagnosis and management. *Curr Infect Dis Rep* 2009;**11**:289–95.

29. Galgiani JN, Ampel NM, Blair JE *et al.* Coccidioidomycosis. *Clin Infect Dis* 2005;**41**:1217–23.

30. Perfect JR, Dismukes WE, Dromer F *et al.* Clinical practice guidelines for the management of cryptococcal disease: 2010 update by the Infectious Diseases Society of America. *Clin Infect Dis* 2010;**50**:291–322.

31. Johnson RH and Einstein HE. Coccidioidal meningitis. *Clin Infect Dis* 2006;**42**:103–7.

32. Tunkel AR. Brain abscess. In GL Mandell, JE Bennett and R Dolin (eds), *Principles and Practice of Infectious Diseases*, 7th edn, Churchill Livingstone Elsevier, Philadelphia, 2010, pp. 1265–78.

33. Cortez KJ and Walsh TJ. Space-occupying fungal lesions. In: WM Scheld, RJ Whitley and CM Marra (eds), *Infections of the Central Nervous System*, 3rd edn, Lippincott Williams and Wilkins, Philadelphia, 2004, pp. 713–34.

34. Al Masalma M, Armougom F, Scheld WM *et al.* The expansion of the microbiologic spectrum of brain abscess with use of multiple 16S ribosomal DNA sequencing. *Clin Infect Dis* 2009;**48**:1169–78.

35. Walsh TJ, Anaissie EJ, Denning DW *et al.* Treatment of aspergillosis: clinical practice guidelines by the Infectious Disease Society of America. *Clin Infect Dis* 2008;**46**:327–60.

36. Tunkel AR. Subdural empyema, epidural abscess and suppurative intracranial thrombophlebitis. In GL Mandell, JE Bennett and R Dolin (eds), *Principles and Practice of Infectious Diseases*, 7th edn, Elsevier Churchill Livingstone Elsevier, Philadelphia, 2010, pp. 1279–87.

37. Nathoo N, Nadvi SS, Gouws E and van Dellen JR. Craniotomy improves outcomes for cranial subdural empyemas: computed tomography-era experience with 699 patients. *Neurosurgery* 2001;**49**:872–8.

38. Darouiche RO. Spinal epidural abscess. *N Engl J Med* 2006; **355**:2012–20.

39. Tunkel AR, Glaser CA, Bloch KC *et al.* The management of encephalitis: clinical practice guidelines by the Infectious Diseases Society of America. *Clin Infect Dis* 2008;**47**:303–27.

40. Whitley RJ. Herpes simplex virus. In: WM Scheld, RJ Whitley and CM Marra (eds), *Infections of the Central Nervous System*, 3rd edn, Lippincott Williams and Wilkins, Philadelphia, 2004, pp. 123–44.

41. Nash D, Mostashari F, Fine A *et al.* The outbreak of West Nile virus infection in the New York City area in 1999. *N Engl J Med* 2001;**344**:1807–14.

42. Sejvar JJ, Haddad MB, Tierney BC *et al.* Neurologic manifestations and outcome of West Nile virus infection. *JAMA* 2003;**290**:511–5.

43. Modlin JF and Coffey DJ. Poliomyelitis, polio vaccines and the postpoliomyelitis syndrome. In: WM Scheld, RJ Whitley and CM Marra (eds), *Infections of the Central Nervous System*, 3rd edn, Lippincott Williams and Wilkins, Philadelphia, 2004, pp. 95–110.

44. Janka J and Maldarelli F. Prion diseases: update on mad cow disease, variant Creutzfeldt–Jakob disease and the transmissible spongiform encephalopathies. *Curr Infect Dis Rep* 2004; **6**:305–15.

SECTION 15

Special Issues

CHAPTER 118

Elder abuse: a UK perspective

Claudia Cooper and Gill Livingston
University College London, London, UK

History of elder abuse management in the UK

In 1975, when Alex Baker coined the phrase 'granny battering', there was relatively little interest in elder abuse in the UK.[1] By 1989, professionals were becoming interested and the first multidisciplinary conference on elder abuse in the UK was held by the British Geriatrics Society.[2] By 1991, Virginia Bottomley, the then Minister for Health, was still informing the House of Commons that it was not a major issue. The UK charity Action on Elder Abuse was formed in 1993 and the Department of Health issued guidance on elder abuse in 2000 (*No Secrets*[3]). In 2004, a House of Commons Health Committee report proposed changes to care home inspection, regulation of care staff and the introduction of mandatory training in elder abuse recognition for professionals working with older people.[4]

In England and Wales, guidance on management of abuse is outlined in *No Secrets*[3] and *In Safe Hands*[5], respectively. In 2008–09, the Department of Health launched a consultation into this guidance, asking whether adult safeguarding should be placed on a statutory footing. In Scotland, the Adult Support and Protection Act (2007) has already made adult protection statutory. This Act created new measures to protect adults believed to be at risk of harm. These include rights of entry to places where adults are thought to be at risk, a range of protection orders including assessment, removal of the adult at risk and banning of the person causing the harm; and supporting the creation of multidisciplinary adult protection committees. In Northern Ireland there is no specific guidance or legislation relating to the management of suspected elder abuse.

Defining elder abuse

Elder abuse is defined as a violation of a vulnerable older person's human and civil rights by another person(s).[3,5] This definition specifies that these acts are abuse when they happen to a 'vulnerable person'. Older people are more likely to be vulnerable due to more physical and cognitive impairments, but there is nothing inherently different about how abuse should be identified and managed in younger and older adults, and they are protected by the same guidelines and legislation.[4] Like domestic violence, elder abuse can also occur in an older person who is physically well and has mental capacity.

Different types of abuse are recognized. Verbal or psychological abuse encompasses acts such as screaming and shouting at an older person, calling them names, threatening, humiliating or 'scapegoating' them. Physical abuse includes non-accidental use of force against an older person, such as hitting, shoving or handling them roughly in other ways, and also inappropriate use of medication, restraint or confinement. The over-prescription and use of as-required medication has attracted considerable attention of late in the UK. Around 100 000 older people in UK care homes are prescribed antipsychotic drugs, often in the absence of psychotic symptoms.

Neglect is defined as ignoring medical or physical care needs, failure to provide access to appropriate health or social care or withholding of the necessities of life, such as medication, adequate nutrition and heating. Financial and sexual abuse involve persuading someone to enter into a financial or sexual transaction to which he or she has not consented or cannot consent. Finally, discriminatory abuse is defined as harassment, slurs or other abusive behaviour towards an older person because of age, race, gender, disability, sexual preferences or other personal characteristics.

Among people providing care, there is often a lack of consensus about what constitutes abuse. While health professionals, family carers and older people are likely to agree that the most serious types of abuse, such as physical violence, should be defined as such, there is often less agreement about other types of behaviour. For example, while locking a person with dementia in their house all day alone to prevent wandering would constitute abuse according to *No Secrets*, less than two-thirds of English family

Principles and Practice of Geriatric Medicine, Fifth Edition. Edited by Alan J. Sinclair, John E. Morley and Bruno Vellas.

carers, medical students and mental healthcare professionals thought that this scenario was abuse when presented with it in a vignette.[6,7]

Most people agree that behaviour has to reach a certain threshold of severity or frequency to constitute abuse. Shouting at someone angrily once, for example, may be accepted within all emotional relationships. Although the parameters change when one member is dependent and vulnerable, this does not mean that such actions automatically constitute abuse. Most abuse measures use cut-points for how frequently a behaviour must be reported to be considered abusive. For example, the Pillemer criteria define abuse caseness as verbal or neglectful acts occurring ≥ 10 times per year and physical or financially abusive acts at least once per year.[8] The Modified Conflict Tactics Scale (MCTS) asks whether abusive acts have happened never, almost never, sometimes, quite frequently or almost always, and defines an 'abuse case' as an abusive act happening at least *sometimes* in the last 3 months.[9]

In clinical practice, standardized measures of abusive behaviour are not generally used and there is variation among clinicians regarding the thresholds for considering behaviour abusive and for acting on these concerns. Thinking about abuse as either happening or not can lead to an 'all or nothing' response (social services referral of only most serious cases and ignoring others). Detecting and actively managing behaviour that is less severe in nature and frequency may lead to help being given before the problem becomes more serious.

Prevalence of elder abuse

Elder abuse is inherently difficult to study. It is a hidden offence, often perpetrated against vulnerable people (many with memory impairment), by those on whom they depend. Prevalence estimates are influenced, and possibly underestimated, by the fact that many older people are unable, frightened or embarrassed to report its presence. Prevalence estimates of abuse vary greatly between studies and this is partly explained by the different thresholds used to define significant abuse. In the 2007 CARD (Caring for Relatives with Dementia) study of family carers of people with dementia recruited from English old-age psychiatric services, the 3 month prevalence of significant abuse reported by carers against the person they were caring for, as defined by a screening instrument, was 34%, but when we asked a panel of old-age psychiatrists to review the carers' responses, they agreed that they would be clinically concerned in 6.8% of cases.[10] The act of abuse does not imply intent and in many cases the carers may not have viewed their own actions in this light.

Rates of abuse are particularly high among vulnerable people, including those with dementia. Around one-quarter of vulnerable older people (e.g. those receiving home care services) reported significant levels of psychological abuse. Rates of elder abuse in UK care homes have not been studied, although in other Western countries, one in six care home staff admit psychologically abusing people in their care and four-fifths observing abuse if asked.

When health professionals or researchers look for evidence of abuse as opposed to asking older people about it, they find less, nearer 5% in vulnerable older people, probably because they are only detecting more serious physical abuse or neglect with physical evidence. The number of abuse cases reported to authorities is low. Unlike in the USA, the UK does not have a system of mandatory reporting of all abuse and neglect cases, so data are not widely available from about the prevalence of cases of elder abuse reported to social services.

The prevalence of abuse in the older general population is lower than in vulnerable groups. Around 5% reported significant abuse over a period of 1 month. Most of this is psychological, verbal and/or financial abuse.[11] In the largest UK survey of elder abuse to date, 4% of older people living in private homes reported abuse. People with cognitive impairment were excluded from this survey.[12]

Risk factors for elder abuse

The causes of abuse are complex and varied. Older people who are more dependent because of physical or cognitive impairment are more at risk of abuse. In addition to requiring more care, they are less able to leave or report an abusive situation. Older people with mental health problems, who are more depressed or have suicidal thoughts, also report more abuse.

Providing care is physically and emotionally demanding. Family carers who are more anxious and depressed are more likely to act abusively towards the person they care for, as are those who use unhelpful coping strategies such as substance use and denial in response to stress or resent their caring role.[13] Family carers who live with the person they care for and have fewer breaks are more likely to report acting abusively.[14] Carer stress is less likely to explain other types of abuse (financial and sexual abuse) which could not be perceived as reactions to the high stress of caring. Professional carers who report high levels of carer stress and burnout are also more likely to report acting abusively.

Abuse is not a one-way phenomenon. Being on the receiving end of abuse is one of the most important predictors of carers acting abusively.[13] Relationships that were previously psychologically or physically violent with acts being perpetuated by both members of the dyad may become abusive if the care recipient no longer has the mental capacity to decide whether or not to stay in a violent relationship or the physical capacity to leave it and live independently. People who lack a close confidant and are socially isolated are more at risk of abuse.

A minority of abuse is sadistic in nature. A few professionals may choose to work in a setting where they have power in order to abuse. There is very little evidence about who is most likely to perpetrate or be a victim of this abuse, which is probably common in the most severe abuse cases. Feelings emanating from the staff member's experiences of caring and being cared for within their own family may affect how they behave in their professional caring role, including whether they behave abusively. Sadomasochistic traits may come to the fore in the unequal power relationship between patients and staff.[15]

Abuse in institutions

The best available evidence for institutional characteristics associated with abuse comes from inquiries conducted into abuse scandals. Prominent inquiries include an investigation into physical and emotional abuse of patients by care staff on Rowan ward in Manchester in 2002[16] and physical mistreatment of older people who were mentally frail by staff at Beech House in London over a 3 year period (1993–96). The following factors were thought to be important in fostering an environment in which abuse could occur and remain undetected for some time: a poor and institutionalized environment, low staffing levels with high use of bank and agency staff and little staff development and poor supervision, a lack of knowledge of incident reporting, closed inward-looking culture, weak management at ward and locality level, low staff morale and lack of involvement by relatives in care delivery, decision-making and evaluation of the service.

Detecting abuse

The best way of detecting verbal, psychological and less severe abuse is to ask older people and their carers about it in a sensitive and non-judgemental way. When we recently asked family carers questions about abuse from the Modified Conflict Tactics Scale, 97% found the questions acceptable.[17] This scale includes questions about psychologically and physically abusive acts.

Screening for objective signs of abuse is only likely to detect the most serious abuse, but this may be abuse that is not volunteered when asked. Detecting abuse is difficult when the victim cannot say what is happening. It is important to take note of changes in behaviour, unusual distress and any previous history of allegations. Unexplained bruising, especially if the distribution is inconsistent with the history or likely causes of accidental bruising, finger marks, burns or untreated sores may be evidence of physical abuse.

More serious neglect is likely to be evident from visiting an older person's home and medical examination. Risk markers include dirty or inappropriate clothing, poor personal hygiene, evidence of malnourishment or dehydration, poor skin integrity, bruising or lacerations, contractures, urine burns/excoriations, diarrhoea or faecal impaction and reports of being left in an unsafe situation or inability to get needed medications.[18] These do not differentiate between a person who has a previously unidentified need for increased care, is refusing to accept care that is offered, and someone who is being neglected, and urgent social investigation will be needed to explore the situation.

Relatives may raise concerns about paid carers or other relatives financially abusing an older person or the older person who does not understand the value of money paying too much or giving away money they cannot afford. Suspicion may be aroused if the older person appears to have financial problems disproportionate to their income, no money available or if a relative appears to be encouraging them to make a financial transaction (e.g. selling their house) which appears unwise.

Abuse is often known about by other professionals or family members. It may go unacknowledged if they feel there are no better management options. In a recent meta-analysis, only one-third of professionals working with older people had detected a case of abuse in the last year and only half of detected abuse was reported.[19] This is surprisingly low given that one-quarter of vulnerable adults report abuse in surveys. Staff who detect abuse may not report it because they are unclear about the procedures to do so or because they empathize with the perpetrator, fear recrimination or believe that procedures designed to deal with it are inappropriate and punitive.[20] Inquiries into abuse scandals have found that abuse was known about and sometimes reported months or years before decisive action was taken to stop it.

It is important that staff are trained about what constitutes abuse, how to recognize it and who to report it to. In a study based in a London mental health trust, an educational intervention increased staff knowledge about how to detect and manage abuse, whereas giving staff the same information in a written format did not.[21] Having whistle-blowing policies that are well publicised can also help to increase detection of abuse in care organizations. In UK law there is no protection of anonymity for staff who raise concerns about malpractice at work (whistle-blowing), but there is protection against victimization and loss of employment as a result of raising a genuine concern.

Management of abuse

All health and social care professionals have a responsibility to act on any suspicion or evidence of significant abuse or neglect. They should contact the local social services to make an 'adult protection' referral. Arrangements are in place throughout the UK for responding to all allegations of abuse against 'vulnerable' adults. Some types of abuse, including assault (sexual or physical), theft and fraud, are criminal offences under UK law and should be reported to the police. Professionals should refer all cases where they think significant harm might be occurring or there is a future risk of significant harm. The UK law commission suggests that 'harm' should be taken to include not only ill treatment (including sexual abuse and all forms of ill treatment that are not physical), but also the impairment of, or an avoidable deterioration in, physical or mental health.

Patients should usually be informed that a referral is to be made to social services if they are able to understand this, unless doing so would increase their distress or the risk of harm to them. Occasionally they may object, in which case professionals should consider whether they have the capacity to make this decision. Any intimidation, misuse of authority or undue influence will have to be assessed in making this judgement. Even if an adult has the capacity to refuse consent for an investigation into any alleged abuse, it may still be necessary to override this if other vulnerable adults are at risk. An initial rejection of help should not always be taken at face value.

Once an adult protection referral is received, social services will record the precise factual details of the alleged abuse, coordinate the investigation and come to a decision. Decisions may be made at a case conference. Actions as a result of an investigation may be supportive or therapeutic, disciplinary action or deregistration for professionals or, in a small minority of very serious cases, criminal prosecution. In England and Wales, the Mental Capacity Act (2005) introduced a new, arrestable criminal offence of ill-treatment or neglect of a person without capacity.

Social services seek the least disruptive, safe option for the older person in managing abuse, and where abuse is less severe, support services may be increased or the carer referred for support in their own right to see if this alleviates the situation. It is logical that if abuse often arises from stress among family carers, then interventions to reduce stress may reduce abusive behaviour. A handful of studies have sought to reduce abuse in this way, but as yet there have been no randomized controlled trials that would provide good evidence that this approach works.

Older people with capacity may decline assistance and refuse interventions deemed appropriate, such as moving to alternative accommodation. People with capacity have the right to make decisions that involve risk. Services have a responsibility in these circumstances to ensure that such risk is recognized and understood by all concerned and minimized whenever possible.

In addition to social services, allegations of abuse made against care professionals are also investigated by the Social Care Inspections bodies (Care Quality Commission in England, Scottish Care Commission, Care and Social Services Inspectorate for Wales and the Northern Ireland Department of Health, Social Services and Public Safety) or for NHS services, the Primary Care Trust. The Protection of Vulnerable Adults (POVA) scheme was introduced for registered care homes and domiciliary care services in 2004 in England and Wales. If there are reasonable grounds to suspect that an employee or ex-employee is guilty of harming or placing at risk of harm a vulnerable adult, a POVA list referral should be made by their employer. This is in addition to usual disciplinary procedures. If appropriate, this person will then be put on the POVA list, to prevent them securing further work with vulnerable adults. Similarly, if there are reasonable grounds to suspect that a health or social care professional has placed a vulnerable adult at significant risk of harm, this should be reported to their regulatory body. Abuse (including physical, verbal or sexual abuse of patients and theft from patients) currently constitutes just under one-third of fitness to practice charges reported to the Nursing and Midwifery Council.

Preventing abuse

It is now policy that all new staff working with children and vulnerable adults in England, Wales and Northern Ireland have a Criminal Records Bureau (CRB) check to ensure that there is no known reason why an individual should not work with these client groups. In Scotland, these disclosures are managed by Disclosure Scotland. Work is under way to register all people working in domiciliary or residential care settings with vulnerable adults with the UK General Social Care Councils for England, Wales, Scotland and Northern Ireland, which were set up in 2001. They facilitate training and enforce their code of practice. Alongside the POVA list, registration will help prevent people who have been found guilty of abuse or neglect being retained in the workforce.

Regular training and supervision of staff help prevent abuse. This is both because people are less likely to commit abusive acts if they are likely to be detected, but also because staff who are referred for disciplinary procedures due to allegations of abuse often do not know their acts would be perceived in this light or may have wanted help but not known who to turn to.

Conclusion

About 5% of elderly people aged 65 years and over and one-quarter of vulnerable elderly people report a recent episode of elder abuse. Older people who are dependent on care from others or live in care homes are at particular risk. When a carer feels stressed they are more likely to abuse the elderly person for whom they are caring. There are currently no evidence-based interventions to reduce abusive behaviours by family carers and we think that the development of these is an urgent next step.

Since the early 1990s, awareness of the prevalence of elder abuse has grown. Prevention initiatives include the registration of all people working in domiciliary or residential care settings with vulnerable adults with the General Social Care Councils and the Protection of Vulnerable Adults list to prevent professionals who abuse from working elsewhere. Social services are the lead agency for managing elder abuse throughout the UK. Reporting of elder abuse is not mandatory in the UK so there are no national figures for the number of cases reported to adult social services, but it is very likely that reported cases are 'the tip of the iceberg'.

Key points

- Elder abuse is defined as a violation of a vulnerable older person's human and civil rights by another person(s).
- In contrast, neglect is defined as ignoring medical or physical care needs, failure to provide access to appropriate health or social care or withholding of the necessities of life, such as medication, adequate nutrition and heating.
- Older people who are more dependent because of physical or cognitive impairment are more at risk of abuse.
- Abuse is often known about by other professionals or family members.

References

1. Baker AA. Granny battering. *Mod Geriatr* 1975;**8**:20.
2. McAlpine CH. Elder abuse and neglect. *Age Ageing* 2008;**37**:132–3.
3. Department of Health. *No Secrets. Guidance on Developing and Implementing Multi-agency Policies and Procedures to Protect Vulnerable Adults from Abuse.* Department of Health, London, 2000.
4. House of Commons Health Committee. *Elder Abuse, Second Report of Session 2003–04*, The Stationery Office, London, 2004.
5. National Assembly for Wales. *In Safe Hands – Implementing Adult Protection Procedures in Wales*, Welsh Government, Cardiff, 2000.
6. Selwood A, Cooper C and Livingston G. What is elder abuse – who decides? *Int J Geriatr Psychiatry* 2007; **22**:1009–12.
7. Thompson-McCormick J, Jones L, Cooper C and Livingston G. Medical students' recognition of elder abuse. *International Journal of Geriatric Psychiatry* 2009;**24**:770–7.
8. Pillemer K and Moore DW. Abuse of patients in nursing-homes – findings from a survey of staff. *Gerontologist* 1989;**29**:314–20.
9. Beach SR, Schulz R, Williamson GM *et al.* Risk factors for potentially harmful informal caregiver behavior. *J Am Geriatr Soc* 2005;**53**:255–61.
10. Cooper C, Maxmin K, Selwood A *et al.* The sensitivity and specificity of the Modified Conflict Tactics Scale for detecting clinically significant elder abuse. *Int Psychogeriatr* 2009;**21**:774–8.
11. Cooper C, Selwood A and Livingston G. The prevalence of elder abuse and neglect: a systematic review. *Age Ageing* 2008;**37**:151–60.
12. O'Keeffe M, Hills A, Doyle M *et al. UK Study of Abuse and Neglect of Older People*, National Centre for Social Research, London, 2007.
13. Cooper C, Selwood A, Blanchard M *et al.* The determinants of family carer's abusive behaviour to people with dementia: results of the CARD study. *J Affect Disord* 2010;**121**:136–42.
14. Cooney C, Howard R and Lawlor B. Abuse of vulnerable people with dementia by their carers: can we identify those most at risk? *Int J Geriatr Psychiatry* 2006;**21**:564–71.
15. Royal College of Psychiatrists. *Institutional Abuse of Older Adults*, Council Report CR84, Royal College of Psychiatrists, London, 2000.
16. Commission for Health Improvement. *Investigation into Matters Arising from Care on Rowan Ward, Manchester Mental Health and Social Care Trust*, Commission for Health Improvement, London, 2003.
17. Cooper C, Manela M, Katona C and Livingston G. Screening for elder abuse in dementia in the LASER-AD study: prevalence, correlates and validation of instruments. *Int J Geriatr Psychiatry* 2008;**23**:283–8.
18. Fulmer T, Paveza G, Abraham I and Fairchild S. Elder neglect assessment in the emergency department. *J Emerg Nurs* 2008;**26**:437–43.
19. Cooper C, Selwood A and Livingston G. Knowledge, detection and reporting of abuse by health and social care professionals: a systematic review. *Am J Geriatr Psychiatry* 2009;**17**:826–38.
20. Kitchen G, Richardson B and Livingston G. Are nurses equipped to manage actual or suspected elder abuse? *Prof Nurse* 2002,**17**:647–650.
21. Richardson B, Kitchen G and Livingston G. The effect of education on knowledge and management of elder abuse: a randomized controlled trial. *Age Ageing* 2002;**31**:335–41.

CHAPTER 119

Good quality care: abuse

Jean-Pierre Aquino[1] **and Geneviève Ruault**[2]

[1]Clinique Médicale de la Porte Verte, Versailles, France

[2]French Society of Geriatrics and Gerontology, Suresnes, France

The empire of old age is spreading its influence. But beyond increased life expectancy at birth, some new situations are emerging. Through medical progress, some deadly diseases have become chronic illnesses (e.g. cancer, AIDS), but other conditions have made themselves at home, such as disabling illnesses and Alzheimer's disease. This epidemiological admission must be completed by an understanding of the problems that handicapped ageing raises.

The insufficient financial resources of some pensioners represent another characteristic. In France, the average pension of a retiree is 1100 euros per month, but the average cost in a retirement home is between 2200 and 2500 euros per month.

Medical and economic factors can contribute to vulnerable situations, which can lead to maltreatment. This has been the French experience.

Definitions

Abuse is an acknowledged deviance. According to the Council of Europe's definition, 'Abuse consists of all and any acts or omissions, which endanger one's life, threatens bodily or psychological integrity or infringes one's liberty or compromises personality development and/or seriously undermines financial security'.

As is well known, those who are vulnerable represent the usual target. Handicapped and dependent people and especially cognitive disorders represent vulnerable clinical situations.

The fight against abuse of the vulnerable elderly has become a social and ethical issue. On a semantic level, 'good quality care' is not the opposite of 'abuse'. Good quality care is based on humanist values. It is an action which promotes quality care and prevents abuse, while developing human relations. It implies particular attention to people's needs and takes professional practices into account.

With regard to the ill elderly, good quality care is expressed in two essential and complementary aspects: the quality of care and the quality of care giving. Quality of life is certainly the pursued objective.

Both at home and in a retirement home, good quality care implies several actions:

- Locate, evaluate and treat pain, which is not always easy when verbal expression is lacking.
- Diagnose depression while considering the risk of suicide.
- Maintain mobility, compensate for functional deficiencies.
- Prevent and treat malnutrition.
- End-of-life care and symptom relief.
- Provide, whatever the need, care quality and continuity, without abandoning technical aspects, while respecting the person's choice.

In retirement homes, the prevalence of dependence, multipathology and, in particular, cognitive disorders in 50–80% of residents; which gives these actions their great importance.

A reminder of the main ethical principles

In a preventive approach, we should recall fundamental ethical principles that must guide geriatricians in their daily practice of caring for vulnerable people:

- *Principle of humanity and dignity*. Everyone, whatever their condition, situation and personal history, has the quality of being human and therefore belongs to a community of human beings. It is a universal and inalienable principle.
- *Principle of solidarity*. People belonging to the same human community are bound by a collective responsibility to grant mutual aid and help to those afflicted by the misfortunes of life.

Principles and Practice of Geriatric Medicine, Fifth Edition. Edited by Alan J. Sinclair, John E. Morley and Bruno Vellas.

• *Principle of fairness and justice*. This principle requires, for every person, the recognition and respect of their rights. Thus, age must not be a pretext to refuse access to diagnostic methods and/or to care, while appreciating, of course, the necessity to avoid relentless therapy.
• *Principle of autonomy*. This principle requires that each individual can freely rule their own life and make their own decisions concerning it.

Multidimensional aspects of abuse

Abuse expresses itself in various ways. The Council of Europe (1992) proposed the following classification. Abuse can be of various natures:
• Physical: blows, bodily cruelty, contention.
• Psychological: verbal violence, insults, familiarity, infantilization, threat of violence, deprivation of visits.
• Financial and material: theft or misappropriation of money, coerced signed cheques, anticipated inheritance.
• Medical: deprivation of medicine and care, lack of basic care, inappropriate care, no treatment information, neuroleptic abuse, no pain relief, lack of care coordination, and so on.
• Infringement of people's rights, their identity, their liberty to come and go, deprivation of the exercise of civic rights and the right to choose, religious practice, abusive use of legal protection.

However, it is necessary also to distinguish situations characterized by negligence:
• Active negligence corresponds to deprivation of indispensable daily care (eating, drinking, receiving visits, etc.), to defective aid leading to unacceptable hygiene, to abandonment, to putting the person in danger.
• Passive negligence results from forgetfulness: there is no intention to harm. It is a result of a lack of aid in getting up, putting to bed, grooming, dressing, walking, and so on. This attitude is a matter of ignorance and inattention to one's duty. Thus in retirement homes, the staff may be negligent because of a lack of training, a shortage in the workforce or ill-adapted working conditions.

The reality in the field teaches us that situations are often intricate, associating medical, psychological, social and economic issues, creating a complex scenario whose analysis proves difficult.

What are the clinical signs which lead us to suspect abuse? The presence of bruises, repetitive unexplained traumatic lesions, pelvic pains or genital bleeding, muteness or agitation on the part of the elderly person in front of a family or professional carer, malnutrition, deficient hygiene, regular trips to the emergency room of a neighbouring hospital, must draw professionals' attention. However, one needs to be careful of elderly people who say they are being abused but who, in fact, live in a delirium of persecution.

But who abuses?

Several situations involve some risk of progressing towards abuse. They must be known, in order to employ preventive measures, both at home and in care establishments. Thus, recent female widowhood, functional dependence, physical problems with urinary incontinence, psychological dependence and behavioural disorders (e.g. Alzheimer's disease) represent factors linked directly to the elderly person.

In the private sphere, the aggressor may be one or more family members, a neighbour, a 'friend'. They are often characterized by overt alcoholism, a difficult social and financial situation or a psychiatric illness. Ignorance of the illness, its non-acceptance, fear of dependence, exhaustion, isolation with a refusal of outside help, all aggravate the context.

The cohabitation of victim and aggressor in a small home facilitates abuse. In a care establishment, staff shortages, lack of trained teams, emotional exhaustion and professional attrition contribute to this failing. We therefore understand the importance of the establishment's project and the managing team's motivation, responsible for maintaining working conditions. However, ill-adapted premises and facilities and poorly used space present security risks for the residents and also represent a kind of abuse.

Conduct to embrace

Preventing abuse situations must be a priority in caring for elderly vulnerable people. It is the role of public authorities, associations and professionals that work in the geriatric field. This prevention calls for information, training and organizing effective measures.

In cases of abuse, either established or suspected, the priority is to protect the victim, in addition to taking into account the person's wishes. Often, hospitalization is the required solution, taking the person away from their presumed aggressor.

In other situations corresponding to suffering or exhaustion of care givers, it is necessary to break the isolation of the victim–aggressor couple, by the intervention of professionals at home, by temporary lodging, by protective legal measures, and so on.

French law stipulates that any qualified abuse offence must be brought to the judicial authority's attention (state prosecutor). The physician is no longer bound by professional confidentiality. Confirming abuse is a matter for penal jurisdiction.

Article 434-3 of the Penal Code

The Article states: 'The fact, for whoever having had knowledge of deprivations, abuse or sexual harassment inflicted on a minor under fifteen or a person who cannot protect himself because of his age, an illness, an infirmity, a physical or psychological deficiency or pregnancy and not having informed the judicial or administrative authorities is punishable by up to 3 years' imprisonment and a 45 000 euro fine'.

Any complaint of abuse must be heard by trained and experienced people and must be discreetly investigated to confirm or invalidate its authenticity.

The laws

Several years ago, France created certain laws to promote good treatment and thus prevent abuse.

The democracy health law (2002) not only recognizes individual patients' rights, but also the collective rights of associations and their users: the right to respect and dignity, to care aimed at relieving pain, rejecting discrimination in access to prevention or care.

It is stipulated that 'anyone over 18 can designate a trustworthy individual, who will be consulted and receive the necessary information to make decisions on behalf of the person in the event that he, one day, becomes incapable of expressing his will. This designation must be made in writing; it revocable at any time'.

The Leonetti law (2005), relating to patients' rights at the end of life, specifies that 'anyone over 18 can write anticipated instructions in case this person should, one day, become incapable of expressing his will. These anticipated instructions indicate the relative end-of-life wishes of the person concerning the conditions of limiting or stopping treatment. They are revocable at any time. Provided that they have been established at least 3 years before the person lapses into a state of unconsciousness, the physician takes this into account before any decision is made concerning an investigation, intervention or treatment.

'The physician protects the dying person's dignity and assures the quality of his end of life'. Important progress has been made in respecting the autonomy of ill people in the sense of respecting their life choices.

The plan for developing good quality care and reinforcing the fight against abuse was launched in 2007 by the Ministry of Health. With 10 measures, this plan of action aims to develop a culture of good quality care in establishments and reinforce the fight against abuse. Created in the framework of this plan is the National Agency of Social and Medico-Social Evaluation, qualified by the Minister of the 'Quality Care Agency'.

Establishments are encouraged to implement a method of improving quality: self-evaluation of their practices, definition of objectives to improve them and external controls. Abuse prevention becomes an element in the quality approach.

This plan also oversees the diffusion of good professional practices, elaborated by the National Agency of Social and Medico-Social Evaluation, intended for staff members. It is also interested in the residents' living environment.

Further, reporting cases of abuse is encouraged, thanks to an SOS abuse hotline and an information campaign communicating the telephone number. The designation of an abuse 'telephone contact' in every French Department allows for the coordination of information from different public services. The number of inspections in establishments has doubled, with sanctions included.

The expertise of the National Committee of Vigilance against abuse is extended to the handicapped.

The 2007 law on structural reform of legal protection for adults (future protective mandate, limitation of tutelages for people medically acknowledged to be incapable of exercising their rights) takes part in the fight against financial abuses.

It is in the framework of these missions that the National Agency of Social and Medico-Social Evaluation elaborated and distributed several recommendations for good professional practices, which include:

- Good quality care: definition and references for its implementation.
- Establishment manager's mission and supervisory role in abuse prevention and treatment.
- The person's expectations and personalized project.
- Implementation of an adaptation strategy for the staff's use with regard to accompanied people.
- The medico-psycho-social accompaniment of people suffering from Alzheimer's disease or related disorders.

In 2008, the Ministry reinforced measures in favour of good quality care for the elderly and handicapped in establishments by increasing unplanned inspections in lodging establishments for dependent elderly persons and renewed support for the national hotline dedicated to the fight against abuse. Every year establishments are obliged to address an internal 'good quality care' evaluation questionnaire to public authorities, completed and viewed by the management team and the President of the Social Life Council. In the absence of a self-evaluation or manifest incoherence in filling in the questionnaire, a flash investigation is carried out in order to identify the problems met by the establishment.

Staff training in the techniques of personalized accompaniment is supported and prefects are solicited to organize departmental 'good quality care' meetings.

After a first report on these measures in favour of good quality care, the Minister declared, 'The culture of good quality care is a collective approach aiming to assure the best possible accompaniment for the elderly, at home or in an establishment, respecting their choices and adapting to their needs. Actions carried out in the framework of operating good quality care in establishments and the opening of a hotline number to fight against all forms of abuse concerning the elderly or handicapped prove that good quality care is a functioning reality mobilizing professionals and public authorities in a voluntary and permanent way'. The social service hotline number received 63 858 calls between 5 February 2008 and 15 April 2009; 81% pertained to problems of abuse, 25.3% of which were psychological abuse; 80% of the controls carried out in medico-social establishments were unplanned verifications.

Finally, the training process of the establishments' staff has a good quality care approach and is engaged in the objective 'to train 100% of retirement home managers in a good quality care culture and organize training for the entire staff'. In 2010, the Minister reinforced the operation again, insisting especially on training intervening parties, professionals and family carers. For abuse predominantly occurring at home, he proposed, regarding family accompaniment, the concept of 'short training sessions' to 'help carers, preparing, enlightening and supporting them'.

Concerning care establishments, the evaluation of quality is reinforced. Some of them received a compliance request. Public authorities are very vigilant concerning formulated request applications (for example, the obligation for medicalization because of the dependent people concerned). Non-conforming establishments, within 3 months, run the risk of being closed down.

Other contributions

Indirect contributions of different public health plans include the pain management improvement plan, the quality of life of people presenting chronic affection plan, the Alzheimer's plan and the palliative care plan.

However, the mobilization of the High Health Authority reinforces the certification requirements of hospitals with the implementation of a complaint management system, the implementation of patients' end-of-life rights and the implementation of a promotional approach for good quality care.

This approach is based on an engagement on behalf of the management and establishment authorities, in particular from the Relations Commission with the Users and the Quality of Care to promote good quality care; training and professional awareness; abuse prevention actions; but also concrete and various actions centred on the daily experience of users, aiming to improve reception, efficient implementation of rights and meeting the needs of people.

MobiQual – mobilization for the improvement of the quality of professional practices

The objective of this national action, implemented by the French Society of Geriatrics and Gerontology, on the initiative of the Ministry of Health and supported by the National Solidarity for Autonomy Fund, is to improve professional practices in retirement homes, in health establishments and in private homes. This approach mobilizes all the actors concerned: public authorities, establishment and service federations, scholarly societies and voluntary service professionals, in the name of quality care and to take care of the elderly and handicapped. It rests on a common base, one of good quality care and specific themes: pain, depression, palliative care, end-of-life accompaniment, nutrition, Alzheimer's disease and risk of infection. It provides useful tools for all professionals: collective reflection guides helping institutional projects develop; professional training to strengthen theoretical and practical knowledge; help in decision-making and practice for quality and harmonious multidisciplinary practice; and cooperative link supports to strengthen the collective expertise. These tools are given to all voluntary establishments to use, in return for a charter attesting to their proper use.

This action includes an implementation and follow-up system: a national team project, guaranteeing the method of diffusion and integrating public authorities, references for each tool, establishment and service federations and a national coordinator for follow-up and evaluation.

The action therefore aims to make the staff aware of EHPAD (établissements d'hébergement pour personnes agées dépendantes), carers and non-carers, to a method of good quality care, while helping them to spot and prevent risky situations and proposing good quality care evaluation tools.

The approach consists of proposing voluntary EHPAD a good quality care kit, accompanied by awareness/training action intended for all professional actors intervening in EHPAD.

MobiQual

'What is good quality care on the institutional level, in the establishment where I work?'

'What is good quality care for me, who works in this establishment?'

'What is good quality care for the person living in the establishment where I work?'

'What is good quality care for the entourage of people living in the establishment where I work?'

> *Good quality care is an interrogation and must be reinvented, starting from some fundamentals, by each establishment and service.*
>
> National Agency of Social and Medico-Social Evaluation.

It is necessary to develop training, but also to give staff time to discuss and reflect. It is necessary to recognize and to evaluate the level of reflection of most carers, because one can only give good treatment if one is treated well.

A temporary report, written at the beginning of 2010, specifies that more than 9000 tools have been distributed to establishments, corresponding to about 245 000 professionals concerned.

The objective the French Society of Geriatrics and Gerontology is to pursue and to develop the programme, in a period of 3 years, starting in 2010, thanks to financial support from the National Solidarity for Autonomy Fund, the Ministry's involvement and the mobilization of geriatricians in the regions.

Further comments

- In France, good quality care is henceforth at the heart of public policies and evaluation methods and improved practices in the socio-medical sector. This approach aims to compel organizations to be more considerate of the needs and expectations of people, to promote the person's wellbeing and keep in mind the risks of abuse.
- Progressively, these developments are also taking hold in the health and hospital fields.
- Coherent public policy on this good quality care theme is a major issue for the French Society of Geriatrics and Gerontology, which endeavours to carry its deliberations to the highest state level.
- Since 2007, some considerable progress has been made, providing an indisputable consistency to the following dynamic: from the priorities for training decreed by the Ministry, to recommendations by agencies, good quality care established as an indicator of quality for professional practices, but also for health and socio-medical establishments.

Conclusion

The mission of developing good quality care in health and socio-medical establishments is now entrusted to Regional Health Agencies, created by the Hospital, Patient, Health and Territories law (2009). It is a signal of transformation. Therefore, let us hope that the twenty-first century will be the one for rights of the elderly, like the twentieth century was for childrens' rights.

However, this aspiration will not fully materialize unless society progressively changes its outlook on the elderly and ageing.

Key points

- Medical and economic factors can contribute to vulnerable situations, which can lead to maltreatment.
- In a preventive approach, we should recall fundamental ethical principles that must guide geriatricians and other healthcare professionals in their daily practice of caring for vulnerable people.
- Preventing abuse situations must be a priority in caring for elderly vulnerable people. It is the role of public authorities, associations and professionals who work in the elderly care field.

Suggested reading

1. Laroque G. Good and adequate care/abuse and neglect: what is the situation in France? *Gerontol Société* 2010;**133**:63–8.
2. Moulias R, Busby F, Hugonot R and France A. A methodology for the management of elder abuse. *Gerontol Société* 2010;**133**:89–102.
3. Ruault G, Aquino JP and Doutreligne S. Good and adequate care of dependent older people: the good care kit of the national MobiQual programme. *Gerontol Société* 2010;**133**:159–69.
4. *Loi No. 2002-303 du 4 mars 2002 relative aux droits des malades et à la qualité du système de santé* (JORF No.54 du 5 Mars 2002).
5. *Loi No. 2005-370 du 22 avril 2005 relative aux droits des malades et à la fin de vie* (JORF No. 95 du 23 avril 2005).
6. *Loi No. 2007-308 du 5 mars 2007 portant réforme de la protection juridique des majeurs* (JORF No. 56 du 7 mars 2007).
7. *Plan de développement de la bientraitance et de renforcement de la lutte contre la maltraitance.* Ministère Délégué à la Sécurité Sociale, aux Personnes âgées, aux Personnes Handicapées et à la Famille, Paris, 2007, http://www.personnes-agees.gouv.fr/point_presse/d_presse/bientraitance_maltraitance/presentation_plan.pdf (last accessed 13 October 2011).
8. *Plan d'amélioration de la prise en charge de la douleur 2006–2010.* Ministère de la Santé et des Solidarités, Paris, 3 mars 2006, http://www.sante-sports.gouv.fr/la-douleur-plan-d-amelioration-de-la-prise-en-charge-de-la-douleur.html (last accessed 13 October 2011).
9. *Plan Qualité de vie des personnes atteintes de maladies chroniques 2007–2011.* Ministère de la Santé et des Solidarités, Paris, avril 2007, http://www.sante.gouv.fr/htm/dossiers/plan_maladies_chroniques/sommaire.htm (last accessed 13 October 2011).
10. *Plan Alzheimer et maladies apparentées 2008–2012.* Présidence de la République, Paris, 1 février 2008, www.elysee.fr/president/root/bank . . . /08-02-01-Dp-Plan-Alzheimer.pdf (last accessed 13 October 2011).
11. *Plan de développement des soins palliatifs 2008–2012.* Présidence de la République, Paris, 13 juin 2008, www.sfap.org/pdf/0-K2-pdf.pdf (last accessed 13 October 2011).

CHAPTER 120

Alcohol consumption and cognition

Luc Letenneur and Jean-François Dartigues

INSERM Unit 897, and Université Bordeaux Segalen, Bordeaux, France

Cognitive impairment is a public health concern for ageing adults. Some of the detrimental effects of heavy alcohol use on brain function are similar to those observed with Alzheimer's disease. Ethanol and acetaldehyde are toxins that negatively affect neural tissues and chronic heavy intake of ethanol is associated with an increased risk of alcohol-related central nervous system disease. Although the toxic effects of long-term, heavy alcohol intake on the central nervous system are well known, there is emerging evidence to suggest that moderate alcohol intake (one to three standard drinks per day) may be associated with a reduced risk of developing cognitive impairment.

Evidence from studies

In a cross-sectional population based study,[1] better global cognitive functioning assessed through psychometric tests such as the Mini Mental State Examination (MMSE) was associated with moderate wine consumption [odds ratio (OR) = 0.62; 95% confidence interval (CI), 0.48–0.81; $p = 0.0004$]. This association disappeared, however, when controlled for age, gender, educational level and occupational category, showing that confounding is a major issue in the study of alcohol consumption. Prospective studies also analysed the association between alcohol consumption and cognitive decline. A subsample of 387 survivors of 1083 subjects recruited between 1983 and 1985 in the cognitive substudy of the Medical Research Council treatment trial of hypertension was examined 9–12 years after the initial visit to assess cognition.[2] Poorer cognitive outcome was associated with abstinence from alcohol prior the age of 60 years.

In a randomly selected sample of 333 men living in Zutphen, The Netherlands, and followed for 8 years, low-to-moderate alcohol intake had a significantly lower risk for poor cognitive function (MMSE <25) than abstainers (OR of 0.3 for less than one drink and 0.2 for one to two drinks per day).[3] However, alcohol intake was not associated with cognitive decline. In women, alcohol consumption was also shown to be associated with a reduced risk of cognitive decline. Data from the Women's Health Initiative Memory Study of postmenopausal combination hormone therapy were used to assess cross-sectional and prospective associations of self-reported alcohol intake with cognitive function.[4] Compared with no intake, intake of ≥1 drink per day was associated with higher baseline modified MMSE scores ($p < 0.001$) and a covariate-adjusted OR of 0.40 (95% CI, 0.28–0.99) for significant decline in cognitive function over 3 years. Associations with incident probable dementia were of similar magnitude but were not statistically significant after covariate adjustment.

In the MoVIES project, cognitive functions and self-reported drinking habits were assessed at 2 year intervals over an average of 7 years of follow-up.[5] Trajectory analyses identified latent homogeneous groups with respect to frequency of alcohol use over time and their association with average decline over the same period in each cognitive domain. Three homogeneous trajectories were defined and were characterized as no drinking, minimal drinking and moderate drinking. Compared with no drinking, minimal drinking was associated with lesser decline on the MMSE (OR = 0.05; 95% CI, 0.01–0.26) and Trail Making Tests (OR = 0.02; 95% CI, 0.001–0.22), that evaluated executive functions. The same trends were observed for moderate drinking (MMSE, OR = 0.27; 95% CI, 0.09–0.84; Trail Making Test, OR = 0.15; 95% CI, 0.03–0.79). Minimal drinking was also associated with lesser decline in tests of learning and naming. These associations did not change on comparing current drinkers with former drinkers (quitters) and with lifelong abstainers.

Prospective evidence

The first prospective study to explore the association between alcohol intake and dementia was the PAQUID programme.[6] A sample of 3777 subjects aged 65 years or older was followed for 3 years and 99 incident cases of

Principles and Practice of Geriatric Medicine, Fifth Edition. Edited by Alan J. Sinclair, John E. Morley and Bruno Vellas.

dementia were diagnosed. Alcohol consumption data were collected at baseline, with wine being the main type of alcohol consumed, usually on a daily basis. Four categories of individuals were defined: non-drinkers, mild drinkers (consuming up to 0.25 l of wine, i.e. two drinks per day), moderate drinkers (consuming up to 0.5 l of wine, i.e. three to four drinks per day) and heavy drinkers (consuming more than four drinks per day). Lower risks of developing dementia were found among drinkers compared with non-drinkers, but the relationship was significant only for moderate drinkers [mild drinkers, risk ratio (RR) = 0.81; moderate drinkers, RR = 0.19; heavy drinkers, RR = 0.31]. No modification effect was found according to gender and the association did not change after adjusting for age, gender, education, occupation and baseline cognition. After 10 years of follow-up, the association between baseline alcohol consumption and incident dementia remained significant, although the risk ratios tended to increase toward unity (mild drinkers, RR = 0.89, 95% CI, 0.70–1.15; moderate drinkers, RR = 0.56; 95% CI, 0.36–0.92).[7]

The Rotterdam Study followed 5395 subjects aged 55 years or older over a period of 6 years; 197 incidents cases of dementia were diagnosed.[8] The number of drinks of alcohol (beer, wine, fortified wine or spirits) was collected at baseline and five categories of intake were studied: no drinks consumed; less than one drink per week; more than one drink per week but less than one per day; one to three drinks per day; more than three drinks per day. The risk of developing dementia was lower among drinkers compared with non-drinkers (Table 120.1) and was significant in the 1–3 drinks per day category. The pattern was different in men and women. No association was found in women, whereas a lower risk was found for men drinking 1–3 drinks per day. A modification effect was found when the apolipoprotein E4 allele (ApoE4) was taken into consideration: the risk was lower among drinkers with an ApoE4 allele, whereas it was less clear for drinkers without the ApoE4 allele (Table 120.1). No difference was found according to beverage type, although beer tended to give marginally lower risk than wine.

In a prospective study of elderly people living in North Manhattan,[9] 2126 subjects were followed for 4 years and 260 incident cases of dementia were diagnosed. The number of drinks per week was collected at baseline and subjects were classified as non-drinkers, light drinkers (less than one drink per month to six drinks per week), moderate drinkers (one to three drinks per day) and heavy drinkers (more than three drinks per day). Light and moderate categories were aggregated because of the small number of moderate drinkers; in this sample, 70% of the subjects were non-drinkers. On analysing the association between each alcoholic beverage type and dementia, wine was significantly associated with a lower risk among light to moderate drinkers [hazard ratio (HR) = 0.64; $p = 0.018$]. On analysing the risk of Alzheimer's disease adjusted for age and gender, a decreased risk was observed in wine drinkers (HR = 0.59; $p = 0.018$), but the association became insignificant when education and the ApoE4 genotype (HR = 0.69; $p = 0.11$) were included. The risk ratios were >1 for light to moderate beer or spirits drinkers (beer, HR = 1.39; $p = 0.094$, spirits, HR = 1.34; $p = 0.152$). When wine, beer and spirits were analysed simultaneously with full adjustment, the risk for Alzheimer's disease was lower in wine drinkers (HR = 0.55; $p = 0.015$), but higher for beer (HR = 1.47; $p = 0.065$) or spirits (HR = 1.51; $p = 0.062$) drinkers. A modification effect was found with the ApoE4 genotype. A significantly lower risk of dementia was found in light to moderate wine drinkers without an ApoE4 allele (HR = 0.44; $p = 0.004$) compared with non-drinkers, whereas the association disappeared for ApoE4 allele bearers (HR = 1.10; $p = 0.093$). No modification effect by gender was found.

The association between alcohol intake and risk for dementia was also examined in studies originally designed to explore cardiovascular events. During follow-up, cognitive functioning was explored and nested case–control studies were performed. In the Copenhagen City Heart study,[10] a nested case–control included 83 cases of dementia and 1626 controls. Alcohol intake was collected in two ways: the number of drinks per week (<1, 1–7, 8–14, 15–21, 22 or more) and the frequency of intake (never/hardly ever, monthly, weekly, daily). No association was found between the number of drinks of alcohol consumed per week and the risk of dementia. When beer, wine and spirits intake were analysed simultaneously, a reduced risk was observed only for wine drinkers (monthly, HR = 0.43; 95%

Table 120.1 Hazard ratios (with 95% CI) of dementia according to alcohol consumption in the Rotterdam Study.

Group	No alcohol	<1 drink per week	≥1 drink per week but <1 per day	1–3 drinks per day	≥4 drinks per day
Total	1.00	0.82 (0.56–1.22)	0.75 (0.51–1.11)	0.58 (0.38–0.90)	1.0 (0.39–2.59)
Men	1.00	0.60 (0.27–1.34)	0.53 (0.28–1.0)	0.40 (0.21–0.74)	0.88 (0.32–2.44)
Women	1.00	0.91 (0.58–1.44)	0.91 (0.55–1.49)	0.85 (0.47–1.57)	–
ApoE4 absent	1.00	1.26 (0.67–2.37)	1.39 (0.73–2.64)	0.67 (0.31–1.46)	–
ApoE4 present	1.00	0.69 (0.35–1.34)	0.46 (0.23–0.94)	0.60 (0.30–1.21)	–

CI, 0.23–0.82; weekly, HR = 0.33; 95% CI, 0.13–0.86; daily, HR = 0.57; 95% CI, 0.15–2.11). Beer drinkers tended to have a higher risk (monthly, HR = 2.28; 95% CI, 1.13–4.60; weekly, HR = 2.15; 95% CI, 0.98–4.78; daily, HR = 1.73; 95% CI, 0.75–3.99) and no clear association was found in spirits drinkers (monthly, HR = 0.81; 95% CI, 0.42–1.57; weekly, HR = 1.65; 95% CI, 0.74–3.69; daily, HR = 1.12; 95% CI, 0.43–2.92). No difference was found between men and women.

Another nested case–control study was performed within the Cardiovascular Health Study, which included 373 cases of dementia and 373 controls.[11] Levels of alcohol intake were defined as 0, <1, 1–6, 7–13 and 14 or more drinks per week. The association between alcohol intake and the risk of dementia followed a J-shaped curve, with a nadir for the category of 1–6 drinks per week (Table 120.2). The pattern was different for men and women: all drinker categories were associated with a lower risk in women, whereas a J-shaped curve was found for men (Table 120.2). A modification effect by ApoE4 was observed: when the ApoE4 allele was absent, the risk was significantly lower among subjects who consumed 1–6 drinks per week. When the ApoE4 allele was present, the HR was below 1.00 only for light drinkers and above 1.00 for heavier drinkers (Table 120.2). The odds of dementia were lower (although not significantly) for wine drinkers (<1 drink per week, HR = 0.72; 95% CI, 0.46–1.11; 1–6 drinks per week, HR = 0.72; 95% CI, 0.39–1.33; >6 drinks per week, HR = 0.62; 95% CI, 0.25–1.50). However, the trend was not the same for beer (<1 drink per week, HR = 0.84; 95% CI, 0.48–1.47; 1–6 drinks per week, HR = 0.74; 95% CI, 0.36–1.54; >6 drinks per week, HR = 1.96; 95% CI, 0.71–5.4]) or spirits drinkers (<1 drink per week, HR = 0.84; 95% CI, 0.48–1.45; 1–6 drinks per week, HR = 1.17; 95% CI, 0.59–2.30; >6 drinks per week, HR = 1.08; 95% CI, 0.55–2.13).

Several other prospective studies have reported an association between alcohol consumption and dementia. A Canadian study[12] reported that at least weekly consumption of alcohol was associated with a decreased risk of Alzheimer's disease (OR = 0.68; 95% CI, 0.47–1.00). In Sweden,[13] the risk of dementia was estimated to be 0.5 (95% CI, 0.3–0.7) among light to moderate drinkers (1–21 drinks per week in men, 1–14 drinks per week in women). In China,[14] light to moderate drinkers (1–21 drinks per week in men, 1–14 drinks per week in women) had a lower risk (RR = 0.52; 95% CI, 0.32–0.85) than non-drinkers, but a non-significant increased risk was observed in heavy drinkers (RR = 1.45; 95% CI, 0.43–4.89). A greater reduction of risk was observed for men (RR = 0.37) than for women (RR = 0.76).

All these studies tend to show the same result: *light to moderate alcohol consumption is associated with a lower risk of developing dementia*. Which mechanisms may be involved in the risk reduction of dementia? One possibility is that alcohol might act by reducing cardiovascular risk factors, either through an inhibitory effect of ethanol on platelet aggregation or through alteration of the serum lipid profile. A second possibility is that alcohol might have a direct effect on cognition through the release of acetylcholine in the hippocampus. Finally, another possible mechanism is through the antioxidant activity of alcoholic beverages, particularly wine, which has been found to have important antioxidant effects.

However, the definition of light to moderate alcohol intake varies considerably across the studies reviewed. The classification of drinking as moderate ranges from monthly or weekly drinking to 3–4 drinks per day, and many studies reported an association for an intake of less than one drink per day. As alcohol intake is self-reported, it is also expected to be under-reported. However, neither a linear dose–response nor a J-shaped curve were systematically found over all studies and the association sometimes differed according to gender. The type of alcohol does not appear to be consistent across studies, yet wine intake is systematically associated with lower risk. If alcohol *per se* were associated with a decreased risk of developing dementia, the same pattern would be expected for beer and wine drinkers, yet beer has been found to be associated with higher risk in several studies.

Table 120.2 Odds (with 95% CI) of incident dementia according to alcohol consumption (drinks per week) in the Cardiovascular Health Study.

Group	None	<1	1–6	7–13	≥14
Total	1.00	0.65 (0.41–1.02)	0.46 (0.27–0.77)	0.69 (0.37–1.31)	1.22 (0.60–2.49)
Men	1.00	0.82 (0.38–1.78)	0.36 (0.17–0.77)	1.42 (0.58–3.48)	2.40 (0.86–6.64)
Women	1.00	0.52 (0.30–0.90)	0.57 (0.28–1.17)	0.23 (0.09–0.61)	0.39 (0.14–1.10)
ApoE4 absent	1.00	0.56 (0.33–0.97)	0.37 (0.20–0.67)	0.64 (0.30–1.38)	0.60 (0.24–1.51)
ApoE4 present	1.00	0.60 (0.24–1.52)	0.62 (0.21–1.81)	1.49 (0.33–6.65)	3.37 (0.67–17.1)

Conclusion

When analysing these results and discrepancies, one can wonder about the nature of the association between alcohol consumption and the risk of dementia. It can be hypothesized that alcohol intake (especially light to moderate intake) is only a marker of a broader psychosocial behaviour that is associated with a decreased risk of developing dementia. However, the analyses were controlled for many other risk factors and the association with alcohol was still significant. It is possible that important confounders (not yet identified) were not considered, which might explain some of the discrepancies between optimal intake, gender or type of alcohol. Light to moderate wine drinkers may prove to be moderate with regard to other risk factors of dementia and alcohol intake would only be an indicator of such behaviour.

Until such factors have been identified, we must be careful in how we interpret results relating to alcohol consumption. We have recently reanalysed the data of the PAQUID study with 20 years of follow-up. Among the 3676 non-demented subjects at the baseline screening, 830 developed dementia during the follow-up. After adjustment for age, gender and education, taking non-drinkers as the reference, the risk of dementia was lower in mild drinkers (HR = 0.85; 95% CI, 0.73–0.9), but failed to reach statistical significance for moderate drinkers (HR = 0.79; 95% CI, 0.60–1.04) and was neutral for heavy drinkers (HR = 1.01; 95% CI, 0.63–1.62). In the same cohort, during the 15 first years of follow-up, 2422 died. With the same adjustment and the same category of reference (non-drinkers), the risk of dying was weakly lower in mild drinkers but failed to reach statistical significance (HR = 0.94; 95% CI 0.86–1.03) and was neutral for moderate drinkers (HR = 1; 95% CI, 0.87–1.15) and for heavy drinkers (HR = 1.06; 95% CI, 0.83–1.36). That means that if a protective effect of mild wine consumption cannot be excluded, the impact of this effect was certainly weak and did not justify recommendations for prevention. People should not be encouraged to drink more in the belief that this will protect them against dementia. However, elderly people who drink mild to moderate amounts of alcohol have no clear reason to stop this little pleasure during ageing.

Key points

- There is emerging evidence to suggest that *moderate* alcohol intake (one to three standard drinks per day) may be associated with a reduced risk of developing cognitive impairment.
- In studies examining the relationship between alcohol intake and risk of dementia, when beer, wine and spirits intake were analysed simultaneously, a reduced risk was observed systematically for wine drinkers.
- There is evidence that among the apoE4 allele bearers, alcohol intake may reduce the risk of dementia in light drinkers compared with non-drinkers.

References

1. Letenneur L, Dartigues JF and Orgogozo JM. Wine consumption and cognitive deficit in elderly individuals from the Bordeaux area. *Ann Intern Med* 1992;**118**:317–8.
2. Cervilla J, Prince M, Joels S *et al.* Long-term predictors of cognitive outcome in a cohort of older people with hypertension. *Br J Psychiatry* 2000;**177**:66–71.
3. Launer LJ, Feskens E, Kalmijn S and Kromhout D. Smoking, drinking and thinking. *Am J Epidemiol* 1996;**143**:219–27.
4. Espeland M, Gu L, Masaki K *et al.* Association between reported alcohol intake and cognition: results frome the Women's Health Initiative Memory Study. *Am J Epidemiol* 2005;**161**:228–38.
5. Ganguli M, Vander Bilt J, Saxton J *et al.* Alcohol consumption and cognitive function in late life. A longitudinal community study. *Neurology* 2005;**65**:1210–7.
6. Orgogozo JM, Dartigues JF, Lafont S *et al.* Wine consumption and dementia in the elderly: a prospective community study in the Bordeaux area. *Rev Neurol* 1997;**153**:185–92.
7. Larrieu S, Letenneur L, Helmer C *et al.* Nutritional factors and risk of incident dementia in the PAQUID longitudinal cohort. *J Nutr Health Aging* 2004;**8**:150–4.
8. Ruitenberg A, van Swieten JC, Witteman JC *et al.* Alcohol consumption and risk of dementia: the Rotterdam Study. *Lancet* 2002;**359**:281–6.
9. Luchsinger J, Tang MX, Siddiqui M *et al.* Alcohol intake and risk of dementia. *J Am Geriatr Soc* 2004;**52**:540–6.
10. Truelsen T, Thudium D and Gronbaek M. Amount and type of alcohol and risk of dementia. The Copenhagen Heart Study. *Neurology* 2002;**59**:1313–9.
11. Mukamal K, Kuller L, Fitzpatrick A *et al.* Prospective study of alcohol consumption and risk of dementia in older adults. *JAMA* 2003;**289**:1405–13.
12. Lindsay J, Laurin D, Verreault R *et al.* Risk factors for Alzheimer's disease: a prospective analysis of the Canadian Study of Health and Aging. *Am J Epidemiol* 2002;**156**:445–53.
13. Huang W, Qiu C, Winblad B and Fratiglioni L. Alcohol consumption and incidence of dementia in a community sample aged 75 years and older. *J Clin Epidemiol* 2002;**55**:959–64.
14. Deng J, Zhou D, Li J *et al.* A 2-year follow-up study of alcohol consumption and risk of dementia. *Clin Neurol Neurosurg* 2006;**108**:378–83.

CHAPTER 121

Drug misuse and the older person: a contradiction in terms?

Antoine Piau and Fatima Nourhashemi

Toulouse University Hospital Toulouse, France

Introduction

There are two possible definitions of 'drug misuse'. The first, obvious, definition is 'drug abuse' with the term 'drug' used to cover illicit substances, but also non-compliant use of prescription drugs such as psychotropic medications and opioids. This drug abuse, which is not peculiar to older people, results from a complex interaction between a substance, a patient and its environment. However, older people are also exposed to another great danger: adverse drug reactions, with the term of 'drug' used to cover licit medication prescribed in agreement with basic medical rules. Here comes the second definition. Avoidable adverse drug reactions result from another interaction, as complex as the first one, involving a substance, a patient and its environment and the medical practitioner. For dementia, it could be even more complex, in part because of cognitive disorder, but also because of another factor that should be taken into account: the professional or informal stakeholder. For example, this one could ask for sedative medication prescription, not only for the direct patient benefit but also for their own quality of life. Both definitions have several meeting points, in particular for psychotropic medications: addiction, dependence, abstinence syndromes and health problems. In both definitions, it is, in most cases, an inappropriate response to a real issue. Consequently, to limit avoidable adverse drug reactions, we need to greatly change the way in which we prescribe for older people.

Drug abuse

For coverage on this subject, see Chapter 122, The use and abuse of prescribed medicines.

Medications and the elderly: geriatric characteristics, adverse drug reactions and drug misuse

Medications and the elderly: characteristics

Benefit–risk evaluation of medications in the elderly

The elderly and clinical trials

Phase III

When a medication has been shown to be effective in the young adult, it is also conventionally accepted that it is generally effective in the elderly. However, such an assertion can be discounted. For example, O'Hare *et al.*[1] carried out a literature review of the indications of angiotensin-converting enzyme (ACE) inhibitors and angiotensin II-receptor antagonists (AIIRA) in chronic kidney disease in the elderly. They came to the conclusion that the recommendations were based on data that are not relevant to the elderly, because of differences in the causes of chronic kidney disease. Similarly, the SENIORS study, performed to determine the effect of nebivolol as add-on therapy in elderly patients with heart failure, regardless of ejection fraction,[2] found that, *a priori*, efficacy was lower than in the young adult.

Medication risks are very poorly evaluated before market authorization, for three essential reasons. First, non-inclusion in Phase III trials of subjects with several concomitant disorders and receiving several medications: very elderly persons are among the populations excluded from clinical trials, including trials that include patients over 65 years of age, if these subjects present comorbid conditions. Several years ago, attention was drawn to this point by international recommendations that have not yet been implemented. Second, inadequate

Principles and Practice of Geriatric Medicine, Fifth Edition. Edited by Alan J. Sinclair, John E. Morley and Bruno Vellas.

collection of adverse effects is also a great limitation. Third, premarketing trials, although they can evaluate the efficacy of a medication in a controlled setting, only detect adverse drug reactions (ADRs) when these occur in more than one case in 100 and are not limited to a particular subgroup. This being so, they yield only relatively restricted information on safety of use (including in the young adult). The denominator of the benefit–risk balance in the elderly patient can only be known through information gained in Phase IV.

Phase IV

In the USA, over a 25 year period, 10% of new drugs were withdrawn from the market or were the subject of major alerts and half of the withdrawals occurred within 2 years of drug introduction.[3]

Through pharmacovigilance, Phase IV notably allows the collection of information on drug-related risk. However, spontaneous notification, which is the cornerstone of pharmacovigilance, principally yields information on type B adverse effects (bizarre or idiosyncratic effects, dose independent and unpredictable) and not on type A adverse effects (augmented pharmacological effects, dose dependent and predictable) which have the dual specificity of being more frequent and also of often being avoidable.

In practice

As the complete information needed to determine the benefit–risk ratio in elderly patients is not available and as the treatment decision cannot be based only on expected efficacy, guidelines with regard to this frail elderly population are often based on low levels of evidence, notably concerning insufficiency of treatment (see the section Classification of the various types of suboptimal prescription) and so affect the expected benefit–risk ratio.

Age and adverse drug reactions

Elderly persons may be more at risk of ADRs due to physiological age-related changes that influence the pharmacodynamics and pharmacokinetics of drugs.[4] These reactions are more frequent after the age of 65 years. However, once confounding factors have been taken into account, age does not seem to be an independent risk factor for ADRs[5] but it is a factor of gravity of such events.

Polypharmacy and adverse drug reactions

Polymorbidity leads to polypharmacy, which may be expected to yield certain benefits. However, polypharmacy, because of disease–disease and drug–disease interactions, may in fact decrease the benefit–risk balance of the treatments given. There are two possible definitions of polypharmacy.[6] The first is concomitant use of several medications. However, although some investigators used a threshold of 3–5 medications, no exact figure has been clearly established. A second definition is overuse or use of more medications than is clinically necessary (see the section Classification of the various types of suboptimal prescription). This definition carries the negative connotation of suboptimal prescription, but without fixing an arbitrary threshold.

Polypharmacy (in the sense of the total number of medications taken) is an independent risk factor of iatrogenic events that is constantly found in the literature. In a study by Gallagher and O'Mahoney, patients taking more than five medications were at greater risk of hospital admission because of inappropriate prescription.[7] Mackinnon and Hepler developed a set of indicators of avoidable ADR[8] and applied it retrospectively to a hospital database.[9] One of the main risk factors was found to be the number of medications (>5). A recent review of the literature showed that polypharmacy is increasing and is a risk factor for morbidity and mortality.[10] The use of an arbitrary number as a cut-off is, however debatable. Viktil *et al.*[11] carried out a hospital-based multicentre prospective study of 827 patients, aiming to determine whether polypharmacy defined as a given number of drugs is a suitable indicator for describing the risk of ADRs. The number of ADRs per patient increased in an almost linear manner with the number of medications at admission. One unit increase in number of drugs increased the incidence of ADRs by 8.6% [95% confidence interval (CI), 1.07–1.10]. The most appropriate definition of polypharmacy in geriatrics therefore seems to be the accumulation of medications considered useless and/or likely to lead to drug interferences.

Several studies found an association between the number of medications and use of inappropriate medications,[12] including an important retrospective study of 2707 elderly patients receiving home care in eight European countries.[13]

Disease–drug interactions, risk factors for iatrogenic events

In this section, we will not address 'classic' disease–drug interactions, such as chronic obstructive pulmonary disease (COPD) and beta-blockers, which are not specific to geriatrics.

Some elderly persons are at increased risk of iatrogenic events. Some authors[14] suggest that the following comorbid conditions should be considered as increasing the risk of ADR: frailty, renal insufficiency and cognitive impairment. As the incidence of ADRs is higher in women, female gender is a potential iatrogenic risk factor. In the study of Gallagher and O'Mahoney, for example, women were twice as likely as men to be admitted to hospital due to inappropriate prescription.[7] With regard to comorbid conditions, an Australian cohort study found that cardiac failure, chronic pulmonary disease, diabetes, renal or liver failure, rheumatological disease and cancers were associated with greater risk of repeated admissions for ADRs.[15] Mackinnon and Hepler, in their retrospective study,[9] found that the number of comorbid conditions was among the main risk factors for avoidable ADRs.

With regard to cognitive impairment, publications are sparse. In a prospective study of patients with Alzheimer's disease, medications were a contributory factor to admission in 25% of cases.[16] In another French cohort[17] of 80 patients with dementia, 37% of short-stay hospital admissions were secondary to an ADR and 57% of admissions were due to potentially avoidable ADRs. About 20% of the ADRs observed were falls and the medications most often involved were psychotropic agents. There appears to be an excess risk of iatrogenic events in persons with dementia. The extent of avoidable iatrogenic events and inappropriate prescriptions is still very poorly known in this population.

Drug–drug interactions

Use of several medications and more numerous comorbid conditions are associated with increased risk of a potential interaction.

Drug interactions in the elderly patient fall into three main categories.[18] Conventionally, these involve drugs with a narrow therapeutic window such as digoxin, phenytoin and warfarin. These interactions are often well known, monitoring tests are available and they are detected by all prescribing software programs. The second category concerns complex interactions; patients with nine medications or more or with numerous comorbid conditions are often in this category. The choice of each medication in isolation is generally appropriate. The third category is the prescribing cascade: an ADR is interpreted as a new independent disease state for which another medication is prescribed and the patient is then susceptible to present with other ADRs because of this unnecessary medication. We can cite, as an example, patients receiving cholinesterase inhibitors who are more at risk of receiving an anticholinergic drug for new-onset incontinence.

A Swedish study of the elderly population showed an increase in polypharmacy and potentially clinically significant interactions between 1992 and 2002.[19] The proportion of elderly persons exposed to potentially clinically significant interactions rose from 17 to 25% in the 10 year period.

Clinical manifestations of drug interactions

A French study[20] analysed for one year the medications taken by elderly patients admitted to a geriatric unit: of the 894 patients (89.4%) who took at least two medications, 538 (60.2%) were exposed to 1087 potential interactions. Clinical or biological effects were observed in 130 patients (14.5% of patients taking two or more medications). A review of the literature from 1990 to 2006 relating to drug interactions in the general population suggests that although potential drug interactions are frequent, they rarely lead to hospital admission. However, this rate seems to increase with age, rising from 0.57 to 4.8% of admissions of elderly patients.[21] Juurlink *et al.*[22] carried out a 7 year case–control study of all patients aged 66 years or over living in Ontario, Canada, and treated with glyburide, digoxin or ACE inhibitors. In the week before admission, patients receiving glyburide and admitted for hypoglycaemia were six times more likely to have taken cotrimoxazole, patients receiving digoxin admitted for ADR were 12 times more likely to have been treated with clarithromycin and patients receiving ACE inhibitors and admitted for hyperkalaemia were 20 times more likely to have been treated with a potassium-sparing diuretic.

In practice

It is not realistic to think that physicians know and recognize all drug interactions. Prescribing software programs can help to reduce interactions but they raise the problem of numerous irrelevant alerts that are ultimately ignored by the prescriber, of significant but unrecognized interactions and updates that are not carried out. The problem is made more complex by the fact that it is difficult to know, among the potential interactions, which ones will be have a clinical expression. It therefore seems necessary to concentrate on monitoring the medications with a narrow therapeutic window, to look for potential interactions when a new co-medication is introduced and to consider the possibility of an ADR when in the presence of symptoms of recent onset, in order to avoid the prescribing cascade.

Medications and the elderly: iatrogenic consequences

A large prospective study[23] showed, in a population that was not specifically geriatric, a 6.5% prevalence of hospital admissions secondary to an ADR. The drugs most often implicated were low-dose aspirin, diuretics (27%), warfarin and non-steroidal anti-inflammatory drugs (NSAIDs). The most common reaction was gastrointestinal bleeding, which was responsible for half of the deaths due to ADRs. These results, however, have to be adjusted for the consumption rates of these drugs. The mean age of subjects admitted for ADRs was 76 years (compared with 66 years for all admissions). Of these ADRs, 72% were considered to be avoidable.

The rate of ADR-related hospitalization appears higher in elderly than in younger adults. A meta-analysis of 17 observational studies estimated the mean rate of ADR-related admissions in elderly subjects as 16.6%.[24] A considerable proportion of these were judged to be avoidable. A cohort study of 30 397 persons followed for 1 year in an ambulatory setting found an overall rate of ADRs of 50 per 1000 patient-years, of which 27.6% were considered to be avoidable.[25] More than one-third of these ADRs (38%) were judged to be severe, life-threatening or fatal and a higher proportion (42.2%) were avoidable. In an institutional setting, the incidence of ADRs varied according to the method of identification used, ranging from 1.19 ADRs for 100 patient-months to 7.26 ADRs for 100 patient-months with a computerized detection system.[26] Between 10 and 45% of the ADRs were considered severe.

Finally, ADRs are a frequent, or even the most frequent, cause of hospital admissions in the elderly. One-third to half of these reactions are severe and on average half could have been avoided.

Medications and the elderly: drug misuse or suboptimal prescribing

Classification of the various types of suboptimal prescription

The appropriateness of prescription reflects its quality. Terms such as optimal or suboptimal may also be used. Several types of suboptimal prescription in elderly subjects are classically described: excess treatment (overuse), inappropriate prescription (misuse) and insufficient treatment (underuse).[6] The indicators defined in Anglo-Saxon countries for assessing prescription quality for the elderly generally employ these three types. To sum up, for a given patient, certain treatments can be considered inappropriate and others insufficiently prescribed. Although it is legitimate in a quantitative approach to seek to reduce the number of medications taken by a patient, close qualitative analysis cannot be dispensed with. For this reason, the number of medications is not a good judgement criterion.

Excess treatment or overuse

This concerns the use of medications prescribed in the absence of an indication (the indication has never existed or no longer exists) or prescription of medications whose efficacy is not proven (insufficient medical service rendered).

Inappropriate prescription or misuse

This relates to use of medications whose risks exceed the expected benefits. This concept was first introduced by Beers, who established a list of drugs to avoid. The list has since been adapted for ambulatory patients and updated.[27]

Insufficient treatment or underuse

This is defined as the absence of initiation of an effective treatment in subjects with a condition for which one or several drug classes have demonstrated their efficacy.

As the frail elderly are generally excluded from clinical trials, a drug–indication pair must fulfil several conditions in order to comply with the definition of underuse:

- It must have a benefit–risk balance that is unquestionably favourable in a population of robust younger adults.
- This benefit, observed in a robust subject, should *a priori* be found in an elderly subject.
- It must not present major excess risk in the frail elderly population (which means that safety data on its use after marketing authorization need to be available).
- It should, to some extent, have been the object of clinical studies revealing increased overall mortality in undertreated patients, but these are observational data that are generally biased.

Four risks can easily be identified:

1 Risk of being satisfied with a debatable diagnosis. Some authors speak of 'underuse' abusively, for example in basing the indication of antidepressant treatment on administration of the short version of the Geriatric Depression Scale. Insufficiency of prescription is related to the quality of the diagnostic investigations which may not have been carried out because of an at-risk comorbid condition.

2 Risk of not taking into account the potential contraindications to the treatment or any other well-founded decision not to treat, such as refusal by the patient.

3 In the absence of relevant clinical trials, the risk of being satisfied with a mediocre level of proof. An example is hormone replacement therapy in the indication of treating cognitive disturbances (on the basis of observational data).

4 The risk of basing treatment indication on data from clinical trials in robust subjects and so concerned only with potential benefit and not risk. An example is hypertensive treatment, which was cited as underprescribed treatment at a time when data on the benefit–risk balance were not available. Robust elderly subjects, finally, are not geriatric subjects.

Relations between the different types of suboptimal prescription (Figure 121.1)

A medication may be underprescribed, for example antidepressants in atypical depression of the elderly person, and at the same time could raise the problem of inappropriate prescription, such as when antidepressants are prescribed for life after an episode of reactive depression.

A study by Steinman *et al.*[28] found a constant rate of underuse whatever the total number of medications

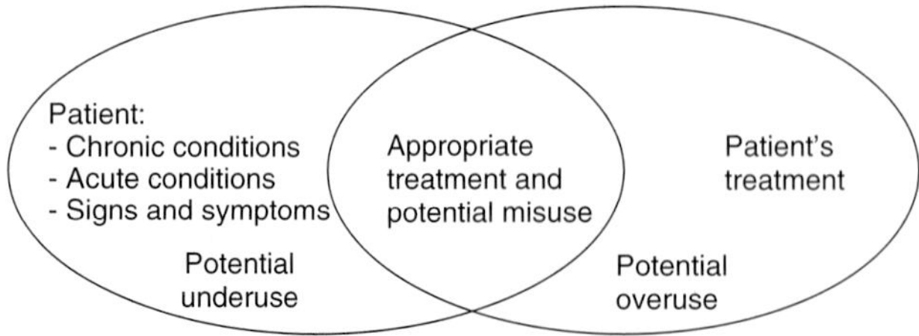

Figure 121.1 Different types of suboptimal prescription.

taken. Polypharmacy carries the risk of an increase in inappropriate prescriptions, while it does not restrict underuse. One possible interpretation of these findings is that polypharmacy is not a protection against underuse and that it is pertinent to restrict the number of medications to those which are strictly necessary by ranking the indications in order of importance.

What is the quality of prescription in the elderly when evaluated according to the different types of suboptimal prescription?

Overuse and inappropriate prescriptions

Examples of inappropriate prescriptions in the elderly are many. Among them are proton pump inhibitors (PPIs) prescribed for banal upper gastrointestinal symptoms or unduly prolonged after gastric ulcers. We may also cite overprescription of digoxin, notably in subjects living in institutions, which are responsible for a large number of serious adverse reactions, and some prescriptions of neuroleptics in nursing homes. Benzodiazepines are also prescribed in excess for insomnia or for anxiety which masks an unrecognized depressive syndrome. In the Three-City study, representative of the population aged 65 years and over living at home, 21.7% of elderly subjects were receiving an inappropriate medication:[12] 5.4% were taking dextropropoxyphen, 6.4% an anticholinergic medication and 9.2% benzodiazepines with a long half-life (more than 20 h). Studies assessing the rate of inappropriate prescriptions in Europe, as defined by the lists of Beers or McLeod, found rates ranging from 10 to 20%. [13,29] In nursing homes, the rate of inappropriate prescriptions is much higher and may be related to the risk of hospitalization and death.[30] A French prospective study carried out in a geriatric short-stay unit[14] showed that 66% of patients had at least one inappropriate medication at admission. Cerebral vasodilators were the most common, followed by long half-life benzodiazepines, dextropropoxyphen, anticholinergic antidepressants and the use of two or more psychotropic drugs of the same class.

Insufficient prescription

Numerous disorders may be undertreated in the elderly, bearing in mind all the limitations that we discussed in the preceding sections. The main disorders cited are systolic arterial hypertension above 160 mmHg, coronary insufficiency with underprescription of platelet anti-aggregants and beta-blockers, cardiac failure with systolic dysfunction and underprescription of ACE inhibitors,[31,32] atrial fibrillation with underprescription of AVK,[33] depression with underprescription of antidepressants and osteoporosis with fractures with underprescription of calcium, vitamin D and bisphosphonates. The authors of the evaluation tool for underuse START (see the section Analysis of available tools for evaluation of prescription quality)[34] applied their screening tool in a population of 600 patients aged over 65 years hospitalized for an acute medical problem : at least one potentially useful medication had been omitted in 57.9% of patients, in the absence of any contraindication. This rate reached 72.2% in patients aged over 85 years and women were twice as much at risk as men. The medications omitted mainly concerned cardiovascular disorders: statins in atherosclerotic disorders (26%), vitamin K antagonists in atrial fibrillation (9.5%), platelet anti-aggregants in arterial disease (7.3%), but also vitamin and calcium supplementation in osteoporosis with fractures (6%).

One study has shown that restricting access to certain medications for Medicaid patients in the USA more than doubled their rate of admission to an institution.[35] For certain medications, inadequate prescription could be associated with clinical criteria such as excess morbidity or mortality. We may also cite beta-blockers and ACE inhibitors.

Studies carried out on beneficiaries of the Medicare system throughout the USA examined the quality of the care received by these patients.[36] Of the 22 indicators of quality of care applied on a national level, nine concerned underuse. It was demonstrated, at a 2 year interval, that there was room for improvement in the prescription of essential medications such as beta-blockers and platelet anti-aggregants after myocardial infarction.[37]

Medication and the elderly: influence of suboptimal prescription in iatrogenic events in the elderly

Inappropriate medications versus inappropriate prescriptions

Some studies did not reveal an increase in ADRs associated with the medications on the Beers list.[14] Other authors concluded that these medications are responsible for only a small proportion of ADRs.[38] A longitudinal Swedish cohort (1995–98) of 785 patients aged over 75 years showed an excess risk (after adjustment for confounding factors) of at least one hospital admission with an odds ratio (OR) of 2.72 (95% CI, 1.64–4.51) in patients with inappropriate medications at baseline (according to a modified list of Beers criteria and evaluation of potential interactions in particular). No association was found with mortality.[39] In nursing homes, the rate of inappropriate prescriptions is high and appears to be linked with the risk of hospitalization and death.[30] An Irish study has also shown that 12% of hospital admissions were secondary to ADRs related to inappropriate prescriptions named on the STOPP list and 6% were related to medications named on the Beers list.[7] In a study by Budnitz *et al.*,[38] 3.6% of emergency admissions of elderly patients after an ADR were due to medications considered to be always inappropriate according to the Beers criteria, 5.2% to medications potentially inappropriate in certain conditions, and 33.3% followed the use of three other medications: warfarin (17.3%), insulin (13%) and digoxin (3.2%). When frequency of prescription of these medications was taken into account, the risk of emergency hospitalization after their use was 35 times greater than the risk related to use of medications considered as always inappropriate. A limitation of Budnitz *et al.*' study is the fact that laboratory tests make attribution of imputability easier with AVK, insulin, diuretics or digoxin in particular, whereas the imputability of psychotropic agents, for example, is generally less simple. A study by Pirmohamed *et al.*,[23] even though it did not specifically concern a geriatric population, found similar results with the following medications being most commonly implicated: low-dose aspirin, diuretics, warfarin and NSAIDs, which are not considered inappropriate in the elderly.

In an ambulatory cohort of 30 397 persons followed for 1 year,[25] the majority of errors associated with avoidable ADRs occurred at the monitoring stage (60.8%) before prescription (58.4%). Cardiovascular medications (24.5%), diuretics (22.1%), non-opiate analgesics (15.4%), hypoglycaemic agents (10.9%) and anticoagulants (10.2%) were most often implicated. In an institutional setting,[26] the majority of errors also occurred at the monitoring stage (70–80%) before prescription (60–70%).

It seems more relevant to encourage good prescribing practices with the aim of reducing avoidable iatrogenic events than to stigmatize inappropriate treatments. These events appear to be due above all to defective monitoring rather than to an inopportune choice of medication. The association between inappropriate medications and undesirable events is no longer open to doubt,[30] but the importance of their role in iatrogenic events in the elderly is debated.

Clinical efficacy of interventions for treatment optimization

Few studies of treatment optimization have shown their efficacy in improving clinical criteria. In 2007, Spinewine *et al.*[30] reviewed the literature on inappropriate prescriptions in the elderly. Of 14 interventional studies, two showed an improvement in clinical criteria such as reduction of severe ADRs or better pain control and fewer hospital admissions. The authors of one study obtained improvements in the Medication Appropriateness Index score (MAI) in two studies and decreased hospital usage in one of them and some others a reduction in the number of falls. In some cases, withdrawal of medications judged not indispensable in the elderly person can have secondary benefits such as a reduction in falls and improvement of cognitive disturbance when a psychotropic agent is discontinued.

This type of study appears to have several evident limitations, in particular because of the focus on medications termed inappropriate and not on the quality of prescription. In addition, identifying at-risk situations by observation is very different from preventing them before they occur.

Prevention of iatrogenic incidents in practice: general rules for individual prescription

Risks are related to the medications themselves, but above all to the way in which they are used. This point is dealt with in extensively the section Inappropriate medications versus inappropriate prescriptions. Application of the general rules of prescription in the elderly person is of major importance in order to limit avoidable iatrogenic events.

Taking the conventional definition of non-optimal prescriptions in the elderly person and extending it, we can propose a broader definition of optimal treatment. It is a question of adapting, taking into account the present state of scientific knowledge, the patient's treatment for his or her disorders in the wider sense of the term:

- chronic conditions (such as dementia, COPD)
- acute conditions requiring overall reassessment of treatment (such as dehydration, falls, confusion)
- signs and symptoms (such as pain, constipation)
- overall gerontological evaluation (such as cognitive function, risk of falls, autonomy),

while ensuring at the same time treatment follow-up according to pre-established criteria of efficacy and risk. Obviously, this is a dynamic process which does not end with the initial act of prescription.

Starting treatment

Diagnostic stage

The first phase of prescription is diagnosis. In a frail geriatric population, the physician sometimes hesitates to carry out the appropriate investigations. However, the risk may be less than that of exposing the patient to blind treatment which will probably not be of any benefit. In these situations of uncertainty, we can sometimes see a tendency to treat with medications that render low medical service but that have the reputation of being well tolerated, rather than by first-line treatments. However, as the benefit gained is generally nil, the risk incurred is not tolerable.

Evaluation of benefit

Once the diagnosis has been made, the potential benefit of the treatment must be determined according to the precise context: reduction of morbidity and mortality, improved comfort and so on. The opinion of the patient and their caregiver must be sought. For example, a high proportion of patients do not know they are receiving antidepressants.

The choice must obviously go to first-line treatments with a maximum level of proof in the robust subject.

Evaluation of risk

As we are dealing with a non-ideal population that is at risk of iatrogenic events, the second stage is to identify at-risk subpopulations. The decision not to treat may be made because of:

- interactions with essential medications (such as NSAIDs associated with ACE inhibitors)
- interactions with comorbid conditions (such as AChE inhibitors and severe COPD)
- an at-risk context (such as digoxin in a demented patient living at home)
- disagreement of the patient or their caregiver because of the potential risks.

If the decision to treat is made, it is necessary to assess drug–drug and drug–disease interactions. Some patients are receiving inappropriate doses of renally excreted drugs and inadequate dose adjustment, in particular for renal function, is the cause of a considerable number of ADRs.

Lastly, scheduling treatment over time is part of the initiation stage. Information on the starting date of an antidepressant treatment is generally not found. Discontinuation must also be scheduled, both in the medical record and with the patient, right from the time the treatment is introduced. For hypnotic agents, benzodiazepines in particular, as soon as treatment is started it is necessary to schedule its discontinuation in conjunction with the patient.

It is noteworthy that one of the main avoidable risk factors of ADRs is the number of prescribing physicians.[9]

Treatment follow-up, adverse drug reaction alert

Time schedule

Treatment follow-up requires that a time schedule should have been determined as soon as treatment was started: start date and end date (e.g. PPI, antidepressants), date for evaluation of efficacy (e.g. antidepressant at 4–6 weeks) and date of safety evaluation (e.g. ACE inhibitors and serum creatinine at 10 days).

Tools for monitoring treatment efficacy

To monitor treatment efficacy, the target indicators must have been identified: clinical criteria (DSM-IV target criteria in depression, for example), biological criteria (serum digoxin, INR) and also target criteria for safety. If treatment fails, compliance should always be checked (beware of escalation of antihypertensive drugs).

Tools for risk prevention and control

As we have seen, treatment follow-up is the cornerstone of prevention of iatrogenic events. At-risk situations can be identified by target indicators of safety or adverse drug reaction alerts. These indicators may be patient dependent, in which case they require identification of at-risk populations (see the section Disease–drug interactions, risk factors for iatrogenic events): women, elderly patients with several comorbid conditions, renal failure, dementia or malnutrition and also patients at risk of falls. The indicators may be dependent on drug-related factors: polypharmacy, medications with a narrow therapeutic window (such as AVK, diuretics, digoxin), psychotropic or cardiovascular drugs, newly marketed drugs. Lastly, they may be dependent on intercurrent events, such as water and salt depletion or introduction or discontinuation of a medication. The role of intercurrent events is particularly important, whether introduction or discontinuation of a medication that is a source of drug interactions or the onset of an additional acute condition (such as diarrhoea, vomiting and dehydration) or variations in climate.

The authors of a retrospective Italian study[40] analysed the records of 16 037 patients (mean age 53.1 years). With regard to monitoring, 28% of patients who had been taking both digoxin and diuretics for at least 5 months had had no control tests and only 11% had had an ECG and serum digoxin and also potassium measurement. Of patients who had been receiving digoxin and amiodarone/verapamil/propafenone for at least 5 months, 36% had had no test. In France, a study by the national health insurance organisation (Caisse Nationale de l'Assurance Maladie) showed that 22.8% of patients aged over 75 years taking diuretics for 12 months had had no laboratory tests during this time. With regard to drug-related factors, the patients who had received the least monitoring were those receiving a fixed diuretics combination.

Global re-evaluation of treatment

Finally, the entire treatment must be reassessed: this must be done when there is an intercurrent event and when a new drug is introduced, and also systematically, for instance once per year (Table 121.1). Periodical review of treatment, for example by a clinical pharmacist or a multidisciplinary team, seems to reduce inappropriate treatments.

Treatment discontinuation

When a medication is not or is no longer indicated, withdrawal rarely seems to be a problem. However, caution is still needed in some situations: beta-blockers and coronary insufficiency, long-term high-dose benzodiazepines and insomnia, corticosteroids and Horton's disease, antiepileptic drugs and epilepsy, anti-Parkinson drugs and Parkinson's disease and so on. More anecdotal is the potential treatment imbalance when an enzyme inducer or inhibitor is discontinued or during changeover between two drugs with a risk of interaction (e.g. the interval of 15 days between discontinuation of a MAOI and starting an SRI). Withdrawal is easier when full information was given when the drug was started, for benzodiazepines for example.

Table 121.1 Example of monitoring criteria for treatment follow-up.

Indication	Drug name	Introduction date	Posology	Duration	Monitoring criteria	
					Efficacy	Security
Heart failure	Enalapril	yyyy/mm/dd	mg per day	Lifetime	Dyspnoea	Kalaemia Serum creatinine Orthostatic hypotension

In some cases, discontinuation of medications considered as not absolutely necessary in the elderly person can be done without major risk – as in withdrawal of an antihypertensive agent which is no longer indispensable – and it may even have secondary benefits, such as a reduction in falls and improved cognition after a psychotropic agent is withdrawn.

Prevention of iatrogenic incidents in practice: tools for collective evaluation

General considerations

Concerning collective evaluation, with regard to prescription quality in the elderly, the potential avoidable ADR to be targeted must correspond to an explicit definition;[8] for example, the adverse event must have been foreseeable, its pre-existing drug-related origin must be identifiable from the information available (the patient's medical record) and the event must be preventable by changing the drug treatment. They also should:

- be well referenced
- be common in the population considered
- have a moderate to severe effect.

It also seems essential that these tools refer to the conventional modalities of non-optimal prescription, whose implication in avoidable iatrogenic events is no longer in doubt, and should include general prescribing rules which are of more importance in avoiding such events.

These evaluation tools are potentially useful to assess prescription quality at a collective level, but some of them could also be useful at an individual level.

Analysis of available tools for evaluation of prescription quality

Classic evaluation tools

Beers

The first to consider the concept of misuse was Beers, who established a list of medications to be avoided in the institutionalized elderly after carrying out a literature review and applying the Delphi method. The list has since been adapted for ambulatory patients and updated.[27] It is a tool which is more suitable for collective than individual evaluation. A revised French version of the list has been developed for application in the cohort of elderly subjects followed in the Three-City (3C) study.[12] The 1997 list was revised by a panel of experts in order to take French characteristics specifically into account.

IPET

Similar initiatives have been undertaken in Canada with the development, by a panel of experts, of a list of indicators divided into three categories: medications generally contraindicated in the elderly, drug–disease interactions and drug–drug interactions. An alternative is proposed for each indicator. This list has been adapted and evaluated by Naugler *et al.* to develop the Improving Prescribing in the Elderly Tool (IPET).[41]

START

This list of 22 clinical indicators, developed by Irish geriatricians, links a clinical situation with an appropriate prescription.[34] This tool, which can detect prescribing omissions, was validated using the Delphi method 'on the basis of the most recent evidence'. However, the studies which served as a basis for this list are not cited. The authors applied their screening tool to a population of 600 patients aged over 65 years hospitalized for an acute condition. In the absence of a contraindication, at least one potentially useful medication had been omitted in 57.9% of patients. This rate reached 72.2% in patients aged over 85 years and the risk was twice as great in women than in men.

STOPP

The authors developed a list of 65 criteria, aiming to identify potentially inappropriate prescriptions, through use of the Delphi method.[7] These criteria are intended to take different clinical situations into account better than the Beers list, for example in the prescription of tricyclic antidepressants (sometimes indicated at a low dose in neuropathic pain). Secondarily, they examined the performances of the STOPP tool compared with the updated Beers list[27] of 68 criteria, for detection of potentially inappropriate prescriptions and their associated ADRs in 715 elderly patients admitted to acute care units. The ADRs that contributed, directly or indirectly, to the reason for admission were identified subjectively (not by application of an algorithm of imputability). An ADR was identified in this way in 90 patients (12.5%), of which 91% were identified by STOPP and 48% by Beers. The inappropriate prescriptions detected by STOPP contributed to 11.5% of admissions, compared with 6% for Beers. According to the authors, these results are in favour of the use of STOPP at an individual level to identify potential ADRs when the clinical presentation is non-specific such as falls or delirium, and they also act as a reminder to bear constantly in mind the possibility of a drug-related origin. With regard to the feasibility of using START, the investigators applied the grid in less than 3 min, once the list of the various conditions and treatments had been established.

Other tools

Mackinnon and Hepler in the USA developed a set of indicators of avoidable ADR using the Delphi method.[8] Their work has the advantage of being based on a clear definition of avoidable ADRs. The participants considered a clinical scenario as an indicator only if it first corresponded to the definition of an avoidable ADR. This explicit definition of avoidability consists of four points: for an undesirable event, a possible pre-existing drug-related origin must be (1) *recognizable*, the undesirable event or treatment failure must have been (2) *foreseeable* and the causes of the drug-related problem and the causes of the event must have been (3) *identifiable* and (4) *controllable*. The experts were therefore asked to respond to these four questions for each clinical scenario:

- In the majority of patients, should health professionals be capable of *identifying* a problem in therapeutic management?
- Should they be capable of *foreseeing* the possibility of this event if the problem is not solved?
- Should they be capable of seeing how management could be changed in order to *prevent* this event?
- Should they modify their management?

This list has the major advantage of including the three conventional types of suboptimal prescription, and also treatment monitoring. The authors retrospectively applied their set of indicators in order to determine the incidence of avoidable ADRs and to identify risk factors.[9] They found an incidence of 28.8 per 1000 avoidable ADRs with the principal risk factors being number of comorbid conditions, number of prescribers and number of medications (>5). These indicators, initially developed in the USA, were secondarily adapted to Canadian practice.

Other authors have established a list of 'positive' medications in geriatrics, restricted to medications with high medical service rendered, of which the prescriber could make better use in order to limit iatrogenic events. Such a list could be of service at a time when, in some European countries, care homes for the dependent elderly are called upon to set up their own internal pharmacy and so to make a choice of medications for priority use.

Limitations

The Beers list has been criticized:

- Concerning its relevance at an individual level. However, Beers and his co-workers never proposed that this list should be applied to individuals.
- Because it does not sum up all cases of inappropriate prescription and in particular does not take account of underuse.
- Because it includes certain medications such as nitrofurantoin or amiodarone,[7] whatever the situation in which they are used.
- Because few studies have reported a clinical benefit resulting from use of these criteria.[30]

These limitations also concern in part the other lists.

The major differences between the American and Canadian lists also raise a problem, as few of the criteria overlap. In a European study using a combination of the criteria of Beers and McLeod, about half the medications were not available in the majority of European countries.[13] Practice indicators need to be adapted to local conditions. For example, some indicators that are relevant in the USA may not be so in the UK because of differences in clinical practices. On the other hand, they can serve as a starting point for developing a more appropriate set, for example using the Delphi method.

We have already discussed the low correlation found between these scores and clinical criteria. We may also add that it is a very different matter to identify at-risk situations by observation and to prevent them beforehand.

Global evaluations tools

The previous lists have been criticized because they do not take into account all cases of inappropriate prescription and they only refer to treatment and not to general prescription rules, monitoring and so on. Some authors have tried to develop more comprehensive tools to assess prescription quality.

MAI

The Medication Appropriateness Index (MAI)[42] offers a more global evaluation of pharmacological management. The MAI incorporates explicit criteria and makes use of implicit instructions. Ten criteria are evaluated for each medication:

1. indication
2. efficacy
3. dosage
4. correct mode of administration
5. practical mode of administration
6. drug interactions
7. interactions with comorbid conditions

8 overlapping medications
9 duration
10 cost (e.g. the existence of an equivalent drug at least 25% less costly).

Each criterion can be weighted with a score of 0–18 per medication, giving a summated quality score. The MAI has been used in certain interventions for treatment optimization.[30] It gives a more global evaluation of the prescription but does not assess all modalities of non-optimal prescription, in particular insufficient prescription. It does not take treatment follow-up into account, especially monitoring of ADRs (only duration of treatment is taken into account after the initial prescription).

ACOVE

The most wide-ranging project, the Assessing Care of the Vulnerable Elder (ACOVE) project, is based on a systematic review of publications analysed by a group of experts in order to develop a set of indicators of quality of care that are relevant to frail elderly subjects. About one-third of indicators refer to medications.[43] The ACOVE indicators have several advantages:

- They include specifically geriatric situations (dementia, falls).
- They refer to treatment, prevention, education and diagnostic documentation.
- They include the three types of non-optimal prescriptions, in addition to monitoring.
- The majority of the indicators are applicable to patients with advanced dementia or an unfavourable prognosis.

However, the ACOVE publications are of uneven quality and their recommendations are sometimes in contradiction with analysis of the literature. These publications may also be considered as a collection of recommendations rather than indicators of clinical practice as such.

Key points

- Two possible meanings of 'drug misuse' are 'drug abuse' such as consumption of illicit substances or incorrect use of prescription drugs and suboptimal prescribing such as licit medication prescribed in an inappropriate way or considered insufficiently prescribed.
- Optimizing treatment consists in adapting the patient's treatment to their disorders: chronic conditions, acute conditions requiring overall reassessment of treatment, signs and symptoms and overall gerontological evaluation, taking into account the present state of scientific knowledge.
- Adverse drug reactions in the elderly appear to be due above all to defective monitoring rather than to an inopportune choice of medication. Consequently, it is more relevant to encourage good prescribing practices such as ensuring treatment follow-up and scheduling treatment over time than to stigmatize inappropriate treatments.

References

1. O'Hare AM, Kaufman JS, Covinsky KE *et al.* Current guidelines for using angiotensin-converting enzyme inhibitors and angiotensin II-receptor antagonists in chronic kidney disease: is the evidence base relevant to older adults? *Ann Intern Med* 2009;**150**:717–24.
2. Flather MD, Shibata MC, Coats AJ *et al.* Randomized trial to determine the effect of nebivolol on mortality and cardiovascular hospital admission in elderly patients with heart failure (SENIORS). *Eur Heart J* 2005;**26**:215–25.
3. Lasser KE, Allen PD, Woolhandler SJ *et al.* Timing of new black box warnings and withdrawals for prescription medications. *JAMA* 2002;**287**:2215–20.
4. Mangoni AA and Jackson SH. Age-related changes in pharmacokinetics and pharmacodynamics: basic principles and practical applications. *Br J Clin Pharmacol* 2004;**57**:6–14.
5. Gurwitz JH and Avorn J. The ambiguous relation between aging and adverse drug reactions. *Ann Intern Med* 1991; **114**:956–66.
6. Hanlon JT, Schmader KE, Ruby CM and Weinberger M. Suboptimal prescribing in older inpatients and outpatients. *J Am Geriatr Soc* 2001;**49**:200–9.
7. Gallagher P and O'Mahony D. STOPP (Screening Tool of Older Persons' potentially inappropriate Prescriptions): application to acutely ill elderly patients and comparison with Beers' criteria. *Age Ageing* 2008;**37**:673–9.
8. Mackinnon NJ and Hepler CD. Preventable drug-related morbidity in older adults. 1. Indicator development. *J Manage Care Pharm* 2002;**8**:365–71.
9. Mackinnon NJ and Hepler CD. Indicators of preventable drug-related morbidity in older adults. 2. Use within a managed care organization. *J Manage Care Pharm* 2003;**9**:134–41.
10. Hajjar ER, Cafiero AC and Hanlon JT. Polypharmacy in elderly patients. *Am J Geriatr Pharmacother* 2007;**5**:345–51.
11. Viktil KK, Blix HS, Moger TA and Reikvam A. Polypharmacy as commonly defined is an indicator of limited value in the assessment of drug-related problems. *Br J Clin Pharmacol* 2007;**63**:187–95.
12. Lechevallier-Michel N, Gautier-Bertrand M, Alpérovitch A *et al.* Frequency and risk factors of potentially inappropriate medication use in a community-dwelling elderly population: results from 3C study. *Eur J Clin Pharmacol* 2005;**60**:813–9.
13. Fialová D, Topinková E, Gambassi G *et al.* Potentially inappropriate medication use among elderly home care patients in Europe. *JAMA* 2005;**293**:1348–58.

14. Laroche ML, Charmes JP, Nouaille Y *et al.* Is inappropriate medication use a major cause of adverse drug reactions in the elderly? *Br J Clin Pharmacol* 2007;**63**:177–86.
15. Zhang M, Holman CD, Price SD *et al.* Comorbidity and repeat admission to hospital for adverse drug reactions in older adults: retrospective cohort study. *BMJ* 2009;**338**: a2752.
16. Nourhashémi F, Andrieu S, Sastres N *et al.* Descriptive analysis of emergency hospital admissions of patients with Alzheimer disease. *Alzheimer Dis Assoc Disord* 2001;**15**:21–5.
17. Granjon C, Beyens MN, Frederico D *et al.* Existe-t-il un sur-risque d'accidents médicamenteux chez les sujets âgés atteints de troubles cognitifs? A propos de 82déments hospitalisés. *Neurologie-Psychiatrie-Gériatrie* 2006;**6**(35):21–8.
18. Mallet L, Spinewine A and Huang A. The challenge of managing drug interactions in elderly people. *Lancet* 2007; **370**:185–91.
19. Haider SI, Johnell K, Thorslund M and Fastbom J. Trends in polypharmacy and potential drug–drug interactions across educational groups in elderly patients in Sweden for the period 1992–2002. *Int J Clin Pharmacol Ther* 2007;**45**:643–53.
20. Doucet J, Chassagne P, Trivalle C *et al.* Drug–drug interactions related to hospital admissions in older adults: a prospective study of 1000 patients. *J Am Geriatr Soc* 1996;**44**: 944–8.
21. Becker ML, Kallewaard M, Caspers PW *et al.* Hospitalisations and emergency department visits due to drug–drug interactions: a literature review. *Pharmacoepidemiol Drug Saf* 2007; **16**:641–51.
22. Juurlink DN, Mamdani M, Kopp A *et al.* Drug–drug interactions among elderly patients hospitalized for drug toxicity. *JAMA* 2003;**289**:1652–8.
23. Pirmohamed M, James S, Meakin S *et al.* Adverse drug reactions as cause of admission to hospital: prospective analysis of 18 820 patients. *BMJ* 2004;**329**:15–9.
24. Beijer HJ and de Blaey CJ. Hospitalisations caused by adverse drug reactions (ADR): a meta-analysis of observational studies. *Pharm World Sci* 2002;**24**(2):46–54.
25. Gurwitz JH, Field TS, Harrold LR *et al.* Incidence and preventability of adverse drug events among older persons in the ambulatory setting. *JAMA* 2003;**289**:1107–16.
26. Handler SM, Wright RM, Ruby CM and Hanlon JT. Epidemiology of medication-related adverse events in nursing homes. *Am J Geriatr Pharmacother* 2006;**4**:264–72.
27. Fick DM, Cooper JW, Wade WE *et al.* Updating the Beers criteria for potentially inappropriate medication use in older adults: results of a US consensus panel of experts. *Arch Intern Med* 2003;**163**:2716–24.
28. Steinman MA, Landefeld CS, Rosenthal GE *et al.* Polypharmacy and prescribing quality in older people. *J Am Geriatr Soc* 2006;**54**:1516–23.
29. Pitkala KH, Strandberg TE and Tilvis RS. Inappropriate drug prescribing in home-dwelling elderly patients: a population based survey. *Arch Intern Med* 2002;**162**:1707–12.
30. Spinewine A, Schmader KE, Barber N *et al.* Appropriate prescribing in elderly people: how well can it be measured and optimised? *Lancet* 2007;**370**:173–84.
31. Soumerai SB, McLaughlin TJ, Spiegelman D *et al.* Adverse outcomes of underuse of beta-blockers in elderly survivors of acute myocardial infarction. *JAMA* 1997;**277**:115–21.
32. Masoudi FA, Rathore SS, Wang Y *et al.* National patterns of use and effectiveness of angiotensin-converting enzyme inhibitors in older patients with heart failure and left ventricular systolic dysfunction. *Circulation* 2004;**110**:724–31.
33. Mendelson G and Aronow WS. Underutilization of warfarin in older persons with chronic nonvalvular atrial fibrillation at high risk for developing stroke. *J Am Geriatr Soc* 1998;**46**:1423–4.
34. Barry PJ, Gallagher P, Ryan C and O'Mahoney D. START (screening tool to alert doctors to the right treatment) – an evidence-based screening tool to detect prescribing omissions in elderly patients. *Age Ageing* 2007;**36**:632–8.
35. Soumerai SB, Ross-Degnan D, Avorn J *et al.* Effects of Medicaid drug-payment limits on admission to hospitals and nursing homes. *N Engl J Med* 1991;**325**:1072–7.
36. Jencks SF, Cuerdon T, Burwen DR, *et al.* Quality of medical care delivered to Medicare beneficiaries: a profile at state and national levels. *JAMA* 2000;**284**:1670–6.
37. Jencks SF, Huff ED and Cuerdon T. Change in the quality of care delivered to Medicare beneficiaries, 1998–1999 to 2000–2001. *JAMA* 2003;**289**:305–12. Erratum: *JAMA* 2002;**289**: 2649.
38. Budnitz DS, Shehab N, Kegler SR and Richards CL. Medication use leading to emergency department visits for adverse drug events in older adults. *Ann Intern Med* 2007;**147**:755–65.
39. Klarin I, Wimo A and Fastbom J. The association of inappropriate drug use with hospitalisation and mortality: a population-based study of the very old. *Drugs Aging* 2005;**22**:69–82.
40. Magro L, Conforti A, Del Zotti F *et al.* Identification of severe potential drug–drug interactions using an Italian general-practitioner database. *Eur J Clin Pharmacol* 2008;**64**:303–9.
41. Naugler CT, Brymer C, Stolee P and Arcese ZA. Development and validation of an improving prescribing in the elderly tool. *Can J Clin Pharmacol* 2000;**7**:103–7.
42. Hanlon JT, Schmader KE, Samsa GP *et al.* A method for assessing drug therapy appropriateness. *J Clin Epidemiol* 1992;**45**:1045–51.
43. Shekelle PG, MacLean CH, Morton SC and Wenger NS. Acove quality indicators. *Ann Intern Med* 2001;**135**(8 Pt 2):653–67.

CHAPTER 122

The use and abuse of prescribed medicines

Abdi Sanati[1] and Mohammed T. Abou-Saleh[2]

[1]Southwest London and St George's NHS Trust, Sutton Hospital, Sutton, UK
[2]St George's, University of London, London, UK

Introduction

Substance misuse occurs mainly in young adults, with most research focusing on this group. Several factors, however, suggest a growing trend towards substance misuse in the elderly, while a generation of lifetime drug users are now entering old age.[1] Along with the increase in ageing of European and North American populations, the number of older adults requiring treatment for substance misuse is predicted to double between 2001 and 2020.[2] The need for age-appropriate treatment interventions has never been greater.

Use and harmful use

When considering drug use among the elderly, it is helpful to consider substances of misuse in three broad categories: medications, both prescribed and non-prescribed; socially sanctioned psychoactive substances; and illicit substances. Self-evidently this classification will differ between countries due to religious, cultural and legal differences.[3] Among the elderly, drugs from the medicines category are over-represented in people with harmful use when compared with other age groups.[4] This reflects the increased access to medicines among this group, allied to the physical and social barriers that make accessing other drugs harder for this group.

This chapter focuses on drug misusers who display 'harmful use', which is defined as 'a pattern of psychoactive drug use that causes damage to health, either mental or physical'.[5] The damage may be physical (as in cases of hepatitis from the self-administration of injected psychoactive substances) or mental (e.g. episodes of depressive disorder secondary to heavy consumption of alcohol).[6] It excludes cases where omission of a psychoactive medication may be harmful, for example, in cases of underuse of antidepressants.

Pharmacology

While drug absorption shows little variation with age, ageing results in an increase in the percentage of body fat, a reduction in lean body mass and a fall in total body water. Hydrophilic drugs, such as alcohol, are distributed in body water, such that with increasing age the volume of distribution falls and the peak concentration for a given dose may rise by 20%,[7] resulting in lower levels of intake giving the same intoxicant effect. Conversely, lipophilic drugs, such as benzodiazepines, that are stored in fatty tissue will remain in the body for longer, which could cause prolonged clinical symptoms such as disturbed cognition and mood.[8] A fall in plasma albumin in old age results in increased bioavailability of protein-bound drugs, such as warfarin and diazepam.

Drug elimination, through direct excretion or metabolism, is reduced in the elderly. Glomerular filtration rates fall steadily in old age, leading to the accumulation of renally excreted drugs. This may be compounded by renal damage due to drug misuse, for example, analgesic abuse.[9] Hepatic metabolism is reduced due to a reduced liver mass and blood flow, which may also be compounded by toxic drug effects. The efficiency of microsomal oxidation also falls with age, leading to reduced drug excretion of hepatically metabolized drugs.[10] The combination of these effects may greatly alter pharmacokinetics in the elderly. For example, the half-life of diazepam in the very elderly has been shown to be over 3 days, compared with 20 h in younger subjects.[11]

Multiple drug use complicates the pharmacokinetics of a substance, due to competition for binding sites and metabolic pathways. Polypharmacy has different effects, depending on whether it is acute or chronic. Alcohol will inhibit microsomal enzyme activity in acute use, while prolonged administration will induce the same enzymes. Hence alcohol will acutely raise concentrations of benzodiazepines, while lowering them if used chronically.[12]

Principles and Practice of Geriatric Medicine, Fifth Edition. Edited by Alan J. Sinclair, John E. Morley and Bruno Vellas.

Pharmacodynamics also alter in the elderly. Few studies of age-related changes in the brain have focused on how these changes affect the function of the reward system and/or its sensitivity to drugs of abuse.[13] There are documented changes in the neurotransmitter systems (dopaminergic, glutamatergic and serotonergic) in the ageing brain. There is a reduction in dopamine receptor binding in the striatum, frontal cortex, anterior cingulated gyrus, temporal insula and thalamus plus the same change in *N*-methyl-D-aspartate (NMDA)-type glutamate receptors in the cortex, striatum and hippocampus.[13]

Prevalence and correlates

The elderly may display harmful use of any psychoactive substance. Illicit drug use is not commonly observed in the elderly, but numbers are on the rise.[14] Shah and Fountain identified the following as factors associated with illicit drug use in the elderly: male gender, 'young old' age group, belonging to the post-War cohort, African-American ethnicity, prior convictions, diagnosis of mental illness or alcohol misuse, serious medical illness and past history of substance misuse with onset before age of 30 years.[15]

Benzodiazepines

Benzodiazepines are the most frequently abused prescribed medication in elderly people.[16] Chronic use may contribute to toxic effects, including cognitive impairment, poor attention and anterograde amnesia, cerebellar signs such as ataxia,[17] dysarthria, tremor, impaired coordination and drowsiness,[18] depression and cognitive decline.[13] Increased falls and hip fractures are associated with benzodiazepine use in the elderly.[16,19–21] The risk is especially high within the first few weeks of use.

Withdrawal may be accompanied by rebound insomnia, agitation, convulsions and an acute confusional state. If benzodiazepines are required for the elderly, then short-acting drugs (i.e. with half-life less than 24 h) at the lowest effective dose may be used for a short duration.[22] There is no 'safe' period of use but tolerance and dependence levels increase with prolonged use.[23]

Prevalence of benzodiazepine use

Establishing levels of benzodiazepine amongst the elderly is problematic. National prescription audits can reflect trends in use but are unhelpful when considering particular population subgroups.

Following the publication of guidance for the appropriate use of benzodiazepines by the Committee on Safety of Medicines (CSM) UK in 1988,[24] prescribing of benzodiazepines has fallen dramatically. In England and Wales, prescriptions fell by 32% from 1987 to 1996.[25] Of concern, however, is that 30% of prescriptions were for long-term treatment and 56% of prescriptions for the three most commonly prescribed benzodiazepines were issued to patients over the age of 65 years.[26]

A community follow-up study of 5000 over-65s in Liverpool[17] revealed that 10% were using benzodiazepines on first assessment and that of these about 70% were taking a benzodiazepine 2 years and 69% 4 years later. Women were twice as likely to be taking a benzodiazepine as men at any stage in the study. In the USA, a study found 6.3% of a large sample of over-65s used a hypnotic, one-third of these daily and nine-tenths for at least 1 year.[27]

Use of benzodiazepines in institutional cohorts has traditionally been higher and associated with female gender, greater age, bereavement and poor health.[28] Chronic benzodiazepine use in older adults in nursing homes has been associated with depression, sleep disturbances and demand for medication.[21] In the USA, a study found that one-quarter of nursing-home residents were prescribed a benzodiazepine and nearly 10% of all residents had chronic benzodiazepine use.[29] Studies from other countries revealed similarly high levels of benzodiazepine use among institutionalized older adults.[29]

Psychiatric morbidity

Significantly high rates of psychiatric disorder have been described among elderly benzodiazepine users.[30] Benzodiazepine misuse happens in comorbidity with anxiety disorders[31,32] and affective and sleep disorders.[32] The incidence of comorbid alcohol abuse has not been consistently shown to be significantly greater among benzodiazepine misusers.[31] However, more recent research suggests that a prior history of alcoholism may predispose to later benzodiazepine misuse in the elderly.[16] Benzodiazepines are also used to reduce the undesirable effect of those substances.[32]

An all-age study found that DSM-III-R Axis I comorbidity existed in all cases of a sample of benzodiazepine-dependent users in Spain.[32] The commonest diagnoses were insomnia, anxiety disorders and affective disorders. Obsessive–compulsive, histrionic and dependent personality disorders were found in half of cases and physical problems in one-third of cases.

Depression can occur during the use and anxiety during the withdrawal. During use and withdrawal, some patients can suffer from psychotic episodes with hallucinations and delusions; nocturnal restlessness, paradoxical excitement and delirium.[33] The risk of suicide also increases.[8]

Gender and age

Benzodiazepine use is over-represented among women of all ages. The likelihood of use of a benzodiazepine increases with age. There is little evidence that this gender divide narrows on reaching old age. Legislative approaches and prescribing guidelines have made some inroads into the over-representation of prescribing to the elderly.[34] Increasing public awareness of the side effects of benzodiazepines and an increase in advocacy services for the elderly are likely to have a similar effect.

Illicit drug misuse

Unfortunately, the prevalence of substance misuse in the elderly has not been investigated thoroughly, partly because substance misuse had not been considered to be a common health problem in this population. Overall, the prevalence of illicit drug use in the elderly is low compared with younger people.[15]

In the Epidemiological Catchment Area (ECA) Study, only 0.1% of elderly subjects met the criteria for drug abuse of an illicit substance in the previous month. Lifetime prevalence was 1.6% for over-65s.[35] Figures from the 2005 and 2006 National Survey on Drug Use and Health found similar low rates in the elderly along with higher rates in the middle aged, lending further evidence to the suggestion that prevalence rates may rise in the elderly as the younger cohort ages.[36] It has been estimated that as the baby boom generation reach older age, the number of elderly drug users will also increase in the Western world. Gfroerer and co-workers predicted that, compared with 2000, by 2020 there will be a 50% increase in number of older adults and a 70% increase in treatment need among them.[14] These predictions were replicated in other studies.[37]

In the UK, few cases of illicit drug use among the over-65s have been reported in the literature; one exception is a series of seven elderly subjects reported to have initiated injecting heroin in later life. They attributed their behaviour to a combination of loneliness and depression.[38]

In the USA, in a study of a Veterans' Administration old age psychiatry inpatient facility, 3% of the patients were found to have a primary drug misuse disorder involving prescribed medication, while 1% were addicted to illicit substances.[16] Also in the USA, attendance at methadone maintenance clinics by the elderly is reported to be rising, although over-60s still form only 2% of those attending.[4] Similarly, a number of elders are reported to continue their use of cannabis into late life.[39]

Explanations for the lower prevalence of drug misuse among the elderly include increase mortality among younger substance misusers, maturation out of substance misuse habit, poor identification of elderly cases and low acceptability of substance misuse among elderly people.[15]

Aetiology

There is a significant difference between the elderly drug user and the younger generation which leads to further marginalization of this group. The concept of marginality is introduced in this context to describe this group who live at the periphery of two cultures and do not belong to either, that is, they are marginal among a marginal group.[40] The result is a feeling of loneliness and the potential of being targeted in these 'old school' substance misusers. As they grow older, the nostalgia and idealization of the past feed back to this sense of loneliness. The role of drugs as a means of coping with loss (of loved ones, of children leaving home, retirement) has also been proposed.[13]

There are several theories on the aetiological role of the psychosocial factors.[41] They include:

1 *Social Control Theory:* Weakness of the strong social bonds that promote engagement in responsible behaviour precipitates engagement in undesirable behaviour, such as substance misuse. According to Moos,[41] the elements in operation in this model include weak attachment to existing social standards along with inadequate monitoring and goal direction.

2 *Social Learning Theory:* The attitude and behaviour of people who serve as the individual's role models play a crucial part in this model. Observing substance misuse by one's role models promotes the same behaviour in the individual through psychological processes of modelling and reinforcement.

3 *Behavioural Economics or Behavioural Choice Theory:* This approach identifies the importance of the social context. Lack of alternative rewards for activities other than substance misuse contributes towards its initiation and maintenance. Those activities include educational, social and also physical activities.

4 *Stress and Coping Theory:* Stressful life operates through increasing distress and alienation to increase the risk of substance misuse. Different stressors have been identified, such as childhood abuse and conflicts. Stress affects a person's self-confidence. Substance misuse is employed as a way of avoidance of coping.

Polysubstance misuse

The elderly have access to a variety of drugs of misuse. In many cases they may misuse one drug without misusing others. This is often the case with prescribed medication, where one medication is overused whereas compliance with the prescription is maintained for the others. Where non-prescribed substances become involved, the possibility of abuse of more than one substance is elevated. Finlayson and Davis [30] found that 15% of over-65s requiring inpatient detoxification from alcohol were also dependent upon a second substance, usually a hypnotic, anxiolytic or analgesic. The phenomenon of cross-tolerance must also be considered. Psychoactive substances may have a cumulative effect, due to either a shared outcome effect or to different drugs acting as interchangeable substitutes for one another (cross-tolerance). Cross-tolerance exists within each class of drug, such that the clinician should always consider the total benzodiazepine or opioid dose, using class-specific equivalence charts.[42] Cross-tolerance for some drugs may also occur outside the class, most notably for alcohol and benzodiazepines. While this phenomenon is widely exploited for detoxification, failure to consider the clinical possibility may lead to cases of dependence being overlooked.

Detection

Self-presentation by elders may be limited by a number of factors.[43,44] Elders may not realize that they are ill or may not realize that the medical profession identifies substance misuse as an illness and will offer help. Also, the elderly are more likely to under-report their substance misuse.[45] Traditional forms of service promotion may fail to reach the elderly, and a service staffed by young professionals may seem intimidating or inappropriate for someone much older, particularly if their substance misuse is associated with a high degree of shame. Greenwood[46] argued that substance misusers, and the elderly in particular, suffer as a result of stigmatization, as their disorder is perceived as self-inflicted. This stigma may be reflected in a clinician's reluctance to become involved by acknowledging the problem. Unfortunately there is evidence that physicians find it hard to discuss substance misuse with the elderly.[13]

If self-presentation is unlikely, then the number of professional caregiver contacts that the elderly have provides a further opportunity for education about the problem and potential sources of help. This resource appears underdeveloped at present, with a need for better training for carers in identification of at-risk individuals and in appropriate actions once misusers have been identified.[47]

Detection of benzodiazepine use

Appropriate prescribing of sedatives for time-limited periods should be accompanied by vigilance for drug-seeking behaviour. Such behaviour includes early requests for repeat prescriptions or requests for increased doses. The elderly may also receive medication from multiple sources. Careful exchange of clinical information is vital in such settings. With these considerations in mind, the need for dependence-inducing drug prescriptions should be regularly reviewed and comorbid contributory conditions, such as depression, should be actively treated. Changes in legislation on prescribing practice may reduce the opportunity for drug misuse.[34]

The Severity of Dependence Scale has been validated as a screening tool for benzodiazepine dependence:[48]

1 Did you think your use of tranquillizers was out of control?

2 Did the prospect of missing a dose make you anxious or worried?

3 Did you worry about your use of tranquillizers?

4 Did you wish you could stop?

5 How difficult would you find it to stop or go without your tranquillizers?

Each of the items is scored on a four-point scale (items 1–4, 0 = never/almost never, 1 = sometimes, 2 = often, 3 = always/nearly always; item 5, 0 = not difficult, 1 = quite difficult, 2 = very difficult, 3 = impossible). A total score of 6 or more indicates problematic use, with a specificity of 94.2% and a sensitivity of 97.9%.[48]

Treatment

Treatment of substance misuse is a multistage process involving the integrated use of physical, psychological and social interventions. These interventions should, where possible, run concurrently as opposed to consecutively and must be provided in a form that is acceptable to the individual and sensitive to the specific needs of the elderly.[45] Amongst this client group, individuals rarely present complaining directly of a substance misuse disorder, but may present with associated physical problems. The first step of treatment is the identification of cases. This requires clinical observation allied to sensitive yet persistent enquiry. The routine use of standardized screening tools may help to focus clinical impression more accurately. Once identified as potential candidates for treatment, the patient's attitude towards their substance misuse requires examination. Exploration of the risks and a discussion of potential avenues for change may help to establish or reinforce the motivation to change. Drugs that cause significant physical dependence may necessitate detoxification regimens, while comorbid conditions such as depression that perpetuate the disorder need to be adequately treated. Social issues, such as housing and a social network that consists mainly of substance misusers, may perpetuate the problem and need to be examined for opportunities to change. The individual requires psychological rehabilitation to address the issues that may have contributed to the uncontrolled use of substances and to provide future coping.

Initiating treatment

There are no published data about the level of uptake of offers of help once elders abusing substances have been identified. However, elders do achieve equivalent or better results than younger adults when they do enter treatment.[2] Unfortunately, the pessimistic attitudes held by many professionals and carers towards the likelihood of successful resolution of the problem are frequently also held by the individual also. A fatalistic resignation to a life of substance misuse is often reported, particularly by long-term users, whereas more recent onset users may express greater motivation for treatment.[49]

Once long-term use of benzodiazepines is established, dose reduction can be difficult to achieve. Withdrawal insomnia and rebound anxiety make patient motivation difficult to achieve. Where abstinence is desired, a conversion to a longer acting benzodiazepine and a gradual reduction in dosage over the course of months are advisable.[43] Rapid detoxification is associated with breakthrough withdrawal symptoms and may be complicated by convulsions. If a rapid withdrawal is necessary, it is best conducted in an inpatient setting if severe dependency is suspected. As with alcohol, the withdrawal period for the elderly is more likely to be complicated by confusion than in younger adults. Longer term prescribing of benzodiazepines should adhere to the following general principles: clear indication of benzodiazepine dependence, clear intermediate treatment goals, regular review and methods to prevent diversion.[50]

Psychological techniques, such as relaxation training and educative initiatives in the areas of sleep hygiene and correct medication use, may also prove valuable. Cormack *et al.*[51] demonstrated that writing to benzodiazepine users in primary care urging them to reduce their medication use resulted in a fall in total use by one-third over the next 6 months. Treatment of other forms of drug misuse in the elderly is under-researched. Misuse of analgesics may require formal detoxification if opioids are involved or physical dependence has developed. More often the patient requires information to allow them to make an informed choice about drug use and an alternative form of treatment for their condition. Still less information is available on the treatment of illicit drug use in the elderly, although several key publications argue for age-appropriate services for the elderly.[2,45] These services should pay particular attention to comorbid health problems and should provide basic-level medical services.[2] Severe or complex health problems should be identified and referred to appropriate specialist services.

Psychological interventions

Once a patient is detoxified, rehabilitation is necessary to address the issues behind their substance use and to foster coping strategies for the future. Few studies have examined the particular needs of the elderly in a rehabilitation setting and have mostly focused on alcohol. Janik and Dunham reported on comparative outcomes for over 3000 over-60-year-olds and younger entrants into alcohol treatment programmes.[52] Outcomes after 6 months showed no differences between the groups.

Psychological programmes designed specifically with the elderly in mind may be more appropriate for consideration. Some success has been claimed for models encouraging the development of social networks with self-management skills.[53] Kofoed *et al.*,[54] in a small study, reported that retention in outpatient treatment of older adults was greater in an age-specific treatment group that focused on socialization and minimal confrontation (a mainstay of many programmes), compared with older patients in a mixed-age treatment group. At 1 year follow-up, the effect was lost.

Variations of the Alcoholics Anonymous 12-step model tailored to the needs of elders have been reported in the USA, with varying degrees of success.[55] Models low on confrontation, traditionally regarded as fundamental to overcoming denial on the part of the patient, appear to be supported by the work of Kashner *et al.*,[56] who found that 1 year follow-up of elders in a confrontational programme revealed half the levels of abstinence compared with a group in a programme where self-esteem, tolerance and peer relationships were promoted. Behavioural approaches, including cue identification and avoidance, have also been reported to be of clinical benefit.[53]

Even fewer age-specific studies are available to guide the clinician in the provision of aftercare to the elderly non-alcoholic drug user. An avoidance of drugs that have a dependence potential is advisable, if practical. Adequate rehabilitation and continuing support of the individual are indicated. This may be provided through generic old age psychiatry services or through specialist drug services, depending upon which service appears best able to cater for the specific needs of the user. The choice of service provider should reflect the lifestyle of the patient, as opposed to being a decision based solely on chronological as opposed to biological age. Further services may also be available in the form of mutual support groups similar to those available for alcohol.

Prognosis

In a survey by Moos *et al.*, it was found that although the standardized mortality ratio (SMR) reduces with age among elderly people with substance misuse, it remains high, 1.66 in those >75 years of age.[57] They also found that patients with no outpatient mental health after discharge from inpatient intervention had a higher mortality, and in fact, intensive outpatient aftercare reduced the mortality rate in this group of patients. The effect could be through adherence to treatments (both psychiatric and medical), better housing and nutrition and better access to other forms of medical care.

Conclusion

Substance misuse and old age psychiatry have long been unpopular choices for specialization. Both fields are known for providing challenging patients with differing priorities to those of the clinician. Research in either field is hampered by the difficulty in obtaining reliable clinical data on conditions for which few empirical measures exist. The field of old age substance misuse has suffered to some extent in clinical practice, where patients do not fit neatly into either service and are welcomed by neither. It is clear, however, that there exists a significant morbidity due to drug use in the elderly. The problem may be iatrogenic and autogenic in origin. Increased life expectancy and the cohort effect of generations of recreational drug users reaching old age are likely to intensify the problem. Adequate research to identify at-risk individuals and the provision of appropriate and accessible treatment services for the elderly drug misuser remain among the major challenges to healthcare providers.

Key points

- There is a growing trend towards substance misuse in the elderly, while a generation of lifetime drug users are now entering old age.
- When considering drug use among the elderly, it is helpful to consider substances of misuse in three broad categories: medications, both prescribed and non-prescribed; socially sanctioned psychoactive substances; and illicit substances.
- Treatment of substance misuse is a multistage process involving the integrated use of physical, psychological and social interventions.

References

1. Patterson TL and Jeste DV. The potential impact of the baby-boom generation on substance abuse among elderly persons. *Psychiatr Serv* 1999;**50**:1184.
2. European Monitoring Centre for Drugs and Drug Addiction. *Substance Use Among Older Adults: a Neglected Problem*, Office for Official Publications of the European Communities, Luxembourg, 2008, pp. 1–4.
3. Murphy JT, Harwood A, Götz M and House AO. Prescribing alcohol in a general hospital: 'not everything in black and white makes sense'. *J R Coll Physicians London* 1998;**32**:358.
4. Pascarelli EF. Drug abuse and the elderly. In: JH Lowinson and P Ruiz (eds), *Substance Abuse: Clinical Problems and Perspectives*, Williams and Wilkins, Baltimore, 1981, pp. 752–7.
5. United Nations International Drug Control Programme. *World Drug Report*, Oxford University Press, Oxford, 1997.
6. World Health Organization. *The ICD-10 Classification of Mental and Behavioural Disorders: Clinical Descriptions and Diagnostic Guidelines*, WHO, Geneva, 1992.
7. Dunne FJ and Schipperheijn JAM. Alcohol and the elderly. *BMJ* 1989;**298**:1660–1.
8. Miller NS, Belkin BM and Gold MS. Alcohol and drug dependence among the elderly: epidemiology, diagnosis and treatment. *Comp Psychiatry* 1991;**32**:153–65.
9. Ghodse AH. Substance misuse leading to renal damage. *Prescrib J* 1993;(33):151–3.
10. Sheehan O and Feely J. Prescribing considerations in elderly patients. *Prescriber* 1999;**10**:75–82.
11. Klotz U, Avant GR, Hoyumpa A *et al*. The effects of age and liver disease on the disposition and elimination of diazepam in adult man. *J Clin Invest* 1975;**55**:347.
12. Lisi DM. Alcoholism in the elderly. *Arch Intern Med* 1997; **157**:242.
13. Dowling GJ, Weiss SRB and Condon TP. Drugs of abuse and the aging brain. *Neuropsychopharmacology* 2008;**33**:209–18.
14. Gfroerer J, Penne M, Pemberton M and Folsom R. Substance abuse treatment need among older adults in 2020: the impact of the aging baby-boom cohort. *Drug Alcohol Depend* 2003;**69**:127–35.
15. Shah A and Fountain J. Illicit drug use and problematic use in the elderly: is there a case for concern? *Int Psychogeriatr* 2008;**20**:1081–9.
16. Edgell RC, Kunik ME, Molinari VA *et al*. Nonalcohol-related use disorders in geropsychiatric patients. *J Geriatr Psychiatry Neurol* 2000;**13**:33–7.
17. Taylor S, McCracken CF, Wilson KC and Copeland JR. Extent and appropriateness of benzodiazepine use. *Br J Psychiatry* 1998;**173**:433–8.
18. World Health Organization Programme on Substance Abuse. *Rational Use of Benzodiazepines*, WHO, Geneva, 1996.
19. McCree DH. The appropriate use of sedatives and hypnotics in geriatric insomnia. *Am Pharmacol* 1989;(5):49.
20. Neutel CI, Hirdes JP, Maxwell CJ and Patten SB. New evidence on benzodiazepine use and falls: the time factor. *Age Ageing* 1996;**25**:273–8.
21. Svarstad BL. Effects of residents' depression. Sleep and demand for medication on benzodiazepine use in nursing homes. *Psychiatr Serv* 2002;**53**; 1159–65.
22. Fick DM, Cooper JW, Wade WE *et al*. Updating the Beers criteria for potentially inappropriate medication use in older adults: results of a US consensus panel of experts. *Arch Intern Med* 2003;**163**:2716.
23. Grantham P. Benzodiazepine abuse. *Br J Hosp Med* 1987; **37**:292.
24. CSM/MCA. Benzodiazepines, dependence and withdrawal symptoms. *Curr Problems Pharmacovig* 1988;(21):1–2.
25. Milburn A. *House of Commons Written Answers*, 6 May 1998.
26. Department of Health. *Patient Safety: Benzodiazepine Warning, Issued by Chief Medical Officer, England and Wales*, CMO Update 37, Department of Health, London, 2004.
27. Stewart RB, May FE, Hale WE and Marks RG. Psychotropic drug use in an ambulatory elderly population. *Gerontology* 1982;28:328–35.
28. Morgan K. Sedative–hypnotic drug use and ageing. *Arch Gerontol Geriatr* 1983;**2**:181.
29. Opedal K, Schjøtt J and Eide E. Use of hypnotics among patients in geriatric institutions. *Int J Geriatr Psychiatry* 1998;**13**:846–51.

30. Finlayson RE and Davis LJ Jr. Prescription drug dependence in the elderly population: demographic and clinical features of 100 inpatients. *Mayo Clin Proc* 1994;**69**:1137–45.

31. Van Balkom A, Beekman ATF, De Beurs E *et al*. Comorbidity of the anxiety disorders in a community-based older population inThe Netherlands. *Acta Psychiatr Scand* 2000;**101**:37–45.

32. Martinez-Cano H, de Iceta Ibáñez de Gauna M, Vela-Bueno A and Wittchen HU. DSM-III-R co-morbidity in benzodiazepine dependence. *Addiction*. 1999; 94:97–107.

33. Weedle PB, Poston JW and Parish PA. Use of hypnotic medicines by elderly people in residential homes. *J R Coll Gen Pract* 1988;**38**:156–8.

34. Brahams D. Benzodiazepine overprescribing: successful initiative in New York State. *Lancet* 1990;**336**:1372.

35. Regier DA, Farmer ME, Rae DS *et al*. One-month prevalence of mental disorders in the United States and sociodemographic characteristics: the Epidemiologic Catchment Area study. *Acta Psychiatr Scand* 1993;**88**:35.

36. Blazer DG and Wu LT. The epidemiology of substance use and disorders among middle aged and elderly community adults: national survey on drug use and health. *Am J Geriatr Psychiatry* 2009;**17**:237.

37. Colliver JD, Compton WM, Gfroerer JC and Condon T. Projecting drug use among aging baby boomers in 2020. *Ann Epidemiol* 2006;**16**:257–65.

38. Frances J. Pain killer. *Commun Care* 1994;(December):15–21.

39. Solomon K, Manepalli J, Ireland GA and Mahon GM. Alcoholism and prescription drug abuse in the elderly: St. Louis University grand rounds. *J Am Geriatr Soc* 1993;**41**:57–69.

40. Anderson, TL and Levy JA. Marginality among older injectors in today's illicit drug culture: assessing the impact of aging. *Addiction* 2003; 98:761–70.

41. Moos RH. Active ingredients of substance use-focus self-help groups. *Addiction* 2008;**103**:387–96.

42. Taylor D, Paton C and Kerwin R. *The Maudsley Prescribing Guidelines*, 9th edn, Informa Healthcare, London, 2007.

43. Ward M and Goodman C. *Alcohol Problems in Old Age*, Staccato, Birmingham, 1995.

44. Wesson J. *The Vintage Years: Older People and Alcohol*, Aquarius, Birmingham, 1992.

45. Rockett IR, Putnam SL, Jia H and Smith GS. Declared and underclared substance use among emergency department patients: a population based study. *Addiction* 2006;**101**: 706–12.

46. Greenwood J. Stigma: substance misuse in older people . *Geriatr Med* 2000;**30**(4):43–9.

47. Herring R and Thom B. The role of home carers: findings from a study of alcohol and older people . *Health Care Later Life* 1998;**3**:199–211.

48. Cuevas CDL, Sanz EJ, Padilla J and Berenguer JC. The Severity of Dependence Scale (SDS) as screening test for benzodiazepine dependence: SDS validation study. *Addiction* 2000;**95**:245–50.

49. Schonfeld L and Dupree LW. Alcohol abuse among older adults. *Rev Clin Gerontol* 1994;**52**:217–25.

50. Department of Health. *Drug Misuse and Dependence: UK Guidelines on Clinical Management*, Department of Health, London, 2007.

51. Cormack MA, Sweeney KG, Hughes-Jones H and Foot GA. Evaluation of an easy, cost-effective strategy for cutting benzodiazepine use in general practice. *Br J Gen Pract* 1994;**44**:5–8.

52. Janik SW and Dunham RG. A nationwide examination of the need for specific alcoholism treatment programs for the elderly . *J Stud Alcohol* 1983;**44**:307–17.

53. Dupree LW, Broskowski H and Schonfeld L. The Gerontology Alcohol Project: a behavioral treatment program for elderly alcohol abusers . *Gerontologist* 1984;**24**:510.

54. Kofoed LL, Tolson RL, Atkinson RM *et al*. Treatment compliance of older alcoholics: an elder-specific approach is superior to 'mainstreaming'. *J Stud Alcohol* 1987;**48**:47.

55. Schonfeld L and Dupree LW. Antecedents of drinking for early- and late-onset elderly alcohol abusers. *J Stud Alcohol* 1991;**52**:587.

56. Kashner TM, Rodell DE, Ogden SR *et al*. Outcomes and costs of two VA inpatient treatment programs for older alcoholic patients. *Psychiatr Serv* 1992;**43**:985.

57. Moos RH *et al*. Diagnostic subgroups and predictors of one-year re-admission among late middle-aged and older substance abuse patients. *J Stud Alcohol* 1994;**55**:173–83.

CHAPTER 123

Transportation, driving and older adults

Desmond O'Neill[1] and David Carr[2]

[1]Trinity College Dublin, Dublin, Ireland

[2]The Rehabilitation Institute of St Louis, St Louis, MO, USA

Introduction

The importance of transportation to health and social inclusion has been under-recognized in both the medical and the gerontological literature. Transportation is a crucial factor in maintaining older adult independence and the car is the most important source of transportation for older people.[1] Not only is community mobility a major priority for older people, but also problems with transportation have been recognized as barriers to access to healthcare for older people.[2] Concerns over access to adequate transportation among older people has been voiced by a number of international agencies, including the Organization for Economic Cooperation and Development (OECD)[3] and the Conference of the European Ministers for Transport.[4] This has been augmented by major national reviews which have also emphasized the need to adapt transportation systems to the needs of older people.[5]

However, the major emphasis of much of the medical literature on transportation and ageing is disproportionately skewed towards risk and crashes. This is particularly unfortunate, as older adults are the safest group of drivers[6] and even the often quoted increased crash risk per mile is an artefact due to limited exposure or fewer miles driven per year. A number of studies have shown that the apparent increased crash risk disappears when one controls for mileage.[7] However, a major issue for older adults is an increase in crash fragility. Whether as car occupants[8] or as pedestrians, older people are more likely to suffer serious injury or death than middle-aged individuals given the same crash severity. In traffic terms, older adult fragility exposes weaknesses in the design of the traffic environment and vehicle. This clearly requires a societal response, in particular attention to in-car safety measures, which recognizes the altered physiology and increased frailty of older people. A good analogy can made with the danger posed by airbags for children who are front seat passengers: the response was not to stop children riding in cars, but rather to adapt the injury control measure (placing the children in the back seat, making occupants use seat belts).

For pedestrians, several responses are possible. Possibly the most important of these is to ensure that we do not unnecessarily turn older people into involuntary pedestrians through inappropriate driver screening programmes. There is evidence that this phenomenon underlies the negative impact of medically screening older drivers in Finland and Australia.[9–11] Other approaches include radically modifying traffic speed, allowing for the time needed for pedestrians to cross busy intersections, construction of safety barriers such as islands or walkbridges, better organization where vulnerable road users (pedestrians and cyclists) share the road with vehicular traffic and educating other road users to exercise caution in environments shared with older pedestrians.[12]

Illness and transportation

The most important impact of age-related illness on transportation is likely to be a reduction of personal mobility. This has been demonstrated for people with dementia,[13] but also happens with other illnesses. Older people report that impaired health is the most common reason for driving cessation.[14,15] However, patients rarely discuss this radical decision with a healthcare provider.[16] Physicians dealing with older adults need to be aware of these limitations and to be able to support their patients to maintain their independence.

The issue of crash risk has been overstated but sadly forms a negative public backdrop to our professional practice: a study of British and Irish media showed an overwhelmingly negative portrayal of older drivers, despite their excellent safety record.[17] Physicians must not allow a negative but inaccurate popular perception to interfere with their task of assessing, treating and advising older people in relation to their independence. This extends to the interpretation of studies on crashes: for example, certain illnesses are more common in older people who have crashes.[18]

Principles and Practice of Geriatric Medicine, Fifth Edition. Edited by Alan J. Sinclair, John E. Morley and Bruno Vellas.

However, since older people have lower crash rates, the likelihood of effective public health interventions to reduce this low rate further are unrealistic and may cause further problems (e.g. driving retirement) recognized with screening of older drivers.

Clearly, for individual patients the maintenance of autonomy must be balanced with public safety to an extent consistent with that applied to the rest of the population. Age-related visual and cognitive diseases, in particular macular degeneration, Alzheimer's disease (AD), stroke and Parkinson's disease,[19] are likely to be the conditions most often associated with mobility and safety problems. Our main ethical prerogative is to preserve a sense of dealing with the issue in a hierarchical fashion common to good practice for all healthcare conditions. This emphasizes in turn the World Health Organization approach of health gain, health maintenance, compensation and finally palliation.[20]

The Older Drivers Project, an initiative between the American Medical Association and the US National Highway Traffic Safety Administration, has reaffirmed this principle, stating that a primary objective of its approach involves helping older drivers stay on the road safely to preserve their mobility and independence.[21] The Older Drivers Project recommends that this can be accomplished through three methods: (1) optimizing the driver, (2) optimizing the driving environment and (3) optimizing the vehicle. In this approach, driving cessation is recommended only after the safety of the driver cannot be secured through any other means.

Clinicians may be reluctant to address the driving issue in the office practice setting. There is a clear need for education in the assessment of mobility and driving: the good news is that such education appears to be effective.[22] Evaluating driving skills should not be viewed differently from the evaluation of risk for falls or other risk for injuries in older adults. Clinicians should consider the recommendation for driving retirement in older adults in a similar way to the decision that a previously ambulatory patient is now wheelchair bound for life: efforts should be made to preserve mobility when possible.

Definitive guidelines on how clinicians can intervene effectively to ensure adequate mobility, driving safety or effect driving cessation in impaired older adults are still needed, but current evidence and available resources indicate a general approach to this issue. There is an increasing body of evidence on the subject and some helpful guides.[23] In addition, the relatively broad approach to Comprehensive Geriatric Assessment means that geriatricians will better understand the limitations of a predominantly cognitive approach to driving assessment, even in conditions characterized by cognitive decline. A good proxy is entry to nursing home care, which is poorly predicted by individual's neurocognitive testing, but better matched by behavioural and functional limitations.[24]

Table 123.1 Schematic outline of driving assessment.

History
- Patient, family/informant
- Driving history

Examination
Functional status
Other illnesses and drugs
Vision
Mental status testing
Diagnostic formulation and prioritization
Disease severity and fluctuations
Remediation
Re-assess
± In-depth cognitive/perceptual testing
± On-road assessment
Overall evaluation of hazard
- Strategic
- Tactical
- Operational

Advice to patient/carer ± DMV/DVLA
If driving too hazardous, consider alternative mobility strategies

Of particular importance has been the recognition that a relatively wide number of interventions can improve driving ease and safety (Table 123.1). It is also remarkable that most reviews on medications and driving emphasize possible negative effects on driving, rather than reflecting that anti-inflammatory, anti-parkinsonian and antidepressant medications might actually improve driving ability and comfort! The possibility that cholinesterase inhibitors might improve or maintain driving skills in dementia is an interesting possibility.[25] Assistive technologies, such as global position system (GPS) devices, may assist some older adults with geographic orientation. Crash warning systems may also be of benefit. Preliminary data support cognitive stimulation[26] and exercise interventions[27] directed at driving-related cognitive abilities in older adults as being potentially beneficial. More intervention studies are sorely needed in these areas.

What do we need to know to assess our older patients?

Physicians assessing older people for transport/driving capability need to know:

1 How does the older adult meet their transportation needs?

2 What intrinsic factors contribute to driving ability and how can we assess them?

3 What common illnesses in later life can impair traffic skills?

4 What, if any, interventions should office-based clinicians pursue?

5 What is the physician's responsibility with regard to driver licensing and insurance authorities?

Taking a driving/transportation history

The interested clinician can check static visual acuity (Snellen chart), hearing (whisper test or hand-held audiometry), attention and reaction time (Trail Making Test A or B), visual spatial skills (clock drawing task), judgment, insight, joint range of motion and muscle strength.[40–43] Many of these tests were recently included in an American Medical Association resource on older drivers as reasonable for assessing and counselling older adult drivers and are available on their web site along with evidence-based medicine references. These tests are probably more important for gaining an overall perspective on the patient's abilities and disabilities, rather than relying overly on the performance of any one component.

Although it may seem obvious that transportation should figure in a comprehensive assessment, this is not necessarily the case. An extreme example of this is the failure of the referring physician to advise on driving restriction for a significant number of people referred to a syncope clinic.[28] It is also likely that many patients do not obtain formal advice or assessment about driving after stroke.[29] As there is potential to improve driving and transportation options, there is also a need to discuss restrictions or planned withdrawal from driving for many patients. There are data to suggest that license restriction is associated with lower crash risks.[30] Thus, a graduated driving reduction may be a viable option rather than driving cessation.

The patient's own assessment of driving should be assessed and a promising approach in this regard is the Adelaide Self-Efficacy Scale.[31] It is encouraging that self-assessed driving skills in mild cognitive impairment seem preserved.[32] A collateral (witness) history of driving abilities is important, given the often collaborative nature of driving in later life,[33] but cognizant of the conflict of interest of a spouse who does not drive.[34] Recent data indicate that informants are able to recognize impaired driving behaviour in some older adults with medical illness.[35]

What factors are important in driving assessment?

The greatest advance in this area has been the understanding that a purely cognitive model of driving ability does not adequately reflect the complexity and hierarchical nature of the driving task.[36] Psychometric approaches have generally been disappointing for a number of reasons[37] and efforts to find a best cognitive battery resemble the alchemist's search for transforming base metal into gold rather than a carefully thought out scientific endeavour. However, recent efforts have pushed correct classification rates in demented samples to 80%, which is encouraging.[38]

Currently, many prediction efforts have focused on heterogeneous groups of older adults during licence renewal. However, the crash rate of this group is already low (e.g. like the odds ratios for predicting crashes) and it is unlikely that any set of tests in this arena will be useful for the prospective prediction of driving safety. Further success at developing fitness-to-drive models will likely need to focus on specific groups of medically impaired older adults that are homogenous in their specific cognitive or visual domains (e.g. dementia with a specific subtype such as AD). In addition, these models will likely need to incorporate additional measures or proxies such as lifelong driving habits (e.g. history of tickets, crashes, abnormal driving behaviours), personality characteristics (e.g. too aggressive or too passive), traffic density and perhaps other measurement concerns such as test anxiety or confidence issues.

The most common model for driver assessment would involve a combination of physician, occupational therapist, neuropsychologist, specialist driving assessor and/or social worker. Not all disciplines will be needed by all patients: a patient with severe dementia clearly cannot drive and simply a referral to the social worker to plan alternative transportation is appropriate. Equally, a mild cognitive defect may only require a review by the physician and occupational therapist. The overall interdisciplinary assessment should attempt to provide solutions to both maintaining activities and exploring transport needs. However, even in a skilled rehabilitation setting, the predictive value of team assessments may be low for diseases such as stroke[39] and the on-road test is the current best assessment available.

The on-road test may be helpful, as it may demonstrate impairments to a patient or caregiver who is ambiguous about the patient stopping driving. At a therapeutic level, members of the team may be able to assist the patients in coming to terms with the losses associated with stopping driving. The occupational therapist may be able to maximize activities and function and help focus on preserved areas of achievement, while the social worker can advise on alternative methods of transport. This approach should save time and valuable resources for occupational therapy, neuropsychology and on-road driver assessors.

In addition to the usual work-up, the medical assessment should include a driving history from patient and ideally (with the patient's permission) also from a caregiver or informant. The physician needs to weigh judiciously the collateral history, taking into account whether or not the carer is also dependent on the patient operating a motor vehicle. Physicians should also inquire about new unsafe driving behaviours. These behaviours can be apparent in mild dementia and would raise concerns about continuing driving privileges. It is important to recognize that these behaviours represent a *change* from baseline. They include becoming lost in familiar areas, driving too fast, reacting too slowly, consistently making poor judgments, failure to notice street signs, having more accidents, receiving indecent gestures from other drivers, miscalculating speed and distances, new dents on the car, knocking off rear-view mirrors, showing poor judgment when making turns or impaired ability to recognize or understand road or traffic signs.

The next stage of testing includes evaluations from occupational therapists and/or neuropsychologists. None of the studies have been sufficiently large to have a reasonable predictive value or to determine cut-off points on neuropsychological test batteries. This situation is paralleled in memory clinics where there is a wide variation in test batteries used: it is likely that the important elements of successful assessment are choice of key domains, familiarity with a test battery and the development of an understanding and close liaison between the physician and the occupational therapist and/or neuropsychologist. In addition, a recent review indicated that to date, there is little evidence to support the use of performance based road tests.

A wide range of tests have been correlated with driving behaviour but few have been sufficiently robust to calculate cut-off points for risky driving. All of these tests can be criticized for taking an over-cognitive view of the driving task.[44] A comprehensive review of tests is available from the US National Highway Transportation Safety Administration[45] and a recent meta-analysis limited to traditional neuropsychological tests indicated that visuospatial skill impairment was the cognitive ability with the strongest association with impaired driving in studies with dementia.[46]

The other interesting aspect is that there may be a disparity between scores on a test battery and the clinical assessment of the neuropsychologist. In a short paper by Fox *et al.*, the neuropsychology test scores and the neuropsychology prediction were found not to be significantly associated, suggesting that the clinicians made their decisions on items not formally measured in the neuropsychology test battery.[47] In conjunction with the clinical assessment and collateral history, these tests will guide the physician as to which patients require on-road testing, and also those who are likely to be dangerous to test!

At present, simulators of sufficient sophistication are not widely available but may represent opportunities for both driver rehabilitation[48] (analogous to training aeroplane pilots) and assessment. The main benefit of large, sophisticated simulators such as the Iowa simulator has been to try to develop and understand neuropsychological and behavioural test batteries in a safe and reliable method and to correlate them with unsafe driving behaviour and crashes. The classic paper by Rizzo *et al.* in 1997 revealed that 29% of AD patients experienced crashes in the simulator versus none of 18 control participants.[49] The drivers with AD were also more than twice as likely to experience 'close calls'. There was also evidence that some drivers with mild AD did not crash and showed fair control of their vehicles compatible with the idea that some patients with mild dementia should be allowed to continue to drive.

On-road driver testing is the gold standard and should be offered to all patients who are not clearly dangerous when driving. The assessor will require a full clinical report and may choose to use one of the recently developed scoring systems for on-road testing of patients with dementia. At least three different road tests have been devised specifically for dementia, although the numbers put through these in published series are still relatively small, with 27 patients in the Sepulveda Road Test,[50] 65 in the Washington University Road Test[51] and 100 in the Alberta Road Test.[52] The tests should ideally involve some degree of cognitive loading, which will tend to bring out the degree and extent to which the older driver can manage complex situations safely.[53]

The quantification, operationalization and validation of these road tests need to be done repeatedly in environments other than that of the originators of the test. The current reliability of standardized tests seems promising.[54] An additional spin-off may well be that just as the simulators may provide information on which behavioural or neuropsychological tests might be helpful in deciding which drivers are safe to drive, so too may road test schedules help in the development of neuropsychological tests. Psychological batteries have been developed from both the Sepulveda and Alberta Road Tests.

There are certain limitations with road tests. Expenses for driving evaluations may vary from $200 to $500 and health insurance or government health providers may not cover the cost. In addition, they often occur in an unfamiliar environment and in an unfamiliar car. However, professional organizations representing geriatricians need to undertake advocacy to ensure that on-road testing is available, of a high standard and affordable to our patients.

What risks are associated with common diseases of later life?

Whereas early papers on dementia and driving emphasized the potential risks from those with dementia, subsequent research has not shown unequivocally that drivers with dementia pose a public health hazard. The precise contribution of the dementias to overall crash hazard is uncertain. Although Johansson *et al.* suggested a major role for dementia as a cause of crashes among older drivers on neuropathological grounds,[55] subsequent interview with families did not reveal significant problems with memory or activities of daily living.[56] The Stockholm group also showed that older drivers who had a high level of traffic violations had a high prevalence of cognitive deficits.[57]

Retrospective studies of dementia and driving from specialist dementia clinics tend to show a high risk,[58–60] whereas those which are prospective and which look at the early stages of dementia show a less pronounced pattern of risk. In the first 2 years of dementia, the risk approximates that of the general population.[61,62] Controlled longitudinal studies of crashes and dementia showed no increase in crash rates for drivers with dementia.[63,64] Likely causes for this counterintuitive finding include a lower annual mileage, using state records for crash data and restriction of driving by the patient, family and physicians. Mild cognitive impairment (MCI), short of dementia, in some studies does not appear to have a significant impact on driving skills.[65,66] For MCI and impaired driving, see Frittelli *et al.* and Wadley *et al.*[100a,b]

Extrapolating from special populations may skew predictions of risk. For example, epilepsy, for which there are relatively clear-cut guidelines in most countries, would seem to pose a clear threat to driving ability as viewed from a clinic setting. Recent population-based studies seem to suggest that the increased risk is relatively low.[67] In a population renewing their licences in North Carolina, the lowest decile had a relative crash risk of 1.5 in the 3 years previous to the cognitive testing.[68] A somewhat reassuring finding from this cohort is that those with the poorest scores for visual and cognitive function also drove less and avoided high-risk situations.[69] A reasonable conclusion from these studies is that dementia among drivers is not yet a public health problem. Although increasing numbers of older drivers may change this situation, it is also possible that 'Smeed's law' will operate, whereby increasing numbers of drivers among a defined population are associated with a drop in fatality rates per car.[70]

Older drivers report less driving at night or during adverse weather conditions and avoid rush hour or congested thoroughfares. Most importantly, cognitively impaired older adults who renewed their licence appear to restrict their exposure even further, many to less than 3000 miles per year.[69] Demented drivers may further limit their exposure when compared with age-matched controls.[71] The data on exposure will require some confirmation, since there certainly are questions raised regarding the accuracy of reporting mileage in any cognitively impaired group. However, decreased exposure may explain why many crash studies have not observed major differences in crash rates from controls when comparing rates on the number of crashes per year and not factoring in total mileage.[72]

Polypharmacy is common in older adults and medication may be additive to crash risk in older adults with cognitive impairment. This is a complex area and it can be difficult to tell whether it is the illness or the medication which is causing the problem. There are many medication classes that have been studied and noted to impair driving skills when assessed by simulators or road tests, although these decrements may not translate into increased safety risk. These include, but are not limited to; narcotics, benzodiazepines, antihistamines, antidepressants, antipsychotics, hypnotics, alcohol and muscle relaxants. Very few studies have focused on the older adult driver. However, long-acting benzodiazepines have been associated with increased crash rates.[73] Another report suggests that there may be a significant number of older adults driving while intoxicated or under the influence of other medications.[74,75] Clinicians should review medications closely with each individual and attempt to discontinue medications that have the potential to affect cognition adversely when appropriate. Screening for alcohol abuse or misuse is also reasonable.

What interventions can we make?

Depending on the illnesses present, there is potentially a wide range of interventions that we can undertake (Table 123.2). Adaptation of the car, following advice from the occupational therapist, physiotherapist or specialist driving assessor, can improve driving comfort and safety. A follow-up review should be organized for those with progressive illness such as dementia and parkinsonism.[76] A review period of 6–12 months would seem to be reasonable with a progressive neurodegenerative dementia.[77] However, patients and carers should be asked to seek an earlier review if they perceive a significant decline in the status of the dementia or in driving abilities. Although some studies have concluded with recommendations that all older adults with dementia should refrain from driving,[58] the majority of clinicians would likely base this decision on dementia severity[78] or a demonstration of impaired driving competence.[79] The American Academy of Neurology guidelines, proposing that no-one with a Clinical Dementia Rating (CDR) Scale of 1 should drive, have been superseded by research that judged 41% of those with a CDR 1 as safe (19% were considered to be marginal and 41% to be unsafe).[77] This reinforces the need for a full assessment and appropriate follow-up.

For progressive neurological conditions, the physician needs to help the patient and their family prepare for eventual withdrawal from driving. Early and appropriate diagnosis disclosure is likely to be important here.[80] A helpful description of this process is the modified Ulysses contract,[81] after the hero who made his crew tie him to the mast on the condition that they did not heed his entreaties to be released when seduced by the song of the sirens. It forms the basis of a useful patient and carer brochure from the Hartford Foundation, which is also available online.[82]

The very act of highlighting the potential of compromised driving ability may have a therapeutic benefit, promoting increased vigilance on the part of the patient and carers that their social contract for driving privileges is not the same as that of the general public. Support is given to this concept by the success of restricted licensing for people

Table 123.2 Sample diseases for which appropriate assessment and remediation may be of benefit.

Neuropsychiatric	
Stroke	Driving-specific rehabilitation[89]
Parkinson's disease	Maximizing motor function, treatment of depression, assessment of cognitive function[90]
Delirium	Treatment and resolution
Depression	Treatment: if antidepressant, choose one with least potential of cognitive/motor effects [91]
Mild dementia	Assess, treat depression, reduce/eliminate psychoactive drugs, advice not to drive alone[92]
Cardiovascular	
Syncope	Advice pending investigation: treat cause[93]
Respiratory	
Sleep apnoea	Treatment of underlying disease[94]
Vision	
Cataract	Surgery, appropriate corrective lens and advice about glare[95]
Metabolic	
Diabetes	Direct therapy to avoid hypoglycaemia[96]
Musculoskeletal	
All arthritides	Driving-specific rehabilitation programme[97]
Iatrogenic	
Polypharmacy	Rationalize medications[98]
Psychoactive medication	Rationalize, minimize[99]

with medical illnesses in the State of Utah.[83] While the effect might arise from the restrictions (avoidance of motorways, night-time driving), it is also possible that the very act of labelling these drivers may heighten self-awareness.

A clear recommendation should be made to the patient and recorded in the medical record; this should include advice to inform their insurance company of relevant illnesses, and also any statutory requirement to inform their driver licensing authority.

When driving is no longer possible, alternative options should be discussed with the patient. For the fortunate minority who have access to a paratransit system (tailored, affordable personal transportation systems[84]), the graduation may be more easy. For the rest, although public transportation systems[85] may have reduced fares for senior citizens, the very disabilities that prevented driving also render such services sub-optimal.[86] Due to restricted sites and cognitive limitations of our older drivers, these services are typically underutilized, and simply not practical. State or locally sponsored services may provide door-to-door transport for older adults in large vans, many of which are lift-equipped. Local communities, societies, retirement centres or local church groups may use funds or volunteers to provide services to physician offices, shops and meetings. Transportation is often provided by family members once the older adult can no longer perform the task.[87,88] More unique and novel transportation services are needed and those such as Independent Transportation Network America (www.itnamerica.org) give promise to future older adults that have lost their privilege to drive.

What is the physician's responsibility with regard to driver licensing and insurance authorities?

In general, the welfarist role of the physician extends to reminding the patient that most insurance companies require disclosure by the driver of 'illnesses relevant to driving' when they arise. Two issues arise: the medical advisers of the insurance companies may not make calculations of insurance rates (or continued insurance) on the basis of reason and evidence but rather on ageist grounds and prejudice against disability. We may be unwittingly exposing the patient to this prejudice. The answer to this lies in continued advocacy efforts of professional groups at a societal level and also support by the physician in individual cases if the assessment supports preserved driving skills. A second issue is whether it is sufficient to recommend disclosure to someone who will not remember this advice. However, the physician's role is primarily to ensure safe mobility. In general, it is reasonable to assume that removal of insurance coverage is a secondary matter in such cases. It is reasonable to share the disclosure information with the carers.

The actual process of breaking confidentiality in the event of evidence of hazard to other members of the public is almost universally supported by most codes of medical practice – but it is to whom this should be reported that poses some ethical challenges. The traditional route of reporting to driver licensing authorities [DMV (USA), DVLA (UK)] may have relatively little benefit – removal of a driving licence is a dramatic event and may possibly be remembered by even a driver with moderate dementia. It is important that this disclosure has some likelihood of impact and results in the least traumatic removal of the compromised older driver from the road. In such instances, the family may be able to intervene in terms of disabling the car and providing alternative modes of transport. In our own experience, we rarely have to invoke official intervention, but find that a personal communication with a senior police officer in the patient's locality may result in a sensitive visit to the patient and cessation of driving.

Mandatory reporting represents a different ethical challenge. It has not been shown to be of benefit and, unless significant benefit can be shown in future studies, the profession should resist the introduction of such schemes. For individual practitioners in jurisdictions where such regulations exist, a twin-track approach is probably necessary – professional advocacy with law-makers and a considered approach as to whether disclosure is in the patient's best interests on a case-by-case basis. If the physician is confident that the state or province has a mechanism for fair assessment and an enlightened approach to maintaining mobility, compliance is not difficult. If the assessment is cursory and aimed at unduly restricting mobility, physicians may be faced with a problem recognized with other laws, which may put patient's welfare at risk and where professional obligations may require non-compliance with an unfair law.

Conclusion

Transportation and driving assessment have become an integral part of the assessment of older people. Geriatricians, appropriately supported by their interdisciplinary team and specialist on-road assessment, can help to support safe mobility and social inclusion in later life. There is a need for more research to clarify further the most appropriate and economical assessments and interventions which further this end.[3]

Key points

- Transportation is an important component of well-being for older people.
- In contrast to previous attitudes which prioritized risk over mobility, current thinking and practice promote the optimization of mobility for older people.
- Geriatricians, appropriately supported by their interdisciplinary team and specialist on-road assessment, can help to support safe mobility and social inclusion in later life.

References

1. Mezuk B and Rebok GW. Social integration and social support among older adults following driving cessation. *J Gerontol B Psychol Sci Soc Sci* 2008;**63**:S298–303.
2. Okoro CA, Strine TW, Young SL *et al.* Access to health care among older adults and receipt of preventive services. Results from the Behavioral Risk Factor Surveillance System, 2002. *Prev Med* 2005;**40**:337–43.
3. OECD. *Ageing and Transport: Mobility Needs and Safety Issues*, OECD, Paris, 2001.
4. CEMT. *Report on Transport and Ageing of the Population*, Report No. CEMT/CM(2001)16, CEMT, Paris, 2001.
5. Committee for the Safe Mobility of Older People. *Transportation in an Aging Society, a Decade of Experience*, Transportation Research Board, Washington, DC, 2004.
6. Fain MJ. Should older drivers have to prove that they are able to drive? *Arch Intern Med* 2003;**163**:2126–8; discussion, 32.
7. Hakamies-Blomqvist L, Ukkonen T and O'Neill D. Driver ageing does not cause higher accident rates per mile. *Transport Res Part F Traffic Psychol Behav* 2002;**5**:271–4.
8. Braver ER and Trempel RE. Are older drivers actually at higher risk of involvement in collisions resulting in deaths or non-fatal injuries among their passengers and other road users? *Inj Prev* 2004;**10**:27–32.
9. Hakamies-Blomqvist L, Johansson K and Lundberg C. Medical screening of older drivers as a traffic safety measure – a comparative Finnish–Swedish Evaluation study. *J Am Geriatr Soc* 1996;**44**:650–3.
10. Langford J, Fitzharris M, Koppel S and Newstead S. Effectiveness of mandatory license testing for older drivers in reducing crash risk among urban older Australian drivers. *Traffic Inj Prev* 2004;**5**:326–35.
11. Langford J, Fitzharris M, Newstead S and Koppel S. Some consequences of different older driver licensing procedures in Australia. *Accid Anal Prev* 2004;**36**:993–1001.
12. O'Neill D. Re: preventing injuries and fatalities among older pedestrians. *Age Ageing* 2010;**39**:406.
13. Taylor BD and Tripodes S. The effects of driving cessation on the elderly with dementia and their caregivers. *Accid Anal Prev* 2001;**33**:519–28.
14. Edwards JD, Ross LA, Ackerman ML *et al.* Longitudinal predictors of driving cessation among older adults from the ACTIVE clinical trial. *J Gerontol B Psychol Sci Soc Sci* 2008;**63**:P6–12.
15. Sims RV, Ahmed A, Sawyer P and Allman RM. Self-reported health and driving cessation in community-dwelling older drivers. *J Gerontol A Biol Sci Med Sci* 2007;**62**:789–93.
16. Johnson JE. Rural elders and the decision to stop driving. *J Community Health Nurs* 1995;**12**:131–8.
17. Martin A, Balding L and O'Neill B. A bad press: older drivers and the media. *BMJ* 2005;**330**:368.
18. McGwin G Jr, Sims RV, Pulley L and Roseman JM. Relations among chronic medical conditions, medications and automobile crashes in the elderly: a population-based case–control study. *Am J Epidemiol* 2000;**152**:424–31.
19. Wood JM, Worringham C, Kerr G *et al.* Quantitative assessment of driving performance in Parkinson's disease. *J Neurol Neurosurg Psychiatry* 2005;**76**:176–80.
20. World Health Organization. *International Classification of Functioning, Disability and Health*, WHO, Geneva, 2001.
21. Wang CC and Carr DB. Older driver safety: a report from the older drivers project. *J Am Geriatr Soc* 2004;**52**:143–9.
22. Meuser TM, Carr DB, Berg-Weger M *et al.* Driving and dementia in older adults: implementation and evaluation of a continuing education project. *Gerontologist* 2006;**46**:680–7.

23. American Medical Association. *Assessing Fitness to Drive in Older People*, AMA, Chicago, 2003.
24. Miller EA and Weissert WG. Predicting elderly people's risk for nursing home placement, hospitalization, functional impairment and mortality: a synthesis. *Med Care Res Rev* 2000;**57**:259–97.
25. Daiello LA, Festa EK, Ott BR and Heindel WC. Cholinesterase inhibitors improve visual attention in drivers with Alzheimer's disease. *Alzheimer's Dementia* 2008;**4**(4,Suppl 1):T498.
26. Lockett D, Willis A and Edwards N. Through seniors' eyes: an exploratory qualitative study to identify environmental barriers to and facilitators of walking. *Can J Nurs Res* 2005;**37**:48–65.
27. Marmeleira JF, Godinho MB and Fernandes OM. The effects of an exercise program on several abilities associated with driving performance in older adults. *Accid Anal Prev* 2009;**41**:90–7.
28. MacMahon M, O'Neill D and Kenny RA. Syncope: driving advice is frequently overlooked. *Postgrad Med J* 1996;**72**:561–3.
29. Fisk GD, Owsley C and Pulley LV. Driving after stroke: driving exposure, advice and evaluations. *Arch Phys Med Rehabil* 1997;**78**:1338–45.
30. Nasvadi GC and Wister A. Do restricted driver's licenses lower crash risk among older drivers? A survival analysis of insurance data from British Columbia. *Gerontologist* 2009;**49**:474–84.
31. George S, Clark M and Crotty M. Development of the Adelaide driving self-efficacy scale. *Clin Rehabil* 2007;**21**:56–61.
32. Okonkwo OC, Griffith HR, Vance DE *et al*. Awareness of functional difficulties in mild cognitive impairment: a multidomain assessment approach. *J Am Geriatr Soc* 2009;**57**:978–84.
33. Vrkljan BH and Polgar JM. Driving, navigation and vehicular technology: experiences of older drivers and their co-pilots. *Traffic Inj Prev* 2007;**8**:403–10.
34. Adler G, Rottunda S, Rasmussen K and Kuskowski M. Caregivers dependent upon drivers with dementia. *J Clin Geropsychol* 2000;**6**:83–90.
35. Croston J, Meuser TM, Berg-Weger M *et al*. Driving retirement in older adults with dementia. *Top Geriatr Rehabil* 2009;**25**:154–62.
36. Fuller R. Towards a general theory of driver behaviour. *Accid Anal Prev* 2005;**37**:461–72.
37. Ranney TA. Models of driving behaviour: a review of their evolution. *Accid Anal Prev* 1994;**26**:733–50.
38. Carr D and Ott BR. The older adult driver with cognitive impairment: 'it's a very frustrating life'. *JAMA* 2010;**303**:1632–41.
39. Akinwuntan AE, Feys H, DeWeerdt W *et al*. Determinants of driving after stroke. *Arch Phys Med Rehabil* 2002;**83**:334–41.
40. Reuben DB. Assessment of older drivers. *Clin Geriatr Med* 1993;**9**:449–59.
41. Underwood M. The older driver. Clinical assessment and injury prevention. *Arch Intern Med* 1992;**152**:735–40.
42. Foley KT and Mitchell SJ. The elderly driver: what physicians need to know. *Cleve Clin J Med* 1997;**64**:423–8.
43. Marottoli RA, Cooney LM Jr, Wagner R *et al*. Predictors of automobile crashes and moving violations among elderly drivers . *Ann Intern Med* 1994;**121**:842–6.
44. De Raedt R and Ponjaert-Kristoffersen I. The relationship between cognitive/neuropsychological factors and car driving performance in older adults . *J Am Geriatr Soc* 2000;**48**:1664–8.
45. Staplin LS, Lococo KH, Stewart J and Decina LE. *Safe Mobility for Older People Notebook*, Report No. DTNH22-96-C-05140, National Highway Traffic Safety Administration, Washington, DC, 1999.
46. Reger MA, Welsh RK, Watson GS *et al*. The relationship between neuropsychological functioning and driving ability in dementia: a meta-analysis. *Neuropsychology* 2004;**18**:85–93.
47. Fox GK, Bowden SC, Bashford GM and Smith DS. Alzheimer's disease and driving: prediction and assessment of driving performance. *J Am Geriatr Soc* 1997;**45**:949–53.
48. Akinwuntan AE, De Weerdt W, Feys H *et al*. Effect of simulator training on driving after stroke: a randomized controlled trial. *Neurology* 2005;**65**:843–50.
49. Rizzo M, Reinach M, McGehee D and Dawson J. Simulated car crashes and crash predictors in drivers with Alzheimer disease. *Arch Neurol* 1997;**54**:545–51.
50. Fitten LJ, Perryman KM, Wilkinson CJ *et al*. Alzheimer and vascular dementias and driving. A prospective road and laboratory study. *JAMA* 1995;**273**:1360–5.
51. Hunt LA, Murphy CF, Carr D *et al*. Reliability of the Washington University Road Test. A performance-based assessment for drivers with dementia of the Alzheimer type. *Arch Neurol* 1997;**54**:707–12.
52. Dobbs AR, Heller RB and Schopflocher D. A comparative approach to identify unsafe older drivers. *Accid Anal Prev* 1998;**30**:363–70.
53. Uc EY, Rizzo M, Anderson SW *et al*. Driver route-following and safety errors in early Alzheimer disease. *Neurology* 2004;**63**:832–7.
54. Akinwuntan AE, DeWeerdt W, Feys H *et al*. Reliability of a road test after stroke. *Arch Phys Med Rehabil* 2003;**84**:1792–6.
55. Johansson K, Bogdanovic N, Kalimo H *et al*. Alzheimer's disease and apolipoprotein E E4 allele in older drivers who died in automobile accidents. *Lancet* 1997;**349**:1143.
56. Lundberg C, Johansson K, Bogdanovic N *et al*. Follow-up of Alzheimer's disease and apolipoprotein E E4 allele in older drivers who died in automobile accidents. In: *Proceedings of International Conference on the Older Driver, Health and Mobility*, ARHC Press, Dublin, 1999.
57. Lundberg C, Hakamies-Blomqvist L, Almkvist O and Johansson K. Impairments of some cognitive functions are common in crash-involved older drivers. *Accid Anal Prev* 1998;**30**:371–7.
58. Lucas-Blaustein MJ, Filipp L, Dungan C and Tune L. Driving in patients with dementia. *J Am Geriatr Soc* 1988;**36**:1087–91.
59. Friedland RP, Koss E, Kumar A *et al*. Motor vehicle crashes in dementia of the Alzheimer type. *Ann Neurol* 1988;**24**:782–6.

60. O'Neill D. Driving and dementia. *Alzheimer Rev* 1993;**3**:65–8.

61. Drachman DA and Swearer JM. Driving and Alzheimer's disease: the risk of crashes. *Neurology* 1993;**43**:2448–56; erratum, *Neurology* 1994;**44**:4.

62. Carr DB, Duchek J and Morris JC. Characteristics of motor vehicle crashes of drivers with dementia of the Alzheimer type. *J Am Geriatr Soc* 2000;**48**:18–22.

63. Trobe JD, Waller PF, Cook-Flannagan CA *et al.* Crashes and violations among drivers with Alzheimer disease. *Arch Neurol* 1996;**53**:411–6.

64. Ott BR, Heindel WC, Papandonatos GD *et al.* A longitudinal study of drivers with Alzheimer disease. *Neurology* 2008;**70**:1171–8.

65. Frittelli C, Borghetti D, Iudice G *et al.* Effects of Alzheimer's disease and mild cognitive impairment on driving ability: a controlled clinical study by simulated driving test. *Int J Geriatr Psychiatry* 2009;**24**:232–238.

66. Wadley VG, Okonkwo O, Crowe M *et al.* Mild cognitive impairment and everyday function: an investigation of driving performance. *J Geriatr Psychiatry Neurol* 2009;**22**(2):87–94.

67. Drazkowski JF, Fisher RS, Sirven JI *et al.* Seizure-related motor vehicle crashes in Arizona before and after reducing the driving restriction from 12 to 3 months. *Mayo Clin Proc* 2003;**78**:819–25.

68. Stutts JC, Stewart JR and Martell C. Cognitive test performance and crash risk in an older driver population. *Accid Anal Prev* 1998;**30**:337–46.

69. Stutts JC. Do older drivers with visual and cognitive impairments drive less? *J Am Geriatr Soc* 1998;**46**:854–61.

70. Smeed R. Variations in the patterns of accident rates in different countries and their causes. *Traffic Eng Control* 1968;**10**:364–71.

71. Dubinsky RM, Williamson A, Gray CS and Glatt SL. Driving in Alzheimer's disease. *J Am Geriatr Soc* 1992;**40**:1112–6.

72. Ross LA, Clay OJ, Edwards JD *et al.* Do older drivers at-risk for crashes modify their driving over time? *J Gerontol B Psychol Sci Soc Sci* 2009;**64**:163–70.

73. Hemmelgarn B, Suissa S, Huang A *et al.* Benzodiazepine use and the risk of motor vehicle crash in the elderly. *JAMA* 1997;**278**:27–31.

74. Higgins JP, Wright SW and Wrenn KD. Alcohol, the elderly and motor vehicle crashes. *Am J Emergency Med* 1996;**14**:265–7.

75. Johansson K, Bryding G, Dahl ML *et al.* Traffic dangerous drugs are often found in fatally injured older male drivers [letter]. *J Am Geriatr Soc* 1997;**45**:1029–31.

76. Martin AJ, Marottoli R and O'Neill D. Driving assessment for maintaining mobility and safety in drivers with dementia. *Cochrane Database Syst Rev* 2009;(1): CD006222.

77. Duchek JM, Carr DB, Hunt L *et al.* Longitudinal driving performance in early-stage dementia of the Alzheimer type. *J Am Geriatr Soc* 2003;**51**:1342–7.

78. Dubinsky RM, Stein AC and Lyons K. Practice parameter: risk of driving and Alzheimer's disease (an evidence-based review): report of the Quality Standards Subcommittee of the American Academy of Neurology. *Neurology* 2000;**54**:2205–11.

79. Drachmann DA. Who may drive? Who may not? Who shall decide? *Ann Neurol* 1988;**24**:787–8.

80. Bahro M, Silber E, Box P and Sunderland T. Giving up driving in Alzheimer's disease – an integrative therapeutic approach. *Int J Geriatr Psychiatry* 1995;**10**:871–4.

81. Howe E. Improving treatments for patients who are elderly and have dementia. J *Clin Ethics* 2000;**11**:291–303.

82. Hartford Foundation. *At the Crossroads: a Guide to Alzheimer's Disease, Dementia and Driving,* Hartford Foundation, Hartford, CT, 2000.

83. Vernon DD, Diller EM, Cook LJ *et al.* Evaluating the crash and citation rates of Utah drivers licensed with medical conditions, 1992–1996. *Accid Anal Prev* 2002;**34**:237–46.

84. Freund K. Independent Transportation Network: alternative transportation for the elderly. *TR News* 2000;(206):3–12.

85. Roper TA and Mulley GP. Caring for older people: public transport. BMJ 1996;**313**:415–8.

86. O'Neill D. Predicting and coping with the consequences of stopping driving. *Alzheimer Dis Assoc Disord* 1997;**11**(Suppl 1):70–2.

87. O'Neill D, Bruce I, Kirby M and Lawlor B. Older drivers, driving practices and health issues. *Clin Gerontol* 2000;**10**:181–91.

88. Johnson JE. Informal social support networks and the maintenance of voluntary driving cessation by older rural women. *J Community Health Nurs* 2008;**25**:65–72.

89. O'Dwyer C and O'Neill D. Driving after stroke. *Geriatr Med* 2007;**9**:111–2.

90. O'Neill D. Driving and safe mobility in Parkinson's disease. In: J Playfer and J Hindle (eds), *Parkinson's Disease in the Older Patient*, Radcliffe Publishing, Oxford, 2008, pp.239–52.

91. Rubinsztein J and Lawton CA. Depression and driving in the elderly. *Int J Geriatr Psychiatry* 1995;**10**:15–7.

92. O'Neill D. Dementia and driving: screening, assessment and advice. *Lancet* 1996;**348**:1114.

93. Sorajja D, Nesbitt GC, Hodge DO *et al.* Syncope while driving: clinical characteristics, causes and prognosis. *Circulation* 2009;**120**:928–34.

94. Alvarez FJ, Fierro I, Gomez-Talegon MT *et al.* Patients treated with obstructive sleep apnea syndrome and fitness to drive assessment in clinical practice in Spain at the medical traffic centers. *Traffic Inj Prev* 2008;**9**:168–72.

95. Monestam E and Wachtmeister L. Impact of cataract surgery on car driving: a population based study in Sweden. *Br J Ophthalmol* 1997;**81**:16–22.

96. Stork AD, van Haeften TW and Veneman TF. The decision not to drive during hypoglycemia in patients with type 1 and type 2 diabetes according to hypoglycemia awareness. *Diabetes Care* 2007;**30**:2822–6.

97. Jones JG, McCann J and Lassere MN. Driving and arthritis. *Br J Rheumatol* 1991;**30**:361–4.

98. Ray WA, Thapa PB and Shorr RI. Medications and the older driver. *Clin Geriatr Med* 1993;**9**:413–38.

99. Ray WA, Gurwitz J, Decker MD and Kennedy DL. Medications and the safety of the older driver: is there a basis for concern? *Hum Factors* 1992;**34**:33–47; discussion, 9–51.

100a. Frittelli C, Borghetti D, Iudice G *et al*. Effects of Alzheimer's disease and mild cognitive impairment on driving ability: a controlled clinical study by simulated driving test *Int J Geriatr Psychiatry* 2009;**24**:232–8.

100b. Wadley VG, Okonkwo O, Crowe M *et al*. Mild cognitive impairment and everyday function: an investigation of driving performance. *J Geriatr Psychiatry Neurol* 2009;**22**:87–94.

CHAPTER 124

Smart homes

Roger Orpwood
University of Bath and Royal United Hospital, Bath, UK

Introduction

Smart homes have been in existence for many years, primarily pursued by those with a love of high-tech living environments. However, despite their rather pretentious label, this technology can provide many benefits to support elderly people and there is a growing body of experience which demonstrates its potential. This chapter looks at the ways in which smart homes can provide support based on the experiences of a number of groups. It considers the issues that have to be addressed if it is to be successful, together with some of the growing evidence for its effectiveness and it concludes with a look at the future of this work.

What is a smart home?

The term 'smart home' has been confused by some by using it to describe technology that relies on sensors in the home that can send messages to call centres. Such technology is really telecare and will be referred to as such in this chapter. The primary property that endows a house with the smart home label is its ability to support the user in an autonomous fashion. In other words, it can monitor the user's activities and the way they interact with appliances in the home, but it is also able to supply a response itself to support the user. For example, if a smart home detects a running bath being nearly full it will respond by turning off the taps rather than calling for someone to come and intervene.

What needs to be incorporated in a house to enable it to qualify for this lofty label? A smart home requires three facilities to be installed in order to operate (see Figure 124.1). First, it requires sensors that can monitor the occupant's behaviour and activities as described above, for example, by sensing the water level in a bath. Second, it requires a series of support devices so that it can autonomously provide the backup needed to support the user, for example, means for automatically turning off the bath water. Third, the particular feature that distinguishes a smart home, it requires a means whereby all the sensors and the support devices can talk to each other. This facility is achieved through the use of a communication bus, which is conventionally a form of wiring that enables messages to be sent between the sensors and the support devices, although increasingly it is embodied in a wireless form. The communication bus is linked to a computer or other logic controller that can see all the information being provided by the sensors and which can then make judgements about the user's behaviour. If it decides some action is needed, then it can initiate the activities of the relevant support device.

Hence there is nothing particularly complicated about smart technology. It has been around for a long time in installations in larger public buildings such as airports and hotels. In such buildings, the technology primarily enables environmental control to be provided autonomously so that the building is able to ensure that appropriate temperatures, ventilation and so on are maintained automatically. The communication bus, a key feature of such installations, has been the subject of some standardization so that different manufacturers' components can talk to each other. Many of the components developed for these purposes, such as lighting controls, can be directly applied to usage in domestic homes (Figure 124.2).

Applicability to elderly people

Given the ready availability of smart home components, a number of groups have explored the possibility of using them in a domestic setting to provide support that augments the help received from carers. A lot of work has been carried out to see if people with physical disabilities can be supported. The Edinvar Housing Association in Edinburgh undertook pioneering work to explore the potential of this technology. The Joseph Rowntree Foundation (JRF) has provided a number of installations in York with a fair amount of success. The JRF has published a number of guides about the technology.[1,2] Some

Principles and Practice of Geriatric Medicine, Fifth Edition. Edited by Alan J. Sinclair, John E. Morley and Bruno Vellas.

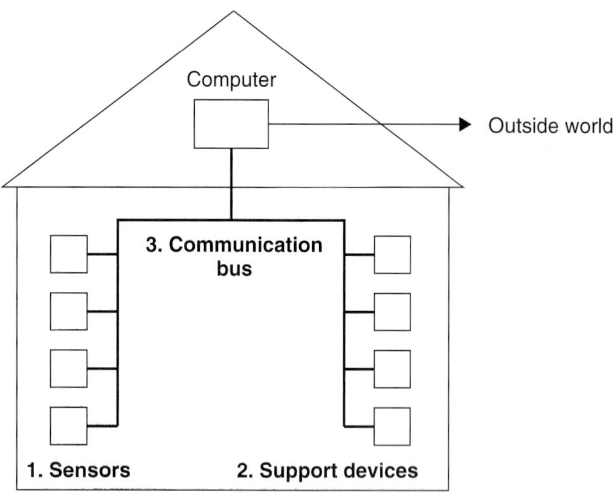

Figure 124.1 Components of a smart house system.

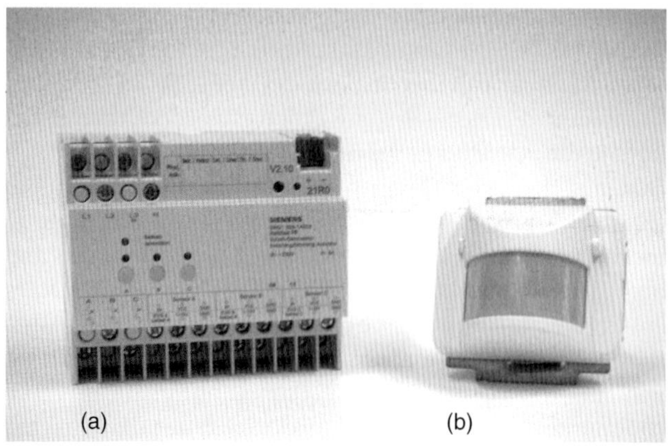

Figure 124.2 Standard commercially available smart home components: (a) a light fader unit and (b) a passive infrared sensor.

pioneering work in Norway has also explored the potential of this technology to support people with dementia.[3] The installations have primarily used commercial smart home components developed for public buildings and configured them in a form that allows their use in a domestic environment. More recently, purpose-designed technology has been developed, such as work at Brunel University on the Millennium Homes project,[4] which enabled the home to give voice prompts to the user to check if they needed outside support.

The majority of these installations have used the ready availability of smart home components to provide the technology that is used. For lighting and ventilation, these components are very appropriate. However, there are a number of situations where such technology is not so appropriate and where support devices need to be better tailored to the needs of the end user. A typical example is the use of commercially available technology to provide tap control. Several installations have used taps controlled by an infrared sensor that could be very useful for someone with poor hand function. All the user has to do is wave their hands in front of the sensor, usually mounted just underneath the tap, and water will be provided while the hands are in position. However, this operation is somewhat unnatural and for someone with a cognitive problem such taps would be totally confusing. These kinds of installations take a somewhat technology-led approach to their design. In other words, the installations start from looking at what technology is available and then configuring it in a form that seems to be close to providing the support needed.

The work carried out at the Bath Institute of Medical Engineering on the Gloucester smart house project explores these issues from a somewhat different perspective.[5] This project is aimed specifically at supporting people with dementia and uses a design technique that is very user-led. In other words, user needs are explored initially to provide a definition of the kind of problems that have to be supported by the technology. Having made these definitions, the design work then moves on to create purpose-designed devices that provide the care needed.

Ensuring user friendliness

There is, of course, a spectrum of reaction to technology on the part of elderly people in the same way as there is for any other age group, and some elderly people are very excited and very proficient in using equipment such as computers. However, there is no doubt that interaction with sophisticated technology can cause a lot of anxiety, which may deter many people from using it. Consequently, when it comes to providing supportive technology for the majority of users, it is preferable that the cognitive load on the user is kept as low as possible. The technology should really provide support with as little intervention as possible from the user.

The problems of designing user-friendly installations are exacerbated when it comes to providing support for people with dementia. For such a user group, having to learn new skills or make sense of a new piece of technology is out of the question. The technology really does have to be invisible and just intervene and provide support when the house deems it to be necessary. The technology has to be totally in the background, where the home appears to be just the same as any other home, where the user does not have to learn any new skills or interact with the new technology. But such installations are also going to be very user friendly for more cognitively able users and will be suitable for those who are less able to cope with new technology. Design approaches that embody this approach have been published.[6,7]

The individual nature of the problems faced by older people has a big impact on the installation of smart home systems. As with all assistive technology, any means of tailoring it to the needs of the individual will make it more effective. Smart home technology is inherently flexible in that the way in which a system responds depends on the control software and this in turn can be easily configured for the individual. Ideally, installations need to be set up for an individual client by a non-technical professional such as an occupational therapist (OT), and this in turn means that such configuring interfaces also need to be user friendly.

Some examples of usage

A few examples can illustrate how new technology can be supportive of someone but require little or no learning. A situation that causes a lot of concern is the problem of an elderly person getting out of bed at night and finding the toilet. For someone who may be unsteady on their feet, rising from lying down to standing is particularly dangerous. The problem is exacerbated by the fact that they are probably in a dark environment. How can smart home technology assist in this situation? First, the house can know whether it is dark or not through ambient light sensors. It can also detect whether someone is in bed and about to get up by means of bed-occupancy sensors. These can be placed underneath the bed legs or across the mattress to detect a weight change (see Figure 124.3). Sometimes pressure-sensitive mats are used on the floor next to the bed, although experience has shown that some users will make a point of not treading on the mat once they have learnt that it is there. Given this information, the house can ensure that when someone gets out of bed in the dark the bedroom light or a bedside lamp is turned on. To reduce the possibility of alarming the user, the light can be activated through faders so that they fade up to a fairly low level in a gentle manner (Figure 124.4). In this way, the user is

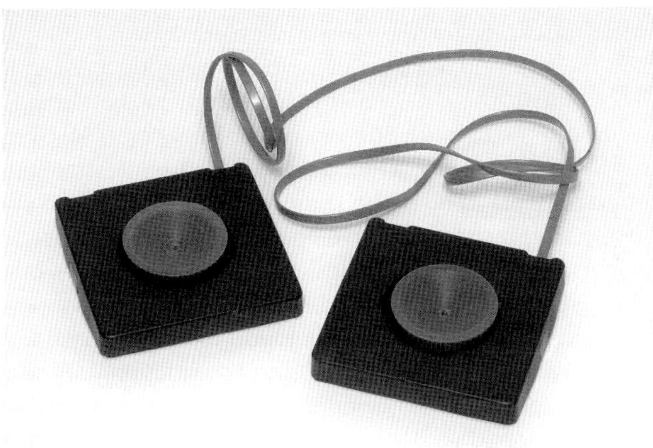

Figure 124.3 A bed-occupancy sensor that fits under a bed leg.

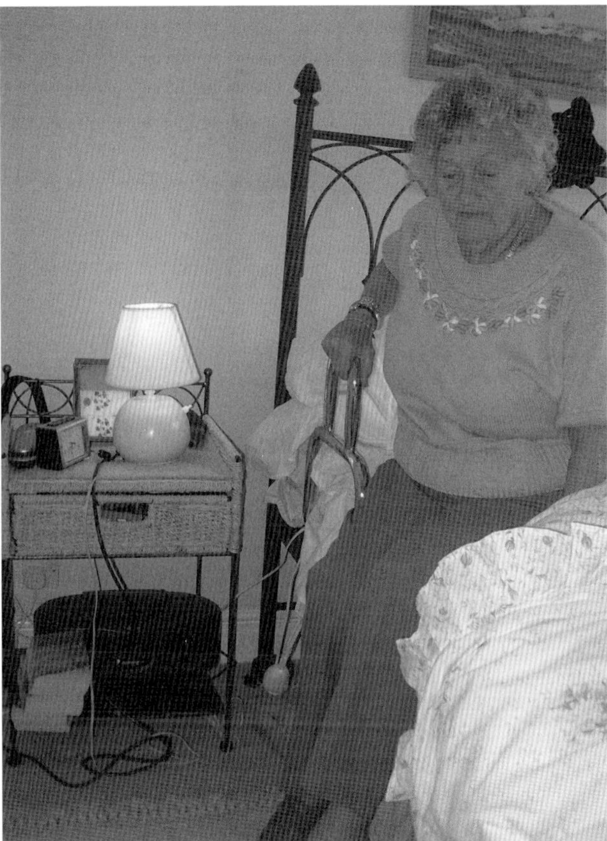

Figure 124.4 An automatic bedside lamp in use.

provided with lighting to help them orientate more easily and move around without tripping or bumping into things. The process can also be reversed. If the user gets back into bed but forgets to turn off the light, the house can again detect that this has happened and can turn the lights off automatically.

This simple use of smart home technology can be taken further. The movements of an occupant about a room can be easily and reliably detected using passive infrared sensors (PIRs). These are the kind of sensors that are used in most home security systems and burglar alarms. It is easy to arrange for lights to come on automatically as the user moves around the house, again ensuring that they have illumination and help reduce falls. If the user has got out of bed and begins to go out of the bedroom, the house could make an initial assumption that they probably want to go to the toilet. It could then fade up the toilet lights and fade down the bedroom lights. In this way, it provides guidance to the toilet for the user. When the user has finished in the toilet and begins to go out of the bathroom, the house could reverse its response, fading up the bedroom light again and fading down the toilet one. In this way, the house can provide guidance to the user moving around the house in addition to providing illumination.

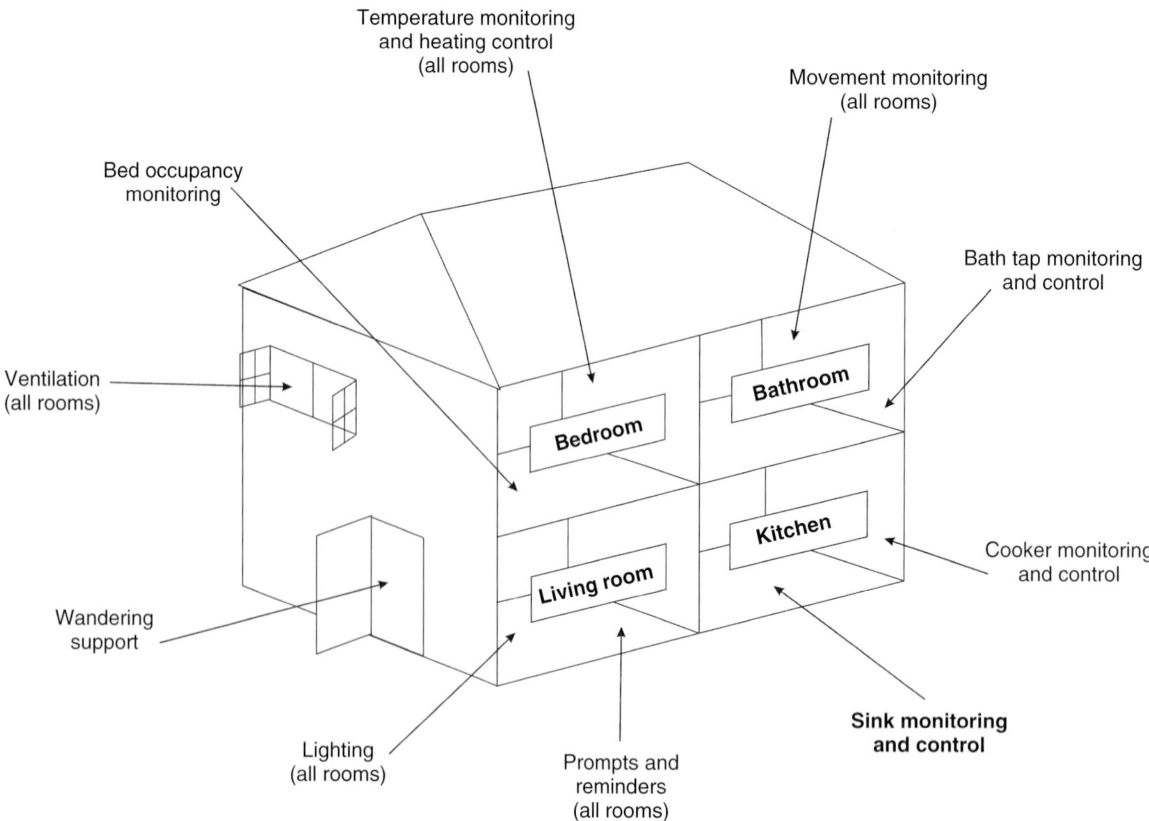

Figure 124.5 Possible support that can be provided by a smart home installation.

There are many other ways that smart house technology can provide support to the occupant (see Figure 124.5). For example, the house can detect if something slightly dangerous has been done, say in the kitchen, and then provide prompts and support. In a similar way, the use of other domestic appliances such as the bath and the kitchen sink can be backed up by keeping water temperatures safe and turning off taps as described above. For people with dementia, the house can keep an eye on wandering tendencies and try to discourage going out of the house and calling for help if it occurs. The house can also provide prompts for activities that need to be carried out such as taking medication or provide a form of day diary to remind people of visitors or mealtimes or even a favourite TV programme. In many ways, the house acts like an extra carer, but one that acts for 24 h per day without becoming tired or frustrated. However, of course it can never supply the qualities of personal human care and it is crucial that installers bear this in mind and do not just see smart homes as a cheap replacement for normal caring.

Appropriate design

Simple application of smart home technology can, in the ways illustrated, provide a lot of support for the user. However, if it is to be effective it has to be designed from a close understanding of the issues that are likely to arise and the way in which users are likely to interact with the technology. A very useful rule of thumb that was used in the development of technology within the Gloucester smart house project was to try to design new support equipment that reacted in a way that emulated the behaviour of personal carers. The reasoning behind this approach was that in many circumstances a personal carer is likely to be the person who best understands what works in caring for the person they are looking after. If they have developed a strategy that works for them, it is likely that any new technology that reacts in a similar way is going to be helpful. Surveys of personal carers showed that there was often a good consensus about strategies found to work. This understanding was a starting point for the new technology developed by the team for use in a smart home. During the design and development work, whenever a situation arose where it was not clear how the technology should react, it was found to be very useful to ask, 'What would the carer do in this situation?'. In this way, the technology is being designed to act as a kind of invisible carer that is ever present, just looking over the user's shoulder, checking that things are alright and just providing help when needed.

A good example of the use of the 'carer emulation' approach is provided by the designs used to control a bath. It would be easy to install a bath water-level sensor that shuts off the water supply when the bath is nearly full. Such a facility would ensure that a forgetful user did not flood the bathroom. However, if they came back to add some more hot water or they let out the water and wanted to run a bath the next day, they would find that the taps did not work because the water had been shut off. A key element in maintaining quality of life for someone with a cognitive problem is to enable them to feel they are still in control of their lives, and finding that their house is taking that control away from them would be counterproductive. How would a carer react to the problem of someone forgetting they were running a bath? It was found that, in these kinds of situations, the carer would follow a simple three-stage response. They would first provide a reminder, 'Don't forget you've got the bath running'. If that did not do the trick, they would then intervene to turn off the bath (or the cooker or other appliance). However, they would turn off the tap in the usual way, which would mean that it could still be used subsequently. Third, they would provide some reassurance to the user, such as, 'I've turned off your bath. It's ready now', so that the user knew why something had happened.

All these actions can be emulated by the smart home, but there is a need for some additional technology. There is a need for a means of communicating with the user, to provide prompts and reminders, and this was done through the use of voice recordings. There is also a need for a means of turning off the bath taps in such a way that the user can still carry on using it themselves (Figure 124.6). The redesigned taps had their insides removed and a new shaft was provided that was rotated when the tap was turned. The shaft was linked to a sensor that could monitor how far the tap had been turned. Hence all the new tap did was to sense how far the user had opened the tap. Depending on this information, an electric valve would open to let the water through at an equivalent rate. If the house needed to shut off the water, it could turn off the electric water valve and then apply an electric brake to the tap shaft. In this way, so far as the user was concerned, the tap felt like it had been turned off. The house would then reset the rotation sensor back to zero. If the user subsequently came to operate the tap, it would first of all feel like someone had turned it off, but it would also activate the sensor in the usual way and the electric valve would supply water. This novel tap design was not just an engineer's good idea about a new tap design, it was completely led by an understanding of the issues involved and the way in which the user was likely to respond through emulating the reaction of carers.

Other techniques have been used to gain a better understanding of what is needed for new designs where there is a very intimate interface with the user. A European Commission-funded project, ENABLE, which evaluated the impact of assistive technology on people with dementia and their carers, placed a lot of emphasis on focus groups and other meetings with professional carers.[8] These sessions were very useful to explore solutions in an interactive manner. Another successful technique pioneered by researchers at Dundee University is the use of actors to provide a bridge between users and researchers.[9] The Dundee team explored the issue of falls in the elderly. They used actors to simulate situations where falls occur. These were useful both to get comments and feedback about situations and strategies and also as tests for the sensing technology they were developing.

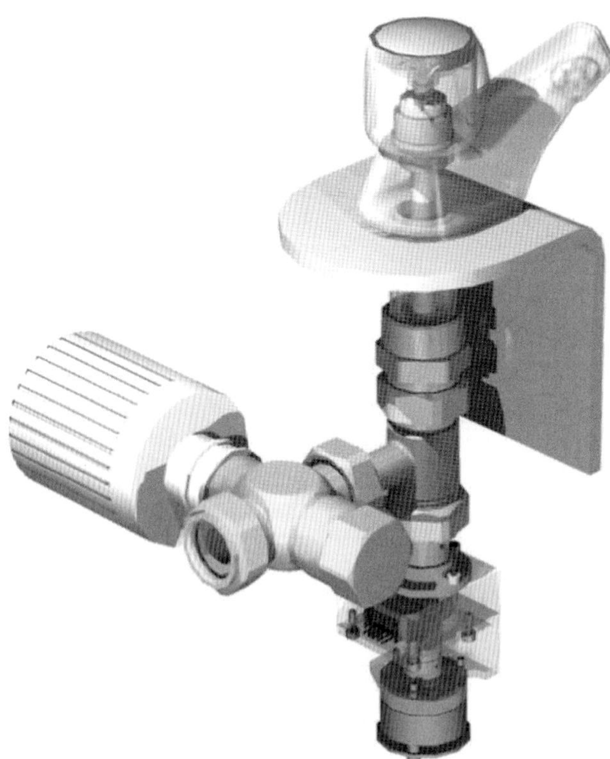

Figure 124.6 Diagram of the tap developed to enable the water supply to be turned off without taking control away from the user.

The difficulty of behaviour monitoring

The main role of sensors in a smart home environment is to allow judgements to be made about user behaviour. Some aspects, such as whether someone has just come out of a toilet or not, are fairly easy to sense and make judgements about. Most aspects, however, are surprisingly difficult to judge, even for simple behaviours, where complications can arise from inevitable variations in the way in which different people act. For example, the work described above on bed-occupancy systems showed that the house cannot just turn the light off as soon as someone gets back into bed. Users were found often to sit on the bed before getting back in, perhaps to remove slippers or dressing gown. If the lights went out straight away it caused some confusion, so a carefully judged delay was introduced to ensure that the user was fully back and settled in bed before turning off the lights. These may seem like minor points in the use of such technology but they can be major factors in the confidence that their users have in them and therefore their acceptance.

Bed-occupancy sensors would superficially seem to be very straightforward. A weight sensor can tell the difference between whether someone is in bed or out of it. However, such a sensor will also be activated by someone turning over in bed or moving from one side to the other. It also has to deal with situations that occur such as someone going to stand up from a bed and then not quite making it and falling back on to the bed before finally getting to their feet. The algorithms (simple computer programs) that use the raw sensor data and make conclusions and judgements based on it have to deal with all these variants of user behaviour (Figure 124.7). To ensure they are effective, a lot of raw data have to be collected so that all the variations can be seen. An effective algorithm can then be developed to deal with them.

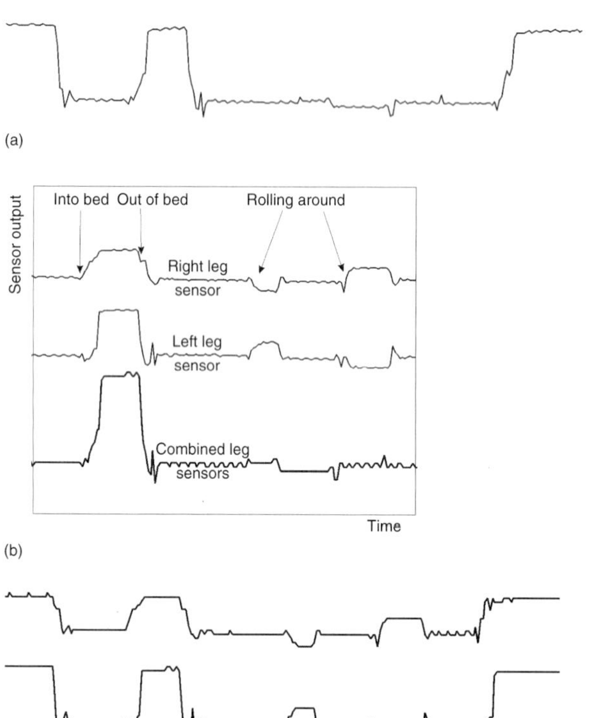

Figure 124.7 Raw data from a bed-occupancy sensor. Traces (a) and (b) show the output from the sensors fitted to both legs at the head end of the bed and trace (c) shows how the summed output can differentiate between getting in and out of bed and simply rolling around.

If the house gets it wrong with a bed-occupancy sensor, it is not so crucial. If it gets it wrong with, say, a gas cooker monitor, then the outcome could be much more serious. Making judgments about human behaviour based on simple sensor data is always going to be probabilistic. For example, with the gas cooker monitor developed for the Gloucester smart house, one of the sensors used was a simple infrared temperature sensor that was mounted at the side of the cooker and could detect the temperature of the pan or kettle. The data from the sensor were to be used to detect whether a pan had boiled dry or not, because then its outside temperature would increase very rapidly. However, users do not just leave a pan alone once it is in use on the cooker. They will very likely turn the gas up and down according to how the cooking was going. They may well move a pan around to different rings on the cooker. Such activities can make it very difficult to judge what is going on from the simple sensor data. A lot of cooking activities were monitored until it was felt that for about 80% of the time a pan could be reliably detected as having boiled dry. However, the other 20% of circumstances had to be dealt with in some way. It was decided to try and ensure that any errors were false positives. In other words, the cooker may on 20% of occasions turn off when it did not really need to do so. However, these false-positive activations proved to be irritating to users during evaluations. The exercise underlined the probabilistic nature of making judgements about user behaviour.

The level of errors could be reduced by incorporating information processing systems with learning capabilities, but it would still not reduce them to zero. Clearly, in these kinds of situations where there is potential danger there has to be some kind of backup. In the case of the cooker monitor, the device had a facility for shutting down the gas supply to the cooker if it continued to sense danger after responding to a danger signal. It also would call for assistance from outside the house in such situations. This is an important conclusion for smart house installations. Some aspects of the support that they provide are fairly safety critical. In these situations, it must be recognized that the house may make a false judgement about the user's behaviour and means for providing some kind of backup and a means for calling for outside assistance are essential.

The importance of communication with the user

It has already been stressed that communication with the user within the smart house is important. The smart house is an intelligent and autonomous care provider and, like any other carer, it needs to communicate with the person for whom it is caring. Voice communication is, of course, very flexible and has the advantage that it reflects the kind of interactions provided by a human carer, but it does have some disadvantages. The communications that it provides are transient. If the user is forgetful, then a message that encourages them, for example, to take some medication may be registered but then forgotten a few minutes later. For users with severe memory problems, such as those with dementia, this problem is exacerbated. In addition, the very fact that voice messages are very anthropomorphic means that users may well treat them emotionally and get angry or irritated when prompted to do something.

When voice prompts were first proposed, some professional carers felt that this might not work for people with dementia because the person may well become very anxious by the use of disembodied voices, particularly people with conditions such as Lewy body disease where they tend to hallucinate and hear voices anyway. The other concern raised was that if the voice is recognized, the person with dementia may well think the owner of the voice is in the building and go looking for them. To try to address the first concern, the designers in the Gloucester smart house project made sure that any voice messages came from devices that normally had voices coming from them, such as the TV or radio. It was also decided to use a voice that was a warm anonymous one.

Most of the project's experience of voice prompts came from the use of a wander reminder for people with dementia. This device sits by the main door and if it detects someone in its vicinity at night-time it plays a voice prompt that says something like, 'It is still night-time, Joan. I should go back to bed' (Figure 124.8). If the user still goes out of the house, this is detected and an alarm is sent to a carer to alert them to the fact. Most of the users have been mild to moderate in their degree of dementia. The results have been very positive, with less wandering reported in most cases and no wandering in several. However, some carers have reported that the user just swears at the voice box!

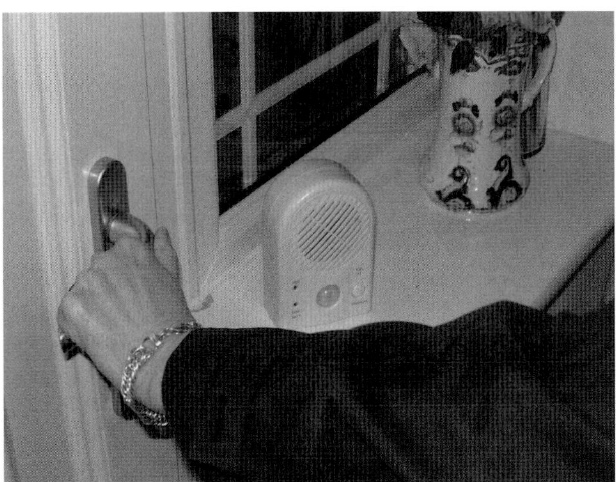

Figure 124.8 A wander reminder fitted near an exit door.

The fact that the voice was disembodied does not seem to have been a problem. It would appear that people are used to voices coming out of little boxes from their lifetime experience of radio, tape recorders and so on, and it seems completely normal. Interestingly, there was some evidence of habituation to the message and the carer was encouraged to change the message from the anonymous one to recording a message of their own. One unexpected outcome from these changes was that it was reported that users seemed to respond better to a voice they recognized and trusted to give them good advice. All voice prompting systems subsequently used by the Bath team have used recorded voices from a close and trusted personal carer.

Other means for communication are being explored. As mentioned above, it would help to use messages that remain for a longer period for people with memory problems or who are forgetful. Simple hand-written text messages are often used by carers of people with dementia. For example, carers might use Post-Its around the house to remind the user not to touch certain appliances or to remind them to take medication and so on. Automated text messages on a small screen on the wall, which can be activated by the house in appropriate situations, are being explored. A further development of this idea that has been successfully tested is the use of simple pictures or graphics in addition to the written message. There is scope for providing these messages on the TV, where simple animation or even small video clips can be used.

Quality of life issues

It has been commented that smart home technology has primarily been used to support safety and security issues and not very much for other activities such as leisure.[10] The technology is ideal for monitoring activities such as cooker, fire and tap usage, to ensure appropriate temperatures and ventilation, to help prevent wandering or disorientation at night and so on. The impact that it has on quality of life is less clear and yet as far as the users themselves are concerned, it is maintenance of or improvement in their quality of life that is all important. Are there ways in which this technology can have an impact on quality of life?

Some work recently completed in the UK explored whether it is possible for smart home technology to have a more direct impact on quality of life.[11] The project, labelled INDEPENDENT, used grounded-theory qualitative techniques to tease out from interviews with people with dementia those aspects of their lives that had the most impact on their quality of life. A wish-list of 11 topics was compiled from this work, covering such aspects as reminiscence, relationship with family, access to music and social isolation. A number of topics were explored from the perspective of technologies that could be included in a smart home environment. A useful example was the issue of reduction of social isolation, which was a key component of the wish-list. The study explored the use of video links between an elderly person and their family. It developed a very intuitive control interface based on the normal social etiquette of visiting someone. For example, the touch screen used for the user's control interface had a knock-on-the-door facility so that the elderly user could request a virtual visit with their family. The success of this work demonstrates that there is a lot of scope for these kinds of uses of technology, but it is in a complex area of human–technology interaction and to be successful it is important that it is led by an understanding of user needs rather than by the availability of technology. There is some indication from other work that even simple phone or video conference chats can provide a sense of social inclusion.[12] The often reported habit of TVs being left on in an otherwise empty home to provide a sense of social involvement gives an indication of the complex way in which people can interact with technology.

A key quality of life issue is, of course, that of independence and for the user to have a sense of being in control of their lives. It is for this reason that so much emphasis had been placed in the Gloucester smart house project on empowering the user and not letting the house take control away from them. Many issues that have an impact on quality of life are very personal to the individual. There can often be some barrier for a given individual that prevents them from doing something that may not seem that important to an outsider, such as being able to cook a simple meal for oneself. If such barriers can be identified and removed through the use of some technology, it could provide a big increase in their personal quality of life.

Links with the outside world

As was mentioned above, the major factor differentiating smart home technology from telecare systems is its ability to act autonomously. However, there is an important need for communication with the outside world. Already mentioned is the need for backup in the event of an emergency. The house needs channels of communication that can alert the carer and others to the fact that the house is not able to cope on its own. The Bath work, for example, used an SMS link to call for assistance. If the gas cooker monitor decided that there was still some danger despite it having turned off the cooker knobs, then it would shut down the gas supply and send a text message to the mobile phones of several carers, advising them to come and check and to turn the gas back on again. This system worked very well. Such links could be provided via landline phones and perhaps to a call centre. It would also be possible to send messages via a web server to appear on a remote monitor.

The external support described could provide details that would enable a care professional to make judgments about the impact of the technology. This is a difficult ethical area that needs much further exploration. On the one hand it might be seen to be useful for an OT just to check on how often one of her clients had used the toilet in case there was evidence of a urinary tract infection, for example. But is such personal intrusion really ethically acceptable? On the other hand, it would make sense for the house itself to flag a warning if it detected anomalous behaviour that might indicate excessive anxiety or to let OTs know if the gas cooker had to turn itself off more than 10 times in a week or if the refrigerator had not been opened for several days. Hence these links to the outside world seem to make sense if they can be preset to draw attention to some trend in the house, but it becomes much more ethically contentious when it is used as a tool to check and pry.

The importance of providing information to the outside world was underlined by the evaluations of smart installations where it was clear that there was an important need for carers, both professional and family, to know how the user was getting on. This was needed both to reassure the carer but also to let professional carers know whether adjustments they have made to the installation are effective or not. However, it is not clear just what kind of information needs to be provided. The raw sensor data are far too detailed to give carers a sense of how the user is doing, but a simple high-level indication, such as an okay/not-okay message, is not adequate. Carers require some interpretation of the raw data that can provide information about how they are sleeping and eating, whether there are any signs of anxiety or distress, and so on. Such interpretation is difficult to provide in an autonomous fashion. Some work has been completed exploring lifestyle monitoring. These techniques try to correlate sensor data with direct behaviour monitoring. They often use the norms of behaviour that have been learnt by the installation and which can then be used to check for changes. For example, simple movement around the living environment can be averaged to provide a measure of 'normal' movement. If there is a sudden increase in this activity it could be interpreted as a sign of increased restlessness or anxiety. This work is an important current research topic and so far has shown that human behaviour is actually very varied and difficult to pin down to norms of behaviour for a given individual.[13]

Having made judgements about how someone is getting on, the system then needs to present this to the carer. For professional carers, with perhaps many clients to oversee, this information needs to be presented in a very succinct fashion. It is likely that the system will alert carers to problems that have arisen rather than provide continuous data and then enable them to gain access and look at the more detailed information. Again, this is a key current research topic.

Experience of usage

A lot of work has been completed on experimental smart home systems, including much work in conjunction with elderly people. The key issue, however, is how users actually manage when using these kinds of installations in the longer term and experience of this usage is starting to accrue. As an illustration of the impact of the technology, some results from a year-long evaluation carried out in London are described below.[14] This work was carried out in a care home so that there was good backup in the event of any problems arising with technology that was still experimental.

The London installation was provided for a man with a moderate dementia, who had a Mini Mental State Examination (MMSE) score of 10 and whose OT assessment showed that he had a continence problem and a tendency to wander at night. A full set of support equipment was installed, to cover lighting, use of his cooker and taps, dealing with wandering, with sensors for movement, bed occupancy, use of equipment and with a complete voice prompt system using recorded messages from his daughter (his primary carer up to that point). Prior to turning on the installed support technology, the sensors were used to monitor his behaviour for the first month to provide some baseline data. The sensors showed that in addition to the problems highlighted by his initial OT assessment, he also had a major sleep problem. On average he was getting about $3\frac{1}{2}$ h sleep per night. He also seemed confused about where he was in the flat, often wandering around various rooms before getting to the toilet at night. Consequently, when the support equipment was configured, these observations were also taken into account. To support his incontinence, which primarily occurred at night, if he got out of bed the bedroom and toilet light were turned on. His daughter's recorded voice would inform him that the toilet light had been tuned on for him. When he finished in the toilet but did not go back to bed, his daughter's voice would encourage him to return to bed. This would be repeated at intervals three times and if he still wandered around the apartment the system would call for assistance from the night care staff. This simple intervention had a major impact on his life. The guidance to the toilet at night enabled him to become completely dry. The encouragement back to bed increased his sleep time up to around 6 h per night. He also had a system installed to discourage him from going out at night and this reduced these wandering incidents to around 20% of their previous level. Interviews with him and the care staff showed he was content and able to cope with most of his life.

This is just one example from a growing body of evidence that is showing the real impact of this technology. It is clear that to be effective it does need to be configured to suit the particular needs of a user, and this requirement complicates the configuration of installations. Such configurations need to be carried out by non-technical staff and so need to be simple to carry out, and make it essential that such staff receive good feedback about how their client is getting on. But the message that is developing is that these kinds of smart installations can enable users to be independent and safe.

The largest usage of smart homes for elderly people is in The Netherlands. Their Smart Home project has been under way for many years and involves many thousands of homes.[15] The installations are fairly basic and not really tailored to the needs of the individual, but they do include automatic lighting, monitoring of the outside door and a central home-locking facility. These approaches have recently been extended to explore their application to people with dementia.

Infrastructure needed for introduction

A lot of the work carried out so far on the use of smart homes for elderly and disabled people has been on very small-scale installations. They have been more akin to research projects to explore the potential of the technology. As evidence mounts that there are distinct personal benefits to the clients and as evidence also mounts as to the cost-effectiveness of the technology, there is an expectation that the technology can be rolled out to be used throughout the community. However, there are a number of infrastructural requirements that are needed to be satisfied before such a major step.

First, any such technology can only be used following an extensive assessment of the user's needs by a care professional, probably an OT. The OTs involved need to be knowledgeable about what assistive devices are available and their potential to provide support. In this way, they can match the needs of the individual to a prescription of the mix of technology that would best suit the client at that time.

Second, there needs to be a knowledgeable set of contractors, either employed by the company manufacturing the assistive technology or able to work for a number of different companies, to carry out the actual installations and configure them according to the results of the assessment process. As with environmental control technology, the commissioning process is complicated because it needs to involve a mix of technical people and OTs.

Third, there needs to be system of operational backup, as described above, in the event of emergencies arising. Such backup may well be provided by call centres, but there is no reason why this cannot be provided via care professionals directly or personal carers, particularly through web-based technology.

Fourth, there needs to be a well thought through system of technical maintenance that can be activated at very short notice. It is clear from the work of projects such as ENABLE that users of sophisticated technology can become very anxious when it does not seem to be operating as they expect and they can quickly reject the technology if it appears to have gone wrong. Such backup would ideally be provided by manufacturers, but a front line of quick-reaction local technical support would probably be essential.

All the infrastructures described above would have to be in place before any large-scale installation of this technology. Similar facilities are also needed, of course, for telecare systems and these have been mostly put in place with remarkable efficiency over the last few years in the UK. Hence there is every reason to expect that such infrastructures can be put in place, particularly once the benefits of using this technology become more widely accepted.

Future trends

There is an important need for much more evaluation of smart home installations to get a better indication of the ways in which it supports users and indeed the ways in which it does not. Evidence is emerging as to those key features that are of most benefit, but much more work needs to be done in this area. In addition, the new support devices developed specifically for the elderly now need to be developed to a more mature state. As has been said, there are many items such as lighting controls that are already available off the shelf. Others such as cooker controllers and reminding devices are less so and need to achieve the same level of maturity. The main area where there is still a lot of work to do is in terms of the actual physical installations. The logic needed to control even a single home or apartment in a care home can be complex, particularly if it has to be able to be configured to suit a range of different users and deal with power cuts and computer crashes. If installations are to be plug-and-play, which they need to be, then the logic element that controls the system and provides the link to the outside world also needs to be plug-and-play. The software needed to configure a system for an individual needs to be developed so that it is very user friendly and can be used by care professionals.

For installations that are provided in care homes and sheltered housing schemes, then, the use of hard-wired communication buses is probably going to be the first choice. Such buses can provide excellent and well-proven reliability and they can provide the low power needed for many components of an installation. For builders of new housing schemes, it makes sense to install the bus cabling during the build, even if it is not being connected to support installations straight away, because it is very cheap to install at that time. For a retrofit installation, however, especially for those used in people's own homes, the use of hard-wired buses is much less suitable. It is very disruptive and time consuming to install and therefore expensive. For people who are likely to be anxious anyway, such as those with dementia, such installations can hardly be justified ethically. In these situations, radio-based buses or buses using mains wiring are much more appropriate. A number of radiofrequency buses are in use already and some modern developments such as the Ziggbee radio bus seem to have the right mix of range and bandwidth and power handling capabilities.

There is a need for further work on support devices and sensors, particularly those that can provide support that improves leisure and quality of life more generally. Finally, the technology to provide background behaviour monitoring, which has been a research topic for some years, is likely to provide added benefits. Such technologies should provide better judgements of complex behaviours that might reflect anxiety levels or specific issues such as falls. An extra topic that has been explored by several academic groups[16] is to see if the technology can be better tailored to the needs of the individual user by allowing it to learn the typical behaviour of the occupant. The house, through its sensors, can acquire a lot of information about the use of various appliances and the patterns of activity within the home. Once this information has been acquired, the house can adjust the settings according to how the user has been getting on. Such adaptive properties will also enable the installation to adapt to changes in the user's behaviour and learn the subtleties of an individual's requirements.

The installations that have been discussed throughout this chapter have been looking at home support technology that can act as a kind of extra care helper. However, the technology also has potential for linking in to other kinds of technological support and may well become integrated with them. For example, the burgeoning developments in telehealth technology could well use some of the same infrastructure as smart homes. If smart homes have appropriate links to the outside world and can sense user behaviour, then there is no reason why they cannot also report health issues resulting from the physiological and other sensors used by telehealth systems. There is also research going on looking at telerehabilitation, where home exercises and physiological responses can be remotely monitored in the same way as telehealth systems.

Conclusion

The application of smart home technology to support elderly and disabled people has developed rapidly over the last few years. Recent work has been much more user-led and aimed at supporting people with a wide variety of abilities, including those with dementia. Evidence is mounting that such systems can provide real benefits to the user and would also appear to have benefits from a cost point of view. There is still much work to be done, particularly with respect to improving quality of life and leisure activities.

However, provided that the relevant infrastructure can be put in place to support the technology, there is no reason why installations in both care homes and people's private homes cannot be a major feature of the support provided to elderly and disabled people in the very near future.

Key points

- The primary property that endows a house with the smart home label is its ability to support the user in an autonomous fashion.
- The main role of sensors in a smart home environment is to allow judgements to be made about user behaviour.
- The application of smart home technology to support elderly and disabled people has developed rapidly over the last few years, but more research is needed.

Acknowledgements

Much of the work reported in this chapter has been made possible through grants from the Engineering and Physical Sciences Research Council in the UK and from the European Commission. I express my gratitude to them and to the many elderly volunteers who have worked with us to ensure the effective development of this promising technology.

References

1. Gann D, Barlow J and Venables T. *Digital Futures: Making Homes Smarter*, Chartered Institute of Housing, Coventry, 1999.
2. Pragnell M, Spence L and Moore R. *The Market Potential for Smart Homes*, Joseph Rowntree Foundation, York, 2000.
3. Bjoerneby S. *The BESTA Flats in Tonsberg. Using Technology for People with Dementia*, Human Factors Solutions, Oslo, 1997.
4. Lines L and Hone KS. Millennium homes: a user centred approach for system functionality, In: *Proceedings of CWUAAT 1st Cambridge Workshop on Universal Access and Assistive Technology*, Cambridge University, 2002, pp. 91–2.
5. Orpwood R. The Gloucester smart house. *J Dementia Care* 2001;**9**:28–31.
6. Orpwood R, Faulkner R, Gibbs C and Adlam T. A design methodology for assistive technology for people with dementia. In: GM Craddock, LP McCormack, RB Reilly and HTP Knops (eds), *Assistive Technology – Shaping the Future*, IOS Press, Amsterdam, 2003, pp.766–70.
7. Orpwood R, Gibbs C, Adlam T *et al*. The Gloucester smart house for people with dementia – user-interface aspects. In: S Keates, J Clarkson, P Langdon and P Robinson (eds), *Designing a More Inclusive World*, Springer, London, 2004, pp.237–45.
8. Orpwood R, Bjoerneby S, Hagen I *et al*. User involvement in dementia product design. *Dementia* 2004;**3**:263–79.
9. Marquis-Faulkes F, McKenna SJ, Gregor P and Newell AF. Scenario-based drama as a tool for investigating user requirements with application to home monitoring for elderly people. *HCI Int* 2003;**3**:512–6.
10. Marshall M. Dementia and technology. In: SM Peace and C Holland (eds), *Inclusive Housing in an Ageing Society*, Policy Press, Bristol, 2001, pp.125–144.
11. Sixsmith A, Orpwood R and Torrington J. Quality of life technologies for people with dementia. *Top Geriatr Rehabil* 2007;**23**,85–93.
12. Monk A and Watts L. Peripheral participation in video-mediated communication. *Int J Hum Comput Stud* 2000;**52**: 933–58.
13. Hanson J, Osipovic D, Hine N *et al*. Lifestyle monitoring as a predictive tool in telecare. *Jf Telemed Telecare*, 2007;**13**:26–8.
14. Orpwood R, Adlam T, Evans N *et al*. Evaluation of an assisted-living smart home for someone with dementia. *J Assist Technol* 2008;**2**:13–21.
15. Bierhoff I, van Berlo A, Abascal J *et al*. Smart home environment. In: PRW Roe (ed.), *Towards an Inclusive Future*, COST, Brussels, 2007, pp.110–56.
16. Dewsbury G, Clarke K, Rouncefield M *et al*. Designing acceptable 'smart' home technology to support people in the home. *Technol Disabil* 2004;**15**:191–201.

CHAPTER 125

Skin disorders

Robert A. Norman[1] and Jaffer Babaa[2]
[1]Dr Robert A. Norman & Associates, Tampa, FL, USA
[2]University of South Florida, pre-medical student, Tampa, FL, USA

As the population continues to age, and the number of elderly persons increases, geriatric medicine. and more specifically geriatric dermatology. become an increasingly relevant specialty. With the progression of age, the incidence of dermatological diseases and disorders tend to increase.[1] This can be due to intrinsic ageing, skin ageing due to normal factors of maturity, which can be found in all of the ageing population, and extrinsic ageing, which is due to external factors such as smoking, environmental pollutants and exposure to UV light. Furthermore, factors that are more common in the elderly, such as decreased mobility, the increase of certain chronic diseases or an increase in a drug that can cause skin disorders as a side effect, all increase the risk of developing many dermatological diseases.[2]

Disorders which hinder vascular efficiency and immune response, such as diabetes mellitus, HIV, congestive heart failure and artherosclerosis, are all examples of diseases that can often cause skin disease or exacerbate already detrimental skin conditions. As people age, many changes take place in the ageing of their skin. Melanocytes decline, while photoageing causes density to double; Langerhans cells decrease in both density and responsiveness, and collagen decreases in density and in elastic papillary dermis tissue.[3]

The skin begins to thin and lose elasticity, resulting in wrinkling, irregular pigmentation, ease of tearing, neoplasia and several other like conditions. Photoageing accelerates and causes many conditions, such as actinic keratoses, wrinkling and telangiectasia, among other things. Likewise, nerves, circulation and sweat glands tend to begin a downward spiral in the path towards decreased ability to regulate temperature and skin sensitivity to burning. Nail health also weakens as the nails thin and become ridged and split and subcutaneous layers of fat atrophy and hypertrophy in their respective regions of the ageing body. Many of the common dermatological conditions developed in geriatric patients who are living in nursing homes or assisted living communities could be prevented with care given to the patient's medical history, medications, allergies, nutritional state, mental state, physical limitation and personal hygiene.[3]

Decubitus ulcers or 'pressure ulcers' are extremely common in the elderly, particularly in patients with illnesses that require them to be bedridden, immobile or in a wheelchair. These ulcers are often found over bony prominences, such as, but not limited to, elbows, ankles, heels and shoulders. Ischaemia and tissue damage result from the extended pressure on tissue for significant durations of time. As the pressure against the skin reduces blood flow to the region, it causes the tissue to die.[3–5]

Decubitus ulcers are organized in stages from Stage I, the first signs, to Stage IV, the worst in severity. The stages can be categorized as follows:

- *Stage I:* Changes in intact skin such as redness or blue or purple hues in darker pigmented skin and also temperature, sensation or consistency changes. The area may be painful or itchy with increased warmth or coolness in temperature and a spongy or firm consistency. Stage I ulcers usually disappear with relief of pressure and are fairly mild.
- *Stage II:* Necrosis in the epidermis and/or dermis accompanied by abrasions, blistering and other superficial ailments to the skin.
- *Stage III:* Deep necrosis to the subcutaneous layer of fat and/or fascia, perichondrium or periosteum. The underlying tendons, muscles, bone and cartilage are not exposed.
- *Stage IV:* Severe necrosis through fascia, exposing tendons, muscles, bone and/or cartilage. Decubitus ulcers of this stage and severity increase the risk for osteomyelitis.[3–5]

There are multiple causes of pressure ulcers, such as constant pressure, friction and shear. Continuous pressure restricts blood flow and deprives the tissue of oxygen whereas friction can damage the skin and thereby make it more likely to develop a pressure ulcer. Likewise, 'shearing', in which underlying bone moves in one direction while the skin moves in another, can cause cell

Principles and Practice of Geriatric Medicine, Fifth Edition. Edited by Alan J. Sinclair, John E. Morley and Bruno Vellas.

wall and blood vessel tearing. This can happen even with slight movements, such as sliding down in bed. Pressure ulcers can result in severe and sometimes even life-threatening complications such as cellulitis that can also lead to meninigitis, bone (osteomyelitis) and joint infections (infectious or septic arthritis), cancer and sepsis.[3]

Diagnosis is usually possible simply by physical examination; however, blood tests are usually ordered to evaluate the patient's nutritional state and health and decide whether further testing is necessary. In cases of infection where antibiotics are to be used, Gram stain cultures should be taken. If the sores do not improve with treatment or are recurring, a biopsy may be done to check for cancer, fungi or abnormal bacteria.[3,4]

There are multiple treatment options, depending mainly on the stage and severity of the ulcers. First, for all decubitus ulcers, the pressure that caused the condition should be relieved. This can be done through the use of support surfaces such as special cushions or mattresses, rotating positions at 15 min intervals for wheelchair-bound patients and once every 2 h for bedridden patients. Other treatments include cleaning, with water and a mild soap for Stage I ulcers and saline solution for open sores, tissue debridement through surgical, mechanical, autolytic or enzymatic debridement, stage-appropriate dressing (such as no dressing for Stage I ulcers, hydrocolloid dressing for Stage II sores, etc.), hydrotherapy, oral antibiotics for infection, nutrition improvement and vitamin therapy such as vitamins A, C and K and zinc, which increase the speed of healing, and prescription of muscle relaxants to relieve muscle spasms. Other treatments include surgical repair and flap reconstruction and experimental treatments such as electrotherapy, hyerbaric oxygen and topical application of human growth factors.[3–5]

Prevention of decubitus ulcers is key. Proper nutrition, reduction of skin-to-skin contact, daily skin examinations for high-risk patients, reduction of pressure and shearing factors, proper hygiene, mobility improvement and introduction of repositioning schedules are all important methods of ulcer prevention. In long-term care facilities, such as hospices and nursing homes, decubitus ulcers are extremely common, generally estimated to have an incidence between 2.4 and 23%. New ulcers have an incidence of 12% over a 6 month period. Furthermore, it was found that there was an increasing number of discharged hospital patients with decubitus ulcers, likely due to the increased frailty and susceptibility to illness of the geriatric patients being treated in such a setting. The transfer of these patients into long-term care facilities explained up to 63% of the decubitus ulcers pre-existing admission.[3,5]

Eczematous dermatitis is a category that contains multiple types of eczema, including seborrheic dermatitis, gravitational eczema, autoeczematization eczema, psychogenic dermatitis, nummular eczema and asteatotic eczema, many of which are often found in the elderly population. Nummular eczema causes sometimes scaly coin-shaped lesions and pruritus, usually on the trunk, lower legs, upper extremities and dorsal surface of the hands. It is usually treated with topical steroids and emollients. Related infections are treated with antibiotics such as cephalexin or dicloxacillin.[3,6]

Stasis dermatitis is accompanied by varicose veins, pedal oedema and venous insufficiency and can cause an increased likelihood of developing cellulitis or ulceration. A 'flare-up' of stasis dermatitis can cause autosensitization dermatitis or an 'id' reaction, thereby causing a secondary distribution, acute and papulovesicular in nature. Seborrheic dermatitis involves erythematous and xerotic skin on the face, scalp, anogenital and trunk areas. The condition's severity may be influenced by the central nervous system as seborrheic dermatitis is found in greater incidence in those with quadriplegia and Parkinson's disease. *Pityrosporum ovale* is also thought to play a role in the illness. Seborrheic dermatitis should be treated with ciclopirox or ketoconazole applied topically daily. In cases of increased severity, oral ketoconazole or fluconazole may be used alongside anti-staphylococcal antibiotics when there is a secondary infection.[3,6]

Psychogenic dermatitides are comprised of multiple disorders including lichen simplex chronicus, neurotic excoriations (see Figure 125.1), delusions of parasitosis and prurigo nodularis. Scaly, red, sharply defined, lichenified plaques are a major signal of lichen simplex chronicus lesions and are often caused by patients who are atopic and overly concerned about pruritic lesions, and who rub and scratch an itchy area until the lichenification is seen. The condition is treated with water soaks, behaviour modification and steroids applied topically to the lesions, and also Kenalog injections in the scalp and clobetasol or fluocinonide solutions on lesions that are resistant.[3,6]

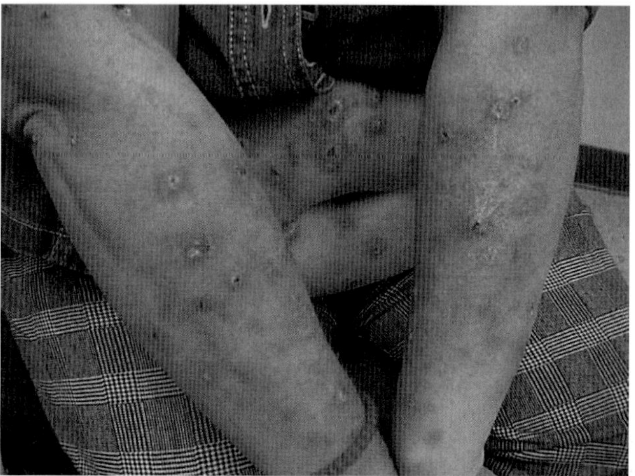

Figure 125.1 Neurotic excoriations of the arms and upper body. See plate section for a colour version of this image.

Prurigo nodularis is also a result of continual rubbing, scratching and picking and can be a result of stress. The nodules that characterize prurigo nodularis are erythematous and generally dispersed with keratotic nodules on the extremities. Treatment includes the topical application of triamcinolone acetonide or another corticosteroid or even a stronger steroid such as betamethasone. Alternative treatments include corticosteroid tape.

Similar treatments are applied for excoriated papules in post-inflammatory scarring at different points of healing. These neurotic excoriations may be found in patients whose condition does not fall into a normal pattern and who use their skin as a tool on which to release stress. Psychotherapeutic treatment plans are recommended by Truensgaard.[3,7] This can include strengthening the relationship between the patient and doctor, introducing alternative tactics to avoid scratching, identifying and reducing causes of stress and identifying triggers.

Delusion of parasitosis is a symptom of psychosis in which the patient complains of the feeling of parasites crawling on them when there is no evidence to support this as being true. Related factors include nutritional deficiency, arteriosclerosis, toxins and drug addiction. Depressive patients are usually treated with fluoxetine or doxepin, alprazolam or hydroxyzine for anxiety and pimozide or haloperidol for delusions. Alternative treatments may be used alongside anti-psychotics. Zyprexa may also be used.[3,6,7]

Fungal infections are also commonplace in the elderly community. These can include candidiasis, tinea pedis, tinea cruris and onychomycosis. *Candida* thrives in warm, moist environments where there is skin-to-skin contact and is a dispersed, bright red eruption with leaking pustules. When examined through a microscope, one can observe spores and pseudohyphae. Candidiasis is often associated with diabetes and oral antibiotic therapies. Treatment usually involves cold compress application with Burrow's solution, topical application of antifungal creams such as econazole or miconazole and, after the eruption is cleared, absorbent powder.[3]

Tinea pedis, also known as 'athlete's foot', infects the foot, appearing as erythematous dermatitis with a scaly and macerated presentation and, in some cases, ulceration and fissures. It can also appear alongside a secondary bacterial infection. Tinea pedis can be prevented with topical applications of benzoyl peroxide post-bathing and the wearing of shower shoes. It is treated with an imidazole such as clotrimazole, econazole or ketoconazole or an allylamine. Resistant infections may be treated with oral itraconazole, fluconazole or terbinafine.[3,8,9]

Tinea cruris, also known as 'jock itch', affects the groin region, in an erythematous, scaly, itchy eruption and is most commonly seen in males. Reduction of moisture is integral to the treatment of the condition and an antifungal cream is usually applied topically as treatment. Severe infection may be treated with oral antifungals. A betamethasone dipropionate–clotrimazole mixture may also be applied topically to areas of inflammation for limited periods of time.[3,9]

Almost half of patients exceeding 70 years of age suffer from onychomycosis, usually caused by tinea unguium, *Candida* or moulds. Symptoms include pain, ulcerations within the nail bed and secondary bacterial infection. The most frequently seen form of onychomycosis, distal and lateral subungual onychomycosis (DLSO), often appears first as just a white spot on a nail that then darkens, causing the nail to become thick and crack. Treatment usually involves debridement, systemic treatment, topical treatment, benzoyl peroxide washes and improvement of hygiene.[3,10]

As malnourishment and malnutrition, disease and trauma, among other things, cause changes and weakness in the skin's makeup, skin infections become a common occurrence in the elderly. Likewise, some forms of dermatitis and insect bites and stings can reduce the skin's natural resistance and thereby allow entrance to infections such as *Staphylococcus* and *Streptococcus*. These strains can cause impetigo in bullous or non-bullous form and, although it is often self-limiting, treatment should still be applied owing to the risk of complications such as post-streptococcal glomerulonephritis.[3,11]

The bullous form of impetigo is a result of the site of the infection producing epidermolytic toxins and is defined by bullae containing cloudy or clear fluid that can burst and leave a hyperpigmented rim surrounding the lesions and honey-coloured crusted exudates. The non-bullous form of impetigo presents as pustules that can rupture, leaving a red, swollen base and a yellowish crust. This comprises 10% of impetigo and is of some resemblance to the reaction to poison ivy.[3,12]

There may be some 'honey crusting' inside the bulla. Usually before impetigo, *Staphylococcus aureus* invades the nose and affects the areas around the nose and mouth and also on the limbs. Group A beta-haemolytic streptococci (GAS) occur on the intact skin and after abrasion, cut or other trauma, they enter the wound and cause infection. Treatment is usually with oral antibiotics such as cephalexin, dicloxacillin or cloxacillin or a 5 day course of azithromycin at 500 mg for the first day and half that amount on subsequent days. Mupirocin is also applied topically three times per day for the lesions.[3,11,12]

Parasitic diseases such as scabies and pediculosis are common in the elderly. Head, body and pubic lice, accompanied by pruritic papules, can be transmitted through direct contact with the infected person. Diagnosis is often carried out through examination and finding of nits. Lice are initially treated with permethrin and combing of nits. In persistent cases, treatment with malathion lotion or lindane may be given.

Scabies is characterized by burrows alongside papules and vesicles. It is diagnosed through the analysis of skin scrapings and finding of ova, mites or faeces. Scabies is often found in the male genitalia or female areolas of the nipples and can also be seen on the scalp. In keratotic scabies, thousands of mites infest the skin, a considerably larger number than the average 3–50 mites. Treatment involves oral ivermectin in 12 mg doses, one week apart, and thorough cleaning of fomites.[3,13,14]

Herpes zoster or 'shingles' is a common affliction in the geriatric community, often waiting in a dormant stage within cutaneous neurons for significant periods of time and reappearing in times where the immune system is weak or the patient is undergoing significant stress. Herpes zoster usually manifests with pruritus, burning or pain before an eruption and, in some cases, lymphadenopathy. Other symptoms may include fever, lethargy or headaches. Shingles is characterized by clusters of vesicles containing clear fluid that quickly become pyogenic and later dry up and crust over. Related pain ranges from mild to severe and can last even years after the physical signs of the condition have faded.

Herpes zoster is managed with prevention by vaccination against varicella zoster. If the condition has already been contracted then antiviral therapy is begun immediately using acyclovir, valacyclovir or another similar medication, preferably within 72 h of the appearance of the first vesicle. Symptoms are managed with bed rest, opioid analgesics, capsaicin cream, NSAIDs, tricyclic antidepressants and, in severe cases of pain, nerve blocks. Ophthalmologist referral may be necessary when there the trigeminal nerve is affected.[3,15]

Another condition seen in the geriatric population is molluscum contagiosum, characterized by dome-shaped, umbilicated papules, and can be transferred by direct skin contact. The condition is more common in HIV patients, which has now become more of a chronic disease and in those who are immunocompromised by a variety of diseases. Treatment usually involves 5% imiquimod cream applied topically, but may also include electrodesiccation, curettage, laser surgery or cryotherapy. It is not uncommon for molluscum contagiosum to be misdiagnosed as warts, sebaceous hyperplasia or skin cancer.

Nutritional deficiencies often play a large role in dermatological disorders within the geriatric population. Scurvy is a result of vitamin C deficiency. Gingival and dermatological haemorrhages and the formation of hyperkeratotic papules surrounding hair follicles are also commonly seen. Pellagra is caused by vitamin B deficiency or niacin deficiency and can cause the skin to develop extreme photosensitivity. Dietary improvement and vitamin supplementation should be utilized as treatment for these deficiencies and also a thorough analysis of underlying and pre-existing causes and illnesses that may play a role in malnourishment.

Vascular disorders such as chronic venous insufficiency can be inherited in addition to being caused and exacerbated by continuous standing or venous thrombosis. Symptoms include oedema, varicose veins, pigment discoloration and venous ulcers. Leg elevation, support stockings, exercise, corticosteroids and surgery are used in treating vascular disorders.[3]

Tumours, both benign and malignant, are a common dermatological finding in the elderly. Benign tumours include leukoplakia, seborrheic keratosis, actinic keratosis, cherry angioma and keratoacanthoma. Malignant tumours include basal cell carcinoma (see Figure 125.2), squamous cell carcinoma and melanoma. Cherry angiomas are a primarily cosmetic concern and are treated with lasers or electrocoagulation. Leukoplakia is found on mucosal surfaces and is related to the use of tobacco and alcohol. A premalignant neoplasm, leukoplakia can turn into an invasive carcinoma. Leukoplakia is treated with topical application of 5-fluorouracil and electro- or cryosurgery. In severe cases, excision may be necessary.[3,16]

Seborrheic keratoses are frequently found in geriatric patients as dark papules 'stuck' on to the skin. In dark or irregular lesions, a biopsy should be taken to eliminate the possibility of melanoma and treatment should include electrocautery or cryosurgery. Actinic keratosis may be accompanied by a burning and stinging sensation and a red–brown papule. High-risk individuals with multiple actinic keratoses have progression rates to squamous cell carcinoma as high as 30% over three years. Treatment options include cryosurgery, electrodesiccation, curettage, blue light therapy and topical 5-fluorouracil.[17]

Basal cell carcinoma (BCC) is the most frequently found malignant tumour in humans and can appear superficial, nodular-ulcerative or morpheaform. Nodular-ulcerative

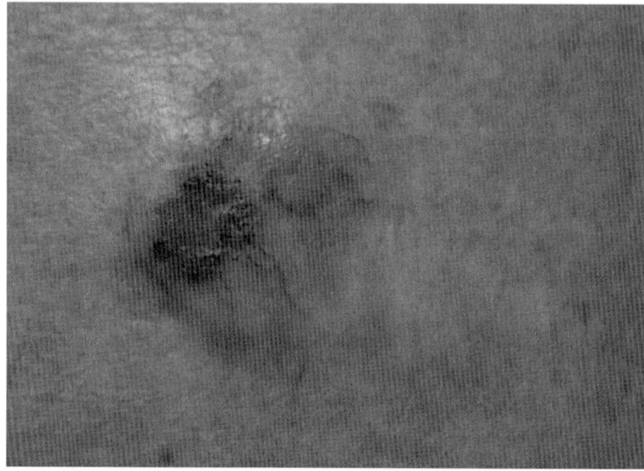

Figure 125.2 Basal cell carcinoma. See plate section for a colour version of this image.

BCC appears red with telangiectasia. Morpheaform lesions tend to have yellow–whitish plaque and superficial BCC has swollen, hyperpigmented lesions. UV exposure and ionizing radiation therapy are major risk factors for BCC. Treatment varies according to the region affected and severity of the BCC and can include excision, electrosurgery, radiation and Mohs micrographic surgery.

Squamous cell carcinoma (SCC) is a result of human papillomavirus (HPV) or UV exposure, the latter being the more frequently seen cause in the elderly. SCC often manifests as scaly, defined plaque and ranges from soft and poorly defined to firm and clearly defined. SCC is generally treated through the use of cryotherapy and 5-fluorouracil applied *in situ*. In severe cases, the lesion may be excised.

Malignant melanoma is occurring with increased incidence, especially with rising age. Types include superficial spreading melanoma, lentigo maligna, nodular melanoma and acral lentiginous melanoma. Superficial spreading melanoma occurs in about 70–80% of the patients with melanoma. Lentigo maligna is most often found in Caucasians who have exposed themselves to large amounts of sun and is asymmetric with abnormal borders. Acral lentiginous melanoma is found more often in individuals with darker shades of skin and can be found in the hands, feet and even the nails. The lesion tends to appear as a brown macule and slowly becomes larger over time.[3,17]

When assessing a prognosis for those who have melanoma, one must measure the depth. Those with a depth of less than 1 mm have a 5 year survival rate of >85% or more whereas those who have melanoma >4 mm in depth have a 5 year survival rate of <50%. With melanoma diagnosis, a biopsy is necessary. A punch biopsy should be used to measure the depth adequately. Melanomas are treated with lesion excision in the subcutaneous fat, close observation, investigation of spread to the lymph nodes and screening of immediate relatives.[3]

Purpura is a result of thrombocytopenia, vascular defect, drug reaction, trauma or platelet abnormality. Due to the loss of blood vessels and elasticity in the skin along with loss of fat and dermal collagen, the skin tends to thin and become increasingly exposed to external trauma. A large proportion of the geriatric population is taking medication which cause thrombocytopenia. Recommended treatment includes identification of initial cause, prescription of oral glucocorticoids and immunoglobulins and platelet transfusions as needed.[18]

A common dermatological disorder within the geriatric population that is not often realized by many to be 'dermatological' in nature is hair loss. Although hair does tend to thin and reduce with age, many in the geriatric population, men and women alike, find themselves with mild to severe hair loss and, as a result, a decreased sense of confidence and self-value. Conditions such as androgenetic alopecia, cicatricial alopecia and alopecia areata can signal an entrance to a stage in life in which one's physical strength and beauty have diminished and mortality and the passage of time are an all too real concern. There are a number of treatments for each of the conditions and also several others that are still in the experimental stage to help with this transition.[19]

Geriatric dermatology is a very broad topic covering many diseases and conditions. This chapter has outlined key, commonly seen illnesses from various categories to give brief snapshots of the bigger picture. However, when considering the depth and breadth of the field that is geriatric dermatology, one must examine multiple facets, from the physical to psychological, and also the underlying factors, including poor hygiene, caregiver neglect, drug reaction or a pre-existing medical cause. Although it is a field that primarily involves the skin, deeper investigation shows that one's dermatological condition is not a shallow field made up only of rashes, xerosis or eczema, but a canvas that can also showcase one's physical state from an internal standpoint, whether it be a decline in health due to diabetes mellitus, HIV or heart failure.

Key points

- Skin disorders increase with ageing.
- Shingles is a common affliction in older persons.
- High-risk patients with multiple actinic keratoses may progress to squamous cell carcinoma.
- Dermatological conditions showcase one's underlying physical status.

References

1. Jackson SA. The epidemiology of aging. In: WR Hazzard, JP Blass, WH Ettinger Jr *et al.* (eds), *Principles of Geriatric Medicine and Gerontology*, 4th edn, McGraw-Hill, New York, 1999, pp. 203–25.
2. Norman R. The aging of the world's population. In: R Norman (ed.), *Geriatric Dermatology*, Parthenon, New York, 2001, pp. 1–4.
3. Norman R. Geriatric dermatology. *Dermatol Ther* 2003; **16**:260–8.
4. Berlowitz D. *Pressure Ulcers: Staging; Epidemiology; Pathogenesis; Clinical Manifestations*, http://www.uptodate.com/home/index.html (last accessed 23 September 2011).
5. Merck. *Pressure Ulcers. The Merck Manuals: The Merck Manual for Healthcare Professionals*, http://www.merck.com/mmpe/sec10/ch126/ch126a.html (last accessed 23 September 2011).
6. Webster GF. Common skin disorders in the elderly. *Clin Cornerstone* 2001;**4**(1):39–44.
7. Truensgaard K. Psychotherapeutic strategy and neurotic excoriations. *Int J Dermatol* 1991;**20**:198–203.
8. Habif TP. Superficial fungal infections. In: TP Habif (ed.), *Clinical Dermatology: a Color Guide to Diagnosis and*

Therapy, 4th edn, Mosby, Philadelphia, 2004; http://www.mdconsult.com/das/book/body/104355536-2/742469442/1195/81.html?printing=true (last accessed 23 September 2011).

9. Goldstein AO *et al. Dermatophyte (Tinea) Infections*, http://www.uptodate.com/home/index.html (last accessed 23 September 2011).
10. Onychomycosis. *The Merck Manuals: The Merck Manual for Healthcare Professionals*, http://www.merck.com/mmpe/sec10/ch125/ch125c.html?qt=nail%20fungus&alt=sh (last accessed 23 September 2011).
11. Habif TP. Bacterial infections. In: TP Habif (ed.), *Clinical Dermatology: a Color Guide to Diagnosis and Therapy*, 4th edn, Mosby, Philadelphia, 2004; http://www.mdconsult.com/das/book/body/103909824-2/0/1195/53.html?tocnode=51440785&fromURL=53.html#4-u1.0-B0-323-01319-8..50011-X_938 (last accessed 23 September 2011).
12. Cole C, Gazewood J. Diagnosis and treatment of impetigo. *Am Fam Physician* 2007;**75**:859–64, 868.
13. Centers for Disease Control and Prevention. *Scabies*, http://www.cdc.gov/scabies/index.html (last accessed 23 September 2011).
14. American Academy of Dermatology. *Scabies*, http://www.aad.org/public/publications/pamphlets/common_scabies.html (last accessed 27 January 2010).
15. Albrecht MA. Epidemiology and pathogenesis of varicella-zoster virus infection: herpes zoster, http://www.uptodate.com/contents/topic.do?topicKey=ID/8292 (last accessed 13 September 2011).
16. Sciubba JJ. Oral mucosal lesions. In: CW Cummings (ed.), *Otolaryngology: Head and Neck Surgery*, 4th edn, Mosby, St Louis, MO, 2005; http://www.mdconsult.com/das/book/body/101896247-4/735379012/1263/585.html#4-u1.0-B0-323-01985-4..50067-8–cesec8_2400 (last accessed 23 September 2011).
17. Habif TP. Premalignant and malignant nonmelanoma skin tumors. In: TP Habif (ed.), *Clinical Dermatology: a Color Guide to Diagnosis and Therapy*, 4th edn, Mosby, Philadelphia, 2004; http://www.mdconsult.com/das/book/body/109438622-3/768950956/1195/158.html#4-u1.0-B0-323-01319-8..50023-6–cesec43_2631 (last accessed 23 September 2011).
18. Rodeghiero F. Idiopathic thrombocytopenic purpura: an old disease revisited in the era of evidence-based medicine. *Haematologica* 2003;**88**:1081–7.
19. Norman R. *Geriatric Dermatology*. Informa HealthCare, London, 2001, pp.35–8.

CHAPTER 126

The prevention and management of pressure ulcers

David R. Thomas
Saint Louis University Health Sciences Center, St Louis, MO, USA

Pressure ulcers are the visible evidence of pathological changes in the blood supply to dermal tissues. Pressure ulcers are rare, affecting only about 0.5% of the total population. The distribution is clustered into two groups, peaking once in younger, mostly neurologically impaired persons, and again in older persons. The cluster in the geriatric population accounts for about 70% of all pressure ulcers.[1]

The chief cause has historically been attributed solely to pressure or force per unit area, applied to susceptible tissues. In this view, external pressure is viewed as the chief cause in the development of a pressure ulcer. Although it is recognized that other contributing or confounding factors are also associated with development of a pressure ulcer, these factors are often downplayed or disregarded.[2] Pressure is concentrated wherever weight-bearing points come in contact with surfaces. Muscle tissue, subcutaneous fat and dermal tissue are differentially affected in that order. The differential effect of pressure on the tissue layers suggests that injury occurs first in muscle before changes are observed in the skin, the so-called deep tissue injury. Pressure ulcers are classified in stages defined by the visible layers of tissue damaged from the surface towards the bone. Current research clearly demonstrates that a bottom-to-top pathogenesis is commonplace. In many cases, the changes visible at the surface of the tissue are minor compared with the damage seen at the deepest layers of tissue. This differential tissue susceptibility suggests that a number of factors are involved in the development of pressure ulcers, including the type of pressure load and biochemical changes in the tissue due to reperfusion injury or tissue compression.[2]

Provocative research into human skin blood flow may shed some light on the development of pressure ulcers. Skin blood flow before and during surgery was monitored in subjects selected because of lengthy abdominal or spine surgical procedures.[3] Pressure ulcers developed in 36% of these subjects. Contrary to the hypothesis that prolonged pressure reduces skin blood flow, an increase in skin blood flow was observed in most subjects during surgery. However, in the persons who developed a pressure ulcer, the skin blood flow decreased to half of the preoperative levels, whereas skin blood flow in persons who did not develop a pressure ulcer increased to 500% of maximum baseline value. These data suggest that individual tissue response is more important than externally applied pressure.

Other studies have suggested that sacral skin blood flow is higher than blood flow over the gluteus maximus,[4] and that a decrease in skin blood flow may be more serious in the sacral area than in other areas. Sacral pressure ulcers are common, but gluteal pressure ulcers are rare. The neural response to cold stimulation produces differences in skin blood flow among older subjects who do or do not develop pressure ulcers. There was a positive correlation between the blood flow response time over the greater trochanter and the development of pressure ulcers.[5]

The measure of skin blood flow is technically difficult, with a high degree of variability. However, these data suggest that individual factors may act in concert with external pressure in the development of pressure ulcers.

About 95% of pressure ulcers occur in the lower part of the body. The sacral and coccygeal areas, ischial tuberosities and greater trochanteric areas account for the majority of pressure ulcer sites.[6] The sacrum is the most frequent site (36% of ulcers). The heel is the next most common site (30%), with other body areas each accounting for about 6% of pressure ulcers.[7,8]

Clinical staging of pressure ulcers

Several differing scales have been proposed for assessing the severity of pressure ulcers. The most common staging, recommended by the National Pressure Ulcer Task Force and nursing home guidelines, derives from a modification of the Shea Scale.[9] Under this schematic, pressure ulcers

Principles and Practice of Geriatric Medicine, Fifth Edition. Edited by Alan J. Sinclair, John E. Morley and Bruno Vellas.

are divided into four clinical stages. The staging system for pressure ulcers relies on a description of the depth of the wound. An evolutionary process in the understanding of tissue injury has led to an expansion into six stages in the USA and recent attempts to reach consensus on clinical description (see Table 126.1).

This staging system for pressure ulcers has several limitations. The primary difficulty lies in the inability to distinguish progression between stages. Pressure ulcers do not progress absolutely through Stage I to Stage IV, but may appear to develop from 'the inside out' as a result of the initial injury. Healing from Stage IV does not progress through Stage III to Stage I, but rather heals by contraction and scar tissue formation. Since pressure ulcers heal by contraction and scar formation, 'reverse staging' is inaccurate in assessing healing. Thus, improvement or deterioration between clinical stages cannot be determined. Clinical staging is inaccurate unless all eschar is removed, since the staging system only reflects depth of the ulcer.

No single measure of wound characteristics has been useful in measuring healing.[10] Several indexes have been proposed, but lack validation. The Pressure Ulcer Status for Healing (PUSH) tool was developed and validated to measure healing of pressure ulcers. The tool measures three components, size, exudate amount and tissue type, to arrive at a numerical score for ulcer status. In clinical development and validation studies, the PUSH tool adequately assesses ulcer status and is sensitive to change over time.[11,12] In the USA, the PUSH tool is incorporated into the Minimum Data Set version 3.0. The PUSH tool is shown in Figure 126.1.

Prevention of pressure ulcers

Despite considerable attention to and research on the prevention of pressure ulcers, the prevalence and incidence of pressure ulcers have changed little over the last decade,[13] even in the face of improved application of prevention modalities. The incidence of pressure ulcers as a primary diagnosis in hospital settings varied from 7.0 to 8.3 per 100 000 population but did not change from 1987 to 2000.[14] In another hospital setting, the point prevalence of Stage II or higher pressure ulcers was 33.3% in 2002 and 28.2% in 2004. The point prevalence decreased in surgical care units (from 26.8 to 17.3%) and increased in medical care units (from 23.6 to 26.7%), despite demonstrated increases in prevention measures.[15] Similar stability has been observed in other populations, indicating that reducing pressure ulcer prevalence rates remains a challenge.

Recognizing patients at risk

Comorbid conditions, especially those resulting in immobility or paralysis or reduced tissue perfusion, such as hypoxia due to respiratory or cardiac disease, greatly increase the risk of developing pressure ulcers. In theory, persons who are at high risk for developing pressure ulcers can be identified and increased effort can be directed to preventing ulcers in these persons.

Considerable effort has been directed towards risk assessment. The classical risk assessment scale is the Norton Score, developed in 1962 and still widely used. Patients are classified using five risk factors graded from one to four. Scores range from 5 to 20, with higher scores indicating lower risk. In the initial study, 48% of patients who scored less than 12 developed pressure ulcers, compared with only 5% of those who scored above 18. The generally accepted at-risk score is 14 or less and patients with scores below 12 are at particularly high risk. The Norton score has been expanded into the Waterlow Scale in the UK.

A commonly used risk assessment instrument in the USA is the Braden Scale. This instrument assesses six items: sensory perception, moisture exposure, physical activity, mobility, nutrition and friction/shear force. Each item is ranked from one (least favourable) to three or four (most favourable) for a maximum total score of 23. A score of 16 or less indicates a high risk. A comparison of the instruments is shown in Table 126.2.

Both the Norton Score and the Braden Scale have good sensitivity (73–92 and 83–100%, respectively) and specificity (61–94 and 64–77%, respectively), but both have poor positive predictive value (around 37% when the pressure ulcer incidence is 20%). In populations with an incidence of pressure ulcers less than 20%, such as nursing homes, the same sensitivity and specificity would produce a positive predictive value of 2%. The Norton Score and Braden Scale show a 0.73 kappa statistic agreement among at-risk patients, with the Norton Score tending to classify patients as at risk when the Braden Scale classified them as not at risk. The net effect of poor positive predictive value means that many patients who will not develop pressure ulcers will receive expensive and unnecessary treatment. Risk factor assessment illustrates the concept that individual patient factors interact with pressure in the aetiology of pressure ulcers.

A systematic review of 33 clinical trials of risk assessment found no decrease in pressure ulcer incidence that could be attributed to the use of an assessment scale.[16] However, the use of a risk assessment scale tended to increase the intensity of prevention interventions. The Braden Scale offered the best balance between sensitivity and specificity and the best risk estimate compared with other scales. In this review, both the Norton Score and Braden Scale were observed to be more accurate in predicting pressure ulcer risk than nurses' clinical judgement. These results agree with other systematic reviews showing no evidence that risk assessment scales are independently effective for pressure ulcer prevention.[17,18]

Table 126.1 Clinical staging of pressure ulcers.[a]

Stage	NPUAP	EPUAP
Stage/Category I	Intact skin with non-blanchable redness of a localized area usually over a bony prominence. Darkly pigmented skin may not have visible blanching; its colour may differ from the surrounding area	Intact skin with non-blanchable redness of a localized area usually over a bony prominence. Darkly pigmented skin may not have visible blanching; its colour may differ from the surrounding area. The area may be painful, firm, soft, warmer or cooler compared with adjacent tissue. Category I may be difficult to detect in individuals with dark skin tones. May indicate 'at risk' persons
Stage/Category II	Partial thickness loss of dermis presenting as a shallow, open ulcer with a red–pink wound bed, without slough. May also present as an intact or open/ruptured serum-filled blister	Partial thickness loss of dermis presenting as a shallow open ulcer with a red–pink wound bed, without slough. May also present as an intact or open/ruptured serum-filled or sero-sanginous filled blister. Presents as a shiny or dry, shallow ulcer without slough or bruising. This category should not be used to describe skin tears, tape burns, incontinence-associated dermatitis, maceration or excoriation
Stage/Category III	Full thickness tissue loss. Subcutaneous fat may be visible but bone, tendon or muscle are not exposed. Slough may be present but does not obscure the depth of tissue loss. May include undermining and tunnelling	Full thickness tissue loss. Subcutaneous fat may be visible but bone, tendon or muscle are not exposed. Slough may be present but does not obscure the depth of tissue loss. May include undermining and tunnelling. The depth of a Stage/Category III pressure ulcer varies by anatomical location. The bridge of the nose, ear, occiput and malleolus do not have (adipose) subcutaneous tissue and Stage/Category III ulcers can be shallow. In contrast, areas of significant adiposity can develop extremely deep Stage/Category III pressure ulcers. Bone/tendon is not visible or directly palpable
Stage/Category IV	Full thickness tissue loss with exposed bone, tendon or muscle. Slough or eschar may be present on some parts of the wound bed. Often include undermining and tunnelling	Full thickness tissue loss with exposed bone, tendon or muscle. Slough or eschar may be present. Often includes undermining and tunnelling. The depth of a Stage/Category IV pressure ulcer varies by anatomical location. The bridge of the nose, ear, occiput and malleolus do not have (adipose) subcutaneous tissue and these ulcers can be shallow. Stage/Category IV ulcers can extend into muscle and/or supporting structures (e.g., fascia, tendon or joint capsule) making osteomyelitis or osteitis likely to occur. Exposed bone/muscle is visible or directly palpable
Suspected deep tissue injury (used in USA)	Purple or maroon localized area of discoloured intact skin or blood-filled blister due to damage of underlying soft tissue from pressure and/or shear. The area may be preceded by tissue that is painful, firm, mushy, boggy, warmer or cooler as compared with adjacent tissue	Purple or maroon localized area of discoloured intact skin or blood-filled blister due to damage of underlying soft tissue from pressure and/or shear. The area may be preceded by tissue that is painful, firm, mushy, boggy, warmer or cooler compared with adjacent tissue. Deep tissue injury may be difficult to detect in individuals with dark skin tones. Evolution may include a thin blister over a dark wound bed. The wound may further evolve and become covered by thin eschar. Evolution may be rapid, exposing additional layers of tissue even with optimal treatment
Unstageable (used in USA)	Full thickness tissue loss in which the base of the ulcer is covered by slough (yellow, tan, grey, green or brown) and/or eschar (tan, brown or black) in the wound bed	Full thickness tissue loss in which actual depth of the ulcer is completely obscured by slough (yellow, tan, grey, green or brown) and/or eschar (tan, brown or black) in the wound bed. Until enough slough and/or eschar are removed to expose the base of the wound, the true depth cannot be determined; but it will be either a Stage/Category III or IV. Stable (dry, adherent, intact without erythema or fluctuance) eschar on the heels serves as 'the body's natural (biological) cover' and should not be removed

[a]A comparison of the National Pressure Ulcer Advisory Panel (NPUAP) and the European Pressure Ulcer Advisory Panel (EPUAP) clinical staging systems. In the USA, the convention is to use the term 'Stage' whereas in Europe the term 'Category' is preferred.
Adapted from European Pressure Ulcer Advisory Panel and National Pressure Ulcer Advisory Panel. *Prevention and Treatment of Pressure Ulcers: Quick Reference Guide*. National Pressure Ulcer Advisory Panel, Washington, DC, 2009.

Patient Initials:________________________________ Date:

DIRECTIONS: Observe and measure the pressure ulcer. Categorize the ulcer with respect to surface area, exudate, and type of wound tissue. Record a sub-score for each of these ulcer characteristics. Add the sub-scores to obtain the total score. A comparison of total scores measured over time provides an indication of the improvement or deterioration in pressure ulcer healing.

	0	1	2	3	4	5	
	0 cm^2	< 0.3 cm^2	0.3-0.6 cm^2	0.7-1.0 cm^2	1.1-2.0 cm^2	2.1-3.0 cm^2	
Length x Width		6 3.1- 4.0 cm^2	7 4.1-8.0 cm^2	8 8.1-12.0 cm^2	9 12.1-24.0 cm^2	10 >24.0 cm^2	**Sub-score**
Exudate Amount	0 None	1 Light	2 Moderate	3 Heavy			**Sub-score**
Tissue Type	0 Closed	1 Epithelial Tissue	2 Granulation Tissue	3 Slough	4 Necrotic Tissue		**Sub-score**
							Total score

Length x Width: Measure the greatest length (head to toe) and the greatest width (side to side) using a centimeter ruler. Multiply these two measurements (length times width) to obtain an estimate of surface area in square centimeters (cm^2). Caveat: Do not guess! Always use a centimeter ruler and always use the same method each time the ulcer is measured.
Exudate Amount: Estimate the amount of exudate (drainage) present after removal of the dressing and before applying any topical agent to the ulcer. Estimate the exudate (drainage) as none, light, moderate, or heavy.
Tissue Type: This refers to the types of tissue that are present in the wound (ulcer) bed. Score as a "4" if there is any necrotic tissue present. Score as a "3" if there is any amount of slough present and necrotic tissue is absent. Score as a "2" if the wound is clean and contains granulation tissue. A superficial wound that is reepithelializing is scored as a "1". When the wound is closed, score as a "0".

4 - **Necrotic Tissue (Eschar):** black, brown, or tan tissue that adheres firmly to the wound bed or ulcer edges and may be either firmer or softer than surrounding skin.
3 - **Slough:** yellow or white tissue that adheres to the ulcer bed in strings or thick clumps, or is mucinous.
2 - **Granulation Tissue:** pink or beefy red tissue with a shiny, moist, granular appearance.
1 - **Epithelial Tissue:** for superficial ulcers, new pink or shiny tissue (skin) that grows in from the edges or as islands on the ulcer surface.
0 - **Closed/Resurfaced:** the wound is completely covered with epithelium (new skin).

Figure 126.1 PUSH Tool Version 3.0. Adapted from Stotts *et al.*[12]

Whether prevention measures should begin as soon as the person has a high risk assessment score or after the development of non-blanchable erythema (a Stage I pressure ulcer) was observed in a randomized controlled trial. All subjects were observed daily for incident Stage I pressure ulcers and a Braden risk assessment scale was obtained every 3 days. Subjects received identical prevention measures, including turning every 4 h in combination with either polyethylene–urethane mattress or an alternating pressure air mattress. In the experimental group, the intervention was started when a Stage I pressure ulcer appeared. In the control group, intervention began when the Braden Score was 17 or less. In the experimental group, 16% of patients received preventive measures, whereas 32% of the risk score assessment group received preventative measures. The pressure ulcer incidence (Stages II–IV) was not significantly different between the experimental group (6.8%) and control group (6.7%). Significantly fewer patients needed preventive measures when preventative measures were postponed until a Stage I pressure ulcer was present, but those patients did not develop more pressure ulcers than patients who received prevention measures based on the standard risk assessment method.[19]

Relieving pressure, friction and shear force

In those patients at risk, the first preventive action targets reduction in the effect of pressure, friction and shear forces. The most commonly recommended method for reducing pressure is frequent turning and positioning. A 2 h turning schedule for spinal injury patients was deduced empirically in 1946.[20] The exact interval for optimal turning for the prevention of pressure ulcers is unknown, but the interval may be shortened or lengthened by host factors. In healthy older

Table 126.2 Comparison of risk assessment scales.

Variable	Norton	Braden	Waterlow
Mobility	×[a]	×	×
Moisture exposure	×	×	×
Physical activity	×	×	
General condition	×		×
Nutrition		×	
Appetite			×
Friction/Shear force		×	
Sensory perception		×	
Mental status	×		
Skin type			×
Medication			×
Weight			×
Age			×
Gender			×
Other (e.g. disease)			×

[a] × = Scale contains this item.

volunteers, intervals of 1–1.5 h rather than the traditional 2 h schedule were required to prevent skin erythema on a standard mattress.[21]

Turning the patient to relieve pressure may be difficult to achieve despite best nursing efforts and is very costly. Despite common-sense approaches to turning, positioning and improving passive activity, no published data support the view that pressure ulcers can be completely prevented by passive positioning.[22,23]

Pressure-reducing surfaces

Because of the limitations and cost of turning schedules, a number of pressure-reducing devices have been developed for prevention of pressure injury. The theoretical goal is to reduce tissue pressure below a capillary closing pressure of 32 mmHg.

Devices can be defined as pressure-relieving (consistently reducing interface pressure below 32 mmHg) or pressure-reducing (less than standard support surfaces, but not below 32 mmHg). The majority of devices are pressure-reducing. Pressure-reducing devices can be further classified as static or dynamic. Static surfaces are stationary and attempt to distribute local pressure over a larger body surface. Examples include foam mattresses and devices filled with water, gel or air. Dynamic devices use a power source to produce air currents and promote uniform pressure distribution over body surfaces. Examples include alternating pressure pads, air suspension devices and air-fluidized surfaces. When compared with a standard hospital mattress, a number of pressure-reducing devices lower the incidence of pressure ulcers by about 60%.[24]

The capability of devices to reduce pressure differs depending on body site. Sacral pressure reduction can be achieved in healthy volunteers by several devices. Three dynamic air support systems lower pressure at the trochanter compared with a conventional mattress. However, no device reduced pressure over the trochanter to physiological levels.[25,26] Few currently marketed devices, including air-fluidized beds, will consistently reduce heel pressure below the minimum capillary pressure.[27] It is important to note that although some dynamic air mattresses and flotation systems can reduce pressure to near physiological levels, all benefit is lost if the head of the bed is elevated to 30°, such as for tube feedings.[28]

Comparison between different devices to reduce pressure remains confusing. No statistically significant difference has been found between alternating pressure, constant low pressure, foam overlays, silicone overlays or air- or water-filled devices.[24] Therefore, a pressure-reducing device should be selected on the basis of cost and ease of use. The cost of pressure-reducing devices varies considerably, with air-fluidized and low-air-loss systems the most expensive and static support overlays the least expensive. Dynamic devices are often noisy and disturbing to patients. Mechanical difficulties are frequent with all types of devices. The data also demonstrate that pressure ulcers develop in some patients in spite of the use of pressure-reducing devices. Overall, the data suggest that patients likely to develop a pressure ulcer should be treated with a pressure-reducing device, although no one device appears to be superior to another.

Combinations of turning/positioning and pressure-reducing surfaces

When a pressure-reducing device is combined with turning and positioning, the effective interval for turning may be reduced. In a randomized controlled trial in high-risk nursing home residents, four different turning schedules were used. Subjects were either turned every 2 h on a standard institutional mattress, or turned every 3 h on a standard institutional mattress, or turned every 4 h on a viscoelastic foam mattress, or turned every 6 h on a viscoelastic foam mattress. The incidence of non-blanchable erythema (a Stage I pressure ulcer) was not different between the groups (35–38%). However, the incidence of a Stage II and higher pressure ulcers was 3% in the 4 h turning interval group, compared with incidence figures in the other groups varying between 14 and 24%. Turning every 4 h on a viscoelastic foam mattress resulted in a significant reduction in the number of higher stage pressure ulcer lesions and suggests that less frequent turning in combination with a pressure-reducing mattress is effective and feasible.[29,30]

The effect of different body positions was evaluated in another randomized controlled trial. Subjects who had non-blanchable erythema (Stage I pressure ulcer) were assigned to either of two groups. In the experimental group, patients were repositioned 2 h in a lateral position alternating with 4 h in a supine position. In the control group, patients were repositioned every 4 h. Both groups received a pressure-reducing mattress. The sitting protocol was identical in both groups. It was found that 16% of subjects in the experimental group and 21% of subjects in the control group ($p = 0.40$) developed an incident Stage II–IV pressure ulcer. Neither the severity, location nor time to development of the pressure ulcers differed between groups. It was difficult to maintain subjects in a lateral position between the turning intervals. The authors concluded that more frequent repositioning on a pressure-reducing mattress does not necessarily lead to fewer pressure ulcer lesions and consequently cannot be considered as a more effective preventive measure.[31] Other trials have found similarly high incidence despite various interventions.[32–34]

A systematic review of published prevention strategies for prevention of pressure ulcers up to June 2006 found only 59 randomized controlled trials, 48 addressing impaired mobility, five addressing nutrition, three addressing impaired skin condition and three addressing turning and positioning.[35] The data confirmed that pressure-reducing devices appear to have an advantage over standard beds, but little difference has been shown between devices. No trial of measures for impaired skin met criteria for study design and only one trial of turning and positioning suggested a reduction in pressure ulcer incidence.

Nutrition in preventing pressure ulcers

Nutritional status has been thought to influence the incidence, progression and severity of pressure sores.[36] Experimental studies in animal models suggest a biologically plausible relationship between undernutrition and development of pressure ulcers. When pressure was applied for 4 h to the skin of both well-nourished and malnourished animals, pressure ulcers occurred equally in both groups. However, the degree of ischaemic skin destruction was more severe in the malnourished animals. Epithelialization of the pressure lesions occurred in normal animals at 3 days post-injury, whereas necrosis of the epidermis was still present in the malnourished animals.[37] This data suggest that although pressure damage may occur independently of nutritional status, malnourished animals may have impaired healing after a pressure injury.

The primary link between pressure ulcers and nutritional status derives from epidemiological observational studies. For example, at hospital admission, patients who are defined as undernourished are twice as likely to develop pressure ulcers as non-undernourished patients.[38] In a long-term care setting, 59% of residents were diagnosed as undernourished on admission. Among these residents, 7.3% were classified as severely undernourished. Pressure ulcers occurred in 65% of these severely undernourished residents. No pressure ulcer developed in the mild to moderately undernourished or well-nourished groups.[39]

Recent advances in the understanding of nutritional deficiencies have given rise to a re-examination of these observational data. The association of undernutrition with pressure ulcers is problematic, because there is no accepted gold standard for the diagnosis of undernutrition. Body weight loss and reductions in acute-phase hepatic proteins are often used as criteria for the diagnosis of undernutrition. However, the markers used for the diagnosis of nutritional status may reflect underlying disease rather than undernutrition in older ill persons. Cachexia and wasting diseases also produce weight loss and decreases in acute-phase reactants such as albumin and prealbumin.[40]

This critical distinction between undernutrition and the effect of wasting diseases is important because undernutrition due to starvation can be reversed by provision of adequate nutrients. Cachexia and wasting diseases are remarkably resistant to hypercaloric feeding.[41] This overlap between undernutrition and cachexia may account for the disappointing results of nutritional interventions in the prevention of pressure ulcers. A systematic review of nutritional intervention for prevention of pressure ulcers found only one of four trials suggesting that nutritional supplements may reduce the incidence of pressure ulcers in critically ill older persons.[42] In the single positive trial, two drinks of a mixed nutritional supplement produced a modest effect size at 15 days. The cumulative incidence of pressure ulcers was 40% in the nutritional supplemented group compared with 48% in the control group.[43]

Pressure ulcer incidence as a quality of care indicator

If pressure ulcers can be prevented, then the presence of a pressure ulcers may be an indicator of quality of care.[44,45] However, if adequately applied prevention interventions are not effective, the link between pressure ulcer incidence and quality of care is severed.[46]

In surveys of prevention practices among hospitalized Medicare beneficiaries, there was no link between documentation of a quality indicator and the incidence of pressure ulcers. In a multicentre retrospective cohort study of 2425 patients aged 65 years and older discharged from acute care hospitals, six processes of care for prevention of pressure ulcers were evaluated, including use of daily skin assessment, use of a pressure-reducing device, documentation of being at risk, repositioning for a minimum of 2 h, nutritional consultation initiated for patients with nutritional risk factors and staging of pressure ulcer. In fact, older adults who had documentation of being at risk and/or who received a pressure-reducing device and/or were turned every 2 h had a higher incidence of pressure ulcer development.[47]

Compliance with quality indicators in 16 nursing facilities in California was assessed after dividing the homes into those with the highest or the lowest quartile incidence of pressure ulcers. The homes in the lowest quartile had a 2.7–5.5% incidence of pressure ulcers whereas the high quartile nursing facilities had a 16.6–29.8% incidence of pressure ulcers. Sixteen process of care quality indicators were assessed, including 10 specific to pressure ulcers. No differences in the pressure ulcer quality indicators derived from the Minimum Data Set was observed between nursing facilities with low and high pressure ulcer incidence. Moreover, there was no difference in direct clinical observation of processes of care between nursing facilities with low and high pressure ulcer incidence.[48]

In 20 facilities with Medicare-certified beds, 12 quality indicators were derived from expert opinion and data available in the Minimum Data Set. An intensive intervention included education, direct facility assistance and multiple site visits by study personnel. The result of the intervention was positive, that is, the facilities showed improvement in eight out of 12 quality indicators. The trial suggests that nursing facility can improve documentation of care in relationship to pressure ulcers. However, there was no improvement in four of the 12 quality indicators. Most importantly, there was no improvement in the incidence of pressure ulcers despite the relatively intense intervention. No difference was observed in the proportion of low-risk residents who developed a pressure ulcer during their stay or in the proportion of high-risk residents who developed a pressure ulcer during their stay.[49]

In a study of 35 self-selected nursing homes, an educational intervention improved compliance with pressure ulcer risk assessment (from 87 to 99%) and weekly wound assessment (from 45 to 67%). There was little change in the incidence of Stage II pressure ulcers (from 2.6 to 2.0 per 100 occupied beds per month) but the incidence of Stage II–iv pressure ulcers declined from 3.2 2.3 per 100 occupied beds per month from the first 3 months to the last 3 months over an 11 month period. The median per facility incidence of Stage III and IV pressure ulcers declined from 0.31 pressure ulcers per 100 occupied beds per month in the first 3 months to 0 per 100 beds per month in the last 3 months of observation. Nevertheless, of the 35 study facilities, an incident Stage III or IV pressure ulcer developed in 28 of the facilities.[50]

These data suggest that the development of pressure ulcers may not be as tightly linked to quality of care processes as has been suggested. Systematic efforts at education, heightened awareness of pressure ulcer prevention and specific interventions by interdisciplinary wound teams suggest that a high incidence of pressure ulcers can be reduced. Over time, reductions in incidence of pressure ulcers of 25–30% have been reported.[51,52] The reduction may be transient, unstable over time, vary with changes in personnel or occur due to random variation.[53] However, no trial has reported an elimination of pressure ulcers over time and a 'floor effect' for pressure ulcer incidence has been noted, despite aggressive measures for prevention.[54] These data confirm a growing body of evidence that severs the hypothesized link between pressure ulcer incidence and quality of care indicators. The data suggest that pressure ulcers can be, but not always are, measures of quality of care.

Treatment of pressure ulcers

Pressure ulcers are chronic wounds. Acute wounds proceed to healing through a well-researched sequential progression towards healing. Pressure ulcers, like other chronic wounds (diabetic ulcers, venous stasis ulcers and arterial ulcers), fail to proceed through an orderly and timely process to produce anatomical or functional integrity.

Normally, fibroblasts and epithelial cells grow rapidly in skin tissue cultures, covering 80% of *in vitro* surfaces within the first 3 days. In contrast, biopsy specimens from pressure ulcers usually do not grow until much later, covering only 70% of surfaces by 14 days.[55] The result is slow healing. About 75% of Stage II pressure ulcers healed in 8 weeks, but only 17% of Stage III or IV pressure ulcers healed in that time.[56] About 23% of Stage II pressure ulcers remained unhealed at 1 year and 48% of Stage IV pressure ulcers were unhealed at 1 year. At 2 years, 8% of Stage II pressure ulcers, 29% of Stage III pressure ulcers and 38% of Stage IV pressure ulcers remained unhealed.[57] The considerable length of time to healing increases the morbidity and cost of treating pressure ulcers and is often frustrating to the patient and caregivers.

Relieving pressure, friction and shear

Although there is clear evidence that pressure reduction leads to a decrease in pressure ulcer incidence, few trials have examined the effect of pressure reduction on the healing of pressure ulcers. Two short-duration trials of air-fluidized therapy have been associated with improved rates of closure of pressure ulcers in hospital settings, but not in longer duration home trials. A low-air-loss bed is superior to a convoluted foam mattress. Other trials directly comparing different devices for improved healing have not shown a difference among devices.[58] Given the data on pressure ulcer prevention, it is reasonable to conclude that pressure-reducing devices may improve healing of pressure ulcers.

Topical dressings and local wound care

Local wound treatment is directed at providing an optimum wound environment and improving host factors. The most commonly used dressing for pressure ulcers at hospital discharge in the USA is dry gauze.[59] The use of dry gauze persists despite clear data suggesting that it results in delayed healing. Compared with wet-to-dry gauze dressings, moist dressings are clearly superior. Moist wound healing allows experimentally induced wounds to resurface up to 40% faster than air-exposed wounds.[60]

The concept of a moist wound environment led to the development of occlusive dressings. The term 'occlusive' describes the inability of a dressing to transmit moisture vapour from the wound to the external atmosphere. The degree to which dressings dry the wound can be measured by the moisture vapour transmission rate (MVTR). An MVTR of less than 35 g of water vapour per square meter per hour is required to maintain a moist wound environment. Woven gauze has an MVTR of $68\,\mathrm{g\ m^{-2}\,h^{-1}}$ and impregnated gauze has a MVTR of $57\,\mathrm{g\ m^{-2}\,h^{-1}}$ In comparison, hydrocolloid dressings have an MVTR of $8\,\mathrm{g\,m^{-2}\,h^{-1}}$.[61]

Occlusive dressings can be divided into broad categories of polymer films, polymer foams, hydrogels, hydrocolloids, alginates and biomembranes. Each has several advantages and disadvantages. The available agents differ in their properties of permeability to water vapour and wound protection. Understanding these differences is the key to planning for wound management in a particular patient.[62]

Comparative qualities among available agents are shown in Table 126.3. Most of the occlusive dressings offer pain relief. Only absorbing granules fail to reduce pain. Polymer films are impermeable to liquid but permeable to gas and moisture vapour. Because of low permeability to water vapour, these dressings are not dehydrating to the wound. Non-permeable polymers such as polyvinylidine and polyethylene can be macerating to normal skin. Polymer films are not absorptive and may leak, particularly when the wound is highly exudative. Most films have an adhesive backing that may remove epithelial cells when the dressing is changed. Polymer films do not eliminate deadspace and do not absorb exudate.

Hydrocolloid dressings are complex layered dressings. They are impermeable to moisture vapour and gases and are highly adherent to the skin. Their adhesiveness to surrounding skin is higher than that of some surgical tapes, but they are non-adherent to wound tissue and do not interfere with epithelialization of the wound. The adhesive barrier of a hydrocolloid dressing can be overcome in highly exudative wounds. Excessive exudate may be overcome with an absorptive dressing such as calcium alginate.

Hydrogels are three-layer hydrophilic polymers that are insoluble in water but absorb aqueous solutions. They are poor bacterial barriers and are non-adherent to the wound. Because of their high specific heat, these dressings are cooling to the skin, aiding in pain control and reducing inflammation. Most of these dressings require a secondary dressing to secure them to the wound.

Alginates are complex polysaccharide dressings that are highly absorbent in exudative wounds. This high absorbency is particularly suited to exudative wounds. Alginates are non-adherent to the wound, but if the wound is allowed to dry, damage to the epithelial tissue may occur with removal. Alginates can be used under a number of dressings to control exudate, including hydrocolloids.

Hydrocolloid dressings and biomembranes do not allow bacteria on the surface of the dressing to penetrate to the wound. Biomembranes are tissue-derived dressings designed to cover the wound and provide potential wound healing factors. The biomembranes are very expensive and not readily available.

Table 126.3 Comparison of occlusive wound dressings.

Item	Moist saline gauze	Polymer films	Polymer foams	Hydrogels	Hydrocolloids	Alginates, granules	Biomembranes
Pain relief	+	+	+	+	+	±	+
Maceration of surrounding skin	±	±	–	–	–	–	–
O_2 permeable	+	+	+	+	–	+	+
H_2O permeable	+	+	+	+	–	+	+
Absorbent	+	–	+	+	±	+	–
Damage to epithelial cells	±	+	–	–	–	–	–
Transparent	–	+	–	–	–	–	–
Resistant to bacteria	–	–	–	–	+	–	+
Ease of application	+	–	+	+	+	+	–

Adapted from Helfman T, Ovington L and Falanga V. Occlusive dressings and wound healing. *Clin Dermatol* 1994;**12**:121–7 and Witkowski JA and Parish LC. Cutaneous ulcer therapy. *Int. J Dermatol* 1986;**25**:420–6.

The dressings differ in the ease of application. This difference is important in pressure ulcers in unusual locations or when considering home care. Dressings should be left in place until wound fluid is leaking from the sides, a period of days to 1 week.

A meta-analysis of five clinical trials comparing a hydrocolloid dressing with a dry dressing demonstrated that treatment with a hydrocolloid dressing resulted in a statistically significant improvement in the rate of pressure ulcer healing (odds ratio 2.6).[63] Hydrocolloid dressings demonstrated higher healing rates compared with moist gauze in four of the five trials. Topical application of collagen showed no significant differences in healing compared with a hydrocolloid. Collagen was more expensive and offered no major benefits to patients otherwise eligible for hydrocolloid treatment.[64]

A systematic review of published trials on topical wound dressings for pressure ulcers up to 2003 found only 21 published randomized controlled trials.[65] Hydrocolloid wound dressings were superior to saline dressings in six trials, whereas comparisons in five trials using other treatment modalities (dextranomer beads, paraffin gauze, polyurethane dressing, amorphous hydrogel) showed no differences compared with saline gauze. In nine trials comparing hydrocolloid dressings with various other advanced dressings, no difference was observed between the intervention and comparison groups. A trial comparing two different polyurethane dressings showed no difference.

A number of growth factors have been demonstrated to mediate the healing process, including transforming growth factor alpha and beta, epidermal growth factor, platelet-derived growth factor, fibroblast growth factor, interleukin 1 and 2 and tumour necrosis factor alpha.[66] Accelerating healing in chronic wounds by using these acute wound factors is attractive. In pressure ulcers, platelet-derived growth factor failed to produce complete healing,[67] although improved time to closure of wounds has been shown with PDGF-BB and basic fibroblast growth factor.[68,69] Topical nerve growth factor is superior to vehicle-only treated patients for pressure ulcers of the foot. Complete healing of a pressure ulcer occurred in eight subjects in the active treatment group but in only one subject in the vehicle control group. Improvement was greater (based on wound size) in the active treatment group than in the vehicle-only group.[70] The development of wound healing factors is still in its infancy but shows great promise.[71]

Vacuum-assisted closure has been used in both acute and chronic wounds. Only two randomized controlled trials on pressure ulcers have been reported. A total of 22 patients with 35 pressure ulcers were randomized to the vacuum-assisted closure device or a system of wound gel products for 6 weeks. Two patients in the vacuum-assisted closure group and two patients in the wound gel group showed complete healing. There was no difference in reduction in ulcer volume between groups.[72] Vacuum-assisted closure was compared with gauze moistened with Ringer's solution in a small trial of pressure ulcer treatment. The time to reach 50% of the initial wound volume was 27 days in the vacuum-assisted group and 28 days in the moist gauze-treated group.[73] Overall, seven randomized controlled trials have compared vacuum-assisted closure in various types of chronic wounds. Four trials compared gauze soaked in either normal saline or Ringer's solution. A further three trials compared vacuum therapy with hydrocolloid gel plus gauze, a papain–urea topical treatment and cadexomer iodine or hydrocolloid, hydrogels, alginate and foam. The results did not show that vacuum-assisted closure significantly increases the healing rate of chronic wounds.[74]

A review of various pressure ulcer treatments was performed over a 6 month period across several healthcare settings. The analysis focused on complete healing as the primary outcome measure. Not surprisingly, those patients with larger ulcer size and a higher wound severity score healed less often than others. Surprisingly, the use of a pressure-relieving device, documentation of a turning schedule or the use of nutritional supplements was associated with less likelihood of healing. Furthermore, the application of topical antiseptics, use of enzymatic debridement and administration of antibiotics all significantly reduced the chances of healing. Pressure ulcers that healed in this study used more 'modern' dressings (such as a hydrocolloid dressing), used more exudate management dressings, had fewer wound debridements (especially mechanical debridement) and had fewer changes in dressing type over the course of healing. Patients residing at a nursing home had more enzymatic debridement and more were given antibiotics, despite having fewer documented infections. Despite these differences in management, the rate of healing in the nursing home population was not different from that in the community-dwelling patients. The multivariate analysis of factors associated with healing demonstrated that patients having Medicaid coverage, cardiovascular disease, frequent changes of dressing type, application of a topical antiseptic, received antibiotics or who used a pressure-relief device had a reduced likelihood of healing. Only the use of an exudate absorptive dressing was associated with an increased likelihood of healing.[75] These data are likely confounded by more severe wounds receiving more complex interventions, but no clear benefit was demonstrated for any specific modality.[76]

Nutritional interventions for healing

Nutritional interventions for the healing of pressure ulcers rests on the theory that undernourished patients do not ingest sufficient energy, proteins, vitamins or minerals to provide for adequate wound healing. Based on this assumption, a number of nutritional interventions have been trialled in the healing of pressure ulcers. The results have been uniformly disappointing.[77]

An optimum dietary protein intake in patients with pressure ulcers is unknown, but may be higher than current adult recommendations of 0.8 g kg^{-1} per day. Half of the chronically ill elderly persons are unable to maintain nitrogen balance at this level.[78] Increasing protein intake beyond 1.5 g kg^{-1} per day may not increase protein synthesis and may cause dehydration.[79] A reasonable protein requirement is therefore between 1.2 and 1.5 g kg^{-1} per day. Specific amino acids such as arginine and branched-chain amino acids have not demonstrated an effect on pressure ulcer healing.[77]

The deficiency of several vitamins has significant effects on wound healing. However, supplementation of vitamins to accelerate wound healing is controversial. High doses of vitamin C have not been shown to accelerate wound healing.[80] In a 12 week study of 88 patients who received either 10 or 500 mg of ascorbic acid twice daily, the healing rates and the healing velocity of their pressure ulcers were not different in the higher dosed group.[81] Zinc supplementation has not been shown to accelerate healing except in zinc-deficient patients.[82] High serum zinc levels interfere with healing and supplementation above 150 mg per day may interfere with copper metabolism.[36]

The use of enteral feeding has been disappointing. In a study of enteral tube feedings in long-term care, 49 patients were followed for 3 months.[83] Patients received 1.6 times basal energy expenditure daily, 1.4 g of protein per kilogram per day and 85% or more of their total recommended daily allowance. At the end of 3 months, there was no difference in number or healing of pressure ulcers. In a study of survival among residents in long-term care with severe cognitive impairment, 135 residents were followed for 24 months.[84] The reasons for the placement of a feeding tube included the presence of a pressure ulcer. Having a feeding tube was not associated with increased survival; in fact, the risk was slightly increased. These data suggests that the effectiveness of enteral feeding in treating pressure ulcers is not established.

Wound debridement

Necrotic debris increases the possibility of bacterial infection and delays wound healing in animal models.[85] This delay in healing results from slow removal of debris required by phagocytosis. Although widely recommended, it remains unclear whether wound debridement is a beneficial process that results in a greater frequency of complete wound healing.[86] There are no studies that compared debridement with no debridement as the control in wound healing. The use of debridement can result in a shorter time to a clean wound bed in anticipation of surgical therapy.

Options for debridement include sharp surgical debridement, mechanical debridement with dry gauze dressings, autolytic debridement with occlusive dressings or application of exogenous enzymes. Surgical sharp debridement produces the most rapid removal of necrotic debris and is indicated in the presence of infection. Surgical or mechanical debridement can damage healthy tissue or fail to clean the wound completely. Mechanical debridement can be easily accomplished by letting saline gauze dry before removal, but may produce pain with removal. Re-moistening of gauze dressings in an attempt to reduce pain can defeat the debridement effect.

Thin portions of eschar can be removed by occlusion under a semi-permeable dressing. Enzymatic debridement can dissolve necrotic debris but possible harm to healthy tissue is debated. Penetration of enzymatic agents is limited in eschar and requires either softening by autolysis or cross-hatching by sharp incision prior to application. Both autolytic and enzymatic debridement require periods of several days to several weeks to achieve results.

The only enzyme product available in the USA for topical debridement is collagenase. Formerly used papain–urea and a papain–urea–chlorophyll combination is unavailable. A trial in 21 patients with pressure ulcers found a greater reduction in necrotic tissue using papain–urea (95.4%) compared with collagenase (35.8%) at 4 weeks, but the rate of complete healing was not different between groups.[87]

A total of five trials have not shown that enzymatic agents increased the rate of complete healing in chronic wounds compared with control treatment.[86] One trial showed an increase in wound size with both collagenase and the control treatment, but the increase was significantly less in the enzyme-treated group. Only one trial out of four that compared a hydrogel with a control treatment found a statistically significant difference between treatments. The single favourable trial suggested a small benefit from treatment with a hydrogel compared with a hydrocolloid dressing. In a single trial comparing different hydrogels, no statistically significant difference was seen between the two hydrogels.

Trials of other debridement agents have shown mixed results. Three trials of dextranomer polysaccharide found a statistically significant difference compared with control, and two trials found the control treatment to be more effective. A hydrogel significantly reduced the necrotic wound area compared with dextranomer polysaccharide paste in one trial, but not in another. Dextranomer polysaccharide was not better than an enzymatic agent in two trials.

A number of heavy metal-impregnated dressings or solutions have been evaluated for chronic wounds, based on the hypothesis that an antimicrobial effect would enhance wound healing. Topical silver and silver-impregnated dressings have been evaluated in three trials of mixed-type wounds suspected of being infected.

Only one trial included pressure ulcers as a wound type. In that trial, there was no difference in complete healing or absolute or relative wound size, but a small effect was calculated for healing rate per day.[88,89]

Conclusion

The accumulating data for the prevention and management of pressure ulcers permit an outline of clinical strategies. Risk assessment remains problematic because of poor predictive validity and an apparent floor effect in preventing all pressure ulcers, but can highlight patient-specific risk factors for development of a pressure ulcer. Pressure-reducing devices are clearly superior to a standard hospital mattress in preventing pressure ulcers. However, it is difficult to distinguish superiority among various devices. The impact of nutrition on the prevention of pressure ulcers remains controversial. Limited data suggest than nutritional supplementation may have an effect on reducing incidence. Nutritional status should be evaluated in all clinical settings as a process of good care.

Limited evidence and clinical intuition support pressure-reducing devices in improving the healing rate of pressure ulcers. The amount of dietary protein intake seems to be linked to improved rates of healing, but the results of enteral feeding to achieve this result are disappointing. Other nutritional interventions, including specific amino acids and vitamin or mineral supplements, have not shown an effect on healing rate.

Local wound treatment should aim at maintaining a moist wound environment. Options include hydrocolloid dressings and other occlusive moist dressings. The choice of a particular dressing depends on wound characteristics such as the amount of exudate, deadspace and wound location. Debridement by any of several methods may improve the time to a clean wound bed, but the effect of debridement on time to healing remains to be demonstrated. The use of topical growth factors in improving healing rates is in its infancy but has not been remarkably effective thus far.

Key points

- Pressure ulcers are related to pathological changes in the blood supply to the tissues.
- Pressure relief prevents and helps with healing of pressure ulcers.
- Hydrocolloid wound dressings are superior to saline dressings.
- There is weak evidence to support supplemental nutrition interventions to improve pressure ulcer healing rates.

References

1. Whittington K., Patrick M. and Roberts JL. A national study of pressure ulcer prevalence and incidence in acute care hospitals. *J Wound Ostomy Continence Nurs* 2000;**27**:209–15.
2. Thomas DR. Does pressure cause pressure ulcers? An inquiry into the etiology of pressure ulcers. *J Am Med Dir Assoc* 2010; **11**:397–405.
3. Sanada H, Nagakawa T, Yamamoto M *et al*. The role of skin blood flow in pressure ulcer development during surgery. *Adv Wound Care* 1997;**10**:29–34.
4. Mayrovitz HN, Sims N and Taylor MC. Sacral skin blood perfusion: a factor in pressure ulcers ? *Ostomy Wound Manage* 2002;**48**:34–8,40–2.
5. Van Marum RJ, Meijer JH and Ribbe MW. The relationship between pressure ulcers and skin blood flow response after of local cold provocation. *Arch Phys Med Rehabil* 2002;**83**:40–3.
6. Vasconez LO, Schneider WJ and Jurkiewicz MJ. Pressure sores. *Curr Problems Surg* 1977;**62**:83–9.
7. Meehan M. National pressure ulcer prevalence survey. *Adv Wound Care* 1994;**7**:27–37.
8. Barbenel J. The prevalence of pressure sores. In: *National Symposium on the Care, Treatment and Prevention of Decubitus Ulcers. Conference Proceedings*, 1984, pp.1–9.
9. National Pressure Ulcer Advisory Panel. Pressure ulcers: incidence, economics, risk assessment. Consensus development conference statement. *Decubitus* 1989;**2**:24–8.
10. Thomas D. Existing tools: Are they meeting the challenges of pressure ulcer healing ? *Adv Wound Care* 1997;**10**:86–90.
11. Thomas DR, Rodeheaver GT, Bartolucci AA *et al*. Pressure ulcer scale for healing: Derivation and validation of the PUSH tool. *Adv Wound Care* 1997;**10**:96–101.
12. Stotts N, Rodeheaver G, Thomas DR *et al*. An instrument to measure healing in pressure ulcers: development and validation of the pressure ulcer scale for healing (PUSH). *J Gerontol A Biol Sci Med Sci* 2001;**56** M795–9.
13. Thomas DR. Are all pressure ulcers avoidable? *J Am Med Dir Assoc* 2001;**2**:297–301.
14. Scott JR, Gibran NS, Engrav LH *et al*. Incidence and characteristics of hospitalized patients with pressure ulcers: State of Washington, 1987 to 2000. *Plast Reconstr Surg* 2006;**117**:630–4.
15. Gunningberg L. EPUAP pressure ulcer prevalence survey in Sweden: a two-year follow-up of quality indicators. *J Wound Ostomy Continence Nurs* 2006;**33**:258–66.
16. Pancorbo-Hidalgo PL, Garcia-Fernandez FP, Lopez-Medine IM and Alvariex-Nieto C. Risk assessment scales for pressure ulcer prevention: a systematic review. *J Adv Nurs* 2006;**54**: 94–110.
17. Cullum N, Deeks J, Fletcher A *et al*. The prevention and treatment of pressure sores: how useful are the measures for scoring people's risk of developing a pressure sore? *Effect Health Care* 1995;**2**,1–18.
18. McGough A. A systematic review of the effectiveness of risk assessment scales used in the prevention and management of pressure sores. In J. Rycroft-Malone and E. McInnes (eds), *Pressure Ulcer Risk Assessment and Prevention, Technical Report*. Royal College of Nursing, London, 2000, pp.84–99.
19. Vanderwee K, Grypdonck M and Defloor T. Non-blanchable erythema as an indicator for the need for pressure ulcer

prevention: a randomized-controlled trial. *J Clin Nurs* 2007; **16**:325–35.

20. Kenedi RM, Cowden JM and Scales JT (eds). *Bedsore Biomechanics*, University Park Press, Baltimore, 1976.
21. Knox DM, Anderson TM and Anderson PS. Effects of different turn intervals on skin of healthy older adults. *Adv. Wound Care* 1994;**7**:48–56.
22. Bliss MR and McLaren R. Preventing pressure sores in geriatric patients. *Nurs Mirror* 1967;**2**:405–8.
23. Clark M. Repositioning to prevent pressure sores – what is the evidence ? *Nurs Stand* 1998;**13**:56–64.
24. McInnes E, Jammali-Blasi A, Bell-Syer SE, *et al.* Support surfaces for pressure ulcer prevention. The Cochrane Wounds Group, *Cochrane Database Syst Rev* 2011;(4): CD001735.
25. Maklebust J, Mondoux L and Sieggreen M. Pressure relief characteristics of various support surfaces used in prevention and treatment of pressure ulcers. *J Enterost Ther* 1986;**13**:85–9.
26. Krouskop TA, Williams R, Krebs M *et al.* Effectiveness of mattress overlays in reducing interface pressures during recumbency. *J Rehabil Res* 1985;**22**:7–10.
27. Guin P, Hudson A and Gallo J. The efficacy of six heel pressure reducing devices. *Decubitus* 1991;**4**:15–23.
28. Mulder GD and LaPan M. Decubitus ulcers: update on new approaches to treatment. *Geriatrics* 1988;**43**:37–50.
29. Defloor T, Bacquer DD and Grypdonck MHF. The effect of various combinations of turning and pressure reducing devices on the incidence of pressure ulcers. *Int J Nurs Stud.* 2005;**42**:37–46.
30. Defloor T. Less frequent turning intervals and yet less pressure ulcers. *Tijdschr Gerontol Geriatr* 2001;**32**:174–7 (in Dutch).
31. Vanderwee K, Grypdonck MHF, DeBacquer D and Defloor T. Effectiveness of turning with unequal time intervals of the incidence of pressure ulcer lesions. *J Adv Nurs* 2007;**57**:59–68.
32. Vanderwee K, Grypdonck M and Defloor T. The effectiveness of alternating pressure air mattresses for the prevention of pressure ulcers. *Age Ageing* 2005;**34**:261–7.
33. Stapleton M. Preventing pressure sores – an evaluation of three products. *Geriatr Nurs (Lond)* 1986;**6**:23–5.
34. Gebhardt KS, Bliss MR, Winwright PL and Thomas J. Pressure-relieving supports in an ICU. *J Wound Care* 1996; **5**:116–21.
35. Reddy M, Gill SS and Bouchon PA. Preventing pressure ulcers: a systematic review. *JAMA* 2006;**296**:974–84.
36. Thomas DR. The role of nutrition in prevention and healing of pressure ulcers. *Geriatr Clin North Am* 1997;**13**:497–512.
37. Takeda T, Koyama T, Izawa Y *et al.* Effects of malnutrition on development of experimental pressure sores. *J Dermatol* 1992;**19**:602–9.
38. Thomas DR, Goode PS, Tarquine PH and Allman R. Hospital acquired pressure ulcers and risk of death. *J Am Geriatr Soc* 1996;**44**:1435–40.
39. Pinchcofsky-Devin GD and Kaminski MV Jr. Correlation of pressure sores and nutritional status. *J Am Geriatr Soc* 1986;**34**:435–40.
40. Thomas DR. Distinguishing starvation from cachexia. *Geriatr Clin North Am* 2002;**18**:883–92.
41. Thomas DR. Loss of skeletal muscle mass in aging: examining the relationship of starvation, sarcopenia and cachexia. *Clin Nutr* 2007;**26**:389–99.
42. Langer G, Knerr A, Kuss O *et al.* Nutritional interventions for preventing and treating pressure ulcers. The Cochrane Wounds Group. *The Cochrane Database of Systematic Reviews* 2003;(4): CD003216.
43. Bourdel-Marchasson I, Barateau M, Rondeau V *et al.* A multi-center trial of the effects of oral nutritional supplementation in critically ill older inpatients. GAGE Group. Groupe Aquitain Geriatrique d'Evaluation. *Nutrition* 2000;**16**:1–5.
44. Requirements for Long Term Care Facilities. *Fed Regist* 1991; **56**:48867–925.
45. Audit Commission. *The Virtue of Patients: Making the Best Use of Ward Nurse Resources*, The Audit Commission for Local Authorities and the National Health Service in England and Wales, London, 1991.
46. Thomas DR and Osterweil D. Is a pressure ulcer a marker for quality of care ? *J Am Med Dir Assoc* 2005;**6**:228–9.
47. Lyder CH, Preston J, Grady JN *et al.* Quality of care for hospitalized Medicare patients at risk for pressure ulcers. *Arch Intern Med* 2001;**161**:1549–54.
48. Bates-Jensen BM, Cadogan M, Osterweil D *et al.* The minimum data set pressure ulcer indicator: does it reflect differences in care processes related to pressure ulcer prevention and treatment in nursing homes? *J Am Geriatr Soc* 2003; **51**:1203–12.
49. Abel RL, Warren K, Bean G, Babbard G *et al.* Quality improvement in nursing homes in Texas: results from a pressure ulcer prevention project. *J Am Med Dir Assoc* 2005; **6**:181 8.
50. Lynn J, West J, Hausmann S *et al.* Collaborative clinical quality improvement for pressure ulcers in nursing homes. *J Am Geriatr Soc* 2007;**55**:1663–9.
51. Berlowitz DR, Bezerra HQ, Brandeis GH *et al.* Are we improving the quality of nursing home care: the case of pressure ulcers. *J Am Geriatr Soc* 2000;**48**:59–62.
52. Hopkins B, Hanlon M, Yauk S *et al.* Reducing nosocomial pressure ulcers in an acute care facility. *J Nurs Care Qual* 2000;**14**:28–36.
53. Richardson GM, Gardner S and Frantz RA. Nursing assessment: impact on type and cost of interventions to prevent pressure ulcers. *J Wound Ostomy Continence Nurs* 1998; **25**:273–80.
54. Hagisawa S and Barbenel J. The limits of pressure sore prevention. *J R Soc Med* 1999;**92**:576–8.
55. Seiler WO, Stahelin HB, Zolliker R *et al.* Impaired migration of epidermal cells from decubitus ulcers in cell culture: a cause of protracted wound healing? *Am J Clin Pathol* 1989;**92**:430–4.
56. Ferrell BA, Osterweil D and Christenson P. A randomized trial of low-air-loss beds for treatment of pressure ulcers. *JAMA* 1993;**269**:494–7.
57. Brandeis GH, Morris JN, Nash DJ *et al.* The epidemiology and natural history of pressure ulcers in elderly nursing home residents. *JAMA* 1990;**264**:2905–9.
58. Cullum N, Deeks J, Sheldon TA *et al.* Beds, mattresses and cushions for pressure sore prevention and treatment. *Cochrane Database Syst Rev* 2004;(3): CD001735.
59. Ferrell BA, Josephson K, Norvid P and Alcorn H. Pressure ulcers among patients admitted to home care. *J Am Geriatr Soc* 2000;**48**:1165–6.

60. Eaglstein WH and Mertz PM. New method for assessing epidermal wound healing. The effects of triamcinolone acetonide and polyethylene film occlusion. *J Invest Dermatol* 1978;**71**:382–4.

61. Bolton L, Johnson C and van Rijswijk L. Occlusive dressings: therapeutic agents and effects on drug delivery. *Clin Dermatol* 1992;**9**:573–83.

62. Thomas DR. Issues and dilemmas in managing pressure ulcers. *J Gerontol Med Sci* 2001;**56**: M238–340.

63. Bradley M, Cullum N, Nelson EA *et al.* Systematic reviews of wound care management: dressings and topical agents used in the healing of chronic wounds. *Health Technol Assess* 1999;**3**(17 Part 2):1–135.

64. Graumlich JF, Blough LS, McLaughlin RG *et al.* Healing pressure ulcers with collagen or hydrocolloid: a randomized, controlled trial. *J Am Geriatr Soc* 2003;**51**:147–54.

65. Bouza C, Saz Z, Munoz A and Amate J. Efficacy of advanced dressings in the treatment of pressure ulcers: a systematic review. *J Wound Care* 2005;**14**:193–9.

66. Thomas DR. Age-related changes in wound healing. *Drugs Aging* 2001;**18**:607–20.

67. Robson MC, Phillips LG, Thomason A *et al.* Recombinant human derived growth factor-BB for the treatment of chronic pressure ulcers. *Ann Plast Surg* 1992;**29**:193–201.

68. Robson MC, Phillips LG, Thomason A *et al.* Platelet-derived growth factor BB for the treatment of chronic pressure ulcers. *Lancet* 1992;**339**:23–5.

69. Robson MC, Phillips LG, Lawrence WT *et al.* The safety and effect of topically applied recombinant basic fibroblast growth factor on the healing of chronic pressure sores. *Ann Surg* 1992;**216**:401–8.

70. Landi F, Aloe L, Russo A *et al.* Topical treatment with nerve growth factor for pressure ulcers: a randomized controlled trial. *Ann Intern Med* 2003;**139**:635–41.

71. Thomas DR. The promise of topical nerve growth factors in the healing of pressure ulcers. *Ann Intern Med* 2003; **139**:694–5.

72. Ford CN, Reinhard ER, Yeh D *et al.* Interim analysis of a prospective, randomized trial of vacuum-assisted closure versus the healthpoint system in the management of pressure ulcers. *Ann Plast Surg.* 2002;**49**:55–61.

73. Wanner MB, Schwarzl F, Strub B *et al.* Vacuum-assisted wound closure for cheaper and more comfortable healing of pressure sores: a prospective study. *Scand J Plast Reconstr Surg Hand Surg* 2003;**37**:28–33.

74. Ubbink DT, Westerbos SJ, Evans D *et al.* Topical negative pressure for treating chronic wounds. The Cochrane Wounds Group. *Cochrane Database Syst Rev* 2008;(3): CD001898.

75. Jones KR and Fennie K. Factors influencing pressure ulcer healing in adults over 50: an exploratory study. *J Am Med Dir Assoc* 2007;**8**:378–87.

76. Thomas DR. Managing pressure ulcers: learning to give up cherished dogma. *J Am Med Dir Assoc.* 2007;**8**:347–8.

77. Thomas DR. Improving the outcome of pressure ulcers with nutritional intervention: a review of the evidence. *Nutrition* 2001;**17**:121–5.

78. Gersovitz M, Motil K, Munro HN *et al.* Human protein requirements: assessment of the adequacy of the current Recommended Dietary Allowance for dietary protein in elderly men and women. *Am J Clin Nutr* 1982;**35**:6–14.

79. Long CL, Nelson KM, Akin JM Jr *et al.* A physiologic bases for the provision of fuel mixtures in normal and stressed patients. *J Trauma* 1990;**30**:1077–86.

80. Vilter RW. Nutritional aspects of ascorbic acid: uses and abuses. *West J Med* 1980;**133**:485–92.

81. ter Riet G, Kessels AG and Knipschild PG. Randomized clinical trial of ascorbic acid in the treatment of pressure ulcers. *J Clin Epidemiol* 1995;**48**:1453–60.

82. Sandstead HH, Henriksen LK, Greger JL *et al.* Zinc nutriture in the elderly in relation to taste acuity, immune response and wound healing. *Am J Clin Nutr* 1982;**36**(Suppl):1046–59.

83. Henderson CT, Trumbore LS, Mobarhan S *et al.* Prolonged tube feeding in long-term care: nutritional status and clinical outcomes. *J Am Coll Clin Nutr* 1992;**11**:309–25.

84. Mitchell SL, Kiely DK and Lipsitz LA. The risk factors and impact on survival of feeding tube placement in nursing home residents with severe cognitive impairment. *Arch Intern Med* 1997;**157**:327–32.

85. Constantine BE and Bolton LL. A wound model for ischemic ulcers in the guinea pig. *Arch Dermatol Res* 1986;**278**:429–31.

86. Bradley M, Cullum N and Sheldon T. The debridement of chronic wounds: a systematic review. *Health Technol Assess* 1999;**3**:1–78.

87. Alvarez OM, Fenandez-Obregon A, Rogers RS *et al.* Chemical debridement of pressure ulcers: a prospective, randomized, comparative trial of collagenase and papain/urea formulations. *Wounds* 2000;**12**:15–25.

88. Vermeulen H, van Hattem JM, Storm-Versloot MN and Ubbink DT. Topical silver for treating infected wounds. Cochrane Wound Group, *Cochrane Database Syst Rev* 2007;(1): CD005486.

89. Meaume S, Vallet D, Morere MN and Teot L. Evaluation of a silver-releasing hydroalginate dressing in chronic wounds with signs of local infection. *J Wound Care* 2005;**14**:411–9.

CHAPTER 127

Perioperative and postoperative medical assessment

Milta Oyola Little
Saint Louis University Medical Center, St Louis, MO, USA

Introduction

Since 1850, life expectancy has increased linearly.[1] With increase in life expectancy comes an increase in medical needs for adults in late life, including surgical procedures. In 2006, inpatient procedures were performed on 4358 per 10 000 patients over the age of 65 years. Surgeons have seen an increase in the rates of certain procedure types over the last decade in this age group. As an example, the rate of total knee replacements increased from 60 per 10 000 population in 2000 to 88 per 10 000 population in 2006.[2] It is estimated that more than half of people currently over the age of 65 years will undergo at least one surgical procedure.[3] As the population grows and ages, the need for specialized surgical care of the elderly will grow. The role of the consulting geriatric specialist is to assist the surgeon in maximizing preoperative function, minimizing the effect of comorbid diseases and preventing or managing postoperative complications.[4]

The approach to perioperative management of the geriatric patient begins with an understanding of age-related changes in physiology and how these changes affect stress responses. Preoperatively, the consultant should identify patients at risk for adverse outcomes, with the intent of maximizing function and minimizing risk. Although often not modifiable, intraoperative factors, such as type of procedure, type of anaesthesia and occurrence of complications, may affect the outcome in elderly patients. Prior to surgery, ways to minimize procedure length and complications should be considered by the operative team, which includes the surgeon, anaesthesiologist and consulting geriatrician. Anticipation of potential postoperative complications leads to early identification and management of adverse outcomes. The most common postoperative complications are cardiac, pulmonary and neurological in origin. Strategies to minimize the risk to these organ systems have been studied and some guidelines exist to assist with management. Prevention and treatment of infection and venous thromboembolism begin in the preoperative period and can also greatly improve outcome. Several other problems can occur postoperatively and the consulting geriatric specialist can help ameliorate those problems with simple multidisciplinary interventions.

The aim of this chapter is to guide the geriatric specialist in perioperative risk assessment and reduction with the goal of lowering complications and improving outcomes. It focuses on evaluation and management of the geriatric patient undergoing non-cardiac surgery. For a discussion on cardiac surgery in the elderly, see Chapter 42.

Outcomes of surgery in the elderly

Survival curves from the UK show an increase in life expectancy with a continual rightward shift since 1850[1] (see Figure 127.1).[5] This argues against the theory of a biologically determined limit to life. However, as mortality shifts, epidemiologists have observed a decompression of morbidity. This means that humans are living longer with more years lived in poor health.

Studies of elderly surgical patients consistently showed poorer outcomes in people over the age of 65 years versus their younger counterparts.[4,6,7] However, when adjusted for comorbid conditions, type and length of procedure or preoperative physical state [as assessed using American Society of Anesthesiologists' (ASA) classification or similar grading tool], the risk of adverse outcomes attributed to age alone is significantly diminished.[4,6] A description of the ASA classification system can be found on the ASA website.[8] A retrospective study carried out at the end of the twentieth century showed a postoperative complication rate of 25% in patients over the age of 80 years, consistent with other studies. Although this number may be troubling, 74% of the cohort did well, with no complications, and the mortality rate was only 4.6%,

Principles and Practice of Geriatric Medicine, Fifth Edition. Edited by Alan J. Sinclair, John E. Morley and Bruno Vellas.

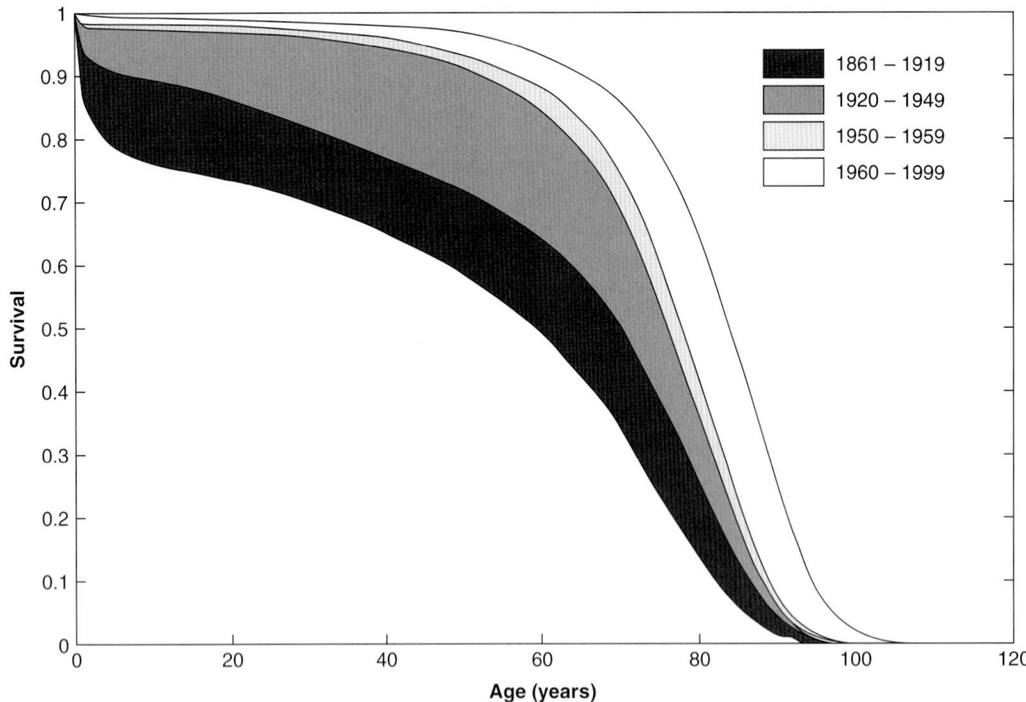

Figure 127.1 Survival curves in Sweden over the last 140 years. Initial survival improvement trends showed a rectangularization of the survival curve, followed by parallel rightward shifts. Reprinted from Smetana,[4] Copyright 2003, with permission from Elsevier.

down from 20% in the 1960s.[9] For this reason, surgery should not be denied based solely on age. Instead, a comprehensive preoperative assessment that determines risk and maximizes function should drive decisions to proceed with surgery, even in the oldest old.

Ageing physiology

Normal physiological changes occur with ageing. These changes should not be viewed as pathological conditions since under normal circumstances the body is able to compensate. During periods of stress, such as surgery or trauma, the ageing body is less able to counter the insult and complications may ensue.[3] An understanding of normal age-related physiological changes helps the geriatric specialist to maximize functional reserve and provide adequate physiological support perioperatively. Note that although these organ system changes occur consistently with ageing, they do not occur at the same rate in each individual, such that there is often a discrepancy between the chronological age and biological age. Therefore, perioperative management must be individualized.

Age-related changes in the cardiovascular system

As humans age, the physiology of the cardiovascular system undergoes numerous changes that affect vascular compliance, blood pressure and myocardial contractility. Blood vessels lose compliance due to calcification, tunica media thickening and elastic fracturing. As a result, systolic blood pressure is often elevated. However, a blunted response to baroreceptor activity predisposes the elderly to orthostatic hypotension. Changes in the peripheral vascular system cause an increase in afterload leading to myocardial hypertrophy. Cellular hypertrophy, along with calcification and fibrosis, brings about diastolic dysfunction and damage to pacemaker cells. As the ventricles stiffen, left ventricular end diastolic volume and cardiac output diminish. Increased preload with atrial enlargement compensates for the reduced cardiac output; therefore, losing atrial contraction as a result of atrial fibrillation can lead to cardiac decompensation.[3,10] Cardiovascular response to stress is also altered with age. Older people have blunted beta-adrenergic sensitivity and also reduced basal vagal tone with an inability to lower vagal tone further, leading to an inappropriate heart rate response to stress.[3]

Age-related changes in the pulmonary system

As in the vascular system, changes in the pulmonary system associated with ageing are largely due to loss in elasticity. This loss of elastic recoil of the lungs decreases oxygen transfer and air trapping. Muscle atrophy and joint damage impair chest wall movement, further reducing ventilation and oxygenation. Vital capacity and FEV1 are decreased, in addition to ciliary function. An increase in residual volume leads to an increase in dead space during normal breathing. These age-related changes increase risk of atelectasis, aspiration and pneumonia postoperatively.[3,10]

Age-related changes in the renal system

Reduced cardiac output, reduced renal mass and glomerulosclerosis cause a decrease in renal plasma flow and glomerular filtration rate (GFR) with age. Renal clearance is slowed, affecting drug elimination and acid excretion. Patients with renal insufficiency are at higher risk of volume overload, electrolyte imbalances and drug accumulation. However, ageing kidneys also have a reduced capacity to concentrate urine, even when fluid intake is inadequate, predisposing the person to dehydration. Creatinine clearance must be calculated prior to surgery for appropriate administration of fluids, anaesthesia and pain medication.[3,10] Laboratory estimates of GFR may not be accurate in elderly populations.

Age-related changes in the neurological system

The major change associated with ageing of the nervous system is loss of neuronal substance, with a decrease in brain weight. Peripheral neurons also decrease in number. This age-related loss of neuronal mass may explain the increased sensitivity to opioids and anaesthetics seen in elderly patients.

Emergency surgery

Emergency surgery has long been associated with increased mortality rates over elective surgery.[11,12] The questions remain of whether age further increases mortality, when emergency surgery should be denied or delayed for resuscitation and if any interventions instituted prior to surgery could ameliorate the risk of mortality in the elderly.

Several observational studies have been carried out to identify the risk factors for mortality in patients undergoing emergency surgery.[11–13] Most were orthopaedic, trauma or general surgery. Mortality rates were consistently higher for elderly patients and those with high ASA classes (three or higher). The leading causes of death were malignancy and septic or cardiac complications. Orthopaedic patients tended to have a more favourable outcome than general surgery patients because limb procedures are less likely to produce cardiopulmonary, metabolic or gastrointestinal (i.e. ileus) complications. Additionally, they were often labelled as 'urgent', meaning the operations took place within 24 h as opposed to immediate (within 1–2 h), allowing some time for stabilization and preparation.[11,12] Current guidelines recommend avoiding night-time operations; however, recent studies suggest that this may be unfounded as no association was found between late-night surgery and increased mortality.[11,12]

A study restricted to elderly patients (50% over the age of 80 years) undergoing emergency abdominal surgery found that mortality rates were affected by preoperative risk (increase in comorbid conditions, high ASA class), delay in diagnosis and surgical treatment and conditions only allowing palliative surgery or non-therapeutic laparotomy. After adjusting for these conditions, age alone did not affect mortality, morbidity or length of stay.[13] Emergency surgery should not be denied to patients strictly based on age.

The above studies suggest that perioperative interventions (particularly during and immediately after surgery), such as appropriate antimicrobial prophylaxis, limiting surgery length and a consideration to delay surgery for stabilization of patients with ASA class 4 or 5, *may* improve outcomes. Prospective studies assessing these interventions are needed.

Preoperative medical assessment of the geriatric patient

Multiple studies have been done to assess the perioperative risks of elderly patients. Several are reviewed in this chapter, with emphasis on current guidelines and recommendations. It is worth noting that although identification of factors associated with postoperative complications is helpful for risk stratification, they are often not modifiable. Additionally, although as a group patients at high surgical risk have far more complications than those at low risk, risk indices cannot predict which *individual* will have a poor outcome. Many patients at high risk have uneventful surgical courses. Continued research to delineate cost-effective interventions most likely to reduce adverse events that can be widely applied to the elderly surgical patient is needed.

Review of data reveals that postoperative complications, including cardiopulmonary events, neurological events or death, are more likely to occur in the setting of poor premorbid function or emergency surgery.[10] Preoperative factors most likely to increase risk of morbidity and mortality include the following:[9,10,14,15]

1 severe systemic disease (ASA Class III–V)
2 acute or chronic renal failure
3 history of chronic obstructive pulmonary disease (COPD) or congestive heart failure
4 recent (within 6 months) myocardial infarction (MI)
5 low albumin level ($<3.5\,g\,dl^{-1}$)
6 anaemia (haemoglobin $<8\,g\,dl^{-1}$)
7 poor functional status (bedridden, assistance with ADL or inability to perform 2 min on a supine bicycle exercise test)
8 impaired sensorium or cognition.

Based on the above factors, preoperative medical evaluation begins with a thorough history emphasizing comorbid diseases and functional status. The physical examination should focus on signs of active cardiopulmonary disease (such as jugular venous distension, rales, an S3 gallop, oedema and wheezing) and evaluation of cognitive status. Basic laboratory evaluation and radiological procedures should be obtained based on history and examination findings.[10,16] For most patients, the initial preoperative workup includes a complete blood count, electrolyte levels, renal function and electrocardiogram (ECG). It should be noted that although several sensitive risk indices exist to predict potential postoperative complications, the risk criteria are not specific. Many patients with multiple risk factors will have uncomplicated operative courses.[14]

Cardiac risk assessment

The most widely published topic in preoperative surgical evaluation is cardiac risk assessment. A PubMed search for 'perioperative cardiac risk assessment' brings up over 1000 articles and nearly 300 reviews. When limited to articles addressing cardiac risk in patients over 65 years of age, 500 articles and 20 reviews are listed. Current guidelines exist to aid the clinician in cardiac risk evaluation, including the 2007 American College of Cardiology/American Heart Association (ACC/AHA) Preoperative Cardiac Risk Assessment.[16] The ACC/AHA guideline utilizes the Revised Cardiac Risk Index (derived from Goldman *et al.*[17] and Lee *et al.*[18]) for stratification and is the most widely used.

The purpose of a cardiac evaluation prior to surgery is threefold:

1 To identify patients with active unstable cardiac disease, for whom surgery ought to be delayed or cancelled for medical management.

2 To identify patients at high risk for postoperative cardiac complications in order to devise interventions to modify and minimize the risk.

3 To identify patients with risk factors for coronary artery disease who should undergo preoperative cardiac testing and receive perioperative beta-blockers.

Table 127.1 lists unstable cardiac conditions that require stabilization prior to non-emergent surgery and strategies for management of surgical patients requiring revascularization.[16]

Goldman *et al.*[17] devised and validated the first Cardiac Risk Index based on 13 parameters in six categories (including history, physical, electrocardiogram, general health status and type of operation). This index was revised in 1999 and included in the ACC/AHA guidelines for evaluation of cardiac risk. The Revised Cardiac Risk Index is based on six clinical parameters that carry postoperative prognostic significance:[18] high-risk surgery, history of ischaemic heart disease, history of or active heart failure, history of cerebrovascular disease, diabetes mellitus requiring insulin therapy and renal insufficiency (serum creatinine $>2.0\ \mathrm{mg\ dl^{-1}}$). Preoperative functional status can also be used to identify risk for cardiac complications.[10,16,18]

Figure 127.2 outlines an approach to evaluating and managing cardiac risk based on the Revised Goldman Cardiac Risk Index and the 2007 ACC/AHA Guidelines.[16,18]

Once it has been determined that non-invasive cardiac stress testing is needed, the consultant must decide which test to perform. The test of choice for ambulatory patients is exercise ECG testing.[16] Exercise testing provides information on cardiac ischaemia and functional status, both predictive of surgical outcomes. Its safety is established[16]

Table 127.1 Management in non-emergent surgery for unstable cardiac conditions.

Defer surgery for management of:	Myocardial infarction within 30 days
	Unstable or severe angina
	Decompensated heart failure
	Severe aortic stenosis (pressure gradient >40 mmHg, valve area <1 cm^2 or symptoms)
	Symptomatic mitral stenosis
	Significant unstable arrhythmias
Refer for PTCA or CABG if:	Stable angina and significant left main disease
	Stable angina and triple-vessel disease
	Stable angina and two-vessel disease *with* proximal LAD lesion and EF <50% or ischaemia on testing
	Unstable angina (UA) or non-ST-segment elevation myocardial infarction (NSTEMI)
	ST-segment elevation myocardial infarction (STEMI)
Defer elective surgery post-PTCA for:	<14 days from balloon angioplasty
	<30 days from bare metal stent placement
	<12 months from drug-eluding stent placement

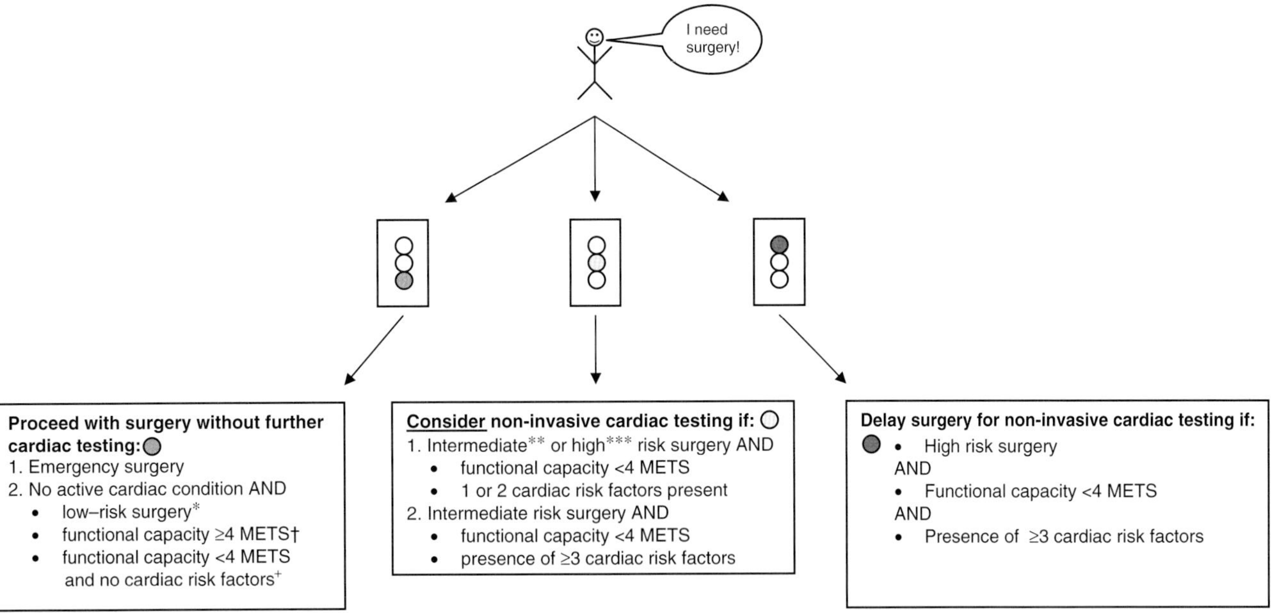

Figure 127.2 Decision tree for evaluation of cardiac risk prior to surgery. See plate section for a colour version of this image.

and studies on elderly patients have shown that a simple supine bicycle exercise test can predict exercise capacity and perioperative cardiac complications better than more expensive and complicated cardiac testing.[14]

If abnormalities exist on baseline resting ECG (e.g. left bundle-branch block, LV hypertrophy with 'strain' pattern or digitalis effect) or if patients are unable to exercise, pharmacological stress cardiac imaging is recommended.[16]

If non-invasive cardiac testing is positive, the patient ought to be referred for percutaneous transluminal coronary angioplasty (PTCA). Following PTCA, the patient is at high risk for restenosis and cardiac decompensation under stressful conditions. Additionally, patients who undergo revascularization require dual antiplatelet therapy to reduce the risk of restenosis. For these reasons, surgery should be delayed, if possible, for a period of time after PTCA. The length of time depends on the method of relieving the vessel obstruction. Table 127.2 outlines the management of the surgical patient following PTCA.[16]

Cardiac events following non-cardiac surgery have been reported to occur at rates of 1–5% and as high as 30% in vascular surgery.[19] Once a patient has been deemed medically appropriate to proceed with surgery, the consulting geriatrician must decide which interventions, if any, could modify perioperative risk and lower the chance of postoperative cardiac complications. One such intervention that has been highly debated is the use of perioperative beta-blocker therapy.

Currently, the ACC/AHA Guidelines recommend initiation of beta-blockers if evidence of cardiac ischaemia is found on preoperative testing or coronary disease and more than one cardiac risk is present in patients undergoing vascular or intermediate-risk surgeries. No recommendation (uncertain usefulness) is given for patients without evidence of ischaemia or with less than two cardiac risks.[16]

Table 127.2 Management of surgical patients after percutaneous coronary angiography (PTCA).

Procedure	Days post-PTCA			
	<14	14–29	30–365	>365
Balloon angioplasty	–[a]	Aspirin[b]	Aspirin[b]	Aspirin[b]
Bare metal stent	–[a]	–[a]	Aspirin[b]	Aspirin[b]
Drug-eluding stent	–[a]	–[a]	–[a]	Aspirin[b]

[a]Defer surgery.
[b]Proceed with surgery with aspirin alone as antiplatelet agent.

A 2005 meta-analysis evaluating cardioselective beta-blocker use in patients over the age of 65 years found an overall protective effect of beta-blocker therapy for perioperative cardiac mortality, long-term overall and cardiac mortality and myocardial infarction (MI) or ischaemia. The largest effect was seen for postoperative myocardial ischaemia with a number needed to treat (NNT) of 6.[19]

In 2008, another meta-analysis showed different results. Overall, use of perioperative beta-blockade was associated with a 35% decrease in non-fatal MI (NNT 63) and 64% decrease in myocardial ischaemia (NNT 16), but it was also associated with a 116% increase risk of non-fatal strokes and *no* reduction in all-cause or cardiovascular mortality.[20]

A large proportion of the data from the second meta-analysis was derived from the landmark PeriOperative ISchemic Evaluation (POISE) trial, which randomized over 8000 patients with or at risk for atherosclerosis to receive extended-release metoprolol or placebo. Patients already on beta-blockade were excluded. Treatment was initiated 2–4 h prior to surgery, titrated to 50% of maximum dose, and was continued for 30 days postoperatively. The researchers found that metoprolol administration was associated with a reduction in the rate of MI, cardiac revascularization and clinically significant atrial fibrillation; however, the same group had significantly more all-cause mortality, stroke, hypotension and bradycardia.[21] Critics of the POISE trial argue that the relatively high doses of metoprolol and initiation of therapy close to surgery (within hours) led to the high number of adverse outcomes.[22] Still, these findings have spurred much debate on the safety of perioperative beta-blocker use.

Currently, experts recommend continuation of beta-blockers in patients on long-term therapy. Additionally, based on studies examining beta-blockers started 30 days prior to surgery, one may consider initiation of low-dose therapy (2.5 mg per day of bisoprolol and 25 mg per day of metoprolol) well in advance (2–4 weeks) of planned, elective surgery.[22]

Other interventions to reduce risk of perioperative cardiac complications should be individualized based on the preoperative evaluation.

Pulmonary risk assessment

Much emphasis has been placed on perioperative cardiac risk assessment; however, postoperative pulmonary complications are as common (and, in some case series, more common) as cardiac complications and equally predict perioperative mortality.[4] A reduction in lung volume occurs during surgery, which in older patients compounds the age-related changes in the pulmonary system, leading to atelectasis and other complications. Clinically important pulmonary complications are pneumonia, atelectasis, bronchospasm, respiratory failure with prolonged mechanical ventilation and exacerbation of COPD.[4] Risk factors for pulmonary complications can be divided into patient-related and procedure-related.

Patient-related risk factors include COPD (most important patient-related factor, increasing risk by 3–4-fold), cigarette use (increases risk by threefold), smoking cessation in the 1–2 months prior to surgery, ASA class >2, poor exercise tolerance (measured by an inability to perform supine bicycle exercise test for 2 min), albumin levels $<3\,g\,dl^{-1}$ and blood urea nitrogen levels $>30\,mg\,dl^{-1}$.[4,14,23]

Procedure-related risk factors include type and length of surgery, long hospital stay, anaesthesia type (lower risk with spinal or epidural) and long-acting neuromuscular blockade (pancuronium).[4,14,23]

The single strongest predictor of postoperative pulmonary complications, outweighing all patient-specific factors, is surgical site.[4] Thoracic and upper abdominal surgeries (closest to the diaphragm) carry the highest risk. Neurological, peripheral vascular, abdominal aortic aneurism and neck surgeries also carry a high risk, presumably owing to the increased length of these procedures and a higher incidence of smoking and COPD in patients undergoing them.[4]

A multifactorial risk index for predicting postoperative respiratory failure has been developed; however, its use for risk reduction is limited by the fact that none of the factors are modifiable in the immediate preoperative period.[7] The utility of preoperative pulmonary function testing for predicting outcome and perioperative management is not supported by evidence and is not routinely recommended.[4]

Interventions to reduce risk of pulmonary complications can be effective. Preoperatively, pulmonary status should be optimized. If elective surgery is planned 8 or more weeks in advance, the geriatrician ought to encourage smoking cessation, teach lung expansion manoeuvres and refer for pulmonary rehabilitation with a focus on improving exercise capacity. If surgery is planned within 1–2 months, patients should not be encouraged to quit smoking, as this can actually increase the risk of postoperative pulmonary complications.[4,10] Exacerbations of COPD or asthma and lower respiratory tract infections should be treated prior to proceeding with surgery.

Intraoperative risk reduction strategies, such as shorter surgical durations and avoidance of pancuronium, require the consulting geriatric specialist to collaborate with the surgeon and anaesthesiologist.[4]

Postoperative risk reduction strategies focus on lung expansion. Incentive spirometry, deep breathing and early ambulation are simple, low-risk, inexpensive and effective methods to avoid atelectasis and pneumonia. Adequate pain control is essential to prevent splinting and maximize lung expansion manoeuvres.[4,10]

Neurocognitive risk assessment

Perioperative neurological complications are common in elderly surgical patients and include cerebral vascular accident or transient ischaemic attack, delirium and neurocognitive disorder. The most common is postoperative delirium (PD).[9,10] Neurological complications increase morbidity, mortality and length of hospital stay.[9,24]

PD is distinguished from postoperative cognitive disorder (POCD) in its time course and manifestation. Delirium is defined by acute, fluctuating changes in memory, consciousness and perception. It is identified using DSM IV or Confusion Assessment Method (CAM) criteria. The incidence of PD in the literature varies widely, from 3 to 61%, with increased incidence in orthopaedic and aortic surgeries.[10,15,24] Major factors predisposing to delirium are increasing age, mild cognitive impairment (MCI), frailty and dementia. Modifiable risk factors for PD include intraoperative blood loss, postoperative anaemia (haematocrit <30%), electrolyte imbalances, sepsis, use of a bladder catheter, physical restraints, poor postoperative mobility and polypharmacy.[10,15] Preoperative evaluation begins with cognitive assessment for MCI, dementia and pre-existing delirium. Examples of assessment tools are given in other chapters of this book (see Section 7, Dementia and Cognitive Disorders, for more details on geriatric cognitive assessment). The geriatric consultant should then assess the patient for the presence of the modifiable risk factors listed above. Geriatrics consultation was shown to reduce PD in a group of elderly hip fracture patients.[25]

Using a structured protocol, a consulting geriatrician made individualized recommendations that addressed modifiable risks for PD. The results were compared with a control group who received usual care by the orthopaedic surgical team. The most frequently followed recommendations were transfusion to keep haematocrit >30%, removal of indwelling urinary catheters by postoperative day two and discontinuing or limiting the use of psychoactive medications. In the geriatric consultation group, no difference in delirium duration or length of stay was noted; however, there was a statistically significant reduction in the incidence of delirium with an NNT of 5.6.[25]

Multidisciplinary non-pharmacological interventions targeting modifiable factors have been shown to decrease delirium;[26] however, research continues in order to find effective pharmacological therapy for the prevention and treatment of PD. A blinded, randomized, placebo-controlled trial evaluated the use of low-dose haloperidol for prophylaxis against PD in a cohort of 430 hip surgery patients. The incidence of delirium did not differ between the groups; however, the severity was lower and duration of delirium and hospital length of stay were shorter in the group given haloperidol.[26] Unfortunately, this study was underpowered and further study is needed before recommendations can be made for pharmacological prophylaxis of PD.

In contrast to PD, POCD manifests days or weeks after surgery and is characterized by impaired concentration, language comprehension, social integration and ability to learn new information that can persist for months to years. The literature suggests a prevalence rate of 15–25% and is most common after coronary artery bypass grafting.[27] The exact aetiology of POCD is unclear, but some perioperative risk factors have been identified, including age, duration of surgery, lack of education, postoperative infection or inflammation, hyperglycaemia and hyperthermia.[10,28] Some evidence for cholinergic and dopaminergic imbalance has been suggested. Of note, general anaesthesia has *not* been associated with increased rates of POCD or PD.[27] Management of POCD has not been well established and largely focuses on supportive care.

Postoperative management of the geriatric patient

The role of the geriatric specialist to improve postoperative outcomes begins before surgery but continues until discharge. There are seven common postoperative problems that if not prevented or managed appropriately can lead to physical decline and poor outcomes (see Box 127.1).[29]

Immobility

Bed rest is bad. The multiple complications of immobility include ulcer formation, bone loss, muscle weakness, psychosocial decline, atelectasis, aspiration, urinary retention, constipation, venous thrombosis and orthostatic hypotension.[29] The effects are even more profound in patients who were frail prior to surgery. The effects of bed rest are easily counteracted by early mobility and rehabilitation. For mobilization to occur successfully, the entire medical team, including doctors, nurses and physical and occupational therapists, must formulate a rehabilitation plan and encourage patient participation.

Box 127.1 The 'Dirty Seven'

Seven barriers to a successful postoperative course

- Immobility
- Infection
- Venous thromboembolism
- Malnutrition
- Pain
- Ileus/constipation
- Urinary retention/incontinence

Infection

The three most common sites of postoperative infection in the elderly are urinary tract, surgical site and respiratory tract.[29] Interventions aimed at preventing infections should focus on those areas. To limit the rate of urinary tract infections, use of indwelling bladder catheters ought to be discouraged. If urinary retention is present, intermittent catheterization with mobilization and a commode toileting schedule is preferable. Aggressive pulmonary toilet and avoiding bed rest can decrease atelectasis and aspiration, which are significant risk factors for postoperative pneumonia. The surgical incision site needs to be examined frequently for signs of infection. Surgical site infections have been shown to increase mortality, hospital length of stay and cost in the elderly.[30] Close surveillance and adequate prophylaxis are particularly needed for patients coming from other healthcare facilities, including long-term care. In a group of elderly orthopaedic surgery patients, admission from a healthcare facility increased the risk of infection.[30] Antimicrobial prophylaxis should be administered 1 h prior to surgery and possibly continued 24 h postoperatively depending on surgical type The choice of antibiotic should be tailored to the institution's antibiogram to include appropriate coverage of the most common organisms.[29]

Venous thromboembolism

Several guidelines exist for the prophylaxis of venous thromboembolic phenomena (VTE). The most comprehensive guideline is from the American College of Chest Physicians (ACCP), last updated in 2008.[31] All surgical patients require prophylaxis against VTE. The type and duration of VTE prophylaxis depend on three factors: (1) surgical risk category, (2) presence of significant comorbid disease (e.g. cancer, renal insufficiency) and (3) bleeding risk. Tables 127.3 and 127.4 summarize the ACCP recommendations for perioperative VTE prophylaxis.[31,32]

Without prophylaxis, the rate of DVT in general surgery patients is estimated to occur at 10–40%; however, the incidence of DVT in orthopaedic surgery patients is much higher at 40–60%.[31] For this reason, the recommendation for VTE prophylaxis differs for orthopaedic patients. Table 127.5 gives a summary of the recommendations.[31,32]

Before initiating anticoagulation for VTE prophylaxis, an estimation of renal function is critical. Geriatric patients experience age- and disease-related reductions in renal function and creatinine clearance. It is essential to calculate creatinine clearance using the Cockroft–Gault or MDRD (Modification of Diet in Renal Disease) equation as creatinine levels may be deceptively normal. This is especially relevant for anticoagulant use as low-molecular weight heparins and fondaparinux are primarily renally eliminated. Reduced renal function leads to reduced drug clearance and increased serum drug concentrations.[32] Options for patients with renal insufficiency include the use of twice daily unfractionated heparin or reduced-dose enoxaparin (30 mg per day s.c.). Note that fondaparinux is contraindicated in patients with renal impairment.[32]

Table 127.3 Surgical risk categories for VTE.

Low risk	Minor or same-day surgery Age <40 years No additional VTE risk factors[a]
Moderate risk	Age <60 years Gynaecological or laparoscopic surgery ≤1 VTE risk factor[a]
High risk	General, colorectal, gynaecological, urological, bariatric or laparoscopic surgery Age >60 years ≥2 VTE risk factors[a]
Very high risk	Cancer surgery

[a]VTE risk factors include congestive heart failure, severe respiratory disease, immobility, active cancer and/or treatment for cancer, previous VTE, sepsis, acute neurological disease, inflammatory bowel disease, advanced age, obesity, central venous catheter and nephrotic syndrome.

Malnutrition

Presurgical nutritional status, classically assessed using serum albumin, predicts surgical outcomes in the elderly.[10] Preoperative optimization of nutrition with supplements may improve outcomes, but it is also important to ensure adequate nutrition postoperatively.[29] Registered dieticians can aid in assessing protein–calorie requirements and recommending appropriate supplementation.

Pain

For various reasons, elderly patients communicate pain less than younger patients, leaving them undertreated.[10] As mentioned previously, changes in the renal and neurological systems with ageing affect sensitivity to and serum concentrations of opioids. This has been shown to manifest as a decreased need for opioids several days following surgery in patients over the age of 70 years compared with younger patients. In the immediate postoperative period, however, the requirements are similar and intravenous doses of morphine and patient-controlled analgesia can be safely used.[10] For more information on the use of opioid medications in the elderly, see Chapter 135: End of life and palliative care

Table 127.4 Recommendations for perioperative VTE prophylaxis.

Risk category	Initiation	Duration	Prophylactic strategy
Low risk	Immediate	Indefinite	Early ambulation
Moderate risk	Within 12–24 h of surgery	7–10 days	Mechanical compression if bleeding risk Unfractionated heparin: 5000 U s.c. b.i.d. LMWH: Enoxaparin 40 mg per day s.c. Dalteparin 5000 IU per day s.c. Enoxaparin 60 mg s.c. b.i.d. (BMI >50 kg m^{-2}) Factor Xa inhibitor: Fondaparinux 2.5 mg per day s.c.
High risk	Within 12–24 h of surgery	7–10 days	Unfractionated heparin: 5000 U s.c. t.i.d. LMWH: Enoxaparin 40 mg per day s.c. Dalteparin 5000 IU per day s.c. Enoxaparin 60 mg s.c. b.i.d. (BMI >50 kg m^{-2}) Factor Xa inhibitor: Fondaparinux 2.5 mg per day s.c. Consider combination of anticoagulation and mechanical compression
Very high risk	2–12 h before or 12–24 h after surgery	≥7–10 days with consideration to extend up to 4 weeks	Unfractionated heparin: 5000 U s.c. t.i.d. LMWH: Enoxaparin 40 mg per day s.c. Dalteparin 5000 IU per day s.c. Tinzaparin 3500 IU per day s.c. Factor Xa inhibitor: Fondaparinux 2.5 mg per day s.c. Consider combination of anticoagulation and mechanical compression

Table 127.5 Recommendations for VTE prophylaxis in the orthopaedic surgical patient.

Type of surgery	Duration	Prophylactic strategy
Knee arthroscopy	Throughout hospital stay	Early ambulation LMWH if additional VTE risk factors are present
Hip fracture repair	10–35 days Initiate preoperatively if surgery delayed	LMWH: Enoxaparin 40 mg per day s.c. Enoxaparin 30 mg s.c. q12 Dalteparin 5000 IU per day s.c. Factor Xa inhibitor: Fondaparinux 2.5 mg per day s.c. Unfractionated heparin 5000 U s.c. b.i.d. or t.i.d. Adjusted-dose warfarin to INR 2.0–3.0
Total hip replacement	10–35 days	LMWH: Enoxaparin 40 mg per day s.c. Enoxaparin 30 mg s.c. q12 Dalteparin 5000 IU per day s.c. Factor Xa inhibitor: Fondaparinux 2.5 mg per day s.c. Adjusted-dose warfarin to INR 2.0–3.0
Total knee replacement	10–35 days	LMWH: Enoxaparin 30 mg s.c. q12 Factor Xa inhibitor: Fondaparinux 2.5 mg per day s.c. Adjusted-dose warfarin to INR 2.0–3.0

Constipation and ileus

Abdominal surgeries, bed rest and poor oral intake all contribute to ileus and constipation. For non-intestinal surgeries, bowel function should be stimulated early to prevent complications. Non-pharmacological strategies include mobilization and increase in fluid intake.[29] Pharmacological strategies include the use of stimulant laxatives. Stool softeners, such as docusate, do not work to stimulate bowel function postoperatively and are not recommended.

Urinary retention and incontinence

Urinary retention and incontinence are not normal signs of ageing. They can occur as a consequence of surgery-related factors, such as immobility, anticholinergic medications, postoperative delirium, indwelling catheters, faecal impaction and urinary tract infection. These causes should be investigated when abnormal urination occurs following surgery. A scheduled toileting plan should be instituted along with avoidance of indwelling catheters and early mobilization.[29]

Conclusion

Comprehensive perioperative management of the geriatric patient is crucial as the population ages and requires more surgical interventions. The perioperative course can be improved with geriatric consultation. Ideally, preoperative assessment and management would begin months in advance of elective surgery to improve premorbid functioning and minimize comorbid conditions. Smoking cessation, nutritional supplementation and improvement in exercise tolerance can all reduce the impact of age-related disease states on postoperative outcomes. Preoperative cardiac, pulmonary and neurological assessments can help identify patients at high risk of related complications and interventions aimed at reducing risk can be instituted. Postoperative problems can be prevented or ameliorated by early mobility, adequate pain control, toileting schedules, VTE prophylaxis and medication review. A multidisciplinary approach is necessary for successful implementation of risk-reduction strategies in the elder surgical patient.

Key points

- Focus on improving premorbid functioning prior to surgery.
- Smoking cessation improves outcomes.
- Peri- and postoperative involvement of a geriatrician can improve outcomes.

References

1. Westendorp RG. What is healthy aging in the 21st century? *Am J Clin Nutr* 2006; **83**: 404S–9S.
2. DeFrances CJ, Lucas CA, Buie VC and Golosinskiy A. 2006 National Hospital Discharge Survey. *Natl Health Stat Rep* 2008; **30**: 1–20.
3. Tonner PH, Kampen J and Scholz J. Pathophysiological changes in the elderly. *Best Pract Res Clin Anaesthesiol* 2003; **17**: 163–77.
4. Smetana GW. Preoperative pulmonary assessment of the older adult. *Clin Geriatr Med* 2003; **19**: 35–55.
5. Yashin AI, Begun AS, Boiko SI *et al.* New age patterns of survival improvement in Sweden: do they characterize changes in individual aging? *Mech Ageing Dev* 2002; **123**: 637–47.
6. Polanczyk CA, Marcantonio E, Goldman L *et al.* Impact of age on perioperative complications and length of stay in patients undergoing noncardiac surgery. *Ann Intern Med* 2001; **134**: 637–43.
7. Arozullah AM, Daley J, Henderson WG and Khuri SF. Multifactorial risk index for predicting postoperative respiratory failure in men after major noncardiac surgery. The National Veterans Administration Surgical Quality Improvement Program. *Ann Surg* 2000; **232**: 242–53.
8. ASA. Physical status classification system, 2009, http://www.asahq.org/clinical/physicalstatus.htm (last accessed 16 September 2011).
9. Liu LL and Leung JM. Predicting adverse postoperative outcomes in patients aged 80 years or older. *J Am Geriatr Soc* 2000; **48**: 405–12.
10. Loran DB, Hyde BR and Zwischenberger JB. Perioperative management of special populations: the geriatric patient. *Surg Clin North Am* 2005; **85**: 1259–66, xi.
11. Cook TM, Britton DC, Craft TM *et al.* An audit of hospital mortality after urgent and emergency surgery in the elderly. *Ann R Coll Surg Engl* 1997; **79**: 361–7.
12. Neary WD, Foy C, Heather BP and Earnshaw JJ. Identifying high-risk patients undergoing urgent and emergency surgery. *Ann R Coll Surg Engl* 2006; **88**: 151–6.
13. Arenal JJ and Bengoechea-Beeby M. Mortality associated with emergency abdominal surgery in the elderly. *Can J Surg* 2003; **46**: 111–6.
14. Gerson MC, Hurst JM, Hertzberg VS *et al.* Prediction of cardiac and pulmonary complications related to elective abdominal and noncardiac thoracic surgery in geriatric patients. *Am J Med* 1990; **88**: 101–7.
15. Dasgupta M and Dumbrell AC. Preoperative risk assessment for delirium after noncardiac surgery: a systematic review. *J Am Geriatr Soc* 2006; **54**: 1578–89.
16. Fleisher LA, Beckman JA, Brown KA *et al.* ACC/AHA 2007 guidelines on perioperative cardiovascular evaluation and care for noncardiac surgery: a report of the American College of Cardiology/American Heart Association Task Force on Practice Guidelines (Writing Committee to Revise the 2002 Guidelines on Perioperative Cardiovascular Evaluation for Noncardiac Surgery): developed in collaboration with the American Society of Echocardiography, American Society

of Nuclear Cardiology, Heart Rhythm Society, Society of Cardiovascular Anesthesiologists, Society for Cardiovascular Angiography and Interventions, Society for Vascular Medicine and Biology and Society for Vascular Surgery. *Circulation* 2007; **116**: e418–99.

17. Goldman L, Caldera DL, Nussbaum SR *et al.* Multifactorial index of cardiac risk in noncardiac surgical procedures. *N Engl J Med* 1977; **297**: 845–50.
18. Lee TH, Marcantonio ER, Mangione CM *et al.* Derivation and prospective validation of a simple index for prediction of cardiac risk of major noncardiac surgery. *Circulation* 1999; **100**: 1043–9.
19. McGory ML, Maggard MA and Ko CY. A meta-analysis of perioperative beta blockade: what is the actual risk reduction? *Surgery* 2005; **138**: 171–9.
20. Bangalore S, Wetterslev J, Pranesh S *et al.* Perioperative beta blockers in patients having non-cardiac surgery: a meta-analysis. *Lancet* 2008; **372**: 1962–76.
21. Devereaux PJ, Yang H, Yusuf S *et al.* Effects of extended-release metoprolol succinate in patients undergoing non-cardiac surgery (POISE trial): a randomised controlled trial. *Lancet* 2008; **371**: 1839–47.
22. Poldermans D and Devereaux PJ. The experts debate: perioperative beta-blockade for noncardiac surgery – proven safe or not ? *Cleve Clin J Med* 2009; **76**(Suppl 4): S84–92.
23. Garibaldi RA, Britt MR, Coleman ML *et al.* Risk factors for postoperative pneumonia. *Am J Med* 1981; **70**: 677–80.
24. Andersson EM, Gustafson L and Hallberg IR. Acute confusional state in elderly orthopaedic patients: factors of importance for detection in nursing care. *Int J Geriatr Psychiatry* 2001; **16**: 7–17.
25. Marcantonio ER, Flacker JM, Wright RJ and Resnick NM. Reducing delirium after hip fracture: a randomized trial. *J Am Geriatr Soc* 2001; **49**: 516–22.
26. Kalisvaart KJ, de Jonghe JF, Bogaards MJ *et al.* Haloperidol prophylaxis for elderly hip-surgery patients at risk for delirium: a randomized placebo-controlled study. *J Am Geriatr Soc* 2005; **53**: 1658–66.
27. Bryson GL and Wyand A. Evidence-based clinical update: general anesthesia and the risk of delirium and postoperative cognitive dysfunction. *Can J Anaesth* 2006; **53**: 669–77.
28. Martin JF, Melo RO and Sousa LP. Postoperative cognitive dysfunction after cardiac surgery. *Rev Bras Cir Cardiovasc* 2008; **23**: 245–55.
29. Beliveau MM and Multach M. Perioperative care for the elderly patient. *Med Clin North Am* 2003; **87**: 273–89.
30. Lee J, Singletary R, Schmader K *et al.* Surgical site infection in the elderly following orthopaedic surgery. Risk factors and outcomes. *J Bone Joint Surg Am* 2006; **88**: 1705–12.
31. Geerts WH, Bergqvist D, Pineo GF *et al.* Prevention of venous thromboembolism: American College of Chest Physicians Evidence-Based Clinical Practice Guidelines (8th Edition). *Chest* 2008; **133**(6 Suppl): 381S–453S.
32. Muntz JE and Michota FA. Prevention and management of venous thromboembolism in the surgical patient: options by surgery type and individual patient risk factors. *Am J Surg* 2010; **199**(1 Suppl): S11–20.

CHAPTER 128

Anaesthesia

Suzanne Crowe
Adelaide Meath and National Children's Hospital, Dublin, and University of Dublin, Ireland

Introduction

Elderly surgical patients present a specific challenge to anaesthesiologists and may be at greater risk of an adverse outcome.[1] This is accounted for by a reduced ability to maintain or restore physiological homeostasis in the face of surgical and medical disease. This is exacerbated further by the presence of medical comorbidity such as cardiac or pulmonary disease or diabetes mellitus.[2] The statistical likelihood of having a coincident medical pathology increases with advancing years. The elderly have a higher rate of mortality associated with anaesthesia and surgery than their younger counterparts. Postoperative adverse events on the cardiac, pulmonary, renal and cerebral systems are the main concerns for older surgical patients at high risk. The very fact that the patient requires hospital admission for their surgery exposes them to risk, with familiar hazards including nosocomial infection, administration of the wrong drug and side effects of certain procedures and investigations. Elderly patients are more likely to experience an adverse event during their hospital stay. The reduction of iatrogenic injury is one of the stated aims of the World Health Organization.[3]

The elderly, in particular those older than 85 years, are the fastest growing segment of the European and North American populations.[4] Accordingly, overall life expectancy and active life expectancy have increased.[4] The number of older patients presenting for surgery and anaesthesia is increasing and should not be a bar to surgery.[5] The complexity of surgical procedures is also expanding. In 2001, the Association of Anaesthetists of Great Britain and Ireland called for this expansion to be recognized and incorporated into service provision. They also called for greater availability of 24 h recovery facilities, High Dependency Unit (HDU) and Intensive Therapy Unit (ITU) beds for these patients.[6]

The National Confidential Enquiry into Perioperative Deaths[7] highlighted the importance of availability of high dependency and intensive care facilities for the safe care of older patients: 'the decision to operate includes the commitment to provide appropriate supportive care'.

This chapter elaborates on some of the risks to the elderly patient during the perioperative period and how they may be managed in order to minimize postoperative morbidity and mortality in this vulnerable patient group.

Outcome of surgery and anaesthesia in the elderly

Mortality after surgery and anaesthesia is defined as the death rate within 30 days.[7] The outcome of older patients from surgery, in general terms, has been studied by several groups in the past two decades,[8–10] suggesting that healthcare practitioners have anecdotally identified areas for potential clinical improvement for many years. However, there are no recent surgical outcome studies for older patients. These early studies suggest that older patients have acceptable rates of perioperative mortality. There have been many advances in surgery and anaesthesia, such as laparoscopic surgery, ultra-short-acting anaesthetic medications, regional pain management and more extensive use of critical care services, over the past two decades, reducing mortality rates (Table 128.1, Figure 128.1). Higher mortality rates are associated with higher American Association of Anesthesiologists (ASA) grade of physical status grade and emergency procedures.[11] ASA is an independent predictor of mortality (Table 128.2). The highest risk surgical procedure in older patients is an exploratory laparotomy, because of the high risk of bowel infarction and disseminated carcinomatosis.

The presence of preoperative renal, liver and central nervous system impairment was a predictor of poorer outcome. Albumin, a marker of nutritional status, may serve as a surrogate marker for the preoperative health status of the surgical geriatric patient.[12]

Principles and Practice of Geriatric Medicine, Fifth Edition. Edited by Alan J. Sinclair, John E. Morley and Bruno Vellas.

Table 128.1 Mortality associated with surgery and anaesthesia.

Age (years)	Mortality rate (%)	Ref.
General population	1.2	13
60–69	2.2	13
70–79	2.9	13
>80	5.8–6.2	10
>90	8.4	9
>95	13	10

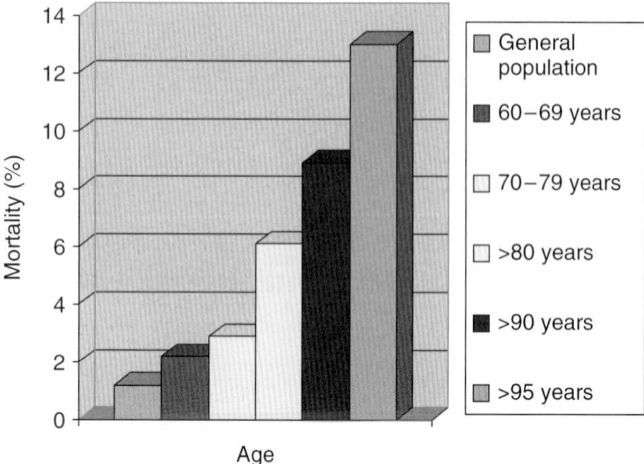

Figure 128.1 Mortality associated with surgery and anaesthesia.

Table 128.2 ASA grading of physical status.[11]

Grade	Status
I	Normal healthy patient
II	Patient with mild systemic disease
III	Patient with severe systemic disease
IV	Patient with severe systemic disease which presents a constant threat to life
V	Moribund patient not expected to survive without operation

Reproduced by permission of the American Society of Anaesthesiologists, Inc.

Cardiovascular morbidity associated with surgery and anaesthesia

The age-related changes that occur within the cardiovascular system are responsible for the higher incidence of perioperative myocardial infarction, cardiac failure and arrhythmias in this age group. There is a reduction in the sensitivity of the parasympathetic system to changes in baroreceptor stretch, blood pressure and heart rate. The sensitivity of the sympathetic system also declines. This diminishes the body's ability to compensate for sudden change. There is a progressive stiffening of both the arterial and venous vessels, again reducing capacity for vasoconstriction or dilatation in the face of loss of intravascular volume. Stiffening of the myocardium also occurs, affecting diastolic relaxation and filling pressures. This may lead on to diastolic dysfunction with an increase in left atrial pressure and pulmonary congestion.

Superimposed on physiological change, anaesthetic agents cause peripheral vasodilatation, with a decrease in systemic vascular resistance. As many elderly patients have a contracted intravascular volume secondary to diuretic therapy, this can mean a sudden fall in tissue perfusion pressure. Anaesthetic agents are myocardial depressants, particularly in higher doses, and have the capacity to affect cardiac output adversely. Preoperative assessment is focused on identifying those risk factors that have been identified in studies as being predictive of adverse postoperative outcome (Table 128.3).[13,14] Following the initial interview, the patient's baseline level of function is assessed. If there are no significant predictors in the history, evaluation may be safely confined to detailed physical examination and a 12-lead electrocardiogram (ECG). The ECG will identify patients with left ventricular hypertrophy or ST segment depression. These patients may require further investigation with an exercise ECG, depending on the surgical procedure planned. Determination of the anaerobic threshold for each patient using cardiopulmonary exercise testing is now considered a sensitive tool for determining patients at high risk.[15] Patients who cannot exercise because of claudication or arthritis may be assessed with a dobutamine stress echocardiograph. Coronary angiography is reserved for patients with angina at rest or unstable angina. On the basis of the results, preoperative revascularization may be warranted. Clinically detected cardiac murmurs and features of congestive cardiac failure are further evaluated using echocardiography.

Preoperative valve replacement is indicated for patients with severe disease. Less severe valve lesions or those

Table 128.3 Predictive factors for postoperative cardiovascular morbidity.

Myocardial infarction within previous 3 months
Decompensated congestive cardiac failure
Arrhythmia (except premature atrial contractions)
Unstable angina or angina at rest (New York Heart Association Grade IV)
Uncontrolled hypertension
Severe valvular disease
Poor general medical condition
Poor exercise capacity
Diabetes mellitus
History of stroke

following valve surgery require prophylactic antibiotic administration. Arrhythmia detected at rest or during exercise should be treated if possible before surgery. If sinus rhythm is not achieved, rate control with anticoagulation is acceptable. Type II or type III heart block requires insertion of a temporary or permanent pacemaker. Using the information gained from the history, examination and further investigations, the anaesthetic management is aimed at maximizing myocardial perfusion through maintenance of tissue perfusion pressure and oxygenation throughout the intra- and postoperative period. Postoperative admission to the HDU or intensive care unit (ICU) should be anticipated for elderly patients with significant cardiac symptoms, especially those undergoing abdominal or thoracic procedures. Invasive monitoring of blood pressure and central venous pressure is commenced early and continued throughout the perioperative period. Regional anaesthesia provides superior analgesia postoperatively and may reduce the incidence of adverse cardiac events in certain patients, such as vascular and abdominal surgery. The institution of perioperative β-receptor blockade has been shown to reduce the risk of myocardial ischaemia and is generally well tolerated by older patients.[16] β-Blockade is thought to increase the time spent in diastole, increasing filling and increasing time for coronary artery perfusion. A combination of intravenous fluid infusion and vasopressor agents is used to maintain mean arterial blood pressure within 20% of the patient's baseline, awake blood pressure. Episodes of hypotension must be managed promptly and oxygenation increased during the period of reduced flow.

Postoperatively, the patient requires a similar level of care and monitoring. Supplemental oxygen therapy, optimum analgesia, rate control and judicious blood transfusion will assist in maximizing myocardial oxygen supply. Particular attention should focus on the first 3 days, when myocardial infarction is most likely to occur. Many episodes of ischaemia in this age group may be silent and may not be associated with the development of Q waves on the ECG. A low index of suspicion, the presence of new ST changes, in combination with serial estimations of serum troponin T and I concentrations, will assist in early diagnosis.

Respiratory morbidity associated with surgery and anaesthesia

The physiological changes associated with ageing predispose the older patient to respiratory complications after surgery and anaesthesia. A mixed obstructive–restrictive pattern develops from the decrease in total lung capacity, elastic recoil of the thorax, pulmonary parenchymal compliance and vital capacity. Decreased compliance and muscle power mean a fall in forced expiration and a reduced capacity to cough and clear secretions. Closing capacity, dead space and residual volume increase so that the lungs of the supine patient become atelectatic. These changes do not occur in a uniform manner throughout the lungs, resulting in areas of good ventilation in combination with underventilated segments. A decrease in pulmonary blood flow combined with progressive loss of alveolar surface area diminishes the resting arterial oxygen tension from 95 ± 2 mmHg at age 20 years to 73 ± 5 mmHg at age 75 years. Occurring in tandem, there is an age-associated loss of central nervous system sensitivity to changes in arterial oxygen and carbon dioxide tensions. The physiological and structural changes cause an increase in ventilation–perfusion mismatch. This is exacerbated by the effect of anaesthesia, in particular, general anaesthesia. In addition, general anaesthesia reduces reflex pulmonary hypoxic vasoconstriction. Regional anaesthesia impacts less on the respiratory system as it does not necessitate intubation of the trachea, avoids the effect of intermittent positive pressure ventilation and provides highly effective postoperative pain relief.

Preoperative preparation of the patient involves a detailed history and examination in combination with functional assessment. Taking the patient for a walk, including two flights of stairs, during the preoperative visit provides a useful measure of the patient's baseline physiological status. Smoking cessation for at least 8 weeks is to be recommended.[17] Chest physiotherapy in the 24 h preceding surgery provides some physical benefit and facilitates instruction for deep breathing and coughing postoperatively. Patients with active pulmonary infection require more postponement of surgery and more aggressive medical treatment. The anaesthetic technique should employ regional analgesia/anaesthesia where possible. Short-acting agents such as propofol, remifentanil, sevoflurane and atracurium are most suitable for general anaesthesia. Muscle relaxants should always be reversed at the end of the procedure. Invasive monitoring may be used to advantage to guide fluid therapy as the older patient will tolerate rapid expansion of intravascular and extravascular volumes poorly due to the changes in pulmonary compliance, perfusion and renal function. This may be continued into the postoperative period in the context of ICU or HDU admission. Postoperatively, oxygen supplementation and chest physiotherapy should be continued for a minimum of 5 days as this is the greatest period of risk of nocturnal hypoxia and the onset of pneumonia.

Central nervous system morbidity associated with surgery and anaesthesia

Elderly patients are at risk of serious central nervous system morbidity and mortality due to neuronal loss associated with ageing, the presence of coincident pathology such as cerebrovascular atherosclerosis and a reduction in neurotransmitter concentrations. This makes them less able to adapt successfully to the challenges imposed by surgery and anaesthesia. The morbidity associated with anaesthesia and surgery in the older patient most commonly takes the form of postoperative confusion (POC) or stroke.

Postoperative confusion

The risk factors for the development of POC are listed in Table 128.4. POC is associated with an increased rate of morbidity, delayed return to baseline function and delayed discharge home from hospital. To date, there is little evidence for an overall strategy to reduce the incidence in surgical patients, but some general recommendations may be made.

Consideration should be given to admitting the patient as a daycase, as elderly patients become less disorientated when in familiar surroundings with familiar carers. The preoperative assessment should highlight particular issues that could be modified or pre-empted, such as alcohol withdrawal depression. Hearing aids and spectacles should be left with the patient until induction of anaesthesia and returned to the patient as soon as possible. Medications listed in Table 128.3 should be avoided. Intraoperative monitoring of blood pressure, ventilation and oxygenation requires a meticulous approach.

Table 128.4 Risk factors for the development of postoperative confusion.

Preoperative factors
Older age
Depression/anxiety
Dementia
Preoperative sensory deficit in hearing or vision
Alcohol withdrawal/sedative withdrawal
Preoperative use of multiple medications
Intraoperative factors
Hypoxia
Hypocarbia
Hypotension
Postoperative factors
Inadequate analgesia
Perioperative factors
Sepsis
Surgical procedure
Cardiac surgery
Orthopaedic surgery, especially joint replacement
Perioperative medications
Anticholinergics: atropine, scopolamine. Glycopyrrolate to a lesser extent
Barbiturates
Benzodiazepines
Antihistamines

Hypoxaemia and hypercarbia should be avoided. The minimum number of medications possible should be employed. Regional analgesic techniques should be employed where possible to reduce the use of sedating narcotics in the postoperative period. There is no difference in the incidence of POC between the intraoperative use of general anaesthesia and spinal or epidural anaesthesia.[18] A geriatrician should be involved in the care of the patient at high risk of confusion. Postoperatively, if the patient is confused, they should be nursed in a quiet, dark room. Organic causes should be treated promptly. Haloperidol 0.25–2 mg orally at night may be useful. Low doses of diazepam or chlorpromazine may be used as adjuncts if the patient does not respond to simple measures. Physical restraints usually serve to antagonize the patient further and should not be used. Referral to the occupational therapy and social work departments will be necessary to assist with cognitive assessment, follow-up and discharge planning.

Long-term cognitive impairment has been documented by the International Study of Postoperative Cognitive Dysfunction (ISPOCD).[19] About 10% of patients were found to have cognitive deficits 3 months after surgery, with age as the only significant predictive factor.

Postoperative stroke

There have been few studies to determine the incidence of stroke occurring after surgery and anaesthesia. The incidence from small retrospective studies seem to suggest that the incidence is low, in the order of 0.25% when a patient is undergoing non-carotid vascular surgery.[20] Stroke most commonly occurs between days 5 and 26 postoperatively. Risk factors for postoperative stroke are given in Table 128.5.[21]

Patients with poorly controlled preoperative hypertension should have their surgery postponed to allow time to institute adequate pharmacological control. Patients with clinically detected carotid bruits should have further investigations and, if necessary, referral to a vascular surgeon before their intended procedure. The severity of the neurological deficit and the potential for rehabilitation after perioperative stroke vary enormously and therapy must be directed at the individual patient.

Renal morbidity associated with surgery and anaesthesia

Renal function is known to deteriorate with age and, therefore, greater care will be needed to maintain renal function perioperatively. Decline in numbers of the functional unit, the glomerulus, with age means that glomerular filtration

Table 128.5 Risk factors for postoperative stroke in the elderly.

Preoperative factors
Pre-existing cerebrovascular disease
Ischaemic cardiac disease
Atherosclerosis
Carotid occlusion
Preoperative vascular disease
Hypertension
Diabetes mellitus
Physical inactivity
Intraoperative and postoperative factors
Haemodynamic instability
Hypoxaemia

Reproduced by permission of Oxford University Press/ *British Journal of Anaesthesia* from Jin and Chung.[21] Copyright The Board of Management and Trustees of the *British Journal of Anaesthesia*.

rate (GFR) falls from 125 ml min^{-1} in the young adult to 80 ml min^{-1} in the older individual. As this fall in GFR is usually accompanied by a decrease in muscle mass, there is rarely an increase in serum creatinine. During the perioperative period, the kidney will be exposed to many challenges: rapid fluid shifts in the intravascular and extravascular compartments, numerous medications administered simultaneously, electrolyte changes and acid–base abnormalities. In the face of these challenges, the underlying loss of function becomes exposed, leading to the development of postoperative renal failure. Atherosclerosis of the vascular supply of the kidney and coincident disease due to diabetes mellitus or hypertension further complicate the situation. In addition, the elderly patient tends to be taking a greater number of prescribed medications that have the potential to interact with anaesthetic agents and conditions arising during surgery, such as hypotension. Anaesthetic drugs have little direct effect on renal function. Anaesthetic agents reduce cardiac output with subsequent renal vasoconstriction, which may cause a fall in renal perfusion. Enflurane and isoflurane produce fluoride when metabolized, which may cause renal injury if the anaesthesia is very prolonged. Sevoflurane produces a substance known as compound A at low fresh gas flows, which is nephrotoxic if not removed by effective scavenging of waste anaesthetic gases.[22] It is unusual for either of these chemical entities to present a problem in the clinical context.

Management of the patient starts with a high index of suspicion. Following a detailed preoperative review, fluid and electrolyte status should be closely monitored in the pre-, intra- and postoperative periods. Nephrotoxic medications should be stopped preoperatively if possible. Medications that deplete the intravascular volume and lead to electrolyte loss should be reviewed in the context of the patient's state of hydration and the planned surgical procedure. For example, a patient taking a loop diuretic scheduled for elective inguinal hernia repair should probably continue taking the medication, whereas a patient with low urinary output scheduled for emergency laparotomy for bowel obstruction should have the loop diuretic reviewed by the anaesthesiologist. The dosing intervals of medications excreted by the kidney such as aminoglycosides may need to change and doses titrated to plasma levels. The development of perioperative renal failure increases the requirement for renal replacement, intensive care admission and mortality. Acute tubular necrosis accounts for the majority of cases of renal failure. Prevention is based on optimizing the circulation preoperatively, close haemodynamic monitoring perioperatively and maintenance of adequate perfusion pressures, including the judicious use of inotropes. Intraoperative low-dose dopamine infusion promoting renal vasodilatation and the use of mannitol as a free radical scavenger have been advocated.[23,24]

Perioperative hypothermia

Elderly patients are at a greater risk of developing perioperative hypothermia than younger patients, owing to a number of factors. They have a reduced muscle mass, with a lower basal metabolic rate. This is often accompanied by reduced fat stores secondary to malnutrition. The shivering mechanism occurs later in response to cooling. In young patients, shivering begins peripherally at 1°C less than the normal core temperature of 36.5°C. As patients age, this may not occur until their core temperature has fallen by 2°C. Shivering increases cellular oxygen demands by 20–30%, increasing myocardial oxygen consumption, which may be deleterious for the older patient with cardiovascular pathology. Less vasoconstriction occurs in the older patient for a given fall in temperature, meaning that more heat is lost to the environment.

Surgery and anaesthesia have a detrimental effect on thermoregulation. Anaesthetic agents cause peripheral vasodilatation with abolition of the shivering mechanism so that patients lose the ability to compensate for cooling. The opening of major cavities such as the abdomen and thorax increases the amount of heat lost to the environment. The effects of perioperative hypothermia are listed in Table 128.6. Prevention of hypothermia is more efficient and cost-effective than warming the patient postoperatively. Patients should be kept in a warm room with blankets during their admission to the operating department. Induction of anaesthesia should take place in a similar environment. Anaesthetic gases should be warmed and humidified.

Intravenous fluids should be warmed. Sterile preparation of the operative site should take place using warmed sterile solutions. A warm ambient temperature of the operating room should be maintained until the patient is draped. Forced air warming blankets may be placed under the

Table 128.6 Effects of perioperative hypothermia.

- Increased cardiac morbidity
- Increased incidence of cardiac arrhythmias
- Altered platelet function
- Increased blood loss
- Increased blood viscosity – combined with vasoconstriction may cause a higher incidence of deep venous thrombosis
- Shift of oxygen dissociation curve to the left with less oxygen released by haemoglobin to the tissues
- Inhalation of cold gases causes reduction in protective reflexes in the respiratory tract through effects on cilia motility
- Increased incidence of postoperative wound infection
- Increased incidence of postoperative decubitus ulcers
- Decreased drug metabolism, resulting in longer recovery times
- Prolonged hospitalization

drapes. At the end of the procedure, warm blankets should be placed over the patient during their transfer to the post-anaesthetic care unit.

Preoperative assessment

When carrying out a preoperative assessment of the older patient, it is important to place the function of the cardiovascular and respiratory systems into the context of the whole patient. It must be remembered that patients may have mild cognitive impairment affecting their memory or they may be embarrassed and unwilling to admit disability. Answers may be slow as information is recalled. The history may be extensive and complicated and so sufficient time should be allotted to the interview. The clinical presentation of disease may differ greatly from that in younger patients. Conditions such as hyper- and hypothyroidism are notoriously difficult to diagnose in the older patient. It is best if the assessment takes place several days before the planned surgery to allow enough time for further investigations if necessary.

Attendance at a preanaesthetic outpatient clinic will mean that the patient can meet all of the multidisciplinary team members together, providing enhanced perioperative and discharge planning. Following the interview, the anaesthesiologist must review the patient's medical chart and carry out a comprehensive physical examination. Keeping in mind the demands and implications of each surgical procedure, the anaesthetic plan will then be made and discussed with the patient. The anaesthesiologist should expect much variation between each elderly patient. Routine investigations based on age alone are not warranted and should be directed by the clinical evaluation.[25]

Particular issues to be addressed over the course of the assessment are the following:

1 The planned surgery.
2 The cognitive status of the patient. Does the patient answer questions in a coherent manner? Will they be suitable for ambulatory admission or a regional anaesthetic technique?
3 The baseline function of the patient. Can they dress themselves, do the shopping, walk up a short flight of stairs?
4 Does the patient have symptoms suggestive of cardiac disease? Remember, patients may not report symptoms because of reduced mobility.
5 Does the patient have signs or symptoms of respiratory disease? Shortness of breath at rest is an important prognostic sign.
6 What are the patient's current medications and their compliance with them?
7 Previous anaesthetic experiences.
8 Vital signs on examination, especially blood pressure, pulse rate and rhythm.

Meticulous attention to detail when planning the perioperative care of the patient can reduce the incidence of minor morbidity. Reduction of minor incidents may prevent escalation into life-threatening events.

Pain assessment and management in the elderly

Pain assessment

Effective pain management in the elderly is subject to all of the usual barriers to pain management, such as fear of addiction. With the older surgical patient, there are additional problems to be overcome. The assessment of pain forms the basis of successful pain relief. It is necessary to obtain a baseline measure of pain before instituting pharmacological measures to reduce that pain. Assessment allows the treatment to be evaluated and the need for further pain relief established.[26]

Conventional pain scores such as the visual analogue score (VAS) have limited application in this age-group due to the prevalence of mild/moderate cognitive impairment, hearing difficulties and poor eyesight. The older patient may differ significantly in their cultural interpretation of pain and pain relief.[27] Reporting of pain may be altered in this age group because of the misperception among older patients that it is necessary for pain to follow surgery and that staff are doing all that they can to relieve it. They may also fear reporting that they have pain in case this means something has gone wrong or that they may be seen as being 'difficult'. Healthcare staff may mistake patients who do not report pain for patients who do *not* have pain. Attempts have been made to validate other scoring systems in older adults, but at present there is no single system suitable for all elderly patients.[28] The accuracy of pain assessments may be increased by making the assessment more frequently, particularly following the administration of each analgesic dose. Another hurdle to achieving adequate pain relief is the assumption that elderly patients do not experience pain to the same extent as younger patients. There is very little evidence for this misperception.[29]

Effect of pain in older surgical patients

The consequences of pain in surgical patients include the following:[30]

- sympathetic hyperactivity, producing tachycardia, myocardial ischaemia, hypertension via the adrenal hormonal axis;
- decreased pulmonary function with atelectasis and hypoxaemia, as a result of poor cough and reduced mobility;
- increased risk of deep venous thrombosis (DVT), as a result of reduced mobility;
- potential development of a chronic pain state through sensitization of pain pathways;
- postoperative delirium, which is particularly the case in patients who have predisposing risk factors for delirium such as visual, hearing or cognitive deficit;
- increased length of stay.

Adequate pain relief in all patients may reduce postoperative morbidity.[30] The preoperative assessment visit should be used as an opportunity to discuss with the patient the postoperative analgesia pertinent for their procedure, particularly when regional analgesic techniques are planned. Education and reassurance may be provided to the patient and their family, diminishing their concerns regarding addiction and side effects. Instruction may be given on the use of equipment for patient-controlled analgesia (PCA), which may be reinforced later by a visit from the acute pain team.

Pharmacological management of pain

A continuous, multimodal approach to postoperative pain management is indicated for elderly patients because it minimizes potential adverse effects from high doses of any single agent. Changes in drug absorption, distribution, metabolism and elimination may affect the eventual plasma level and effect of a given analgesic drug. Increased gastric pH and decreased gastric motility reduce or delay drug absorption. The volume of distribution of drugs changes because of an increase in total body fat and a decrease in body water. Water-soluble opiates such as morphine have a smaller volume of distribution and therefore can produce higher plasma levels. Lipid-soluble drugs, such as fentanyl, have a larger volume of distribution and can produce a prolonged duration of action in older patients. Reduced serum albumin concentrations and other plasma proteins from chronic illness or poor nutrition will reduce drug distribution, increasing the potential for adverse affects. Concurrent medical conditions, for example, renal impairment, may reduce excretion of the drug from the body. Liver disease may reduce drug metabolism and lead to accumulation of active drug and active drug metabolites.

Reduced muscle mass leads to unpredictable absorption of drugs administered by the intramuscular route. The pharmacological analgesic options available are listed in Table 128.7. The key to effective pain management in patients of all ages is regular and appropriate assessment, combined with regular administration of multimodal analgesic agents.

The role of regional analgesia

The intraoperative use of regional anaesthetic techniques either in combination with general anaesthesia or alone has been shown to reduce short- and long-term mortality in the elderly following total hip arthroplasty, vascular surgery and abdominal surgery. It is thought to do this by sympatholysis, attenuating the stress response and improving myocardial oxygenation. Regional analgesia continued into the postoperative phase provides more profound analgesia with lower doses of narcotics than intravenous opioid administration, thus minimizing the potential for sedation, respiratory depression and ileus. It decreases the incidence of respiratory complications in patients undergoing abdominal and thoracic procedures and decreases admission rates to the intensive care unit and overall length of stay. Regional analgesia decreases the rate of postoperative DVT due to relative vasodilatation of the venous plexus in the lower limbs and by decreasing the time to mobilization. Continuous epidural analgesia postoperatively can cause hypotension and lower extremity motor and sensory deficits. For this reason, nursing and medical staff require training in the recognition and management of potential complications of regional analgesic techniques.

The role of patient-controlled analgesia (PCA) in the elderly

Intravenous PCA has been shown to be safe in elderly patients,[31] but healthcare staff frequently hesitate to prescribe it because of the concern that it may cause confusion or inadequate analgesia in the older patient. Older patients should not be automatically excluded from using PCA, via either the intravenous or the epidural route. The cognitive state and physical abilities of each patient should be assessed on an individual basis.

Ethical considerations for perioperative care of the elderly

Decisions regarding surgery and anaesthesia become more complicated in the older patient, particularly when their ability to make a competent decision is compromised

Table 128.7 Pharmacological analgesic options.

Agent	Advantages	Side effects
Acetaminophen (paracetamol)	Oral, intravenous and rectal routes Opioid sparing	Hepatotoxicity, do not exceed 4 g per 24 h
NSAIDs[a]	Oral, rectal, and parenteral routes Opioid sparing	Gastric irritation Renal toxicity Antiplatelet effects
COX-II[a] inhibitors	Oral and parenteral routes Opioid sparing	Gastric irritation Renal toxicity Less severe gastric irritation and renal toxicity than NSAIDs Possible cardiac effects
Opioids	Oral, rectal, parenteral, spinal and epidural routes Profound analgesia Available as short- and long-acting preparations	Sedation/confusion/dysphoria Respiratory depression Metabolites may be toxic, e.g. normeperidine Nausea/vomiting Ileus Pruritus Urinary retention when administered into CSF/epidural space Bradycardia Hypotension, especially if patient is dehydrated

[a]NSAID, non-steroidal anti-inflammatory drug; COX-II, cyclooxygenase-II.

through cognitive impairment or illness. Paternalism on the part of the physician does not respect the patient's fundamental right to autonomy. Patients must be provided with the information they require, in a suitable format, to empower them with decision-making capacity. Informed consent leading to the choice of a treatment option or informed refusal of a treatment option must be respected by all professionals. If there is concern regarding the older patient's ability to assimilate information and decide, then further advice should be taken before deeming the patient 'incompetent'. Formal assessment of mental state may be necessary. If legal incompetence is concluded, decisions about the cessation or instigation of treatment may be taken by a proxy. This is often a family member. However, it may not be valid to assume that the proxy knows the wishes of a patient as they may never have discussed issues such as withdrawal of treatment. The proxy may be appointed on a formal basis through enduring power of attorney or the patient may make their wishes known through an advanced directive. The legal standing of advanced directives varies across legal jurisdictions. If there is no proxy available, doctors may make decisions about care 'in the best interests' of the patient. Efforts should be made early in the patient's admission to anticipate important decisions about medical care so that the patient may be involved as much as possible and proxy decision-making is avoided. The patient's current and potential quality of life may impact on the decision to proceed to surgery or not.

Previously made decisions concerning resuscitation, often referred to as do-not-resuscitate (DNR) orders, should be revised before a patient is admitted to the operating department for surgery. The outcome of cardiac arrest differs greatly from that on the general ward, with 60% of patients surviving to hospital discharge compared with 7–17% of patients who sustain cardiopulmonary arrest on the ward.[32] This because cardiac arrest in the operating theatre is monitored and witnessed, whereas a patient may be arrested on the ward for a variable length of time before resuscitation efforts begin. In addition, cardiac arrest in the operating theatre is often due to reversible causes such as arrhythmia, medication administration or hypovolaemia, which, when promptly managed, restore adequate circulation to the patient. In the light of this, a patient with a terminal process such as pancreatic cancer, with a DNR order on the ward, may have this decision reversed during the period they are in the operating theatre for palliative ileostomy, if that is what the patient wishes following informed consent.

Strategy to reduce postoperative morbidity and mortality in the elderly

Reductions in anaesthesia- and surgery-related morbidity and mortality involve a strategy that encompasses both individual organ systems and a wider view of the perioperative process (Table 128.8).

Table 128.8 Summary of the anaesthetic management of elderly patients.

Preoperative assessment for identifying high-risk patients
Careful history
Physical examination
12-lead ECG
Functional status assessment
Nutrition assessment
Preoperative preparation
Effective control of coexisting disease
Stopped smoking for 8 weeks
Training in cough and lung expansion techniques
Chest physiotherapy for elderly at risk of pulmonary complications
Correction of malnutrition
Routine precautions for major surgery
Temperature monitoring and control
Ripple mattress
DVT prophylaxis
Intra-arterial pressure monitoring
Haemodynamic stability
Combination of anaesthetic and vasopressor, β-blockers and vasodilatation
Avoid fluid overload
Quick recovery from anaesthesia
Use short-acting anaesthetic agents
Combine epidural anaesthesia with GA for major abdominal and thoracic surgery
Antagonize neuromuscular blocking drugs
Postoperative period
Prevent hypoxaemia: supplemental oxygen, reversal of neuromuscular drugs
Prevent hypothermia: keep warm perioperatively
Effective postoperative pain control: regular multimodal analgesia

Preoperative nutritional supplementation

Up to 40% of older patients admitted to hospital are malnourished.[33] Elderly patients with malnutrition are poor candidates for surgery and anaesthesia, as it places them at particular risk from hypothermia, decubitus ulcers, drug overdose, local and systemic infection, anaemia and wound breakdown. The most common form of malnutrition in this age group is protein–calorie malnutrition. Low protein intake is associated with low intakes of calcium and vitamin D, both of which are necessary in the formation of callus after fracture. Loss of muscle secondary to malnutrition increases fatigability, decreases strength and reduces the ability to maintain adequate ventilation. The evidence from various studies, including a Cochrane review,[34] suggests that nutritional supplementation should be confined to those patients who are malnourished, in order to achieve an acceptable risk–benefit ratio, where side effects to the patient are balanced against a demonstrable clinical effect. The evidence to date suggests that simple oral supplements are the optimum method of supplementation as oral supplementation is more cost-effective, more tolerable and psychologically more acceptable to patients than nasogastric or parenteral nutrition. It has not been extensively studied, however. Simple qualitative assessment of nutritional status on admission to hospital may be carried out as part of the routine nursing assessment. Because of the prevalence of poor nutrition in older patients presenting for surgery, prompt preoperative referral to a dietician of all patients who are deemed malnourished on nursing assessment should take place. This will facilitate early institution of simple oral supplementation in the postoperative phase, with nasogastric supplementation in patients who are severely malnourished. The emphasis should be on restoring function and decreasing perioperative morbidity rather than rapid weight gain.

Prevention of perioperative decubitus ulcers

The older surgical patient presents a unique challenge to the perioperative care team in the prevention of pressure ulcers. It is suggested that 25% of pressure ulcers are acquired intraoperatively. For many patients, pressure ulcers mean increased pain, longer hospital stays and reduced quality of life. A pressure ulcer can be defined as an area of localized damage to the skin and underlying tissue, caused by a disruption in the blood supply, preventing oxygen and vital nutrients from reaching the cells.[35] A pressure sore begins in the operating theatre, developing initially in muscle and the subcutaneous tissues before progressing outwards to the dermis and epidermis. This causes an erythematous area, which may be mistaken for a burn. This may go on to become an established pressure sore. Pressure sores occurring in surgical patients are often not attributed to their time spent in theatre, as the initial damage may not be apparent until several hours or days have passed.

The development of a pressure ulcer is considered to be largely preventable with the implementation of an effective preventive strategy,[35] and the occurrence of pressure ulcers has been used as a proxy measurement of quality care. Anaesthetized patients are subjected to prolonged pressure on dependent body parts as neither the position nor duration of surgery can be altered. Duration of surgery is a major risk factor in pressure ulcer formation, in conjunction with the patient's level of tissue tolerance and the support surface. Other risk factors for pressure ulcer formation have been well established (Table 128.9). A constellation of these features is frequently found in the older patient presenting for surgery. On the basis of the literature

Table 128.9 Risk factors for the development of perioperative decubitus ulcers.

Extrinsic
Pressure
Shear
Friction
Moisture
Intrinsic
Age (>40 years)
Nutritional status
Body mass index
Comorbidity
Core temperature
Low diastolic pressure
Low serum albumin
Immobility prior to surgery
Operating room factors
Duration of surgery
Surgical position
Type of mattress
Positioning devices
Warming devices
Epidural anaesthesia/analgesia
Anaesthetic agents
Type of surgery
Extracorporeal circulation
Inappropriate manual handling

to date, prevention of decubitus ulcers in the perioperative period should concentrate on the following points:

- early assessment of risk factors, combined with full history and clinical examination;
- meticulous attention during manual handling, particularly after the patient has been anaesthetized;
- caution during positioning for surgery;
- use of specialized table mattresses such as alternating air devices or gel overlays for patients at particular risk;
- maintaining normothermia;
- maintaining diastolic blood pressure above 35 mmHg;
- low-dose local anaesthetic infusions for regional analgesic techniques;
- frequent re-evaluation.

The role of daycase admission

There is no upper age limit for daycase admission and older patients may benefit cognitively from reduced disruption to their daily environment and routine. Prior consultation at the preoperative assessment clinic should screen patients for suitability. Patients should be medically stable and able to understand simple instructions with regard to medications and fasting. A reminder telephone call the evening before surgery is useful in encouraging compliance. Patients require a responsible companion to accompany them home and to stay overnight. It is this issue that most often causes difficulty. Community services and follow-up need to be in place before the patient leaves the hospital.

Safe sedation of the older patient

Ventilatory responses to hypoxia and hypercarbia are reduced in the geriatric patient with greater risks for apnoea. Changes in volume of distribution, bioavailability and receptor sensitivity lead to alterations in pharmacodynamics for most drugs. Limitations in renal clearance and hepatic function require attenuation of dosage. Since many elderly have prolonged circulation time, longer periods are required for interval dosing. Therefore, titration to effect is an important principle in applying clinical judgment to the geriatric patient. When sedating the geriatric patient, the agent of choice should have a short half-life, with minimal active metabolites and limited side effects. One should avoid using standard dosages calculated on a mg kg^{-1} basis. These boluses frequently produce unwanted respiratory depression and hypotension. Likewise, slower administration of an agent and allowing more time for peak effects often achieve the desired goals with less overall dose.[36]

Choice of surgical approach

The appropriateness of the surgery may need to be reviewed in older patients who, because of their preoperative baseline, are at particular risk of a poor outcome. Unnecessary surgery that exposes the patient to a high risk–low benefit ratio should not be undertaken without expert opinion and full informed consent from the patient. If possible, a less invasive surgical approach may be utilized, for example, thoracoscopic evacuation of haemothorax or laparoscopic-assisted colonic resection. These techniques result in less pain, a quicker recovery and a shorter hospital stay.

Early access to critical care

Although questioned in the past, there are good data in the USA that critical care improves outcome in the elderly and that age should not be used arbitrarily to withhold admission. There are also increasing data which indicate that early, direct ICU admission for some critically ill elderly patients not only prevents a later transfer from the general ward, but also favourably impacts survival.[37]

Perioperative audit

There is an important role for perioperative audit in the care of the older surgical patient. Attendance at preoperative assessment clinics, proportion of patients cancelled for medical reasons on the morning of surgery, unplanned admission to the ICU, incidence of postoperative myocardial infarction, patient satisfaction and 30 day mortality are just a few examples of outcome measures that may provide scope for audit and implementation of change in individual surgical units.

Conclusion

Good anaesthetic care of the older person involves an assiduous approach to both minor and major elements of the perioperative process. The preparation of the patient begins early and is best carried out in a multidisciplinary unit that is focused on the needs of the elderly. Most information required to plan the anaesthetic may be gained from a detailed history and clinical examination of the patient. Occasionally, special investigations or preparatory procedures are required. Short-acting agents and/or regional anaesthesia are recommended, provided that there are no special indications for general anaesthesia or contraindications to regional techniques. Provision of adequate pain relief with regular assessment and formal charting of pain scores should be adopted as routine practice. Fluid and electrolyte management should not be left to the most junior member of the team – consideration of the fluid, electrolyte and nutritional needs of the patient should be a priority throughout the perioperative course. Oxygen supplementation should be continued routinely to reduce the incidence of hypoxaemia preoperatively and postoperatively.

Key points

- Advanced age is not a barrier to anaesthesia and surgery.
- Anaesthesia should be carried out, or closely supervised, by an anaesthesiologist with sufficient experience of anaesthesia in elderly patients.
- Adequate time must be allocated for a detailed preoperative assessment.
- Invasive monitoring and regional anaesthesia should be utilized liberally.
- Intraoperative anaesthesia care should be viewed as part of a continuum, with therapy such as oxygen supplementation, analgesia and fluid management continued into the postoperative period.

References

1. Kazmers A, Perkins AJ and Jacobs LA. Outcomes after abdominal aortic aneurysm repair in those >80 years of age: recent veterans affairs experience. *Ann Vasc Surg* 1998; **12**:106–12.
2. Eagle KA, Brundage BH, Chaitman BR *et al.* Report of the American College of Cardiology/American Heart Association Task Force on Practice Guidelines. Committee on Perioperative Cardiovascular Evaluation for Noncardiac Surgery. Guidelines for perioperative cardiovascular evaluation for noncardiac surgery. *Circulation* 1996;**93**:1278–317.
3. Haynes AB, Weiser TG, Berry WR *et al.* Safe Surgery Saves Lives Study Group. A surgical safety checklist to reduce morbidity and mortality in a global population. *N Engl J Med* 2009;**360**:491–9.
4. Hall WJ. Update in geriatrics. *Ann Intern Med* 1997;**127**: 557–64.
5. Crosby DL, Rees GAD and Seymour DG (eds). *The Ageing Surgical Patient: Anaesthetic, Operative and Medical Management*, John Wiley & Sons, Ltd, Chichester, 1992.
6. The Association of Anaesthetists of Great Britain and Ireland. *Anaesthesia and Peri-Operative Care of the Elderly*, AAGBI, London, 2001.
7. Department of Health. *National Confidential Enquiry into Peri-Operative Deaths*, Department of Health, London, 1999.
8. Chelluri L, Pinsky MR and Grenvik AN. Outcome of intensive care of the 'oldest old' critically ill patients. *Crit Care Med* 1992;**20**:757–61.
9. Hosking MP, Lobdell CM, Warner MA *et al.* Anaesthesia for patients over 90 years of age. Outcomes after regional and general anaesthetic techniques for two common surgical procedures. *Anaesthesia* 1989;**44**:142–7.
10. Djokovic JL and Hedley-Whyte J. Prediction of outcome of surgery and anesthesia in patients over 80. *JAMA* 1979;**242**: 2301–6.
11. American Society of Anesthesiologists. New classification of physical status. *Anesthesiology* 1963;**24**: 11.
12. Gibbs J, Cull W, Henderson W *et al.* Preoperative serum albumin level as a predictor of operative mortality and morbidity: results from the National VA Surgical Risk Study. *Arch Surg* 1999;**134**:36–42.
13. Pedersen T, Eliasen K and Henriksen E. A prospective study of mortality associated with anaesthesia and surgery: risk indicators of mortality in hospital. *Acta Anaesthesiol Scand* 1990;**34**:176–82.
14. Goldman L, Calderal DL and Nussbaum SR. Multifactorial index of cardiac risk in non-cardiac surgical procedures. *N Engl J Med* 1977;**297**:845–50.
15. Smith TB, Stonell C, Purkayastha S and Paraskevas P. Cardiopulmonary exercise testing as a risk assessment method in non cardio-pulmonary surgery: a systematic review. *Anaesthesia* 2009;**64**:883–93.
16. Poldermans D, Boersma E, Bax JJ *et al.* Dutch Echocardiographic Cardiac Risk Evaluation Applying Stress Echocardiography Study Group. The effect of bisoprolol on perioperative mortality and myocardial infarction in high-risk patients undergoing vascular surgery. *N Engl J Med* 1999 **341**:1789–94.
17. Smetana GW. Preoperative pulmonary evaluation. *N Engl J Med* 1999;**340**:937–44.

18. Chung F, Meier R, Lautenschlager E *et al*. General or spinal anesthesia: which is better in the elderly? *Anesthesiology* 1997;**67**:422–7.

19. Moller JT, Cluitmans P, Rasmussen LS *et al*. Long-term postoperative cognitive dysfunction in the elderly ISPOCD1 study. ISPOCD Investigators. International Study of Postoperative Cognitive Dysfunction. *Lancet* 1998;**351**:857–61.

20. Larsen SF, Zaric D and Boysen G. Postoperative cerebrovascular accidents in general surgery. *Acta Anaesthesiol Scand* 1988;**32**:698–701.

21. Jin F and Chung F. Minimizing perioperative adverse events in the elderly. *Br J Anaesth* 2001;**87**:608–24.

22. Conzen PF, Kharash ED, Czerner SF *et al*. Low flow sevoflurane compared with low flow isoflurane anesthesia in patients with stable renal insufficiency. *Anesthesiology* 2002; **97**:578–84.

23. Kellum JA and Decker JM. Use of dopamine in acute renal failure: a metaanalysis. *Crit Care Med* 2001;**29**:1526–31.

24. Lameire NH, De Vriese AS and Vanholder R. Prevention and nondialytic treatment of acute renal failure. *Curr Opin Crit Care* 2003;**9**:481–90.

25. Fleisher LA. Routine laboratory testing in the elderly: is it indicated? *Anesth Analg* 2001;**93**:249–50.

26. Cook AKR, Niven CA and Downs MG. Assessing the pain of people with cognitive impairment. *Int J Geriatr Psychiatry* 1999;**14**:421–5.

27. Severn AM and Dodds C. Cognitive dysfunction may complicate assessment of pain in elderly patients. *BMJl* 1997;**315**: 551.

28. Herr KA, Mobilly PR, Kohout FJ and Wagenaar D. Evaluation of the Faces Pain Scale for use with the elderly. *Clin J Pain* 1998;**14**:29–38.

29. Oberle K, Paul P and Wry J. Pain, anxiety and analgesics: a comparative study of elderly and younger surgical patients. *Can J Aging* 1990;**91**:13–22.

30. Ballantyne JC, Carr DB, deFerranti S *et al*. The comparative effects of postoperative analgesic therapies on pulmonary outcome: cumulative meta-analyses of randomized, controlled trials. *Anesth Analg* 1998;**86**:598–612.

31. Egbert AM, Parks LH, Short LM and Burnett ML. Randomized trial of postoperative patient-controlled analgesia vs. intramuscular narcotics in frail elderly men. *Arch Intern Med* 1990;**150**:1897–903.

32. Martin RL, Soifer BE and Stevens WC. Ethical issues in anesthesia. Management of the do-not-resuscitate patient. *Anesth Analg* 1991;**73**:221–5.

33. McWhirter JP and Pennington CR. Incidence and recognition of malnutrition in hospital. *BMJl* 1994;**308**:945–8.

34. Avenell A and Handoll HH. Nutritional supplementation for hip fracture aftercare in the elderly. *Cochrane Database Syst Rev* 2000;(4): CD001880.

35. European Pressure Ulcer Advisory Panel. A policy statement on prevention of pressure ulcers. *Br J Nurs* 1998;**7**:888–90.

36. Darling E. Practical considerations in sedating the elderly. *Crit Care Nurs Clin North Am* 1997;**9**:371–380.

37. Rady MY, Ryan T and Starr NJ. Perioperative determinants of morbidity and mortality in elderly patients undergoing cardiac surgery. *Crit Care Med* 1998;**26**:225–35.

CHAPTER 129

Health issues in the ageing female

Carolyn D. Philpot
Saint Louis University Medical Center St Louis, MO, USA

Cancer

Cancer is one of the leading causes of death in women.[1] The ageing female is at risk for endometrial, ovarian, breast, cervical, vulvar and vaginal cancer. Since there is risk with increasing age, reviewing the risk factors is important to help promote a good quality of life. Proper screening, early detection, treatment and management of comorbidities are essential.

Endometrial cancer

Endometrial cancer is the fourth most common malignancy in women after breast cancer, colorectal and lung cancer. Peak incidence occurs in women between 50 and 60 years of age and the incidence appears to be climbing. The 5 year survival rate for all stages of endometrial cancer has been estimated at 65%.

Risk factors include nulliparity, obesity and prolonged use of unopposed exogenous estrogens. The most common symptom is postmenopausal vaginal bleeding.

Besides a physical examination and Pap smear, a pelvic ultrasonography and either an endometrial biopsy or dilatation and curettage (D & C) is required for diagnosis or exclusion of diagnosis of endometrial cancer. [a positive Papanicolaou (Pap) test for endometrial cancer will only show in 35–50% of the cases and should not be the only determinant in diagnosis.] Optimal treatment is a hysterectomy with bilateral oophorectomy and dissection of retroperitoneal lymph nodes in the pelvic and para-aortic region.[2] Additional treatment, such as chemotherapy, radiation or both, may also be indicated in advanced stages of cancer and discussion is needed with the patient's oncologist and geriatrician to weigh the risks against the benefits.

Ovarian cancer

After endometrial cancer, ovarian cancer is the second most common gynaecological malignancy. Peak incidence occurs in women aged between 50 and 60 years. Risk factors included uninterrupted ovulation (nulliparity or contraceptive usage) and inherited genetic mutations.

Symptoms usually are non-specific. Abdominal pain, abdominal distension and gastrointestinal disturbances are complaints sometimes voiced by women with ovarian cancers, but symptoms may not develop until late in the disease process. Screening, except for high-risk patients, may include ultrasonography and tumour markers; however, it is thought to be of limited value.

Ovaries are generally small and not palpable in postmenopausal women and if upon physical examination an ovary is able to be palpated, immediate evaluation is warranted since it is suggestive of ovarian cancer. Initial treatment involves surgical removal of the tumour. Chemotherapy may be considered depending on the tumour stage, the patient's comorbidities and benefits versus risks. Since most ovarian cancers are detected when the tumour is advanced, long-term prognosis is usually poor.

Breast cancer

Approximately 50% of all new breast cancer cases occur in women over the age of 65 years. The incidence of breast cancer increases up to the age of 80 years, levels out between the ages 80 and 85 years and then is thought to decline. It is difficult to evaluate those over 85 years of age owing to limited data. Risk factors for developing breast cancer may include personal or family history of breast cancer and/or colon or endometrial cancer in the first-degree relatives, nulliparity or late first pregnancy at 31 years of age or older, late menopause, early menarche, abdominal obesity, estrogen replacement therapy and history of atypical hyperplasia on biopsy for benign breast disease.[3]

Screening for breast cancer in a postmenopausal woman includes monthly self-breast examinations, an annual physical examination by a physician or other healthcare provider and a mammogram, yearly or every 2 years. Research has

Principles and Practice of Geriatric Medicine, Fifth Edition. Edited by Alan J. Sinclair, John E. Morley and Bruno Vellas.

shown that screening for breast cancer in women aged 50–70 years has improved survival by early detection. There are many doctor s who feel that mortality could be reduced by 25–30% if all women received proper mammographic screening. There are limited data on breast screening in women over 70 years of age, but it is though that mammography is of benefit. Since 10–20% of all breast cancers are not picked up on mammography, physical examination is also important.

Fewer than 50% of all women aged 65 years or older have ever had a mammogram and those who have obtained one on a routine basis. There has been argument by physicians against instituting routine screening for breast cancer in elderly women, stating that disability and shorter life expectancy may have a direct effect on the desirability and cost-effectiveness of screening. On the other hand, the life expectancy of a healthy woman in her mid- to late-70s is approximately 10 more years and for a healthy woman 85 years of age it is 7 more years. Hence screening appears to be warranted.

The clinical characteristics of breast cancer are the same, despite the age of the individual. Cancer is generally suspected when breast lesions palpated feel firm or abnormalities are detected on mammography. A palpable breast mass in a postmenopausal woman requires immediate attention, since most palpable masses are malignant. All breast masses in this age-group should have a biopsy whether the mass was palpated and/or detected on mammography.

Prognosis is determined by the stage of the disease. Owing to lack of clinical studies, it is unclear whether women over the age of 65 years have the same clinical course as younger women. The course of treatment is prompted by the stage of the disease. Until recently, many elderly women with breast cancer were not aggressively treated; however, today many older women are working with their oncologists and geriatricians discussing various treatment options.

Cervical cancer

Cervical cancer occurs in women of all ages but its incidence peaks in women 40–50 years of age.[4] Symptoms may vary and hinge on the stage of the tumour. Some women may be asymptomatic, whereas others may show clinical signs of postmenopausal or postcoital bleeding. Routine Pap testing is the best method of screening. If the Pap testing is positive, colposcopy-directed biopsies and endocervical curettage are used to establish diagnosis.

Radical hysterectomy is the recommended treatment for cervical cancer. Adjuvant radiation or chemotherapy may also be used. The combined cure rate for cervical cancers is 50–60%.

Vulvar cancer

Vulvar cancer accounts for approximately 3–4% of all gynaecological malignancies in the USA.[5] The average age at diagnosis is 70 years and the incidence increases with age. The most common symptoms exhibited in vulvar cancer are vulvar pruritus, pain and a palpable vulvar lesion; however, many women are asymptomatic.[6] A discharge may be present. Histology generally reveals squamous cell carcinoma. Biopsy may be indicated for diagnosis. Treatment is generally surgical and, for extensive lesions, a radical vulvectomy with unilateral or bilateral inguinal lymphadenectomy is recommended. Radiation and chemotherapy may also be considered adjuvant therapy. Prognosis for early-staged lesions is generally favourable. The 5 year survival rate is 80–90% if there is no metastasis to the lymph node and 16–30% if lymph node metastasis is present.

Vaginal cancer

Vaginal cancer is relatively rare.[7] The average age at diagnosis is 60–65 years. It is estimated that 95% of these lesions are squamous cell carcinomas. Vaginal bleeding or discharge is an early symptom. Pain or post-coital bleeding may be exhibited in sexually active women. Where the tumour involves the anterior vaginal wall, it may cause dysfunction with voiding, since the vaginal wall may invade into the urethra. Biopsy is indicated for diagnosis. Radiation is the main choice of treatment; however, surgery and chemotherapy may be utilized in specific cases. Prognosis is dependent upon the size and location of the tumour. The 5 year survival rate for all types is estimated to be 25–48%.

Menopause

Menopause is the permanent cessation of menses as a result of ovarian ageing. It is clinically diagnosed after 12 months of amenorrhoea. The average age in the USA at which menopause occurs is 51 years. The perimenopausal transition is defined as the time prior to permanent cessation of menses and is identified with irregular menstrual cycles. Transitional time has been shown to vary in length from 2 to 8 years.

Early symptoms of menopause include irregular menstrual cycles, headaches, fatigue, changes in mood and cognition, insomnia and hot flashes (Table 129.1). Some women may experience vertigo, heart palpitations and tachycardia. A later clinical presentation may include urinary incontinence, dry skin, breast changes, genital atrophy with dyspareunia, vaginitis and cystitis.

Early symptoms of menopause are often associated with irregular menstrual periods. They may vary in frequency,

Table 129.1 Signs and symptoms of menopause.

Irregular menstrual cycle
Insomnia
Hot flashes
Mood swings
Cognitive changes
Skin changes
Genitourinary atrophy
Headache
Fatigue
Vertigo
Heart palpitations/tachycardia

duration and blood flow amount. Menstrual bleeding that is unusually heavy, lasting more than 10 days or that occurs more often than once every 3 weeks should be clinically evaluated for possible neoplasms.

Another early symptom of menopause is hot flashes. About 80% of all perimenopausal women report hot flashes and up to 50% of these women may continue to have symptoms for up to 5 years. Hot flashes may also occur after surgical menopause. Research shows that short-term use of hormone replacement therapy (HRT) will help relieve severe vasomotor symptoms, but will not abolish symptoms.

Women who have had bilateral salpingo oophorectomy are at high risk for cardiovascular disease. This is especially true if HRT was not initiated. Early natural menopause is also at high risk.

Diagnosing menopause may be determined by elevated serum levels of follicle-stimulating hormone. Estrogen replacement therapy is the best treatment for symptoms of menopause. Duration of estrogen replacement therapy is controversial and each case should be reviewed for risk versus benefit.

Postmenopausal vaginal bleeding

About 20–30% of postmenopausal vaginal bleeding is due to atypical adenomatous endometrial hyperplasia or endometrial cancer. It may also be caused by the use of estrogens or progesterone or by genital atrophy resulting from low estrogen levels.

History taking should include past and present gynaecological problems. A drug history should indicate whether any exogenous estrogens were used. A pelvic and bimanual examination should be performed to rule out any trauma, tumours or bleeding from atrophic sites. A Pap test should also be performed to aid in diagnosis. Transvaginal ultrasonography may be useful for diagnosis. If the endometrial thickness is less than 5 mm, cancer or endometrial hyperplasia is doubtful. Endometrial thickness over 5 mm is suspicious for malignancy and further work-up is promptly warranted. Endometrial biopsy may then be indicated as well as a full fractional D & C.

If postmenopausal bleeding is found to be cancerous, then treatment should be tumour specific. If cancer is not detected, estrogen treatment is indicated because it may be secondary to atrophy. For those women taking exogenous hormones, the estrogen dosage may need to be decreased and that of progesterone increased. If bleeding continues, a more aggressive work-up is needed.

Postmenopausal hormone replacement therapy

Approximately 6 million women in the USA are taking HRT. The use of estrogen therapy ranges from relief of postmenopausal symptoms to what were assumed, until recently, to be long-term health benefits. Until recently, it was felt that estrogen replacement therapy had a protective effect against cardiovascular disease. From the data collected by the Heart and Estrogen/Progestin Replacement Study Follow-up (HERS II) trial and other recent secondary prevention studies, the new recommendations are against initiating or continuing its use for primary prevention of cardiovascular disease. The Women's Health Initiative (WHI) study stated that estrogen and progestin therapy should not be initiated or continued for the primary prevention of coronary heart disease and it was suggestive that it may stimulate breast cancer growth and hinder breast cancer diagnosis. This condition of hormone replacement also showed an increase in pulmonary embolus.

Sexual dysfunction in the menopausal women

Many women have experienced a lack of interest (decreased libido) or arousal in sexual activity (sexual arousal disorder), achieving orgasm (female orgasmic disorder) or have had pain prior to or during sexual activity (dyspareunia).[8,9] When one or more of these symptoms occur, causing anguish and interference with interpersonal relationships, it is diagnosed as female sexual dysfunction (FSD). The exact prevalence is unknown; however, one survey found that more than 40% of women aged 18–59 years alluded to having sexual dysfunction. It has also been suggested that the prevalence of FSD increases while women are going through the menopause transition.

Peri- and postmenopausal women have repeatedly reported they have lost interest in sex and do not find sex 'pleasurable'. Studies have shown that there has been a decline in sexual functioning from early to late

Table 129.2 Screening questions for female sexual dysfunction.

1 Are you currently involved in a sexual relationship? With men? With women? Both? Multiple partners?
2 How often do you engage in sexual activity? Intercourse? Masturbation?
3 Do you feel that your sex drive has changed? Less? Same? Increased?
4 Do you have difficulty in obtaining an orgasm? Inability? Pain with?
5 Are you satisfied with your current sexual relations?
6 Do you have sexual concerns that you would like to discuss?

perimenopausal. In late perimenopausal to postmenopausal women, studies reveal that there is a decrease in libido and sexual responsitivity, an increase in dyspareunia and a decline in sexual activity. Screening questions that are useful are given in Table 129.2.

The causes of FDS are multifactorial. Hormonal, physical and psychosocial changes are key components of FDS.

Hormonal changes

There is a decline of circulating androgens during the late reproductive years. Androgen deficiency is associated with a decline in libido, arousability and sensitivity to sexual stimulation.

Estrogen deficiency can cause changes in the genitourinary system. Estrogen therapy, both topical and systemic, has been shown to improve vaginal atrophy, increase blood flow to the vagina and increase lubrication.

Physical changes

In addition to the hormonal changes that occur in the genitourinary system, other conditions can contribute to FDS. Limited movement or pain from arthritis may be a factor. Recent pelvic surgery or trauma is another. Some medications, such as antihistamines, antidepressants and blood pressure medication can lead to a decreased libido and inability to achieve orgasm.

Psychosocial changes

A woman may have concerns over the wellbeing of her sexual partner. If she or her sexual partner is ill or have a debilitating disease, it can have a direct impact on sexual function. Women, who live longer than men, are often without a sex partner. Not having a sex partner does not mean that they are no longer in need of nurturing, affection and physical contact. Depression and anxiety can contribute to FDS.

Research has shown that only 14% of Americans aged 40–80 years have been asked by their doctor if they had any sexual problems within the past 3 years. Since this number is relatively small, the physician or healthcare provider needs to remember to inquire about the patient's sexual health along with the history taking during the physical examination.

Data from a large survey have indicated that 68% of men and women thought their physician would be uncomfortable talking about sex and 71% thought that if sexual problems were disclosed, nothing would be done about the problem. Only 14% out of 1384 women ever reported sexual problems to their healthcare provider in a study conducted by the American Association of Retired Persons. Of those women discussing sexual problems, most confer with their gynaecologist rather than their private medical doctor (primary care provider or PCP). It is felt that physicians do not talk about sex because of a lack of education, comfort and confidence and lack of time and treatment options (Table 129.2).

Osteoporosis

Osteoporosis is a major risk factor for fractures in the older population and is estimated to account for approximately 1.5 million low trauma fractures yearly.[10] The lifetime risk of sustaining a fracture to the spine (symptomatic), hip or distal radius in white women is ~40% (but only 13% in white men) aged 50 years and older. The 6 month mortality rate from a hip fracture is ~10–20%. Of the survivors, about 25% will require assistive or nursing home care and ~50% will require an assistive device to aid in their ambulation. Osteoporotic fractures are associated with annual costs in the USA ranging between 7 and 20 billion dollars. About 1–1.5% of all hospital beds in Europe are occupied by patients with osteoporosis. This European figure is expected to more than double in the next 50 years. In the USA, the estimated prevalence of osteoporosis is 8 million in women and 2 million in men and the estimated related health costs exceed 14 million dollars annually. Primary osteoporosis occurs mainly in older people aged 51–75 years and can be arranged in two groups: postmenopausal osteoporosis and age-related bone loss (senescence). The incidence of primary osteoporosis is six times more common in women than in men. Women are at higher risk because they have a lower peak bone mass than men and have an acceleration of bone loss during menopause.

Primary osteoporosis is thought to be atypical in premenopausal women, while secondary osteoporosis composes only a small amount of elderly women. (Elderly women may have a combination of both primary and secondary osteoporosis.)

Age-related bone loss is complex and multifactorial. As one ages, changes occur in the cortex bone, trabecular bone and bone marrow. Studies show that there is a decline in bone mineral density after the third decade of life and it continues to decline at a rate of approximately 0.5% per year. During menopause, women, however, have an accelerated bone mineral density loss at an estimated rate of 3–5%.

Hormonal changes of vitamin D and reduction of calcium absorption also have an impact on ageing bone. Vitamin D levels decrease with age and vitamin D deficiency in elderly people is common. Absorption rates also decline by 40%. Ageing changes in skin reduce the amount of 7-dehydrocholesterol, the precursor and the rate of conversion of vitamin D_3. Declining renal function leads to a decrease in activity of 1-α-hydroxylase, which is responsible for the activation of vitamin D_3. Lower calcium levels then occur from these changes, causing activation of the calcium sensor receptor in the parathyroid gland. Parathyroid hormone is secreted, stimulating osteoclast activity, which keeps serum calcium levels in homeostasis at the price of bone mineralization. Secondary osteoporosis may also have many other conditions causing bone loss such as various endocrine and neoplastic abnormalities, gastrointestinal disease and drug usage (Table 129.3).

Osteoporosis has no symptoms; therefore, a thorough evaluation is critical for detection of osteoporosis. Assessment begins with a complete history alluding to its risk factors as stated in Table 129.4. Major risk factors for osteoporosis are increased age, female gender, ethnicity and thin body habitus. History of previous fracture(s) needs further assessment, focusing on whether the fracture occurred with only minimal trauma (suggestive of low body density). Physical examination for osteoporosis should look for secondary causes. For example, an ill, cachectic woman may need assessment for malnutrition, malignancy or malabsorption syndrome. A loss of body height may indicate vertebral compression fracture(s) or dorsal kyphosis from osteoporosis may be seen on clinical examination.

Table 129.3 Secondary causes of osteoporosis.

Endocrine:
Hyperthyroidism
Cushing's syndrome
Osteomalacia
Paget's disease
Primary hyperparathyroidism
Gastrointestinal:
Malabsorption syndromes
Alcoholism
Neoplastic states:
Bone metastases
Multiple myeloma
Medication:
Anticonvulsants
Excessive thyroid hormone replacement

Table 129.4 Risk factors for osteoporosis.

Advanced age
Female gender
Race (more prevalent among white, Asian and Hispanic descent)
Heredity (~50–80% of peak bone mass is genetically determined)
Small body size/weight (<127 lb/58 kg)
Smoking
Alcoholism
Sedentary lifestyle/immobility
Low dietary calcium/vitamin D intake
History of previous fractures/falls
Decrease long life exposure to estrogen
Certain medication (anticonvulsants, glucocorticoids, thyroid hormone, barbiturates)
Caffeine use
Early menopause or oophorectomy

Laboratory evaluation should reflect clinical findings. All women with osteoporosis should receive a chemistry profile including electrolytes, kidney and liver function, glucose, calcium, phosphorus and albumin. They should also have a complete blood count to rule out anaemia and malignancy. Thyroid function should be assessed in women over 50 years of age. Other laboratory tests should be ordered as individually warranted, such as 25-hydroxy-vitamin D and parathyroid hormone for those with low serum calcium to look for vitamin D deficiency and secondary hyperparathyroidism.

The combination of history taking, physical examination and laboratory tests will help in diagnosing osteoporosis or other secondary causes.

Bone densitometry is the only test which confirms diagnosis of osteoporosis in the absence of fracture. To confirm diagnosis of primary osteoporosis, one needs to rule out secondary osteoporosis, malignancy and osteomalacia. Although many women have some type of knowledge of osteoporosis, healthcare providers need to educate the general population about the importance of taking certain steps to aid in its prevention. Treatment includes providing calcium and vitamin D supplementation, which can reduce the risk of fracture by up to 30%. The best choice in the treatment of osteoporosis is the use of biphosphonates. This group of drugs increase bone mass, thus decreasing the risk for fractures. Other treatment modalities include exercise with a focus on muscle strengthening, weight bearing and balance. Direct effects on bone may be relatively small but will aid in decreasing the incidence of falls which may lead to fractures.

Key points

- Screening for cancer remains important in older women.
- Female sexual dysfunction is a relatively common problem in older women.
- The Women's Health Initiative has decreased the enthusiasm for hormone replacement therapy in older women.
- Osteoporotic fractures are a major cause of disability and mortality in older women.

References

1. Levi F, Lucchini F, Negri E *et al*. Changed trends of cancer mortality in the elderly. *Ann Oncol* 2001;**12**:1467–77.
2. Geisler JP and Geisler HE. Radical hysterectomy in the elderly female: a comparison to patients age 50 or younger. *Gynecol Oncology* 2001;**80**:258–61.
3. Chlebowski RT, Hendrix SL, Langer RD *et al*. Influences of estrogen plus progestin on breast cancer and mammography in healthy postmenopausal women. *JAMA* 2003; **289**:3243–53.
4. Benedet JI, Odicino F, Maisonneuve P *et al*. Carcinoma of the cervix. FIGO annual report. *J Epidemiol Biostat* 2001:**6**:5–44.
5. Beller U, Sideri M, Maisonneuve P *et al*. Carcinoma of the vulva. FIGO annual report. *J Epidemiol Biostat* 2001:**6**:153–74.
6. Hyde SE, Ansink AC, Burger MP *et al*. The impact of performance status on survival in patients 80 years and older with vulvar cancer. *Gynecol Oncol* 2002;**84**:388–93.
7. Beller U, Sideri M, Maisonneuve P *et al*. Carcinoma of the vagina. FIGO annual report. *J Epidemiol Biostat* 2001:**6**: 141–52.
8. Gutmann JN. Exploring sexual dysfunction in the menopausal woman. *Sexual Reprod Menopause* 2005;**3**:8–11.
9. Kingsburg S. Just ask! talk to patients about sexual function. *Sexual Reprod Menopause* 2004;**2**:199–203.
10. Ribeiro V, Blakeley J and Laryea M. Women's knowledge and practices regarding the prevention and treatment of osteoporosis. *Health Care Women Int* 2000;**21**:347–53.

CHAPTER 130

Antiageing strategies

Ligia J. Dominguez and Mario Barbagallo
University of Palermo, Palermo, Italy

Introduction

The certainty of ageing and death has been a major concern of humans since the beginnings of time, with a consequent never-ending search for methods to combat the consequences of the ageing process and to delay the final moment as long as possible. Current advances in the understanding of the mechanism(s) of the ageing process and the factual extraordinary increase in human life expectancy during the twentieth century worldwide have made it possible to envisage that altering this process and further postponing natural death may actually be plausible in the not too distant future. In addition, not only prolongation of life expectancy is foreseen as the chief aim of research and interventions in the field of gerontology, but also an increase in the number of years without disease and disability, namely, the extension of health expectancy. However, expectations may be higher than what really is scientifically proven. So far, most of the results have been obtained in a wide array of animal models, such as yeasts, worms, flies, mice and primates,[1–4] but the translation of these promising results into humans awaits realistic verification.[5]

Charlatans, swindlers and so-called wise men may take advantage of the incessant wish of people to live longer, proposing miraculous cures and unproven antiageing products that are expensive and very profitable for their proponents but that need to be critically scrutinized. This has led to the concept that antiageing medicine is a fraud and has surrounded the subject with controversy.[6] Conversely, investigators involved in research in the fields of gerontology and geriatrics are making genuine attempts to develop strategies for the prevention and treatment of age-related diseases, functional decline and disability.

The demographic revolution

Human life expectancy increased extraordinarily during the twentieth century worldwide,[7] first because of child mortality reduction and then because of reduced mortality in middle and old age, probably related to medical advances (e.g. antibiotics, vaccinations, improved care of pregnant women, enhanced surgical techniques) and improved socioeconomic conditions during the recovery period after World War II (e.g. improved sanitation, greater food supply, improved work environment and decrease in excessive manual labour). Societal conditions remarkably affect life expectancy, as shown by the rapid increase in life expectancy in East Germany after the fall of the Berlin Wall.[8] Of note, the increase in human life expectancy during the twentieth century took place not only in developed countries, but also in less developed regions, and the pace of the increase was greater in these nations: it is estimated that the over 60-year-old population in China will double in only 27 years.[9] In 1900, 40% of newborns were expected to live beyond age 65 years in developed countries. In contrast, it has been estimated that if the pace of increase in life expectancy over the past century continues through the twenty-first century, most babies born since 2000 in developed countries with long life expectancies will reach 100 years.[10] These dramatic demographic changes will undoubtedly impact societies to a major extent. However, life extension is of little value in the absence of quality of life during the gained years. The imminent rapid increase in numbers of ageing adults will pose major challenges to healthcare systems in the coming years and will have deep consequences for the sustainability of modern society. For instance, the oldest-old group (>85 years), which has been the most rapidly growing segment of the population, is also the most susceptible to disease and disability.[11] Hence now more than ever, the search for ways to prolong health expectancy with effective prevention of disability has become a primary goal in medicine.

The secret to longevity has been related since mediaeval times to a healthy lifestyle and avoidance of excess. As far back as the thirteenth century, Friar Roger Bacon in England stated that in order to live a long life it was necessary to

Principles and Practice of Geriatric Medicine, Fifth Edition. Edited by Alan J. Sinclair, John E. Morley and Bruno Vellas.

follow a controlled diet, proper rest, exercise, moderation in lifestyle, good hygiene and inhaling the breath of a young virgin.[12] The modern equivalent is found in the results of the Norfolk-EPIC study, showing that four simple lifestyle habits (getting some exercise, eating five helpings of fruit and vegetables each day and drinking 1–14 glasses of alcohol per week) were associated with 14 years younger physiological parameters.[13] Another aspect that has been confirmed to be associated with longevity in places such as Japan, Macau and Hong Kong is fatty fish intake, rich in eicosahexanoic and docosahexanoic acids.[14]

Evidence that human ageing can indeed be modified is the fact that disability has decreased in the older population in the USA[15] and Europe.[16] However, recent data suggest that disability rates did not change significantly between 2000 and 2005 among older non-institutionalized Americans.[17] Furthermore, it has recently been suggested that there may be a possible slowing on the pace of life extension observed in the last century because of the poor lifestyle of young people today.[18] The disabled population spends ten times more on care than non-disabled people,[15] hence there are not only important humanitarian but also economic reasons to improve quality of life in old age.

There is currently much promise in research that provides information about the underlying biology of ageing and longevity, which has unveiled possible interventions to slow the ageing process. And a myriad of epidemiological studies have shown that interventions in lifestyle, along with early diagnosis of diseases, appropriate use of advanced medical care and new discoveries that result from basic research may indeed decrease the susceptibility to disease development, increasing longevity and healthspan.

This chapter explores the topic of antiageing therapies from different perspectives. First, it discusses the rationale behind the possible delay of death, disease and disability. Second, some of the advances in biogerontological research in animal models and possible translations into humans are explored. Third, it examines the results of epidemiological studies on lifestyle modification proven to be effective in the promotion of healthy ageing.

What is antiageing medicine?

As far back as the ancients, humans have searched for immortality. Curiously, ancient Egyptians used olive leaves to extend life,[19] while currently there is evidence that virgin olive oil, used as part of the Mediterranean dietary pattern, is associated with longer and healthier lives.[20] Indian ayurvedic medicine has alluded for centuries to 'rejuvenation', developing specific lifestyle rules and herbs to prolong life. One of the most celebrated stories about antiageing is Ponce de León's search for the 'Fountain of Youth' in Bimini, in the Bahamas. Instead, he discovered Florida, where now many American retirees spend their last years in facilities with various amenities and stimulating environments, a true heaven for many elders. The writer James Hilton created in 1933 a place called Shangri-La in his book 'Lost Horizon', which was a paradise where people would not age. Many persons went to search for the fantastic place in the Himalayan Mountains. Even Nobel Prize winners are tempted to believe in magic-bullet remedies for healthy longevity. This is the case of Élie Metchnikoff, who believed that Bulgarians lived extremely long lives due to the use of large amounts of yoghurt in their diets. One of the first books promoting longevity, entitled *Life Extension*, was published by Durk Pearson and Sandy Shaw in 1982. It provided detailed animal experiments and started a long list of self-improvement books that fill the shelves of bookstores worldwide.[6]

Ageing has always been seen as negative since it leads to death. However, now people who have witnessed the recent extraordinary increase in life expectancy want to learn more about what they can do to live longer and healthier lives and to remain vibrant and fit in their later years. As an answer to this widespread ambition, there is a proliferation of antiageing societies, advertisements, products and interventions. The term 'antiageing medicine' was created in 1992 after the foundation of the American Academy of Anti-Ageing Medicine (A4M). Antiageing medicine or interventions are defined by the A4M as 'measures to slow, arrest and reverse phenomena associated with aging and to extend the human lifespan'. It provides a number of certifications in antiageing medicine for physicians, publishes the *International Journal of Anti-Ageing Medicine* and claims hundreds of thousands of members worldwide. Antiageing products have boomed in recent years perhaps due to the ageing of 'baby boomers', who started turning 65 years old around 2010, to the light regulation of antiageing products and easy availability for marketing on the Internet and to the enormous profits that this market can raise. Nevertheless, many of these interventions and products may cause harm, involve economic fraud and may move people away from proved beneficial therapies. Products that claim to reverse ageing mislead the public and impact on the reputation of those doing serious work.

Another example of antiageing initiatives is the Life Extension Foundation, based in Florida and founded by Saul Kent in 1980, which publishes the magazine *Life Extension*, with a readership thought to be ~350 000, and sells dietary supplements by mail order. Two more physicians whose books have promoted antiageing philosophies are Andrew Weil and Deepak Chopra.

Aubrey de Grey, a Cambridge-educated scientist, editor/founder of the journal *Rejuvenation Research* and a regular guest on television programmes, has developed a theory called 'Strategies for Engineered Negligible Senescence' (SENS), which suggests seven types of ageing damage which are readily open to treatment and that will permit unlimited life extension in the near future: cancer mutations, mitochondrial mutations, intracellular junk, extracellular junk, cell loss, cell senescence and extracellular cross-links.[21] The SENS proposal has been widely criticized by gerontologists, especially because it may make the research community dedicated to ageing studies appear exceptionally optimistic and unrealistic in its promises.[22] Olshansky, Hayflick and Carnes have openly and extensively criticized this approach, stating that 'no currently marketed intervention has yet been proved to slow, stop or reverse human ageing. . . . The entrepreneurs, physicians and other health care practitioners who make these claims are taking advantage of consumers who cannot easily distinguish between the hype and reality of interventions designed to influence the aging process and age-related diseases'.[23]

Numerous concerns about antiageing products have been raised in recent years. One of them entails human growth hormone (HGH), one of the oldest and still most popular antiageing treatments. HGH has been used widely since an article by Rudman *et al.*[24] in the *New England Journal of Medicine* catapulted it to the forefront as a major breakthrough in ageing research in the eyes of the lay public. Several studies on animal models have supported a role for HGH in longevity.[25–28] Nevertheless, a recent meta-analysis showed that the changes in body composition are small and the rate of adverse events is high, including cancer development, weight gain, high blood pressure and diabetes.[29] In addition, studies in mice, flies and nematodes suggest a harmful role.[30,31] Mice genetically modified to produce more HGH live shorter lives than controls,[32,33] whereas mice producing less GH live longer; GH-deficient mice such as Snell mice (pit-1 gene mutation), Ames mice (PROP-1 gene mutation) and Laron mice (GM receptor knockout) live longer than controls. Patients with Laron syndrome (isolated IGF-1 syndrome) have lifespans into their eighties or nineties[34] and receptor mutations in IGF-1, which lead to reduced activity, are more common in centenarians.[35] An extreme example of scam is the HGH nasal preparation advertised and sold on the Internet.

Can death be delayed?

Ageing is a progressive process, universal and irreversible, that takes place at different levels, affecting practically all living organisms, and is the greatest risk factor for death. Ageing and death have been viewed conventionally as programmed events, a kind of immutable biological clock for each individual. However, in several animal models genetic manipulation[25,26] and caloric restriction (CR) without malnutrition[2] have repeatedly been shown to increase the lifespan vs. control littermates fed *ad libitum*, but there is little evidence that this can be translated to humans.[5] On the other hand, numerous studies on dietary patterns[20,36,37] have shown that balanced diets rich in foods of vegetable origin and fish, such as the Mediterranean diet, decrease overall mortality and mortality-associated with cardiovascular disease and cancer, and hence increase longevity. In addition, a high total energy expenditure in 70–80 year olds leads to increased longevity[38] with climbing stairs being the major factor that resulted in an increased total energy expenditure. In fact, there is growing evidence that modifiable lifestyle factors may interact with the ageing process and may alter the susceptibility of an individual to develop age-associated diseases, which are the major causes of mortality.[39] For instance, the best example of healthy ageing is given by exceptionally long-lived persons whose ability to survive appears to be the result of a complex combination of genetics, lifestyle, environmental and psychological factors and chance.[40]

Can the course of disability and functional dependence be reversed?

As age advances, functional capacity reserve decreases and susceptibility to diseases and functional limitations/disability increases. Disability and functional dependence can be reversible to some extent; however, when the functional reserve becomes extremely depleted, the restoration of normal function is no longer possible but the prediction or identification of the 'point of no return' is not yet clear. The development of biotechnological devices, such as the 'exoskeletons' (lifesuits),[41] nanotechnology[42] or bionic implants (e.g. Advanced Bionics cochlear implants),[43] suggests that technology will continue to push that point further away.

Can disability and functional dependence be delayed?

Since the main goal is not only to extend life but also (if not more so) to decrease disability, this is a key question. Indeed, this is the area of geriatrics that has been investigated most intensely, given epidemiological data for a factual decrease in disability in developed countries,[15,16] and the results from numerous studies showing that the onset of disease and disability may in fact be delayed by adopting a healthy lifestyle, by managing chronic conditions such as diabetes and hypertension and by detection and treatment of cancer at an early stage. The recently published INVADE study (intervention project on cerebrovascular diseases and dementia in the district of Ebersberg, Bavaria) demonstrated that moderate to high physical activity is associated with a reduced incidence of cognitive impairment, an important cause of disability, in a large population of older adults.[44] Likewise, the LIFE pilot study found that the rate of onset of mobility disability was lower among a group of older adults who engaged in a structured exercise programme for 1 year compared with a group of seniors who took part in a health education programme for the same time period.[45] Compression of morbidity and of disability rather than prolongation of survival may be one of the main goals of disease management in the older patient.[46]

Caloric restriction (CR)

Several studies in a wide array of species (e.g. yeasts, worms, flies, mice) have shown that animals under CR without malnutrition have a longer lifespan than control littermates fed *ad libitum*.[1] The first of these studies was published in 1935 by Clive McKay at Cornell University, showing that limiting the food intake of laboratory rats (dietary restriction) resulted in prolongation of their lifespan. Subsequent studies in mice and rats supported the idea that CR delays the ageing process.[2] CR can increase the lifespan of mice by as much as 40% and even greater increases have been reported in non-mammalian models.[3] Recently, striking results from a study in primates were published showing that 50% of *ad libitum*-fed animals survived compared with 80% of CR animals; in addition, CR delayed the onset of age-associated diseases (e.g. cardiovascular disease, diabetes, cancer).[4] However, other studies in monkeys have shown that even if dietary restriction improves metabolic profiles (e.g. glucose, cholesterol)[47] and may attenuate Alzheimer's-like amyloid changes in their brains,[48] these animals also show an increased propensity for bone loss and for the development of hip fractures. In addition, CR fails to extend life in older animals.[33,49] Furthermore, CR does not enhance longevity in all species.[5] Species living in a fairly constant environment will have little opportunity to develop mechanisms to respond to food shortages; this may help to explain why tropical squirrel monkeys respond less to CR than the temperate Rhesus monkey. Also, medflies and some desert-living species (e.g. the spiny mouse) able to depress their metabolism while remaining active in response to food shortage fail to increase lifespan with CR.[5] Several conditions in the laboratory environment may contribute to make the results very variable, even at the same laboratory when studying strains with uncontrolled genetic differences.[50] A recent study found no increase in mean lifespan in wild-derived mice, which had a longer lifespan and lower food intake than the laboratory counterparts. Natural enemies, including pathogens, are greatly reduced in the laboratory and there is a superabundance of food and little opportunity for exercise, which make laboratory animals quite different from animals in the wild and more respondent to CR.[50]

In humans, some studies suggest that CR has a protective effect against atherosclerosis, beneficial effects on cardiac function and some benefits in reducing weight and adiposity,[51] although the benefits were similar to those obtained by exercising. The observation that reducing calories is beneficial to overweight patients is not surprising. A high-calorie diet is unhealthy for most people and a well-known risk factor for the development of atherosclerosis and type 2 diabetes, but the demonstration of a true delay of ageing in humans is not yet viable. Whether CR may also benefit lean people who already have a healthy lifestyle is questionable. Furthermore, CR may have important side effects, such as chronic lack of energy sensation, sexual dysfunction, infertility and mental stress for controlling hungry that may lead to depression and to anorexia.

An organization called the Caloric Restriction Society, founded in 1984 by Ray and Lisa Walford and Brian Delaney, have members who observe CR to varying degrees. Studies in this group, funded by the Nutritional Institutes of Health, have shown that the middle-aged among the members have lower blood pressure, glucose and cholesterol values[52]. However, multiple studies have shown that weight loss increases mortality, institutionalization and hip fractures in persons over 60 years of age.[53] Hence CR may be harmful in elders who are at particular risk of malnutrition.[54]

There are currently several CR-type diets advertised to the public as a method of prolonging life. The CRON diet (Caloric Restriction with Optimal Nutrition), developed by the founders of the above-mentioned society, recommends a 20% CR based on individual basal metabolic rate. The Okinawa diet, a low-calorie, nutrient-rich diet, is founded on the original diet of people living on the Japanese island of Okinawa (Ryuku Islands), which has the highest concentration of centenarians in the world. The diet has fewer calories than a traditional Japanese diet and consists mainly of vegetables (especially sweet potatoes), a half serving of fish per day, legumes and soy. It is low in meat, eggs and dairy products. Other diets based on similar food combinations, such as the New Longevity Diet, have been developed. None of these diets have been proven to extend longevity and Roy Walford, a major proponent of dietary restriction, died at 79 years of age of amyotrophic lateral sclerosis (ALS). Of note, animal studies have suggested that CR is especially hazardous for animals with ALS.

Numerous mechanisms have been proposed to explain why CR may promote longevity. One of these mechanisms is autophagy or cellular self-digestion, involved in protein and organelle degradation. A common characteristic of ageing cells is the accumulation of damaged proteins and organelles that predispose the cells to a pathogenic phenotype with aggregate-prone mutant proteins. These deposits of altered components are particularly detrimental in non-dividing differentiated cells, such as neurons and cardiomyocytes, where the age-dependent functional decline usually manifests. It is proposed that the decreased autophagy with age may play a major role in functional deterioration. CR seems to improve autophagy induction, possibly owing to lower levels of insulin, an autophagy inhibitor.[55] Another mechanism proposed to explain CR effects is hormesis, which states that CR represents a low-level stress that allows the animal to develop enhanced defences and to slow the ageing process.[56] It has also been suggested that CR reduces oxidative damage, enhances insulin sensitivity and decreases tissue glycation.[57]

CR mimetics

Current efforts aim to reproduce or mimic the beneficial effect of CR, without its side effects. Interest is particularly high with regard to CR mimetics as possible therapies for obesity. Autophagy induction has been tested through the use of antilipolytic drugs, which mimic the starvation state induced by CR.[55] Another CR mimetic, which upregulates autophagy, is rapamycin (sirolimus) or its analogue everolimus.[58] It has recently been demonstrated that treatment with this antibiotic delays ageing and extends lifespan in yeast,[59] *Caenorhabditis elegans*[60] and mice.[61] The 'silent information regulator' (Sir) gene is upregulated by CR in yeast and in mammals and sirtuin-activating compounds (STACs) are under development. Resveratrol, an antioxidant component in red wine, is a STAC that has been shown to extend lifespan in yeast, flies and worms[62,63] and to modulate insulin secretion and action.[64] Although it is possible that resveratrol is healthy, just as other antioxidants contained in vegetables and fruits, or may have a positive effect on the prevention of age-related diseases such as diabetes, there is at present no evidence that it can delay, even slightly, the human ageing process.

Epigenetics

This is a field that has recently been linked to longevity. Epigenetics refers to changes in gene expression caused by mechanisms other than changes in the underlying DNA. These changes may remain through cell divisions for the remainder of the cell's life and may also be transferred to the next generation. For example, nutrition might induce epigenetic changes that could be transmitted to the next generation, impacting on health. It has been shown that the ancestors' food availability and nutrition during the slow growth period before the prepuberal peak is followed by different transgenerational responses, which are the main influence on longevity.[65]

Translation of results into humans

Can the results of biogerontological research in experimental models be extended to humans? This is an unresolved question. There have been attempts to search for similarities in the IGF-1/insulin signalling (one of the main regulators implicated in the ageing process) in *C. elegans* and humans.[66] A 6.4-fold increase in lifespan in *C. elegans* was first reported secondary to a single base mutation in daf-2, the equivalent of IGF-1 receptor in humans,[67] but the relationship between insulin signalling and ageing seems to be more complicated in mammals: insulin-receptor knockout mice die in early neonatal life of diabetic ketoacidosis.[68]

Even though genetically modified animals such as dwarf mice have shown extreme lifespans[25,26] and rats bred to have high aerobic capacity had fewer cardiovascular risk factors than control rats,[69] the identification of genetic determinants of human longevity is still inconclusive. Although many plausible candidate genes have been proposed, only one finding [apolipoprotein E (Apo-E)] has so far been replicated.[66] The initial expectation that a few rate-limiting targets modulate ageing has been contrasted with the finding that over 100 gene manipulations may increase longevity in *C. elegans*.[66] Another important downside in the search for longevity determinants is that mortality trends seem to be stochastic in nematodes[70] and in humans,[66] with enormous variations in lifespan.

Stem cell ageing

It has been proposed that age-related defects in stem cells can limit proper tissue maintenance and contribute to a shortened lifespan.[71] In competitive repopulation experiments, there was little difference in haematopoietic stem cell (HSC) activity 4 weeks after transplantation in young versus old HSCs. However, at 8 and 16 weeks post-transplantation, old HSCs showed a reduced contribution compared with young control HSCs.[71]

It has been suggested that stem cell ageing may determine the ageing process, but the connections at different levels are complex. At the genomic level, both internal and environmental factors may cause alterations in individual or groups of genes through epigenetic changes with direct damage to DNA. However, it is not clear whether age-related epigenetic changes render DNA more susceptible to damage or DNA damage underlies epigenetic changes.[72]

The emergence of possible therapies with stem cells in order to regenerate tissues, for example the heart, has created a fair amount of hope. However, the response to stem cell therapies has been shown to be different in aged as compared with younger animals. In an animal model of induced myocardial infarction, cardiac structure and function were reversed dramatically in young animals treated with granulocyte colony-stimulating factor and stem cell factor, but old animals did not show any benefit.[73] On the other hand, stem cells with a muscle-specific IGF reversed the muscle loss (sarcopenia) seen in ageing mice[74] and a major predictor of disability.[75] A recent review of the possible role of stem cell ageing as a determinant of human ageing concluded that a more precise mechanistic understanding is needed before it can be translated into human antiageing therapies. The authors recommend adhesion to a healthy lifestyle (smoking cessation, a balanced diet and regular exercise) as the most clinically validated advice at the moment.[76]

Nevertheless, the colossal advances in stem cell research in the past few years cannot be ignored. Induced pluripotent stem (iPS) cells created from skin cells first in mice[77] and then in humans[78] and the induction of insulin secretion in iPS mouse cells[79] may open paths for future potential therapeutic possibilities, provided that they prove to be safe.

The hormonal fountain of youth

Towards the end of the nineteenth century, Brown-Séquard suggested that a testicular extract produced remarkable antiageing effects. The powerful effect of placebo was demonstrated, since it is unlikely that his extract had any testosterone. Many wealthy men in Europe and the USA received monkey testicular implants and claimed that they had rejuvenation effects. Brinkley in the USA pioneered the use of 'goat gland' extracts, which were equally ineffective, but made him a rich man. Subsequently, almost every hormone has been publicized as having antiageing effects. The case of HGH, with many rich persons paying exorbitant amounts of money to attain everlasting youth, has already been mentioned. Dehydroepiandrosterone (DHEA) is similarly promoted for antiageing therapy. Despite positive animal studies,[80] well-controlled human studies have failed to show any beneficial effects.[81,82] DHEA replacement showed to increase bone mineral density in a randomized controlled trial, but the effect was relatively small compared with traditional osteoporosis therapies.[83] Likewise, 2 years of DHEA supplementation did not change body composition, muscle strength, insulin sensitivity or quality of life. DHEA may improve some metabolic parameters and measures of psychological wellness in subjects with adrenal insufficiency, but the benefit is not consistently sustained in long-term therapy.[84]

Of the hormones, the best available positive data are for vitamin D. A meta-analysis showed that vitamin D replacement decreases mortality,[85] improves function, decreases falls and prevents hip fracture in persons with 25-hydroxy-vitamin D levels below 30 ng ml^{-1}.[86] There is agreement about the need for older persons either to get regular skin exposure (15–30 min per day) without sun block or to take 800–1000 IU of vitamin D per day. All persons over 70 years of age should have their 25-hydroxy-vitamin D levels measured at least yearly (preferably in winter) and, when needed, have their level raised above 30 ng ml^{-1}.

Similarly to HGH, testosterone levels decline with ageing (in both men and women). Some, but not all, studies have shown that low testosterone is associated with increased mortality in males, but the findings are confounded by the decrease in testosterone levels induced by illness.[87–92] Meta-analyses have shown that testosterone improves sexual function and muscle mass and strength in older men.[93,94] Bone mineral density in hypogonadal men increases under testosterone substitution.[95] However, fracture data are not available, hence the long-term benefit of testosterone warrants further investigation. In oophorectomized women, testosterone enhances sexual function.[96] This has led to the development of selective androgen receptor molecules, which appear to improve power in older males and females.[97] The role of testosterone in older persons is established for the treatment of sexual dysfunction (both low libido and in some cases erectile problems).[98] A recent consensus statement from diverse international scientific societies has provided valuable guidelines for the diagnosis of age-associated testosterone deficiency syndrome, for treatment with testosterone supplementation and for the identification of possible adverse effects and contraindications of such treatment.[99] A careful selection of candidates, an appropriate dosing of hormonal supplementation and an attentive clinical follow-up are crucial instruments for the correct use of testosterone replacement therapy.

Even though short-term estrogen/progesterone replacement therapy (HRT) to treat severe menopause-related symptoms and to reduce osteoporotic fracture risk in selected postmenopausal women is well established, its long-term use for disease prevention has generated extensive debate. Studies conducted in the USA[100,101] and the UK[102,103] showed no effect on protection against cardiovascular disease and even suggested that this therapy may increase the risk. Recent reanalysis of these trial results supports positive cardiovascular outcomes provided that HRT is initiated within 10 years since menopause. The favourable benefit–risk ratio for HRT decreases with ageing and with time since menopause.[104] Moreover, HRT seems to increase the incidence of dementia when initiated in women aged 65 years and older.[104] Hence current guidelines recommend HRT use close to menopause, when indicated, for the shortest time and at the lowest dose possible.

Anabolic steroids are emerging as possible candidates for adjuvant therapy during rehabilitation, and it is possible that they will play a role in improving healthspan. However, their potential harmful prostatic effects[105] suggest that they possibly will not be used as longevity agents.

Studies by Morley and co-workers in mice have shown that pregnenolone is a potent memory enhancer.[80] Nevertheless, results in humans have been largely negative, hence at present pregnenolone should not be used as a memory enhancer or an antiageing hormone.[106]

The hormone melatonin, produced by the pineal gland, also declines with ageing. Although it has antioxidant properties and has hypnotic effects, overall it appears to have minimal effects as an antiageing agent.

Most of data available for antiageing interventions relate to hormonal replacement treatments. However, despite initial promising results in the past decades, currently available data do not validate an extensive use of hormones in order to reverse or delay the ageing process, with the exception of vitamin D. Despite these facts, many unscrupulous charlatans prescribe and probably will continue to prescribe and supply hormones inappropriately and ageing people will continue to use them avidly with the dream of eternal youth. In reality, the search for a hormonal fountain of youth has been as disappointing as Ponce de León's search for a fountain of youth.

Preventive gerontology

Ageing is by far the main risk factor for a wide range of clinical conditions that are at present the most frequent causes of morbidity and mortality. It is now widely accepted that ageing is the result of the sum of damage during the course of life, with consequent alterations in several functions of the organism that may favour the development of diseases commonly observed in old age. One of the most accepted mechanisms, among over 300, to explain the ageing process is the excessive mitochondrial production of free oxygen radicals [reactive oxygen species (ROS)] – called oxidative stress – with damage to cellular structure and subsequent inflammation.[107,108] Oxidative stress accumulates when pro-oxidants overwhelm the antioxidant defence mechanisms and has been implicated in diverse age-associated chronic diseases, including atherosclerosis, cardio- and cerebrovascular disease, cardiometabolic syndrome, obesity, type 2 diabetes, osteoporosis and osteoarthritis, neurodegeneration (Alzheimer's disease, Parkinson's disease), cancer, depression, sarcopenia and frailty.[109,110] ROS serve as precursors to the formation of oxidized low-density lipoprotein (LDL), essential to the formation of atherosclerotic plaques.[110] Elevated ROS have also been associated with an increased expression of pro-inflammatory cytokines such as tumour necrosis factor (TNF)-α, plasminogen activator inhibitor (PAI)-1 and interleukin (IL)-6.[111] Chronic inflammation has been associated with a broad spectrum of degenerative diseases of ageing, including Alzheimer's disease, Parkinson's disease, amyotrophic lateral sclerosis and age-related macular degeneration, and has been also proposed as one of the main causes of frailty in older persons.[112] This concept has led researchers to seek factors that may reduce or contrast the cellular damage or enhance the repair mechanisms, hence delaying the beginning of diseases and improving the quality of life in older age.

Antioxidants

It is now widely accepted that consumption of fruits and vegetables, natural products that are rich in antioxidants, appear to prevent multiple diseases. However, there is no evidence that persons taking vitamin supplements have a longer life than those who do not take supplements. Studies on vitamin E and cardiovascular disease in humans have found that supplementation either has no effect or is harmful.[113] Similarly, studies of the effects of vitamin E on cancer have shown mixed results. Vitamin E had minimal effects on persons with Alzheimer's disease.

The ATBC trial demonstrated that β-carotene supplementation was associated with an increased incidence of lung, prostate and stomach cancer.[114] The CARET study also resulted in an increase in lung cancer mortality in persons previously exposed to asbestos who received β-carotene preparations.[115] No effects with β-carotene supplementation have been also demonstrated for cardiovascular disease in a number of studies.[116] Similarly, vitamin C has been shown to have minimal beneficial effects. α-Lipoic acid, a powerful antioxidant, has been proved to be useful in the treatment of diabetic neuropathy.[117] It reversed memory disturbances in SAMP8 mice, a partial model of Alzheimer's disease,[118] but it seemed to increase mortality rate in mice. A recent Cochrane review concluded that multivitamin/mineral supplements conferred no benefit in preventing cardiovascular disease.[119] In summary, human studies do not support the use of antioxidant vitamin supplementation.

Lifestyle

Numerous epidemiological studies have shown that interventions in lifestyle (e.g. smoking cessation, a balanced diet, regular physical and mental activity) may decrease the susceptibility to disease development, increasing longevity and healthspan. A healthy lifestyle has demonstrated positive effects on longevity also in older populations. As mentioned, centenarians have generally adhered to a healthy lifestyle. A prospective study conducted in 2357 men showed that modifiable biological and lifestyle factors, assessed at a mean age of 72 years, were associated with exceptional longevity of 90 or more years and with high functional status in late life.[120] The EPIC-Norfolk study showed that not smoking, getting some exercise, eating five helpings of fruit and vegetables each day and drinking 1–14 glasses of alcohol per week[13] provided an estimated 14 year improvement in chronological age. Thus, encouraging favourable lifestyle behaviours, including smoking abstinence, weight management, blood pressure control and exercise, may not only enhance life expectancy but may also reduce morbidity and functional decline in later years.

Exercise

A growing body of evidence has accumulated in the past two decades confirming that promotion of physical activity is perhaps the most effective prescription that physicians can formulate to promote ageing successfully. Practically all age-related diseases leading to physical disability during late life are linked in some way to a sedentary lifestyle. Indeed, exercise in moderation appears to be a cornerstone of longevity. Mice with an excess of phosphoenolpyruvate carboxykinase (PEPCK-C) in their skeletal muscle are more active than their controls and can run for 5 km at a speed of 20 m min^{-1} compared with 0.2 km for control mice.[121] These mice live longer than controls and females remain reproductively active until 35 months of age.

Observational studies in humans have strongly suggested that those who are physically active live longer. It has been shown that high total energy expenditure in 70–80 year olds leads to increased longevity,[38] with climbing stairs being the major factor that resulted in increased total energy expenditure. Fries found that older runners had 13 years delay in the development of disability compared with a group of sedentary older persons.[122] Likewise, the LIFE-Pilot study demonstrated that a structured physical activity programme significantly improved functional performance, measured with the Short Physical Performance Battery, which includes walking, balance and chair stands tests, and the 400 m walking speed, suggesting that this type of intervention may offer benefit on more distal health outcomes, such as mobility disability.[45] Walking speed is associated with decreased disability and physical activity is associated with decreased dysphoria. Persons aged 50 years of age who exercise regularly are less likely to develop Alzheimer's disease as they age.[123] In addition, it has been reported that regular physical activity reduces the rate of deterioration in persons with dementia.[124]

Diet

A myriad of studies have shown that different components of a balanced diet may contribute to decrease the incidence of cardiovascular disease, diabetes mellitus and some types of cancer. There is mounting evidence that a dietary pattern similar to that followed by traditional populations living in the Mediterranean basin during the post-World War II period, based on bread, grains, olive oil, legumes, fruits, fresh vegetables, nuts and fish, has remarkable effects in reducing total mortality, cardiovascular mortality and cancer-related mortality.[16,36,37,125–134] The Mediterranean diet includes a significantly large amount of plant foods rich in antioxidant compounds, which may help to explain its multiple benefits. A study conducted in 74 607 subjects without coronary artery disease, stroke or cancer at enrolment recruited from 10 European countries concluded that every 2 unit increment in a score constructed with the above-mentioned elements of the Mediterranean diet conferred a reduction of 8% in overall mortality.[36] In patients with coronary heart disease at baseline, the reduction in overall mortality was even higher, with a 27% reduction in mortality.[37] The Mediterranean diet has also been demonstrated to decrease the incidence of diabetes mellitus in different populations[135,136] and to decrease the need for hypoglycaemic therapy for newly diagnosed diabetics.[137] A recent meta-analysis of 12 large studies including a total of over 1.5 million subjects confirmed a significant reduction in all-cause mortality associated to increases in Mediterranean diet score adherence.[20] The meta-analysis also included recent studies demonstrating a reduction in the risk of developing Parkinson's[138] and Alzheimer's[139] disease. Also, the incidence of depression has been shown to decrease with increased adherence to this dietary pattern.[140] All the studies on the Mediterranean diet emphasize the effects of the whole dietary pattern with the combination of different nutrient-rich and antioxidant foods rather than individual elements. In fact, the effects of the combination of components of a balanced diet may potentiate the effect of single elements, as shown by the effects of a 'polymeal' on cardiovascular events frequency. Analyses of data from the Framingham heart study and the Framingham offspring study showed that combining different foods with well-known evidence of cardioprotection (wine, fish, dark chocolate, fruits, vegetables, garlic and almonds) would reduce cardiovascular events by 76%.[141]

Ethical issues

Antiageing medicines raise a number of ethical issues. For instance, in a society with limited resources, is extending the life of older populations appropriate? How would one approach the question of life extension if it is associated with cognitive impairment? Is extending life duration without improvement in quality appropriate? Will it be possible for most people? How long is it appropriate to extend life for: 5, 10, 50 years, ..., or is it appropriate to think about a future life extension of 100 years? There are no simple answers to these questions and certainly they belong not only to scientific and philosophical areas, but also to ethics, fiscal regulations and religious beliefs.

Another concern is the use of technological advances. Technology may make our life better, but the price paid sometimes is high and a world that depends completely on technology may be a world of slaves. It is essential that well-controlled human trials are carried out so that we do not end up shortening rather than prolonging lifespan. In addition, technological advances may not be available for the majority of people, which may generate rising discrimination and inequality issues.

What should be considered as successful ageing? The measures for successful ageing entail physiological parameters such as disease incidence, mobility and mental acuity, but also important psychological determinants, including resilience, emotional wellbeing, connectedness and spirituality. In fact, psychological factors such as sociality, conflict avoidance and adaptiveness seem to be associated with exceptional longevity,[142] and resilience, or the ability to cope with adversity and losses, has been associated with healthy longevity.[143] With respect to older patients, the multidimensional aspects are even broader and may include, for instance, having autonomy over the place and manner of the final days.[144] With these concepts in mind, it is possible that the achievement of disease/disability avoidance and life extension may have less value if other determinants of wellbeing are not taken into account.

Conclusion

Who does not hope for longevity combined with good health in later years? However, since ageing is so complex, it is unlikely that one pill or a single magic bullet procedure can slow the ageing process. In recent decades, striking advances in the understanding of the ageing process have come from studies of animal models, but the translation of positive results to humans is not yet realistic. Therapies that are highly effective in animals can be highly toxic in humans. Even if simple solutions that may require some physical labour are not easy to put in practice, a balanced diet of moderate proportions, in addition to regular exercise, today remains the best clinically validated advice, namely, the only proven fountain of youth.

Demographic changes will mould new contexts of societies and of developments around the world and will test the capacity of health systems to provide quality of life for millions of older persons. Support systems from governments and social agencies will be needed to cope with the tough challenges of these new societies that should focus on the promotion of healthy ageing. The factual prolongation of the 'active life expectancy' of the population in past decades suggests that disease and disability may indeed be delayed. Compression of morbidity and of disability rather than prolongation of survival may be one of the main goals of disease management in the older patient.

The geriatrician may play an important role in educating older persons about the positive and negative faces of antiageing strategies. It cannot be ignored that in the future stems cells, information/communication technology, nanotechnology and robotics will change the practice of medicine. The potential for these strategies, such as stem cells to rejuvenate diverse tissues, cochlear implants and retinal computer chips, is enormous, but their application to humans is only just starting.

Continuous advances in medical knowledge contribute to increased longevity and improved quality of life. Even taking into consideration the possible negative sides, medical advances are at present the strongest antiageing medicine. However, the ageing public continues to spend billions of dollars on antiageing remedies of unproven value. Geriatricians have an essential role as educators on how to age successfully.

Key points

- Interventions in lifestyle (e.g. a diet rich in fruit and vegetables, low in saturated fats, salt and sweetened drinks, without *trans*-fatty acids; regular moderate exercise; smoking cessation; drinking 1–2 glasses of alcohol daily; fish consumption) decrease the susceptibility to age-associated disease development and mortality, and hence delay ageing.
- Animal studies reporting interventions that increase longevity are often assumed to be directly applicable to humans before appropriate clinical trials have been performed.
- There is no evidence that hormones, vitamins or antioxidant supplementation prolong life.
- Vitamin D replacement, in persons with low 25-hydroxy-vitamin D levels, decreases hip fractures, decreases fall incidence, improves muscle strength, enhances function and decreases mortality.
- Antiageing medicine has been taken over by swindlers who promote unproven, potentially dangerous and expensive remedies to a credulous ageing public.

References

1. Narasimhan SD, Yen K and Tissenbaum HA. Converging pathways in lifespan regulation. *Curr Biol* 2009;**19**:R657–66.
2. Weindruch R, Walford RL, Fligiel S and Guthrie D. The retardation of aging in mice by dietary restriction: longevity, cancer, immunity and lifetime energy intake. *J Nutr* 1986;**116**:641–54.
3. Johnson TE. *Caenorhabditis elegans* 2007: the premier model for the study of aging. *Exp Gerontol* 2008;**43**:1–4.
4. Colman RJ, Anderson RM, Johnson SC *et al*. Caloric restriction delays disease onset and mortality in rhesus monkeys. *Science* 2009;**325**:201–4.
5. Shanley DP and Kirkwood TB. Caloric restriction does not enhance longevity in all species and is unlikely to do so in humans. *Biogerontology* 2006;**7**:165–8.
6. Fisher A and Morley JE. Antiaging medicine: the good, the bad and the ugly. *J Gerontol A Biol Sci Med Sci* 2002;**57**:M636–9.
7. Kirkwood TB. A systematic look at an old problem. *Nature* 2008;**451**:644–7.
8. Nolte E, Shkolnikov V and McKee M. Changing mortality patterns in East and West Germany and Poland. II: short-term trends during transition and in the 1990s. *J Epidemiol Community Health* 2000;**54**:899–906.

9. Dominguez LJ, Galioto A, Ferlisi A *et al.* Ageing, lifestyle modifications and cardiovascular disease in developing countries. *J Nutr Health Aging* 2006;**10**:143–9.
10. Christensen K, Doblhammer G, Rau R and Vaupel JW. Ageing populations: the challenges ahead. *Lancet* 2009;**374**: 1196–208.
11. Berlau DJ, Corrada MM and Kawas C. The prevalence of disability in the oldest-old is high and continues to increase with age: findings from The 90+ Study. *Int J Geriatr Psychiatry* 2009;**24**:1217–25.
12. Chase P, Mitchell K and Morley JE. In the steps of giants: the early geriatrics texts. *J Am Geriatr Soc* 2000;**48**:89–94.
13. Khaw KT, Wareham N, Bingham S *et al.* Combined impact of health behaviours and mortality in men and women: the EPIC-Norfolk prospective population study. *PLoS Med* 2008;**5**:e12.
14. Yamori Y. Food factors for atherosclerosis prevention: Asian perspective derived from analyses of worldwide dietary biomarkers. *Exp Clin Cardiol* 2006;**11**:94–8.
15. Manton KG, Gu X and Lamb VL. Change in chronic disability from 1982 to 2004/2005 as measured by long-term changes in function and health in the U.S. elderly population. *Proc Natl Acad Sci USA* 2006;**103**:18374–9.
16. Knoops KT, de Groot LC, Kromhout D *et al.* Mediterranean diet, lifestyle factors and 10-year mortality in elderly European men and women: the HALE project. *JAMA* 2004;**292**:1433–9.
17. Fuller Thomson E, Yu B, Nuru Jeter A *et al.* Basic ADL disability and functional limitation rates among older Americans from 2000–2005: the end of the decline? *J Gerontol A Biol Sci Med Sci* 2009;**64**:1333–6.
18. Stewart ST, Cutler DM and Rosen AB. Forecasting the effects of obesity and smoking on U.S. life expectancy. *N Engl J Med* 2009;**361**:2252–60.
19. Morley JE. A brief history of geriatrics. *J Gerontol A Biol Sci Med Sci* 2004;**59**:1132–52.
20. Sofi F, Cesari F, Abbate R *et al.* Adherence to Mediterranean diet and health status: meta-analysis. *BMJ* 2008;**337**:a1344.
21. Anonymous. Abstracts of Strategies for Engineered Negligible Senescence (SENS) Fourth Conference, Cambridge, United Kingdom, September 3–7, 2009. *Rejuvenation Res* 2009;**12**(Suppl)1: S17–59.
22. Warner H, Anderson J, Austad S *et al.* Science fact and the SENS agenda. What can we reasonably expect from ageing research? *EMBO Rep* 2005;**6**:1006–8.
23. Olshansky SJ, Hayflick L and Carnes BA. Position statement on human aging. *J Gerontol A Biol Sci Med Sci* 2002;**57**:B292–7.
24. Rudman D, Feller AG, Nagraj HS *et al.* Effects of human growth hormone in men over 60 years old. *N Engl J Med* 1990;**323**:1–6.
25. Liang H, Masoro EJ, Nelson JF *et al.* Genetic mouse models of extended lifespan. *Exp Gerontol* 2003;**38**:1353–64.
26. Flurkey K, Papaconstantinou J, Miller RA and Harrison DE. Lifespan extension and delayed immune and collagen aging in mutant mice with defects in growth hormone production. *Proc Natl Acad Sci USA* 2001;**98**:6736–41.
27. Al-Regaiey KA, Masternak MM, Bonkowski M *et al.* Long-lived growth hormone receptor knockout mice: interaction of reduced insulin-like growth factor I/insulin signaling and caloric restriction. *Endocrinology* 2005;**146**:851–60.
28. Sun LY, Al-Regaiey K, Masternak MM *et al.* Local expression of GH and IGF-1 in the hippocampus of GH-deficient long-lived mice. *Neurobiol Aging* 2005;**26**:929–37.
29. Liu H, Bravata DM, Olkin I *et al.* Systematic review: the safety and efficacy of growth hormone in the healthy elderly. *Ann Intern Med* 2007;**146**:104–15.
30. Dong MQ, Venable JD, Au N *et al.* Quantitative mass spectrometry identifies insulin signaling targets in *C. elegans*. *Science* 2007;**317**:660–3.
31. Flatt T, Min KJ, D'Alterio C *et al.* *Drosophila* germ-line modulation of insulin signaling and lifespan. *Proc Natl Acad Sci USA* 2008;**105**:6368–73.
32. Bartke A, Chandrashekar V, Turyn D *et al.* Effects of growth hormone overexpression and growth hormone resistance on neuroendocrine and reproductive functions in transgenic and knock-out mice. *Proc Soc Exp Biol Med* 1999; **222**:113–23.
33. Forster MJ, Morris P and Sohal RS. Genotype and age influence the effect of caloric intake on mortality in mice. *FASEB J* 2003;**17**:690–2.
34. Laron Z. Do deficiencies in growth hormone and insulin-like growth factor-1 (IGF-1) shorten or prolong longevity? *Mech Ageing Dev* 2005;**126**:305–7.
35. Suh Y, Atzmon G, Cho MO *et al.* Functionally significant insulin-like growth factor I receptor mutations in centenarians. *Proc Natl Acad Sci USA* 2008;**105**:3138–42.
36. Trichopoulou A, Orfanos P, Norat T *et al.* Modified Mediterranean diet and survival: EPIC-elderly prospective cohort study. *BMJ* 2005;**330**:991.
37. Trichopoulou A, Bamia C and Trichopoulos D. Mediterranean diet and survival among patients with coronary heart disease in Greece. *Arch Intern Med* 2005;**165**:929–35.
38. Manini TM, Everhart JE, Patel KV *et al.* Daily activity energy expenditure and mortality among older adults. *JAMA* 2006;**296**:171–9.
39. Perls TT. The different paths to 100. *Am J Clin Nutr* 2006;**83**:484S–7S.
40. Galioto A, Dominguez LJ, Pineo A *et al.* Cardiovascular risk factors in centenarians. *Exp Gerontol* 2008;**43**:106–13.
41. Ferris DP, Sawicki GS and Daley MA. A physiologist's perspective on robotic exoskeletons for human locomotion. *Int J HR* 2007;**4**:507–28.
42. Fernandez PL. Nanotechnology, nanomedicine and nanopharmacology. *An R Acad Nac Med (Madr)* 2007;**124**: 189–200; discussion 200–1 (in Spanish).
43. Perreau A, Tyler RS and Witt SA. The effect of reducing the number of electrodes on spatial hearing tasks for bilateral cochlear implant recipients. *J Am Acad Audiol* 2010;**21**:110–20.
44. Etgen T, Sander D, Huntgeburth U *et al.* Physical activity and incident cognitive impairment in elderly persons: the INVADE study. *Arch Intern Med* 2010;**170**:186–93.
45. Pahor M, Blair SN, Espeland M *et al.* Effects of a physical activity intervention on measures of physical performance: results of the lifestyle interventions and independence for Elders Pilot (LIFE-P) study. *J Gerontol A Biol Sci Med Sci* 2006;**61**:1157–65.

46. Fries JF, Green LW and Levine S. Health promotion and the compression of morbidity. *Lancet* 1989;**i**:481–3.
47. Anderson RM and Weindruch R. Calorie restriction: progress during mid-2005–mid-2006. *Exp Gerontol* 2006;**41**: 1247–9.
48. Qin W, Chachich M, Lane M *et al.* Calorie restriction attenuates Alzheimer's disease type brain amyloidosis in Squirrel monkeys (*Saimiri sciureus*). *J Alzheimers Dis* 2006;**10**:417–22.
49. Lipman RD, Smith DE, Bronson RT and Blumberg J. Is late-life caloric restriction beneficial? *Aging (Milano)* 1995; **7**:136–9.
50. Partridge L and Gems D. Benchmarks for ageing studies. *Nature* 2007;**450**:165–7.
51. Fontana L and Klein S. Aging, adiposity and calorie restriction. *JAMA* 2007;**297**:986–94.
52. Fontana L, Meyer TE, Klein S and Holloszy JO. Long-term calorie restriction is highly effective in reducing the risk for atherosclerosis in humans. *Proc Natl Acad Sci USA* 2004;**101**:6659–63.
53. Morley JE. Weight loss in older persons: new therapeutic approaches. *Curr Pharm Des* 2007;**13**:3637–47.
54. Morley JE, Chahla E and Alkaade S. Antiaging, longevity and calorie restriction. *Curr Opin Clin Nutr Metab Care* 2010; **13**:40–5.
55. Mizushima N, Levine B, Cuervo AM and Klionsky DJ. Autophagy fights disease through cellular self-digestion. *Nature* 2008;**451**:1069–75.
56. Rattan SI. The science of healthy aging: genes, milieu and chance. *Ann N Y Acad Sci* 2007;**1114**:1–10.
57. Gugliucci A, Kotani K, Taing J *et al.* Short-term low calorie diet intervention reduces serum advanced glycation end products in healthy overweight or obese adults. *Ann Nutr Metab* 2009;**54**:197–201.
58. Inuzuka Y, Okuda J, Kawashima T *et al.* Suppression of phosphoinositide 3-kinase prevents cardiac aging in mice. *Circulation* 2009;**120**:1695–703.
59. Alvers AL, Wood MS, Hu D *et al.* Autophagy is required for extension of yeast chronological life span by rapamycin. *Autophagy* 2009;**5**:847–9.
60. Hansen M, Chandra A, Mitic LL *et al.* A role for autophagy in the extension of lifespan by dietary restriction in *C. elegans*. *PLoS Genet* 2008;**4**:e24.
61. Harrison DE, Strong R, Sharp ZD *et al.* Rapamycin fed late in life extends lifespan in genetically heterogeneous mice. *Nature* 2009;**460**:392–5.
62. Howitz KT, Bitterman KJ, Cohen HY *et al.* Small molecule activators of sirtuins extend *Saccharomyces cerevisiae* lifespan. *Nature* 2003;**425**:191–6.
63. Wood JG, Rogina B, Lavu S *et al.* Sirtuin activators mimic caloric restriction and delay ageing in metazoans. *Nature* 2004;**430**:686–9.
64. Frojdo S, Durand C and Pirola L. Metabolic effects of resveratrol in mammals – a link between improved insulin action and aging. *Curr Aging Sci* 2008;**1**:145–51.
65. Kaati G, Bygren LO, Pembrey M and Sjostrom M. Transgenerational response to nutrition, early life circumstances and longevity. *Eur J Hum Genet* 2007;**15**:784–90.
66. Christensen K, Johnson TE and Vaupel JW. The quest for genetic determinants of human longevity: challenges and insights. *Nat Rev Genet* 2006;**7**:436–48.
67. Partridge L and Gems D. Mechanisms of ageing: public or private? *Nat Rev Genet* 2002;**3**:165–75.
68. Russell SJ and Kahn CR. Endocrine regulation of ageing. *Nat Rev Mol Cell Biol* 2007;**8**:681–91.
69. Wisloff U, Najjar SM, Ellingsen O *et al.* Cardiovascular risk factors emerge after artificial selection for low aerobic capacity. *Science* 2005;**307**:418–20.
70. Herndon LA, Schmeissner PJ, Dudaronek JM *et al.* Stochastic and genetic factors influence tissue-specific decline in ageing *C. elegans*. *Nature* 2002;**419**:808–14.
71. Chambers SM, Shaw CA, Gatza C *et al.* Aging hematopoietic stem cells decline in function and exhibit epigenetic dysregulation. *PLoS Biol* 2007;**5**:e201.
72. Brunet A and Rando TA. Ageing: from stem to stern. *Nature* 2007;**449**:288–91.
73. Lehrke S, Mazhari R, Durand DJ *et al.* Aging impairs the beneficial effect of granulocyte colony-stimulating factor and stem cell factor on post-myocardial infarction remodeling. *Circ Res* 2006;**99**:553–60.
74. Musaro A, Giacinti C, Borsellino G *et al.* Stem cell-mediated muscle regeneration is enhanced by local isoform of insulin-like growth factor 1. *Proc Natl Acad Sci USA* 2004; **101**:1206–10.
75. Morley JE, Baumgartner RN, Roubenoff R *et al.* Sarcopenia. *J Lab Clin Med* 2001;**137**:231–43.
76. Sharpless NE and DePinho RA. How stem cells age and why this makes us grow old. *Nat Rev Mol Cell Biol* 2007;**8**:703–13.
77. Yamanaka S Takahashi K. Induction of pluripotent stem cells from mouse fibroblast cultures. *Tanpakushitsu Kakusan Koso* 2006;**51**:2346–51 (in Japanese).
78. Yamanaka S. Strategies and new developments in the generation of patient-specific pluripotent stem cells. *Cell Stem Cell* 2007;**1**:39–49.
79. Zhou Q, Brown J, Kanarek A *et al.* *In vivo* reprogramming of adult pancreatic exocrine cells to beta-cells. *Nature* 2008;**455**:627–32.
80. Flood JF, Morley JE and Roberts E. Memory-enhancing effects in male mice of pregnenolone and steroids metabolically derived from it. *Proc Natl Acad Sci USA* 1992;**89**: 1567–71.
81. Percheron G, Hogrel JY, Denot-Ledunois S *et al.* Effect of 1-year oral administration of dehydroepiandrosterone to 60- to 80-year-old individuals on muscle function and cross-sectional area: a double-blind placebo-controlled trial. *Arch Intern Med* 2003;**163**:720–7.
82. Baulieu EE, Thomas G, Legrain S *et al.* Dehydroepiandrosterone (DHEA), DHEA sulfate and aging: contribution of the DHEAge Study to a sociobiomedical issue. *Proc Natl Acad Sci USA* 2000;**9**:4279–84.
83. Nair KS, Rizza RA, O'Brien P *et al.* DHEA in elderly women and DHEA or testosterone in elderly men. *N Engl J Med* 2006; **355**:1647–59.
84. Bhagra S, Nippoldt TB and Nair KS. Dehydroepiandrosterone in adrenal insufficiency and ageing. *Curr Opin Endocrinol Diabetes Obes* 2008;**15**:239–43.

85. Autier P and Gandini S. Vitamin D supplementation and total mortality: a meta-analysis of randomized controlled trials. *Arch Intern Med* 2007;**167**:1730–7.

86. Morley JE. Should all long-term care residents receive vitamin D? *J Am Med Dir Assoc* 2007;**8**:69–70.

87. Morley JE, Kaiser FE, Perry HM III *et al.* Longitudinal changes in testosterone, luteinizing hormone and follicle-stimulating hormone in healthy older men. *Metabolism* 1997; **46**:410–3.

88. Khaw KT, Dowsett M, Folkerd E *et al.* Endogenous testosterone and mortality due to all causes, cardiovascular disease and cancer in men: European prospective investigation into cancer in Norfolk (EPIC-Norfolk) Prospective Population Study. *Circulation* 2007;**116**:2694–701.

89. Laughlin GA, Barrett-Connor E and Bergstrom J. Low serum testosterone and mortality in older men. *J Clin Endocrinol Metab* 2008;**93**:68–75.

90. Shores MM, Matsumoto AM, Sloan KL and Kivlahan DR. Low serum testosterone and mortality in male veterans. *Arch Intern Med* 2006;**166**:1660–5.

91. Araujo AB, Kupelian V, Page ST *et al.* Sex steroids and all-cause and cause-specific mortality in men. *Arch Intern Med* 2007;**167**:1252–60.

92. Morley JE and Melmed S. Gonadal dysfunction in systemic disorders. *Metabolism* 1979;**28**:1051–73.

93. Bolona ER, Uraga MV, Haddad RM *et al.* Testosterone use in men with sexual dysfunction: a systematic review and meta-analysis of randomized placebo-controlled trials. *Mayo Clin Proc* 2007;**82**:20–8.

94. Isidori AM, Giannetta E, Gianfrilli D *et al.* Effects of testosterone on sexual function in men: results of a meta-analysis. *Clin Endocrinol (Oxf)* 2005;**63**:381–94.

95. Amory JK, Watts NB, Easley KA *et al.* Exogenous testosterone or testosterone with finasteride increases bone mineral density in older men with low serum testosterone. *J Clin Endocrinol Metab* 2004;**89**:503–10.

96. Morley JE and Perry HM III Androgens and women at the menopause and beyond. *J Gerontol A Biol Sci Med Sci* 2003;**58**:M409–16.

97. Morley JE and Thomas DR. Cachexia: new advances in the management of wasting diseases. *J Am Med Dir Assoc* 2008;**9**: 205–10.

98. Nieschlag E, Swerdloff R, Behre HM *et al.* Investigation, treatment and monitoring of late-onset hypogonadism in males. *Aging Male* 2005;**8**:56–8.

99. Wang C, Nieschlag E, Swerdloff R *et al.* Investigation, treatment and monitoring of late-onset hypogonadism in males: ISA, ISSAM, EAU, EAA and ASA recommendations. *Eur Urol* 2009;**55**:121–30.

100. Hulley S, Grady D, Bush T *et al.* Randomized trial of estrogen plus progestin for secondary prevention of coronary heart disease in postmenopausal women. Heart and Estrogen/progestin Replacement Study (HERS) Research Group. *JAMA* 1998;**280**:605–13.

101. Rossouw JE, Anderson GL, Prentice RL *et al.* Risks and benefits of estrogen plus progestin in healthy postmenopausal women: principal results from the Women's Health Initiative randomized controlled trial. *JAMA* 2002;**288**:321–33.

102. Clarke SC, Kelleher J, Lloyd-Jones H *et al.* A study of hormone replacement therapy in postmenopausal women with ischaemic heart disease: the Papworth HRT atherosclerosis study. *BJOG* 2002;**109**:1056–62.

103. Cherry N, Gilmour K, Hannaford P *et al.* Oestrogen therapy for prevention of reinfarction in postmenopausal women: a randomised placebo controlled trial. *Lancet* 2002;**360**: 2001–8.

104. Utian WH, Archer DF, Bachmann GA *et al.* Estrogen and progestogen use in postmenopausal women: July 2008 position statement of The North American Menopause Society. *Menopause* 2008;**15**:584–602.

105. Calof OM, Singh AB, Lee ML *et al.* Adverse events associated with testosterone replacement in middle-aged and older men: a meta-analysis of randomized, placebo-controlled trials. *J Gerontol A Biol Sci Med Sci* 2005;**60**: 1451–7.

106. Horani MH and Morley JE. Hormonal fountains of youth. *Clin Geriatr Med* 2004;**20**:275–92.

107. Harman D. Free radical theory of aging: dietary implications. *Am J Clin Nutr* 1972;**25**:839–43.

108. Terzioglu M and Larsson NG. Mitochondrial dysfunction in mammalian ageing. *Novartis Found Symp* 2007;**287**:197–208; discussion 208–13.

109. Ames BN, Atamna H and Killilea DW. Mineral and vitamin deficiencies can accelerate the mitochondrial decay of aging. *Mol Aspects Med* 2005;**26**:363–78.

110. Sigurdardottir V, Fagerberg B and Hulthe J. Circulating oxidized low-density lipoprotein (LDL) is associated with risk factors of the metabolic syndrome and LDL size in clinically healthy 58-year-old men (AIR study). *J Intern Med* 2002;**252**:440–7.

111. Furukawa S, Fujita T, Shimabukuro M *et al.* Increased oxidative stress in obesity and its impact on metabolic syndrome. *J Clin Invest* 2004;**114**:1752–61.

112. Ferrucci L and Guralnik JM. Inflammation, hormones and body composition at a crossroad. *Am J Med* 2003;**115**:501–2.

113. Bjelakovic G, Nikolova D, Gluud LL *et al.* Antioxidant supplements for prevention of mortality in healthy participants and patients with various diseases. *Cochrane Database Syst Rev* 2008;(2): CD007176.

114. Virtamo J, Pietinen P, Huttunen JK *et al.* Incidence of cancer and mortality following alpha-tocopherol and beta-carotene supplementation: a postintervention follow-up. *JAMA* 2003;**290**:476–85.

115. Smigel K. Beta carotene fails to prevent cancer in two major studies; CARET intervention stopped. *J Natl Cancer Inst* 1996;**88**:145.

116. Roychoudhury P and Schwartz K. Antioxidant vitamins do not prevent cardiovascular disease. *J Fam Pract* 2003; **52**:751–2.

117. Ziegler D. Treatment of diabetic neuropathy and neuropathic pain: how far have we come? *Diabetes Care* 2008; **31**(Suppl 2): S255–61.

118. Farr SA, Poon HF, Dogrukol-Ak D *et al.* The antioxidants alpha-lipoic acid and *N*-acetylcysteine reverse memory impairment and brain oxidative stress in aged SAMP8 mice. *J Neurochem* 2003;**84**:1173–83.

119. Huang HY, Caballero B, Chang S *et al*. Multivitamin/mineral supplements and prevention of chronic disease. *Evid Rep Technol Assess* 2006;**139**:1–117.

120. Yates LB, Djousse L, Kurth T *et al*. Exceptional longevity in men: modifiable factors associated with survival and function to age 90 years. *Arch Intern Med* 2008;**168**:284–90.

121. Hanson RW and Hakimi P. Born to run; the story of the PEPCK-Cmus mouse. *Biochimie* 2008;**90**:838–42.

122. Fries JF. Measuring and monitoring success in compressing morbidity. *Ann Intern Med* 2003;**139**:455–9.

123. Larson EB, Wang L, Bowen JD *et al*. Exercise is associated with reduced risk for incident dementia among persons 65 years of age and older. *Ann Intern Med* 2006;**144**:73–81.

124. Rolland Y, Pillard F, Klapouszczak A *et al*. Exercise program for nursing home residents with Alzheimer's disease: a 1-year randomized, controlled trial. *J Am Geriatr Soc* 2007;**55**:158–65.

125. Knoops KT, Groot de LC, Fidanza F *et al*. Comparison of three different dietary scores in relation to 10-year mortality in elderly European subjects: the HALE project. *Eur J Clin Nutr* 2006;**60**:746–55.

126. Trichopoulou A. Traditional Mediterranean diet and longevity in the elderly: a review. *Public Health Nutr* 2004;**7**:943–7.

127. Rimm EB and Stampfer MJ. Diet, lifestyle and longevity – the next steps? *JAMA* 2004;**292**:1490–2.

128. Psaltopoulou T, Naska A, Orfanos P *et al*. Olive oil, the Mediterranean diet and arterial blood pressure: the Greek European Prospective Investigation into Cancer and Nutrition (EPIC) study. *Am J Clin Nutr* 2004;**80**:1012–8.

129. Trichopoulou A, Costacou T, Bamia C and Trichopoulos D. Adherence to a Mediterranean diet and survival in a Greek population. *N Engl J Med* 2003;**348**:2599–608.

130. Covas MI, Marrugat J, Fito M *et al*. Scientific aspects that justify the benefits of the Mediterranean diet: mild-to-moderate versus heavy drinking. *Ann N Y Acad Sci* 2002;**957**:162–73.

131. Hu FB. The Mediterranean diet and mortality – olive oil and beyond. *N Engl J Med* 2003;**348**:2595–6.

132. Kok FJ and Kromhout D. Atherosclerosis – epidemiological studies on the health effects of a Mediterranean diet. *Eur J Nutr* 2004;**43**(Suppl 1): I/2–5.

133. Esposito K, Marfella R, Ciotola M *et al*. Effect of a mediterranean-style diet on endothelial dysfunction and markers of vascular inflammation in the metabolic syndrome: a randomized trial. *JAMA* 2004;**292**:1440–6.

134. Kris-Etherton P, Eckel RH, Howard BV *et al*. AHA Science Advisory: Lyon Diet Heart Study. Benefits of a Mediterranean-style, National Cholesterol Education Program/American Heart Association Step I Dietary Pattern on Cardiovascular Disease. *Circulation* 2001;**103**:1823–5.

135. Martinez-Gonzalez MA, de la Fuente-Arrillaga C, Nunez-Cordoba JM *et al*. Adherence to Mediterranean diet and risk of developing diabetes: prospective cohort study. *BMJ* 2008;**336**:1348–51.

136. Mozaffarian D, Marfisi R, Levantesi G *et al*. Incidence of new-onset diabetes and impaired fasting glucose in patients with recent myocardial infarction and the effect of clinical and lifestyle risk factors. *Lancet* 2007;**370**:667–75.

137. Esposito K, Maiorino MI, Ciotola M *et al*. Effects of a Mediterranean-style diet on the need for antihyperglycemic drug therapy in patients with newly diagnosed type 2 diabetes: a randomized trial. *Ann Intern Med* 2009;**151**:306–14.

138. Gao X, Chen H, Fung TT *et al*. Prospective study of dietary pattern and risk of Parkinson disease. *Am J Clin Nutr* 2007;**86**:1486–94.

139. Scarmeas N, Stern Y, Tang MX *et al*. Mediterranean diet and risk for Alzheimer's disease. *Ann Neurol* 2006;**59**:912–21.

140. Sanchez-Villegas A, Delgado-Rodriguez M, Alonso A *et al*. Association of the Mediterranean dietary pattern with the incidence of depression: the Seguimiento Universidad de Navarra/University of Navarra follow-up (SUN) cohort. *Arch Gen Psychiatry* 2009;**66**:1090–8.

141. Franco OH, Bonneux L, de Laet C *et al*. The Polymeal: a more natural, safer and probably tastier (than the Polypill) strategy to reduce cardiovascular disease by more than 75%. *BMJ* 2004;**329**:1447–50.

142. Darviri C, Demakakos P, Tigani X *et al*. Psychosocial dimensions of exceptional longevity: a qualitative exploration of centenarians' experiences, personality and life strategies. *Int J Aging Hum Dev* 2009;**69**:101–18.

143. Inui TS. The need for an integrated biopsychosocial approach to research on successful aging. *Ann Intern Med* 2003;**139**:391–4.

144. McCann Mortimer P, Ward L and Winefield H. Successful ageing by whose definition? Views of older, spiritually affiliated women. *Australas J Ageing* 2008;**27**:200–4.

CHAPTER 131

Ethics in geriatric medicine

François Blanchard
Hôpital Maison Blanche, Reims, France

Scenes from everyday life in the Geriatrics Unit, or how do you do what's right?

A selection of scenes (case histories)

Mrs A

Mrs A, 90 years old, is admitted after a fall. She lives at home alone, but was able to call for help thanks to her remote alarm device. This is the third time in six months that she has been admitted for a fall. No particular cause could be identified, apart from moderate balance disorders.

Mrs A has two sons, one is a surgeon and the other a lawyer. Naturally worried about their mother, they refused to let her return home and raised the idea of nursing home placement. They said that if she was allowed to go home, they would hold the physician responsible for the accident that, in their view, would inevitably ensue.

Mrs A does not see things in the same light. A former militant in the women's lib movement, with a strong character, she decidedly wants to go home. She also has mild cognitive decline, some memory difficulties that she denies and a Mini Mental State Examination (MMSE) score of 24/30. What should you do?

Mr B

Mr B is 75 years old, a former metallurgy worker, with polyvascular disease and several risk factors (former smoker, hypercholesterolaemia). He had a heart attack three years previously, followed by a variety of complications. He now has a pacemaker for permanent systolic pacing. He has stage IV lower limb arteriopathy, with early-stage necrosis of the right toe. After a consultation in vascular surgery, Mr B accepted to undergo transmetatarsal amputation, which was scheduled rapidly. He was supported and encouraged in this decision by his family. However, the day before the scheduled operation, he suffered a left sylvian stroke with hemiplegia and aphasia.

What is the right decision? Should the operation go ahead? What should you do?

Mr C

Mr C is 81 years old, a former gymnast, physical education teacher and amateur opera singer. He suffers from severe dementia. He had just moved to a new nursing home, after his family suspected some elder abuse in the previous one. He has considerable behavioural problems and every evening at nightfall he gets agitated and shouts, with the shouting increasing in intensity if he is locked in his room. He tends to roam and wanders into the other residents' rooms, making them afraid of him. The families of other residents are complaining about him. The manager of the nursing home asks the doctor to give Mr C something to calm him. What should you do?

Mr D

Mr D is aged 85 years, a former marketing director, and up to now had been enjoying an active retirement, dividing his time between his grandchildren, his activities in various associations and some travelling. He was found lying on the ground in his house, 3 h after a fall from which he was unable to get up. In the Emergency Department, the cause of the fall was found to be a silent infarction with probable paroxysmal cardiac arrhythmia. The cardiac care unit refused to take him on the grounds that they only had one bed free, which 'had to be reserved' for a potentially younger patient. In the end, he was admitted to the geriatrics unit and the cardiac threat passed, but he developed acute renal insufficiency due to 'crush syndrome' brought on by the fall. The nephrology intensive care unit is reluctant to take him for haemodialysis because of his advanced age and the cardiac risk.

Should the physician insist? What should you do?

The approach to ethical debate

The above four situations clearly introduce an ethical debate: how do you do what is right?

General ethical reflection based on moral philosophy filters down into these situations, where decisions are

Principles and Practice of Geriatric Medicine, Fifth Edition. Edited by Alan J. Sinclair, John E. Morley and Bruno Vellas.

difficult because there is a conflict of values. Morals, law and ethics are intimately related. Moral philosophy tries to define universally what is right, what is good and what is evil through imperatives, and tries to act fairly. The law fixes rules, duties and limits for life in society. Heteronomous law applies to everyone from the outside and in a formal manner. Ethics is a process of questioning, in special situations, with a view to doing what is right for others and what is good in general and making fair and efficacious decisions. It could be defined as 'philosophical wisdom that guides practical existence towards the representation of good' in specific situations. Through the questions that it raises, medical ethics seeks to determine what is right, taking into account the state of scientific knowledge and also the constraints related to the patients and their psychological, social and economic environment.

There are no ethics specific to advanced age. Conversely, in elderly populations, there are particular situations that call for increased ethical vigilance.

The primary ethical principle, around which all the others are based, is the principle of humanity and dignity. From birth to the grave, every person belongs to a community of human beings and, as such, possesses a unique quality that cannot be estimated, measured or compared. As stated by Kant, dignity is essential, superior at all costs and can stand neither equivalent nor quantification, comparison nor commerce.

These reflections on general ethics have particularly concrete applications in ethics as applied to healthcare. For example, a patient with advanced Alzheimer's disease, bedridden and mute, has no less value or dignity than the physician caring for him or than the politician shaping the laws governing the management of this patient's dependence.

Similarly, very elderly persons are citizens in their own right, who can and should be able to state their opinion. These persons have stood the test of time and, in many cases, possess a wisdom that merits respect. Their rights and duties should by no means be rescinded (except in special clinical circumstances).

However, it is obvious that although the principles are straightforward, their application in daily life is often problematic: on the one hand, because of the attitude of our society towards elderly people – our productivist society exalts youth and decries old age, which incites fear – and, on the other hand, because of the frailty and vulnerability of many elderly people, often also compounded by cognitive decline that can alter their judgement.

Obstacles and restraints

The obstacles and restraints that prevent us from having an ethical attitude towards elderly people are manifold. It is useful to distinguish between obstacles that arise from the organization of the healthcare system and health professionals' behaviour and those that arise from the frailty of the patients themselves. The former are manifested by 'ageism', which is reflected by forms of exclusion based solely on age. This form of exclusion is all the more hypocritical since it is rarely labelled as such.

Restrictions on access according to age are the most visible form of this phenomenon, such as limited access to prevention, refused access to certain diagnostic or therapeutic techniques or even refused access to certain hospital units. While it is important that there be a thorough reflection on the risk–benefit ratio, frailty and prognosis when justifying the use of therapy that can often be highly invasive, it is nonetheless unacceptable that age alone be a justification for excluding fully independent elderly people.

On the other hand, many medications are prescribed in elderly people. They may appear to be useful, but their efficacy is often unproven. The side effects can be numerous, but poorly documented, since frail elderly patients are excluded from most randomized clinical trials that are the basis for approval of drugs for release on to the market.

This situation therefore calls for vigilance and citizenly commitment to the ethics of responsibility on the part of all health professionals (physicians, nurses, nurses' aids, administrators, etc.). As Emmanuel Levinas reminds us, the human part of man is his responsibility for others. The physician cannot simply diagnose, treat or prognosticate, but must take a stand on behalf of the patient, all the more so when this vulnerable and elderly person has trusted him.

Lack of competence or negligence by health professionals constitutes a further obstacle to an ethical attitude. This is particularly true in the field of geriatric medicine, where scientific knowledge and management practices are rapidly evolving.

One of the primary ethical requirements for health professionals is the duty to update their knowledge regularly, to maintain an acceptable level of competence.

Let us consider a few examples:

- Nowadays, how can we imagine telling an elderly person who is complaining of moderate memory problems that 'it's only natural, it's your age', without proposing appropriate assessment of cognitive function? Especially when there is a risk that, a few months or years later, the patient will be diagnosed with Alzheimer's disease that could have been detected much earlier?
- How is it possible that, according to some studies, almost half of the cases of Alzheimer's disease will never be diagnosed, including (and especially) when the disease causes the patient to be placed in a nursing home?
- How we can explain the frequency of iatrogenic disease, which often reaches dramatic proportions in these polypathological patients? Iatrogenic diseases could

often be avoided if the physicians had been sufficiently knowledgeable about drug–drug interactions and the specific modalities of prescription in frail elderly patients.

• How many dependent, elderly patients, through lack of information, do not receive the material or financial aid that they require?

Hence among situations where there is an ethical dilemma regarding elderly persons, we must distinguish between the ethical risk that comes from the outside (societal views, institutional constraints, economic pressures, attitude of health professionals and/or their level of competence, etc.) and the risk that is related to the patient themselves.

Fit elderly persons who have aged successfully should be treated in the same manner as their younger counterparts. Fit elderly persons make up a considerable proportion of the population, but since they rarely make use of health-care services, they are never really the topic of much discussion.

Conversely, a sizeable proportion of the elderly population is characterized by its frailty and vulnerability. The exhaustion of the physical reserves required to deal with perturbations and stress, and also frequent polypathologies, quickly draw these subjects into a downward spiral.

The presence of cognitive decline with alteration of judgement further complicates the decision-making process, in which many of these subjects are no longer able to participate. Instruments for reflection, as proposed by Renée Sebag-Lanoë and later Jean-Marie Gomas, become indispensable in these situations, where it is important to adopt an ethical approach.

When the situation is complex and ambiguous, the best solution is not always immediately obvious. An ethical debate should then be initiated. According to the fundamental principles of humanity and dignity, Childress and Beauchamps, in the earliest days of bioethics, proposed four principles (without any particular hierarchy), namely autonomy, beneficence, non-maleficence and, finally, justice and equality. We might also add the principle of solidarity.

These principles are moral values that have been formulated explicitly, but numerous other moral values come into consideration and competition implicitly when there is an ethical debate, such as freedom, truth, privacy, honesty, integrity, respect, security, fraternity, protection of the weak, and so on. There is no hierarchy, either formal or explicit, between these values. Each person will implicitly create their own hierarchy of values, based on their history, their experience in life, their philosophical concepts, their religious beliefs or their professional and/or institutional position. Indeed, the choice of the values to prioritize could even change depending on the context or the person's relation with the patient. This personalization of the criteria serves to enhance the utility of ethical debate, where there are no 'good guys' or 'bad guys', since no one is either right or wrong. Institutional conflicts, conflicts of interest, family conflicts or economic pressures also often compound the complexity of the debate.

The 10-point approach

In this context, it is important to distinguish the moral values at stake on the one hand and the underlying conflicts on the other, as there are no 'ready-made' solutions. A 10-point approach can be proposed and requires multidisciplinary consultation.

'The patient is a person'

The most important point is to restore the patient to their status as a 'vulnerable person' and restore their humanity. This implies listening to the patient, looking at them, asking their opinion, which is of vital importance (according to the tenets of the so-called 'Kouchner' law of 4 March 2002), asking the patient what they understand about their situation and what their wishes are.

Even a person in cognitive decline can express their wishes, if the available alternatives are proposed in a simple fashion.

The conflict of values

Subsequently, the situation can be examined from an ethical point of view, that is, every effort must be made to identify the moral values at stake and consider all the possible outcomes.

Collect additional information

• What is this patient's main disease? (Incomplete diagnosis? Stage of evolution? Prognosis? Any open therapeutic options? Iatrogenia?).

• Does the patient suffer from any other diseases and, if so, how are they interlinked with the primary disease? Possibility of a downward spiral? Prognosis?

• Know your patient: what do they know about their disease, what are their desires to live, fight, cooperate, consent to care? What does their body language express? Are they suffering (note the utility of visual analogue scales and, for non-communicative patients, non-verbal scales such as Doloplus, Algoplus and EPCA).

• What do we know about the patient's environment? Living conditions? Family circle or extra-familial circle? Personal relationships? Mode of relations? Desires? What can be learned from the patient's previous decisions in their personal relations or from their life story?

The family

The family has to be taken into consideration. Do they regularly come to visit the patient? Did someone meet the family to inform them about the patient's situation? What do they think of the situation? All these points must be taken into account, albeit without placing the burden of decision on the family.

Initiate debate within the team

Initiating the debate implies finding the time to bring together all the members of the caregiving team and those who take care of the patient on a daily basis, in order to give their opinion about how they see the situation and what they know of the patient. Confronting all these points of view can often be very informative.

Often, it is also necessary to include outside experts in the debate, to acquire a wider range of viewpoints. Such outside contributors could include a psychologist or the palliative care team when end-of-life situations are being considered. If there is enough time, an Ethics Committee could also be asked for advice.

Identify the ethical risks

- Lack of knowledge regarding the disease, the patient, the family, and so on.
- Difficulty controlling fantasies and projections, particularly in end-of-life situations.
- Lack of multidisciplinary consultation.
- Failure to take into consideration the patient's family and environment.

Take sufficient time

Real emergency situations are few and far between. Generally, the emergencies are more of a psychological nature. Taking sufficient time to reflect provides an opportunity to step back, escape the pressure and analyse and reflect appropriately.

There are more solutions than problems

The team discussions and multidisciplinary consultations in the previous steps should produce a range of proposed solutions. A certain amount of imagination is required. A single solution is often the wrong one. A two-sided solution is often restrictive. Finding three or even four alternatives gives the impression that a real choice is available.

Naturally, it is then necessary to assess the feasibility, acceptability, legal suitability and potential cost of each proposed solution, in order to establish a hierarchy among the possibilities. The final choice will often be made in the end by trying to find the best balance between beneficence (doing the most good, often including the most risky solution) and non-maleficence (doing the least harm, including the least risky solution).

Take responsibility for the decision and explain the choice

Someone has to make the final decision and take responsibility for it. This is the role of the physician caring for the patient (general practitioner or hospital physician). Although the discussion must be open, the decision cannot be collective. Once a final decision has been made, the physician should make sure that the patient consents to the proposed solution and then explain the modalities of implementation to the family.

Take notes and re-evaluate

Every decision must be clearly documented and notified in the patient's medical file and be signed by the physician who made the decision, with mention of all the people who participated in the decision-making process. This documentation can be used as a reference. In this file, it should always be specified at what time point in the future this decision should be reviewed, in order to ensure that the decisions remain appropriate even when the patient's situation has evolved.

Conclusion

The main aim of this reflection on the ethics related to frail, elderly patients is to maintain or restore the patient's basic dignity as a human being. It also reminds caregivers of the fundamental values that underlie their profession, based on respect and solidarity for all, and can give their work new meaning thanks to the changes brought about by this new ethical vision.

Key points

- Morals, law and ethics are intimately related.
- Decisions that are expected to be taken by doctors are often difficult because there may be a conflict of values.
- The application of medical ethics is intended to seek to determine what is right, taking into account the state of scientific knowledge and also the constraints related to the patients and their psychological, social and economic environment.
- This situation therefore calls for vigilance and citizenly commitment to the ethics of responsibility on the part of all health professionals.

Further reading

Bergeret-Amselek C (ed.). *La Cause des Aînés*, Desclée de Brouwer, Paris, 2010.

de Klerck-Rubin V. *Validation: la Méthode de Naomi Feil pour Aider et Accompagner les Grands Vieillards Désorientés*, Lamarre, Paris, 2010.

Feil N. *Validation Mode d'Emploi: Techniques Élémentaires de Communication avec les Personnes Atteintes de Démence*, Pradel, Paris, 1994.

Fiat E and Geoffroy M. (eds). *Question d'Amour. De l'Amour dans la Relation Soignante*, Lethielleux, Paris, 2009.

Henrard J-C. *Les Défis du Vieillissement*, La Découverte, Paris, 2002.

Kübler-Ross E. *Accueillir la Mort*, Du Rocher, Paris, 1998.

Kübler-Ross E. *La Mort est une Question Vitale*, Albin Michel, Paris, 2010 [In English: *Questions and Answers on Death and Dying*, Simon and Schuster, 1997.].

Levine S. *Who Dies? An Investigation of Conscious Living and Conscious Dying*, Gateway Books, Bath, 1986.

Ploton L. *Ce que Nous Enseignent les Malades d'Alzheimer*, 2nd edn, Chronique Sociale, Lyon, 2011.

Ricoeur P. *Vivant Jusqu'à la Mort*, Du Seuil, Paris, 2007.

Ricot J. *Ethique du Soin Ultime*, Presses de l'EHESP, Rennes, 2010.

CHAPTER 132

Participation of older people in clinical trials

Nicola Coley and Sandrine Andrieu
University of Toulouse III, INSERM Unit 1027, Toulouse, France

Introduction

The need for clinical trials involving older people

The ageing of the global population has brought about a greater need to understand the health status, underlying risk factors and prevention and care needs of older people.[1] Observational epidemiological studies on ageing, such as the Baltimore Longitudinal Study on Aging, Women's Health and Aging Study, Health Aging and Body Composition Study, Rotterdam Study and PAQUID, are now well established and have shown that the recruitment and retention of older adults in clinical studies are clearly feasible.

The most reliable evidence regarding the efficacy of interventions aimed at preventing, curing or managing a disease or health status comes from randomized controlled trials. However, traditionally, older people have been excluded from such studies,[2] meaning that the level of participation in clinical trials is highly disproportionate to the level of health burden, healthcare expenditure and prescription drug use in this population.[3] For example, in cancer trials, only around one-third of participants are thought to be elderly, whereas over 60% of incident cancers occur in elderly persons.[4,5] Older adults are even under-represented in trials for diseases that almost exclusively affect older people, such as osteoarthritis[6] and dementia.[7] Aside from the evident need to test treatments for specific age-related diseases, such as dementia, age-related macular degeneration, osteoporosis or cataracts, in elderly populations, another important reason for conducting clinical trials on older people is that in this population drug doses may need to be adapted to physiological changes associated with old age in order to avoid serious adverse events, and also the high level of comorbidities and concomitant medications must be taken into account.

Why are older people excluded from clinical trials?

There are various potential reasons for the exclusion of elderly people from clinical trials, for example, patient fear and misunderstanding of research, physician bias against suggesting enrolment in trials (perhaps through fear that elderly people will not be able to withstand aggressive therapies) or too rigorous exclusion criteria that eliminate many potential participants.[8,9] Although age in itself is not now generally used as an exclusion criterion, older people may be excluded from trials on the basis of haematological, hepatic, renal or cardiac abnormalities that may be widespread in this population. Furthermore, trial participants may be required to be ambulatory, to be able to walk and to be able to carry out activities of daily living independently, thus excluding further categories of older people. The use of strict inclusion and exclusion criteria for clinical trials is favoured by researchers since it ensures a more homogeneous study population, which may facilitate demonstration of efficacy. However, trials based on such populations provide little indication of real-life effectiveness.

Even if the inclusion and exclusion criteria allow their participation, investigators may be deterred from enrolling older subjects due the numerous methodological difficulties of conducting research with older people, for example, high rates of dropout or death, selection bias and the presence of comorbidities and multiple medicines (polypharmacy). Rates of attrition (or 'dropout') are higher in trials carried out in older populations than those carried out in younger individuals,[10] which reduces the statistical power of trials to detect treatment effects and can affect the validity of the results obtained. High attrition rates can be brought about in trials of older adults due to death, worsening health, decreasing autonomy, institutionalization and refusal to continue trial participation, often because of the perceived burden of study visits. Also, trials for older people often require the participation of another family member or close friend, at the very least in order to transport or accompany the participant to study visits, but in some cases to act as a proxy in order to give information about the patient's health status and/or quality of life if the patient is incapable of giving this information him- or herself. This may impact on attrition bias, since if the family member cannot or does

Principles and Practice of Geriatric Medicine, Fifth Edition. Edited by Alan J. Sinclair, John E. Morley and Bruno Vellas.

not want to participate, then the participant will have to withdraw from the study. There may also be problems with the validity of using information gained from proxies since one cannot be sure that it is a valid or reliable measure of the patient's actual health status. A further problem in trials of older people is selection bias, since older individuals who participate in research studies are generally healthier than those in the general population. Finally, elderly people are likely to have a high rate of comorbidities and risk factors for various diseases, which bring about risks of drug interactions, side effects, death and hospital admission, all of which may be seen as having negative influences on trial findings.

Consequences of the exclusion of older adults from clinical trials

The exclusion of older people from clinical trials limits the generalizability of their findings, since there will be insufficient data about positive or negative effects of treatment in this specific population, which may well contain individuals with the greatest need for new treatments.[5] This can result in suboptimal treatment for older people – either through not receiving potentially useful therapies because of a lack of evidence or through exposure to unnecessary risks because of a lack of information on adverse events in older people of therapies tested in trials involving primarily younger subjects.[11]

There are therefore now calls for trial participants to be more representative of the patient population for the disease under study;[12] for many chronic diseases, this will require the inclusion of significantly more older people. Despite the methodological complexities highlighted above, it has been demonstrated that clinical trials can be successfully carried out both in healthy older subjects[13] and also in those with serious illnesses.[14] Furthermore, it has been shown that older people are willing to participate in clinical trials.[11]

Given the projected increases in the number of older adults in the coming years, there is an urgent need to develop new interventions for the prevention, treatment or management of age-related syndromes and diseases. It is therefore important to increase the participation of older adults in clinical trials.

Summary of existing clinical trials involving older people

Clinical trials reported in the literature

A search was carried out in the PubMed database in order to quantify the number of clinical trials for older people reported in the literature since 1990. The total number of articles per year indexed in the database and classed as randomized controlled trials has tripled in the last two decades, gradually increasing each year from ~6700 papers in 1990 to ~18 000 papers per year in 2007–2009 (Figure 132.1). The proportion of these trials conducted specifically in older populations has also increased over time from ~3% per year in the 1990s to ~5% per year since 2003 (Figure 132.2).

Clinical trials recorded in an online registry

Another source of information about clinical trials is the online clinical trials registry ClinicalTrials.gov. A search in August 2010 showed that there were 266 intervention trials specifically for 'seniors' registered in the database. These studies represented 0.4% of the total number of registered intervention trials.

The earliest registered trial that was specifically for seniors began in 1990, but there were only two such trials prior to 1997. Between 1998 and 2002, there were between 4 and 10 trials per year for seniors and since 2003 there have been more than 20 trials per year (Figure 132.3). Since 1997, these trials have generally represented less than 0.5% of all intervention trials per year (Figure 132.3).

Of the 266 seniors trials identified, 156 were ongoing or not yet started as of August 2010 (recruitment status: 'Recruiting'; 'Enrolling by invitation'; 'Active, not recruiting'; or 'Not yet recruiting'). Most of these trials were focused on a specific condition such as cancer ($N = 63$) or cardiovascular disease ($N = 20$), whereas others were targeted towards more general syndromes of ageing, such as frailty and sarcopenia ($N = 12$) or 'healthy ageing' or the prevention of disability ($N = 4$) (Figure 132.4).

Most of these trials for seniors are taking place in Europe ($N = 93$) and North America ($N = 56$), with other regions clearly under-represented, participating in at most 12 trials (Figure 132.5). Africa is the least represented region in clinical trials for seniors and is only participating in one trial at the present time.

Determinants of participation of older people in clinical trials

The factors that motivate older adults to participate in clinical trials may differ from those that motivate younger individuals. The specific identification of barriers and motivators that prevent or facilitate the enrolment of older adults in clinical trials, and also factors that are predictive of enrolment, can inform the development of strategies aimed at increasing the participation of this population of individuals in future trials.

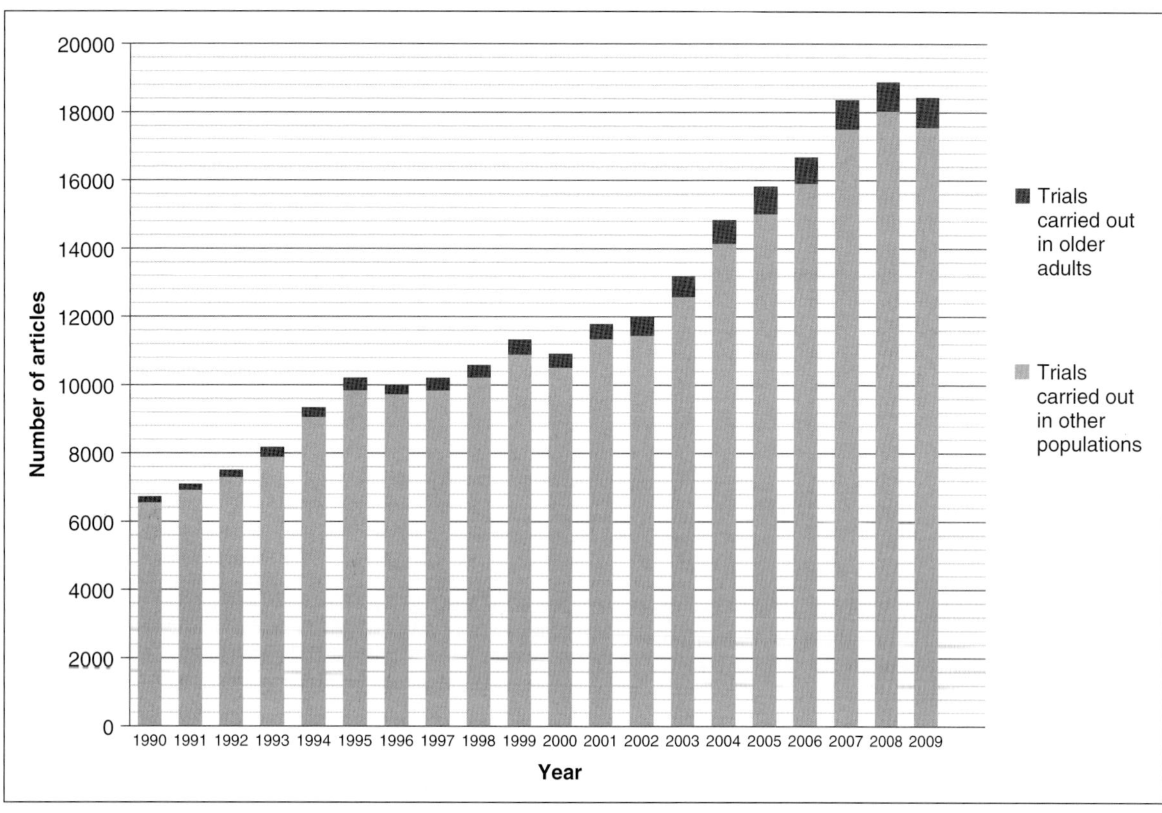

Figure 132.1 Number of articles indexed in PubMed reporting randomized controlled trials, by year of publication.

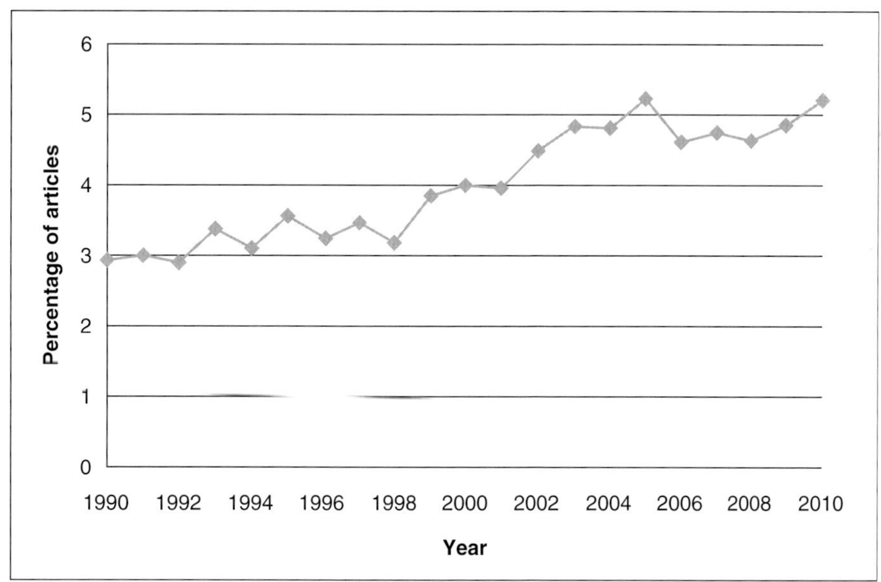

Figure 132.2 Percentage of articles indexed in PubMed reporting randomized controlled trials carried out specifically in older subjects, by year of publication. Results for 2010 do not include the whole year (search carried out in August 2010).

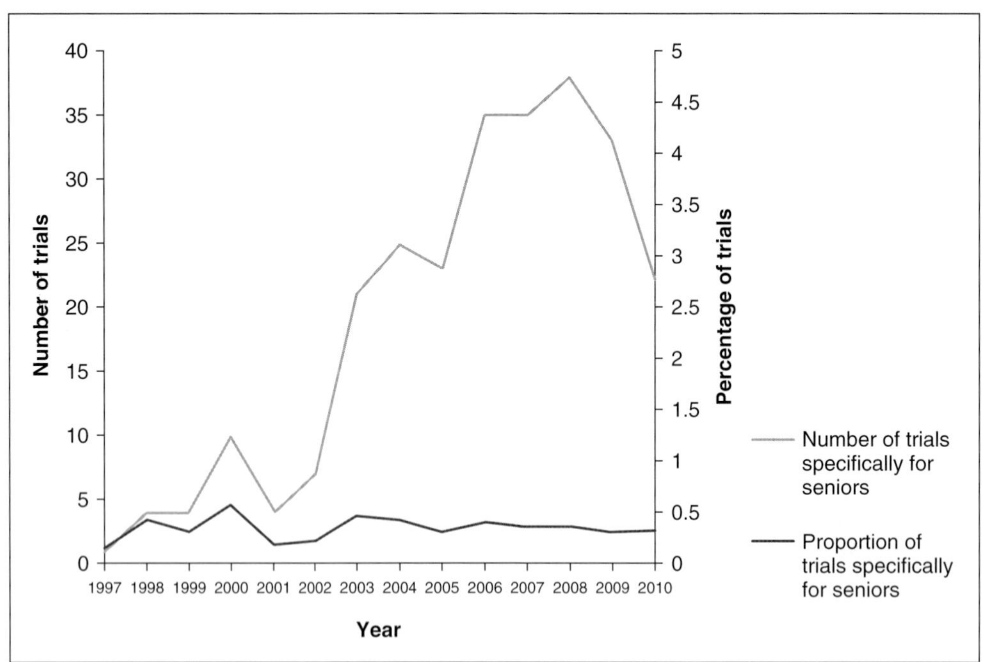

Figure 132.3 Number (grey line) and percentage (black line) of intervention trials specifically for seniors registered in the ClinicalTrials.gov database, by trial start year. Results for 2010 do not include the whole year (search carried out in August 2010).

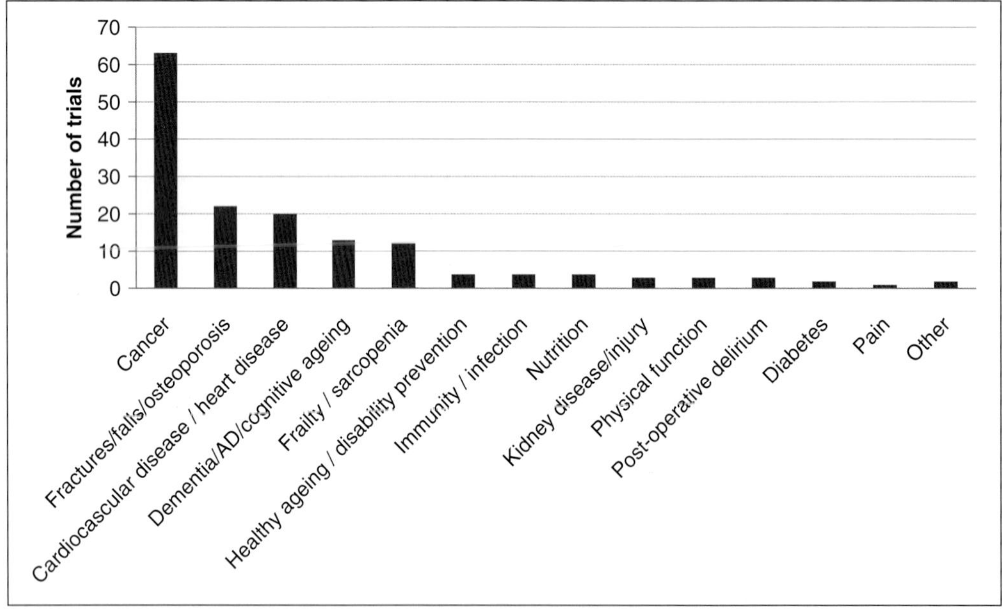

Figure 132.4 Primary conditions targeted by the 156 ongoing clinical trials specifically for seniors registered in the ClinicalTrials.gov database.

Patient factors

Patient factors associated with participation or non-participation

There are few studies that have made a detailed comparison of the characteristics of older people who enrol in clinical trials with those who do not enrol, perhaps due to the ethical difficulties of obtaining detailed information from non-participants. Other studies have assessed factors associated with willingness to participate in a clinical trial, often in a hypothetical situation, rather than actually comparing those who do and do not participate in an actual trial.

Sociodemographic factors

Whereas some studies have found no difference in terms of demographic characteristics between older adults participating in certain trials and those not participating,[15,16] others have suggested that age and level of education or socioeconomic status can affect older adults' participation in clinical trials. A review of the literature noted that older people with a lower level of education or lower socioeconomic status are less likely to want to participate in research or actually do so.[11] Indeed, non-participants in a lifestyle intervention trial for patients with stable cardiovascular disease had a lower level of education than participants,[17] as did non-participants in an intervention study on successful ageing for people aged 65 years compared with participants in this study.[18]

Even for clinical trials specifically targeting older adults, age seems to be predictive of trial participation. For example, in a primary prevention trial for Alzheimer's disease for people aged 75 years or older, persons under age 85 years were more likely to enrol than those aged over 85 years.[19] Also, participants in an intervention study on successful ageing for people aged 65 years or more were younger than non-participants[18] and non-participants in a lifestyle intervention trial for patients with stable cardiovascular disease were older than participants.[17]

There is little information regarding gender differences between participants and non-participants in clinical trials for older adults, although it was noted that men were more likely to enrol than women in a primary prevention trial for Alzheimer's disease.[19]

Disease severity and general health status

There is little information regarding the relationship between disease severity and trial participation in older adults.

General health status may affect older adults' participation in clinical trial since it was found that participants in an intervention study on successful ageing had better physical status and functional abilities and fewer depressive symptoms than non-participants.[18] Another study showed that while eligible refusers and participants (from the usual care control group only) in a disability prevention trial in older adults were similar in terms of self-perceived health at baseline, refusers had a significantly higher rate of mortality [adjusted relative risk (RR) 1.49; 95% confidence interval (CI) 1.15–1.93; $p = 0.002$] during 3 years of follow-up.[16]

Other factors

Other factors that may be associated with trial participation amongst older adults include prior experience or knowledge of clinical trials,[11] the person giving the informed consent for participation (the patient him/herself or a proxy if the patient is incapable of giving their own consent) and marital and working status. For example, patients themselves were more likely to accept to participate in an acute stroke trial than proxies (if the patient was incapable of giving informed consent)[15] and non-participants in a lifestyle intervention trial for patients with stable cardiovascular disease were more likely to be single and less likely to be working, compared with participants.[17]

Patient-related motivators for participation

As a complement to the identification of patient characteristics associated with participation in clinical trials, some studies have attempted to determine the reasons driving older adults' participation in clinical trials.

Personal benefit

The potential for personal benefit is clearly a strong motivator for the participation of older adults in clinical trials. Personal gain (feeling better or living longer due to the treatment) was amongst the most frequent reasons likely to influence the willingness of older cancer patients to participate in clinical trials,[20] and personal health benefits were the most common motivation for postmenopausal women to participate in a cardiovascular trial.[21] Similarly, for older women with breast cancer, the most common reasons for participating in a trial were that it would provide access to the best treatment available and bring about an improvement in their health.[22]

The reasons rated most highly for participation in a cardiovascular lifestyle intervention trial were having poor health and willingness to change lifestyle to improve health,[17] indicating a desire for personal benefit through taking part in the trial.

Interest in research

An interest in or desire to support research also seems to be a common reason for older adults to participate in clinical trials. For example, participants in a trial of statins for older adults with vascular disease or risk factors most commonly stated that curiosity/interest in the study and wanting to support research were the factors motivating them to respond to an initial invitation letter about the study.[23] Also, more than 40% of postmenopausal women who indicated

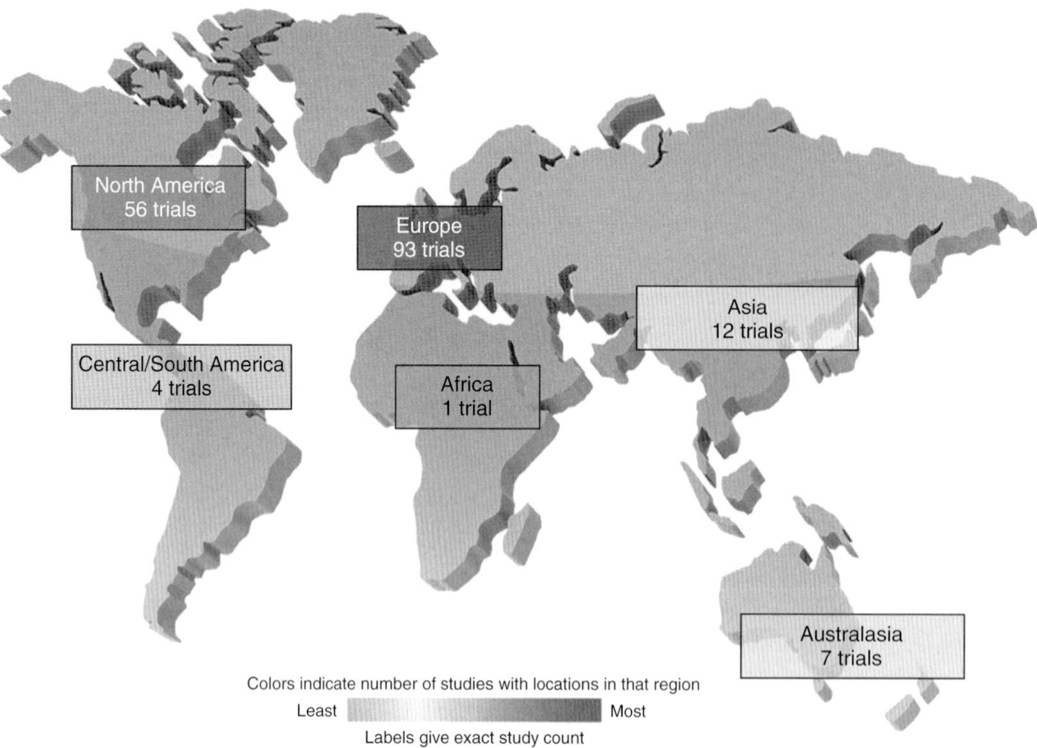

Figure 132.5 Participation by region in ongoing clinical trials specifically for seniors registered in the ClinicalTrials.gov database.

that they would participate in a cardiovascular clinical trial stated that an interest in research was one of their motivations.[21]

Altruism

A desire to help others and to give something back to the healthcare system is also a common motivator for participation in clinical trials. The possibility of benefiting society was given as a motivation to participate in a cardiovascular trial by around one-third of postmenopausal women who indicated that they would participate in clinical research,[21] and for older people taking part in a nutrition trial the most important reasons reported for taking part in the trial were helping the research team and medical knowledge and helping other older people.[24]

Patient-related barriers to participation

Finally, the determination of older adults' reasons for not participating in clinical trials can help to identify the barriers preventing the broader inclusion of this population in clinical trials.

Financial costs/time investment

The financial costs associated with participation and the time investment required are important barriers to the participation of older adults in clinical trials; these were the main barriers reported by non-participants in a cardiovascular disease lifestyle intervention trial.[17]

Lack of interest in research/negative perceptions

A lack of interest in the trial was the primary reason for refusal to participate in a prevention trial for Alzheimer's disease involving people aged 75 years and older.[23] Reluctance to participate in a research project was also the primary reason for non-participation in a randomized controlled trial of influenza vaccination in fit, healthy individuals aged 65–74 years.[25]

Poor self-perceived health

Poor health seems to be a common reason for older adults not to participate in clinical trials, especially for primary or secondary prevention trials. For example, self-perceived poor health was the second most common reason for refusal to participate in a primary prevention trial for Alzheimer's disease,[19] and personal illness was the most common reason given by postmenopausal women for not participating in a cardiovascular clinical trial.[21] About 15% of respondents in this study were also reluctant to increase their medication intake.

Comment

A number of patient-related factors have therefore been identified which seem to facilitate or prevent the participation of older adults in clinical trials. It is interesting to note that one study[16] showed that refusers may be a relatively heterogeneous group of people who refuse participation for different reasons, which could explain the differences between studies in terms of the characteristics of refusers and trial participants. The authors identified four separate groups of adults aged 75 years and older who had refused to take part in a disability prevention trial: those who did not participate because they considered themselves 'too healthy', those who thought they were 'too ill', those who had 'no interest' in taking part and those with 'other' reasons for not taking part, with relatively different baseline characteristics.[16] The medical and demographic characteristics of refusers were associated with their reason for refusal. For example, those who had refused because they were 'too healthy' ($N = 105/401$ refusers) had better perceived health, were less likely to receive home-help care and were less likely to have seen a physician during the 6 months prior to baseline compared with trial participants. On the other hand, those who refused because they were 'too ill' ($N = 51$) were older, had poorer self-perceived health, were more likely to received home-help care and more likely to have seen a physician during the 6 months prior to baseline than participants. Also, overall, refusers were found to have a higher rate of mortality than trial participants during 3 years of follow-up after the study inclusion, but a subgroup analysis showed that in fact it was only the 'too ill' and the 'no interest' subgroups that had a higher risk.[16]

Furthermore, different factors may be related to participation at different stages of the recruitment process for clinical trials (e.g. initial contact, presence at screening visits, uptake of intervention).[26] The nature of the trial and its intervention is also likely to be important and there may be differences between older people who accept to take part in primary prevention trials and those who take part in a treatment trial for a specific disease. The nature of the disease (e.g. life-threatening or not, disease burden, chronicity) and the nature of the intervention (e.g. lifestyle intervention versus pharmacological treatment, high-risk versus low-risk surgery) are also likely to play important roles. Indeed, a study of patients with primary and secondary colorectal cancer showed that patients with different stages of the same disease had very different fears and anticipations of drug trials (e.g. patients in the secondary stages of the disease were more motivated by altruism, whereas patients in primary stages were more motivated by personal benefits).[27]

Physician factors

In addition to factors related to older adults themselves, physician-related factors also can also play a role in the participation of older adults in clinical trials.

Physicians can play a major role in determining whether or not older adults will participate in a clinical trial. For example, recommendations from a cancer doctor for or against participation were the highest ranked reasons for older cancer patients' decisions to participate or not in a clinical trial.[20] Also, in the same study, a recommendation from the family doctor was more important for trial participation than recommendations from family or friends.

Older adults may have greater confidence in physicians involved in their everyday care than physicians carrying out research studies: nearly one-third of healthy older individuals questioned about their reasons for not participating in a trial of influenza vaccination stated that they would prefer their own doctor to give the vaccine.[25]

Effect of patient characteristics

In addition to giving their opinions about trial participation, another aspect of physicians' roles in determining the participation of older adults in clinical trials is their attitude and preferences towards 'offering' clinical trial options to individuals.[28] However, there has been relatively little research into this subject. One study showed that breast cancer patients aged 65 years or older were less likely to be offered trial participation than younger patients in one study.[22] Also, a study of the willingness of primary care providers to encourage enrolment of hypothetical patients into cancer prevention trials showed that geographic location, younger vignette patient age (65 versus 80 years) and higher trust score were significantly and independently predictive of primary care providers recommending trial enrollment.[29] Factors that were not associated were: existing breast cancer chemoprevention trials, knowledge of the outcome of a different trial testing the same drug, experience of using the study drug and perceived changes to control in patient care.

Barriers to the participation of older adults in clinical trials, according to physicians

Physicians' opinions about the barriers to the participation of older adults in clinical trials can help us to understand why they may not bring up the subject of clinical trial with certain patients. A review[30] of physician-perceived barriers to the inclusion of older adults in cancer trials highlighted the following factors: comorbid conditions and toxicity of the treatment; lack of support for the older patient to manage side effects at home; patient preference and influence of their families; transportation needs; patient difficulty in understanding the trial; excessive time required to enrol older patients; lack of coverage for certain healthcare costs related to clinical trial participation; physicians' personal bias that one arm of the trial was not effective or unacceptable; perceptions that the best treatments for their patients were not included in the trial; that the life expectancy of some patients was too short to justify participation in clinical trials; or that the likelihood of success was low in many trials. Significant barriers to Alzheimer's disease clinical trial referral also included physician concerns about exposure of patients to uncomfortable tests and procedures and a lack of time to discuss research participation.[31]

Physician characteristics and knowledge

Certain physician characteristics, such as specialty, age, gender and percentage of patients older than 65 years, may not be associated with their likelihood of offering clinical trial participation to older patients,[22,31] although physicians who were more likely to refer patients to Alzheimer's disease clinical trials saw greater benefits to patients, families and their practice compared with physicians who were less likely to refer.[31]

A further reason for physicians not discussing trial participation with their patients is that they may not be aware that a trial is available.[30] A study of factors affecting primary care providers' referral of patients with cancer to clinical treatment trials showed that attendance by the primary care provider at clinical trial educational sessions was a consistent predictor of referral.[32] Close proximity to a specialist Alzheimer's Disease Research Centre was the strongest predictor of referral by community physicians of patients to a clinical trial for Alzheimer's disease,[31] perhaps because physicians working closer to specialist research centres are more aware of ongoing trials than other community physicians.

Environmental/logistical factors

Finally, environmental or logistical factors, including characteristics of the trial, may affect the participation of older adults in clinical trials.

Transportation and distance to the study centre

Transportation can be a major barrier to participation in clinical trials for many elderly people,[11] either through reduced physical mobility or inability to continue driving. Transportation issues were cited as a reason for non-participation in a cardiovascular trial by nearly one in five of the postmenopausal women who declined to participate in the trial.[21] It is also unsurprising that the distance to the research institution can also play a major role in determining older adults' participation in clinical trials.[11] Non-participants in a cardiovascular disease lifestyle intervention trial, for example, cited distance to the study centre as an important reason for non-participation (even though on average they lived the same distance from study centres as trial participants).[17]

Incentives/cost

Although older people do not rate material gain highly as a reason for participating in research,[11] and may therefore be less susceptible to incentives than younger participants, they may be unwilling to support additional costs for taking part in a trial, such as transportation costs and healthcare insurance (in some countries). Indeed, costs were amongst the main barriers reported by non-participants in a cardiovascular disease lifestyle intervention trial.[17] Revision of the US Medicare system in 2000 allowed coverage of trial visit costs, but it is unclear if this has affected the number of older adults participating in clinical trials.[11]

Trial characteristics

There has been little study of the effect of trial characteristics in relation to the participation of older adults. Research has mainly been focused on the risk of the intervention and potential side effects. For example, participation in an acute stroke trial was inversely related to the risk of the proposed trial intervention.[15] In trials of pharmacological interventions, the risk of side effects is clearly an important factor. Postmenopausal women invited to take part in a cardiovascular trial gave concern about adverse health effects as one of their reasons for not participating,[21] and older adults approached to take part in an influenza vaccine trial were also concerned about side effects.[25]

Communication

One-quarter of people questioned about their reasons for not participating in a trial of influenza vaccination in healthy older individuals stated that they objected to the term 'geriatric medicine' on the letter of invitation,[25] suggesting that the way in which trials are presented to older adults, including the language used, is also an important influence on participation. A lack of interest in clinical trials could be driven by negative media stories about medical research abuses or concerns about commercially driven motives for trials.[23]

Facilitating the access of older people to clinical trials

The review of patient, physician and environmental factors associated with the participation of older adults in clinical trials shows that there are numerous modifiable barriers which could be targeted. In order to demonstrate the evidence of strategies aiming to remove such barriers, randomized controlled trials are needed, but so far very few have tested the efficacy of an intervention aimed at increasing the participation of older adults in clinical trials.

Table 132.1 Other proposed strategies.

Theme	Strategy
Exclusion criteria	Relaxation of exclusion criteria affecting older adults: • Avoidance of upper age limit • Use of medical exclusion criteria only when justified Sensitization of ethics committees to the problem of unjustified exclusion of older people from clinical trials

Primary healthcare providers' awareness of clinical trials	Neither primary healthcare providers nor older patients may be actively seeking clinical trials:
	• Inform and educate clinicians and primary healthcare providers about the existence of clinical trials for ageing and age-related diseases
	  • Educational seminars and materials for physicians
	  • Development and promotion of clinical trial registries
	  • Encourage physicians to discuss clinical trial participation with eligible patients

Recruitment strategies	Tailor recruitment strategies for older people: • Mass media may not be appropriate for trials for specific conditions • Face-to-face contact is important for older adults • Telephone contact may also be useful, but may not be suitable in all instances, e.g. for older adults with hearing problems • Other recruitment methods should be investigated, such as home visits and referrals by primary healthcare providers
Presentation of clinical trials to potential participants	Sufficient time must be set aside to explain clinical trials to older adults and for their decision-making process: • Older adults may not be familiar with the concept of clinical trials, so the general aim of clinical trials should be explained (with a clear explanation of issues such as randomization or blinding) • The details of specific trials should be clearly explained, including the risks and benefits • Written materials should be tailored towards older adults, bearing in mind that some may have a relatively low level of education. Prejudicial language such as 'geriatric' or 'elderly' should be avoided • If physicians themselves do not have enough time to discuss trial participation with their patients, other personnel should be made available for this purpose • Family members should be included in enrolment discussions if possible (even if a repeat visit is required) • Material should be provided with information about the trial relative to carers and family members who may help in the decision-making process for older adults • Give sufficient time for older adults to discuss participation with their families and close friends
Participant costs (time and financial)	Personal costs (both time and money) should be minimized. Transport problems should be addressed: • Free transport (such as a minibus or taxi) could be provided to bring participants to the study centre • Travel costs could be reimbursed • Family members or friends who drive participants to trial visits should be thanked • Home visits could be offered as an alternative, although they may not be acceptable to all participants The burden of study visits should also be kept to a minimum: • Avoid redundant or unnecessary evaluations
Maintaining communication	• It is important to maintain good communication between participants and trial staff throughout the study • Consultation with older people can improve recruitment strategies and overcome barriers to participation for future trials • Feedback of the results of a trial could provide an opportunity to interact with the older adults and may encourage them to participate in future trials Trial researchers should also engage with clinicians who work with older adults on a daily basis in order to inform the design and implementation of research involving older people

Strategies tested in randomized controlled trials

Two randomized trials have assessed the effects of different recruitment methods on the recruitment rate of older adults into clinical trials. One found that telephone contact significantly increased the recruitment of older adults to a physical activity study compared with methods without telephone contact,[33] and the second, focused on the recruitment of older African-American men for a cancer screening trial, found that the strategy with the highest rate of face-to-face contact with study participants produced the highest recruitment yield.[34] A third trial assessed whether a comprehensive educational intervention (involving standard information plus an educational seminar, educational materials, a list of available protocols for use on charts, a monthly e-mail and mail reminders for 1 year and a case discussion seminar) directed to physicians and other members of the medical and research team would improve the accrual of older persons to cancer treatment trials.[35] No effect of this intervention could be demonstrated. The authors suggested several reasons for the inefficacy of the programme, such as low intervention intensity, high baseline accrual rates (all of the centres in the trial belonged to a cancer network) and closure of several high-accruing protocols during the study. No other trials were identified that have tested a strategy specifically aiming to improve the involvement of older adults in clinical trials.

Other proposed strategies

Table 132.1 summarizes some of the other strategies, not yet tested in randomized controlled trials, that could be used to improve the participation of older adults in clinical trials based on the barriers identified in the previous section and other suggestions from the literature.[11,30,36–38]

Conclusion

Older adults need to be included in clinical trials so that treatments can be adapted to the physiological changes and comorbidities commonly present in this population and to study the prevention, management and treatment of age-related syndromes or diseases. Currently, older adults are under-represented in clinical trials and so their rate of participation needs to be increased. Further work is required to identify strategies that may facilitate the participation of older people in clinical trials. This will require further determination of the differences between study participants and non-participants and identification of modifiable barriers or facilitators to participation. The effectiveness of new strategies aiming to increase enrolment or participation must be tested in randomized controlled trials.

Key points

- Traditionally, older people have been excluded from clinical trials.
- The level of participation of older adults in clinical trials is highly disproportionate to their level of health burden, healthcare expenditure and prescription drug use.
- Even if the inclusion and exclusion criteria allow their participation, investigators may be deterred from enrolling older subjects due the numerous methodological difficulties of conducting research with older people, for example, high rates of dropout or death, selection bias and the presence of comorbidities and multiple medicines (polypharmacy).
- The effectiveness of new strategies aiming to increase enrolment of older adults or their participation must be tested in randomized controlled trials.

References

1. Fried LP. Epidemiology of aging. *Epidemiol Rev* 2000;**22**: 95–106.
2. Van Spall HG, Toren A, Kiss A and Fowler RA. Eligibility criteria of randomized controlled trials published in high-impact general medical journals: a systematic sampling review. *JAMA* 2007;**297**:1233–40.
3. Herrera AP, Snipes SA, King DW *et al.* Disparate inclusion of older adults in clinical trials: priorities and opportunities for policy and practice change. *Am J Public Health* 2010;**100**(Suppl 1):S105–12.
4. Hutchins LF, Unger JM, Crowley JJ *et al.* Underrepresentation of patients 65 years of age or older in cancer-treatment trials. *N Engl J Med* 1999;**341**:2061–7.
5. Lewis JH, Kilgore ML, Goldman DP *et al.* Participation of patients 65 years of age or older in cancer clinical trials. *J Clin Oncol* 2003;**21**:1383–9.
6. Liberopoulos G, Trikalinos NA and Ioannidis JP. The elderly were under-represented in osteoarthritis clinical trials. *J Clin Epidemiol* 2009;**62**:1218–23.
7. Schoenmaker N and Van Gool WA. The age gap between patients in clinical studies and in the general population: a pitfall for dementia research. *Lancet Neurol* 2004;**3**:627–30.
8. McMurdo ME, Witham MD and Gillespie ND. Including older people in clinical research. *BMJ* 2005;**331**:1036–7.
9. Mitka M. Too few older patients in cancer trials: experts say disparity affects research results and care. *JAMA* 2003;**290**:27–8.
10. Gardette V, Coley N, Toulza O and Andrieu S. Attrition in geriatric research: how important is it and how should it be dealt with ? *J Nutr Health Aging* 2007;**11**:265–71.

11. Witham MD and McMurdo ME. How to get older people included in clinical studies. *Drugs Aging* 2007;**24**:187–96.
12. Roehr B. Trial participants need to be more representative of patients. *BMJ* 2008;**336**:737.
13. Dodge HH, Zitzelberger T, Oken BS *et al*. A randomized placebo-controlled trial of *Ginkgo biloba* for the prevention of cognitive decline. *Neurology* 2008;**70**:1809–17.
14. Keime-Guibert F, Chinot O, Taillandier L *et al*. Radiotherapy for glioblastoma in the elderly. *N Engl J Med* 2007;**356**:1527–35.
15. Kasner SE, Del Giudice A, Rosenberg S *et al*. Who will participate in acute stroke trials ? *Neurology* 2009;**72**:1682–8.
16. Minder CE, Muller T, Gillmann G *et al*. Subgroups of refusers in a disability prevention trial in older adults: baseline and follow-up analysis. *Am J Public Health* 2002;**92**:445–50.
17. Lakerveld J, Ijzelenberg W, van Tulder MW *et al*. Motives for (not) participating in a lifestyle intervention trial. *BMC Med Res Methodol* 2008;**8**:17.
18. van Heuvelen MJ, Hochstenbach JB, Brouwer WH *et al*. Differences between participants and non-participants in an RCT on physical activity and psychological interventions for older persons. *Aging Clin Exp Res* 2005;**17**:236–45.
19. Fitzpatrick AL, Fried LP, Williamson J *et al*. Recruitment of the elderly into a pharmacologic prevention trial: the Ginkgo Evaluation of Memory Study experience. *Contemp Clin Trials* 2006;**27**:541–53.
20. Townsley CA, Chan KK, Pond GR *et al*. Understanding the attitudes of the elderly towards enrolment into cancer clinical trials. *BMC Cancer* 2006;**6**:34.
21. Cheung AM, Lee Y, Kapral M *et al*. Barriers and motivations for women to participate in cardiovascular trials. *J Obstet Gynaecol Can* 2008;**30**:332–7.
22. Kemeny MM, Peterson BL, Kornblith AB *et al*. Barriers to clinical trial participation by older women with breast cancer. *J Clin Oncol* 2003;**21**:2268–75.
23. Tolmie EP, Mungall MM, Louden G *et al*. Understanding why older people participate in clinical trials: the experience of the Scottish PROSPER participants. *Age Ageing* 2004;**33**:374–8.
24. Fearn P, Avenell A, McCann S *et al*. Factors influencing the participation of older people in clinical trials – data analysis from the MAVIS trial. *J Nutr Health Aging* 2010;**14**:51–6.
25. Allsup SJ and Gosney MA. Difficulties of recruitment for a randomized controlled trial involving influenza vaccination in healthy older people. *Gerontology* 2002;**48**:170–3.
26. Wittink MN, Oslin D, Knott KA *et al*. Personal characteristics and depression-related attitudes of older adults and participation in stages of implementation of a multi-site effectiveness trial (PRISM-E). *Int J Geriatr Psychiatry* 2005;**20**:927–37.
27. Garcea G, Lloyd T, Steward WP *et al*. Differences in attitudes between patients with primary colorectal cancer and patients with secondary colorectal cancer: is it reflected in their willingness to participate in drug trials ? *Eur J Cancer Care (Engl)* 2005;**14**:166–70.
28. Cox K and McGarry J. Why patients don't take part in cancer clinical trials: an overview of the literature. *Eur J Cancer Care (Engl)* 2003;**12**:114–22.
29. Battaglia TA, Ash A, Prout MN and Freund KM. Cancer prevention trials and primary care physicians: factors associated with recommending trial enrollment. *Cancer Detect Prev* 2006;**30**:34–7.
30. Townsley CA, Selby R and Siu LL. Systematic review of barriers to the recruitment of older patients with cancer onto clinical trials. *J Clin Oncol* 2005;**23**:3112–24.
31. Galvin JE, Meuser TM, Boise L and Connell CM. Predictors of physician referral for patient recruitment to Alzheimer disease clinical trials. *Alzheimer Dis Assoc Disord* 2009;**23**:352–6.
32. Sherwood PR, Given BA, Scholnik A and Given CW. To refer or not to refer: factors that affect primary care provider referral of patients with cancer to clinical treatment trials. *J Cancer Educ* 2004;**19**:58–65.
33. Harris TJ, Carey IM, Victor CR *et al*. Optimising recruitment into a study of physical activity in older people: a randomised controlled trial of different approaches. *Age Ageing* 2008;**37**:659–65.
34. Ford ME, Havstad SL and Davis SD. A randomized trial of recruitment methods for older African American men in the Prostate, Lung, Colorectal and Ovarian (PLCO) Cancer Screening Trial. *Clin Trials* 2004;**1**:343–51.
35. Kimmick GG, Peterson BL, Kornblith AB *et al*. Improving accrual of older persons to cancer treatment trials: a randomized trial comparing an educational intervention with standard information: CALGB 360001. *J Clin Oncol* 2005;**23**:2201–7.
36. Goode PS, Fitzgerald MP, Richter HE *et al*. Enhancing participation of older women in surgical trials. *J Am Coll Surg* 2008;**207**:303–11.
37. Karlawish J, Cary MS, Rubright J and Tenhave T. How redesigning AD clinical trials might increase study partners' willingness to participate. *Neurology* 2008;**71**:1883–8.
38. Kornblith AB, Kemeny M, Peterson BL *et al*. Survey of oncologists' perceptions of barriers to accrual of older patients with breast carcinoma to clinical trials. *Cancer* 2002;**95**:989–96.

CHAPTER 133

Restraints and immobility

Elizabeth A. Capezuti[1], Laura M. Wagner[1] and Kathleen C. Reid[2]

[1]New York University, New York, NY, USA

[2]Women's College Hospital, Toronto, ON, Canada

Introduction

Immobility is strongly associated with functional decline among older adults. Restrictive devices such as physical restraints and siderails deter mobility. Despite a growing body of literature documenting the negative consequences associated with immobilizing older adults with restrictive devices, the practice persists in both acute and long-term healthcare settings, where most healthcare providers continue to believe that restraints are an effective strategy in keeping older adults safe. This chapter provides an overview of the effects of immobility, with emphasis on the consequences of prolonged physical restraint and restrictive siderail usage. Finally, clinical strategies and organizational approaches to replace restraints and restrictive siderails and the evidence to support their use are presented.

Immobility

Immobility is the restriction of time spent out of bed (or chair) by medical orders, restrictive devices, chemical restraints, lack of mobility aids, human assistance or encouragement. Immobility has been correlated with muscle atrophy, loss of muscle strength and endurance, bone loss, joint contractures and problems with balance and coordination that lead to an increased incidence of falls.[1–3] Moreover, reduced bone mass, which is a consequence of decreased weight-bearing and physical activity, can contribute to the increased likelihood that falls will result in serious injury.[4] Other secondary effects of immobility include increased risk of infection, new pressure sores, contractures and functional incontinence. Table 133.1 lists the effects of immobility.[5,6]

It is well documented that functional decline, including new walking dependence, occurs in one-third to half of older hospitalized patients.[7–12] Functional decline or 'deconditioning' refers to the loss of the ability to perform basic activities of daily living. Attributed primarily to the effects of immobilization by 'forced bed rest, immobilizing devices (e.g. catheters), restraint use and lack of encouragement of independence in self-care',[13] functional decline has been correlated with numerous negative consequences. As many as one-third of older patients are restricted to bed rest or chair rest during hospitalization.[7] A systematic review of 30 studies examining correlates of functional decline found that between 15 and 76% of hospitalized elders experience diminished performance in at least one activity of daily living at discharge. Of those with decline at discharge, only half will recover function at 3 months post-discharge and, for many, this decline will result in permanent loss of independent living.[8,12,14–16] Functional decline is considered a profound marker of morbidity and mortality,[17,18] resulting in longer lengths of stay, greater costs and increased rate of nursing home (NH) placement.[8,12,19,20]

One of the most physically debilitating effects of immobility is the development of contractures. The word contracture is used to describe both muscle fixation and joint fixation. Contractures are prevalent in the NH setting, as they are a major consequence of immobility. They develop out of a complex process that involves structural changes that cause shortening in the muscles adjacent to a major joint. Together, the muscles and joint become fixated in a position of flexion. It is thought that this creates a permanent decrease in range of motion.

There is strong support in the literature linking prolonged physical restraint use with the consequences of immobility.[10,19,21,22] This process, labelled 'spiralling immobility' by Tinetti and Ginter,[23] creates a 'catch-22' situation in which an older person, perceived to be at risk of falling, is restrained to prevent falling and is then unable to ambulate again, independently or safely, due to the immobilizing consequences of physical restraint. Other restrictive devices (e.g. full enclosure siderails) or practices (e.g. lack

Principles and Practice of Geriatric Medicine, Fifth Edition. Edited by Alan J. Sinclair, John E. Morley and Bruno Vellas.

Table 133.1 Effects of immobility.

Musculoskeletal
Muscle atrophy
Loss of muscle strength and endurance
Osteoporosis
Joint contractures
Problems with balance and coordination
Gastrointestinal
Constipation
Impaction
Integumentary
Pressure ulcers
Respiratory
Pneumonia
Atelectasis
Cardiovascular
Deep vein thrombosis
Pulmonary embolism
Orthostasis

of assistance out of bed) also contribute to immobilization. Table 133.2 summarizes the effects of physical restraints and siderails.

Physical restraints

Physical restraints are defined as 'any manual method or physical or mechanical device, material or equipment attached or adjacent to the individual's body that the individual cannot remove easily which restricts freedom of movement or normal access to one's body'.[24] Examples of physical restraints include chest/vest, pelvic, combination of wrist, mitt or ankle, and also geriatric chairs with fixed tray tables and cushion tables in wheelchairs. These devices are generally not easily removed by the older adult.[25]

Restraint use in NHs varies widely among countries and institutions. Restraint practice patterns are attributed to cultural backgrounds and ethical views.[26] In general, the restraint use in Denmark, Iceland and Japan is low with less than 9% of NH residents restrained at any time.[26] Between 15 and 17% of residents were restrained in France, Italy and Sweden. Spain demonstrated almost 40% of residents restrained. Similarly, Germany reported restraint use at 26%[27] and Switzerland at 40%.[28] Another study found that 24% of older adults are restrained in Sweden[29] and at least 52% of residents in Dutch NHs are restrained.[30]

Combined with the research and heavy regulatory oversight in the USA, the prevalence of restraint use among NH residents dropped from 9.7% in 2001 to 5.5% in 2007.[31] However, restraint use continues to vary widely throughout the USA,[32] with some regions reporting almost 20% usage[33] while others continue with even higher usage.[34]

Table 133.2 Negative effects of physical restraints and siderails.

Musculoskeletal
Immobility
Contractures
Falls
Decreased muscle mass, tone, strength
Osteoporosis
Fractures
Rhabdomyolysis
Neurological
Brachial plexus injury
Axillary vein thrombosis
Compressive neuropathy
Cardiovascular
Stress-induced cardiac arrhythmias
Orthostasis
Dependent oedema
Psychological
Depression
Agitation
Increased confusion
Integumentary
Pressure ulcers
Skin tears, bruises, abrasions
Cellulitis
Gastrointestinal/genitourinary
Incontinence
Constipation
Infectious disease
Nosocomial infections
Miscellaneous
Strangulation/death
Entrapment
Asphyxiation
Hyperthermia

Spurred by the practice shift in the NH setting, in American hospitals, the prevalence varies from 3.4 to 24.3% in non-intensive and intensive care settings, respectively.[35] The past two decades have shown an overall decrease in physical restraint use in acute care and a change in practice patterns.[36,37] In hospitals, restraint use is more often employed to prevent treatment interference than to avert falls, thus arm/limb restraints prevail over chest/vest restraints.[38–40] A chair that prevents rising is the most common form of restraint while limb restraints are the least commonly used.[41] Trunk restraints are more prevalent in Sweden and the USA than other restraint types.[26] In The Netherlands, Germany and Switzerland, siderails are reported as being the most commonly used form of restraint.[42] In addition to decreased restraint usage over the past 30 years, restraints are now 'less restrictive' compared with previous decades; wheelchair cushions and seat belts are more often used than the more restrictive vest restraints.

Siderails

Siderails, also referred to as bed rails, cotsides, guardrails, safety rails or sideboards, are adjustable metal or rigid plastic bars that attach to the bed and come in a variety of sizes.[25] Beds include bilateral, full-length siderails or four 'half' or 'split' siderails, allowing diverse combinations of rails from one upper rail to both upper and lower rails.[43] Siderails are defined as restraints or 'restrictive' devices when used to impede a patient's ability to get out of bed voluntarily.[44] Since the use of restraints in bed has been drastically reduced in both NHs and hospitals, siderails have become the most frequently used restraint to prevent older adults from independent or accidental egress from bed.[45–47]

Similarly to physical restraints, siderail use varies among countries and institutions. A study conducted in a British hospital reported that 8.4% of patients had full-length siderails raised and a multisite study in English and Welsh hospitals showed full-length siderail use varying between 12.2 and 38.9%.[48] There are no national statistics available for siderail prevalence in American NHs and hospitals;[25] however, several studies report rates of restrictive siderail use ranging from 18 to 64%.[46,49–51] The Royal College of Nursing issued guidelines aimed at further reduction of restraints, and bedrails are listed as the most likely form of restraint.

The continued use of both restraint and siderail usage is based on embedded practices of healthcare providers who for decades have linked these devices to patient safety and protection.[52,53] As a result, efforts to reduce their use have occurred through regulatory oversight and guideline development for the assessment of risk. For example, the US Food and Drug Administration (FDA) has issued several guidelines, including the most recent 'A Guide for Modifying Bed Systems and Using Accessories to Reduce the Risk of Entrapment'.[54] The United States Centers for Medicare and Medicaid Services (CMS) (formerly the Health Care Financing Administration) has guidelines to NHs that classify siderails as restraints when they prevent voluntary egress.[55] These guidelines emphasize that restraints are defined according to their functional application as any device, material or equipment that inhibits mobility or change in position and are not easily removed by the person.[56] Similarly, the 1999 CMS Hospital Conditions of Participation and 2001 JCAHO standards redefined siderail use as restraints for hospitals using this functional definition.[57] Since then, the FDA Hospital Bed Workgroup has created guidelines that describe assessment techniques for implementing siderails, and also developed the Bed Safety Tool Kit, which includes information and tools aimed at reducing the rate of entrapment in siderails.[58] Based on the American guidelines, Canada issued 'Adult Hospital Beds: Patient Entrapment Hazards, Side Rail Latching Reliability and Other Hazards' in 2008, which provides similar recommendations.[59]

Risk factors and justification

Use of restrictive devices depends on three factors: patient characteristics, organizational attributes and healthcare providers' justification. Prevalence of restrictive devices varies with age, functional status and cognition.[60] Greater age, worsened physical health, a previous fall and the presence of depression or other psychiatric disorders have been associated with restraint use.[49,61,62]

Impaired cognition is the most significant patient factor associated with restraint and siderail use.[33,45,53,63,64] Among ambulatory NH residents, a restraint prevalence of 37% was reported in confused residents, whereas non-confused residents were virtually never restrained.[64] Confused older adults and elders are also the most likely to be restrained in hospitals.[65,66]

Castle *et al.* reported that organizational attributes, rather than patient factors, were more predictive of restraint use.[67] These include high nursing aide–patient ratios, reduced occupancy rates and prospective Medicaid reimbursement. Similarly, in hospitals, high utilization of licensed practical nurses rather than registered nurses and nurse staffing patterns on weekend shifts are strongly associated with restraint use.[66] The American statistics are in direct contrast, however, to a recent European study that revealed job characteristics (i.e. high workload) and ward characteristics (i.e. low percentage of nurses) were less significant in predicting restraint use than resident factors.[42] High risk of self-harm or injury to staff is a common reason cited for patient restraint.[68] Other reasons include paradigms that restraint use is generally appropriate and that siderails are only moderately restrictive.[42]

Justification for restraints is also based on the healthcare providers' view that these devices prevent vulnerable older adults from injury secondary to falls, behavioural symptoms or treatment interference. The most common reason cited for restraint and siderail use is prevention of falls,[25] and other common reasons include mobility aid and prevention of wandering.[48] There is no empirical evidence, however, to support the use of these devices to prevent falls.

Numerous studies demonstrate a significant incidence of falls and injury among restrained confused patients in both NH and hospital settings.[64,69–72] In addition, another study examining the relationship between restraint use and falls among NH residents found that restraints were not associated with a significantly lower risk of falls or fall-related injuries.[64]

There is also no evidence to support the use of restrictive siderails to prevent falls. One NH study examined resident outcomes associated with consistent restrictive siderail status when compared with residents with no or non-restrictive siderail use for 1 year.[46] Controlling for cognition, functional and behavioural status, the study found no indication of a decreased risk of falls or recurrent falls with restrictive siderail use. Similarly, a retrospective hospital-based study found that the incidence of falls from bed with siderails elevated was equal to or higher than the outcome when siderails were not elevated. Those patients with impaired cognition status were found to be the most likely to fall from bed when the siderails were elevated.[47]

Another major reason that healthcare providers choose restrictive devices is to reduce or control behavioural symptoms. Interestingly, although restraints are employed to 'treat' these symptoms, the use of these devices is strongly correlated with physical or verbal aggression, especially among those with dementia.[73–76] Delirium has also been found to be highly correlated with restraint use in several large-scale studies.[77–79] The usage of restrictive devices to manage behavioural symptoms in NHs or medical/surgical (non-psychiatric) care settings is strongly prohibited.

Behavioural symptoms, such as anxiety, agitation, physical aggression and delirium, may result in patient interference with medical treatments. Treatment interference refers to both removal and manipulation of a monitoring or treatment device (e.g. feeding tubes, urinary catheters, intravenous lines, oxygen therapy).[80–83] This can be especially dangerous when the treatment or device fulfils a life-saving or life-maintaining function such as mechanical ventilatory support. Hand restraints may not prevent unplanned extubations in agitated patients.[84] Since many of those with unplanned extubations do not require reintubation,[84,85] restraints may be a marker of insufficient sedation that requires more attention to implementation of evidence-based guidelines for sedation of intubated patients.[86,87] The lack of evidence to support routine restrictive device usage to prevent falls and treatment interference or reduce behavioural symptoms is thus compounded by the numerous complications associated with use of these devices.

Complications

The use of restrictive devices is not without risk. In the 1980s and 1990s, research describing the negative physical and psychological sequelae associated with restrictive devices was the major impetus for changing the practice in hospitals and NHs.[88] Psychologically, restrained older adults experience anger, humiliation, depression and low self-esteem.[89–91] Additionally, the use of restraints may convey feelings of punishment, emotional harm and patient suffering.[68]

As described earlier in this chapter, the most common physical consequence of prolonged restraint or siderail use is immobility.[10,19,21,22,33] Other harmful medical outcomes associated with restraint include hyperthermia,[92] rhabdomyolysis,[93] brachial plexus injury,[94] axillary vein thrombosis,[95] compressive neuropathy,[96] Hess's sign[97] and stress-induced cardiac arrhythmias.[98] Furthermore, siderails have been identified as a vector for nosocomial infections. Microbes cultured from siderails have been associated with subsequent integumentary and respiratory ailments.[99–104]

Although less common, restrictive devices have also been associated with fatal outcomes such as thromboembolic disease[105] and strangulation and asphyxiation.[98,106,107] Strangulation can occur due to improper application of a vest restraint or when an older adult with a vest restraint slips between two half rails. Asphyxiation results from gravitational chest compression when an older adult is suspended by a vest or belt restraint in a bed or chair.[108,109] Asphyxiation can also occur if a person is entrapped within siderails or when patients become entrapped between theapeutic overlay air mattresses and siderails.[110]

Entrapments occur through the siderail bars, through the space between split siderails, between the siderail and mattress or between the head or footboard, siderail and mattress.[111] Persons at high risk for entrapment include older adults with pre-existing conditions such as altered mental status (dementia or delirium), restlessness, lack of muscle control or a combination of these factors.[112,113] More recently, cases of asphyxiation deaths due to patients becoming trapped between therapeutic overlay air mattresses and siderails have been reported.[110] These negative consequences associated with restraint use have served as an impetus for research aimed at identifying alternative 'best practices' to restrictive devices.

Outcomes of restrictive device reduction

Several studies have described the relationship between restraint reduction and fall/injury rates. In all of these studies, significant reduction in restraints and siderails occurred without increases in falls or fall-related injuries.[50,70,114–118] Although none of the studies represent a randomized clinical trial, no significant differences were found in the number of patients falling prior to or following the reduction of physical restraint use. Further, the studies demonstrated no statistically significant difference in falls compared with historical controls when restrictive siderails are removed.[119]

Fall-related injuries are rarely examined statistically, since the number of subjects required is often cost prohibitive for most research studies. Fall-related minor injury in older persons, however, has significant implications for morbidity and mortality.[120] Capezuti *et al.* reported that continued restraint use (versus restraint removal) was the only characteristic to increase significantly the risk of fall-related minor injury (bruises, abrasions, certain sprains and other soft tissue injuries that do not result in hospitalization or bed rest).[70] In summary, results from studies of restrictive device reduction efforts have demonstrated that they can be removed without negative consequences.

The positive outcomes associated with restrictive device reduction may represent not only the safe removal of these devices, but also the effectiveness of interventions aimed at decreasing the likelihood of falling and injuries. Both individual alternatives and the most effective strategies used to implement these interventions have been evaluated in NH and hospital settings.

Approaches to reduce restrictive device usage

Optimal resolution requires multiple interventions that rely on coordination via interdisciplinary dialogue and action.[121] Comprehensive assessment, coordinated care management and individualized intervention plans targeting identified risk factors have been found to be the most successful strategies to reduce restrictive devices.

'Best practice' approaches to restrictive device reduction are described in the literature or by professional associations as clinical practice guidelines for use in the NH and acute care hospital.[47,58,108,122–124] Professional standards and governmental and accreditation regulations emphasize that a decision to use physical restraints and/or siderails should only be made after clinical evaluation and interdisciplinary care planning determines the purpose for the intervention. Further, alternatives to restrictive devices should be implemented and evaluated prior to initiating restraints. Thus, a thorough assessment is necessary in the following situations: in patients who are at high risk for application of physical restraints or siderails, prior to and during restraint reduction efforts, or in situations where the provider is assessing the continued need for restrictive devices.

Multidisciplinary collaboration is an important part of any evaluation regarding the use of restraints and siderails. There is also an indication that, due to the differences in staff opinions regarding restraint use, cultural sensitivity is necessary in designing interventions to reduce the use of physical restraints.[42] The following sections describe clinical approaches that reduce the likelihood of restrictive device use.

Promote mobility

Maintaining physical activity in hospitalized elders and NH residents is crucial to preventing the harmful effects of immobility. Careful consideration is warranted when ordering bed rest. The ability to move around in bed and to transfer and ambulate safely is also important to prevent falls and injuries.[125] The assessment should include the patient's ability to perform the skills necessary for safe mobility and transfer, including the need for assistance and assistive devices (e.g. walkers, canes). If there are problems, then a physical or occupational therapist should be consulted. Rehabilitation therapists may suggest transfer devices to enable or assist in safe transfer and promote stability when standing, which may include a trapeze, transfer pole or bar or raised one-quarter or half length siderail directly attached to or adjacent to the top of the bed. These may also serve as assistive bed mobility devices.

Certain activities by nursing staff promote mobility, such as encouraging or assisting patients with changing position in bed, transferring out of bed to chair and ambulating.[126] Organized group walks around the nursing unit at specific times during the day promote mobility, provide diversion and involve the patient in his/her recovery. Bed and toilet seat height should be adjusted to the patient's lower leg height in order to promote safe transfers.[127]

Facilitate observation

Patients at risk for falls or treatment interference should be located in rooms closer to the nurses' station to facilitate observation. Increased time spent out of rooms in hallways, at the nurses' station or in 'day' rooms with other patients facilitates surveillance. Family and friends should be encouraged to visit, especially during mealtimes and treatments and at night to provide both meaningful distraction and assistance to staff. Providing communal dining when possible serves both this purpose and an opportunity for socialization.

Volunteers or paid 'companions' can be an alternative when families are unable to stay with the patient.[128] This, however, can incur significant cost and must be evaluated in relationship to the potential harm of leaving a patient alone. Patients at high risk for restraint require frequent observation, especially in a new environment. Hence these patients may need to be targeted for 'one-on-one' companions if other means of increased staff surveillance are not available.

An open intercom, 'nursery' or 'baby' monitor will promote audio contact between staff and patients. Video monitoring may be an option in some hospitals, and also motion-sensor lights or alarms in rooms that alert staff that the resident is ambulating in their room unassisted. Elopement control devices are used for 'wanderers' who may walk into unsafe areas. They work similarly to department store tag devices. An identification tag placed on the resident's wrist or ankle will signal the detection monitoring device when the resident walks by it, thus setting off the alarm.[129]

Devices such as alarms are useful; however, staff must be available to respond quickly. There are various types of alarms: pressure-sensor activated, cord activated and patient worn.[130] Pressure-sensor activated alarms sound as shifts in weight occur on a pad placed over the mattress or chair cushion. Alarms worn by patients (usually on the thigh) are sensitive to resident position changes (e.g. from lying to standing). A call bell or similar device attached to clothing will sound when the resident rises and disconnects the cord from the socket. Alarms require individualization of delay time to minimize number of 'false' alarms. Also, the occurrence of 'nuisance' sounds may increase agitation in confused patients. Models that sound at the nurses' station, light a hallway call system or activate a staff pager reduce nuisance alarms.[130] Some alarms include a voice 'alarm', that is, a tape recorder that can play an individualized message addressing the resident by name and calmly instructing the resident to remain in his/her chair until the nurse arrives to provide assistance.

Offer activities

It is not surprising that patients will attempt to ambulate without assistance or remove tubes when isolated in a room without meaningful activities. Television is not the solution; it may actually incite agitation. Recreation or activities therapists, if available, should be consulted. Family members can be encouraged to bring in favourite music or videotapes, hobby materials (e.g. knitting) or other items that the patient may enjoy. Staff or volunteers can also provide activities based on the patient's interest and cognitive level, for example, towels to fold, magazines to read and stuffed animals to hold. Activities also serve to distract patients from 'investigating' or disturbing tubes, monitor, leads and dressings.[131]

Maintain continence

Often patients attempt to ambulate unassisted because of an urgent need to void. Assess the patient's ability to use a bedside commode or urinal safely, which may reduce the distance travelled to the bathroom and thus reduce falls. Query the patient or nursing staff regarding a change in toileting patterns, including nocturia and bowel and bladder incontinence, which may require further evaluation by a continence specialist.

Promote comfort

Comfort needs include equipment individualized to a patient's medical/functional condition and appropriate pain management. Providing comfortable and individualized seating is a major challenge, especially in the NH setting. In the NH, most patients spend the majority of their day in a wheelchair.[132] The prevalence of wheelchairs in NHs exceeds 50% and many patients spend their time in chairs that do not fit and are uncomfortable.[133] Wheelchairs were originally designed for transport only, not for long periods of sitting. Their sling-back seats do not provide the appropriate support. Seating problems such as poor back support; wheelchair being too tall, heavy or wide; foot rests too high; and the hammock effect of the sling are all associated with pain and agitation.[134] All these effects increase the risk for falling and use of physical restraints, since the patient may be uncomfortable and attempt to transfer unsafely. Many products are available to adapt the chair to the individual resident's seating needs. Other adaptations for the wheelchair include a wedge cushion inserted under the resident's buttocks and thighs, which tilt the resident backwards. A wedge seat prevents the resident from sliding forward. Similarly, leaning to the side is corrected with lateral supports or cushions. Stroke victims with hemiplegia (one-sided weakness) are at risk for shoulder subluxation if the weakened arm slips off the side of the chair. This can be prevented with devices attached to a wheelchair: an arm trough, elevated armrest, lateral arm support or half tray. Patients who spend a considerable time in a wheelchair are to be referred to a physical or occupational therapist for a seating evaluation.[134,135] The patient's comfort in bed can be improved with an overlay mattress cushion, air mattress or sheepskin mattress pads.[136] Pillows and leg separator cushions can be used to facilitate positioning. Heel pads and/or bed cradles are good choices for those with significant peripheral vascular disease or pressure ulcers. Refer to a wound, ostomy and continence (WOC) nurse or physical therapist for device recommendations. Chronic and acute pain is common in older adults; however, many are inadequately treated. Pain management includes both administration of analgesics and other treatments (e.g. physical rehabilitation exercise, relaxation training, biofeedback, hot packs). Older adults with dementia have the same types of medical conditions as non-demented elders; however, evidence suggests that they are less likely to receive pain treatment.[137] Thus, routinely scheduled analgesia is strongly recommended.[138] Since the patient may not be able to report or describe pain, observation of non-verbal signs of pain is necessary. Indicators of pain in cognitively impaired elders include facial grimacing, physical aggression, pacing, uncooperativeness and restless behaviour.[139]

Investigate mental status changes

It is important to assess changes in mental status since impaired cognitive status is highly associated with increased risk of falling and use of restrictive devices.[140] New behavioural symptoms (e.g. physical aggression) should first trigger a comprehensive evaluation of potential physical and/or environmental causes prior to initiating any physical or chemical restraint. Behaviour can be used to communicate a need, threat to self-esteem, a state of arousal or anxiety.[60] Confused older adults may not be able to express verbally that they are experiencing pain or have the need to use, for example, the toilet and will often act out with some form of behaviour (e.g. anxiety, wandering).[141,142] Complicated cases could require a geriatric psychiatry consultation.

Address fall risk

If a patient has been deemed at risk of falls or has fallen, then a thorough evaluation of amenable risk factors contributing to future risk should be conducted. Falls, especially sudden onset of repeated falls, may indicate underlying acute pathology, such as infection, hypoglycaemia or dehydration.[143] Evaluation of fall risk is addressed by several medical associations and academic institutions, such as the American Geriatrics Society and British Geriatrics Society,[144] American Medical Directors Association and The American Health Care Association,[145] the University of Iowa[146] and Assessing Care of Vulnerable Elders (ACOVE) Project on Falls Prevention.[147]

Medications are associated with an increased risk for falling. All types of psychoactive medications (hypnotics, antidepressants, anxiolytics, benzodiazepines and antipsychotics) have consistently been linked to an increased risk for falling[148] due to the risk for adverse side effects such as syncope and orthostasis.[149–151] Ray *et al.*[152] identified benzodiazepine users in NH residents having a rate of falls 44% greater than those not taking benzodiazepines. Additionally, fall risk increased with a higher dose of benzodiazepine use. Those on antidepressants, both tricyclic antidepressants and selective serotonin-reuptake inhibitors, have a higher risk for falls compared with non-users.[149,153] Therefore, prescription of these medications must be carefully balanced against the risk of falls and related injuries. A general rule of geriatric pharmacology is to minimize the number of medications, assess the risk and benefit of each medication and use those medications with the shortest half-life, least centrally acting or least associated with hypotension and at the lowest effective dose. A pharmacist may be consulted to uncover potential drug–drug interactions and to make suggestions regarding inappropriate drug usage.

Environmental modifications may reduce falls. For example, a non-skid mat placed at the side of the bed and/or toilet and raised-tread socks can reduce the likelihood of slipping.[125] For those patients unable to stand safely but who may accidentally roll out of or unsafely exit from bed, bed bumpers on mattress edges, concave mattresses, pillows, 'swimming pool noodles' or rolled blankets under the mattress edge demarcate bed perimeters.[132]

Reduce injury risk

Since falling on to hard surfaces may increase the likelihood of fractures, a bedside cushion such as an exercise mat or an egg crate foam mattress may be used to reduce impact.[136] Hip protector pads are the best studied single intervention strategy for fall-related injury prevention among high-risk older adults. Hip protectors are pads held in place next to the greater trochanter that reduce the force transmitted in a fall.[154] There are several large-scale, randomized and controlled clinical trials that demonstrate a strong association between reduced hip fracture rates and hip pad usage in community-dwelling elders.[155,156] However, their use in NH settings is more controversial, as the Cochrane Systematic Review on the use of hip protectors suggests that lack of compliance with wearing the hip protector pad is often due to discomfort and thus decreases their potential efficacy in reducing injury.[157] This is consistent with other literature, suggesting that further research into the use of hip protector pads in nursing homes would be helpful.[158] Compliance with wearing the hip protectors is a significant problem due to discomfort and poor fit.[157,158] Incontinent NH residents experience discomfort when wearing the garment.[159,160] For residents with a history of climbing around or over siderails, reducing the risk of an entrapment injury is paramount. Since restraint-related deaths can occur in less than a few minutes, these devices necessitate increased, not decreased, staff observation. Inspect bed frames, siderails and mattresses to identify possible entrapment areas.[58,112]

Address treatment interference

Discomfort caused by unstable tube placement can increase the chances of self-removal or disruption of tube performance. Commercial tube holders to stabilize Foley catheters, intravenous lines and feeding, drainage and endotracheal tubes should be used.[161] Waterproof tape can decrease accidental extubations.[162] Devices can be camouflaged by hiding them under cloth (e.g. abdominal binder), undergarments or clothing, sheets or blankets, to divert the patient's attention from a treatment. Infusion sites can be covered with commercial holders, bandages or stockinettes.[161] For confused patients who 'pick' or who are seeking tactile stimulation, provide fabric, stuffed animals or an activity apron. Finally, periodically assess the need for any treatment such as bladder catheterization or intravenous fluids; determine if it can be discontinued or if a less invasive treatment can replace it.[60]

Advanced practice nursing interventions

Advanced practice nursing (APN) interventions can be effective in reducing or eliminating restrictive restraint use in NH settings.[163,164] Although the APN role can help reduce restraint use, adherence to these policies over an extended period of time is largely influenced by administrative support.[117] The APN can support NHs in reducing restraint use by utilizing individualized assessments and a complex clinical decision-making process. Additionally, APNs can use their roles as staff educators and clinical nursing consultants to help address staff and resident perceptions about the use of restrictive siderails.[163] The presence of research staff in a clinical area and familiarization of nursing staff with current research and best practices can also generate a better understanding of the policies regarding the use of siderails and restraints.[165]

Staff education programmes

The literature on the use of educational interventions to affect staff attitudes and knowledge on the use of physical restraints is conflicting. One cluster-randomized controlled trial showed that a 6 month educational programme for nurses was successful in reducing the use of physical restraints and increasing staff knowledge.[166] However, another similar study showed that a shorter 2 month educational programme combined with nurse specialist consultation does not prevent the use of physical restraints.[167] Short-term educational programmes may only influence restraint use for the length of the study period and may not have any long-term effects.[30] These results indicate that longer educational interventions may be more successful in changing staff attitudes towards restraint use and also lend to the idea that interventions at an organizational level may be necessary in order to instigate change.

The need for long-term organization-level educational programmes is emphasized by an Australian study that focused on educating management personnel on the use of restraints in NHs.[168] This allows for knowledge dissemination to all staff members and encourages the use of current research. Likewise, Moore and Haralambous[169] found that NH staff at all levels require education in evidence-based practice surrounding restraint use.

Conclusion

Physical restraints and restrictive siderails play a limited role in providing medical care to frail older patients. Rather, use of restraints and siderails leads to the harmful effects of immobility. Several studies have demonstrated that restraints and siderails can be removed without negative consequences. Primary care providers can reduce the use of physical restraints and restrictive siderails by conducting a careful assessment and implementing appropriate individualized interventions. The use of non-restrictive measures has been correlated with positive patient outcomes and helps to promote mobility and functional recovery. Most of these products, however, have not been prospectively evaluated in large randomized clinical trials for their individual contribution to reduction of falls or treatment interference.[119,144] Further research on the efficacy of individual interventions that replace restrictive devices and improve mobility is still needed.[170]

Key points

- Immobility is correlated with functional decline, which is considered a profound marker of morbidity and mortality.
- There is strong support in the literature linking physical restraint and restrictive siderail use with the consequences of immobility.
- The continued use of both restraint and siderail usage is based on embedded practices of healthcare providers who for decades have linked these devices to patient safety and protection.
- Restrictive devices are associated with numerous negative outcomes, including strangulation and asphyxiation.
- Research demonstrates that restrictive devices can be safely eliminated.

References

1. Bloomfield SA. Changes in musculoskeletal structure and function with prolonged bed rest. *Med Sci Sports Exercise* 1997;**29**:197–206.
2. Covertino VA, Bloomfield SA and Greenleaf JE. An overview of the issues: physiological effects of bed rest and restricted physical activity. *Med Sci Sports Exercise* 1997;**29**:187–90.
3. Allen C, Glasziou P and Del Mar C. Bed rest: a potentially harmful treatment needing more careful evaluation. *Lancet* 1999;**354**:1229–33.
4. Grisso JA, Kelsey JL, Strom BL *et al.*; NE Hip Fracture Study Group. Risk factors for falls as a cause of hip fracture in women. *N Engl J Med* 1991;**324**:1326–30.
5. Frengley J and Mion LC. Incidence of physical restraints on acute general medical wards. *J Am Geriatr Soc* 1986; **34**:565–8.
6. Robbins L, Boyko E, Lane J *et al.* Binding the elderly: a prospective study of the use of mechanical restraints in the acute care hospital. *J Am Geriatr Soc* 1987;**35**:290–6.
7. Brown CJ, Friedkin RJ, Inouye SK. Prevalence and outcomes of low mobility in hospitalized older patients. *J Am Geriatr Soc* 2004;**52**:1263–70.
8. Fortinsky RH, Covinsky KE, Palmer RM and Landefeld CS. Effects of functional status changes before and during hospitalization on nursing home admission of older adults. *J Gerontol A Biol Sci Med Sci* 1999;**54**:M521–6.
9. Hirsch CH, Sommers L, Olsen A *et al.* The natural history of functional morbidity in hospitalized older patients. *J Am Geriatr Soc* 1990;**38**:1296–303.
10. Mahoney JE. Immobility and falls. *Clin Geriatr Med* 1998; **14**:699–726.

11. Mahoney JE, Sager MA and Jalaluddin M. New walking dependence associated with hospitalization for acute medical illness: incidence and significance. *J Gerontol A Biol Sci Med Sci* 1998;**53**:M307–12.
12. McCusker J, Kakuma R and Abrahamowicz M. Predictors of functional decline in hospitalized elderly patients: a systematic review. *J Gerontol A Biol Sci Med Sci* 2002;**57**:M569–77.
13. Kortebein P, Symons TB, Ferrando A *et al.* Functional impact of 10 days of bed rest in healthy older adults. *J Gerontol A Biol Sci Med Sci* 2008;**63**:1076–81.
14. Brown CJ, Roth D, Allman RM *et al.* Trajectories of life-space mobility after hospitalization. *Ann Intern Med* 2009;**150**(6):372–8.
15. Sager MA, Franke T, Inouye SK *et al.* Functional outcomes of acute medical illness and hospitalization in older persons. *Arch Intern Med* 1996;**156**:645–52.
16. Covinsky KE, Justice AC, Rosenthal GE *et al.* Measuring prognosis and case mix in hospitalized elders. The importance of functional status. *J Gen Intern Med* 1997;**12**:203–8.
17. Thomas DR. Focus on functional decline in hospitalized older adults. *J Gerontol A Biol Sci Med Sci* 2002;**57**:M567–8.
18. Walter LC, Brand RJ, Counsell SR *et al.* Development and validation of a prognostic index for 1-year mortality in older adults after hospitalization. *JAMA* 2001;**285**:2987–94.
19. Inouye SK, Bogardus ST, Charpentier PA *et al.* A multicomponent intervention to prevent delirium in hospitalized older patients. *N Engl J Med* 1999;**340**:669–76.
20. Janelli LM. Physical restraint use in acute care settings. *J Nurs Care Qual* 1995;**9**:86–92.
21. Inouye SK, Bogardus ST, Baker DI *et al.* The hospital elder life program: a model of care to prevent cognitive and functional decline in older hospitalized patients. *J Am Geriatr Soc* 2000;**48**:1697–706.
22. Selikson S, Damus K and Hamerman D. Risk factors associated with immobility. *J Am Geriatr Soc* 1988;**36**:707–12.
23. Tinetti ME and Ginter SF. Identifying mobility dysfunction in elderly patients-standard neuromuscular examination or direct assessment. *JAMA* 1988;**259**:1190–3.
24. Centers for Medicare and Medicaid Services. *Code of Federal Regulations: 42 CFR Part 483.13(a), 1999.*
25. Braun JA and Capezuti EA. The legal and medical aspects of physical restraints and bed siderails and their relationship to falls and fall-related injuries in nursing homes. *DePaul J Health Care Law* 2000;**4**:1–72.
26. Ljunggren G, Phillips CD and Sgadari A. Comparisons of restraint use in nursing homes in eight countries. *Age Ageing* 1997;**26**:43–7.
27. Meyer G and Köpke S. 2007. Restraint use in nursing homes: a multi centre observational study. In: *Abstracts Book 60th Annual Scientific Meeting of the Gerontological Society of America*, San Francisco, 16–20 November 2007.
28. Lindenmann R. Physical restraints: attitudes of nursing staff and prevalence in state-run geriatric institutions in the city of Lucerne. Unpublished Master Thesis, Maastricht University, 2006 (in German).
29. Karlsson S, Bucht G, Eriksson S and Sandman PO. Physical restraints in geriatric care in Sweden: prevalence and patient characteristics. *J Am Geriatr Soc* 1996;**44**:1348–54.
30. Huizing A, Hamers J, Gulpers M and Berger M. Short-term effects of an educational intervention on physical restraint use: a cluster randomized trial. *BMC Geriatr* 2006;**6**:17.
31. Harrington C, Carrillo H and Blank B. *Nursing Facilities, Staffing, Residents and Facility Deficiencies, 2001 Through 2007.* Department of Behavioral and Social Sciences, University of California, San Francisco, 2008.
32. Phillips CD, Hawes C, Mor V *et al.* Facility and area variation affecting the use of physical restraints in nursing homes. *Med Care* 1996;**34**:1149–62.
33. Capezuti E and Talerico KA. Review article: physical restraint removal, falls and injuries. *Res Pract Alzheimer's Dis* 1999;**2**:3–24.
34. Castle NG. Nursing homes with persistent deficiency citations for physical restraint use. *Med Care* 2002;**40**:868–78.
35. Minnick AF, Mion LC, Leipzig R *et al.* Prevalence and patterns of physical restraint use in the acute care setting. *J Nurs Admin* 1998;**28**:19–24.
36. Minnick AF, Mion LC, Leipzig R *et al.* Prevalence and patterns of physical restraint use in the acute care setting. *J Nurs Admin* 1998;**28**:19–24.
37. Minnick AF, Mion LC, Johnson ME, Catrambone C, Leipzig R. Prevalence and variation of physical restraint use in acute care settings in the US. *J Nurs Scholarsh* 2007;**39**:30–7.
38. Frengley J and Mion L. Physical restraints in the acute care setting: issues and future directions. *Clin Geriatr Med* 1998;**14**:727–43.
39. Mion LC. Establishing alternatives to physical restraints in the acute care setting: a conceptual framework to assist nurses' decision making. *AACN Clin Issues* 1996;**7**:592–602.
40. Mion L, Minnick A and Palmer R. Physical restraint use in the hospital setting: unresolved issues and directions for research. *Milbank Q* 1996;**74**:411–33.
41. Centers for Medicare and Medicaid Services. http://www.cms.hhs.gov/media/press/release.asp?Counter=947, 2004.
42. Hamers JPH, Meyer G, Köpke S *et al.* Attitudes of Dutch, German and Swiss nursing staff towards physical restraint use in nursing home residents, a cross-sectional study. *Int J Nurs Stud* 2009;**46**:248–55.
43. Levine JM, Hammond M, Marchello V and Breuer B. Changes in bedrail prevalence during a bedrails-reduction initiative. *J Am Med Dir Assoc* 2000;**1**:34–6.
44. Capezuti E. Preventing falls and injuries while reducing siderail use. *Ann Long-Term Care* 2000;**8**:57–63.
45. O'Keefe S, Jack IA and Lye M. Use of restraints and bedrails in a British hospital. *J Am Geriatr Soc* 1996;**44**:1086–8.
46. Capezuti E, Maislin G, Strumpf N and Evans LK. Side rail use and bed-related fall outcomes among nursing home residents. *J Am Geriatr Soc* 2002;**50**:90–6.
47. van Leeuwen M, Bennett L, West S *et al.* Patient falls from bed and the role of bedrails in the acute care setting. *Aust J Adv Nurs* 2001;**19**:8–13.
48. Healey F, Cronberg A and Oliver D. Bedrail use in English and Welsh hospitals. *J Am Geriatr Soc* 2009;**57**:1887–91.
49. Tinetti ME, Liu WL, Marottoli RA and Ginter SF. Mechanical restraint use among residents of skilled nursing facilities: prevalence, patterns and predictors. *JAMA* 1991;**265**:468–71.

50. Si M and Neufeld RR. Removal of bedrails on a short-term nursing rehabilitation unit. *Gerontologist* 1999;**39**: 611–4.
51. Capezuti E, Bourbonniere M, Strumpf N and Maislin G. Siderail use in a large urban medical center. *Gerontologist* 2000;**40**:117.
52. Brush BL and Capezuti E. Historical analysis of siderail use in American hospitals. *J Nurs Scholarsh* 2001;**33**: 381–5.
53. Strumpf N and Tomes N. Restraining the troublesome patient: a historical perspective on a contemporary debate. *Nurs History Rev* 1993;**1**:3–24.
54. Hospital Bed Safety Workgroup. *A Guide for Modifying Bed Systems and Using Accessories to Reduce the Risk of Entrapment*. US Department of Health and Human Services, Food and Drug Administration, Silver Spring, MD, 2006.
55. Health Care Financing Administration. *HCFA Interpretative Guidelines, Rev. 250. Part II. Guidance to Surveyors for Long-term Care Facilities*, Department of Health and Human Services, Centers for Medicare and Medicaid Services, Woodlawn, MD, 1992, Tag numbers F221–222, pp. 76–8, F320, pp. 131–2.
56. Health Care Financing Administration. *Siderails Guidance. February 4, 1997 and December 1999*, Department of Health and Human Services, Centers for Medicare and Medicaid Services, Woodlawn, MD, 1997 and 1999.
57. Capezuti E and Braun JA. Medico-legal aspects of hospital siderail use. *Ethics Law Aging Rev* 2001;**7**:25–57.
58. Hospital Bed Safety Workgroup. Clinical guidance for the assessment and implementation of bed rails in hospitals, long term care facilities and home care settings. *Crit Care Nurs Qy* 2003;**26**:244–62.
59. Health Canada. *Adult Hospital Beds: Patient Entrapment Hazards, Side Rail Latching Reliability and Other Hazards*; http://www.hc-sc.gc.ca/dhp-mps/md-im/applic-demande/guide-ld/md_gd_beds_im_ld_lits-eng.php, 2008.
60. Strumpf NE, Robinson JP, Wagner JS and Evans LK. *Restraint-Free Care: Individualized Approaches for Frail Elders*, Springer, New York, 1998.
61. Frengley J and Mion LC. Incidence of physical restraints on acute general medical wards. *J Am Geriatr Soc* 1986; **34**:565–8.
62. Berland B, Wachtel TJ, Kiel DP *et al*. Patient characteristics associated with the use of mechanical restraints. *J Gen Intern Med* 1990;**5**:480–5.
63. Castle NG and Mor V. Physical restraints in nursing homes: a review of the literature since the Nursing Home Reform Act of 1987. *Med Care Res Rev* 1998;**55**:139–70.
64. Capezuti E, Evans L, Strumpf N and Maislin G. Physical restraint use and falls in nursing home residents. *J Am Geriatr Soc* 1996;**44**:627–33.
65. Sullivan-Marx EM, Strumpf NE, Evans LK *et al*. Predictors of continued physical restraint use in nursing home residents following restraint reduction efforts. *J Am Geriatr Soc* 1999;**47**:342–8.
66. Bourbonniere M, Strumpf NE, Evans LK and Maislin G. Organizational characteristics and restraint use for hospitalized nursing home residents. *J Am Geriatr Soc* 2003;**51**: 1079–84.
67. Castle NG, Fogel B and Mor V. Risk factors for physical restraint use in nursing homes: pre- and post-implementation of the nursing home reform act. *Gerontologist* 1997;**37**:737–47.
68. Gelkopf M, Roffe Z, Werbloff N and Bleich A. Attitudes, opinions, behaviors and emotions of the nursing staff toward patient restraint. *Issues Mental Health Nurs* 2009;**30**: 758–63.
69. Neufeld RR, Libow LS, Foley WJ *et al*. Restraint reduction reduces serious injuries among nursing home residents. *J Am Geriatr Soc* 1999;**47**:1202–7.
70. Capezuti E, Strumpf NE, Evans LK *et al*. The relationship between physical restraint removal and falls and injuries among nursing home residents. *J Gerontol A Biol Sci Med Sci* 1998;**53**:M47–52.
71. Shorr RI, Guillen MK, Rosenblatt LC *et al*. Restraint use, restraint orders and the risk of falls in hospitalized patients. *J Am Geriatr Soc* 2002;**50**:526–9.
72. Tinetti ME, Liu WL and Ginter SF. Mechanical restraint use and fall-related injuries among residents of skilled nursing facilities. *Ann Intern Med* 1992;**116**:369–74.
73. Talerico KA and Evans LK. Responding to safety issues in frontotemporal dementias. *Neurology* 2001;**56**:S52–5.
74. Talerico KA, Evans LK and Strumpf NE. Mental health correlates of aggression in nursing home residents with dementia. *Gerontologist* 2002;**42**:169–77.
75. Kolanowski A, Hurwitz S, Taylor LA *et al*. Contextual factors associated with disturbing behaviors in institutionalized elders. *Nurs Res* 1994;**43**:73–9.
76. Cohen-Mansfield J and Werner P. Environmental influences on agitation: an integrative summary of an observational study. *Am J Alzheimers Dis Other Demen* 1995;**10**:32–7.
77. Inouye SK and Charpentier PA. Precipitating factors for delirium in hospitalized elderly persons. Predictive model and interrelationship with baseline vulnerability. *JAMA* 1996;**275**:852–7.
78. McCusker J, Cole M, Abrahamowicz M *et al*. Environmental risk factors for delirium in hospitalized older people. *J Am Geriatr Soc* 2001;**49**:1327–34.
79. Morrison A and Sadler D. Death of a psychiatric patient during physical restraint. *Med Sci Law* 2001;**41**:46–50.
80. Bryant H and Fernald L. Nursing knowledge and use of restraint alternatives: acute and chronic care. *Geriatr Nurs* 1997;**18**:57–60.
81. Werner P and Mendelson G. Nursing staff members' intentions to use physical restraints with older people: testing the theory of reasoned action. *J Adv Nurs* 2001;**35**:784–91.
82. Matthiesen V, Lamb KV, McCann J *et al*. Hospital nurses' views about physical restraint use with older patients. *J Gerontol Nurs* 1996;**22**:8–16.
83. Sullivan-Marx EM and Strumpf NE. Restraint-free care for acutely ill patients in the hospital. *AACN Clin Issues* 1996;**7**:572–8.
84. Chevron V, Menard JF, Richard JC *et al*. Unplanned extubation: risk factors of development and predictive criteria for reintubation. *Crit Care Med* 1998;**26**:1049–53.
85. Tung A, Tadimeti L, Caruana-Montaldo B *et al*. The relationship of sedation to deliberate self-extubation. *J Clin Anesth* 2001;**13**:24–9.

86. Slomka J, Hoffman-Hogg L, Mion LC *et al*. Influence of clinicians' values and perceptions on use of clinical practice guidelines for sedation and neuromuscular blockade in patients receiving mechanical ventilation. *Am J Crit Care* 2000;**9**:412–8.
87. Bair N, Bobek MB, Hoffman-Hogg L *et al*. Introduction of sedative, analgesic and neuromuscular blocking agent guidelines in a medical intensive care unit: physician and nurse adherence. *Crit Care Med* 2000;**28**:707–13.
88. Evans LK and Strumpf NE. Tying down the elderly: a review of the literature on physical restraint. *J Am Geriatr Soc* 1989;**37**:65–74.
89. Strumpf NE and Evans LK. Physical restraint of the hospitalized elderly: perceptions of patients and nurses. *Nurs Res* 1988;**37**:132–7.
90. Mion LC, Frengley JD, Jakovcic CA and Marino JA. A further exploration of the use of physical restraints in hospitalized patients. *J Am Geriatr Soc* 1989;**37**:949–56.
91. Happ MB, Kagan SH, Strumpf NE *et al*. Elderly patients memories of physical restraint use in the intensive care unit. *AmJ Crit Care* 2001;**10**:367–9.
92. Greenland P and Southwick WH. Hyperthermia associate with chlorpromazine and full-sheet restraint. *Am J Psychiatry* 1978;**135**:1234–5.
93. Lahmeyer HH and Stock PG. Phencyclidine intoxication, physical restraint and acute renal failure: case report. *J Clin Psychiatry* 1983;**44**:184–5.
94. Scott TF and Gross JA. Brachial plexus injury due to vest restraints. *N Engl J Med* 1989;**320**:598.
95. Skeen MB, Rozear MP and Morgenlander JC. Posey palsy. *Ann Intern Med* 1993;**117**:795.
96. Vogel CM and Bromberg MB. Proximal upper extremity compressive neuropathy associated with prolonged use of a jacket restraint. *Muscle Nerve* 1990;**13**:860.
97. O'Connor B, Moore A and Watts M. Hess'sign produced by bedrail injury. *Ir Med J* 2003;**96**:313.
98. Robinson BE, Sucholeiki R and Schocken DD. Sudden death and resisted mechanical restraint: a case report. *J Am Geriatr Soc* 1993;**41**:424–5.
99. Mayer RA, Geha RC, Helfand MS *et al*. Role of fecal incontinence in contamination of the environment with vancomycin-resistant enterococci. *Am J Infect Control* 2003; **31**:221–5.
100. Noskin GA, Stosor V, Cooper I and Peterson LR. Recovery of vancomycinresistant enterococci on fingertips and environmental surfaces. *Infect Control Hosp Epidemiol* 1995; **16**:577–81.
101. Bonten MJ, Hayden MK, Nathan C *et al*. Epidemiology of colonisation of patients and environment with vancomycin-resistant enterococci. *Lancet* 1996;**348**:1615–9.
102. Podnos YD, Cinat ME, Wilson SE *et al*. Eradication of multi-drug resistant Acinetobacter from an intensive care unit. *Surg Infect* 2001;**2**:297–301.
103. Slaughter S, Hayden MK, Nathan C *et al*. A comparison of the effect of universal use of gloves and gowns with that of glove use alone on acquisition of vancomycin-resistant enterococci in a medical intensive care unit. *Ann Intern Med* 1996; **125**:448–56.
104. Catalano M, Quelle LS, Jeric PE *et al*. Survival of *Acinetobacter baumannii* on bed rails during an outbreak and during sporadic cases. *J Hosp Infect* 1999;**42**:27–35.
105. Dickson B and Pollanen M. Fatal thromboembolic disease: a risk in physically restrained psychiatric patients. *J Forensic Legal Med* 2009;**16**:284–6.
106. Katz L. Accidental strangulation from vest restraints. *JAMA* 1987;**257**:2032–3.
107. Miles SH and Irvine P. Deaths caused by physical restraints. *Gerontologist* 1992;**32**:762–5.
108. Joint Commission on Accreditation of Healthcare Organizations. *Issue 8 Sentinel Event Alert: Preventing Restraint Deaths (November 18, 1998)*, http://www.jcaho.org/pub/sealert/sea8.html, 1998.
109. Miles SH and Irvine PI. Common features of deaths caused by physical restraints. *Gerontologist* 1991;**31**:42.
110. Miles SH. Deaths between bedrails and air pressure mattresses. *J Am Geriatr Soc* 2002;**50**:1124–5.
111. Hospital Bed Safety Workgroup. *Hospital Bed System Dimensional and Assessment Guidance to Reduce Entrapment – Guidance for Industry and FDA Staff*. US Department of Health and Human Services, Food and Drug Administration, Silver Spring, MD, 2006.
112. Parker K and Miles SH. Deaths caused by bedrails. *J Am Geriatr Soc* 1997;**45**:797–802.
113. Todd JF. Hospital bed side rails. Preventing entrapment. *Nursing* 1997;**27**:67.
114. Werner P, Cohen-Mansfield J, Koroknay V and Braun J. The impact of a restraint reduction program on nursing home residents. *Geriatr Nurs* 1994;**15**:142–6.
115. Evans LK, Strumpf NE, Allen-Taylor SL *et al*. A clinical trial to reduce restraints in nursing homes. *J Am Geriatr Soc* 1997;**45**:675–81.
116. Capezuti E, Strumpf N, Evans LK and Maislin G. Outcomes of nighttime physical restraint removal for severely impaired nursing home residents. *Am J Alzheimers Dis Other Demen* 1999;**14**:157–64.
117. Capezuti E, Wagner L, Brush B *et al*. Consequences of an intervention to reduce restrictice side rail use in nursing homes. *J Am Geriatr Soc* 2007;**55**:334–41.
118. Hanger HC, Ball MC and Wood LA. An analysis of falls in the hospital: can we do without bedrails ? *J Am Geriatr Soc* 1999;**47**:529–31.
119. Agostini JV, Baker DI and Bogardus ST. Prevention of falls in hospitalized and institutionalized older people. In: KM McDonald (ed.), *Making Health Care Safer: a Critical Analysis of Patient Safety Practices. Evidence Report/Technology Assessment No. 43*, Agency for Healthcare Research and Quality, Rockville, MD, 2001, Chapter 26.
120. Grisso JA, Schwarz DG, Wolfson V *et al*. The impact of falls on an inner city elderly African-American population. *J Am Geriatr Soc* 1992;**40**:673–8.
121. Tinetti ME, Inouye SK, Gill TM and Doucette JT. Shared risk factors for falls, incontinence and functional dependence. *JAMA* 1995;**273**:1348–53.
122. American Geriatrics Society. *Position Statement: Restraint Use. Developed by the AGS Clinical Practice Committee and Approved May 1991 by the AGS Board of Directors*, 1991,

reviewed 1997 and 2002, http://www.americangeriatrics.org/products/positionpapers/index.html.

123. Happ MB. Using a best practice approach to prevent treatment interference in critical care. *Prog Cardiovasc Nurs* 2000;**15**:58–62.

124. Maccioli GA, Dorman T, Brown BR *et al*. Clinical practice guidelines for the maintenance of patient physical safety in the intensive care unit: use of restraining therapies – American College of Critical Care Medicine Task Force 2001–2002. *Crit Care Med* 2003;**31**:2665–76.

125. Capezuti E, Talerico KA, Strumpf N and Evans LK. Individualized assessment and intervention in bilateral siderail use. *Geriatr Nurs* 1998;**19**:322–30.

126. Resnick B. *Restorative Care Nursing for Older Adults: a Guide for All Care Settings*, Springer, New York, 2004.

127. Capezuti E, Wagner L, Brush B *et al*. Bed and toilet height as potential environmental risk factors. *Clin Nurs Res* 2008;**17**:50–66.

128. Jenson B, Hess-Zak A, Johnston SK *et al*. Restraint reduction: a new philosophy for a new millennium. *J Nurs Admin* 1998;**28**:32–8.

129. Connell BR. Role of the environment in falls prevention. *Clin Geriatr Med* 1996;**12**:859–80.

130. Anonymous. Bed-exit alarms. A component (but only a component) of fall prevention. *Health Devices* 2004; **33**:157–68.

131. Happ MB. Preventing treatment interference: the nurse's role in maintaining technologic devices. *Heart Lung J Acute Crit Care* 2000;**29**:60–9.

132. Capezuti E and Lawson WT. Falls and restraint liability issues. *Nursing Home Litigation Investigation and Case Preparation*, Lawyers and Judges Publishing Company, Tucson, AZ, 1999.

133. Brechtelsbauer DA and Louie A. Wheelchair use among long-term care residents. *Ann Long Term Care* 1999;**7**:213–20.

134. Rader J, Jones D and Miller L. The importance of individualized wheelchair seating for frail older adults. *J Gerontol Nurs* 2000;**26**:24–32.

135. Rader J, Jones D and Miller LL. Individualized wheelchair seating: reducing restraints and improving comfort and function. *Top Geriatr Rehabil* 1999;**15**:34–47.

136. Capezuti E, Talerico KA, Cochran I *et al*. Individualized interventions to prevent bed-related falls and reduce siderail use. *J Gerontol Nurs* 1999;**25**:26–34.

137. Scherder E, Bouma A, Borkent M and Rahman O. Alzheimer patients report less pain intensity and pain affect than non-demented elderly. *Psychiatry* 1999;**62**:265–72.

138. American Geriatrics Society. Pharmacological management of persistent pain in older persons. *J Am Geriatr Soc*, 2009; **57**:1331–46.

139. Decker SA and Perry AG. The development and testing of the PATCOA to assess pain in confused older adults. *Pain Manage Nurs* 2003;**4**:77–86.

140. van Doorn C, Gruber-Baldini AL, Zimmerman S *et al*. Dementia as a risk factor for falls and fall injuries among nursing home residents. *J Am Geriatr Soc* 2003;**51**:1213–8.

141. Talerico KA, Capezuti E, Evans L and Strumpf N. Making sense of behavior: individualized care based on needs of the older adult. *Gerontologist* 1995;**35**:128.

142. Miller LL and Talerico KA. Pain in older adults. *Annu Rev Nurs Res* 2002;**20**:2063–88.

143. Gray-Miceli DL, Waxman H, Cavalieri T and Lage S. Prodromal falls among older nursing home residents. *Appl Nurs Res* 1994;**7**:18–27.

144. American Geriatrics Society and The British Geriatrics Society. *Clinical Practice Guideline for the Prevention of Falls in Older Persons*, http://www.americangeriatrics.org/education/summ_of_rec.shtml, 2010.

145. American Medical Directors Association and The American Health Care Association. *Falls and Fall Risk: Clinical Practice Guideline American Medical Directors Association*, American Medical Directors Association, Columbia, MD, 1998.

146. Ledford L. Prevention of falls research-based protocol. In: MG Titler (ed.), *Series on Evidence Based Practice for Older Adults*, University of Iowa Gerontological Nursing Interventions Research Center Research Dissemination Core (RDC), Iowa City, IA, 1996.

147. Rubenstein L, Powers C and MacLean CH. Quality indicators for the management and prevention of falls and mobility problems in vulnerable elders. *Ann Intern Med* 2001;**135**:686–93.

148. Yip YB and Cumming RG. The association between medications and falls in Australian nursing-home residents. *Med J Aust* 1994;**160**:14–8.

149. Thapa PB, Gideon P, Fought RL and Ray WA. Psychotropic drugs and risk of recurrent falls in ambulatory nursing home residents. *Am J Epidemiol* 1995;**142**:202–11.

150. Beers MH. Explicit criteria for determining potentially inappropriate medication use by the elderly: an update. *Arch Intern Med* 1997;**157**:1531–6.

151. Leipzig RM, Cumming RG and Tinetti ME. Drugs and falls in older people: a systematic review and meta-analysis: I. Psychotropic drugs. *J Am Geriatr Soc* 1999;**47**:30–9.

152. Ray WA, Thapa PB and Gideon P. Benzodiazepines and the risk of falls in nursing home residents. *J Am Geriatr Soc* 2000;**48**:682–5.

153. Thapa PB, Gideon P, Cost TW *et al*. Antidepressants and the risk of falls among nursing home residents. *N Engl J Med* 1998;**339**:875–82.

154. Cameron ID. Hip protectors: prevent fractures but adherence is a problem. *BMJ* 2002;**324**:375–6.

155. Cameron ID, Venman J, Jurrle SE *et al*. Hip protectors in aged-care facilities: a randomized trial of use by individual higher-risk residents. *Age Ageing* 2001;**30**:477–81.

156. Kannus P, Parkkari J, Siemi S *et al*. Prevention of hip fracture in elderly people with use of a hip protector. *N Engl J Med* 2000;**343**:1506–13.

157. Parker MJ, Gillespie LD and Gillespie WJ. Hip protectors for preventing hip fractures in the elderly. *Cochrane Database Syst Rev* 2005;(2): CD001255.

158. Kiel DP, Magaziner J, Zimmerman S, *et al*. Efficacy of a hip protector to prevent hip fracture in nursing home residents. *JAMA* 2007;**298**:413–422.

159. Wallace RB, Ross JE, Huston JC *et al*. Iowa FICSIT trial: the feasibility of elderly wearing a hip joint protective garment to reduce hip fractures. *J Am Geriatr Soc* 1993;**41**:338–40.

160. Ross JE, Wallace RB, Woodworth G *et al*. The acceptance of elderly of a hip joint protective garment to prevent hip fractures: Iowa FICSIT trial. In: *The Second World Conference on Injury Control*, Centers for Disease Control and Prevention, Atlanta, GA, 1993, pp. 90–1.

161. Capezuti E and Wexler S. Choosing alternatives to restraints. In: EL Siegler, S Mirafzali and JB Foust (eds), *A Guide to Hospitals and Inpatient Care*, Springer, New York, 2003.

162. Tominaga GT, Rudzwick H, Scannell G and Waxman K. Decreasing unplanned extubation in the surgical intensive care unit. *Am J Surg* 1995;**170**:586–9.

163. Wagner LM, Capezuti E, Brush B, Boltz M, Renz S and Talerico K. Description of an advanced practice nursing consultative model to reduce restrictive siderail use in nursing homes. *Res Nurs Health* 2007;**30**:131–40.

164. Capezuti E, Taylor J, Brown H *et al*. Challenges to implementing an APN-facilitated falls management program in long-term care. *Appl Nurs Res* 2007;**20**:2–9.

165. Ralphs-Thibodeau S, Knoefel F, Bnejamin K, *et al*. Patient choice: an influencing factor on policy-related research to decrease bedrail use as physical restraint. *Worldviews Evid Based Nurs* 2006;**3**:31–9.

166. Pellfolk T, Gustafson Y, Bucht G and Karlsson S. Effects of a restraint minimization program on staff knowledge, attitudes and practice: a cluster randomized trial. *J Am Geriatr Soc* 2010;**58**:62–9.

167. Huizing A, Hamers J, Gulpers M and Berger M. Preventing the use of physical restraints on residents newly admitted to psycho-geriatric nursing home wards: a cluster-randomized trial. *Int J Nurs Stud* 2009;**46**:459–69.

168. Johnson S, Ostaszkiewicz J and O'Connell B. Moving beyond resistance to restraint minimization: a case study of chance management in aged care. *Worldviews Evid Based Nurs* 2009;**6**:210–8.

169. Moore K and Haralambous B. Barriers to reducing the use of restraints in residential elder care facilities. *J Adv Nurs* 2007;**58**:532–40.

170. Capezuti E. Building the science of falls prevention research. *J Am Geriatr Soc* 2004;**52**:461–2.

CHAPTER 134

Centenarians

Thomas T. Perls
Boston University School of Medicine, Boston, MA, USA

An optimistic view

The prevalent notion that 'the older you get, the sicker you get' often leads the lay public to assume that those who achieve exceptional longevity must have numerous age-related illnesses that translate into a very poor quality of life. Among researchers and clinicians, the observation that the prevalence and incidence of dementia increase with age leads many to assume that dementia is inevitable for those who survive to age 100 years and older.[1,2] For example, the East Boston Study indicated that almost 50% of people over the age of 85 years have Alzheimer's disease.[3,4] Over the past decade or so, however, significant light has been shed on this assumption, with a number of nonagenarian and centenarian studies addressing the prevalence and incidence of dementia amongst the oldest old; these are summarized in Table 134.1.

As most of the studies noted in Table 134.1 indicate, dementia is not inevitable with very old age. Conservatively, ~15–20% of centenarians are cognitively intact. Furthermore, when dementia does occur, it tends to do so very late in life. In one study, over 90% of the centenarians did not experience functional impairment until the average age of 93 years.[18] The Heidelberg Centenarian Study proposed that those who develop dementia at extreme age have a shorter period of functional decline prior to the end of their lives.[16] In their review of the neuropathology literature amongst studies of nonagenarians and centenarians, von Gunten *et al.* concluded that the absence of Alzheimer's-related pathology in some of these individuals indicates that this disease is not a necessary consequence of ageing.[19] There have also been observations by several groups that in some centenarians, there is a disassociation between advanced pathology and clinical presentation, which suggests the presence of functional reserve or some form of adaptive capacity that allows these individuals to do better than expected given the degree of pathology on postmortem examination. The authors conclude that at least some centenarians have some form of resistance to Alzheimer's disease, the underlying cause of which has yet to be determined. Hence centenarians are of interest in the study of dementia not only for the fact that some of them escape dementia, but also because most of them markedly delay the clinical expression of the disease until very late in their exceptionally long lives.

Compression of morbidity versus disability

The compression of functional impairment towards the end of life that is observed among centenarians would at first glance appear to be consistent with James Fries's compression-of morbidity hypothesis.[20] Fries proposed that as the limit of human lifespan is approached, the onset and duration of lethal diseases associated with ageing must be compressed towards the end of life.[21] Although we found that functional impairment was compressed towards the end of life among centenarians, we noted that some centenarians had long histories of an age-related disease. Perhaps an unusual adaptive capacity or functional reserve allowed some of these persons to live a long time with what normally would be considered a debilitating, if not fatal, disease while delaying its attendant disability and death by as much as decades.[22–26]

Consistent with this observed phenomenon of compression of disability, the Danish Centenarian Study accessed 1997 and 2004 data from the Danish Civil Registration System on nearly 40 000 people born in 1905 and found that centenarians had fewer hospitalizations and shorter hospital stays compared with other members of their birth cohort who died at younger ages. It was concluded that centenarians are a useful cohort for the study of healthy ageing.

To explore this hypothesis in our centenarian sample, we conducted a retrospective cohort study exploring the timing of age-related diseases amongst individuals achieving exceptional old age.[27] Three profiles emerged from the analysis of health history data. Some 42% of the participants were 'survivors', in whom at least one of the 12 most

Principles and Practice of Geriatric Medicine, Fifth Edition. Edited by Alan J. Sinclair, John E. Morley and Bruno Vellas.

Table 134.1 Dementia studies of nonagenarians and centenarians.

Study	Comments
Dutch population-based centenarian study	10 centenarians in a population of 100 000 people were all noted to have clinically evident dementia.[5] Expansion of the study to a population of 250 000 led to finding 15 of 17 centenarians as having dementia[6]
Swedish population-based study of people aged ≥77 years	The prevalence of dementia amongst the 94 subjects aged ≥95 years was 48% (30% for men and 50% for women)[7]
Canadian Study of Health and Ageing	Dementia prevalence of subjects aged ≥95 years ($n = 104$) was 58%. The rate of increase in prevalence slowed at very advanced ages[1]
Study of Japanese Americans in King County, Washington	Dementia prevalence for subjects aged ≥95 years was 74%[8]
MRC-ALPHA Study, of older people in Liverpool	Dementia prevalence amongst centenarians was 47%[9]
Northern Italian Centenarian Study	Dementia was diagnosed in 62% of 92 centenarians[10]
Finnish population-based centenarian study	56% of 179 centenarians had cognitive impairment[11]
Meta-analysis of nine epidemiological studies of dementia among people aged ≥80 years	Prevalence of dementia levelled off at around age 95 years at a rate of 40%[12]
New England Centenarian (population-based) Study	Cognitive impairment prevalence was 79%[13]
Danish Centenarian Study	Dementia prevalence was 67%[14]
Coordinated study of dementia prevalence among centenarians in Sweden, Georgia (USA) and Japan	Dementia prevalences ranged from 40 to 63%[15]
Heidelberg Centenarian Study	Cognitive impairment prevalence was 75%[16]
French Centenarian Study	Dementia prevalence was 65% among female and 42% among male centenarians[17]

common age-associated diseases was diagnosed before the age of 80 years; 45% were 'delayers', in whom one of these age-associated diseases was diagnosed at or after the age of 80 years, which was beyond the average life expectancy for their birth cohort; and 13% were 'escapers', who attained their 100th birthday without diagnosis of any of the 10 age-associated diseases studied. That most centenarians appear to be functionally independent through their early 90s suggests the possibility that 'survivors' and 'delayers' are better able to cope with illnesses and remain functionally independent compared with the average ageing population. Therefore, in the case of centenarians, it may be more accurate to note a compression of disability rather than a compression of morbidity. As would be expected, this is not generally the case with illnesses associated with high mortality risks. When examining only the most lethal diseases of the elderly, such as heart disease, non-skin cancer and stroke, 87% of males and 83% of females delayed or escaped such diseases (relatively few centenarians were 'survivors' with such diseases). These results suggest there may be multiple routes to achieving exceptional longevity. The survivor, delayer and escaper profiles represent different centenarian phenotypes and probably also different genotypes. The categorization of centenarians into these and other groupings (for example, cognitively intact persons or smokers without smoking-related illnesses) should prove useful in the study of factors that determine exceptional longevity.

Nature versus nurture

The relative contribution of environmental and genetic influences to life expectancy has been a source of debate. Assessing heritability in 10 505 Swedish twin pairs reared together and apart, Ljungquist *et al.*[28] attributed 35% of the variance in longevity to genetic influences and 65% of the variance to non-shared environmental effects. Other twin studies indicate heritability estimates of life expectancy between 25 and 30%.[29,30] A study of 1655 old order Amish subjects born between 1749 and 1890 and surviving beyond age 30 years resulted in a heritability calculation for lifespan of 0.25.[31] These studies support the contention that the life spans of average humans with their average set of genetic polymorphisms are differentiated primarily by their habits and environments. Supporting this idea is a study of Seventh Day Adventists. In contrast to the American average life expectancy of 80 years, the average life expectancy of Seventh Day Adventists is 88 years. Because of their religious beliefs, members of this religious faith maintain optimal health habits such as not smoking, a vegetarian diet, regular exercise and maintenance of a lean body mass that translate into the addition of 8 years to their average life expectancy as compared with other Americans.[32] Given that in the USA 75% of persons are overweight and one-third are obese,[33] far too many persons still use tobacco[34] and far too few persons regularly exercise,[35] it is no wonder that our average life expectancy is about 8 years less than what our average set of genes should be able to achieve for us.

Of course, there are exceptions to the rule. There are individuals who have genetic profiles with or without prerequisite environmental exposures that predispose them to diseases at younger ages. There is also a component of luck, which good or bad, plays a role in life expectancy. Finally, there is the possibility that there exist genetic and environmental factors that facilitate the ability to live to ages significantly older than what the average set of genetic and environmental exposures normally allow. Because the oldest individuals in the twin studies were in their early to mid-80s, those studies provide information about heritability of average life expectancy, but not of substantially older ages, for example, age 100 years and older. As discussed below, to survive the 15 or more years beyond what our average set of genetic variations is capable of achieving for us, it appears that people need to have benefited from a relatively rare combination of what might be not-so-rare environmental, behavioural and genetic characteristics, which are often shared within families.

Studying Mormon pedigrees from the Utah Population Database, Kerber *et al.*[36] investigated the impact of family history upon the longevity of 78 994 individuals who achieved at least the age of 65 years. The relative risk of survival (λ_s) calculated for siblings of probands achieving the 97th percentile of 'excess longevity' (for males this corresponded to an age of 95 years and for women to an age of 97 years) was 2.30. Recurrence risks among more distant relatives in the Mormon pedigrees remained significantly greater than 1.0 for numerous classes of relatives, leading to the conclusion that single-gene effects were at play in this survival advantage. The Mormon study findings agree closely with a study of the Icelandic population in which first-degree relatives of those living to the 95th percentile of surviving age were almost twice as likely to also live to the 95th percentile of survival compared with controls.[37] Both research groups asserted that the range of recurrent relative risks that they observed indicated a substantial genetic component to exceptional longevity.

To explore further the genetic aspects of exceptional old age, Perls *et al.* analysed the pedigrees of 444 centenarian families in the USA that included 2092 siblings of centenarians.[38] Survival was compared with 1900 birth cohort survival data from the US Social Security Administration. As shown in Figure 134.1, female siblings had death rates at all ages that were about half the national level; male siblings had a similar advantage at most ages, although it diminished somewhat during adolescence and young adulthood. The siblings had an average age of death of 76.7 years for females and 70.4 years for males compared with 58.3 and 51.5 years, respectively, for the general population. Even after accounting for race and education, the net survival advantage of siblings of centenarians was found to be 16 years greater than the general population. An increasing genetic role with increasing age at very advanced ages is further supported by the work of Tan *et al.*, who noted that the power of a genome-wide association study to discover genes associated with exceptional longevity increases with the age of the subjects, for example from 90s to 100s.[39]

Siblings might share environmental and behavioural factors early in life that have strong effects throughout life. It would make sense that some of these effects are primarily responsible for the shared survival advantage up to middle age. Evidence of effects of early life conditions on adult morbidity and mortality points to the importance of adopting a life course perspective in studies of chronic morbidity and mortality in later life and also in investigations of exceptional longevity.[40–47] Characteristics of childhood environment are not only associated with morbidity and mortality at middle age, but have also been found to predict survival to extreme old age.[48,49] Stone[50] analysed effects of childhood conditions on survival to extreme old age among cohorts born during the late nineteenth century. Key factors predicting survival from childhood to age 110+ years for these individuals, most of whom were born between 1870 and 1889, were farm residence, presence of both parents in the household, American-born parents, family ownership of its dwelling, residence in a rural area and residence in the non-South; characteristics similar to those that had been previously shown to predict survival to age 85 years.[48,49]

In general, however, environmental characteristics such as socioeconomic status, lifestyle and region of residence, are likely to diverge as siblings grow older. Thus, if the survival advantage of the siblings of centenarians is primarily due to environmental factors, that advantage should decline with age. In contrast, the stability of relative risk for death across a wide age range suggests that the advantage is due more to genetic than to environmental factors.

Whereas death rates reflect the current death rate at a moment in time, survival probability reflects the cumulative experience of death up to that moment in a cohort's life history. Thus, a relatively constant advantage from moment to moment (as seen in the relative death rates) translates into an increasing survival advantage over a lifetime [as seen in the relative survival probabilities (RSPs)]. This increase is seen in Table 134.2, which shows the RSPs of the male and female siblings of centenarians at various ages.

By the age of 100 years, the relative survival probability for siblings of centenarians is 8.2 for women and 17 for men. From the analysis of death rates, we know that the siblings' survival advantage does not increase as the siblings age. Rather, the siblings' relative probability of survival is a cumulative measure and reflects their life-long survival advantage over the general population born around the same time. The marked increase in relative survival probability and sustained survival advantage in extreme old age could be consistent with the forces of demographic

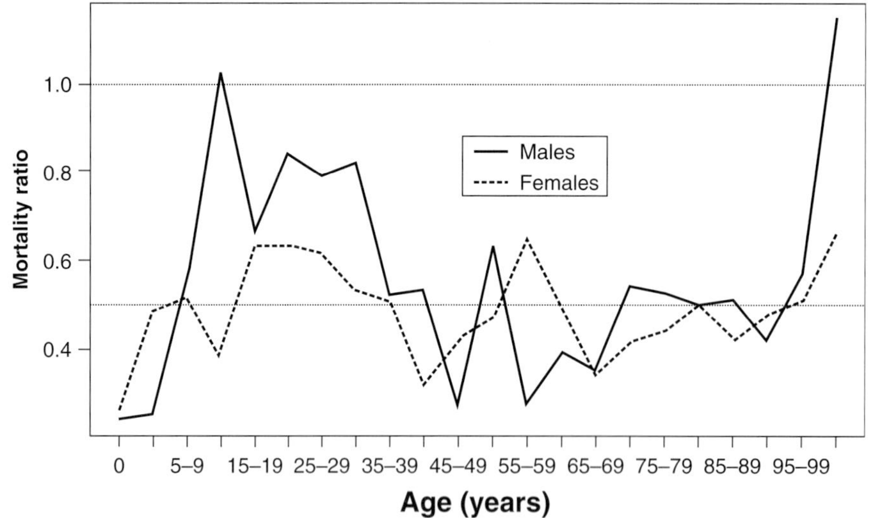

Figure 134.1 Relative mortality of male and female siblings of centenarians compared with birth cohort matched individuals (controls) from the general American population (survival experience of the controls comes from the Social Security Administration's 1900 birth cohort life table).

Table 134.2 Relative survival probabilities (RSP) with 95% confidence intervals (CI) of siblings of centenarians versus the US 1900 birth cohort.

Age	Males			Females		
(years)	RSP	Lower 95% CI	Upper 95% CI	RSP	Lower 95% CI	Upper 95% CI
20	1.00	1.00	1.00	1.00	1.00	1.00
25	1.00	0.99	1.01	1.01	1.00	1.02
60	1.18	1.15	1.21	1.12	1.09	1.14
65	1.29	1.25	1.33	1.16	1.13	1.19
70	1.48	1.42	1.53	1.24	1.21	1.28
75	1.68	1.60	1.77	1.36	1.31	1.41
80	2.03	1.90	2.16	1.54	1.47	1.60
85	2.69	2.47	2.91	1.83	1.73	1.93
90	4.08	3.62	4.54	2.56	2.39	2.74
95	8.35	6.98	9.71	4.15	3.73	4.57
100	17.0	10.8	23.1	8.22	6.55	9.90

selection, in which genes or environmental factors (or both) that predispose to longevity win out over those that are associated with premature or average mortality. The substantially higher relative survival probability values for men at older ages might reflect the fact that male mortality rates are substantially higher than female mortality rates at these ages and, therefore, that men gain a greater advantage from beneficial genotypes than women do. Another possibility is that men require an even rarer combination of genetic and environmental factors to achieve extreme age than women do.[51] Either possibility could explain why men make up only 15% of centenarians.

Centenarian offspring: following in the footsteps of their parents

The familiality of exceptional longevity demonstrated amongst centenarians and their siblings appears to extend also to the offspring of centenarians. Centenarian offspring currently in their 70s and 80s have approximately half the relative prevalence of hypertension, diabetes and cardiovascular disease (including coronary artery disease, myocardial infarction, congestive heart failure and/or arrhythmia) and cardiovascular risk factors compared with controls whose parents died at or before the average life expectancy of their birth cohort or to spousal controls.[52,53]

Among the centenarian offspring who did develop these conditions, the age of onset was significantly delayed compared with the age at onset for controls.[54] Examining the causes of death for deceased centenarian offspring and controls, centenarian offspring had a 62% risk reduction in all-cause mortality, an 85% risk reduction in coronary heart disease-specific mortality and a 71% risk reduction in cancer-specific mortality.[55] Barzilai *et al.*[56] demonstrated that centenarian offspring, when compared with spousal controls, have favourable lipid profiles. These individuals have significantly larger HDL (high-density lipoprotein) and LDL (low-density lipoprotein) particle sizes than controls.[57] The larger particle sizes are associated with lower prevalences of cardiovascular disease, hypertension and metabolic syndrome and are hypothesized to be predictive for longevity.

In addition to lipid profiles, another biomarker, heat shock protein 70 (HSP70), has been examined in the offspring of centenarians compared with spousal controls. Heat shock proteins, which help to chaperone, transport and fold proteins when cells are exposed to a variety of stresses, may protect against or modify the progression of atherosclerosis. In a pilot study of 20 centenarian offspring and nine spousal controls, Terry *et al.*[58] demonstrated a nearly 10-fold difference in levels of circulating HSP70.

Genetic findings

Centenarians may be rare because a complex set of environmental and genetic variables must coexist for such survival to occur. The first genetic association with exceptional longevity, that has also withstood the test of time and numerous studies, has been the observation that the apolipoprotein E epsilon-4 (apo ε-4) allotype is rare amongst centenarians. Individuals who are homozygous for apo ε-4 have a 2.3–8 times greater risk of developing Alzheimer's disease compared with the general Caucasian population.[59,60] The allelic frequency of apo ε-4 drops off dramatically in the oldest age groups, presumably because of its association with Alzheimer's disease and vascular disease.[61] Interestingly, the effect of apolipoprotein E allotype upon Alzheimer's disease incidence appears to decrease with age at these very old ages.[11]

Richard Cutler, in what is now a classic paper in gerontology, proposed that persons who achieve extreme old age do so in great part because they have genetic variations that affect the basic mechanisms of ageing and result in a uniform decreased susceptibility to age-associated diseases.[62] Our studies and those of others researching the oldest old have proposed that persons who achieve extreme old age probably lack many of the variations (the 'disease genes') that substantially increase risk for premature death by predisposing persons to various fatal diseases, both age-associated and non-age-associated.[63] Recently however, both the New England Centenarian Study[64] and the Leiden Longevity Study[65] noted that the extreme old have just as many disease-associated genetic variants as younger subjects. Both groups hypothesize that other genetic variations (so called 'longevity enabling genes') might confer protection against such deleterious variants and also other factors that would otherwise decrease the 'risk' for exceptional longevity.[66]

The elevated relative survival probability values found among the siblings of centenarians support the utility of performing genetic studies to determine what genetic region or regions and ultimately what genetic variations centenarians and their siblings have in common that confer their survival advantage.[67] Centenarian sibships from the New England Centenarian Study were included in a genome-wide sibling-pair study of 308 persons belonging to 137 families with exceptional longevity. According to non-parametric analysis, significant evidence for linkage was noted for a locus on chromosome 4 at D4S1564 with an Maximum LOD Score (MLS) of 3.65 ($p = 0.044$).[68] A detailed haplotype map was created of the chromosome 4 locus that extended over 12 million base pairs and involved the genotyping of over 2000 single-nucleotide polymorphism (SNP) markers in 700 centenarians and 700 controls. The study identified a haplotype, approximating the gene microsomal transfer protein (MTP).[69] All known SNPs for MTP and its promoter were genotyped in 200 centenarians and 200 controls (young individuals). After haplotype reconstruction of the area was completed, a single haplotype, which was under-represented in the long-lived individuals, accounted for the majority of the statistical distortion at the locus (~15% among the subjects versus 23% in the controls). MTP is a rate-limiting step in lipoprotein synthesis and may affect longevity by subtly modulating this pathway. Given that cardiovascular disease is significantly delayed among the offspring of centenarians and that 88% of centenarians either delay or escape cardiovascular disease and stroke beyond the age of 80 years, it makes sense that the frequency of genetic polymorphisms that play a role in the risk for such diseases would be differentiated between centenarians and the general population.[27,53]

Nir Barzilai and his colleagues, studying Ashkenazi Jewish centenarians and their families, found another cardiovascular pathway and gene that is differentiated between centenarians and controls.[57] In Barzilai *et al.*'s study, controls are the spouses of the centenarians' children. They noted that HDL and LDL particle sizes were significantly larger among the centenarians and their offspring and the particle size also differentiated between subjects with and without cardiovascular disease, hypertension and metabolic syndrome. In a candidate gene approach, they then searched the literature for genes that impact upon HDL and LDL particle size, and hepatic lipase and cholesteryl ester transfer protein (CETP) emerged as candidates. Comparing centenarians and their offspring against controls, one variation of CETP was noted to be significantly increased among those with or predisposed for exceptional longevity. Of additional note, a number of groups have observed an association between FOXO3A plus or minus FOXO1A and longevity.[70–75] FOXO3A emerged as a candidate gene for further investigation in centenarian association studies because of findings in lower organism studies that noted a role for FOXO in the insulin signalling pathway and ultimately longevity. As with CETP, the question remains of whether these variants are associated with age-related diseases (e.g. heart disease or diabetes) and/or determinants of human ageing itself.

A proposed multifactorial model for exceptional longevity and exceptional survival phenotypes

The fact that siblings of centenarians maintain half the mortality risk of their birth cohort from age 20 years to extreme age suggests that multiple factors contribute to achieving exceptional longevity. For example, sociodemographic advantages may play key roles at younger ages, whereas genetic advantages may distinguish the ability to go from old age to extreme old age. Undoubtedly, exceptional longevity is much more complicated, with temporally overlapping roles for major genes and polygenic, environmental and stochastic components. Such a scenario would be consistent with a threshold model, where predisposition for the exceptional longevity trait can be measured on a quantitative scale. Figure 134.2 illustrates the standard threshold model proposed by Falconer,[76] where it is predicted that the proportion of affected relatives will be highest among the most severely affected individuals. In the case of exceptional longevity, perhaps severity can be measured by additional years beyond a certain age (threshold) or by additional years of delay in age at onset for disease.

Examples of phenotypes fitting the threshold model are early-onset breast cancer and Alzheimer's disease, where relatives of patients who develop these diseases at unusually young ages are themselves at increased risk or liability. Thus, a 108-year-old's 'liability' or predisposition for exceptional longevity is further beyond the threshold than someone more mildly affected, as for example a person who died at age 99 years. One interpretation of data indicating the higher relative survival probability of male siblings of centenarians compared with female siblings is that the males carry a higher liability for the trait, given the presence of the requisite traits. The model predicts that if a multifactorial trait is more frequent in one gender (as is the case with exceptional longevity, which is predominantly represented by females), the liability will be higher for relatives of the less 'susceptible' gender (males, in the case of exceptional longevity).[77] Although we have not yet looked at the relative survival probability of siblings of male versus female probands (something that certainly needs to be done), these elevated risks for male versus female siblings are interesting in this context. The model also predicts that the risk for exceptional longevity will be sharply lower for second-degree relatives compared with first-degree relatives, another observation that we hope to test by having access to many expanded pedigrees. The ramifications of this model holding true for exceptional longevity (and/or exceptional survival phenotypes) include (1) the older the subject, the better the chances of discovering traits predisposing for exceptional longevity and (2) there are gender-related differences in both relatives and probands in 'liability' for exceptional longevity, given the presence of specific traits conducive to exceptional longevity.

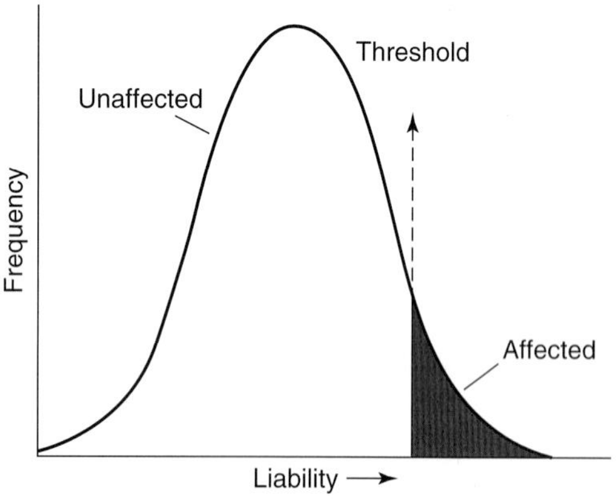

Figure 134.2 Threshold model of a multifactorial trait.

Conclusion

Although centenarians are rare, one per 5000 people in industrialized societies, they are also the fastest growing age category of our population. It is unlikely that they are rare because of any one rare factor. Rather, becoming a centenarian might entail achieving the right combination of genetic and environmental factors, much like winning the lottery requires the right combination of numbers. Each number by itself is not rare, but the right combination of five or six numbers certainly is. Complicating matters, the right combination of factors also likely varies from one person to the next, although there are similarities within families. One reason why the incidence of centenarians is growing may be understood by considering the analogy where the selection of lottery numbers is left less and less to chance. Better health-related behaviours and more effective public health and medical interventions make it significantly more likely for people to reach older age and for some to achieve extreme old age.

With the power of demographic selection, centenarians have already proven helpful in deciphering some polymorphisms and genetic loci associated, positively or negatively, with exceptional old age. The offspring of centenarians, who seem to be following closely in their parents' footsteps, might yield additional discoveries about phenotypic and genetic correlates of successful ageing. Discovering genes that could impart the ability to live to old age while compressing the period of disability towards the end of life should yield important insight into how the ageing process increases susceptibility to diseases associated with ageing and how this susceptibility might be modulated.[18,38] We anticipate that human longevity-enabling genes will be found to influence ageing at its most basic levels, thus affecting a broad spectrum of genetic and cellular pathways in a synchronous manner. Another approach that researchers are in the early stages of understanding is differential gene expression in models known to slow the ageing process, such as caloric restriction.[78] This may be another tool for discovering longevity-enabling genes. The centenarian genome should also be an efficient tool for ferreting out disease genes. Comparison of SNP frequencies implicated in diseases in centenarians and in persons with the diseases should show clinically relevant polymorphisms. The hope, of course, is that these approaches to gene discoveries will help identify drug targets and create drugs that would allow persons to become more 'centenarian-like' by maximizing the period of their lives spent in good health.

Key points

- An optimistic view. Centenarians support the observation 'the older you get, the healthier you've been'.
- Compression of morbidity versus disability. Achieving exceptional old age likely requires a compression of disability, not necessarily morbidity, towards the relative end of life.
- Nature versus nurture. The majority of the variation in average life expectancy is likely related to health-related behaviours. However, there appears to be a strong familial component to exceptional longevity and, for truly extreme old ages, such as >103 years, specific genetic variations may play a prominent role.
- Centenarian offspring. Following in the footsteps of their parents, the offspring of centenarians are a valuable model for the study of environmental and genetic factors related to successful ageing.
- Genetic findings. Reproducible genetic associations with exceptional longevity are still rare, reflecting the likely complex nature of gene–gene and gene–environment interactions that dictate the ability to survive to extreme old age.

References

1. Ebly EM, Parhad IM, Hogan DB and Fung TS. Prevalence and types of dementia in the very old: results from the Canadian study of health and aging. *Neurology* 1994;**44**:1593–600.
2. Thomassen R, van Schaick HW and Blansjaar B. Prevalence of dementia over age 100. *Neurology* 1998;**50**:283–6.
3. Evans DA, Funkenstein HH, Albert MS *et al.* Prevalence of Alzheimer's disease in a community population of older persons. Higher than previously reported. *JAMA* 1989;**262**(18): 2551–6.
4. Hebert LE, Scherr PA, Beckett LA *et al.* Age-specific incidence of Alzheimer's disease in a community population. *JAMA* 1995;**273**:1354–9.
5. Thomassen R, van Schaick HW and Blansjaar BA. Prevalence of dementia over age 100. *Neurology* 1999;**52**:1717.
6. Blansjaar BA, Thomassen R and van Schaick HW. Prevalence of dementia in centenarians. *Int J Geriatr Psychiatry* 2000;**15**:219–25.
7. von Strauss E, Viitanen M, De Ronchi D *et al.* Aging and the occurrence of dementia: findings from a population-based cohort with a large sample of nonagenarians. *Arch Neurol* 1999;**56**:587–92.
8. Graves AB, Larson EB, Edland SD *et al.* Prevalence of dementia and its subtypes in the Japanese American population of King County, Washington state. The Kame Project. *Am J Epidemiol* 1996;**144**:760–71.
9. Copeland JR, McCracken CF, Dewey ME *et al.*, The MRC-ALPHA Study. Undifferentiated dementia, Alzheimer's disease and vascular dementia: age-and gender-related incidence in Liverpool. *Br J Psychiatry* 1999;**175**:433–8.
10. Ravaglia G, Forti P, De Ronchi D *et al.* Prevalence and severity of dementia among northern Italian centenarians. *Neurology* 1999;**53**:416–8.
11. Sobel E, Louhija J, Sulkava R *et al.* Lack of association of apolipoprotein E allele epsilon 4 with late-onset Alzheimer's disease among Finnish centenarians. *Neurology* 1995; **45**:903–7.
12. Ritchie K and Kildea D. Is senile dementia 'age-related' or 'ageing-related'? – Evidence from meta-analysis of dementia prevalence in the oldest old. *Lancet* 1995;**346**:931–4.
13. Silver MH, Jilinskaia E and Perls TT. Cognitive functional status of age-confirmed centenarians in a population-based study. *J Gerontol B Psychol Sci Soc Sci* 2001;**56**:P134–40.
14. Andersen-Ranberg K, Vasegaard L and Jeune B. Dementia is not inevitable: a population-based study of Danish centenarians. *J Gerontol B Psychol Sci Soc Sci* 2001;**56**: P152–9.
15. Hagberg B, Alfredson BB, Poon LW and Homma A. Cognitive functioning in centenarians: a coordinated analysis of results from three countries. *J Gerontol B Psychol Sci Soc Sci* 2001;**56**:P141–51.
16. Kliegel M, Moor C and Rott C. Cognitive status and development in the oldest old: a longitudinal analysis from the Heidelberg Centenarian Study. *Arch Gerontol Geriatr* 2004;**39**:143–56.
17. Robine JM, Romieu I and Allard M. French centenarians and their functional health status. *Presse Med* 2003;**32**: 360–4.

18. Hitt R, Young-Xu Y, Silver M and Perls T. Centenarians: the older you get, the healthier you have been. *Lancet* 1999;**354**:652.
19. von Gunten A, Ebbing K, Imhof A *et al*. Brain aging in the oldest-old. *Curr Gerontol Geriatr Res* 2010; article 358531, doi:10.1155/2010/358531.
20. Vita AJ, Terry RB, Hubert HB and Fries JF. Aging, health risks and cumulative disability. *N Engl J Med* 1998;**338**: 1035–41.
21. Fries JF. Aging, natural death and the compression of morbidity. *N Engl J Med* 1980;**303**:130–5.
22. Lee JH. Genetic evidence for cognitive reserve: variations in memory and related cognitive functions. *J Clin Exp Neuropsychol* 2003;**25**:594–613.
23. Richards M and Sacker A. Lifetime antecedents of cognitive reserve. *J Clin Exp Neuropsychol* 2003;**25**:614–24.
24. Scarmeas N and Stern Y. Cognitive reserve and lifestyle. *J Clin Exp Neuropsychol* 2003;**25**:625–33.
25. Stern Y. The concept of cognitive reserve: a catalyst for research. *J Clin Exp Neuropsychol* 2003;**25**:589–93.
26. Wilson R, Barnes L and Bennett D. Assessment of lifetime participation in cognitively stimulating activities. *J Clin Exp Neuropsychol* 2003;**25**:634–42.
27. Evert J, Lawler E, Bogan H and Perls T. Morbidity profiles of centenarians: survivors, delayers and escapers. *J Gerontol A Biol Sci Med Sci* 2003;**58**:232–7.
28. Ljungquist B, Berg S, Lanke J *et al*. The effect of genetic factors for longevity: a comparison of identical and fraternal twins in the Swedish Twin Registry. *J Gerontol A Biol Sci Med Sci* 1998;**53**:M441–6.
29. Herskind AM, McGue M, Holm NV *et al*. The heritability of human longevity: a population-based study of 2872 Danish twin pairs born 1870–1900. *Hum Genet* 1996;**97**:319–23.
30. McGue M, Vaupel JW, Holm N and Harvald B. Longevity is moderately heritable in a sample of Danish twins born 1870–1880. *J Gerontol* 1993;**48**:B237–44.
31. Mitchell BD, Hsueh WC, King TM *et al*. Heritability of life span in the Old Order Amish. *Am J Med Genet* 2001;**102**:346–52.
32. Fraser GE and Shavlik DJ. Ten years of life: is it a matter of choice ? *Arch Intern Med* 2001;**161**:1645–52.
33. Fontaine KR, Redden DT, Wang C *et al*. Years of life lost due to obesity. *JAMA* 2003;**289**:187–93.
34. Wechsler H, Rigotti NA, Gledhill-Hoyt J and Lee H. Increased levels of cigarette use among college students: a cause for national concern. *JAMA* 1998;**280**:1673–8.
35. Wei M, Kampert JB, Barlow CE *et al*. Relationship between low cardiorespiratory fitness and mortality in normal-weight, overweight and obese men. *JAMA* 1999;**282**:1547–53.
36. Kerber RA, O'Brien E, Smith KR and Cawthon RM. Familial excess longevity in Utah genealogies. *J Gerontol A Biol Sci Med Sci* 2001;**56**:B130–9.
37. Gudmundsson H, Gudbjartsson DF, Frigge M *et al*. Inheritance of human longevity in Iceland. *Eur J Hum Genet* 2000;**8**:743–9.
38. Perls TT, Wilmoth J, Levenson R *et al*. Life-long sustained mortality advantage of siblings of centenarians. *Proc Natl Acad Sci USA* 2002;**99**:8442–7.
39. Tan Q, Zhao JH, Zhang D *et al*. Power for genetic association study of human longevity using the case–control design. *Am J Epidemiol* 2008;**168**:890–6.
40. Barker DJP. *Mothers, Babies and Health in Later Life*, Churchill Livingstone, London, 1998.
41. Blackwell D, Hayward MD and Crimmins EM. Does childhood health affect chronic morbidity in later life ? *Soc Sci Med* 2001;**52**:1269–84.
42. Costa D. Understanding the twentieth century decline in chronic conditions among older men. *Demography* 2000;**37**:53–72.
43. Elford J, Whincup P and Shaper AG. Early life experience and adult cardiovascular disease: longitudinal and case–control studies. *Int J Epidemiol* 1991;**20**:833–44.
44. Elo I. *Childhood Conditions and Adult Health: Evidence from the Health and Retirement Study*, Population Aging Research Center Working Papers, University of Pennsylvania, Population Aging Research Center, Philadelphia, 1998.
45. Hall A and Peekham CS. Infections in childhood and pregnancy as a cause of adult disease: methods and examples. *Br Med Bull* 1997;**53**:10–23.
46. Kuh D and Ben-Shlomo B. *A Life Course Approach to Chronic Disease Epidemiology*, Oxford University Press, Oxford, 1997.
47. Mosley W and Gray R. Childhood precursors of adult morbidity and mortality in developing countries: implications for health programs. In: J Gribble and S Preston (eds), *The Epidemiological Transition: Policy and Planning Implications for Developing Countries*, National Academy Press, Washington, DC, 1993, pp. 69–100.
48. Preston S, Hill ME and Drevenstedt GL. Childhood conditions that predict survival to advanced ages among African Americans. *Soc Sci Med* 1998;**47**:1231–46.
49. Preston S, Elo IT, Hill ME and Rosenwaike I. *The Demography of African Americans, 1930–1990*, Kluwer, Dordrecht, 2003.
50. Stone L. Early life conditions that predict survival to extreme old age. Paper presented at the Annual Meeting of the Population Association of America, Atlanta, GA, 2002.
51. Perls T and Fretts R. *Why Women Live Longer Than Men*, Scientific American Press, New York, 1998, pp. 100–7.
52. Atzmon G, Schechter C, Greiner W *et al*. Clinical phenotype of families with longevity. *Journal of the American Geriatrics Society* 2004;**52**:274–7.
53. Terry DF, Wilcox M, McCormick MA *et al*. Cardiovascular advantages among the offspring of centenarians. *J Gerontol A Biol Sci Med Sci* 2003;**58**:M425–31.
54. Terry DF, Wilcox MA, McCormick MA and Perls TT. Cardiovascular disease delay in centenarian offspring. *J Gerontol A Biol Sci Med Sci* 2004;**59**:M385–9.
55. Terry DF, Wilcox M, McCormick M *et al*. Reduced all-cause, cardiovascular and cancer mortality in centenarian offspring. *J Am Geriatr Soc* 2004;**52**:2074–6.
56. Barzilai N, Gabriely I, Gabriely M *et al*. Offspring of centenarians have a favorable lipid profile. *J Am Geriatr Soc* 2001;**49**:76–9.
57. Barzilai N, Atzmon G, Schechter C *et al*. Unique lipoprotein phenotype and genotype in humans with exceptional longevity. *JAMA* 2003;**290**:2030–40.

58. Terry D, McCormick M, Andersen S *et al*. Cardiovascular disease delay in centenarian offspring: role of heat shock proteins. *Ann N Y Acad Sci* 2004;**1019**:502–5.
59. Corder EH, Saunders AM, Strittmatter WJ *et al*. Gene dose of apolipoprotein E type 4 allele and the risk of Alzheimer's disease in late onset families. *Science* 1993;**261**:921–3.
60. Evans DA, Beckett LA, Field TS *et al*. Apolipoprotein E epsilon4 and incidence of Alzheimer disease in a community population of older persons. *JAMA* 1997;**277**:822–4.
61. Schachter F, Faure-Delanef L, Guenot F *et al*. Genetic associations with human longevity at the APOE and ACE loci. *Nat Genet* 1994;**6**:29–32.
62. Cutler RG. Evolution of human longevity and the genetic complexity governing aging rate. *Proc Natl Acad Sci USA* 1975;**72**:4664–8.
63. Schachter F. Causes, effects and constraints in the genetics of human longevity. *Am J Hum Genet* 1998;**62**:1008–14.
64. Sebastiani P, Solovieff N, Puca A *et al*. Genetic signatures of exceptional longevity in humans. *Science* 2010; published on line 1 July 2010, http://www.sciencemag.org/cgi/rapidpdf/science.1190532?ijkey=su1cvScg1VYF6andkeytype=refandsiteid=sci.
65. Beekman M, Nederstigt C, Suchiman HED *et al*. Genome-wide association study (GWAS)-identified disease risk alleles do not compromise human longevity. *Proc Natl Acad Sci USA* 2010;**107**:18046–9.
66. Perls T, Kunkel L and Puca A. The genetics of aging. *Curr Opin Genet Dev* 2002;**12**:362–9.
67. McCarthy MI, Kruglyak L and Lander ES. Sib-pair collection strategies for complex diseases. *Genet Epidemiol* 1998;**15**:317–40.
68. Puca AA, Daly MJ, Brewster SJ *et al*. A genome-wide scan for linkage to human exceptional longevity identifies a locus on chromosome 4. *Proc Natl Acad Sci USA* 2001;**98**:10505–8.
69. Geesaman BJ, Benson E, Brewster SJ *et al*. Haplotype based identification of a microsomal transfer protein marker associated with human lifespan. *Proc Natl Acad Sci USA* 2003;**100**:14115–20.
70. Koijima T, Kamei H, Aizu T *et al*. Association analysis between longevity in the Japanese population and polymorphic variants of genes involved in insulin and insulin-like growth factor 1 signaling pathways. *Exp Geronotol* 2004;**39**:1595–8.
71. Willcox BJ, Donlon TA, He Q *et al*. FOXO3A genotype is strongly associated with human longevity. *Proc Natl Acad Sci USA* 2008;**105**:13987–92.
72. Flachsbart F, Caliebe A, Kleindorp R *et al*. Association of FOXO3A variation with human longevity confirmed in German centenarians. *Proc Natl Acad Sci USA* 2009;**106**:2700–5.
73. Li Y, Wang WJ, Cao H *et al*. Genetic association of FOXO1A and FOXO3A with longevity trait in Han Chinese populations. *Hum Mol Genet* 2009;**18**:4897–904.
74. Pawlikowska L, Hu D, Huntsman S *et al*. Association of common genetic variation in the insulin/IGF1 signaling pathway with human longevity. *Aging Cell* 2009;**8**:46–72.
75. Zeng Y, Cheng L, Chen H *et al*. Effects of FOXO genotypes on longevity: a biodemographic analysis. *J Gerontol A Biol Sci Med Sci* 2010;**65**:1285–99.
76. Falconer D. The inheritance and liability to certain disease estimated from the incidence among relatives. *Ann Hum Genet* 1965;**29**:51–76.
77. Farrer L and Cupples A. Determining the genetic component of a disease. In: J Haines and MA Pericak-Vance (eds), *Approaches to Gene Mapping in Complex Human Diseases*, Wiley-Liss, New York, 1998.
78. Lee CK, Klopp RG, Weindruch R and Prolla TA. Gene expression profile of aging and its retardation by caloric restriction. *Science* 1999;**285**:1390–3.

CHAPTER 135

End-of-life and palliative care

Rachelle E. Bernacki[1], Ryan Westhoff[2] and Miguel A. Paniagua[3]

[1]Brigham and Women's Hospital, Boston, MA, USA
[2]University of Kansas Medical Center, Kansas City, KS, USA
[3]Saint Louis University School of Medicine, St Louis, MO, USA

Introduction

Palliative care (also known as supportive care) encompasses the assessment and treatment of pain and other non-pain symptoms with the goal of relieving suffering across multiple domains. Palliative care can be provided in conjunction with curative treatment at any point in a disease trajectory, even from the time of diagnosis (see Figure 135.1).

Palliative care assists increasing numbers of people with chronic, debilitating and life-limiting illnesses. A growing number of programmes provide this care in a variety of settings: hospitals, outpatient settings, community programmes within home health organizations and hospices. Within these settings, dedicated teams may include physicians, nurses, social workers, chaplains, counsellors, nursing assistants, rehabilitation specialists, speech and language pathologists and other healthcare professionals. These providers assess and treat pain along with other non-pain symptoms and also facilitate patient-centred communication and decision-making. The ideal palliative care delivery system fosters the coordination of continuity of care across settings throughout the disease continuum (see Figure 135.1). Whereas palliative care refers to an approach to care focused on symptom management and improving quality of life, palliative medicine refers to the medical specialty focused on providing palliative care. Despite the emergence of palliative medicine as a formally recognized medical specialty across the world, all physicians who care for patients with serious and advanced illnesses need to be able to provide appropriate pain and symptom management and identify and treat other sources of suffering in their patients. In order to achieve this goal, all physicians need training in palliative care.[1–3]

Palliative care services and palliative care domains are summarized in Tables 135.1 and 135.2, respectivly.

Palliative and hospice care

Palliative care is not synonymous with hospice care in that hospice utilization in the USA requires that a physician endorse a prognosis of 6 months or less in order for a patient to qualify for services. Enrolment in a hospice programme is but a final piece in what the whole of palliative care provides, ideally from the onset of serious life-threatening illness. The goal of palliative care is to prevent and relieve suffering and to support the best possible quality of life for patients and their families, regardless of the stage of the disease or the need for other therapies. Palliative care is both a philosophy of care and an organized, highly structured system for delivering care. The fundamental elements of hospice and palliative care maintain the following:[4]

1 Pain and symptom control, psychosocial distress, spiritual issues and practical needs are systematically addressed with the patient and family throughout the continuum of care. If present, any conditions are treated based upon current evidence and with consideration of cultural aspects of care.

2 Patients and families acquire ongoing information in a culturally sensitive, appropriate and understandable manner to facilitate the comprehension of the condition and realistic potential of treatment options. In the process, values, preferences, goals and beliefs are elicited over time. The benefits and burdens of treatment are regularly reassessed and the decision-making process about the care plan is sensitive to changes in the patient's condition.

3 Genuine coordination of care across settings is ensured through regular and high-quality communication between providers at times of transition or changing needs and through effective continuity of care and case management.

4 Both patient and family, however defined by the patient, are appropriately prepared for the dying process and for death when it is anticipated. Hospice options are

Principles and Practice of Geriatric Medicine, Fifth Edition. Edited by Alan J. Sinclair, John E. Morley and Bruno Vellas.

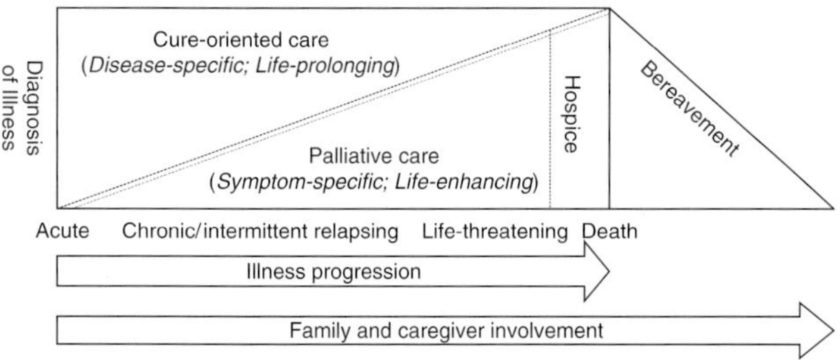

Figure 135.1 Palliative care is most effective for patients and their families when it is integrated across the healthcare continuum. It is optimally initiated in collaboration during the cure-oriented phase, continuing through the course of illness and culminating in end-of-life care (hospice), then bereavement support for family and caregivers. As the disease progresses, more palliative services are integrated into the patient's care as needed. Simultaneously, the emphasis on curative (or life-prolonging) therapies diminishes as the goals of care focus more on palliative care measures (quality-of-life-enhancing).

Table 135.1 Palliative care services.

- Provides relief from pain and other distressing symptoms
- Will enhance quality of life and may also positively influence the course of illness
- Is applicable early in the course of illness, in conjunction with other therapies that are intended to prolong life, such as chemotherapy or radiation therapy
- Includes those investigations needed to understand and manage distressing clinical complications better
- Integrates the psychological and spiritual aspects of patient care
- Offers a support system to help patients live as actively as possible until death
- Affirms life and regards dying as a normal process
- Intends neither to hasten nor to postpone death
- Offers a support system to help the family cope during the patient's illness and in their own bereavement
- Uses a team approach to address the needs of patients and their families, including bereavement counselling, if indicated

Source: information from WHO's *Definition of Palliative Care*, http://www.who.int/cancer/palliative/definition/en/(last accessed 26 November 2011).

explored, opportunities for personal growth are enhanced and bereavement support is available for the family.

Symptom assessment and treatment

Palliative care aims at the relief of suffering caused by physical, psychosocial and spiritual aspects of disease and utilizes an interdisciplinary team to provide care. By focused symptom management and clear goals of care, patients living with advanced illness can improve quality of life and spend valuable time with friends, family and loved ones. One of the core principles of the delivery of end-of-life care is the alleviation of pain and other physical and psychological symptoms. The goal of pain and symptom management is a reduction of the symptoms to a level that the patient defines as satisfactory. Providers should be careful not to state that all symptoms will be completely alleviated, because although this goal is sometimes achievable, more often symptoms, such as pain and nausea, are attenuated to an acceptable level.

Pain

The optimal control of pain in the palliative care patient relies on the understanding of the underlying pathophysiology and mechanisms involved and include somatic, neuropathic and visceral aetiologies. These might include tumour invasion of local tissues or metastatic bone pain (somatic), nerve compression or chemotherapy-related nerve pain (neuropathy) or bowel obstruction (visceral). Therefore, management starts with the evaluation of the causes of the pain by a comprehensive history, physical and directed imaging as indicated by the initial evaluation.[5] Many cases of advanced life-threatening illness require the use of opioids; providers should prescribe opioids in doses sufficient to relieve pain and to acquire skills in the management of predictable opioid side effects. Providers must also anticipate and correct patients' misconceptions about the use of opioids, including side effects, addiction, somnolence and hastening of death. Because patients may become unable to take medications orally, the sublingual, transdermal, rectal and subcutaneous routes may be used. The World Health Organization (WHO) pain relief ladder (see Figure 135.2) is a well-established and reasonable starting point in the management of pain symptoms. If pain occurs, the first step is oral administration of medication in the following order: non-opioids (aspirin and paracetamol); then, as necessary, mild opioids (codeine); then strong opioids such as morphine, until the patient's pain is attenuated. It should be noted that this approach has potential limitations in the context of longer survival and increasing disease complexity if used in isolation and without a comprehensive clinical approach to the pain syndrome. To complement this, combination and adjuvant therapies, including procedural interventions, are used where appropriate, tailored to the needs of an individual with the goals of optimizing pain relief and minimizing adverse effects.[6,7] Furthermore, older and debilitated patients' ability to request 'on demand' (or PRN) medications should compel the provider to consider scheduled dosing, particularly if in a setting such as a long-term care facility where frequent and timely reassessment of pain can be limited by staffing. To maintain freedom from pain, drugs should be given 'by the clock', that is, every 2–6 h, rather than 'on demand'. This three-step approach of administering the right drug in the right dose

Table 135.2 Palliative care domains.

Area	Examples
Physical	Pain, shortness of breath, nausea, fatigue, weakness, anorexia, insomnia, confusion, constipation, treatment side effects, functional capacities, treatment efficacy and alternatives (and patient and family preferences)
Psychological/ psychiatric	Anxiety, depression, care-giving needs or capacity of family; stress; grief and bereavement risks for the patient and family (e.g. depression and co-morbid complications); coping strategies
Social	Family structure and geographic location; cultural concerns and needs; finances; sexuality; living arrangements; caregiver availability; access to transportation; access to prescription and over-the-counter medicines
Spiritual/religious/ existential	Spiritual background, beliefs and practices of the patient and family; hopes and fears; life completion tasks; wishes regarding care setting for death

Source: information from National Consensus Project for Quality Palliative Care, *Clinical Practice Guidelines for Quality Palliative Care*, 2nd edn, 2009, http://www.nationalconsensusproject.org (last accessed 7 November 2011).

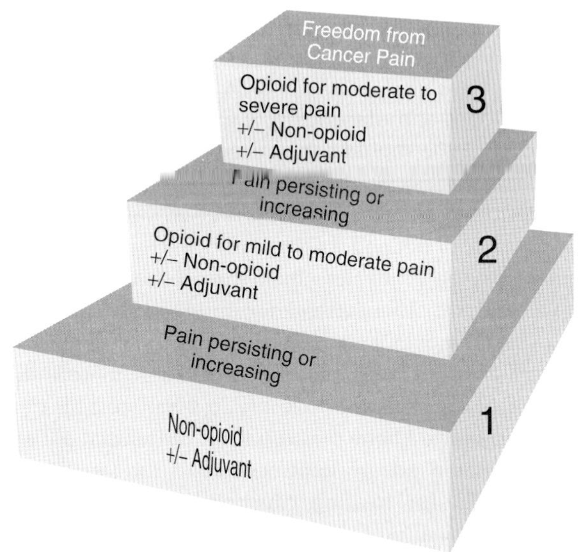

Figure 135.2 *WHO's Pain Ladder*.[8] Reproduced with permission from the World Health Organization from http://www.who.int/cancer/palliative/painladder/en/index.html (last accessed 26 September 2011).

at the right time is inexpensive and 80–90% effective.[8] Surgical intervention on appropriate nerves may provide further pain relief if drugs are not wholly effective (see Figure 135.2).

In essence, the optimal means of providing palliation of pain symptoms is first to consider evaluation and treatment of the underlying removal or minimization of the cause (i.e. disease-directed therapies). For example, in malignant bone pain, surgery, chemotherapy, radiotherapy, and/or bisphosphonates may be used.[9] In infection, antimicrobials or surgical drainage of an abscess may be required. Alongside disease-directed therapy, there are a host of pharmacological and non-pharmacological therapies, which should be used on an individual basis depending on the clinical situation.

Non-pain symptoms

Dyspnoea and respiratory symptoms

Changes in respiratory patterns are common in dying patients. Breathing usually becomes shallow as death nears and periods of apnoea are common. Opioids are the main therapy for treating dyspnoea. Some patients and providers may not be familiar with using opioids for this purpose and should be educated. Secretions that accumulate in the pharynx due to the patient being too weak or unresponsive to swallow or cough can produce a rattling sound that can be distressing to the family. Deep suctioning should be avoided as it can lead to gagging and may be uncomfortable. Atropine, scopolamine or glycopyrrolate (the last does not cross the blood–brain barrier, thereby minimizing contribution to delirium) can be effective in reducing rattle by decreasing the amount of mucus and saliva produced. Rooms should be cool and well ventilated and a fan can aid in reducing the sensation of dyspnoea. It may be appropriate to stop taking blood pressure and monitor only respiratory rate and pulse in order to avoid disturbing the patient or causing alarm to the patient's loved ones.

Gastrointestinal symptoms: nausea and vomiting

Nausea and vomiting are common symptoms in patients with advanced illnesses, including cancer, congestive heart failure, end-stage renal disease and AIDS. For patients and families facing a life-threatening illness, nausea and vomiting can cause substantial distress due to concerns about maintaining adequate nutrition and also fear that these symptoms indicate disease progression.[10] Nausea and vomiting can be triggered by activation of any of four general pathways (Table 135.3).[11]

Each of these four pathways can then activate the vomiting centre, a specific area of the medulla that coordinates the final act of vomiting via the parasympathetic system and gastrointestinal tract. Activation of the vomiting centre is believed to be mediated by histamine (H1) receptors or

Table 135.3 General pathways that can trigger nausea and vomiting.

Area	Activated by	Mediated by
Cortex	Meningeal irritation Increased intracranial pressure Cognitive/emotional factors	Anxiety
Chemoreceptor trigger zone (located in the floor of the fourth ventricle and lacks a blood–brain barrier)	Metabolic abnormalities Toxins Medications	Primarily by the dopamine (D2) receptor, but others include neurokinin-1 (NK1) and serotonin (5HT3)
Vestibular system	Motion or inner ear disease	Via histamine (H1) and muscarinic acetylcholine (ACh) receptors
Peripheral pathways. Signals transmitted along afferent tracts (vagus, glossopharyngeal, splanchnic and sympathetic nerves)	Mechanoreceptors and chemoreceptors in the gastrointestinal tract and heart	5HT3 receptors in the gastrointestinal tract

muscarinic acetylcholine (ACh) receptors.[11,12] Evaluation should include a thorough history and physical examination, with careful attention to common causes of nausea in the terminally ill, including medications (chemotherapy, opioids), constipation, bowel obstruction, electrolyte abnormalities, liver and kidney failure, radiation therapy, CNS lesions and anxiety. Providers should identify the likely mechanism or pathway responsible for a patient's nausea, as this will guide the therapeutic approach.

Non-pharmacological strategies can be helpful for many patients. Patients should eat small, frequent meals as they are able and may need to adjust the types of foods that they eat. Relaxation techniques may be useful for patients with significant anxiety or anticipatory nausea, which occurs prior to chemotherapy sessions due to a conditioned response. Patients with chemotherapy-induced symptoms may consider acupuncture as studies have found that acupuncture-point stimulation appears to reduce the incidence of acute chemotherapy-induced vomiting.[13]

Most patients with nausea or vomiting will need pharmacological therapy. First, determine the clinical aetiology of nausea and select a first-line antiemetic based on the likely mechanism. Then, use the first-line agent on a scheduled basis initially until nausea symptoms are controlled, then consider tapering to as-needed dosing. If symptoms persist, consider adding another agent in a different class while keeping the first-line agent. Nausea is frequently multifactorial and may need therapy directed at multiple sources. Recognize the side effect profiles of different antiemetics and use them to the patient's advantage, not disadvantage (e.g. haloperidol can be useful in patients who also have delirium). Ondansetron causes constipation and would be inappropriate for a patient with nausea due to constipation/obstipation. Finally, avoid using multiple agents in the same class simultaneously (e.g. metoclopramide and prochlorperazine should not be used simultaneously).

Constipation

Constipation is defined as decreased frequency of bowel movements (generally less than three bowel movements per week), hard stool consistency and difficulty with passage of bowel movements.[14] Despite attempts by physicians to describe the characteristics of constipation, there is still a high degree of observer variability in what are considered 'troubling' bowel habits.[15] Ultimately, individual patients' concerns should govern treatment goals for constipation. The strategies for treating constipation are varied and prone to personal preferences of both the patient and the physician;[15] unfortunately, little evidence exists to support rationally choosing any one medication over another.[15,16]

Constipation is a common symptom in chronic disease and can occur from medication used to treat the disease, the debility induced by the disease and the disease itself. The main strategy for treating constipation is prevention. Similarly to other symptom management strategies, chronic use of medications to decrease occurrence combined with strategies to overcome 'breakthrough' symptoms is necessary. The need for rescue medications or laxatives should be anticipated by healthcare providers and included in the care plan.[17] Generally, medications used to treat constipation are divided based on mechanism of action into the following four categories: stimulant laxatives, osmotic laxatives, stool softeners and bulking agents. Combinations of medications with different mechanisms of action are often used to achieve desired bowel function. Stimulant laxatives such as senna and osmotic laxatives such as sorbitol, lactulose and polyethylene glycol are the most common agents. Stool softeners, such as docusate, when used alone are less effective when bowel stimulation is the most likely underlying aetiology for constipation.[18]. Bulking agents, such as psyllium, used in the absence of adequate oral fluid intake can lead to impaction and should not be used in patients at the end of life.

Bowel obstruction

Bowel obstruction in palliative medicine tends to be as a result of malignancy or its treatments, which include surgical, opioid-related impaction or other sources of inflammatory bowel disease. The obstruction can lead to full bowel obstruction with obstipation or partial obstruction with episodic signs and symptoms. These symptoms usually develop over time and, if accompanied by large-volume emesis, tend to be of the upper gastrointestinal tract. With a limited life expectancy, should aggressive medical interventions fail to relieve symptoms, then endoscopic stenting should be considered if available, as it is potentially less invasive and complicating than surgical intervention. If neither of these options is available or feasible, the use of steroids in conjunction with octreotide to decrease secretions is effective.

Agitation and delirium

Agitation, although not common at end of life, is not infrequent and is troubling for patients and families. If the patient is experiencing agitation due to increased pain, pain should be treated with opioids as appropriate, or if thought to be due to dyspnoea, treated with oxygen and opioids. Behavioural interventions such as brushing a patient's hair or providing music therapy can be highly effective in treating agitation. When these measures do not work and the cause is uncertain, agitation should be treated with low doses of neuroleptics, such as haloperidol (or, if more sedation is needed, chlorpromazine). In palliative care, many drugs used for symptom management can cause neuropsychiatric side effects, as they either directly or indirectly affect the central nervous system. If unrecognized, these effects can generate considerable suffering and iatrogenic harm to patients. Side effects of commonly used palliative care medications include delirium, drug-induced parkinsonism, akathisia, serotonin syndrome and neuroleptic malignant syndrome. Antiemetics such as metoclopramide and haloperidol can cause significant levels of neuropsychiatric toxicity and should be carefully monitored and discontinued if necessary. Many drugs induce delirium, including anxiolytics, opioids, antidepressants, antihistamines, steroids, antipsychotics and antibiotics (fluoroquinolones such as ciprofloxacin). Timing of administration of medications can help determine the offending agent. If the offending medication or medications remain necessary to treat other distressing symptoms such as pain, management of delirium with neuroleptics, opioid rotation and hydration may be helpful.

Fatigue

Fatigue is described as a persistent sense of tiredness or diminished energy related to an underlying life-threatening illness (such as cancer) and/or its treatment, which is not relieved by rest and which causes diminution in functional capacity and quality of life. The treatment of fatigue in patients with chronic illness starts with a review of associated symptoms as many common physical and psychological symptoms are associated with fatigue.[19] Adequate treatment of pain, insomnia or depression is necessary as the common medications used to treat fatigue will not appropriately control these symptoms, other than antidepressant medications. A complete evaluation of possible medication side effects for fatigue inducing medications is also necessary.

After attempts to control other associated symptoms, the commonly used medication classes are psychostimulants, antidepressants, glucocorticoids and haematopoietic growth factors.[20] These medications are used to treat physical exhaustion, depressive symptoms and pathophysiological processes associated with fatigue. Unfortunately little strong evidence exists to support choosing one class of medications over another and often there is even a significant response to placebo in trials.[21] Given the unclear benefit from one class to another, methylphenidate is the first choice of therapy and can be considered as initial therapy in geriatric patient populations while monitoring for potential side effects.[22,23] Outcomes have been demonstrated in particular patient populations, such as cancer patients,[20,24,25] but its effectiveness has also been shown in smaller trials in a variety of medical illnesses.[22] Other medication classes are limited to specific clinical circumstances, such as the use of glucocorticoids in the prevention of chemotherapy-related fatigue,[26,27] by concern over serious adverse events such as haematopoietic growth factors or by lack of evidence of their effectiveness for isolated fatigue in placebo-controlled trials, such as antidepressants.[28,29] As with any pharmacological intervention, the main guiding principle should be close monitoring to make certain that the therapy is not causing more problems than the symptom, particularly when treating geriatric patients.

Communication

A key element of palliative care is effective communication in order to elicit a patient's preferences and goals of care.[30] Understanding the needs and goals of the patient and family is essential for providing high-quality palliative care. Palliative care teams provide coordination of care and create plans to deal with potential crises, thereby allowing the patient to remain in their setting of choice. Palliative care providers also need good prognostication skills in order to help patients and families define goals of care and make appropriate decisions and plans.[31,32] For example, when a family calls and states that a patient is eating poorly, it is important to know whether this represents a potentially reversible condition that could be relieved with a treatment or procedure or alternatively is a sign that the patient is approaching the final days to weeks of life. Prognostic information is important in helping patients make treatment decisions. For example, one patient may want treatment order to be able to eat and drink and survive to attend a granddaughter's marriage, while a different patient in a similar clinical situation may decide that they do not want to undergo yet another procedure. When the disease progresses, communication becomes even more important, to ensure that all involved have the same understanding of the prognosis and plan of care. Finally, clinician recognition of the signs and symptoms of the active dying phase of illness is crucial to completing the developmental tasks of the end of life, helping patients and families understand what is happening and what to expect and coordinating care and logistics in the days leading up to death. Although it is impossible to know exactly what will happen to any particular patient, providers can use scored instruments such as the Palliative Performance Scale, Karnofsky, Eastern Cooperative Oncology Group (ECOG) and clinical experience to offer patients and families estimates such as hours to days, days to weeks, weeks to months and months to a year that communicate prognosis while recognizing the inherent uncertainty of such predictions.

Palliative medicine teams formulate and document care plans based on patient wishes, then convey them to patients, family and other providers.[33] Care plans change according to the needs of the patient and family and should involve additional input from other specialists. Functional and cognitive status, disease trajectory, cultural and spiritual preferences and home support must be considered in formulating care plans. For example, a patient may want to remain at home during the final days and weeks of his life, but his wife, who is the primary caregiver, has trouble managing his medications due to mild cognitive impairment. In this situation, home nursing services or hospice can provide a weekly mediset and provide daily telephone call reminders to the wife to ensure administration of the medicines. As death nears, the team may address the possibility of pursuing an inpatient hospice given the wife's limitations.

Psychosocial and spiritual domains

In addition to addressing physical aspects of care, palliative care should address psychological issues and psychiatric needs and support emotional growth.[34,35] Physicians should acknowledge the stress involved in caring for patients with life-threatening illness for both our colleagues and for our patient's family and other caregivers. Caregivers reporting emotional stress have a significantly increased mortality rate; physician identification of vulnerable caregivers and referral to social workers and other community resources can be lifesaving. Physicians must recognize the importance of the time after referral to hospice and understand that patients and families are particularly vulnerable to feeling abandoned at this time by their physicians. Making follow-up appointments for patients and calling on the telephone can help reassure patients that a referral to hospice is not abandonment by the physician. It is important to express thanks and appreciation for the privilege of caring for the patient and, when appropriate, to say goodbye to the patient and their family members. Physicians must also be aware of normal and complicated grief and screen and address those issues appropriately.[36,37] Hospice programmes provide bereavement services and follow-up for 12 months after the death of the patient. Finally, all providers can discuss and offer coping strategies to determine the most constructive approach to dealing with loss based on individual family needs and temperament. Referral to a palliative care social worker can promote access to services, community resources and volunteers that can help patient and family in the home or with transportation. Collaboration with pharmacists can ensure that patients have access to necessary medications; home nursing agencies can ensure that proper equipment is available. Family structure and living arrangements, geographic location, finances and caregiver availability are considered and reflected in the care plan. For example, an older patient with advanced illness may have a partner who is ill and unable to provide care. In such a situation, where the support system is already at its limit, the palliative care team must develop a plan to ensure appropriate care and safety for the patient and their partner.

Sending a patient home without adequate support can often lead to readmission; addressing needs early and activating community support can allow patients to remain at home as long as possible. Different teams may provide these services in differing ways. Some teams have dedicated social workers to address these issues, whereas others may use case managers or nurses to focus on these matters. It is important to realize that the care coordination involved is more than a physician or nurse or social worker can do alone; the interdisciplinary nature of palliative care draws upon the strengths of each field.

Beliefs surrounding illness and death are profoundly influenced by a patient's and family's religious and spiritual values.[38] The salient spiritual needs of patients at the end of life encompass questions of meaning, value and relationship. Physicians can play a key role in helping patients express these needs by asking patients about their religious and spiritual beliefs and practices and how these impact on the patient's view of illness. At a minimum, physicians should recognize these spiritual needs, enquire as to the patient's spiritual roots and offer a referral to the hospital chaplain. Chaplains and other members of the spiritual care service can address such issues in a non-threatening and supportive way and help facilitate religious or spiritual rituals in addition to contacting spiritual communities identified by the patient and family. When religious beliefs appear to be a barrier to providing good end-of-life care, spiritual engagement is the direct approach to resolution. For example, one patient and his family had a strong religious belief in a miraculous cure for metastatic cancer. The palliative care team chaplain explored this belief explicitly and negotiated a treatment plan that was respectful of the family's belief but also realistic and practical. The chaplain articulated that forgoing additional chemotherapy would not change whether or not a miracle was possible. The patient then accepted a referral to hospice care, where he received continued spiritual, emotional and physical support.

Cross-cultural issues

The experience of a serious illness is deeply affected by a patient's and family's cultural values.[39] Culture often defines how patients and families understand illness, suffering and dying. Encounters between physicians and patients of different backgrounds are common given the diversity in the USA and therefore there are many opportunities for cross-cultural misunderstandings.[40] Use of life-prolonging therapies and technology, the locus of decision-making and truth telling are all influenced by cultural norms. While autonomy is the legal basis for medical decision-making in the USA, some cultures prefer that families make medical decisions as a unit. Adult children commonly wish to protect their parent from bad news and may ask the clinician not to tell the truth. Palliative medicine providers often address this issue by helping the family understand that the information will not be imposed but offered only if the patient indicates an explicit desire to know. Asking the patient if they are the kind of person who prefers all the details about their illness or if they would rather hear a general outline or leave the details of decision-making to a family member does this. Such communication can demonstrate respect for the patient's culture without assuming that the patient will conform to their cultural norms. Skilled communication, genuine curiosity and openness to differences can increase the likelihood that patients and families are satisfied with the process and outcomes of care.

Care transitions in end-of-life care

Healthcare organizations are beginning to use palliative care to improve quality, because it is an effective approach to reducing symptoms and improving patient and family satisfaction. In addition, use of palliative care services can improve transitions of care, support timely and successful discharge, avert unnecessary readmissions and contribute to the efficient use of healthcare resources. Care should be provided in the setting that the patient chooses. If it is not possible to provide care in the patient's preferred location, the least restrictive alternative setting should provide flexible visiting hours, adequate space for visitors and sufficient respite for care providers. When the patient cannot be in their choice of setting, creative measures are taken to make the alternative care setting as comfortable and familiar as possible. Prior to discharge from a hospice, evaluation of home safety and equipment needs is required. Necessary supplies including hospital beds, oxygen, commodes and shower chairs should be delivered prior to patient arrival and the hospital team must ensure that a family member or friend is at the home to accept delivery. If the patient requires ambulance transport home, the timing of arrival should be carefully considered (e.g.. time the ambulance to arrive when young children are at school). Most transport companies allow a family member to travel with the patient if going home from a hospice. For opioid prescriptions, the hospital team should confirm who will prescribe opioids for patient after discharge and verify that the patient's pharmacy actually carries the medication. For opioids, a quantity must be specified (e.g. one cannot write 'one month's supply'). Patients on opioids should not be discharged until the prescription is filled and available at home, as it is often difficult to find a pharmacy that carries these medicines, particularly in poor neighbourhoods. Prior authorization from insurance companies may be required for some new medications or large quantities, hence this should be discussed prior to discharge. Finally, it is prudent to discuss prognosis (hours to days, days to weeks and weeks to months) with patient and family. Some patients and families may opt to attempt to have their loved one get home prior to death, even if death is imminent. Other families may choose to remain in the hospital when death is imminent. Families should be guided in the important developmental tasks of this stage of life, including conduct of important conversations while the patient is still able to participate. Many teams provide family members with a written list of Byock's 'Five Things' to think through and discuss as applicable when a loved one is dying: thank you; forgive me; I forgive you; I love you: goodbye. Depending upon their age and wishes, children may visit after preparation for what they will see and encouragement to draw a picture or write a letter to the patient expressing their feelings towards them, as a means of saying goodbye.

Key points

- Palliative care encompasses the assessment and treatment of symptoms with the goal of relieving suffering across multiple domains.

- The ideal palliative care delivery system fosters the coordination of continuity of care across settings throughout the disease continuum.
- The goal of palliative medicine providers in the process of providing symptom management is to alleviate suffering regardless of its cause.
- The optimal control of pain in palliative care requires an understanding of the underlying pathophysiology and mechanisms involved and include somatic, neuropathic and visceral aetiologies.
- Understanding the multidimensional needs and goals of the patient and family is essential in providing high-quality palliative care.
- Use of palliative care services can improve transitions of care, support timely and successful discharge, avert unnecessary readmissions and contribute to efficient use of healthcare resources.

References

1. Block SD, Bernier GM, Crawley LM *et al*. Incorporating palliative care into primary care education. National Consensus Conference on Medical Education for Care Near the End of Life. *J Gen Intern Med* 1998;**13**:768–73.
2. Ferris FD, Bruera E, Cherny N *et al*. Palliative cancer care a decade later: accomplishments, the need, next steps - from the American Society of Clinical Oncology. *J Clin Oncol* 2009; **27**:3052–8.
3. Morrison RS and Meier DE. Clinical practice. Palliative care. *N Engl J Med* 2004;**350**:2582–90.
4. NHPCO. *NHPCO Facts and Figures: Hospice Care in America*, National Hospice and Palliative Care Organization, Alexandria, VA, 2011.
5. Ripamonti C and Bandieri E. Pain therapy. *Crit Rev Oncol Hematol* 2009;**70**:145–59.
6. Raphael J, Ahmedzai S, Hester J *et al*. Cancer pain: Part 1. Pathophysiology; oncological, pharmacological and psychological treatments: a perspective from the British Pain Society endorsed by the UK Association of Palliative Medicine and the Royal College of General Practitioners. *Pain Med* 2010; **11**:742–64.
7. Raphael J, Hester J, Ahmedzai S *et al*. Cancer pain: Part 2. Physical, interventional and complementary therapies; management in the community; acute, treatment-related and complex cancer pain: a perspective from the British Pain Society endorsed by the UK Association of Palliative Medicine and the Royal College of General Practitioners. *Pain Med* 2010;**11**:872–96.
8. World Health Organization. *WHO's Pain Ladder*, WHO, Geneva, 2011, http://www.who.int/cancer/palliative/painladder/en/index.html (last accessed 26 September 2011).
9. Benedetti C, Brock C, Cleeland C *et al*. NCCN Practice Guidelines for Cancer Pain. *Oncology (Williston Park)* 2000; **14**(11A):135–50.
10. Wood GJ, Shega JW, Lynch B and Von Roenn JH. Management of intractable nausea and vomiting in patients at the end of life: 'I was feeling nauseous all of the time . . . nothing was working'. *JAMA* 2007;**298**:1196–207.
11. Ezzo J, Streitberger K and Schneider A. Cochrane systematic reviews examine P6 acupuncture-point stimulation for nausea and vomiting. *J Altern Complement Med* 2006;**12**:489–95.
12. Naeim A, Dy SM, Lorenz KA *et al*. Evidence-based recommendations for cancer nausea and vomiting. *J Clin Oncol* 2008;**26**:3903–10.
13. Streitberger K, Ezzo J and Schneider A. Acupuncture for nausea and vomiting: an update of clinical and experimental studies. *Auton Neurosci* 2006;**129**:107–17.
14. Longstreth GF, Thompson WG, Chey WD *et al*. Functional bowel disorders. *Gastroenterology* 2006;**130**:1480–91.
15. Mihaylov S, Stark C, McColl E *et al*. Stepped treatment of older adults on laxatives. The STOOL trial. *Health Technol Assess* 2008;**12**(13): iii–iv, ix–139.
16. Petticrew M, Watt I and Brand M. What's the 'best buy' for treatment of constipation? Results of a systematic review of the efficacy and comparative efficacy of laxatives in the elderly. *Br J Gen Pract* 1999;**49**:387–93.
17. Miles CL, Fellowes D, Goodman ML and Wilkinson S. Laxatives for the management of constipation in palliative care patients. *Cochrane Database Syst Rev* 2006;(4): CD003448.
18. Petticrew M, Watt I and Sheldon T. Systematic review of the effectiveness of laxatives in the elderly. *Health Technol Assess* 1997;**1**(13): i–iv, 1–52.
19. Yennurajalingam S, Palmer JL, Zhang T *et al*. Association between fatigue and other cancer-related symptoms in patients with advanced cancer. *Support Care Cancer* 2008;**16**: 1125–30.
20. Minton O, Stone P, Richardson A *et al*. Drug therapy for the management of cancer-related fatigue. *Cochrane Database Syst Rev* 2008;(1): CD006704.
21. de la Cruz M, Hui D, Parsons HA and Bruera E. Placebo and nocebo effects in randomized double-blind clinical trials of agents for the therapy for fatigue in patients with advanced cancer. *Cancer* 2010;**116**:766–74.
22. Hardy SE. Methylphenidate for the treatment of depressive symptoms, including fatigue and apathy, in medically ill older adults and terminally ill adults. *Am J Geriatr Pharmacother* 2009;**7**:34–59.
23. Lasheen W, Walsh D, Mahmoud F *et al*. Methylphenidate side effects in advanced cancer: a retrospective analysis. *Am J Hosp Palliat Care* 2010;**27**:16–23.
24. Lower EE, Fleishman S, Cooper A *et al*. Efficacy of dexmethylphenidate for the treatment of fatigue after cancer chemotherapy: a randomized clinical trial. *J Pain Symptom Manage* 2009;**38**:650–62.
25. Hanna A, Sledge G, Mayer ML *et al*. A phase II study of methylphenidate for the treatment of fatigue. *Support Care Cancer* 2006;**14**:210–5.
26. Kawazoe H, Takiguchi Y, Tanaka H *et al*. Preventive effects of low-dose dexamethasone for delayed adverse events

induced by carboplatin-based combination chemotherapy. *Yakugaku Zasshi* 2007;**127**:1001–6.

27. Inoue A, Yamada Y, Matsumura Y *et al*. Randomized study of dexamethasone treatment for delayed emesis, anorexia and fatigue induced by irinotecan. *Support Care Cancer* 2003; **11**:528–32.
28. Moss EL, Simpson JS, Pelletier G and Forsyth P. An open-label study of the effects of bupropion SR on fatigue, depression and quality of life of mixed-site cancer patients and their partners. *Psychooncology* 2006;**15**:259–67.
29. Cullum JL, Wojciechowski AE, Pelletier G and Simpson JS. Bupropion sustained release treatment reduces fatigue in cancer patients. *Can J Psychiatry* 2004;**49**:139–44.
30. Pantilat SZ. Communicating with seriously ill patients: better words to say. *JAMA* 2009;**301**:1279–81.
31. Lamont EB and Christakis NA. Complexities in prognostication in advanced cancer: 'to help them live their lives the way they want to'. *JAMA* 2003;**290**:98–104.
32. Christakis NA and Sachs GA. The role of prognosis in clinical decision making. *J Gen Intern Med* 1996;**11**:422–5.
33. Steinhauser KE, Christakis NA, Clipp EC *et al*. Factors considered important at the end of life by patients, family, physicians and other care providers. *JAMA* 2000;**284**:2476–82.
34. Block SD. Perspectives on care at the close of life. Psychological considerations, growth and transcendence at the end of life: the art of the possible. *JAMA* 2001;**285**:2898–905.
35. Block SD. Psychological issues in end-of-life care. *J Palliat Med* 2006;**9**:751–72.
36. Stroebe M, Schut H and Stroebe W. Health outcomes of bereavement. *Lancet* 2007;**370**:1960–73.
37. Prigerson HG, Maciejewski PK, Reynolds CF III *et al*. Inventory of complicated grief: a scale to measure maladaptive symptoms of loss. *Psychiatry Res* 1995;**59**:65–79.
38. Sulmasy DP. Spiritual issues in the care of dying patients: '. . . it's okay between me and God'. *JAMA* 2006;**296**:1385–92.
39. Crawley LM, Marshall PA, Lo B and Koenig BA; End-of-Life Care Consensus Panel. Strategies for culturally effective end-of-life care. *Ann Intern Med* 2002;**136**:673–9.
40. Kagawa-Singer M and Blackhall LJ. Negotiating cross-cultural issues at the end of life: 'You got to go where he lives'. *JAMA* 2001;**286**:2993–3001.

CHAPTER 136

End-of-life care: special issues

Victoria J. Wheatley[1] and Ilora G. Finlay[2]
[1]Aberdare General Hospital, Aberdare, UK
[2]Cardiff University and Velindre Hospital, Cardiff, UK

Palliative care

The World Health Organization defines palliative care as an approach that 'improves the quality of life of patients and families who face life-threatening illness, by providing pain and symptom relief, spiritual and psychosocial support'.[1] The National Institute for Health and Clinical Excellence (NICE) states that 'patients want to be treated as individuals, with dignity and respect, and to have their voices heard in decisions about treatment and care. Should they need it, they expect to be offered optimal symptom control and psychological, social and spiritual support. They want to be assured that their families and carers will receive support during their illness'.[2]

Most healthcare professionals will at some time during their careers provide care for those who are terminally ill and dying. These professionals will already be providing personalized care with the aim of improving the quality of life of their patients, whether or not the option of life prolongation is available. Those involved in such care will acknowledge the need to relieve psychological distress in addition to physical symptoms and the benefits for the patient of providing support to informal carers. Thus, all healthcare professionals are providing palliative care – sometimes termed 'generic' palliative care – and those providing it should be able to[3]

- Assess the care needs of each patient and their families across the domains of physical, psychological, social, spiritual and information needs.
- Meet those needs within the limits of their knowledge, skills, competence in palliative care.
- Know when to seek advice from or refer to specialist palliative care services.

In addition to the generic palliative care provided by all those with patient contact, specialist palliative care is provided (in some areas of the world) by those who have undergone extensive education and training focusing on the care of patients with terminal illnesses. These specialists will often work exclusively with palliative care patients. Current UK guidance emphasizes the benefits of providing this care by working in multiprofessional teams.[2] The UK's National Council for Palliative Care recommends that 'specialist teams should include palliative medicine consultants and palliative care nurse specialists together with a range of expertise provided by physiotherapists, occupational therapists, dieticians, pharmacists, social workers and those able to give spiritual and psychological support'.[3]

The benefits of a palliative approach

About 1% of the Western population die each year and, although it can be hard to identify those patients who will die, identification of those patients likely to benefit from a palliative approach to their care can improve the experience of the patient and their family at the end of life. Such a palliative approach can help symptom control interventions take priority over those which lengthen life, and also facilitate discussions to inform advance care planning and the provision of care. This approach enables care to be tailored to the needs of the patient, the family and informal carers.

It may be possible to avoid crises and prevent hospital admissions, something that is desirable in view of the fact that studies in the UK reveal that 49–100% of patients with cancer express a wish to be cared for and to die at home,[4] but in 2008 only 26% of cancer deaths and around 20% of all deaths occurred at home.[5,6] More meaningful is the result from an audit in a hospice in England that showed for patients who had a documented preference, the place of death matched the most recently documented preferred place of care in 73%.[7]

Traditionally, cancer patients and those with acquired immune deficiency syndrome (AIDS) have had access to specialist palliative care (SPC) services, whereas those with other terminal diagnoses have tended not to be referred. This may be due, at least in part, to the fact that treatments for cancer and AIDS prolong life at the expense

Principles and Practice of Geriatric Medicine, Fifth Edition. Edited by Alan J. Sinclair, John E. Morley and Bruno Vellas.

of its quality and that hospices were often founded by cancer charities. Another factor favouring implementation of a palliative approach for cancer patients is the prompt to do so provided by the withdrawal of anticancer treatments, when prognosis may still be of the order of weeks to months. In contrast, many interventions for patients with other diagnoses, for example, heart failure and chronic obstructive pulmonary disease, prolong life while at the same time improving symptom control. These treatments are often withdrawn only very shortly before death, (precisely because they provide an element of symptom control) and their withdrawal is therefore not a useful prompt for initiation of a palliative approach.

However, patients with non-malignant terminal diseases have a significant symptom burden[8] and would often benefit from referral to SPC services. Professionals without extensive experience of using symptom control drugs such as opioids, anti-emetics and benzodiazepines are often concerned about their use, particularly about side effects and the potential for harm to the patient. One worry often cited is concern about the sedative and respiratory depressant effect of opioids, especially in frail elderly patients who are likely to have a degree of renal impairment. There is significant evidence that appropriate titration of symptom control drugs (including opioids) does not risk premature death due to sedation and respiratory compromise.[9] There is also much evidence to confirm the beneficial effects of appropriate use of these drugs in these patients, without an excessive burden from side effects.[9,10]

One of the barriers to use of a palliative approach for patients with non-malignant terminal diagnoses is the difficulty in prognosticating for this group of patients. A trajectory of gradual decline in function, punctuated by episodes of acute illness, from which the patient may recover with aggressive treatment, is typical of end-stage chronic obstructive pulmonary disease and heart failure.[11]

For some patients, families and professionals, it can be hard to understand that using a palliative approach to symptom control does not preclude aggressive interventions (including admissions) for acute decompensation. Referral to specialist palliative care teams (SPCTs) can provide a welcome opportunity for discussions about a patient's goals, with clarification of the aims of treatment. Such discussions, if undertaken sensitively and over a period of time, can assist with advance care planning (ACP). Following discussions, patients and families may be empowered to decline admissions in the event of future deteriorations, in preference for treatment in the community. In the absence of these discussions, patients and their relatives are often not aware that there are alternatives to inpatient treatment. In addition, primary care teams may not be aware of how to look after such sick patients in their own homes and may need professional support from the SPCT to show them how to organize care and give them the skills and confidence to offer it.

A third disease trajectory is often demonstrated by patients with advanced dementia and elderly patients with multiple comorbidities.[11] These patients have very low levels of functional ability and suffer from fluctuations in their condition over time. The precipitants for any deterioration may be unclear and may be potentially reversible, for example, a urinary tract infection that can be treated with oral antibiotics. This group of patients can also benefit from ACP (if this is possible) or planning for future care carried out by professionals in collaboration with relatives and informal carers. Use of such a palliative approach for these patients can inform decisions about how far to escalate treatment and give professionals insight into which proposed treatments are really likely to gain the patient any meaningful quality or length of life. These patients are extremely frail and are often cared for in nursing homes or similar facilities.

One of the questions that professionals often fail to consider when a patient's condition deteriorates is, 'Is this patient dying?' Unless this possibility is considered, many of these patients will continue to be removed from their homes and admitted to acute hospitals for their last hours and days of life.

It is therefore clear that many patients with terminal diagnoses would benefit from the use of a palliative approach by their team of healthcare professionals. These benefits include improved symptom control and greater openness about likely prognosis and the aims of medical interventions, which may inform ACP and relieve psychological distress for all involved. Additional benefits of using this approach include provision of support for relatives and informal carers, better coordination of care and tailoring care more closely to the needs of patients and their families.

To help overcome the difficulties of prognosticating for patients with diverse diagnoses, The Gold Standards Framework,[11] developed in England, proposes the use of the following three triggers to identify those patients who would benefit from a palliative approach:[11]

1 The 'surprise' question – Would you be surprised if this patient were to die in the next 6–12 months?
2 Choice/need – The patient with advanced disease makes a *choice* for comfort care only, not 'curative' treatment or is in special *need* of supportive/palliative care.
3 Clinical indicators – Specific indicators of advanced disease for each of the three main end-of-life patient groups as described above.

When to involve SPCTs

One of the questions that those caring for patients with a terminal diagnosis must consider is whether and when to refer to SPC services. Not all patients will benefit from a referral and many patients can be cared for by their usual doctors and nurses, either in the community or as inpatients. When it is clear to the patient, his relatives and informal carers and his professional carers that he is terminally ill, several factors must be considered to determine whether a referral to SPC services will be of benefit.

For some patients, even when their usual team of healthcare professionals has adopted a palliative approach, there is the potential for further improvements in care with the involvement of SPCTs. Sometimes the SPCT can access sources of care and equipment not available to others. Team members may have the luxury of more time to spend with patients and their families than non-specialists. This time is often needed for the delicate nature of discussions relating to ACP, which often develop over the course of several weeks as the patient assimilates information at their own pace. There is also the potential for relief of psychological distress and the facilitation of more open communication between the patient and their family. SPCT doctors and nurses will be much more familiar with pharmacological interventions for symptom control, will have a greater knowledge of the evidence supporting their prescribing and will be able to recommend the use of drugs in ways that minimize the risks and burdens associated with their use. Thus any terminally ill patients with multiple or severe symptoms are likely to benefit from referral to SPC services.

Referral to specialist services should also be considered if the patient's usual team of professionals is not familiar with managing the terminal phase of the disease in question (for example, the incidence of motor neurone disease in the UK is low, so only neurologists, respiratory physicians and SPCTs care for these patients regularly).

Even when professionals recognize the benefits of a palliative approach, a referral may be hindered by the patient's lack of awareness of their terminal condition and the inability of the referring team to acknowledge openly that disease control has failed. Even when patients and families are aware of this, they may block referral to the SPCT because of (incorrect) beliefs that this indicates that they are in the last weeks and days of life. In such circumstances, the professional team should try to initiate sensitive discussions about likely prognosis and the benefits that may be achieved by engagement with SPC services.

Withholding and withdrawing treatment

One of the most important roles of healthcare professionals in any setting is to make assessments of which interventions are likely to be of benefit to each patient and recognize those which are failing to provide benefit. This skill is a key duty and responsibility of healthcare professionals. When any intervention is considered for a patient, the likelihood and magnitude of benefit that the patient can expect to gain must be balanced against the magnitude and likelihood of potential harms and possible risks to the patient. It is only when greater benefits than harms are expected that it is appropriate to offer an intervention to the patient.[12] Similarly, ongoing interventions should be reassessed routinely and the balance of benefits, burdens and risks considered. For palliative care patients with progressive conditions, these may have altered so that when an intervention ceases to have a net overall benefit for the patient, it should be discontinued. For example, when palliative chemotherapy is offered to a patient with metastatic rectal carcinoma, this is done with the hope that the cancer's growth will be slowed, with consequent benefits in length and/or quality of life for the patient. If, after three cycles of chemotherapy, it becomes clear that the patient's disease is progressing despite the treatment and he or she is now suffering from significant side effects, then chemotherapy should be stopped. Such decisions to withhold or withdraw treatment are morally justifiable because they follow from judgements about beneficence and non-maleficence, and also concerns to ensure distributive justice (if resources are consumed in providing expensive, ineffective and harmful chemotherapy for one patient, they are then not available for the provision of effective treatment for another patient).

Implementing these decisions can be particularly challenging if the patient and/or their family wish to continue the ineffective intervention. Many patients (and indeed clinicians) equate ongoing active treatment with hope and fear the destruction of the patient's emotional wellbeing by its withdrawal. The emotional burden of treatment withdrawal is compounded if the patient is told 'there is nothing more that can be done' and to the clinician this sentiment confirms their failure. In fact, it would be much more accurate if clinicians explained to patients and relatives that (to paraphrase a well-known advertising slogan) 'there is nothing more that I can do, but I know a man who can'! It is at this point, when the clinician feels that there is nothing more that can be done, that SPC services should be involved. The approach of specialist palliative care services is that there is *always* something, however small, that can be done for a patient to improve their quality of life. This may involve drug treatments for symptom control or interventions that are not traditionally within the domain of healthcare, such as facilitating the patient's attendance at a family wedding. The authors argue that the cessation of some treatments (although constituting bad news for the patient) does not mean the loss of all quality of life. Instead, such a decision can provide an opportunity for the patient to revisit their priorities and make plans for the time they have left.

This is not to deny the emotional burden on healthcare professionals of making these decisions and then communicating them to patients and relatives. This emotional burden is greater when decisions are made to withdraw a treatment that has already been started than when deciding not to offer a treatment in the first place. This may be partly due to the different types of conversation needed when withdrawing a treatment as opposed to withholding it. In the latter case, the patient and relatives may not be aware of the possible treatment and in these circumstances clinicians often do not feel the need to explain that a treatment is being withheld, which of course makes for an easier dialogue from perspective of the emotional burden on the professional. In all cases where an ineffective and unduly burdensome treatment has been withdrawn or withheld, it is the patient's underlying disease that causes their death. However, this is much more apparent to observers when a treatment has never been started. In contrast, when an ineffective treatment is trialled and then withdrawn, the patient's relatives and some of the professional team may believe that death was caused by the lack of treatment. This is a particular risk when the time between treatment withdrawal and death is short, as often happens when ventilatory support is withdrawn from a ventilator-dependent patient. In such cases, conversations with relatives and between team members in advance of treatment withdrawal should focus on the fact that the particular treatment is not providing any useful benefit for the patient and that it is the underlying disease that will ultimately cause death.

The moral argument for the equivalence of withholding and withdrawing ineffective and unduly burdensome treatments has been made in the preceding paragraphs and is supported by UK law.[13] Thus there is no moral or legal pressure to favour withholding treatment over withdrawing it. This enables clinicians to make decisions in the best interests of patients and to undertake a time-limited trial of any intervention whose effectiveness for the patient in question may be in doubt.

Cardiopulmonary resuscitation (CPR)

CPR is a medical treatment which is no different to any others from an ethical perspective. However, decisions to withhold CPR have attracted much controversy over recent years and these decisions warrant further discussion.[14,15] One of the reasons for clinicians' frequent discomfort about making decisions that CPR would be an inappropriate intervention stems from confusion about the two related but distinct ethical decisions that must be made.

The first decision (as with all other medical treatments being considered for a particular patient) concerns the likelihood and magnitude of benefit that the patient can expect to gain from CPR in contrast to the certain harms and likely risks involved. The chance of CPR having any physiological benefit (the return of a pulse with accompanying cardiac output and spontaneous respiration) is markedly decreased in patients with advanced terminal disease (including cancer, end-stage organ failure and degenerative neurological disease).[16] In the unlikely event of such physiological benefit, the chances of it being sustained and the patient gaining any useful quality of life are miniscule; in one series, none of the terminally ill patients who had CPR performed survived.[17] One of the harms associated with unsuccessful CPR is prevention of a peaceful and dignified death, something that most patients and their relatives would wish for.[18] A thorough ethical analysis of these issues will include consideration of the opportunity costs associated with staff attempting to resuscitate a dying patient. We will address the issue of patient autonomy in later paragraphs.

In making a decision about the prospect of success from CPR, the clinical team is not being asked to judge whether the patient's life has value or what the patient's quality of life is. Only the patient themself can decide whether they have sufficient quality of life to warrant attempts to prolong it. If the multiprofessional team have first decided that CPR carries a realistic prospect of physiological success for a particular patient, discussion with the patient will then be required, to ascertain whether they wish to consent to attempts at CPR in the event of a cardiac arrest.[10]

Should clinicians decide that the likelihood of physiological success from CPR is so slight that it is not appropriate to offer this intervention, they must then address the thorny issue of whether and how to communicate this to the patient and their family. As mentioned above, CPR is (from a moral and legal perspective) a medical intervention like any other. Clinicians are not generally obliged to have an explicit discussion with patients about all possible interventions and why they would be ineffective for that patient. Thus there is no requirement (either legal or moral) to inform a patient that a decision not to attempt CPR (DNACPR) has been made.[19,20]

Sensitive enquiries often ascertain that patients would prefer not to receive bad news, and that at least some patients are content with the professional team making this decision without their involvement.[18] Clinical experience informs us that many patients will become unduly distressed by such a conversation. Although it may not be necessary or desirable to tell all patients that a DNACPR decision has been made, this does not remove the responsibility of professionals to attempt to ensure that the patient and their relatives are aware of the terminal nature of their diagnosis and that the focus of care is on comfort and symptom control, rather than prolongation of life. The Preferred Priorities for Care documentation[21] and (for those in the last days of life) the Liverpool Care Pathway for the Dying Patient[22] will prompt professionals to ensure that patients and their relatives understand the aims of care.

Difficulties around communication of DNACPR decisions arise when a healthcare professional is not clear themself about the stages described above for making and communication these decisions. In such circumstances, it is all too easy to initiate a discussion which appears to give the patient a choice about whether to consent to CPR.[18] These discussions are entirely appropriate when (as considered above) the clinician feels that there is the potential for the patient to benefit from CPR. However, such discussions are not appropriate if the multiprofessional team judges that attempting CPR would be inappropriate for this patient. The patient can be misled into thinking that they have a choice about this intervention and that is has a realistic chance of success and is then upset when they are told that CPR will not be attempted.[18]

One of the reasons why patients and their families may expect CPR (and be upset by a DNACPR decision) is their lack of understanding of what it can achieve. Portrayal of CPR and its success rates in popular medical television dramas show much greater rates of success than actually occur in clinical practice.[23] When patient and relatives are truly aware of the potential harms of CPR, the extremely low chance of meaningful success and understand and accept the terminal nature of their disease, they often concur with a DNACPR decision. The challenge for those clinicians who aspire to an explicit discussion about CPR with all patients is to get the patient to this stage without unnecessary distress – something that it may not be possible to achieve.[18]

Clinicians should also remember that the pathophysiology of death, whether it is expected or sudden, is that of a cardiorespiratory arrest. In inpatient settings and in the community in the UK, the default position is that CPR should be attempted in the absence of a DNACPR decision. This highlights the need for a DNACPR decision to be made and documented for all patients who are expected to die and for whom the aim of care is a peaceful and dignified death.

Artificial nutrition and hydration

Nutrition and hydration needs should be considered separately in clinical decisions. Although people can live for a time with inadequate or almost no nutrition, hydration is essential to maintain life as failing renal function and dehydration can occur rapidly. When a patient cannot swallow oral fluids, maintaining a degree of hydration can be an important comfort measure. A subcutaneous fluid infusion can be set up in almost any environment; it is very simple to administer through a subcutaneous needle in to the abdominal wall, carries a very low risk of any complications and is as effective as intravenous hydration for long-term maintenance.[24] Maintenance of hydration can be an important adjunct to good mouth care, but care must be taken to avoid fluid overload, including in those with cardiac decompensation.

Nutrition is an emotionally charged area. Families often feel an overwhelming desire to try to provide calories, in particular as food, for a person who is dying; dying patients often have no appetite or distorted taste and may have disease-related cachexia. Anorexia can be the first sign of subclinical nausea, so it is important to exclude causes of nausea, such as hypercalcaemia, renal failure and infections, particularly of the urinary tract. In the past, steroids have been advocated as a short-term expedient to stimulate appetite, but their problems are legion. Apart from only having a short-lived effect on appetite, steroids can worsen muscle wasting, precipitate gastrointestinal erosion and bleeding and often have a profoundly disturbing effect on mood.[25] Although a frank steroid psychosis is relatively rare, patients often complain of feeling emotionally labile with impaired sleep. Megestrol acetate appears to have no advantage over glucocorticoids.[26]

Any form of artificial nutrition needs very careful consideration, because in most patients it is unlikely to bring about a benefit either in survival or in quality of life. Nasogastric feeding is very uncomfortable because the tube through the nose is irritating, disfiguring and it carries a significant risk of aspiration pneumonia. Percutaneous endoscopic gastrostomy (PEG) feeding requires a tube to be placed; although this is a relatively simple procedure, it can be most disruptive in someone who is frail; 15% of patients suffer from some side effects such as diarrhoea.[27] Therefore, the patient's informed wishes and the anticipated benefits and potential harms need to be weighed carefully in someone with a short life expectancy, although in the longer term benefit is likely to be seen with PEG feeding.[28]

Care planning

Autonomy

The concept of autonomy is very important in medicine, because it protects patients from interventions to which they do not consent. Autonomy means 'self-governance'; it is our ability to govern ourselves in our daily lives. Respect for autonomy allows each person to be respected as an individual with their own thoughts, wishes, privacy and personal boundaries; it recognizes their relationships with others and the effects of their actions on others. An individual's autonomy is not limitless and should be restricted when it infringes the autonomy of another.

It is a concept that establishes equality in relationships and gives rise to all the principles that underlie consent, particularly that valid consent is informed, voluntary and that the person has the mental capacity (or competence) to make the particular decision.

In care of the elderly, this is precisely why the healthcare professional may be assaulting a person if they assume consent but have ignored the communication needs of the patient. For example, a deaf patient may need a hearing aid in place to be able to understand an explanation; for many elderly people a patient leaflet is no use if the typeface is too small or the patient does not have their reading glasses.

Much of the media refer to autonomy as if it means 'I want therefore I get'. It does not. In a patient with capacity it does mean 'you may not do things to me without my permission' – so even if a patient's refusal of treatment seems unwise but they have capacity, then their refusal stands. In the face of such a decision, the professionals' duty of care does not diminish; all care should continue without prejudice.

In those with reduced capacity, every effort should be made to maximize their capacity for autonomous decision-making before deciding that they are unable to make a decision. At the point that they are deemed to lack capacity for a particular decision, the lead clinician – usually the doctor – must take a decision in the 'best interests' of the patient as a person.

Personhood exists in the patient even in extremis and after losing many functions in life – while still alive they are no less a person even though they may be a different person to the one they were before becoming ill. Once dead, they are no longer a person and have become a corpse, so responsibly for the body falls to the person named as next of kin.

Advance care planning

ACP has recently been adopted in clinical practice as a process of discussing and recording wishes to future care and treatment. Various care planning tools have been developed, but they are no substitute for simple communication with the patient and clear documentation in the clinical record.[29]

Part of the discussion around ACP involves documenting a patient's particular wishes in addition to knowing whether the patient has an advance decision to refuse treatment. Such an advance decision, known as an advance directive in Scotland and colloquially called a living will, is legally binding in UK law provided that it is valid. This means that it must apply to the specific situation being considered, must have been drawn up at a time when the patient had the mental capacity to take such a decision, the decision must have been voluntary and adequately informed and the patient must not have acted to render the advance decision invalid.[30] Whatever is written down, the clinician must check with the patient the nature of their current wishes if the patient has capacity, as advance decisions only come into effect once the patient has lost capacity for making the decisions in question. If the clinician is in doubt over the validity of a documented advance decision and the patient lacks capacity, then the reason why the validity is in doubt must be clearly documented and decision-making reverts to the 'best interests' principle. However, clinicians are still obliged to use the advance decision to inform their best interests decision-making.[30]

Future care planning

Many palliative care patients will not have participated in advance care planning and are not able to be involved in decisions about provision of care. Reasons for this include cognitive impairment, extreme fatigue or preferences for minimal involvement in decision-making. The legal framework outlining the way in which decisions must be made for these patients varies between countries. When making decisions for those without the necessary mental capacity, clinicians must consider what factors should inform their decisions and who should participate in decision-making.

In the UK, there are specific circumstances when decision-making should be undertaken by a proxy previously nominated by the patient. These circumstances are laid out in the relevant legislation. In all other circumstances, decisions should be made by the team of healthcare professionals. In these cases, clinicians should be clear both to themselves and to others that liaison with relatives and informal carers provides valuable information about what might be in the patient's best interests. If relatives are given the (incorrect) impression that decisions about how to proceed are theirs to make, they may suffer significant distress brought about by the emotional burden of decision-making, even if a consensus between different individuals can be reached.

Legislation sets out factors that should inform decisions for patients who lack capacity. In England and Wales, a broad definition of best interests is outlined by the Mental Capacity Act 2005.[31] This encompasses much more than just physical aspects of the patient's care and includes aspects of their psychological wellbeing.

Irrespective of the way in which decisions must be reached, there are benefits for both patients and health services in attempting to make decisions about how and where a patient should be cared for in the future. This is especially true for patients who are expected to die in within weeks to months. We have already cited the example of frail nursing home patients being admitted to hospital for their last hours of life because nobody recognized that they were dying. There is a particularly strong argument to be made for what we shall call 'future care planning' for all nursing home patients. In order to need nursing home care, patients must have a significant disease burden and be sufficiently frail that they need 24 h nursing care. Many of these patients are suffering from one or more progressive conditions which will shorten their life. Many of them will also have a degree of cognitive impairment which is likely to contribute to psychological distress and confusion in the event of a change of environment. In the event of a deterioration in the condition of such a patient, the likelihood of significant gains in quality or length of life from admission to hospital are minimal and the harms and risks are substantial. All healthcare systems have finite resources, so one ought also to consider the opportunity costs of inappropriately aggressive intervention with minimal chance of gain (with other patients not receiving care from which they may have a greater chance of benefit). Hence there is a strong case for collaborative planning of future care for all nursing home residents, involving medical and nursing staff as well as family members. Decisions can be made that some interventions ought not to be considered for particular patients. This might include any investigation or treatment that required hospital admission, including CPR and ventilation. Some interventions that could be administered in the nursing home may also be deemed inappropriate in the light of an analysis of the likely benefits, burdens and risks involved, for example, artificial nutrition for a patient with advanced dementia, whereas others such as antibiotics for a urinary tract infection may remain appropriate for almost all patients.

Future care planning can also be helpful for palliative care patients in settings other than nursing homes. In places where usual care services are only available during the working week (which in the UK constitutes only 24% of the whole week), patients at home and in hospital are very likely to be reviewed by somebody unfamiliar with their case in the event of a deterioration. Without a clearly documented plan for future care (similar to those described above for nursing home patients), decisions may be made to escalate care inappropriately or to restrict care inappropriately. Although good practice with respect to thorough handover and high-quality case notes will reduce the risks of inappropriate decisions, a time of unexpected crisis is not the time for an unfamiliar nurse or doctor to attempt a complex discussion with a patient and their family about the options for care. It is highly likely that better quality decisions and therefore better outcomes will follow decisions about future care that are made by the patient's usual healthcare team and are subject to regular review.

Terminal care

In earlier parts of this chapter, we have considered patients with terminal diagnoses and prognoses of weeks to months. For many terminally ill patients, there is a period of hours to days when it is clear that they are actually dying – the terminal phase. Not all patients have a recognizable terminal phase; instead, some will die very suddenly, for example following a massive pulmonary embolus or terminal haemorrhage. For those patients who have entered the terminal phase, provision of high-quality evidence-based care can be facilitated by using the approach set out in the Liverpool Care Pathway for the Dying Patient (LCP) (or other similar documentation).[22] Care pathways such as these prompt professionals to review the patient's care thoroughly, to continue or initiate parenteral routes for administration of symptom control drugs, to prescribe in anticipation of the development of likely symptoms and ensure the drugs are available, to discontinue ineffective and burdensome interventions and to address relatives' needs for information and support. Use of the LCP and other similar pathways has been shown to improve symptom control for patients in the terminal phase,[32] improve the quality of communication between professionals and relatives[33] and improve nurses' confidence in caring for the dying.[32]

One of the key factors in ensuring that patients benefit from the use of such a pathway is that an informed and considered decision is made before using it to guide care. As is suggested by the name, use of the Liverpool Care Pathway for the Dying Patient only provides prompts to high-quality care for patients who are actually dying. It is imperative that healthcare teams consider and address (as appropriate) any reversible causes for a patient's deterioration before using the care pathway as a tool to guide care.

It is worth noting that the condition of some patients actually improves when their care is guided by an end-of-life care pathway.[32] If it becomes evident that the patient is no longer dying, use of the care pathway should be discontinued and review of the situation may highlight the need to commence (or recommence) additional interventions. One of the reasons why patients may improve in these circumstances is the cessation of medications not strictly necessary for symptom control; in retrospect, it may be clear that such medications were the cause of a patient's deterioration, rather than the underlying disease process.

Terminal sedation

Sedation at the end of life should rarely be necessary. There are a few situations where sedation to decrease conscious levels may be required as a way of controlling difficult symptoms, such as when a patient is exhausted with complex pain or profoundly distressed following a neurological insult. The use of sedation in this way requires patient consent as it is a therapeutic intervention. In the event of the patient lacking capacity, a short period of sedation, for example to control difficult delirium, may be deemed to be in the patient's best interests; such a decision should only be taken with the agreement of the person legally appointed by the patient to have power of attorney for health and welfare decisions or, failing that, following consultation with the patient's preferred proxy decision-maker and other interested parties. Clinicians should consider and review the likely benefits, burdens and risks of ongoing parenteral hydration and enteral nutrition for patients who require sedation for the relief of intractable symptoms.

Sedation with short-acting agents, such as midazolam, can be achieved by carefully titrating up the dose in increments to achieve the desired therapeutic effect. Regular review is essential, so that the dose can be lowered again at the time agreed and the clinical situation reviewed.

In the last days and hours of life, patients may become restless and appear anxious. Small anxiolytic doses of a short-acting benzodiazepine can be helpful to relieve distress, but it is not necessary deliberately to render the patient deeply unconscious. This principle is set out in end-of-life care pathway documentation, such as the LCP.[22]

A protocol for 'terminal sedation' has been devised in The Netherlands and is used as a way to achieve deep sedation which is maintained until death occurs.[34] In this approach, higher doses of sedative drug are given by continuous infusion and nutrition and hydration withheld. It has been suggested that this approach is linked to euthanasia, without incurring the administrative framework for euthanasia required in The Netherlands.

It is possible to achieve clarity about the difference between palliative sedation and deliberate attempts to end the patient's life by considering the following factors. The aim of palliative sedation is to relieve intractable symptoms; this is achieved by careful titration of sedative medications according to their effect on the patient's symptoms and the patient's death occurs as a result of their underlying disease process. In contrast, administration of sedative and other drugs to render a patient deeply unconscious, without titration according to effect and without considering the possibility of ongoing artificial nutrition and hydration appears to be undertaken with the aim of shortening life and may well have this effect.[35]

Assisted dying

Assisted dying is the euphemistic term widely used to cover assisted suicide and euthanasia. There has been extensive debate about 'assisted dying' in many countries in the world, but at the time of writing, Belgium and Luxembourg have legalized euthanasia, Oregon and Washington states in the USA have legalized assisted suicide and The Netherlands has legalized both.

Assisted suicide is where a person supplies the means to help another take their own life; it may involve the prescription of a lethal dose of a drug (physician-assisted suicide) or may involve the supply of other lethal means by someone who is not associated with healthcare (assisted suicide). Euthanasia is the deliberate giving of a lethal drug to bring about a patient's death as rapidly as possible; in the context of this section, the term euthanasia is used as applying to voluntary euthanasia only.

Arguments in favour of assisted suicide/euthanasia revolve around patient autonomy, existential distress and a sense of futility at enduring the course of a final illness. Arguments against assisted suicide/euthanasia focus on public safety, namely the danger to vulnerable patients of coercion, the inability of safeguards to be watertight and the principles around respect for life.[36]

As with any form of consent to an intervention, proposed safeguards around an application for assisted dying require the patient to be fully informed, making a decision of their own free will and with the mental capacity appropriate to the decision being taken. Difficulties with accurate information arise because diagnosis is an imprecise art; a significant proportion of antemortem diagnoses are shown to be inaccurate at postmortem,[36] so patients who believe their life expectancy to be short or with a catastrophic course may be very wrong. Mental capacity must be intact to take such a momentous decision (that of ending one's own life); it is of note that in an in-depth study of 18 patients receiving a prescription for lethal drugs under the Oregon Death with Dignity Act, three were found to have an unrecognized and untreated depression.[37] Detection of coercion is difficult, particularly when internal coercion (feeling a duty to die) rather than external coercion is present.[36]

The UK Director of Public Prosecutions has indicated that any physician or other healthcare worker is particularly likely to be prosecuted for assisting suicide. His guidance on prosecution for assisting suicide also states that underlying disease or disability of the victim is not a mitigating circumstance when considering whether a person assisting a suicide should be prosecuted.[38] Indeed, the law gives a message about how we behave – it gives a clear and strong message that the routinization of assisted suicide (death by appointment) is not condoned. However, in the event of a person assisting the suicide of another in extremis purely out of compassion, the law will be interpreted with compassion too. The medicalization of assisted suicide is particularly dangerous, as recognized in the Director of Public Prosecutions' guidance, and our suicide prevention strategies in society hold good whatever the age or infirmity the patient may be. The importance of all efforts, however small, being made to improve quality of life is no less important when individuals are incurably ill and dying.

When a patient expresses a wish is for assisted suicide or euthanasia, it is important that the clinician considers what the real question is that the patient is asking. Does the patient have a confirmed wish to die or are they asking whether their life is worth carrying on with? The way in which the clinician responds will have an enormous influence on the way in which the patient perceives the future and any hope for quality of life. It is important to remember that many elderly patients dying today have witnessed poor deaths, often without the benefit of any palliative care intervention at all. Up until about 20 years ago, morphine was rarely used with dying patients, through a mistaken belief that morphine would hasten death. The result was that many patients were left with unrelieved pain and distress – a situation witnessed and living on in the memory of those who were bereaved. These experiences will inevitably colour the perception of death and dying of the elderly person who is now the patient.

Bereavement

The process of grief begins from the time that someone's health is deteriorating. For many elderly couples who have lived together for many years, this also marks the beginning of a very painful parting. For the relative who is not dying, the loss of a lifelong partner is equivalent to part of their own personal dying.

The way in which people adapt in grief is influenced by their experience of being bereaved. It is very important that relatives are aware of what is happening, are encouraged to be involved in care and that their concerns are listened to. Even when frail and elderly, they may want to be at the bedside of the person they love; it does them a great disservice to deny them the ability to be present.

There are some factors which are warning signals for complicated grief, suggesting that the bereaved person will find it particularly difficult to adapt to the situation after the death of the person they love. Risk factors include sudden unexpected death, traumatic death, loss of a child and loss of a partner with whom the relationship had been ambivalent ('can't live with, can't live without').[39] Depression is common in the bereaved and associated with the period of increased mortality.[39]

For many children, a grandparent is the most secure adult in their life as social disintegration and mobility may leave the child very dependent on the grandparent. It has been estimated that on average across the UK, in every school class there are approximately two children bereaved of a person close to them such as a grandparent and one child bereaved of a parent or sibling.[40]

Thus the way in which we provide care of the dying patient and their family will influence the next generation's ability to cope with illness and death.

Conclusion

Provision of high-quality care for those nearing the end of life is one of the hallmarks of a civilized society. The way in which we care for the most vulnerable, the way in which we value the individual and work to help them achieve their last goals in life, reflect on us as professionals. The absolute finality of death should never be taken lightly and the importance of care for those left behind is also crucial. The way in which we live and the way in which we die affect all around us and live on in the memory of others for a lifetime.

Key points

- Palliative care improves experiences of persons with terminal illnesses.
- Patients and families should be involved in end-of-life decisions.
- Assisted dying remains a controversial issue.
- There is increased awareness that end-of-life care is appropriate for patients other than those with cancer, for example, patients with heart failure and dementia.

References

1. World Health Organization. *Palliative Care*, http://www.who.int/cancer/palliative/en/ (last accessed 6 June 2010).
2. National Institute for Health and Clinical Excellence. *Guidance on Improving Supportive and Palliative Care for Adults with Cancer*, NICE, London, 2004.
3. National Council for Palliative Care. *Palliative Care Explained*, http://www.ncpc.org.uk/palliative_care.html (last accessed 25 April 2010).
4. Higginson IJ and Sen-Gupta GJ. Place of care in advanced cancer: a qualitative systematic literature review of patient preferences. *J Palliat Med* 2000;**3**:287–300.
5. Office for National Statistics. *Deaths, Place of Occurrence and Sex by Underlying Cause and Age Group, 2008*, http://www.statistics.gov.uk/downloads/theme_health/DR2008/Table12.xls (last accessed 3 May 2010).
6. National Council for Palliative Care. *Changing Gear: Guidelines for Managing the Last Days of Life in Adults*. National Council for Palliative Care, London, 2006.
7. Dorman S. *Auditing Preferred Place of Care – What Are the Benefits and Limitations?*, 2009, http://www.dorothyhouse.co.uk/uploads/downloads/conference/sd_pref_place.pdf, (last accessed 6 June 2010).
8. Addington-Hall J, Fakhoury W and McCarthy M. Specialist palliative care in non-malignant disease. *Palliat Med* 1998;**12**:417–27.
9. Seamark DA, Seamark CJ and Halpin DMG. Palliative care in chronic obstructive pulmonary disease: a review for clinicians. *J R Soc Med* 2007;**100**:225–33.
10. Evans LAM. Cancer isn't the only malignant disease. Competent, compassionate terminal care should be given to everyone. *BMJ* 2002;**324**:1035.
11. The Gold Standards Framework. *Prognostic Indicator Guidance*, http://www.goldstandardsframework.nhs.uk/Resources/Gold%20Standards%20Framework/PIG%20Paper%20v33%20Sept%2008.pdf (last accessed 6 June 2010).
12. Randall F and Downie RS. Choice and best interests: clinical decision-making in end of life care. In: F Randall and RS Downie, *End of Life Choices: Consensus and Controversy*, Oxford University Press, Oxford, 2010, pp. 25–7.
13. British Medical Association. *Withholding and Withdrawing Life – Prolonging Medical Treatment. Guidance for Decision Making*, 3rd edn, Blackwell Publishing, Oxford, 2007, pp. 19–20.
14. NHS Executive. *Resuscitation Policy HSC 2000/028*, Department of Health, London, 2000.

15. Manisty C, Waxman J and Higginson IJ. Doctors should not discuss resuscitation with terminally ill patients. *BMJ* 2003;**327**:614–6.
16. Goodlin SJ, Zhong Z, Lynn J *et al*. Factors associated with use of cardiopulmonary resuscitation in seriously ill hospitalized adults. *JAMA* 1999;**282**:2333–9.
17. Ewer MS, Kish SK, Martin CG *et al*. Characteristics of cardiac arrest in cancer patients as a predictor of survival after cardiopulmonary resuscitation. *Cancer* 2001;**92**:1905–12.
18. Willard C. Cardiopulmonary resuscitation for palliative care patients: a discussion of ethical issues. *Palliat Med* 2000;**14**:308–12.
19. Ginn D and Zitner D. Cardiopulmonary resuscitation. Not for all terminally ill patients. *Can Fam Physician* 1995;**41**: 649–52, 655–7.
20. National Council for Hospice and Specialist Palliative Care Services and Association for Palliative Medicine of Great Britain and Ireland. *Ethical Decision Making in Palliative Care: Cardiopulmonary Resuscitation (CPR) for People Who Are Terminally Ill*. National Council for Hospice and Specialist Palliative Care Services, London, 2002.
21. NHS National End of Life Care Programme. *Preferred Priorities for Care (PPC)*, http://www.endoflifecare.nhs.uk/eolc/ppc.htm (last accessed 6 June 2010).
22. The Marie Curie Palliative Care Institute, Liverpool. *Liverpool Care Pathway for the Dying Patient*, http://www.mcpcil.org.uk/liverpool-care-pathway/ (last accessed 25 April 2010).
23. Diem SJ, Lantos JD and Tulsky JA. Cardiopulmonary resuscitation on television – miracles and misinformation. *N Engl J Med* 1996;**334**:1578–82.
24. Lipschitz S, Campbell AJ, Roberts MS *et al*. Subcutaneous fluid administration in elderly subjects: validation of an under-used technique. *J Am Geriatr Soc* 1991;**39**:6–9.
25. Palliativedrugs.com. *Systemic Corticosteroids*, http://www.palliativedrugs.com/systemic-corticosteroids.html (last accessed 19 June 2010).
26. Leśniak W, Bała M, Jaeschke R *et al*. Effects of megestrol acetate in patients with cancer anorexia–cachexia syndrome – a systematic review and meta-analysis. *Pol Arch Med Wewn* 2008;**118**:636–44.
27. Schoenemann J and Rosée D. Percutaneous endoscopic enterostomy. Advantages and risks. *Med Klin (Munich)* 1996;**91**:753–7.
28. Erdil A, Saka M, Ates Y *et al*. Enteral nutrition via percutaneous endoscopic gastrostomy and nutritional status of patients: five-year prospective study. *J Gastroenterol Hepatol* 2005;**20**:1002–7.
29. Froggatt K, Vaughan S, Bernard C *et al*. Advance care planning in care homes for older people: an English perspective. *Palliat Med* 2009;**23**:332–8.
30. Department for Constitutional Affairs. *Mental Capacity Act 2005 Code of Practice*, The Stationery Office, London, 2007, pp. 158–77, http://www.dca.gov.uk/legal-policy/mental-capacity/mca-cp.pdf (last accessed 19 June 2010).
31. Department for Constitutional Affairs. *Mental Capacity Act 2005 Code of Practice*, The Stationery Office, London, 2007, pp. 64–91, http://www.dca.gov.uk/legal-policy/mental-capacity/mca-cp.pdf (last accessed 19 June 2010).
32. Edmonds P, Burman R and Prentice W. End of life care in the acute hospital setting. *BMJ* 2009;**339**:b5048.
33. Johnstone R, Jones A and Fowell A. *The All-Wales Integrated Care Pathway (ICP) for the Last Days of Life: In-Depth Audit 2009*. Betsi Cadwaladr University Health Board, Bangor, 2010.
34. Rietjens JAC, Buiting HM, Pasman HRW *et al*. Deciding about continuous deep sedation: physicians' perspectives: a focus group study. *Palliat Med* 2009;**23**:410–7.
35. Randall F and Downie RS. Choice and best interests: sedation to relieve otherwise intractable symptoms (terminal sedation). In: F Randall and RS Downie, *End of Life Choices: Consensus and Controversy*, Oxford University Press, Oxford, 2010, pp. 99–112.
36. Finlay IG, Wheatley VJ and Izdebski C. The House of Lords Select Committee on the Assisted Dying for the Terminally Ill Bill: implications for specialist palliative care. *Palliat Med* 2005;**19**:444–53.
37. Ganzini L, Goy ER and Dobscha SK. Prevalence of depression and anxiety in patients requesting physicians' aid in dying: cross sectional survey. *BMJ* 2008;**337**:a1682.
38. Crown Prosecution Service. *Policy for Prosecutors in Respect of Cases of Encouraging or Assisting Suicide*, 2010, http://www.cps.gov.uk/publications/prosecution/assisted_suicide_policy.html (last accessed 6 June 2010).
39. Parkes CM. Coping with loss. Bereavement in adult life *BMJ* 1998;**316**:856–9.
40. Green H, McGinnity A, Meltzer H *et al*. *Mental Health of Children and Young People in Great Britain*, Palgrave Macmillan, London, 2004.

PART 3

Global Healthcare Systems

CHAPTER 137

Improving quality of care

Julie K. Gammack and Carolyn D. Philpot
Saint Louis University Health Sciences Center, and GRECC, St Louis VA Medical Center St Louis MO, USA

Introduction

Throughout most of history, medical care was delivered to an individual patient by an individual clinician. Public health services were rarely available and infection control practices were poorly understood. Institutional care was uncommon and reserved for those with means to afford the medical services. Over the last century, medical care has drastically changed through the development of antibiotics, immunizations, and new surgical techniques. The world's population is now growing rapidly, is ageing, and is requiring more health services. Population-based medicine has become a priority as cost, volume and efficiency became critical issues in meeting the growing healthcare demands of the medical consumer.

From provision of services to meeting standards of practice, the healthcare industry is under increasing pressure to provide the highest level of services to the greatest number of recipients. In an era of limited healthcare dollars, practitioners often must do more with less, yet medical advances and fear of litigation drive the cost of care upward. For these reasons, efficient, high-quality care is of increasing importance. Consumer groups, medical societies and healthcare organizations have been at the forefront in promoting quality in healthcare. With a collective voice, these groups have promoted change in the healthcare system. Although slower than many other industries, the healthcare establishment has recognized the importance of delivering quality goods and services.

With the advent of computers, the growth of the pharmaceutical industry, and advances in diagnostic technologies, the level of medical sophistication has risen dramatically. Clinicians and patients are now afforded a multitude of therapeutic options unavailable only a few years before. As with other industries, however, quantity of services does not automatically equate to quality of services. It is necessary to critically evaluate not only medical treatments and techniques but also the process by which medicine is delivered to the healthcare consumer. Defining quality, measuring performance and changing ineffective practices must now become routine activities as medicine moves toward more efficient and effective methods of healthcare delivery.

The history of quality

The history of quality in business

In 1906, the International Electrotechnical Commission (IEC) was established to provide uniformity to the electrotechnical field. (See Appendix 137.1 for organizational abbreviations.) The IEC promoted quality, safety, performance, reproducibility and environmental compatibility of materials and products. This was the first organization to develop international standards of business practice.

The International Federation of the National Standardizing Association (ISA) was another organization, focused on mechanical engineering, which set standards for industry and trade from 1926–1942. After ISA dissolved, a delegation of 25 countries convened to create a new organization to unify the standards of industry and production practices. In 1947 this organization, the International Organization for Standardization (ISO), was established in the United Kingdom to oversee the manufacturing and engineering trades.

The ISO is a federation of non-governmental agencies with membership from 163 countries across the world.[1] The ISO has developed international standards by which trade, technology and scientific activities can be measured. Companies may choose to be certified by the ISO-9000 quality management system. This certification ensures a minimum standard by which business processes, quality management and safety are maintained.[1] ISO certification is especially important for international and intercontinental business to ensure a uniform delivery of goods and services. The healthcare industry is one of many fields that may be evaluated in the ISO method. At this time ISO has developed 187 work item standards under the technical sector of health, safety and environmental.[2] Although used in some

Principles and Practice of Geriatric Medicine, Fifth Edition. Edited by Alan J. Sinclair, John E. Morley and Bruno Vellas.

countries to evaluate medical practices, it is not the widely accepted model for evaluation of the healthcare system.

Around the same time that ISO was created, Dr W. Edwards Deming, a physicist and statistician from the United States, developed a new process for quality improvement in business. Through this process, all members of a work unit were responsible for continuous monitoring and improvement of products along all steps of production. High frequency errors were identified, corrected, and the resulting outcome monitored for improved quality. Any step in the production process could and would be a continuous target for revision. In this method, focus was shifted from the specific error of an individual to the systemic faults that allowed an error to go unnoticed or proceed uncorrected. The workforce was thus empowered to identify problems and institute a plan of correction. Deming introduced this process which is now known as Continuous Quality Improvement (CQI) and also referred to as Total Quality Management (TQM), Quality Assurance (QA) or Performance Improvement (PI). Used in Japan, TQM quickly led to a revolution in the efficient manufacturing of high-quality goods.

Deming knew that successful management of a complex process or problem required the focused attention of a team of individuals. Although each member was uniquely skilled in a task, the team worked together in developing solutions. The TQM process is well suited for quality improvement in the complex healthcare environment, but has not historically been embraced by the medical establishment. The narrow view that blame for errors be placed on a sole individual and that physicians be allowed autonomous control over medical processes has hindered the acceptance of TQM. This view is changing as organizations realize that medical errors and inefficiencies are usually the result of systemic problems that require multifactorial solutions.

The evolution of quality in healthcare

One of the first efforts to standardize medical delivery occurred in 1917 with the 'Minimum Standard for Hospitals' programme set forth by Drs Franklin Martin and John Bowman of the American College of Surgeons (ACS). A one-page, five-point set of criteria was crafted to assess the quality of hospitals[3] (see Table 137.1). In 1918, only 89 of 692 hospitals surveyed met the minimum criteria.

Table 137.1 The Minimum Standard.

'The Minimum Standard' American College of Surgeons 1917
1 That physicians and surgeons privileged to practice in the hospital be organized as a definite group or staff.
2 That membership upon the staff be restricted to physicians and surgeons who are
a full graduates of medicine in good standing and legally licensed to practice
b competent in their respective fields
c worthy in character and in matters of professional ethics
3 That the staff initiate and, with the approval of the governing board of the hospital, adopt rules, regulations, and policies governing the professional work of the hospital.
4 That accurate and complete records be written for all patients and filed in an accessible manner in the hospital.
5 That diagnostic and therapeutic facilities under competent supervision be available for the study, diagnosis, and treatment of patients.

The ACS was responsible for hospital accreditation until 1952 when the Joint Commission on Accreditation of Hospitals (JCAH) was established to take on this responsibility. Led initially by Dr Arthur W. Allen, the JCAH published standards for hospital accreditation in 1953. The JCAH initiatives were also incorporated outside of the United States with Canada offering its own accreditation through the Canadian Commission on Hospital Accreditation in that same year. Over the next two decades, the JCAH grew to include the review of long-term care facilities in 1966 and subsequently mental health, dental, ambulatory care and laboratory facilities. In 1987 JCAH was renamed the Joint Commission on Accreditation of Healthcare Organizations (JCAHO) to encompass the variety of services and activities offered.[4] The organization was rebranded in 2007 and is now generally referred to as 'The Joint Commission'.

The Joint Commission has been a world leader in healthcare accreditation and a prototype for further development of organizations that monitor and measure the quality of healthcare delivery. Over the past two decades the interest and efforts in healthcare quality have grown exponentially. A variety of national and international organizations have evolved to assist the healthcare industry in meeting new consumer and regulatory demands for high-quality services and programmes.

Organizations leading healthcare quality improvement

In the United States, the Agency for Healthcare Research and Quality (AHRQ), previously the Agency for Healthcare Policy and Research (AHCRP), is a leader in healthcare quality initiatives. Founded in 1989, this agency of the US Department of Health and Human Services has a mission to improve the healthcare quality, safety, efficiency and effectiveness for all Americans. AHRQ awards millions of dollars in grants to further evidence-based, outcomes research related to healthcare quality improvement. Federal legislation authorizes AHRQ to coordinate health partnerships, support research, and advance information and technology systems. Of the many projects that are overseen by AHRQ, the United States Preventive Services

Task Force (USPSTP) and Consumer Assessment of Health Plans (CAHPS) are most prominent. The AHRQ also publishes data on quality and trends in healthcare effectiveness and patient safety. For the past seven years, AHRQ has produced the National Healthcare Quality Report and the National Healthcare Disparities Report.[5]

The USPSTF is a 15-member, private-sector panel of experts, first convened by the United States Public Health Service in 1984 to develop and assess evidence-based preventive service measures. The hallmark publication of this taskforce titled *Guide to Clinical Preventive Services* was published in 1989, with a second edition released in 1996 and third edition in 2002.[6] Although clinicians and healthcare societies do not always agree upon the details, these guidelines are frequently cited as 'best evidence' and considered to represent the 'standard of care' in preventive medicine services. This agency has developed recommendations for adults and children in the clinical areas of: Cancer, Heart and Vascular Diseases, Injury and Violence, Infectious Diseases, Mental Health Conditions and Substance Abuse, Metabolic, Nutritional and Endocrine Conditions, Musculoskeletal Disorders, Obstetric and Gynaecological Conditions, Vision and Hearing Disorders, and Miscellaneous conditions.

CAHPS is an organizational databank of healthcare information used by consumers, employers and health plans in evaluating heath care systems and services. Surveys and reporting instruments are used to collect and present information on healthcare providers such as Medicare and the Federal Employees Health Benefits Program. In the private sector, the National Committee for Quality Assurance (NCQA) reviews the quality of managed care health plans. Established in 1990, this non-profit group also accredits the healthcare organizations.

NCQA uses the Healthcare Effectiveness Data and Information Set (HEDIS) tool to measure and report the performance of health plans and physician practices. More than 90% of US health plans use the HEDIS system which consists of 71 measures and 8 care domains. Such measures could include lead screening in children, blood pressure control and smoking cessation counselling.[7]

The Institute of Medicine (IOM) is another leader in the development of quality healthcare in America. This non-profit organization was chartered in 1970 as a segment of the National Academy of Sciences. The mission of the IOM is to work outside the governmental framework in providing an independent, scientifically based analysis of the healthcare system. 'Quality of Care' was defined by the IOM in 1990 as, 'the degree to which health services for individuals and populations increase the likelihood of desired health outcomes and are consistent with current professional knowledge'.[8]

IOM formally launched the first of three phases of a quality initiative plan, beginning in 1996 with an intensive review of the state of healthcare in America. In a statement declaring 'The urgent need to Improve Health Care Quality', the IOM began focusing on overuse, underuse and misuse in medical care. During Phase Two, the Quality of Health Care in America Committee convened and has since published several reports, including *To Err is Human: Building a Safer Health System*, and *Crossing the Quality Chasm: A New Health System for the 21st Century*. The most recent IOM quality improvement publications have focused on patient safety and performance measures. These titles include: *Rewarding Provider Performance: Aligning Incentives in Medicare; Preventing Medication Errors: Quality Chasm Series;* and *Performance Measurement: Accelerating Improvement*.[9]

The IOM has lobbied for an error reporting system and legislation to protect those who report errors in an effort to promote quality improvement strategies. Twenty 'Priority Areas for National Action' have been established based on diseases or conditions that may be best managed using clinical practice guidelines (see Table 137.2). The IOM has established six 'Aims for Improvement' in health system function. Healthcare should be: (1) safe, (2) effective, (3) patient-centred, (4) timely, (5) efficient, and (6) equitable. The Committee has also identified '10 simple rules for [healthcare system] redesign' which change the focus of healthcare from provider driven to consumer/system driven care (see Table 137.3).

Table 137.2 Health priority areas.

20 priority areas for improvement in healthcare quality
• Care coordination
• Self-management/health literacy
• Asthma
• Cancer – focus on colorectal and cervical cancer
• Children with special healthcare needs
• Diabetes – focus early disease management
• End of life with advanced organ system failure
• Frailty associated with old age
• Hypertension – focus on early disease management
• Immunization – children and adults
• Ischaemic heart disease
• Major depression – screening and treatment
• Medication management – preventing medication errors and antibiotic overuse
• Nosocomial infections – prevention and surveillance
• Pain control in advanced cancer
• Pregnancy and childbirth – appropriate prenatal and intrapartum care
• Severe and persistent mental illness – focus on treatment in the public sector
• Stroke – early intervention and rehabilitation
• Tobacco dependence treatment in adults
• Obesity

Table 137.3 Rules for health system redesign.

Ten rules for health system redesign
1 Care is based on continuous healing relationships.
2 Care is customized according to patient needs and values.
3 The patient is the source of control.
4 Knowledge is shared and information flows freely.
5 Decision making is evidence based.
6 Safety is a system property.
7 Transparency is necessary.
8 Needs are anticipated.
9 Waste is continuously decreased.
10 Cooperation among clinicians is a priority.

In the United Kingdom, healthcare is provided nationally through a national healthcare service programme within each country. In England, the National Health Service (NHS) has received annual reviews since the Commission for Health Improvement (CHI) was established in 1999 by the national government. In April 2004 this organization was replaced by the Healthcare Commission (HC), which was charged with the task of reviewing and improving the quality of healthcare in the NHS and in the private sector. In April, 2009 the Healthcare Commission merged with the Mental Health Act Commission and the Commission for Social Health Inspection to become the Care Quality Commission (CQC). The CQC collects data on quality of healthcare services that are delivered on a local and national level. This data is available for public inspection. On 1 October 2010, legislation established five essential standards of quality and safety that are required for all agencies that provide health services.[10] These standards are as follows:

1 the recipient is informed and involved at all times
2 care and treatment will meet individual needs
3 the recipient will be protected from harm and provided safe care
4 care is provided by qualified individuals
5 care providers will be involved in quality improvement.

This legislation moves the NHS quality assurance process from an inspection-reporting process to a continuous quality improvement process.

Other countries in the United Kingdom have their own regulatory agencies and standards for healthcare services. In Scotland, the Regulation of Care (Scotland) Act 2001 established the Scottish Commission for the Regulation of Care (SCRC) based on a set of National Care Standards. The standards define the expected quality of service that is provided and allows for regulatory reports to be generated for health service agencies. In 2004, the Healthcare Inspectorate Wales (HIW) was established to review the quality and safety of all healthcare provided in this country. In Northern Ireland, the Regulation and Quality Improvement Authority (RQIA) monitors and inspects the Health & Social Care Services in Northern Ireland. This agency was established in 2003.

In Australia, evaluation and accreditation of medical practice takes place through the Australian Council on Healthcare Standards (ACHS) and its subsidiary the Australian Council on Healthcare Standards International (ACHSI). The ACHSI uses Australian standards and modifies these to be culturally and internationally appropriate. ACHSI then works in partnership with healthcare accreditation bodies in Ireland, India, New Zealand, Bahrain and Hong Kong through exchange surveyor programmes.

Established in 1974, ACHS is an independent body comprised of healthcare leaders, governmental representatives and consumers. ACHS accredits programmes using a standardized model called the Evaluation and Quality Improvement Program (EQuIP). EQuIP sets standards in two broad categories: (1) patient care services across the continuum of care, and (2) the healthcare infrastructure. EQuIP standards are revised every four years. On 1 July 2011 the version EQuIP5 will be implemented.

ACHS also provides comparative information on the processes and outcomes of healthcare through the Clinical Indicator Programme. Using 23 Clinical Indicator Sets with over 350 Clinical Indicators, data submitted from a healthcare organization can be quantitatively measured and objectively compared with other organizations and with national aggregate data. Outlying data generates a 'flag', which can alert the organization to quality control problems.[11]

In 2006 the Australian Commission on Safety and Quality in Health Care (ACSQHC) was established to develop a national framework for improving safety and quality across Australia.[12] This commission is charged with:

- identifying priority healthcare issues and setting policy directions
- disseminating knowledge and advocating for heath safety and quality
- public reporting of health safety and quality data
- coordinating and developing national health and safety data bases
- advising Health Ministers
- recommending national safety and quality standards.

Australia is also the original host country of The International Society for Quality in Health Care (ISQua), which moved to Ireland in 2008. This non-profit organization 'Accredits the Accreditors' and provides services and information on healthcare quality to medical providers and consumers. Over 50 healthcare organizations, standards and surveyor programmes are accredited through ISQua.[13] ISQua hosts an annual international summit to discuss performance indicators and promote a multidisciplinary approach to quality improvement programmes. Participants include health policy leaders, researchers, healthcare professionals and consumer organizations. The ISQua also supports the *International Journal for Quality in Health Care*, a peer-reviewed journal in its 22nd year of publication.

Models for evaluating quality

The approach to quality in healthcare bears many similarities to quality improvement in the commercial sector by focusing on key issues of safety, effectiveness, consumer satisfaction, timely results and efficiency. Within Europe, there is much diversity in the oversight and governmental mandates for quality of healthcare practice. Most legislation surrounds the health system and hospital accreditation process, with less emphasis placed on individual clinical practices. Based on the established healthcare and payer system, each country may address quality control quite differently.

To better understand the most common methods of measuring healthcare quality, a survey of European External Peer Review Techniques (ExPeRT) was initiated.[14] The results of this ExPeRT Project, revealed four commonly used quality improvement models: healthcare system accreditation, ISO certification (both discussed previously in this chapter), the European Foundation for Quality Management (EFQM) Excellence Model, and the Visitatie peer review method.

The EFQM is a global non-for-profit foundation founded in 1988 by presidents of leading European companies and which uses the 'EFQM Excellence Model' for assessing the quality of an organization. The framework for this TQM approach includes nine criteria by which an organization is evaluated on 'what it does' and 'what it achieves'. A Quality Award is presented after a process of self-assessment and internal review. Members within the EFQM foundation learn from each other and share best practices for improving the quality of service provided to the consumer.[15]

The Visitatie model originated in the Netherlands and focuses on medical practice specifically, rather than on business practices broadly. Visitatie is a peer review consultation process that uses practice and practitioner-derived guidelines to evaluate patient care. Emphasis is placed on individual and team performance, not organizational structure or outcomes. Unlike other methods, Visitatie does not result in a certification or accreditation award. Because the focus is on improving care through peer feedback, there is no 'pass/fail' or punitive outcome. This model is becoming popular across Europe as a method for personal and peer review of medical care. Groups who have used this consultation approach to practice management reported more success and fewer barriers when implementing quality improvement changes in practice.[16]

Quality improvement in geriatrics

The elderly population is prone to adverse outcomes, especially when healthcare delivery is fragmented. Research has demonstrated that adverse health events are more likely to occur in the elderly population and that the risk of adverse hospital events is twice as high for individuals over age 65.[17,18] Preventive medicine for seniors includes identifying patient safety issues that can lead to functional decline and poor health outcomes. Identifying risk factors for decline and providing early intervention is effectively approached though a healthcare team-based TQM process.

Quality in healthcare has evolved from a reactive Quality Assurance (QA) model (see Figure 137.1), to a proactive TQM model (see Figure 137.2). Instead of focusing on compliance and adherence to external regulations or standards (QA model), TQM focuses on the continuous process of improving care relative to current internal practices. TQM involves not only change in practices on an individual level, but also change in process on a larger scale that can benefit a broader population.

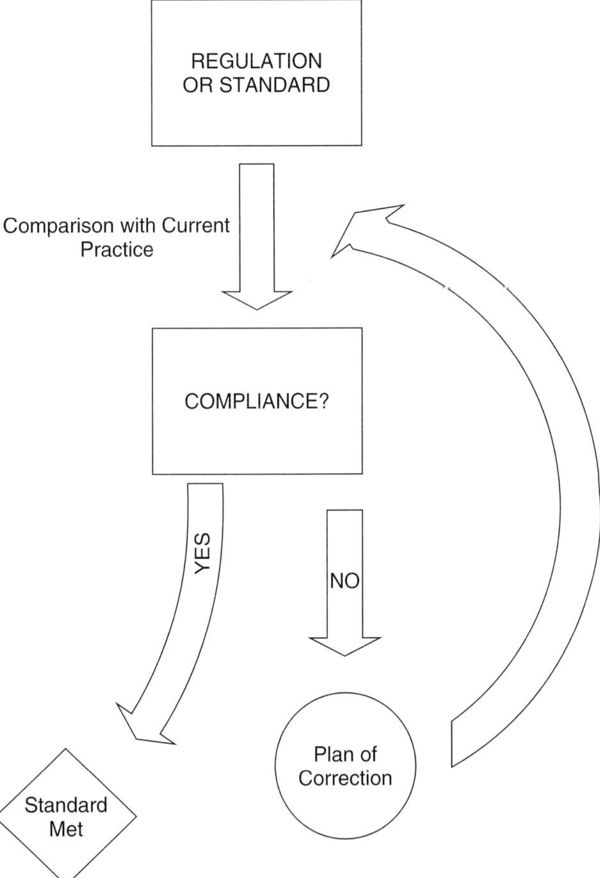

Figure 137.1 Quality Assurance Model.

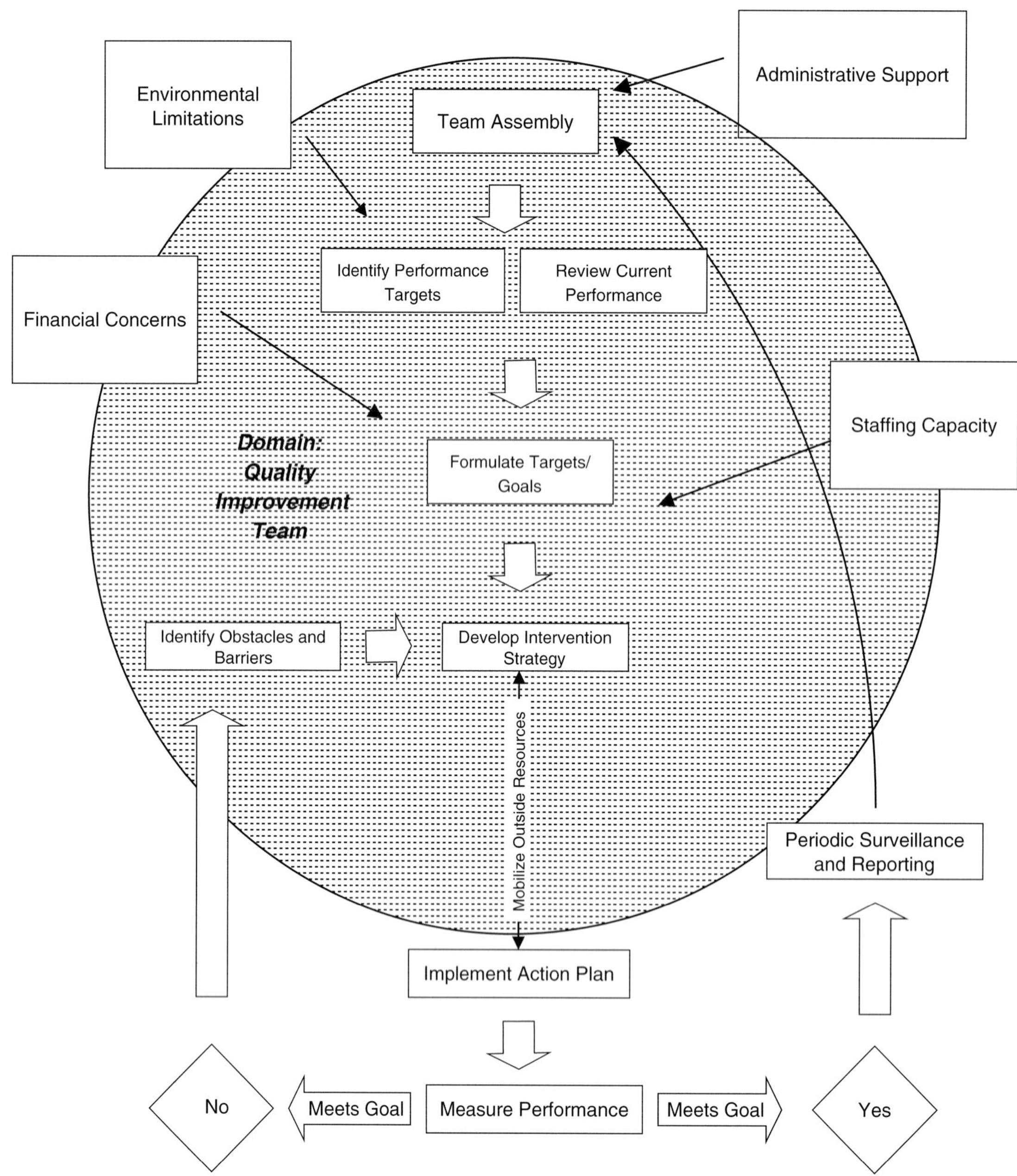

Figure 137.2 Total Quality Management (Continuous Quality Improvement) Model.

In the TQM team process, each discipline reports data collected on patient care since the previous team meeting, as well as areas of ongoing concern or newly identified issues. The team discusses markers (indicators) of quality and establishes targets to achieve by the next meeting. The team then develops a plan for achieving these targets. A method of measuring performance and collecting data is established. An individual or subcommittee is then assigned to carry out the quality improvement protocol and provide a progress report at the next meeting. If the goals are achieved, data continues to be tracked over time to identify trends in performance and to maintain the established goals. If previously established quality targets are not met, barriers or obstacles are explored.

Geriatricians are in a unique position to take a lead in the healthcare quality improvement process. Interdisciplinary management and teamwork are at the core of geriatrics training and practice. Geriatricians are comfortable entrusting responsibility to team members and sharing in the problem-solving process. This is a requirement for the success of TQM programmes. Geriatricians are also more likely than other physicians to have experienced the TQM process, as this is a routine activity in long-term care facilities. Through TQM, data on events such as falls and dehydration are tracked and shared with the staff at regular intervals. Trends are then discussed and solutions proposed when outlying results are identified.

Quality indicators

In the United States, markers for quality in nursing home care, termed 'Quality Indicators' have been developed and tracked by the federal government through the completion of the required Minimum Data Set (MDS) resident evaluation questionnaire[19,20] (see Table 137.4). Quality is assessed on these indicator domains using 'Quality Measures'. These measures include sentinel events such as faecal impaction or dehydration, and incidence/percentage of residents with certain conditions such as indwelling catheters and pressure ulcerations. Data on these measures is collected and reported federally through the MDS, and facilities are then compared against local and national facility averages. Facilities with outlying rates on the quality measures are 'flagged' which may prompt investigation or oversight by the state nursing home regulatory board.

Concerns have been raised about the accuracy and utility of data extracted from the MDS. For this reason, the previous version of MDS 2.0 has recently been replaced by version 3.0, which directly includes nursing home residents in the assessment process and employs more standardized

Table 137.4 Measures of nursing home quality.

Domain/Quality Indicator	Quality Measure
Accidents	• Incidence of new fractures • Prevalence of falls
Behaviour/Emotional Patterns	• Prevalence of behavioural symptoms affecting others (high and low risk individuals) • Prevalence of depression with no antidepressant therapy • Percent more depressed or anxious
Clinical Management	• Use of 9 or more different medications
Cognitive Patterns	• Incidence of cognitive impairment
Elimination/Incontinence	• Prevalence of bladder or bowel incontinence • Prevalence of occasional or frequent bladder or bowel incontinence without a toileting plan • Percent with a catheter inserted • Prevalence of faecal impaction
Infection Control	• Percent given influenza vaccination • Percent given pneumococcal vaccination • Percent with a urinary tract infection
Nutrition/Eating	• Percent with excess weight loss • Prevalence of tube feeding • Prevalence of dehydration
Pain Management	• Percent with moderate to severe pain
Physical Functioning	• Percent spending most of their time in bed or chair • Percent with declining ability to move about their room • Percent with increased activities of daily living needs • Incidence of decline in range of motion
Psychotropic Drug Use	• Prevalence of antipsychotic use in the absence of psychotic conditions (low- and high-risk individuals) • Prevalence of any antianxiety/hypnotic use • Prevalence of hypnotic use more than two times in the last week
Quality of Life	• Percent physically restrained • Prevalence of little or no physical activity
Skin Care	• Percent at high risk with pressure sores • Percent at low risk with pressure sores
Post-Acute Care	• Residents with delirium • Residents with moderate to severe pain • Residents with pressure ulcers

protocols for obtaining resident data. Schnelle and others have published a tremendous body of literature on the care process and health outcomes in nursing homes based on information obtained from the MDS.[21–23] In some cases the quality measures are strongly associated with a positive or negative clinical outcome.[22,23] In other cases, the indicators do not predict an event that might be expected based on the provided data.[21,22] A recent systematic review failed to find strong and consistent evidence that MDS data was a reliable or valid measure of the nursing home quality indicators.[25]

The existing quality indicators do not adequately address quality of life (QOL) and provision of daily care services. To address these issues, an expert panel of geriatricians convened and developed an additional set of quality indicators that complements the existing MDS-derived indicators. These measures may better track the quality of day-to-day care in nursing facilities.[24] The quality indicator domains include (1) preferences for daily life activities, (2) frequency and form of activities of daily living (ADL) assistance, (3) activity, (4) assistive devices, (5) goals of care, and (6) communication. Although considered markers of quality care, many of these QIs are successfully achieved only in 'the best nursing homes'. Thus, although a target to strive for, these QIs may not be attainable for the average facility.

Geriatric medicine organizations focus on quality

Interest groups and specialty organizations such as the American Geriatrics Society (AGS), American Medical Directors Association (AMDA), British Geriatric Society (BGS), and the Australian and New Zealand Society for Geriatric Medicine (ANZSGM) have taken a leadership role in bringing global quality improvement initiatives to the ageing population. These organizations work within the healthcare framework and governmental regulations unique to each country. Whereas national physician organizations focus efforts widely across the healthcare system, these specialty groups address ageing specific healthcare issues.

The ANZSGM has established a series of position papers that outline standards for geriatric care in Australia. The most recent paper is on transitions of care, a process that is especially challenging for older adults.[26] Care transitions are of increasing importance in designing safe and effective health systems for the elderly. The Australian Institute of Health and Welfare has published a systematic review assessing the evidence for transitions in care of people with dementia. This publication addresses care transitions and pathways through the Australian healthcare system.[27]

The British Geriatrics Society has also published numerous position papers, clinical guidelines and best practice guides on the care of elders in the United Kingdom. These papers increasingly focus on safety and quality of care.[28] One way the United Kingdom has addressed the quality of hospital care for seniors with orthopaedic trauma is through the development and expansion of orthopaedic rehabilitation units. These wards provide multidisciplinary care and partnership between geriatric medicine consultants and orthopaedic surgery physicians. Although individual studies have demonstrated some benefits in reducing length of stay and improved functional outcomes, a Cochrane Database analysis on the subject did not find conclusive evidence that coordinated multidisciplinary hip fracture care improved long-term post-surgical outcomes.[29–31] Small benefits have been noted in activities of daily living and mobility in the immediate postoperative period.[32]

In the United States, medical organizations regularly lobby congress on behalf of the geriatric medicine profession and elderly patients. The institution of a prescription drug benefit for Medicare health insurance beneficiaries is one example of the influence of healthcare organizations and consumers on healthcare policy and quality. The American Medical Directors Association (AMDA) has been a tremendous advocate for quality, focusing primarily on the long-term care setting. AMDA has created clinical practice guidelines for nursing home care and has established a certification process for medical directors in these facilities. Within the medical community, AMDA has pressed for a change in approach to long-term care and is viewed as the leading organization in long-term care reform.

From a consumer perspective, the Leapfrog Group is an organization with great potential for influencing the quality of healthcare plans and services. Founded by Fortune 500 executives, this group of over 150 companies aims to improve patient safety by lobbying for computerized physician ordering systems, appropriate patient referrals to subspecialty hospitals, and uniform critical care staffing in intensive care units. The Leapfrog Group represents 37 million healthcare consumers and uses its healthcare benefit purchasing power to influence the insurance industry in delivering healthcare that meets these quality standards.[33]

Quality in the nursing home

When trying to improve quality of care, one must first characterize quality. Quality is the degree to which an outcome measures up to the expected gold standard. In healthcare delivery, a quality process or intervention is measured against a standard practice that is administered to an individual patient, in a given situation, with a particular problem. Deviations from the standard of care affect the quality of care. Patients and their families expect health services to meet or exceed the standard of care but may not understand what constitutes a reasonable standard.

To maintain the highest quality of care, continuous system-wide observation, evaluation and monitoring are needed. Healthcare managers are responsible for establishing performance standards for their staff and ensuring that these standards are met. The employees should feel comfortable providing feedback to the supervisors when aspects of healthcare delivery require improvement. Managers must work with facility administrators to negotiate the resources necessary to allow the staffing team to carry out daily duties in an effective manner. Many quality improvement teams use the term 'continuous quality improvement' to describe this process because maintaining quality is an ongoing activity.

Identifying the problem

Areas of concern are brought to the attention of the healthcare manager through a variety of avenues. In the long-term care setting, a nursing home administrator collects and catalogues this information through direct or indirect contact with residents, their families and the facility staff. Administrators should also expect feedback and performance reports from the medical director and attending physicians working within the facility. Good communication between all members of the facility is essential to ensure a positive resolution to a perceived problem.

Identifying a problem shortly after it occurs and promptly initiating a plan of correction is paramount. Timeliness often affects outcome. First impressions are very important when a patient first enters a long-term care facility. Every effort must be made to ensure that the transitional period is a positive experience. After acclimating to the facility, it is important for the residents to have periodic meetings to discuss the plan of care. These meetings help to maintain a good line of communication and empower the resident to be a participant in the healthcare process.

The nursing home administrator

The nursing home administrator is responsible for the overall care within a facility and must handle all areas of concern that arise. Problems should be examined and categorized to better understand the origin of the difficulty. This information can alert the administrator to potential problems or areas of concern that need to be addressed. Nursing home administrators should to be visible and accessible to families and residents, as well as staff, when responding to facility concerns. When complaints increase, the facility administrator must investigate and take steps to correct the problem.

Nursing care

There are many inter-related components that impact the care provided by facility nursing staff. One of the most important areas, besides ensuring skill proficiency in the nursing staff, is the organization and function of nursing 'systems'. Systems of nursing practice must be in place in order to deliver high-quality care. Two examples of these 'systems' include the structure of the nursing staff and the function of the nursing staff. Critical components of these systems include staffing patterns, delegation of work assignments, supervision and evaluation of performance. Educational programmes for the nursing staff should also be provided on an ongoing basis. The nursing assistants as well as the licensed nurses need to learn and review basic skills as well as specialty techniques necessary for the care for their residents. Ensuring a smoothly running system requires responsibility, good communication, respect and clearly defined expectations. Nurses and administrators must view their interactions as two-way streets in order to build and maintain well-functioning nursing systems within a facility.

To maintain high-quality care, nurses must be able to identify residents 'at risk' for unwanted outcomes. This can be performed during weekly multidisciplinary 'high risk' needs assessment meetings for problems such as skin breakdown, falls and confusion. Because mental status may change quickly and without notice in older adults, medical status must be assessed frequently. Nursing managers should periodically review high-risk individuals to help assure optimal care. Routine nurse manager oversight can address these and other potential problems before serious issues occur.

Quality improvement meetings

Members of the quality improvement team should include pharmacy, lab, attending physicians, the medical director, nursing, therapy, dietary, maintenance, activities, social work, medical records and administration. Many long-term care facilities meet only on a quarterly basis to discuss various issues of quality care. This is not frequent enough. Monthly meetings help improve the communication of information and remind everyone of quality initiatives and areas for improvement.

Pharmacy should present the monthly number or percentage of residents on antipsychotics, anxiolytics and antidepressants. By reassessing the continued need for psychotropic medication in nursing home residents, dosing and prescribing reduction frequently occurs. Pharmacy should also report the incident and type of medication errors and assist in developing methods to reduce errors. To minimize possible drug–drug interactions, a goal of nine medications or less per resident should be a target at the facility.

The laboratory service provider should report the number of microbial cultures performed during that month with those that were negative as well as positive. Organisms that are identified are reviewed along with antibiotic sensitivity patterns. Timeliness of the cultures reported to the facility and institution of appropriate antibiotics are reviewed. Trends in organisms, antimicrobial sensitivity and clustering of infections should be assessed. Laboratory services should also investigate unnecessarily prolonged return of blood work reports and the effectiveness of data transmission to the nursing facility.

Each month, nursing should present the number of residents who developed decubitus ulcers, have indwelling foley catheters, and received physical restraints. To reduce the rate of injuries and falls, each facility should strive to be restraint-free.[34] The rate of facility acquired decubitus and indwelling foley catheters, should be under 5%. If rates rise above 5%, action should be taken to justify or remedy this trend. Weight loss and excessive gain should be reported every month, including a probable cause and a plan of correction. Awareness is key and all disciplines can participate in weight loss prevention protocols.

Incident reports should be reviewed monthly. Investigation of resident incidents should include type, location where the incident took place, time of day (during which shift), weekend versus weekday, and degree of injury or impact. Trends or patterns in this data should be noted and a plan for incident reduction implemented. Employee incidents should also be evaluated. An increase in employee incidents and injuries is often directly related to employee dissatisfaction.

Patient census should be reviewed at each meeting along with admissions, transfers to and from the hospital, discharges to home/another facility and deaths. When looking at nursing home admissions, one should also look at the source of their admission. Was the new admit from a hospital, and if so, which hospital? Are admissions trending up or down? What days and times are the hospital admissions arriving at the nursing home? Transfers to the hospital or emergency department should also be tracked. Was the transfer preventable? Are certain shifts or floors more likely to transfer residents out for urgent evaluation? This valuable information allows the nursing home administrator and director of nursing to identify staffing or skill deficiencies within the facility.

When providing therapy to the long-term care resident, the therapist needs to keep a record of the functional level prior to therapy, the number of days in therapy, the functional level when therapy was discontinued, and disposition upon discharge. It has been demonstrated that extending therapy a few more days often improves overall outcome. Therapy services can use this information as a marketing tool. The department may display, in a graphic format, the functional level or residents prior to illness, upon initiation of therapy and upon discharge of therapy.

The quality improvement process that is discussed and monitored during team meetings should be documented in an organized and systematic manner using a standardized reporting process (see Table 137.5). Topics relevant to patient care quality (e.g. falls) are selected by the team. Indicators of quality (e.g. fall rate, injurious falls, number of fractures) are identified and a target rate for the facility is established (e.g. <5% of falls resulting in injury). Data on patient outcomes is collected within the facility and compared with the established indicator target. If current standards fail to meet the target, areas for improvement (e.g. reducing nighttime falls) are identified and a plan of action established (e.g. scheduled toileting at bedtime). During the follow-up phase, data on the indicators is again collected to determine if the intervention has resulted in successful achievement of the established goals.

Quality in acute care practices

Hospital accreditation

The internationally recognized Joint Commission on Accreditation of Healthcare Organizations (JCAHO) mission is to provide accreditation and performance review for the safety and quality of healthcare facilities. Established over 50 years ago, this independent non-profit organization reviews not only hospitals, but also a variety of healthcare facilities such as nursing homes, home care organizations, healthcare networks, outpatient centres and clinical laboratories. Accreditation is a marker of quality valued by the community and used to promote the excellence of an institution.

Accreditation takes place after undergoing an on-site survey by a team of medical and business professional. All aspects of care are reviewed, including compliance with safety procedures, patient care processes and the work environment. Hospital accreditation is valid for three years. JCAHO uses standardized performance criteria that were developed with the expertise and guidance of healthcare leaders in academic medicine, business and governmental agencies.

In other parts of the world, the hospital evaluation process may take place through national or international regulatory organizations. In Europe, hospital accreditation first was introduced in Spain through the Catalan Hospital Accreditation Programme (CHAP) in the early 1980s.[35] Due to financial setbacks, this programme was not continuously active until 1991. In the United Kingdom, a sustained accreditation programme has been in place since 1990. Results of a 2004 survey indicated that 18 European countries were formally utilizing or implementing a hospital accreditation programme.[36] By 2009, 18 different accrediting organizations were active throughout Europe.[37]

In the United Kingdom, healthcare facility accreditation began in 1989 through two organizations: the Caspe Healthcare Knowledge Systems (CHKS) and the King's Fund Organisational Audit (KFOA). These non-governmental organizations were first developed to oversee the National Health Service hospitals but have grown to include accreditation of public and community healthcare centres. The

Table 137.5 Continuous Quality Improvement Report.

Topic ____________ Dept. ____________
Report Date____________ ________ Initial Report____________ Follow-up

I. Process Planning
Reason for selecting topic____________
Starting Date____________
Frequency of Monitoring____________
Sampling Population____________
Source of Information__________ Records __________ Survey
____________Observation ________ Other
Method for Data Collection____________

II. Indicators and Data Presentation

Indicator	Goal (Frequency or %)	Data (Numerical)	Data (Percent)

Interpretation of Data and Comparison to Established Goals:

III. Analysis and Plan of Improvement

A. Areas for Improvement	Obstacles or Barriers

B. Action Plan	Key Personnel	Initiation Date	Completion Date

IV. Follow-up and Re-evaluation

Indicator	Date to Re-evaluate	Key Personnel	Date for Follow-up Report

Report Prepared and Reviewed by:

Name Title Date

KFOA became the Health Quality Service (HQS) in 1998 and was acquired by CKHS in 2005. Accreditation reports are available for public inspection in the United Kingdom and a handful of other countries, but in general are not available to healthcare consumers in Europe. Although the majority of accredited programmes are hospital-based, evaluations of community and outpatient care centres are evolving in several European countries.

Both JCAHO and CKHS offer international accreditation services. In 1999 JCAHO initiated an international programme for accreditation. To address the international differences in healthcare delivery, a 16-member task force developed 'international consensus standards' for the Joint Commissions International. This task force represents the healthcare concerns, values and governments of countries on six continents. CKHS offers consultation services within and outside of Europe and is accredited by ISQua to provide the ISO 9001 quality management systems for healthcare organizations.

The hospital environment

It has long been known by geriatricians that the hospital is a dangerous place for frail elderly individuals who are at high risk for iatrogenic complications. If immobility, delirium and nutrition are not addressed upon hospitalization, unwanted morbidity and functional decline can rapidly occur.[38,39] Altering the hospital environment to improve outcomes in the elderly has become a focus of research and a measure of quality in healthcare. *US News and World Report* magazine ranks United States hospitals and medical programmes each year. Among a host of factors used to evaluate quality, hospital-based geriatric services are included in this calculation.[40]

Over the past decade, several geriatric services have been developed with demonstrated benefit in reducing the risk of hospital-related morbidity and mortality. These programmes have largely targeted the prevention of delirium and reduction in functional decline. Hospitals are increasingly aware that reducing adverse events in the elderly is important not only for maintaining a positive public reputation, but in reducing healthcare costs.

Acute Care for the Elderly (ACE) units have been shown to decrease discharge to nursing homes and to improve functional outcomes at hospital discharge.[41,42] The general principles of ACE units include an interdisciplinary care approach, tailoring the hospital environment to reduce iatrogenesis, maximizing functional status, daily geriatric assessments with an active involved, specially trained nursing staff and proactive discharge planning. The implementation of ACE units in hospitals is growing.

The Geriatric Evaluation and Mangement Unit (GEMU) is another multidisciplinary care model linked closely to the inpatient hospitalization setting. GEMUs provide subacute care and rehabilitation in a setting that bridges hospital to home. The goals of GEMU care include maximizing functional, social and medical status through comprehensive geriatric assessment. Patients who would otherwise require nursing home placement receive dedicated medical and therapy services to regain lost independence. The GEMU model has demonstrated benefit in reducing rehospitalization, improving physical and cognitive functioning, reducing mortality and increasing the likelihood of living at home after discharge.[43] These outcomes are indicators of the quality and benefit of a multidisciplinary approach to care of the older adult.

Quality in the community setting

Home care

Medical care in the home has shifted from the historical single-provider model of the early 1900s to a team-based service with the advent of home healthcare organizations. This multidisciplinary approach has expanded the access and availability of healthcare services to homebound individuals. Australia has taken home care to an even higher level of sophistication with the 'Hospital in the Home' approach. This model provides hospital-like services to individuals at home who are acutely ill but unwilling to enter the hospital or for whom hospitalization is unlikely to provide any measurable health benefit. The quality of care for Hospital in the Home as measured by cost, patient satisfaction and medical outcomes, is at least equivalent to traditional hospital care.[44,45]

Patient care in the home is of increasing complexity and acuity. For organizations to meet the quality care standards expected by consumers, home-care services must be broad in scope and efficient in delivery. The success of Hospital in the Home and growth of home care is in part due to the advancement of portable medical technologies. Mobile radiology and laboratory services have expanded the diagnostic capabilities of home-care providers. The availability of intravenous access services and infusion devices have allowed more frail and debilitated elders to receive necessary intravenous therapies without transfer to the hospital or nursing home setting. Portable electrocardiogram monitors and serum analysis systems, although not in widespread use, now allow providers a more efficient and expedited evaluation of the home-care patient.

To address the question of how home health services improve the quality of medical care, the Agency for Healthcare Research and Quality, through the Centers for Medicare and Medicaid Services (CMS) in the United States, has developed a Home Health Quality Initiative project. CMS currently provides financial reimbursement for more than half of the home-care expenditures for seniors.[46] A set of 41 quality measures are used to evaluate home-care agency services. These measures are based on outcomes data from the Outcome and Assessment Information Set (OASIS) national standardized home-care database. Quality measures are functionally based, such as improvement in toileting or improvement in bathing, but also include the utilization of emergency or hospital services.[47] Using the reported outcomes on these quality measures, certified home-care agency evaluations can now be reviewed online by the medical consumer.

Home monitoring and telemedicine systems are of increasing interest in the care of chronically ill seniors. A variety of products that record patient information, transmit data to a monitoring centre, or give patient reminders are now commercially available. Remote medical monitoring systems can intermittently or continuously monitor vital signs and disease symptoms using non-invasive and minimally intrusive sensors. These systems use internet, radio, or phone-line transmission of medical information to a hardware- or software-based system that acquires, stores and processes the data. Medical staff can examine the data in real-time or at periodic intervals. Alert parameters can be programmed to immediately notify the provider of abnormal findings. These systems are used almost exclusively in association with home healthcare services. Initial studies suggest that for chronic disease management, electronic home monitoring systems can reduce hospitalization rates and length of stay and improve disease control.[48–51]

The most basic home care technologies include personal alarm systems and emergency response telephones that make a voice connection between the patient and the response centre. This 'lifeline' monitoring system uses a self-activated call button that is often worn as a necklace or bracelet. More expansive and complex systems are being designed to monitor the home and activity of frail elders. The 'smart home' technology utilizes sensors placed throughout the home to track 'normal' daily activity and report potential emergencies by detecting deviations from typical activity patterns. These devices may improve the safety and security of older adults living at home, but conjure up unsettling images of an Orwellian world where 'Big Brother' is watching.

Database analysis in the United States

Large, centralized healthcare organizations, such as health maintenance organizations (HMO) and the Department of Veterans' Affairs Medical Centers (VAMC) in the United States, frequently use health database analysis to track costs, utilization of services and patient care outcomes. Data from these organizations is used for epidemiology studies and for population-based research on disease and healthcare services. Although cost containment may be a driving force in the monitoring of health statistics, these organizations have the infrastructure to use healthcare data for quality improvement purposes.

Because laboratory, radiology and pharmacy services are usually provided within the organization, utilization statistics may be readily available to the clinical and administrative providers. Often this information is tracked electronically within the organization. Practice patterns can be monitored and feedback sent to clinicians or departments to improve the delivery of patient care. Appointment backlogs, vaccination rates and cancer screening rates may be targeted by the organization. Goals for improving the delivery of healthcare can be set and trends measured after instituting a plan of improvement.

There is growing interest in a disease-based team approach to improve health outcomes. Common disorders that require regular monitoring or result in high use of urgent care services, such as diabetes and asthma, are often the target of these efforts. Using nationally developed practice guidelines or internally developed clinical care protocols, centralized healthcare organizations have the infrastructure to implement care processes to improve health outcomes.

Although clinical practice guidelines are not universally agreed upon in every detail, they are generally considered to represent a reasonable and achievable standard of care supported by current evidence-based research. Thus, adherence to practice guidelines may serve as a marker for quality care within an organization or clinical patient base. Pharmacy and clinical laboratory databases are used to provide individual feedback to clinicians on decision-making behaviour, compliance with national guidelines, and improvement in patient outcomes over time. The use of database monitoring to generate electronic reminders that prompt screening and disease management have demonstrated improvement in practitioner adherence to healthcare standards.[52–54]

Although database analysis offers much statistical information, ongoing problems include limitation of content, relative inaccessibility to information, lack of automated data and data mismatches.[55,56] This could be improved through new financial and technical support to HMOs interested in outcomes-based research.

Healthcare audit in the United Kingdom

In the United Kingdom, population-based review is conducted through a process called clinical audit. The National Health Service has used this method of quality improvement for over 20 years. Clinical audit is a 'systematic, critical analysis of the quality of medical care including the procedures used for diagnosis and treatment, the use of resources, and the resulting outcome and quality of life for the patient'.[57] Clinical audit has evolved from a clinician-targeted to a system-targeted review that evaluates the outcomes of a quality improvement process.

Clinical audit is an internal method whereby a clinical practice, such as the frequency of ophthalmologic evaluation in diabetic patients or rate of influenza vaccination, is measured using medical record review. Performance markers are compared to accepted standards, practice guidelines, or previously established audit goals. If performance falls below expectations, a plan for practice revision is established and implemented. Follow-up audit is conducted to assess the success in achieving the targeted practice goals.

Clinical audit is a dynamic process that requires attention to changes in population demographics, health resources and advances in medical knowledge. Comparison of audit results between clinical sites or regions must account for this heterogeneity. The geriatric population itself is a heterogeneous group. For the elderly, important clinical outcomes are linked less to chronological age than to functional ability. A clinical audit outcome measure of cancer screening rates in a healthy 75-year-old population, for example, may be quite different than a chronically ill and debilitated 75-year-old cohort.

The success of a clinical audit requires a well-structured approach, appropriate time and appropriate resources. Too frequently, a problem is identified through the clinical audit but a plan of correction is not implemented or the outcome of the correction is never evaluated. This may be due to a lack of experience and time on the part of the auditors, who are often junior clinicians within the organization. Resources must be available if an organization plans to undergo a systematic review of a clinical issue with the intent to implement a meaningful change in clinical practice.

Large-scale clinical audits can require significant administrative support. Charts must be collected, data extracted and statistical evaluation performed. A protocol for change in practice must be developed with the input and agreement of clinical practitioners. Piloting the proposed change may be necessary to troubleshoot unforeseen barriers before implementing the plan on a larger scale. After an appropriate duration of practice, the clinical issue must be re-evaluated to determine if the new protocol has had an impact on the targeted outcome of the programme.

It is important that a clinical audit be viewed as a quality improvement activity and not as a means to emphasize personal shortcomings or to generate punitive action. The audit should focus on areas in need of general improvement and methods to achieve practice goals of the group or within the organization.[58]

Clinical audit itself is not research, although it may generate research questions. Because an audit reveals epidemiological and demographic information about a clinical practice, the results may lead to publication of healthcare trends or results of a quality improvement process. In an era of increasing attention to patient confidentiality and ethical research practices, approval to conduct an audit may be required by an organization. This is especially true in the United States where academic centres and many healthcare organizations have institutional review boards to ensure the safety and confidentiality of patient information.

Future initiatives in healthcare quality

With the advent of high technology, the perception of quality has expanded to encompass the use and accessibility of electronic and computer-based devices in healthcare. Medical diagnosis, treatment and documentation have advanced in sophistication to a point where electronics are standard and necessary for patient care practices. Healthcare services, communication and reimbursement are expedited with the use of high technology. Individuals and organizations without internet access, electronic medical records, or access to innovative diagnostic/therapeutic devices may be viewed as 'behind the times'. Healthcare consumers have an increasing expectation, well-founded or not, that technology-based initiatives provide superior quality and better medical outcomes.

High technology in medical education

The use of technology has fundamentally altered the format of medical education. Computers have changed the classroom environment and augmented the quality of medical presentations. Lectures now efficiently utilize multimedia resources with the ability to present complex content using sophisticated instructional formats. Internet-ready classrooms allow an educator to conduct a search of the literature and access clinical information in real-time.

Online, as opposed to live in-class lectures are available at many medical schools. In one study, students expended 50 minutes less time to complete an online lecture activity than the live lecture group, but demonstrated equal post-lecture knowledge.[59] Many studies have failed to demonstrate the superiority of internet-based or computer-assisted tutorials over the traditional lecture and textbook format.[60–63] Thus an 'electronic professor' does not replace the need for live interaction with medical educators. Like any instructional tool, electronic and computer-based programmes must be used in the right context, for the right group, and with the appropriate level of 'real-life' interaction.

Subjects with a high degree of visual-spatial complexity such as gross anatomy and histology have seen remarkable benefit from the growth of digital teaching tools. Three-dimensional views and electronically created images have assisted students in understanding anatomical and physiological relationships. Trainees are being exposed to new technologies from the classroom through the clinical years. Teaching tools that did not exist just a few years ago are readily being incorporated into the educational environment.

New methods of medical education using simulation models are of increasing interest in reducing the incidence of procedural complications. In some studies, surgeons who received virtual reality simulator training for laproscopic procedures demonstrated significant improvement in skill performance over those without this training.[64,65] Other research has failed to demonstrate a difference in procedure time and patient discomfort between medical residents trained using a virtual reality-based procedural simulator and traditional bedside teaching techniques.[66] As the use of technology in diagnosis and treatment expands, so will the use of technology-based teaching tools in hopes of improving the quality of medical training.

In an effort to improve the efficiency and safety of patient care, hand-held Personal Digital Assistant (PDA) devices have become increasingly popular in medical practice and medical education. Some medical schools and residency programmes are providing trainees with these devices pre-programmed with educational tools and reference databases. PDAs have demonstrated benefit in reducing adverse medical events and improving the accuracy of medical documentation. Data is most supportive in the reduction of medication errors and identification of medication side effects.[67,68]

Because PDAs now have wireless and Internet access capability, the potential for remote-site electronic access to a central patient care database is being utilized at some institutions. This access can be especially useful for the geriatric medicine practitioner performing house calls, nursing home care and rural community-based care. These sites traditionally have limited access to electronic resources. Several institutions within the United States, including the VAMC system, have employed technologies that allow practitioners to use portable devices for remote access to patient information. Patient confidentiality has been addressed through the use of encryption programs that prevent unauthorized access by wireless users.

PDA programs can be used to track and store patient information. This is especially useful in the immediate and accurate retrieval of patient during after hours, off site and telephone consultation with patients and other medical providers. The applications to patient safety are of growing importance in the quality improvement process at all sites of care. The use PDAs and other portable electronic equipment will continue to grow as the demand for immediate and accurate medical information increases.

Electronic medical records

Electronic documentation of patient information is also of increasing importance in the delivery of quality medical care. The hospital setting currently makes greatest use of electronic records given the volume of information that must be collected and shared among medical practitioners. Whether data is entered electronically by practitioners or accessed in a read-only format, the electronic medical record (EMR) facilitates communication and access to information. Electronic charting has been shown to reduce documentation time and to improve the accuracy of assigning diagnostic codes.[69] The use of computer technology in patient management has repeatedly been associated with a reduction in the frequency of many types of medical errors.[70]

Many electronic record systems operate via an internet-based access system that allows users to enter and access data through any internet-ready computer. Other institutions use onsite computer systems that require users to access data through terminals or workstations networked for this purpose. This system limits access but is potentially a more secure means of maintaining patient confidentiality.

The VAMC in the United States exclusively uses an EMR. This computerized patient record system (CPRS) is the largest EMR in the world. All medical orders, laboratory tests, medical progress notes, medications and other data are entered and viewed electronically by all medical providers. The system can be accessed remotely for those providers located off of the main medical campus. Alerts, prompts and pre-designed order sets have reduced the occurrence of medical errors and improved the efficiency of medical care within the VAMC system. Those countries with national healthcare systems or large health provider groups (such as the VAMC) may be at best advantage to use an all-electronic record system, given the need for a well-structured system to oversee the design and support this form of health information system.

Telemedicine

With the advancement of digital data transfer, the Internet and wireless-based technologies, rapid relay of visual and audio transmissions have led to the development of telemedicine programs between remote geographic locations. Videoconferencing has extensive educational and clinical applications for the healthcare systems. Training can be provided in real-time using interactive video technology that allows remote classrooms sites to see, hear and speak with the instructor. Telemedicine allows primary and specialty care providers to interact with patients and clinicians in geographically isolated or underserved segments of the population.

In a Singapore hospital pilot project, geriatric specialists conducted telerounds with two off-site homes for the elderly.[71] This project was considered a success and was viewed favourably by both patients and clinicians. Improving access to healthcare resources is an area of ongoing interest in the quality improvement process. As the technology improves and hardware costs decline, telemedicine will become an increasingly popular means of providing a broader array of healthcare services to a larger segment of the patient population.

Conclusion

'Quality of care' has been defined as, 'the degree to which health services for individuals and populations increase the likelihood of desired health outcomes and are consistent with current professional knowledge'. Quality in healthcare has become a priority as cost, volume and efficiency became critical issues in meeting the growing healthcare demands of the medical consumer. Over the past two decades, the interest in healthcare quality improvement has grown dramatically. Consumer groups, medical societies and healthcare organizations have actively promoted quality in healthcare. These national and international associations work within the healthcare framework and governmental regulations unique to each country to help meet consumer and regulatory demands for high-quality medical services.

Based on the established healthcare and payer system, each organization may address quality control quite differently. Healthcare facility accreditation is a common means of marking quality and promoting the excellence of an institution. Other groups may choose certification using established standards such as the ISO-9000 process. At the level of the individual provider, performance may be assessed through audit or comparison of practices to established clinical guidelines.

The TQM process is well suited for the complex healthcare environment. This method is used to critically evaluate not only medical treatments and techniques but also the process by which medicine is delivered to the healthcare consumer. Quality improvement may then involve change in practice on an individual level and change in operation on a larger scale that benefits a broader population. Using quality indicators and outcome measures that quantitatively and objectively measure care, outlying data can be used to alert the organization to quality control problems.

Geriatricians are in a unique position to influence the healthcare quality improvement process. Interdisciplinary care and TQM are already familiar practices for most medical practitioners. As medical directors, geriatricians have taken a leadership role in improving institutional and rehabilitation practices. The quality of care for the elderly has been enhanced through new initiatives such as ACE and GEMU models and home-care technologies. Using new technologies, electronic databases and internet resources, care for the older population stands to broaden in scope and sophistication in coming years. Geriatricians will continue to be strong advocates for care practices that improve the process and outcomes of medical care for a growing and ageing population.

Key points

- The process of standardizing healthcare quality has evolved over the last 100 years.
- The Joint Commission on Accreditation of Healthcare Organizations (JCAHO) has accredited hospitals and healthcare facilities for over 50 years.
- Continuous Quality Improvement, also known as Total Quality Management, is a team-based approach used to evaluate and institute system-wide changes.
- Database analysis and healthcare audit are two methods of evaluating quality on a population-based scale.
- The use of computers and electronic communication systems have improved medical efficiency and reduced medical errors.

Appendix 137.1 Healthcare quality organizations.

Abbreviation	Organization	Origin	Created
ACHS	Australian Council for Health Care Standards	Australia	1974
ACHSI	Australian Council on Healthcare Standards International	Australia	2005
ACS	American College of Surgeons	United States	1913
ACSQHC	Australian Commission on Safety and Quality in Health Care	Australia	2006
AGS	American Geriatrics Society	United States	1942
AHRQ	Agency for Healthcare Research and Quality	United States	1999
(AHCPR)	(Previously Agency for Healthcare Policy and Research)		(AHCPR 1989)
AMDA	American Medical Directors Association	United States	1978
ANZSGM	Australian and New Zealand Society for Geriatric Medicine (ANZSGM)	Australia	2006
(ASGM)			1970s
(AGS)	(Previously: Australian Society for Geriatric Medicine, Australian Geriatrics Society, Australian Association of Gerontology)		1960s
BGS	British Geriatric Society	United Kingdom	1947
CAHPS	Consumer Assessment of Health Plans	United States	1999
CHAP	Catalan Hospital Accreditation Programme	Spain	1981
CHI	Commission for Health Improvement	United Kingdom	1999
CHKS	Caspe Healthcare Knowledge Systems	United Kingdom	1989
(HQS)	(Previously Health Quality Service & King's Fund Organisational Audit)		(HQS 1998)
(KFOA)			(KFOA 1989)
CMS	Centers for Medicare and Medicaid Services	United States	2001
(HCFA)	(Previously Health Care Financing Administration)		(HCFA 1977)
CQC	Care Quality Commission	England	2009
EFQM	European Foundation for Quality Management	Europe	1988
HC	Healthcare Commission	England	2004
HIW	Healthcare Inspectorate Wales	Wales	2004
IEC	International Electrotechnical Commission	United States	1906
IOM	Institute of Medicine	United States	1970
ISA	International Federation of the National Standardizing Association	Europe	1926
ISO	International Organization for Standardization	United Kingdom	1947
ISQua	The International Society for Quality in Health Care	Australia	1985
JCAH	Joint Commission on Accreditation of Hospitals	United States	1951
JCAHO	Joint Commission on Accreditation of Healthcare Organizations	United States	1987
NCQA	National Committee for Quality Assurance	United States	1990
NHS	National Health Services	United Kingdom	1948
RQIA	The Regulation and Quality Improvement Authority	Northern Ireland	2003
SCRC	Scottish Commission for the Regulation of Care	Scotland	2001
USPSTP	U.S. Preventive Services Task Force	United States	1984
VAMC	Department of Veterans Affairs Medical Centers	United States	1989
(VA)	(Previously Veterans Administration)		(VA 1930)

References

1. International Organization for Standards. ISO members. http://www.iso.org/iso/about/iso_members.htm (last accessed December 2011).
2. International Organization for Standards. ISO in figures for the year 2010, p. 3. http://www.iso.org/iso/about/iso_in_figures/iso_in_figures_3.htm (last accessed January 2012).
3. Shaw P, Elliott C, Isaacson P *et al. Quality and Performance Improvement in Health Care. A Tool for Programmed Learning*, 2nd edn, American Health Information Management Association, Chicago, IL, 2003. Also available at: http://library.ahima.org/xpedio/groups/public/documents/ahima/bok1_020002.pdf
4. Joint Commission on Accreditation of Healthcare Organizations. The Joint Commission History. Last update 15 July 2010. http://www.jointcommission.org/assets/1/18/Joint_Commission_History_20111.PDF (last accessed December 2011).
5. Agency for Healthcare Research and Quality (ARHQ). United States Department of Health and Human Services. 2009 National Healthcare Quality & Disparities Reports. Last update March 2010. http://www.ahrq.gov/qual/qrdr09.htm (last accessed December 2011).
6. U.S. Preventive Services Task Force. *Guide to Clinical Preventive Services*, 3rd edn: Periodic Updates. U.S. Preventive Services Task Force, October 2002. http://www.uspreventiveservicestaskforce.org/3rduspstf/preface.htm (last accessed December 2011).
7. National Committee for Quality Assurance (NCQA). HEDIS & Quality Measurement. http://ncqa.org/tabid/59/Default.aspx (last accessed December 2011).
8. Richardson WC, Corrigan JM. Shaping the future. The IOM Quality Initiative: A progress report at year six. *The IOM Newsletter* 2002;**1**:1–8.
9. Institute of Medicine of the National Academies. About Reports. Last update 15 December 2011. http://iom.edu/Reports.aspx (last accessed December 2011).
10. Care Quality Commission. The essential standards of quality and safety. http://caredirectory.cqc.org.uk/caredirectory/whathaschanged.cfm (last accessed December 2011).
11. The Australian Council on Healthcare Standards. Updated 22 December 2010. http://www.achs.org.au/ (last accessed December 2011).
12. Australian Commission on Safety and Quality in Healthcare. http://www.achs.org.au/ACSQHC (last accessed December 2011).
13. The International Society for Quality in Health Care (ISQua). Accreditation. http://isqua.org/accreditations.htm (last accessed December 2011).
14. Heaton C. External peer review in Europe: an overview from the ExPeRT Project. *Int J Qual Health Care* 2000;**12**:177–82.
15. European Foundation for Quality Management. About EFQM. http://www.efqm.org/en/tabid/108/default.aspx (last accessed December 2011).
16. Lombarts MJ, Klazinga NS, Redekop KK. Measuring the perceived impact of facilitation on implementing recommendations from external assessment: lessons from the Dutch Visitatie programme for medical specialists. *J Eval Clin Pract* 2005;**11**:587–97.
17. Leap LL, Brennan TA, Laird N *et al*. The nature of adverse events in hospitalized patients. Results of the Harvard Medical Practice Study II. *New Engl J Med* 1991;**324**:277–84.
18. Miller MR, Elixhauser A, Zhan C *et al*. Patient Safety Indicators: using administrataive data to identify potential patient safety concerns. *Health Serv Res* 2001;**36**:110–32.
19. Center for Medicare and Medicaid Services. MDS Quality Measure/Indicator Report. Last update 23 November 2010. http://www.cms.gov/MDSPubQIandResRep/02_qmreport.asp?qtr=22&isSubmitted=qm2 (last accessed December 2011).
20. Zimmerman DR, Karon SL, Arling G *et al*. Development and testing of nursing home quality indicators. *Health Care Fin Rev* 1995;**16**:107–27.
21. Bates-Jensen BM, Alessi CA, Cadogan M *et al*. The minimum data set bedfast quality indicator: differences among nursing homes. *Nurs Res* 2004;**53**:260–72.
22. Schnelle JF, Bates-Jensen BM, Levy-Storms L *et al*. The minimum data set prevalence of restraint quality indicator: does it reflect differences in care? *Gerontologist* 2004;**44**:245–55.
23. Cadogan MP, Schnelle JF, Yamamoto-Mitani N *et al*. A minimum data set prevalence of pain quality indicator: is it accurate and does it reflect differences in care processes? *J Gerontol A Biol Sci Med Sci* 2004;**59**:281–5.
24. Saliba D, Schnelle JF. Indicators of the quality of nursing home residential care. *JAGS* 2002;**50**:1421–30.
25. Hutchinson AM, Milke DL, Maisey S *et al*. The Resident Assessment Instrument-Minimum Data Set 2.0 quality indicators: a systematic review. *BMC Health Serv Res* 2010;**10**:166.
26. Australian & New Zealand Society for Geriatric Medicine. Position Statements. Last updated 15 June 2010. http://www.anzsgm.org/posstate.asp (accessed 6 December 2011).
27. Runge C, Gilham J, Peut A. Transitions in care of people with dementia: A systematic review, AIHW, Canberra, February 2009. http://www.aihw.gov.au/publications/index.cfm/title/11074 (last accessed December 2011).
28. British Geriatrics Society. Resources, 2010. http://www.bgs.org.uk/index.php?option=com_content&view=article&id=34&Itemid=472 (last accessed December 2011).
29. Incalzi RA, Gemma A, Capparella O *et al*. Continuous geriatric care in orthopedic wards: A valuable alternative to orthogeriatric units. *Aging Clin Exp Res* 1993;**5**:207–16.
30. Kennie DC, Reid J, Richardson IR *et al*. Effectiveness of geriatric rehabilitative care after fractures of the proximal femur in elderly women: a randomized clinical trial. *BMJ* 1988;**297**:1083–6.
31. Cameron ID, Handoll HHG, Finnegan TP *et al*. Coordinated multidisciplinary approaches for inpatient rehabilitation of older patients with proximal femoral fractures. *Cochrane Methodology Review* 2003;**4**. http://www.cochrane.org/reviews
32. Handoll HG, Cameron ID, Mak J, Finnegan TP. Multidisciplinary rehabilitation for older people with hip fractures. *Cochrane Database Syst Rev* 2010;**2**.
33. The Leapfrog Group for Patient Safety. The Leapfrog Group Fact Sheet, Washington DC, 2010; http://www.

leapfroggroup.org/media/file/FactSheet_LeapfrogGroup.pdf (last accessed December 2011).

34. Capezuti E, Strumpf NE, Evans LK *et al*. The relationship between physical restraint removal and falls and injuries among nursing home residents. *J Gerontol A Biol Sci Med Sci* 1998;**53A**: M47–52.
35. Shaw CD. External quality mechanisms for health care: summary of the ExPeRT project on visitatie, accreditation, EFQM and ISO assessment in European Union countries. External Peer Review Techniques. European Foundation for Quality Management. International Organization for Standardization. *Int J Qual Health Care* 2000;**12**:169–75.
36. Shaw CD. Accreditation in European health care. *Jt Comm J Qual Patient Saf* 2006;**32**:266–75.
37. Shaw CD, Kutryba B, Braithwaite J, Bedlicki M, Warunek A. Sustainable healthcare accreditation: messages from Europe in 2009. *Int J Qual Health Care* 2010;**22**:341–50.
38. Inouye SK, Peduzzi PN, Robison JT *et al*. Importance of functional measures in predicting mortality among older hospitalized patients. *JAMA* 1998; 279:1187–93.
39. Inouye SK, Rushing JT, Foreman MD *et al*. Does delirium contribute to poor hospital outcomes? A three-site epidemiologic study. *J Gen Intern Med* 1998;**13**:234–42.
40. Comarow, A. *US News and World Magazine* Report: America's Best Hospitals 2010–2011: The Methodology, 14 July 2010. http://health.usnews.com/health-news/best-hospitals/articles/2010/07/14/best-hospitals-2010-11-the-methodology.html (last accessed December 2011).
41. Landefeld C, Palmer R, Kresevic D *et al*. A randomized trial of care in a hospital medical unit especially designed to improve the functional outcomes of acutely ill older patients. *New Engl J Med* 1995;**332**:1338–44.
42. Counsel S, Holder C, Liebenauer L *et al*. Effects of a multicomponent intervention on functional outcomes and process of care in hospitalized older patients. *JAGS* 2000;**48**:1571–81.
43. Stuck AE, Siu AL, Wieland GD *et al*. Comprehensive geriatric assessment: a meta-analysis of controlled trials. *Lancet* 1993;**342**:1032–36.
44. Board N, Brennan N, Caplan GA. A randomised controlled trial of the costs of hospital as compared with hospital in the home for acute medical patients. *Aust N Z J Public Health* 2000;**24**:305–11.
45. Caplan GA, Ward JA, Brennan NJ *et al*. Hospital in the home: a randomised controlled trial. *Med J Aust* 1999;**170**:156–60.
46. The National Association for Home Care and Hospice. Basic Statistics About Home Care, Updated 2010. http://www.nahc.org/facts/10HC_Stats.pdf (last accessed December 2011).
47. Centers for Medicare and Medicaid Services. Background: the Outcome Assessment Information Set (OASIS). Last update 20 December 2010. http://www.cms.gov/OASIS/02_Background.asp#TopOfPage (last accessed December 2011).
48. Kornowski R, Zeeli D, Averbuch M *et al*. Intensive home-care surveillance prevents hospitalization and improves morbidity rates among elderly patients with severe congestive heart failure. *Am Heart J* 1995;**129**:762–6.
49. Mehra MR, Uber PA, Chomsky DB *et al*. Emergence of electronic home monitoring in chronic heart failure. *Congest Heart Fail* 2000;**6**:137–9.
50. Maiolo C, Mohamed EI, Fiorani CM *et al*. Home telemonitoring for patients with severe respiratory illness: the Italian experience. *J Telemed Telecare* 2003;**9**:67–71.
51. Rogers MA, Small D, Buchan DA *et al*. Home monitoring service improves mean arterial pressure in patients with essential hypertension. A randomized, controlled trial. *Ann Intern Med* 2001;**134**:1024–32.
52. Bentz CJ, Davis N, Bayley B. The feasibility of paper-based tracking codes and electronic medical record systems to monitor tobacco-use assessment and intervention in an Individual Practice Association (IPA) Model Health Maintenance Organization (HMO). *Nicotine Tob Res* 2002;**4**(Suppl 1):S9–17.
53. Kitahata MM, Dillingham PW, Chaiyakunapruk N *et al*. Electronic human immunodeficiency virus (HIV) clinical reminder system improves adherence to practice guidelines among the University of Washington HIV Study Cohort. *Clin Infect Dis* 2003;**36**:803–11.
54. Filippi A, Sabatini A, Badioli L *et al*. Effects of an automated electronic reminder in changing the antiplatelet drug-prescribing behavior among Italian general practitioners in diabetic patients: an intervention trial. *Diabetes Care* 2003; **26**:1497–500.
55. Fink R. HMO data systems in population studies of access to care. *Health Serv Res* 1998;**33**:741–59.
56. Mullooly J, Drew L, DeStefano F *et al*. Quality of HMO vaccination databases used to monitor childhood vaccine safety. *Am J Epidemiol* 1999;**149**:186–94.
57. Department of Health. *Working for patients. Medical audit*, HMSO, London, 1989.
58. Dickenson E, Sinclair AJ. Clinical audit of health care. In: MSJ Pathy, *Principles and Practice of Geriatric Medicine*, 3rd edn, John Wiley & Sons, Ltd, Chichester, 1998, pp. 1575–81.
59. Spickard A, Alrajeh N, Cordray D *et al*. Learning about screening using an online or live lecture: does it matter? *J Gen Intern Med* 2002;**17**:540–5.
60. Buzzell PR, Chamberlain VM, Pintauro SJ. The effectiveness of web-based, multimedia tutorials for teaching methods of human body composition analysis. *Adv Physiol Educ* 2002;**26**:21–9.
61. Vichitvejpaisal P, Sitthikongsak S, Preechakoon B *et al*. Does computer-assisted instruction really help to improve the learning process? *Med Educ* 2001;**35**:983–9.
62. Williams C, Aubin S, Harkin P *et al*. A randomized, controlled, single-blind trial of teaching provided by a computer-based multimedia package versus lecture. *Med Educ* 2001;**35**:847–54.
63. Seabra D, Srougi M, Baptista R. *et al*. Computer aided learning versus standard lecture for undergraduate education in urology. *J Urol* 2004;**171**:1220–2.
64. Grantcharov TP, Kristiansen VB, Bendix J *et al*. Randomized clinical trial of virtual reality simulation for laparoscopic skills training. *Br J Surg* 2004;**91**:146–50.
65. Jordan JA, Gallagher AG, McGuigan J *et al*. A comparison between randomly alternating imaging, normal laparoscopic imaging, and virtual reality training in laparoscopic psychomotor skill acquisition. *Am J Surg* 2000;**180**:208–11.

66. Gerson LB, Van Dam J. A prospective randomized trial comparing a virtual reality simulator to bedside teaching for training in sigmoidoscopy. *Endoscopy* 2003;**35**:569–75.

67. Collins MF. Measuring performance indicators in clinical pharmacy services with a personal digital assistant. *Am J Health Syst Pharm* 2004;**61**:498–501.

68. Carroll AE, Tarczy-Hornoch P, O'Reilly E *et al.* The effect of point-of-care personal digital assistant use on resident documentation discrepancies. *Pediatrics* 2004;**113**:450–4.

69. Stengel D, Bauwens K, Walter M *et al.* Comparison of handheld computer-assisted and conventional paper chart documentation of medical records. *J Bone Joint Surg* 2004; **86A**:553–60.

70. Bates DW, Gawande AA. Improving safety with information technology. *N Engl J Med* 2003;**248**:2526–34.

71. Pallawala PM, Lun KC. EMR-based TeleGeriatric system. *Medinfo* 2001;**10**:849–53.

CHAPTER 138

Clinical audit of healthcare

Rhona Buckingham[1], Jonathan Potter[2] and Adrian Wagg[1,3]
[1]Royal College of Physicians, London, UK
[2]Formerly Royal College of Physicians, London, UK
[3]University of Alberta, Edmonton, Alberta, Canada

> In order to work out how to improve we need to measure and understand exactly what we do.
> Making data on how well we are doing widely available to staff, patients and the public will help us understand variation and best practice and focus on improvement.
>
> Lord Darzi, *High Quality Care for All*, Department of Health, 2008.[1]

> At present, PROMs [patient reported outcome measures], other outcome measures, patient experience surveys and national clinical audit are not used widely enough. We will expand their validity, collection and use.
>
> *Equity and excellence: Liberating the NHS*, Department of Health, 2010.[2]

Definition

The Healthcare Quality Improvement Partnership (HQIP) in its *Local clinical audit: handbook for physicians* describes clinical audit as 'an approach to quality improvement based on clinical data collected by clinicians, to support the work of clinicians in improving the quality of care for patients.

Clinical audit is, first and foremost, a professional and clinical tool, not a management or regulatory tool. The General Medical Council (GMC) guidance requires all doctors to seek to improve the quality of care. Clinical audit provides a method for achieving such improvement'.[3]

Clinical audit has many definitions. One definition, internationally recognized and endorsed by the HQIP, comes from the *Principles of Best Practice in Clinical Audit*.[4]

> Clinical audit is a quality improvement process that seeks to improve patient care and outcomes through systematic review of care against explicit criteria and the implementation of change. Aspects of the structure, process and outcomes of care are selected and systematically evaluated against explicit criteria. Where indicated, changes are implemented at an individual, team, or service level and further monitoring is used to confirm improvement in healthcare delivery.

The following chapter will expand on the components of this definition.

Background

Clinical audit and quality of healthcare

Professor Avedis Donabedian introduced the modern era of clinical audit with his seminal works in the 1960s–1980s.[5,6] He introduced a rigorous approach to improving quality in healthcare and developed the concept of measuring structure (what is needed to provide a good service), process (what is done to provide a good service) and outcome (what is expected of a good service) as key elements to evaluating quality of care. In the 1980s Royal Colleges were promoting medical audit as part of good professional practice. Over time, medical audit became clinical audit, recognizing that care is a multidisciplinary process, but audit remained a local activity with modest impact on the service.

In 1997, the new Labour Government introduced a sea change in the role of quality management in the NHS with the White Papers, *The new NHS; modern and dependable*, and *A first-class service: quality in the new NHS*. Quality of care was no longer to be the preserve of individual professionalism but became a matter of management responsibility. The government sought to improve the quality of healthcare by:

- Continual improvement in the overall standards of clinical care;
- Reducing unacceptable variations in clinical practice;
- The best use of resources so that patients receive the greatest benefit.

These aims were to be achieved by:

- Setting, delivering and monitoring quality standards;

Principles and Practice of Geriatric Medicine, Fifth Edition. Edited by Alan J. Sinclair, John E. Morley and Bruno Vellas.

• Making quality of care a management responsibility rather than just a professional commitment.

To execute these changes the government established bodies and programmes as indicated in Table 138.1.

In 2008, the government White Paper, *High Quality Care for All*, authored by Lord Darzi, built on the undoubted success of bodies such as the National Institute for Health and Clinical Excellence (NICE) and the Healthcare Commission in setting standards, monitoring standards and laying the foundation for improved patient care. The White Paper re-emphasized the importance of measuring performance, benchmarking and the use of data to drive change.[1]

In 2010 the White Paper, *Equity and excellence: Liberating the NHS*, provided the new Coalition Government vision for how the changes introduced in 1998 and reinforced by Lord Darzi could be developed further. The role of national audit was strongly endorsed with two particular changes of emphasis:[2]

1 The need to measure outcomes.

Organizational process targets would be downgraded and the emphasis would be on measures of clinical performance that are directly linked the improved health outcomes.

2 The need to embrace the patient perspective of healthcare.

The patient perspective would be incorporated increasingly into measurements of healthcare building on the use of patient satisfaction, patient reported experience measures and patient reported outcome measures.

Quality of healthcare can be broken down into 'domains'. Donabedian proposed two domains: technical quality of care and interpersonal quality of care. More recently the Institute of Health Improvement have proposed widening the concept to include six domains, namely: safety, effectiveness, patient centredness, timeliness, efficiency and equity.[7] Lord Darzi in *High Quality Care for All* emphasizes the importance of safety, effectiveness and the patient experience.[1]

Table 138.1 National developments to implement the quality agenda in healthcare–1997.

Setting standards
- National Institute of Clinical Excellence (NICE)
- National Service Frameworks (NSFs)
- National Clinical Governance Support Team (NCGST)

Delivering improvements in care
- Modernization Agency
- National Information Strategy

Monitoring standards
- Commission for Health Improvement (CHI)
- Performance Frameworks
- Patient Councils

National clinical audit

National audits have demonstrated over time how clinical audit can provide valuable information to address these domains of quality and contribute to improved service provision and patient care. National clinical audits, such as that of stroke[8] and myocardial infarction[9] have demonstrated the great variation in care in hospitals around the country as well as the dramatic changes and improvements in practice that have occurred over time. Data from such audits have had a significant impact on the formulation of national policy for developing services as well as providing local teams with invaluable data with which to seek improvements in care at a local level.

In addition to contributing to improving healthcare, national clinical audits serve other roles including providing a basis for research, education and revalidation.

Local clinical audit

Local clinical audit, while being routinely incorporated into the work requirements of trained doctors and doctors in training, has struggled to maximize its potential. In 2008 the Healthcare Quality Improvement Partnership was commissioned by the Department of Health to not only manage the national clinical audit programme, but also to re-invigorate local audit. The Partnership has initiated many projects to enhance local audit and has provided a much needed champion for all those involved in local audit.

Within the medical specialities, specialist societies have advanced their commitment to clinical audit, seeking to coordinate work, and provide web-based data collection systems to facilitate multisite local audit. Societies such as the British Thoracic Society have been in the vanguard of these developments. Such approaches will help all clinicians maximize the use of local clinical audit for the benefit of patients.

The audit cycle

Planning an audit

Identifying what is to be reviewed

It is sensible, for pragmatic reasons and on the basis of the research evidence relating to effective clinical audit, to focus on topics where there is a perceived inadequacy or variation in patient care or service provision. Professionals with specialized areas of interest may wish to perform an audit of local practice. Audit may be used as part of the clinical governance mechanism to explore aspects of care where there are concerns over the quality of care or where there have been significant numbers of complaints.

The value of an audit can be enhanced if the topic to be evaluated is important to several or many sites. It may be

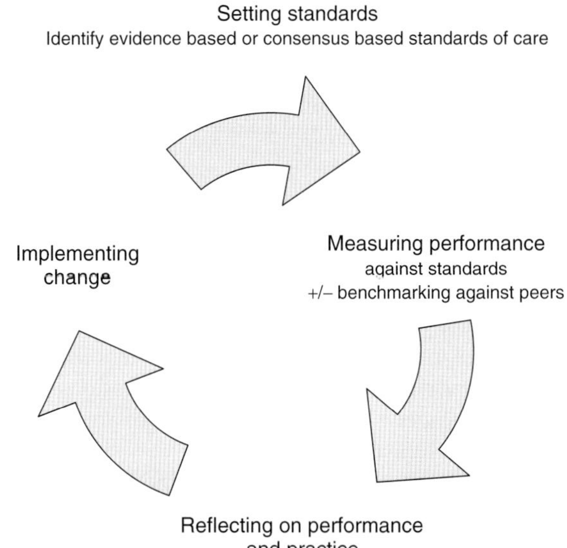

Figure 138.1 The audit cycle.

possible, either on a regional basis or via a specialist society, to coordinate the audit over a number of sites so that the data can be used to 'benchmark' local performance against that achieved by peers elsewhere in the country.

Commitment to audit

The recommendations of the Bristol Inquiry emphasized the importance of clinical audit within the system of local monitoring of performance and the need for trusts to fully support such activity – including access to time, facilities, advice and expertise.[10] These recommendations, welcomed by the government, echo the findings of systematic review, that clinical audit will only be successful if it is adequately resourced and it becomes part of routine practice.

Commitment is not just a clinical matter. It is essential that healthcare organizations as a whole seriously embrace these recommendations so that when results are available clinicians and managers are both willing to respond and jointly plan appropriate changes.

The planning phase needs to look ahead to how the conclusions will be used. This ranges from the need to include variables that allow for useful interpretation of the results as well as quality considerations to ensure the results are valid and reliable. The huge potential of audit for improving care can only be realized if the outcomes of each study are accepted as valid by all parties and thus utilized as the basis for reviewing and adapting practice.

Skills for carrying out audit

The infrastructure required includes access to skilled personnel (with dedicated time for the project) to carry out the work and systems to facilitate audit. Expertise is required in establishing a sound methodology for the work (see the following text) including an understanding of such issues as the size of population required for study, identifying relevant data for collection, the reliability and feasibility of data collection, data analysis, data presentation and implementation of change. Even apparently simple tasks such as setting out a questionnaire are in practice quite difficult. Poorly phrased or ambiguous questions result in data that cannot be interpreted. Therefore, most projects should be performed in conjunction with non-clinical staff with experience and expertise both in the technical aspects and in project management. They need support from professional healthcare workers to ensure the clinical acceptability and credibility and hence the validity of the study. At a local level, clinical teams should, therefore, work with clinical audit departments to ensure issues of methodology and project management are properly addressed. For national clinical audit significant investment in such audit infrastructure is required to ensure effective project delivery.

A multidisciplinary team is required that can effectively oversee and provide advice on the planning, carrying out and dissemination of the results of audit work. The group should include user involvement.

Modern audit has been made possible by the widespread availability of computing systems. They include software that can facilitate data collection, code and encrypt patient identifiable data and do sophisticated analysis. Access to such resources and expertise will enhance the audit process.

Patient and user input

Health services exist to serve the public and any assessment of care quality should include patient and users as full partners at all stages of the assessment process. Feedback from service users may shed a useful light on where services are inadequate, and also on the users' perspective of what is important as opposed to the views of management and professionals. Kelson has provided useful advice as to how user involvement can be achieved.[11]

As well as involving patients in the setting up and running of audits it is increasingly important to ensure that audit evaluates care from the perspective of the patient or user.[12,13] The patient perspective can be measured in terms of:

1 Patient satisfaction measures.

These measures provide a global assessment of the healthcare received [process] or the outcomes of care [outcomes] from the patient perspective. Such measures are helpful in monitoring trends but are very non-specific and provide no insight into the cause of any inadequacy of care.

2 Patient reported experience measures (PREMs).

These gather more specific feedback from patients with regard to the process of care received. These do provide an insight into where deficiencies in service provision lie from the patient perspective. Such measures are useful for assessing care for patients with chronic conditions.

3 Patient reported outcome measures (PROMs).

Such measures are currently much in vogue. There is a disease-specific component and a global component that measure the patient's perception of their health status following an intervention. Currently such measures are developed and in use in the NHS for surgical procedures, for example hip surgery, varicose veins surgery, hernia repair and cataract surgery. PROMs for more medical conditions are in the process of being developed.

Determining standards

As indicated in Figure 138.1, explicit standards of best practice must be established against which to audit. The important first step is to establish a statement or statements of the level of practice against which healthcare is to be assessed. There are two approaches: (1) define a gold standard and assess against that absolute target, or (2) collect comparative data and assess relative performance against the benchmark created by what one's peers are doing. In theory, the gold standard is preferred but often the evidence needed to set that standard is lacking. Furthermore, gold standards can rarely command 100% compliance, for example the Coronary Heart Disease NSF (National Service Framework) target for 30 minutes 'door to needle' for thrombolysis was set at 75% to allow, for example, for those where diagnosis was delayed.[9]

Evidence-based standards

Where possible, such statements of best practice should be derived from evidence-based research. The process calls for careful attention to literature searching, critical appraisal and peer review. The methods used by such bodies as the Cochrane Collaboration, the Scottish Intercollegiate Guideline Network (SIGN), and the National Institute for Health and Clinical Excellence (NICE) all ensure a high degree of credibility in the recommendations derived. Evidence-based audit standards can be determined from such recommendations.

Example: The NICE Clinical Guideline on 'Chronic Obstructive Pulmonary Disease' (COPD) has as an evidence-based recommendation that 'The presence of airflow obstruction should be confirmed by performing spirometry. All health professionals managing patients with COPD should have access to spirometry and be competent in the interpretation of the results'.[14] The audit criterion proposed to complement the recommendation is: 'Percentage of patients with a diagnosis of COPD who have had spirometry performed'.

The role of NICE is becoming increasingly important in not only developing guidelines but also in producing associated quality standards.

Consensus-based standards

Where it is not possible to obtain evidence-based standards consensus techniques should be used.[15] These will enable the best opinion of current health practice to be determined. The challenge in such a process is to ensure that there is no bias due to individual personalities or professions and to ensure that the views of all interested parties are included. Approaches include the following:

Consensus panels: the use of panels who receive expert advice and representation and who then formulate a statement of best practice.

Nominal group techniques: relevant parties are brought together to discuss recommendations. Chairing has to be skilled to ensure that all view points are heard and to ensure that a full range of options are considered. Voting is in a blinded fashion so that personal views are expressed.

Delphi exercises: postal questionnaires are sent to a large range of individuals with a relevant interest. Statements of practice are proposed and voted on. Recommendations are refined and recirculated so that the recommendations move toward a consensus of the views of the group.

Selection of gold standard

In practical terms, healthcare settings will need to determine what aspect of care they wish to audit. They will then need to seek the most appropriate standard(s) against which to audit, which has the authority of being derived from one of the approaches above.

Determining audit criteria

The Donabedian principle of measuring structure, process and outcome remains the basis for selecting the type of audit criteria.

Structure

Measures of the facilities and resources available to a healthcare setting will reflect the potential to provide high-quality care. It is difficult for staff to provide a high-quality service unless they have the resources to do it. Equally, it has to be recognized that high-class care is not guaranteed in premium facilities. Facilities have to be matched with staff who are provided with training and the expertise to carry out the appropriate care.

Example: For coronary heart disease, if a hospital does not have access to immediate coronary angiography it is not possible to provide the highest quality care for people with acute coronary syndromes.

Measures of 'structure' can include facilities, staffing levels, skill mix, access to training, standard use of protocols, mechanisms for advice and information for patients and relatives. Data relating to 'structure' are the easiest of the audit measures to obtain. Such data form the basis of accreditation schemes and systems of this type are widely used internationally and in some parts of the United Kingdom as an indication of service quality.

Process

Audit criteria of 'process' explicitly define key aspects of care that should be provided if high-quality care is to be achieved. Aspects of process measured may include the history, examination, investigation, treatment and follow-up care. The process may also include the involvement of carers. Processes of care need to be clearly defined to ensure reliable comparison between different sites and different data collection episodes.

Example: In stroke care, a swallow assessment is important as a process. The audit has to define what constitutes an appropriate swallow assessment and what detail within the records reliably reflects what was carried out. Process data may be collected retrospectively by reviewing a selected number of cases. Such an approach has significant problems in ensuring that there is no selection bias in the notes that are retrieved. A planned retrospective audit such as the National Sentinel Audit of Stroke[8] (assessing the care of 40 *consecutive* stroke patients in all hospitals in England, Wales and Northern Ireland) reduces the risk of bias. An alternative, but organizationally more challenging, approach is to obtain prospective data with data collection part of routine practice as in the Myocardial Infarction National Audit Project (MINAP).[9] In practice, measurement of process provides a useful reflection of whether care matches up with expected best practice. Data related to process can be more difficult to retrieve than measures of structure but tend to be easier to collect than outcome measures and have the added benefit that they are not dependent on case mix. Structure, process and outcome are all interrelated. Data from the National Stroke audit has demonstrated that settings where good structures are in place presage better processes of care and lead to better outcomes. It is rarely apparent, however, at the outset, which will be the most sensitive measures. Increasing clinical audit experience will help provide an indication of the structures and processes that are important in determining high-quality care. There are problems, however. If specific processes are identified as the markers for quality, departments and services wishing to be seen to provide high-quality care may concentrate purely on the selected process to the detriment of overall care.

Outcomes

Ideally, the quality of healthcare should be evaluated by the outcomes it achieves.

Example: For urinary incontinence, does appropriate assessment and treatment of patients result in a reduction in the prevalence of incontinence?

Outcomes may be recorded as outcome 'measures', for example prevalence of a condition or death at 30 days, or as an outcome 'indicator', for example percentage of asthma patients given a steroid inhaler on discharge. The latter is a process proxy that is linked to risk of readmission but is not in itself an outcome. Outcome 'measures' can be difficult to utilize. Consideration needs to be given as to whether an outcome 'measure' is a true measure or a surrogate measure. For the treatment of osteoporosis, reduced fracture rate is more important than increased bone density, although the latter is easier to measure. When measuring outcomes great care needs to be given to: the definition of terms, clarifying numerator and denominator populations, case mix and sample size (see 'Collecting data' below).

Outcome 'indicators' provide an alternative to outcome 'measures' and have the potential advantage of being (1) measurable and (2) having face validity for those involved in treatment, that is, it is not surprising that giving out an effective therapy works. While it is important to determine whether outcome measures can be used, in practice it may be more pragmatic to use outcome indicators.

Whether 'measures' or 'indicators' are used, it is important to be clear from whose perspective the outcome is being considered, is it that of the professionals, the management, the patients, or the carers? For stroke, professionals may seek the best neurological recovery, the patient may seek the best functional recovery, and the management may seek the most cost-effective recovery, all of which will be measured in different ways. The patient perspective is increasingly important[2] and may be recorded as patient satisfaction, experience or outcome.[12,13]

Outcomes provide data that most directly demonstrate progress with improving healthcare. In the future health outcomes will be increasingly sought as a measure of healthcare performance.[2] However, there are pitfalls in using data in this way that need to be carefully borne in mind. League tables relying on outcome measures have generated some bizarrely anomalous results and are mistrusted. One District General Hospital which was a beacon site for stroke care had a very high stroke death rate (Hospital Standardized Mortality Rate (SMR) was approximately 120) but the district SMR was only 94. As a beacon site, the hospital was keeping all patients with transient ischaemic attacks and mild strokes out of hospital or in intermediate

Table 138.2 Considerations with regard to clinical audit data collection.

Defining terms
Defining populations
Case mix adjustment
Sampling
Data sources
Define data analysis
Consent and confidentiality
Piloting

care facilities – thus the hospital SMR was based upon a different population compared with other hospitals. If public scrutiny of outcome measures is to occur, great care will be required to adjust for the potential confounding factors.

Collecting data

Issues that need to be considered are shown in Table 138.2.

Defining terms

Consistency in data collection requires accurate definition of terms throughout the audit proforma.

In the National Sentinel Stroke Audit (organizational)[16] for example, patients should be managed in a 'stroke unit' but in the absence of an accurate definition of such a unit, responses to audit questions are unlikely to be consistent.

All patients with suspected stroke should have brain imaging and in the majority of cases this needs to be conducted rapidly – within 24 hours after admission. However, if the patient is moribund, this may not be appropriate and thus in collecting data for audit purposes, a 'No but ... ' option will allow the case to be excluded because the standard is not applicable.

The appropriate data to collect from notes must be clear. If a blood pressure measurement is required during a hospital stay, is it the first recorded measure, the mean, or a measure at some specific time point that is required? How does the data collector deal with a comment written in the notes such as 'blood pressure normal' rather than a specific measure?

It is essential that these issues are clearly addressed or there will be considerable variability in the audit data collected from different sites and between different auditors. Advice sheets or notes addressing these issues are extremely helpful to audit teams and should, where possible, be backed up with recourse to the audit developer to clarify specific issues if necessary.

The development of standardized, or national data sets, are also helpful as they establish key data to be collected and identify the problems that may arise in data collection.

Defining populations

Outcome measures are often expressed as prevalence rates.

Good healthcare for urinary incontinence should reduce the prevalence of incontinence. How will the population with urinary incontinence be defined, identified and measured (the numerator)? Is this the population within a ward, a hospital, a general practice list, a Primary Care Trust? Is the prevalence to be determined per 1000 population, per number entering a service or on a GP list (the denominator)? In making comparisons with other healthcare settings it will be important that both the numerator and denominator are comparable.

Again, clear advice to the auditing team from the audit developer is essential.

Case mix adjustment

Comparisons of outcomes between settings will require case mix adjustment.

When planning an audit, the ways in which data will be presented, and to whom, should suggest what objections are likely to be raised to the results. Usually, these will be because a particular confounding factor has not been considered. Adding the appropriate extra variables increases the work of the audit but ensures that the results/comparisons are accepted as valid.

Example: For urinary incontinence when comparing between care in different nursing homes, it will be important to be aware of the physical dependency and cognitive function of people whose care is being assessed. Differences in the numbers of people with dementia and with relevant physical disability such as stroke, will have an important impact on the prevalence and management of continence.

There are many potential factors to take into consideration in case mix adjustment. In practical terms, it is sensible to collect only case mix data that are relevant to the planned presentation and use of the data.

Sampling

The sample size must be determined to ensure that meaningful results are obtained. Numbers will vary according to the measure being audited. These are statistical considerations that will not be described in detail, but intended to ensure that the results of an audit are robust enough to justify changing care practice and are not simply chance findings.

In the National Sentinel Audit of Stroke (clinical),[8] each site retrospectively reviewed a minimum of 20 and a maximum of 60 case notes of patients admitted between 1 April 2008 and 30 June 2008 with a primary diagnosis of stroke. If analysed alone, it would be hard to reach many conclusions but when compared with 11 300+ cases from other hospitals, the statistical power is greatly increased.

For outcome measures, a power calculation is required depending on the degree of change expected. If the desire is to see whether the management of osteoporosis is satisfactory using fractured femur as an outcome measure, many thousands of cases will need to be studied. If the outcome measure is the appropriate prescribing of bisphosphonates to prevent osteoporosis, meaningful results can be obtained with small numbers of subjects and can be achieved within hospital departments or general practices.

It may not be possible or practical to obtain all records and some method of randomization may be required. This may be achieved by collecting all cases over a limited period of time – or by the use of random numbers. Care must be taken to ensure that all randomly identified cases are obtained so that no systematic bias influences the findings. It may, for example, prove difficult to obtain notes when a person has died. Exclusion of such patients may have an important bearing on the evaluation of quality of care.

Data sources

Clinical data are usually obtained from patient records following identification of eligible cases often via coding systems in healthcare organizations, such as Hospital Episode Statistics (HES) in England which capture ICD-10 (diagnosis) and OPCS-4 (procedures and interventions) information, or 'Read Codes' in General Practice.

The difficulty in obtaining reliable data retrospectively from patient records is familiar to most healthcare professionals. Unless there has been a predetermined data set incorporated into the records systems, there will be inherent difficulties in obtaining reliable data. Processes and outcomes of care may occur without being recorded. The data required may not be readily accessible. Different departments and practices use different data record systems.

In order to increase the likelihood of reliable data collection, it is advisable to limit the numbers of items to be collected and to give careful consideration to what is most reliably available and important in the record systems to be reviewed.

For the future, standardized data collection systems in routine practice, for example standardized admission clerking sheets or IT systems, will simplify data collection. Furthermore, the goal should be to incorporate required audit data items into routine collection so that prospective real-time audit data collection becomes possible.

Consent and confidentiality

Issues of consent and confidentiality are complex.

The General Medical Council[17] makes it very clear that patients have a right to have their medical data handled confidentially, but also makes it clear that doctors must keep good records and should actively evaluate the services they deliver. Therefore local audit, that is the evaluation of care quality within the clinician team, is considered a part of direct medical care and does not require specific patient consent nor is it subject to formal ethical approval. Whilst clinical audit does not require formal ethical approval, it must nevertheless be conducted within an ethical framework which means abiding by the principles of the Data Protection Act.

The Data Protection Act in the United Kingdom and parallel European legislation provide important safeguards to individuals to ensure that any data (paper or electronic) held on them is handled in a responsible manner that reflects their wishes.

Many patients have care from different parts of the healthcare system, for example diagnosis of a tumour in a district hospital followed by referral to a tertiary centre for radiotherapy. Within cancer networks both secondary and tertiary units form part of the cancer team, such that when evaluating the effectiveness of care both parts are important. The concept of the 'domain of care' or 'care across interfaces' is more useful than simply considering the institution. While it is permissible to collect data from the records of identified individuals, it is not permissible to identify those individuals in any of the resulting reports or analyses without the specific consent of that individual. A guidance document from the HQIP provides useful information with regard to the Data Protection Act and related issues.[18]

An important feature in the data protection legislation is that patients receiving care should be made aware of how their data are to be used. It has not been routine practice in the United Kingdom to provide leaflets for patients about the use of their data but this is now increasingly required along with information as to how individuals can 'opt out' of allowing their data to be used. The National Diabetes Audit was one of the first to provide such information and to develop a process to manage those patients who chose to opt out.[19]

Many audit studies would like to combine data from more than one unit and thus require local units to submit data to a central analysis system. This can only be done under three very specific conditions:

- If the locally collected data are fully anonymized, that is, all identifiers such as name, date of birth, post code, are removed then the data may be transmitted to a centre to be aggregated and analysed.
- If some of the identifiers are retained within the data but encrypted or 'pseudonymized' in such a way that no one in the central team can 'read' the original, then the data are treated as 'effectively anonymized'. This may be useful if it

is required at a later stage to link the data on an individual across more than one database – an activity that can be performed within the machines via the encrypted identifiers, and without needing central staff to break the code.

• If specific consent has been obtained from each patient to permit the transmission and use of their data.

It is a requirement for every NHS organization to have a Caldicott Guardian.[20] This is normally a senior health professional who oversees all procedures affecting access to person-identifiable health data. Anyone establishing an audit that requires data to be shared beyond the 'clinical domain' should check with the Caldicott Guardian to ensure that all necessary precautions have been taken. Those collecting data must also consider other aspects of confidentiality such as the need to store data files in a secure filing cabinet or on a secure computer, and that data protection duties extend not only to the rights of the patient but also to the rights of the clinicians delivering the services.

Piloting

It is essential to pilot an audit project to test the method for identifying cases, along with the feasibility of collecting information from records and entering them to the data-collection tool, be it paper or electronic. Testing a 10% sample in a pilot phase will provide an opportunity to assess inter-rater reliability by asking more than one person to collect and submit data from the same sample, as well as checking the data to see if they present a reasonable reflection of practice.

An evaluation of the pilot phase should lead to refinements of the methodology, data collection tools and supporting documents prior to the full audit, as appropriate.

Dissemination and change

The benefits of clinical audit as a quality improvement tool can only be realized if there is a mechanism for stimulating change to improve future care where change is required. Knowledge translation (KT), achieving the translation of research evidence into practice is an increasingly well-researched area of which audit and feedback forms just a portion. Unfortunately, the evidence for the impact of audit and feedback alone in promoting change shows only a small effect and needs to be supplemented by other KT techniques to achieve a lasting impact.[21] Certainly the very act of performing the audit serves a function in raising awareness of the subject under study, and any working group involved in putting together the audit can act as champions (see below) for the audit.

It is, in general terms, impossible to over-communicate during the period of the audit to maximize awareness. An integrated approach to communication as the audit progresses is important to keep auditors engaged, deal with problems along the way and keep the process alive. Once the results are available then they must be as widely distributed as possible, and in various forms, depending upon the intended audience. Generating an audit report is really only the first stage in the change process. Feedback to and engagement of clinical teams on the ground is important to begin the process.

Many different techniques have been used and researched to achieve change, such as mentorship and facilitation by an external 'change agent', peer and reminders (see Table 138.3). It is clear, however, that certain elements must be in place to maximize the impact of clinical audit as a tool for quality improvement as achieving change in a complex healthcare system (like the UK National Health Service) is difficult. Relevant factors appear to be: (1) motivation of key stakeholders to achieve the target for change; (2) instrumental, personal and interactive resources for change; (3) motivators outside the service, including the larger healthcare environment and government; and (4) opportunities for change – that is, how key stakeholders understand the change options. Unless these are addressed it is unlikely that improvements in practice, and hence the benefit of audit, will be realized. Likewise, the audit data must be perceived as valid and credible, be presented in a timely fashion to motivate change, be constructive, rather than destructive and complemented by both local ownership and a managerial commitment for change.[22]

Commitment

Clinical teams may accept the findings of an audit but be unable to improve care because they do not have the authority to make the required organizational or financial changes needed to facilitate this. Change therefore requires the active cooperation of both clinical and management teams in order to do this. Each audit project needs to ensure that the results will have sufficient credibility (data reliability, numbers, case mix) and that clinicians will embark on the discussions needed to create change. Planning should ensure that the right data are being collected, that the audit topic is considered important by the end users and that the aims are shared by all parts of the organization before data collection even begins.

The influence of a local champion in achieving change should not be neglected. Diffusion of innovation theory, using a social model[23] indicates that these individuals can have a marked impact upon the adoption of innovations. Published data, however, suggest that such champions have mixed effects on professional practice and that it is not always clear how their characteristics are defined or what they do that causes action.[24]

Table 138.3 Classification of quality improvement strategies (QIS) and their relative effectiveness.

Intervention	Level of effectiveness†
Clinician/patient driven QIS	
Evidence-based medicine	?
Clinical practice guidelines	+++
Care pathways Guideline-based derivative tools that stipulate when certain actions should be taken in the longitudinal care of specific patient groups.	+
Educational outreach Upskilling of clinicians in their usual work environment by specially trained 'academic detailers' or content experts who may use written materials, case conferences, office or clinic visits, and practice reviews and feedback as educational tools.	++
Local opinion leaders Influential and respected clinicians working within local practice environments who encourage others to seek their opinions on best practice and emulate their practice routines.	++
Audit and feedback	+++
Physician practice profiling Internal peer comparisons and feedback based on relative utilization of tests, treatments and procedures, but in the absence of analysing concordance with evidence-based recommendations	++
Peer case reviews Review of individual cases of patient care provided by one clinician (or clinician group) by one or more peers not involved in the care of the original patients	+
Clinical decision support systems Formal manual or computerized systems that prompt, remind and caution clinicians to do, or not do, certain things under specific clinical circumstances.	+++
Continuing medical education	-For most didactic +++ For small group interactive
Professional development and self-directed learning Deliberate processes of reflection, analysis of critical incidents encountered in personal practice, self-assessment and self-audlt, and personalized, self-directed learning based on identified gaps in knowledge and skills.	? Depends on methods
Extended professional roles Extension of professional roles of non-physician clinicians such as hospitalists, nurses, clinical pharmacists and others to include more of the tasks previously undertaken by other disciplines. Synonmys included 'task transfer' or 'task substitution' initiatives.	Clinical pharmacists ++ Other disciplines?
Interdisciplinary collaboration and teamwork	?
Patient-mediated quality improvement strategies	+++
Chronic disease management Programmes intended to manage patients with one or more chronic diseases using systematic, multifaceted interventions comprising multidisciplinary care teams, patient self-management strategies, co-ordinated care teams with delivery system redesign, clinical information systems that track patient progress, care processes and outcomes, and evidence-based decision support.	+++
Specialty outreach programmes Delivery of medical specialist consultative services colocated with primary care and community care settings	+++

(continued overleaf)

Table 138.3 *(continued)*.

Intervention	Level of effectiveness[†]
Multisite quality improvement collaborations The Institute of Healthcare Improvement in the USA, the National Health Service Modernization Agency in the UK and the National Institute of Clinical Studies in Australia have sponsored a number of multisite collaborations in hospital and primary care settings aimed at improving care for specific patient populations.	++
Manager/policy-maker driven QIS	
Continuous quality improvement programmes Programmes aimed at continually improving care delivery aimed at providing a 'good' service that meets or exceeds patient expectations. Attributes of patient safety, convenience, timely access to care and efficiency of service delivery are the primary focus.	+
System re-engineering (or business process redesign) Major structural changes, both clinical and managerial, across whole systems of care delivery aimed at improving care delivery and outcomes. Changes may relate to better use of information technology, measurement and reporting of performance; integration of services; realignment of payment policies; use of disease management strategies; quality and safety improvement programmes; and more efficient management structures.	Varies
Risk and safety management Systems that seek to minimize the frequency of preventable health care-related adverse events and reduce the medicolegal liability of individuals and organizations. Strategies include sentinel incident reporting, root cause analyses, risk registries and open disclosure policies.	?
Adjuvant models of care Models of care that obviate either the need for hospitalization or, if it is required, minimize the length of stay and reduce the need for readmission. Such strategies include formal discharge planning and facilitation procedures (with or without dedicated discharge coordinators), transitional care schemes (such as subacute care wards supervised by nurses for patients who require predischarge convalescent or rehabilitative care), acute care in the home programmes and community or home-based rehabilitation.	+
Public scorecards ad performance reports Many countries including the USA, UK, Canada and Australia have witnessed a growth in public release of hospital 'report cards' or 'scorecards', which, in some cases, have been used to rank hospitals according to performance.	
Pay for performance schemes Key attribute is a defined change in reimbursement to a clinical provider (individual clinician, clinician group or hospital) in direct response to change in one or more performance measures as a result of one or more practice innovations.	++ if directed to clinician groups
External accreditation and quality improvement Formal review of institutional performance by external accreditation agencies, which may or may not be coupled with external quality improvement organizations seeking to improve quality of care.	?
Clinical service networks Networks of like-minded institutions or groups of clinicians, which serve as agents of service change and improvement across large-area jurisdictions, with some acting as budget-holders and assuming purchaser–provider functions	+
Clinical governance Systematic coordination and promotion of activities that contribute to continuous improvement of quality of care: clinical audit; clinical risk management; patient/service user involvement; professional education and development; clinical effectiveness research and development; staff focus; use of information systems; and institutional clinical governance committees.	?

[†]Source: Reproduced from Scott I. What are the most effective strategies for improving quality and safety of health care? *Internal Medicine Journal* 2009;**39**:389–400, Table 2, with permission from Wiley-Blackwell.

Identifying the cause of problems

Where results of the audit show a divergence from accepted best practice, the reasons need to be investigated. Never presume that the observed divergence is the 'fault' of individuals, good staff may be handicapped by inadequate organization, poor facilities or resources available for service delivery, or the problem may relate to poor or outdated clinical practice. Once a cause has been identified, an action plan can be drawn up to address the problems.

Achieving change

Evidence suggests that there is considerable variation in the effectiveness of differing methods of achieving change. Most recent systematic reviews indicate that multifaceted intervention is not necessarily needed so long as one of the more successful targeted approaches is used. Details of the effectiveness of differing interventions are shown in Table 138.3. As noted above, simple feedback of results may not be enough and effects are most often small, although larger changes are noticed when the deviations from the accepted standards are large.[25,26] A recent meta-analysis building on the previous Cochrane review and using a theoretical framework first described in industry concluded that feedback needed to be frequent, non-punitive and individualized at the level of the individual practitioner and paired with goal setting for improvement in practice.[27] There are additionally data from a Cochrane review showing efficacy of printed educational materials in achieving positive change in professional behaviours and patient outcomes.[28]

The UK National Health Service's Institute for Innovation and Improvement (www.institute.nhs.uk) website contains a library of quality improvement and sustainability tools that are applicable to change management following audit and feedback which span every stage of the quality improvement cycle.

Sharing of data

Access to audit data has become an increasingly important issue. With the advent of clinical governance derived from the NHS White Paper *The new NHS: modern and dependable*,[1] audit has become very much part of the management process. Clinical data is increasingly required and used in monitoring the quality of services provided and the individual performance of clinicians. Audit data from multicentre projects are made available at local Hospital and Primary Care Trust level, to strategic health authorities and nationally to the Department of Health and to regulators such as the Care Quality Commission and form part of the annual quality report from each national health service institution. The National Clinical Audit Advisory Group in the UK National Health Service, established to advise the Department of Health with regard to national clinical audit, has recommended that all national clinical audits in England and Wales provide publicly accessible, institution identifiable audit results. Results therefore need to be presented in a manner that is understandable, with an accompanying commentary and will necessarily not include all the details of interest to clinicians. Such data will undoubtedly be used in revalidation of individual clinicians and in fitness to practice assessments as confidence in the quality of the data increases.

While this more open use of data is inevitable and will help drive the benefits of audit, it challenges those performing the audit process (managers and clinicians alike) to ensure that audit data are a true and fair reflection of the service and practice under review. This has implications for institutional support of clinical audit to ensure robust method, often such support at institutional level is lacking.

Re-audit and sustaining improvement

Cyclical re-audit must be carried out to 'close the loop'; to assess whether changes in service have resulted in improvement and to ensure that improvements are maintained. Ideally, with audit data incorporated into routine clinical care, prospective monitoring of performance can be maintained with minimal additional effort, but this is still a rare situation. Where recurrent cross-sectional audits are required, it is challenging for services to maintain continuous audit of one particular subject, particularly as priorities change over time.

Sustainability of change in clinical practice is also difficult and ideally the change required should fulfil the criteria specified by Rogers.[29] Such change should be compatible with existing routines; have relative advantage and not require extensive training; should be simple and customizable and its benefit should be observable to others. It is easy to see why the changes required in clinical practice, as judged by adherence to clinical standards or guidelines often do not meet many of these criteria and thus adoption is far more difficult. The Institute for Health Improvement (http://www.ihi.org/IHI/), based in Cambridge, Massachusetts, an internationally recognized body in the field of healthcare quality improvement, and the NHS Institute for Innovation and Improvement (www.institute.nhs/sustainability) both produce guidance, advice and toolkits for sustainability of change within clinical services, much freely available, which should aid the process.

In general practice other approaches have been adopted. The primary care information service (PRIMIS+) allows practitioners to compare anonymized data on practice performance. Although aimed primarily at enhancing data quality, it is hoped that ultimately patient care will also benefit. The Quality Outcomes Framework, essentially items of service linked to payment, has led to much attention being given to key disease-related indicators. These financial benefits are impossible to replicate at the individual level in the secondary care setting in a social healthcare system without performance billing but the apparent success of these programmes would suggest that a lesson could be learnt which might be applied to hospitals.

In England and Wales, an annual quality report, mandated by the Care Quality Commission, the regulatory body for health and social care is currently under review, but contains elements relating to participation in and acting on results of clinical audit to establish clinical effectiveness. Additionally, clinical revalidation for the UK General Medical Council will require clinicians to produce evidence of participation as part of the process.

Conclusion

There is good evidence that clinical audit performed well can identify substandard care, can stimulate changes that improve care, and can confirm sustained improvement. Although the principles have been known for many years, the use of clinical audit has not been maximized by the professions and only relatively recently has the health service taken clinical audit seriously in order to inform quality assessments. The advent of new information technology should make data collection relatively easy but has yet to reach every clinical setting, particularly in nursing care homes, and as electronic patient records continue to roll out, albeit slowly, so will the opportunities for continuous quality improvement The adoption of the minimum data set, such as the Minimum Data Set – Resident Assessment Index (MDS-RAI) for care home residents, would be a major step forward for the UK. Such datasets have been adopted in many other countries, allowing standardized data to be collected for the benefit of many patients including the frailest in society. Clinicians need to take the opportunities that now exist to contribute to well-designed and targeted clinical audit programmes. Subjects should be chosen which are of priority importance locally and nationally and where there is evidence from other sources that current practice is suboptimal. Clinicians need to be involved with the intention of seeking sustained improvements in the service they provide and all clinicians should seek to ensure that their job specification includes time for audit. Healthcare management needs to be committed to the process, and this is likely to be the case given the drive towards outcomes assessment as the benchmark for clinical performance. This commitment needs to include the infrastructure, in terms of well-established audit departments whose direction is an integral part of the Trust strategy. There should be investment in systems for simplifying data recording and retrieval and there should be a commitment to routine audit data collection. Management also needs to demonstrate willingness to review and improve facilities, resources and staffing if such is required to improve services. Success breeds success. The realization that audit can induce change and improvement would strongly encourage commitment to the process.

Key points

- The clinical audit is a quality improvement tool.
- Clinical audits have demonstrated variances and inadequacies in healthcare.
- Audits can measure structure, processes or outcomes.

References

1. Department of Health. *High Quality Care for All*, HMSO, London, 2008.
2. Department of Health. *Equity and excellence: Liberating the NHS*, HMSO, London, 2010.
3. Healthcare Quality Improvement Partnership (HQIP). *Local clinical audit: handbook for physicians* August 2010 http://www.hqip.org.uk/assets/Guidance/Local-clinical-audit-handbook-for-physicians-August-2010-FINAL.pdf (last accessed 13 January 2012).
4. National Institute for Health and Clinical Excellence (NICE). *Principles for Best Practice in Clinical Audit*, Radcliffe Medical Press, Oxford, 2002.
5. Donabedian A. Evaluating the quality of medical care. *Milbank Memorial Fund Quarterly: Health and Society* 1966;**44**(3 suppl 1):166–206.
6. Donabedian A. The quality of care. How can it be assessed? *JAMA* 1988;**260**:1743–8.
7. Institute for Healthcare Improvement. Improvement methods, 2010. http://www.ihi.org/IHI/Topics/Improvement/caseforimprovement.htm (last accessed 5 December 2011).
8. Royal College of Physicians. *National Sentinel Stroke Audit: Phase II (clinical audit)* 2008. http://www.rcplondon.ac.uk/sites/default/files/stroke-audit-report-2008.pdf (last accessed 5 December 2011).
9. Myocardial Infarction National Audit Project (MINAP), 2009. http://www.ucl.ac.uk/silva/nicor/audits/minap/publicreports/pdfs/minappublicreport2009 (accessed 13 January 2012).
10. Department of Health. *Learning from Bristol: the Report of the Public Inquiry into Children's Heart Surgery at the Bristol Royal Infirmary 1984–1995*. Command paper CM 5207, HMSO, London, 2001.
11. Kelson M. *A Guide to Involving Older People in Local Clinical Audit Activity: National Sentinel Audits Involving Older People*, College of Health, London, 1999.
12. Coulter A, Fitzpatrick R, Cornwell J. *The Point of Care. Measures of patients' experience in hospital: purpose, methods and uses*, The King's Fund, London, 2009.

13. Devlin NJ, Appleby J. *Getting the most out of PROMS: Putting health outcomes at the heart of NHS decision making*, The King's Fund, London, 2010.
14. National Institute for Health and Clinical Excellence (NICE). *Chronic Obstructive Pulmonary Disease: management of chronic obstructive pulmonary disease in primary and secondary care*, NICE, London, 2010. http://www.nice.org.uk/nicemedia/live/13029/49425/49425.pdf (last accessed 5 December 2011).
15. Murphy MK, Black NA, Lamping DL *et al*. Consensus development methods and their use in clinical guideline development. *Health Technology Assessment, NHS R&D HTA Programme*, vol. 2, issue 3, Department of Health, London, 1998.
16. Royal College of Physicians. *National Sentinel Stroke Audit, Phase I (organisational audit)* 2008. http://www.rcplondon.ac.uk/sites/default/files/org-2008-concise-stroke-audit-round-6.pdf (accessed 13 January 2012).
17. General Medical Council. *Good Medical Practice*, 2006. http://www.gmc-uk.org/guidance/good_medical_practice.asp (last accessed 5 December 2011).
18. Harrison W, Sharp H. *An Information Governance Guide for Clinical Audit*, Healthcare Quality Improvement Partnership, London, 2010. http://www.hqip.org.uk/assets/Downloads/Information-Governance-and-Audit-Guide.pdf (last accessed 5 December 2011).
19. What is the national diabetes audit? Information Centre, London, 2010. http://www.ic.nhs.uk/webfiles/Services/NCASP/Other%20related%20documents/142832%20IC%206pp%20Diabetes.pdf (last accessed 5 December 2011).
20. Department of Health. *The Caldicott Guardian Manual*, 2010. http://www.dh.gov.uk/prod_consum_dh/groups/dh_digitalassets/@dh/@en/@ps/documents/digitalasset/dh_114506.pdf (last accessed 5 December 2011).
21. Jamtvedt G, Young JM, Kristoffersen DT *et al*. Audit and feedback: effects on professional practice and health care outcomes. *Cochrane Database Syst Rev* 2003;**3**:CD000259.
22. Bradley EH, Holmboe ES, Mattera *et al*. Data feedback efforts in quality improvement: lessons learned from US hospitals. *Qual Saf Health Care* 2004;**13**:26–31.
23. Rogers EM. *Diffusion of Innovations*, 5th edn, Free Press, New York, 2003.
24. Doumit G, Gattellari M, Grimshaw J, O'Brien MA. Local opinion leaders: effects on professional practice and health care outcomes. *Cochrane Database Syst Rev* 2007;**1**:CD000125.
25. Jamtvedt G, Young JM, Kristoffersen DT *et al*. Audit and feedback: effects on professional practice and health care outcomes. *Cochrane Database Syst Rev* 2006;**2**:CD000259.
26. Jamtvedt G, Young JM, Kristoffersen DT *et al*. Does telling people what they have been doing change what they do? A systematic review of the effects of audit and feedback. *Qual Saf Health Care* 2006;**5**:433–6.
27. Hysong SJ. Meta-analysis: audit and feedback features impact effectiveness on care quality. *Med Care* 2009;**47**:356–63.
28. Farmer AP, Légaré F, Turcot L *et al*. Printed educational materials: effects on professional practice and health care outcomes. *Cochrane Database Syst Rev* 2008;**3**:CD004398.

CHAPTER 139

Carers and the role of the family

Jo Moriarty
King's College London, UK

> I was rung just before Christmas and was told that my mother [aged] 94 was ready for discharge that afternoon. I was also told that no one was available to help me until well after Christmas! I am 70 years old.
>
> Respondent to survey of carers' experiences of hospital discharge[1]

> Carers often have a deep insight into the condition of the person they are caring for ... They need to be treated by professionals as "Partners in Care". [When carers are excluded, this can lead] to poorer outcomes for all and sadly on occasions [put] the person and their carers at risk.
>
> Chief Executive of voluntary organization[2]

Introduction

These opening statements highlight the importance of the role played by carers and families in achieving successful outcomes in geriatric medicine. Without carers' expert knowledge about the person for whom they care and the practical and emotional assistance that they provide, many older people receiving geriatric healthcare might otherwise need to remain in hospital or move into long-term care. Nevertheless, although professionals and policy-makers now possess much greater appreciation of the part played by carers than they did in the past, many carers and families continue to lack all the support that they need.

Over the past 30 years, a substantial literature on caring has developed and this chapter summarizes some of the key studies in the field that have especial relevance for clinicians working in geriatric medicine. It outlines some of the particular issues faced by those caring for an older person and some of the ways of identifying carers whose own health may be put at risk, either because of their own existing health problems or because their caring responsibilities have become too great. Examples of the types of support that carers find beneficial are given. However, it should be recognized that the chapter only provides a brief overview and there is an extensive literature on caring that goes beyond the material presented here.

Definitions of caring

Origins of the terms 'carer' and 'caregiver'

The Oxford English Dictionary reports that the first use of the term 'carer' to describe the unpaid work undertaken by people – generally women – looking after relatives or friends in need of support because of age, disability, or illness occurred in the late 1970s and early 1980s. In North America and Australasia, the term 'caregiver' is used more frequently than 'carer'. Both words share a similar etymological history in that their use can be dated from the time when increases in life expectancy and changes to the organization of systems of care for older people led to greater numbers of older people living at home and a reduction in the number of long-stay institutions. This coincided with wider recognition of the role played by women, in particular, in undertaking unpaid domestic work, often at the expense of their own opportunities for paid employment and for leisure time. Before long, it became clear that carers themselves comprised an extremely heterogeneous group and that this variation would influence their experiences of caring. For example, the terms 'women in the middle' and the 'sandwich generation'[3] were coined to describe the multiple responsibilities of women combining care of older parents or parents in law with other family and employment responsibilities. Other examples of attempts to differentiate between different types of carer include research looking at those caring for someone with a particular health problem, such as dementia,[4] stroke,[5] or Parkinson's disease,[6]

Principles and Practice of Geriatric Medicine, Fifth Edition. Edited by Alan J. Sinclair, John E. Morley and Bruno Vellas.

the impact of kin relationships, such as being a daughter or spouse carer,[7,8] and the ways in which carers' demographic characteristics such as ethnicity[9–11] or sexuality[12] impact upon experiences of caring.

Conceptually, definitions of caring go beyond merely providing assistance with tasks such as shopping or bathing that people are unable to carry out independently by themselves.[13] Caring almost always takes place within pre-existing relationships and there are likely to be strong ties of affection or obligation[14,15] which strongly influence how older people and their carers respond to clinicians' recommendations about future care options, particularly when these involve a possible move into long-term care.

Distinctions between paid and unpaid caring

The appropriation of the term 'carer' or 'caregiver' to describe paid workers has meant that the prefix 'family' is increasingly added to the words carer or caregiver to differentiate between those with paid and unpaid roles. Even when family carers and those for whom they care are not biologically or legally related to each other, they often regard themselves as fictive kin, meaning that they may describe themselves as, for example, husband or wife, as if they had the actual relationship implied by the title. The term 'informal carer' was once used quite widely but family carers and organizations representing family carers criticized its failure to reflect the reality that so-called 'informal' carers provide the overwhelming majority of assistance to those in need of support. This is illustrated by secondary analysis of data on a representative sample of the older UK population which showed that 80% of those needing help with domestic tasks or activities of daily living such as washing or dressing received support only from members of their family, friends or neighbours with just 20% receiving help from any type of paid worker or volunteer.[16]

While this chapter is concerned with the support provided by family carers or caregivers, it should be recognized that blurring between paid and unpaid care does occur. For example, in the case of intergenerational transfers, older people may provide resources to adult children or grandchildren in return for care. Alternatively, a person originally employed to do domestic work may, over time, take on more and more caring tasks should their employer begin to require help with activities of daily living, such as washing and dressing. In instances such as this, the two may develop close ties that go beyond the traditional relationship between employer and employee. The introduction of 'cash for care' schemes through which family carers of older people receive a cash grant which can be used to pay for care in many countries in the more developed world has shifted the boundaries between the two further.[17]

Changes to the way' carer' and 'caring' are conceptualized

More recently, some commentators, especially those associated with the disability movement, have challenged the assumptions underpinning the words 'carer' or 'caring', criticizing its construction of people needing assistance in their daily lives as 'dependants' or 'recipients of care' and calling for new paradigms that reflect the realities of the reciprocities between carers and those for whom they provide support.[18,19] Thus, while 'carer' and 'caring' remain useful shorthand words to describe the range of support that is given in the context of relationships of kinship or affinity, they are not value free and may be interpreted in a variety of ways.

Legal frameworks

As Chapters 143–148 which describe different healthcare systems throughout the world show, variations in legislative and funding arrangements impact upon the type of assistance received by older people and their carers. In some countries, increasing recognition of the role played by carers has resulted in new legislative entitlements. These are not in themselves guarantees that carers will receive all the help that they need but they do influence the type of support that multidisciplinary geriatric teams can call upon when arranging care for their patients. In the UK, three pieces of legislation: the Carers (Recognition and Services) Act 1995; the Carers and Disabled Children Act 2000; and the Carers (Equal Opportunities) Act 2004 have given those defined as providing 'regular and substantial' care the rights to have their needs assessed and to receive services in their own right. In Australia, while there is no national legislation to protect carers, several states have introduced their own legislation, for example the South Australian Carers Recognition Act 2005. In Germany, the introduction of long-term care insurance (*Pflegeversicherung*) has improved the position of carers[20] while, in Finland, carers are entitled to cash benefits in return for a contractual agreement to provide a certain amount of care.[21] Carers may also have rights arising from employment or equalities legislation that protects them from discrimination arising from their status as carers. However, this picture is very variable and much may depend upon the extent to which family members are held legally responsible for the care of their older members and the existence of some policies which can actually penalize those who are providing care because the person for whom they care then loses his or her rights to support from statutory sources.[22]

Assessment of family carers

Even when there is no legal obligation to assess carers' needs, good practice dictates that geriatric assessments also include an assessment of what support is provided by family carers and how they are managing. Carers' assessments need to identify, first, what support carers are providing and secondly, their feelings about how they are managing their caring role.

Typologies of caring

The gerontological and caregiving literature established some time ago[23,24] the nature of the inter-relationships between older people's needs, the extent and type of support they receive from family caregivers, and how its availability affects the need for support from 'formal' services such as home care (home health aides), sheltered accommodation and extra care housing (assisted living) and long-term care. In summary, it demonstrates that while friends and neighbours are likely to provide help with transportation, housework and shopping, it is rare for them to provide support with more intimate or personal activities, such as washing, bathing, or assistance in eating and drinking. Furthermore, where an older person has extensive support needs, for example if they are unable to be left alone for more than a few minutes (sometimes described as 'critical interval needs'),[25] it is generally only those carers who live in the same household as the person for whom they care or who live nearby who are able to provide this level of help. Most often, the majority of caring is undertaken by one person on his or her own (the primary carer), although 'secondary' carers may be involved. The most frequent example of a secondary carer in North American, European and Australasian societies is an adult daughter living apart from her parents but who supports one parent caring for the other. In Asian countries, the role of primary carer would traditionally be taken by the daughter in law. Where carers are providing help without any assistance from other family members or friends they are described as 'sole carers'.

It is important to establish exactly how much help carers provide on a daily basis and if other family or friends are providing any other assistance. As with comprehensive geriatric assessment (see Chapter 112) and assessment of residents in long-term care, carers' assessments need to be multidimensional in order to reflect the profound and far-reaching ways in which caring affects people's lives.

A theory that has been profoundly influential in the literature is the Stress Process Model[26] which distinguishes between *objective* stressors, that is, those factors that are attributable to the disease or disability in the person cared for, for example needing help to get washed or dressed, and *subjective* stressors, the extent to which the carer perceives these problems as causing them stress. The next subsections summarize some of the key areas that have been associated with carer stress. However, it is important to recognize that this process should not merely focus on deficits, such as the absence of social support, but should also take account of the strengths that carers may have,[27] such as their sense of determination or motivation.

Increased risk of psychological ill health

The effects of one person being almost wholly responsible for another person's care over time are considerable. While it is difficult to demonstrate direct causal relationships between caring and psychological health, there is strong evidence from both the United States (US) and the UK that some carers are in poorer psychological health than their age- and gender-matched counterparts in the general population.[28,29] Strikingly, the prevalence of psychological ill health among carers is associated with more intensive forms of caregiving, such as caring for a person in the same household and caring for more than 20 hours a week.[29]

An important message from this research is that clinicians should not assume that *all* family carers are at risk of psychological ill health but should aim to become more effective at identifying those family carers who are *at greater risk* of experiencing difficulties than others. In particular, clinicians need to be aware that while many family carers derive satisfaction and pride from their contribution, and wish to continue caring, there are circumstances in which the difficulties they face may outweigh the positive aspects of caring.

The impact of the cared-for person's health needs

Earlier chapters in this book have described the impact of long-term health problems such as dementia and other cognitive disorders (see Section 7), stroke (see Chapters 57 and 58), and Parkinson's disease (see Chapter 63). In addition to the way that these diseases impact on the lives of those older people directly affected by these conditions, research suggests that high levels of difficulty are reported among those caring for a person with dementia[30] or Parkinson's disease[6] and following a stroke.[31] Where the clinical picture also includes behavioural problems and aggression, then additional stressors may also be experienced.[30]

Physical health

As the opening quotation to this chapter showed, adult child or spousal caregivers of persons receiving geriatric healthcare are themselves likely to be older and at risk of age-associated health problems of their own. Poor physical health in carers does not necessarily result in poor psychological health but the deleterious effects of ill health seem to be most pronounced among older carers who may already be experiencing poor psychological health.[30]

Specific problems reported by carers include acquiring back pain from lifting or aggravating the pain of arthritis as a result of helping someone else wash and dress. Caregiving has also been found to be associated with reduced functioning of the immune system,[32] meaning that carers may be more vulnerable to, or take longer to recover, from illness. However, despite high levels of physical frailty among many family caregivers, healthcare providers may actually have increased expectations about the tasks that they ask family caregivers to provide. There is some evidence that improved health technology has meant that many carers are undertaking tasks that in the past would have been undertaken by nurses or healthcare assistants.[33]

Financial aspects

Efforts have now been made to quantify the contribution made by family carers in terms of the costs of replacing family care with paid care and in the opportunity costs to carers as a result of their reduced opportunities for employment and leisure. For example, a report on dementia expenditure in the UK[34] concluded that dementia cost the UK economy around £19.7 billion per year (approx. US$30 billion). Of this, almost half could be attributed to the contribution made by family carers. On an individual level, carers may incur extra expenditure to pay for equipment, services, heating and clothing. In addition, they may give up paid employment, forego promotion prospects, or retire early. While women are still likely to be affected more severely than men, particularly in terms of being able to build up savings and a pension in retirement, this is an issue for both genders.[35]

Social support

Social isolation and loneliness are frequently reported by carers who may no longer have the time to meet up with family members and friends, or to pursue hobbies or other interests. Carers not only report feelings of loss and social isolation in their relationships with others, their relationship with the person for whom they care may also have altered. Others have argued that levels of *received* (or enacted) social support may not be as important as how carers *perceive* they are supported. Thus, good overall levels of perceived social support may be associated with increased carer well-being.[36] By contrast, if a carer does not feel supported, then he or she may express feelings of distress even if others are providing help.

Coping styles and strategies

Carers use a number of strategies to help them cope with caring[27,37] and these may influence the extent to which they seek and utilize support from others, including support from professionals and other family members. However, the exact nature of the relationship of coping styles to outcomes for carers and the person for whom they care is uncertain, not least because of uncertainties inherent in the disease process itself. Further, the use of coping strategies may reflect patterns developed over the life course which is why it can be valuable to find out how carers and those for whom they care have responded when faced with difficult life events at earlier times in their lives. It can also be helpful in enabling carers to identify the strengths that they bring to their caring experiences.

Screening measures for carers

A number of standardized measures have been developed to help identify problems faced by carers and summaries of the ones that have been used most extensively exist.[38,39] Unfortunately, the majority of these measures were developed for use in research and only a small number have been tested for their suitability in routine clinical settings where speed and ease of administration and scoring are important factors contributing to clinical utility. Examples of comparatively short screening measures designed to identify carer stress that have been psychometrically tested include the *Screen for Caregiver Burden* (SCB)[40] and the *Zarit Burden Interview* (ZBI),[11] also available in shorter 12 and 4-item versions.[42] Both were originally developed for caregivers of people with dementia but have been widely used with other types of carer. However, given that these measures were originally developed with ethnically homogenous, largely white, samples of carers, questions have been raised about their cross-cultural validity and the ethnocentrism of some of the ways in which they conceptualize caring.[43] Although Japanese versions of the ZBI[44] and Chinese versions of the SCB[45] exist, this remains an under-researched issue and it should also be acknowledged that some carers, whatever their ethnic and cultural background, would find the concept of caring as a 'burden' distasteful.

The suite of instruments, the Carers' Assessment of Managing Index (CAMI), Carers' Assessment of Difficulties Index (CADI), and the Carers' Assessment of Satisfactions Index (CASI)[46] were developed as a way of moving away from the concept of burden and incorporating a recognition that caring may bring satisfactions as well as difficulties. However, they are quite long, albeit in a format that is suitable for self-completion by carers who do not have literacy or sight problems prior to a clinical interview. Alternatively, the *Carers of Older People in Europe* (COPE)[47] is shorter, identifies positive as well as negative impacts of caregiving, and has been used in six European Union countries and in New Zealand.[48]

Although instruments such as these can identify carers who are experiencing difficulties with their caring roles, they are not designed to screen for psychological ill health. Clinicians may wish to supplement a screening measure about caring with one of the widely used instruments to detect psychological ill health such as the *General Health Questionnaire* (GHQ)[49] or the *Center for Epidemiological Studies Depression Scale* (CES-D).[50] Alternatively, a measure of health-related quality of life (HRQoL), such as the *SF-36*[51] may also be valuable in identifying carers in need of additional support.

An important consideration for clinicians in geriatric healthcare settings is that carers' needs and QOL may change significantly if the person for whom they care has a progressive illness. Therefore, it is important to re-administer any standardized measures every 6–12 months in order to see if there have been any changes.

Arranging services to support carers

A number of services have been developed aimed at supporting carers, ranging from practical services designed to give carers a break from caring to psychoeducational interventions aimed at helping carers develop strategies to help them cope with different aspects of caring. Most of these will be delivered by other members of the multidisciplinary team including social workers, nurses, occupational therapists and psychologists. However, it can be helpful for clinicians to understand what these services are and why they have been found to be helpful.

In addition to the main interventions to support carers, described below, the interconnectedness of the lives of many carers and the older people for whom they care means that services ostensibly aimed at the older person, such as home care or hospital at home schemes may also be beneficial for carers, indicating that services for older people and services for carers need to be provided in tandem. Another example of the way in which services primarily intended for older people can bring benefits to their carers is the role of telecare (see Chapter 124). Assistive technologies may be particularly valued by carers who do not live in the same household as the person for whom they care.

Information

Satisfaction with information provision contributes to overall ratings of satisfaction among patients and carers. Despite this, the difficulty in accessing appropriate information at the right time is a constant theme within carer research. A Cochrane review of information provision for patients and carers following stroke concluded that while information improved patient and carer knowledge, it had no impact upon carer mood or satisfaction and that further work on the best way to provide information was needed.[52] Carers' accounts suggest that they value information that is timely and provided in both verbal and written forms. They also need a wide range of information, including information on the prognosis, symptoms and treatment for the person for whom they care but also about the services that might be available to them, including welfare benefits and information about financial and legal issues. A study of stroke survivors and their carers found that while carers were generally happy with the information they received about stroke, they were less happy with the provision of information on what community services would be available to them and information on legal and financial planning.[53] As with older people themselves (see Chapter 11), attention needs to be paid to using language that can be understood by a layperson and ensuring that any literacy or language needs on the part of carers are met. Organizations representing the interests of older people or carers have considerable experience in providing information and carers can be directed to the resources that they provide.

Studying recall is an important way of measuring the effectiveness of information provision but unfortunately more research on patients' rather than on carers' recall has been undertaken. However, good practice suggests that it is important to review the information provided to carers at a later date to see how much carers can recall about the information they have been given and whether it has been useful.

Carers' support groups

Support groups for carers generally fall into one of two types: the first is a time-limited intervention in which carers are offered training in how to deliver an aspect of care or in managing their caring roles. These will be described in more detail in the next section. The second offers an ongoing forum for carers to share their experiences and provide mutual support to each other. Long-term groups of this sort are also likely to provide a source of social support and social activities for their members. Although carers attending support groups generally evaluate them positively, not all carers are comfortable with the idea of meeting with others. In addition, substitute care arrangements may need to be made so that the carer is able to leave the person for whom they care.

Although carers' groups offering long-term support are generally open to anyone who wishes to attend, there are instances where attendance is restricted to carers sharing a certain characteristic, for example groups for people caring for someone with a specific disease. Another example is where carers share the same demographic characteristic such as being a member of a minority ethnic group[54] or being a lesbian, gay, bisexual or transgendered (LGBT) carer. In these instances, carers may be more likely to attend groups for specific types of carer because they feel reassured that that they will meet people in a similar position to themselves.

Carer and family support workers

One UK development that combines the role of information and support is that of the family support worker for stroke patients and their families. These workers also liaise with other professionals. They have been positively evaluated by carers with one evaluation suggesting that they can result in demonstrable improvements in QOL for carers.[55]

Carer education and training

A number of studies have looked at the effectiveness of carer education and training programmes. Of these, the majority have looked at the impact of psychoeducational programmes designed to support carers of people with dementia, especially in terms of helping carers develop problem-solving techniques to deal with behavioural problems. Examples include training in cognitive behavioural therapy (CBT)[56] for carers of people with dementia, a psychoeducational programme to help deal with behavioural problems,[57] and a combined educational and support programme supplemented by follow-up telephone support.[58] When combined with cholinesterase inhibitor therapy in the person cared for, one study reported positive effects on the levels of depression among carers from quite moderate levels of input (five sessions of counselling plus ad hoc telephone support).[59] The use of telephone support highlights the potential to use alternative forms of delivery to enhance or replace interventions that are provided face to face.[60]

Positive results have also been reported from interventions designed to support carers of people with a stroke. A UK study looked at the effectiveness of a training programme for carers while the person for whom they cared received rehabilitation after a stroke.[61] At follow-up, carers who had undertaken the training programme had better psychosocial outcomes than the control group who had not. It also resulted in reduced costs of care.

Respite services

Respite is the term used to describe a range of services giving carers a break, ranging from one or two hours in the home to overnight care in care homes or specialist units. As with 'burden', the word respite does carry some negative connotations for the person cared for and the term 'break' is more neutral. As well as services that offer carers a regular break from caring, emergency services are also likely to be needed. Carers of older people are more likely to be sole carers and this means that if they become ill or if a crisis occurs, emergency respite care will be needed, ideally in the person's own home but more probably in the form of temporary admission to a care home.

A number of studies have looked at the impact of respite services but the results present a mixed and sometimes contradictory picture.[62] Partly, this is because the outcome measures used most often (changes in carers' psychological health and reductions in admissions to long-term care) may not be amenable to change from the provision of comparatively small amounts of help. Carers themselves rate respite services highly when they are felt to be of sufficient quality and meet the preferences of both themselves and the person for whom they care. Carers and service providers have different perspectives about what constitutes respite. This means that it is important that respite care is offered in a form that is meaningful to carers. The advent of 'cash for care' schemes may result in more choices for carers about how they find ways of taking a break from caring.

Service effectiveness

One difficulty in evaluating the effectiveness of services for carers has been the continuing variability in the quality of research. There has been little consistency in approaches to sampling and in the selection of outcome measures. Outside the United States, the number of controlled intervention studies remains comparatively low. This means that effectiveness is often judged on the basis of very moderate levels of service input, delivered in differing ways to differing groups of people using outcomes that can be quite intractable to change – such as carers' psychological health – rather than their QOL or their perceptions of benefit. Few studies have included measures of cost effectiveness. There are issues about the cross-national relevance from studies based upon service systems which may be very different. Furthermore, there is a need for new forms of evaluation that take account of the outcomes that are important to carers, not just to service providers, researchers, or policy-makers.

Role of clinicians in service utilization

Classically, models of service utilization have looked at the predisposing, enabling and illness-level determinants in explaining an individual's service utilization.[63] However, this approach has been criticized for failing to take account of carer characteristics, especially among certain types of carer, such as carers from minority ethnic groups[64] who are generally thought to be under-represented in services designed to support carers. An issue that is rarely reported in the literature but exists widely in everyday practice settings is the role played by professionals in helping carers to reach decisions about which services to use. There is now a much greater focus in medical education on enabling clinicians to acquire good skills in communicating with patients but this also needs to be extended to communicating with carers. Although there is now much greater societal recognition of the role of carers, knowledge about what services are available to support carers remains limited. This means that it tends only to be at times of crisis, such as hospital admission, that carers are asked to make important decisions about the sort of services they want and they are very often reliant upon professionals to explain what help is available to them. This highlights the role of clinicians in signposting carers to potential sources of support and in liaising with other members of the multidisciplinary team. Follow-up and outpatient appointments provide a good opportunity to review the support provided to carers, as well as reviewing the treatment of the person for whom they care.

Discussion

Although this chapter has highlighted the diversity to be found among carers and the debates that exist about the effectiveness of different services to support them, a number of clear messages emerge. Many carers caring for older people using geriatric health services are themselves old and are providing considerable amounts of assistance. Although the majority of carers will not experience difficulties with their caring role, a substantial number will and this is usually influenced by the amount of care that they provide and the emotional context in which it is given. Interventions increasingly use a combination of methods and may be based upon the use of new technologies. The amount and type of care that will be required to sustain older people in the future is uncertain. Greater geographical and social mobility, changes in living arrangements with greater numbers of people living on their own and greater geographical distances between family members, may lead to changes in the way that care is provided. At the same time, new technologies offer new opportunities for people to remain in touch and to provide care at a distance. What is certain is that most family members continue to wish to care for their relatives. The challenge for services is in responding to the diversity of caregiving arrangements and in providing help that is acceptable to both carers and to those for whom they care.

Key points

- Carers provide the majority of support to older people needing help with their daily lives. Many of these are spouses with health problems of their own.
- It is possible to identify carers at greater risk of needing support themselves.
- Services need to be more focused upon the sort of help that carers themselves define as useful.

Acknowledgement

The preparation of this chapter was made possible by a grant from the National Institute for Health Research (NIHR) School for Social Care Research on social care practices with carers. The views expressed in this chapter are those of the author and not necessarily those of the NIHR School for Social Care Research or the Department of Health/NIHR.

References

1. Holzhausen E, Clark D. *You can take him home now: Carers' experiences of hospital discharge*, Carers National Association, London, 2001.
2. Standing Commission on Carers. *Report of the Standing Commission on Carers: 2007 to 2009*, Department of Health, London, 2009.
3. Brody EM. *Women in the Middle: Their Parent-Care Years*, 2nd edn, Springer, New York, 2004.
4. Bruce DG, Paley GA, Nichols P *et al*. Physical disability contributes to caregiver stress in dementia caregivers. *J Gerontol A Biol Sci Med Sci* 2005;**60**:345–9.
5. van Exel NJA, Koopmanschap MA, van den Berg B, Brouwer WBF, van den Bos GAM. Burden of informal caregiving for stroke patients. *Cerebrovascular Diseases* 2005;**19**:11–17.
6. McRae C, Sherry P, Roper K. Stress and family functioning among caregivers of persons with Parkinson's disease. *Parkinsonism and Related Disorders* 1999;**5**:69–75.
7. Murray JM, Manela MV, Shuttleworth A, Livingston GA. Caring for an older spouse with a psychiatric illness. *Aging & Mental Health* 1997;**1**:256–60.
8. Schofield HL, Murphy BM, Nankervis JM, Singh BS, Herrman HE, Bloch S. Family carers: women and men, adult offspring, partners, and parents. *Journal of Family Studies* 1997;**3**:149–68.
9. Dilworth-Anderson P, Williams IC, Gibson BE. Issues of race, ethnicity, and culture in caregiving research: A 20-year review (1980–2000). *The Gerontologist* 2002;**42**:237–72.
10. Katbamna S, Ahmad W, Bhakta P, Baker R, Parker G. Do they look after their own? Informal support for South Asian carers. *Health & Social Care in the Community* 2004;**12**:398–406.
11. Pinquart M, Sorensen S. Ethnic differences in stressors, resources, and psychological outcomes of family caregiving: a meta-analysis. *The Gerontologist* 2005;**45**:90–106.
12. Price E. Coming out to care: gay and lesbian carers' experiences of dementia services. *Health & Social Care in the Community* 2010;**18**:160–8.
13. Twigg J, Atkin K. *Carers Perceived: Policy and Practice in Informal Care*, Open University Press, Buckingham, 1994.
14. Finch J, Mason J. *Negotiating Family Responsibilities*, Routledge, London, 1993.
15. Qureshi H, Walker A. *The Caring Relationship: Elderly People and their Families*, Macmillan, Basingstoke, 1989.
16. Pickard L, Wittenberg R, Comas-Herrera A, Davies B, Darton R. Relying on informal care in the new century? Informal care for elderly people in England to 2031. *Ageing & Society* 2000;**20**:745–72.
17. Ungerson C, Yeandle S (eds), *Cash for Care in Developed Welfare States*, Palgrave Macmillan, Basingstoke, 2006.
18. Forbat L. *Talking about Care: Two sides to the story*, The Policy Press, Bristol, 2005.

19. Fine M, Glendinning C. Dependence, independence or inter-dependence? Revisiting the concepts of 'care' and 'dependency'. *Ageing & Society* 2005;**25**:601–21.
20. Schunk MV, Estes CL. Is German Long-term Care Insurance a model for the United States? *International Journal of Health Services* 2001;**31**:617–34.
21. Martimo K. Community care for older people in Finland. In: C Glendinning (ed.), *Rights and Realities: Comparing New Developments in Long-Term Care for Older People*, The Policy Press, Bristol, 1998, pp. 67–82.
22. Glendinning C, Tjadens F, Arksey H *et al*. *Care Provision within Families and its Socio-Economic Impact on Care Providers. Report for the European Commission DG EMPL Negotiated Procedure VT/2007/114*. Working Paper Number EU 2342, Social Policy Research Unit, York, 2009.
23. Wenger GC. A network typology: from theory to practice. *Journal of Aging Studies* 1991;**5**:147–62.
24. Chappell N, Blandford A. Informal and formal care: exploring the complementarity. *Ageing & Society* 1991;**11**:299–317.
25. Isaacs B, Neville Y. The needs of old people: the 'interval' as a method of measurement. *Br J Prev Soc Med* 1976;**30**:79–85.
26. Pearlin LI, Mullan JT, Semple SJ, Skaff MM. Caregiving and the stress process: an overview of concepts and their measures. *The Gerontologist* 1990;**30**:583–94.
27. Nolan M, Lundh U. Satisfactions and coping strategies of family carers. *Br J Community Nurs* 1999;**4**:470–5.
28. Schulz R, Newsom J, Mittelmark M *et al*. Health effects of caregiving: the caregiver health effects study: an ancillary study of the Cardiovascular Health Study. *Annals of Behavioral Medicine* 1997;**19**:110–16.
29. Hirst M. Caring-related inequalities in psychological distress in Britain during the 1990s. *J Public Health* 2003;**25**:336–43.
30. Pinquart M, Sorensen S. Correlates of physical health of informal caregivers: a meta-analysis. *J Gerontol B Psychol Sci Soc Sci* 2007;**62**:126–37.
31. Jones AL, Charlesworth JF, Hendra TJ. Patient mood and carer strain during stroke rehabilitation in the community following early hospital discharge. *Disability & Rehabilitation* 2000;**22**:490–4.
32. Hawkley LC, Cacioppo JT. Stress and the aging immune system. *Brain, Behavior, and Immunity* 2004;**18**:114–19.
33. Schulz R, Martire LM. Family caregiving of persons with dementia: prevalence, health effects, and support strategies. *Am J Geriatr Psychiatry* 2004;**12**:240–9.
34. Luengo-Fernandez R, Leal J, Gray A. *Dementia 2010: The economic burden of dementia and associated research funding in the United Kingdom*, Alzheimer's Research Trust, Cambridge, 2010.
35. Carmichael F, Charles S. The opportunity costs of informal care: does gender matter? *Journal of Health Economics* 2003;**22**: 781–803.
36. Chappell NL, Reid RC. Burden and well-being among caregivers: examining the distinction. *The Gerontologist* 2002;**42**:772–80.
37. Chappell NL, Dujela C. Caregivers – who copes how? *Int J Aging Hum Dev* 2009;**69**:221–4.
38. Deeken JF, Taylor KL, Mangan P, Yabroff KR, Ingham JM. Care for the caregivers: a review of self-report instruments developed to measure the burden, needs, and quality of life of informal caregivers. *Journal of Pain and Symptom Management* 2003;**26**:922–53.
39. Moriarty J. *Assessing the Mental Health Needs of Older People: Systematic Review on the Use of Standardised Measures to Improve Assessment Practice*, Social Care Workforce Research Unit, London, 2002.
40. Vitaliano PP, Russo J, Young HM, Becker J, Maiuro RD. The screen for caregiver burden. *The Gerontologist* 1991;**31**:76–83.
41. Zarit SH, Reever KE, Bach-Peterson J. Relatives of the impaired elderly: correlates of feelings of burden. *The Gerontologist* 1980;**20**:649–55.
42. Bédard M, Molloy DW, Squire L *et al*. The Zarit Burden Interview. *The Gerontologist* 2001;**41**:652–7.
43. Smith A. Cross-cultural research on Alzheimer's disease: a critical review. *Transcultural Psychiatry* 1996;**33**:247–76.
44. Arai Y, Kudo K, Hosokawa T *et al*. Reliability and validity of the Japanese version of the Zarit Caregiver Burden Interview. *Psychiatry and Clinical Neurosciences* 1997;**51**:281–7.
45. Holaday B, Chou K-R. A psychometric assessment of caregiver burden: A cross-cultural study. *Journal of Pediatric Nursing* 1997;**12**:352–62.
46. Nolan M, Grant G, Keady J. *Assessing The Needs of Family Carers: A Guide for Practitioners*, Pavilion Publishing, Brighton, 1998.
47. Balducci C, Mnich E, McKee KJ *et al*. Negative impact and positive value in caregiving: validation of the COPE index in a six-country sample of carers. *The Gerontologist* 2008;**48**:276–86.
48. Roud H, Keeling S, Sainsbury R. Using the COPE assessment tool with informal carers of people with dementia in New Zealand. *NZ Med J* 2006;**119**: 2053–.
49. Goldberg D, Williams P. *A User's Guide to the General Health Questionnaire*, 1st edn, NFER-Nelson Publishing Co. Ltd, Windsor, 1988.
50. Locke BA, Putman P. *Center for Epidemiological Studies Depression Scale (CES-D)*, Epidemiology and Psychpathology Research Branch, Division of Epidemiology and Services Branch, Public Health Service, National Institutes of Mental Health, Bethesda, MD, 1971.
51. Ware J Jr, Kosinski M, Keller SD. A 12-Item Short-Form Health Survey: Construction of scales and preliminary tests of reliability and validity. *Med Care* 1996;**34**:220–33.
52. Forster A, Smith J, Young J *et al*. Information provision for stroke patients and their caregivers. *Cochrane Database Syst Rev* 2008;**2**: CD001919.
53. Simon C, Kumar S, Kendrick T. Formal support of stroke survivors and their informal carers in the community: a cohort study. *Health & Social Care in the Community* 2008;**16**:582–92.
54. Monaghan DJ, Greene VL, Coleman PD. Caregiver support groups: factors affecting use of services. *Social Work* 1992;**37**:254–60.
55. Mant J, Carter J, Wade DT, Winner S. Family support for stroke: a randomised controlled trial. *Lancet* 2000;**356**:808–13.
56. Marriott A, Donaldson C, Tarrier N, Burns A. Effectiveness of cognitive-behavioural family intervention in reducing the burden of care in carers of patients with Alzheimer's disease. *Br J Psychiatry* 2000;**176**:557–62.

57. Ostwald SK, Hepburn KW, Caron W, Burns T, Mantell R. Reducing caregiver burden: a randomized psychoeducational intervention for caregivers of persons with dementia. *The Gerontologist* 1999;**39**:299–309.

58. Brodaty H, Gresham M, Luscombe G. The Prince Henry Hospital Caregivers' Training Programme. *Int J Geriatr Psychiatry* 1997;**12**:183–92.

59. Mittelman MS, Brodaty H, Wallen AS, Burns A. A three-country randomized controlled trial of a psychosocial intervention for caregivers combined with pharmacological treatment for patients with Alzheimer disease: effects on caregiver depression. *Am J Geriatr Psychiatry* 2008;**16**: 893–904.

60. Magnusson L, Hanson E, Nolan M. The impact of information and communication technology on family carers of older people and professionals in Sweden. *Ageing & Society* 2005;**25**:693–713.

61. Kalra L, Evans A, Perez I *et al*. Training carers of stroke patients: randomised controlled trial. *BMJ* 2004;**328**: 1099–101.

62. Arksey H, Jackson K, Croucher K *et al*. *Review of Respite Services and Short-Term Breaks for Carers for People with Dementia*, NHS Service Delivery and Organisation (SDO) Programme, London, 2004.

63. Andersen R, Newman JF. Societal and individual determinants of medical care utilization in the United States. *Milbank Memorial Fund Quarterly Health and Society* 1973;**51**:95–124.

64. Radina ME, Barber CE. Utilization of formal support services among Hispanic Americans caring for aging parents. *Journal of Gerontological Social Work* 2004;**43**:5–23.

CHAPTER 140

Nursing home care

David R. Thomas[1], Yves Rolland[2] and John E. Morley[3]

[1]Saint Louis University Health Sciences Center, St Louis, MO, USA
[2]INSERM Unit 1027, F-31073; University of Toulouse III and Gérontopôle of Toulouse, France
[3]Saint Louis University School of Medicine and St Louis Veterans' Affairs Medical Center, St Louis, MO, USA

Introduction

Nursing home facilities are more unique than similar. The care of elderly persons in institutionalized settings varies by country and region and in societal and cultural factors. Nursing homes also rapidly evolved because the quality of nursing home care has become a growing concern everywhere and because residents are generally showing increasing levels of disability and require increasingly more complex treatments. However, this evolution relies more on empirical practice than research studies. Only 2% of the research into the elderly population concerns nursing home residents.[1]

Approaches to long-term care in various countries include chronic geriatric hospitals, short-stay rehabilitation centres, residential living centres and institutionalized skilled nursing homes. The nomenclature of a facility varies across settings, including 'nursing home' in the United States and 'care home' in the United Kingdom. A 'nursing home' in the USA may refer to a specialized centre for persons on ventilators, with acquired immunodeficiency syndrome or with dementia who need skilled nursing care. A 'care home' in the UK generally refers to a home registered under the Care Standards Act providing personal and residential care for older people and also includes homes that provide nursing care (nursing homes). Not only is the classification confusing, but also the public, and often the professional, view of nursing homes involves a number of misperceptions.

Misperception: most older adults will live for many years in a nursing home and eventually die there. Truth: fewer than 5% of older adults in USA and fewer than 10% in the UK and France reside in resident and nursing home settings.

Misperception: once a person enters a nursing home, they stay there for good. Truth: many older adults who enter a nursing home will recover and leave (short-stay residents), while fewer older adults will remain in a nursing home once admitted (long-stay residents). In France, half of the nursing home residents will also have a hospitalization every year.[1]

Misperception: nursing homes are warehouses for older persons with little or no stimulation: Truth: a good home provides a social environment that often is very comforting for older persons who may have been isolated in previous living environments.

Misperception: no one likes living in a nursing home. Truth: many residents prefer the reassurance of medical care, socialization and a safe environment and find the experience positive.

Facility demographics

In the USA, there are ~16 100 nursing homes with ~1.5 million residents. The number of nursing home beds decreased in the USA from 1999[2] to 2004[3] from 1.9 to 1.7 million beds, respectively. The average number of beds per facility rose to 108 from 105. The occupancy rate (number of residents divided by number of available beds) was 86%. However, the demographics of facilities vary by country. In France, the number of beds in nursing homes is about five times higher (about 10 000 nursing homes for 60 million inhabitants with a bed occupancy close to 97%).

Ownership of most nursing homes in the USA is by for-profit entities (61%); 31% operate as voluntary non-profit facilities and the remaining 8% are owned by governmental entities (Figure 140.1). Half of the nursing homes are public in France. In the USA some 56% of nursing homes are affiliated with other nursing homes in a chain ownership. These facilities account for 57% of all beds, 57% of all residents and 61% of all discharges. Most nursing homes (62%) are located in a metropolitan statistical area.[4] The distribution of nursing homes is uneven, with the midwestern and

Principles and Practice of Geriatric Medicine, Fifth Edition. Edited by Alan J. Sinclair, John E. Morley and Bruno Vellas.

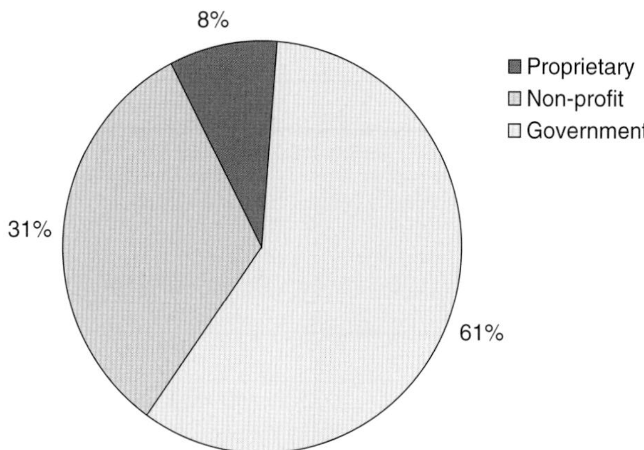

Figure 140.1 Percentage distribution of nursing home facilities by ownership: United States, 2004. Source: Jones AL, Dwyer LL, Bercovitz AR and Strahan GW. The National Nursing Home Survey: 2004 overview. National Center for Health Statistics. *Vital Health Stat* 2009;**13**(167):1–155.

southern US census regions having 34 and 32% of facilities and 32 and 33% of all beds, respectively.

The nursing home industry employs a large number of persons in various occupations (Figure 140.2). The rate of staffing does not appear to vary much by type of nursing home ownership. A major problem for patient care in nursing homes is the high staff turnover rate. A vacancy rate of 19% for nurses has been reported.[5] The turnover rate for nursing assistants has been reported to be as high as 93%.[6] These high vacancy rates disturb continuity and force continuous training of new personnel. This nursing home staff turnover impacts on the quality of care.[7]

Nursing home care is expensive. Residents in US nursing homes use several sources of payment (Figure 140.3). At admission, most residents reported private resources (42%) as a payment source, followed by Medicare (36%) and Medicaid, a means-tested governmental source in the USA (35%). However, during admission, residents using Medicare as a source of payment dropped to 13% of all current residents. Longer term residents reported private sources increasing to 66%, and those with Medicaid rose to 60%. The national cost of nursing home care was $53 billion in 1990 and was the fastest growing component of major healthcare expense in the national budget.[8] The projected cost for 2000 exceeded $140 billion and it may exceed $700 billion by 2030.[9]

These predictions of continued nursing home growth and expenditures are becoming modified by several societal changes. The proportion of Medicaid beneficiaries aged 65–74 years residing in nursing homes remained fairly constant at about 6% from 1999 to 2003, but the percentage of Medicaid recipients aged 85 years and older declined from 48 to 44% from 1999 to 2003. This does not reflect a decrease in Medicaid recipients, who increased from about 4.2 million in 1999 to 4.8 million in 2003.

The growth in community-based care alternatives to nursing homes, such as assisted living and other group residential options, has been suggested as one of the reasons for the shrinking nursing home population in the USA. However, there is considerable variability at the State level in the availability and provision of home- and community-based services to people with long-term care needs.[10] Because of the expense of nursing home care, several States have initiated programmes to favour home-based services financially. These trends will define the future number of nursing home beds required to care for the ageing population.

Nursing homes in other cultural settings differ considerably. For example, the Dutch experience demonstrates that among persons older than 65 years, ~20% had a short

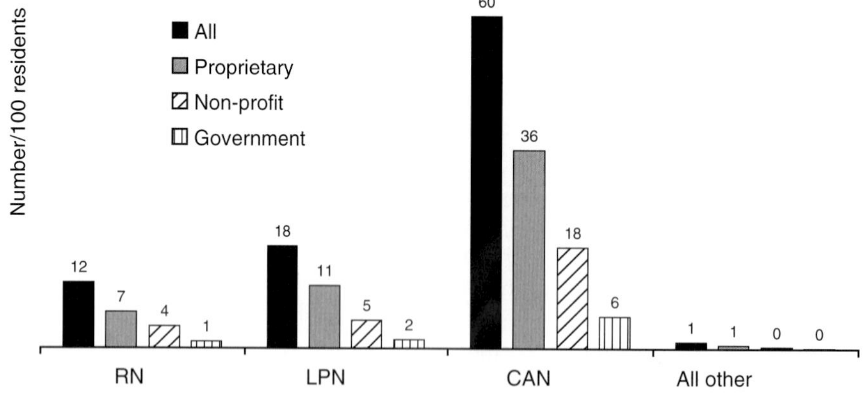

Figure 140.2 Number per 100 residents of full-time equivalent employees by occupational categories and selected nursing home characteristics: United States, 2004. CNA, certified nursing assistant; LPN, licensed practical nurse; RN, registered nurse. Source: Jones AL, Dwyer LL, Bercovitz AR and Strahan GW. The National Nursing Home Survey: 2004 overview. National Center for Health Statistics. *Vital Health Stat* 2009;**13**(167):1–155.

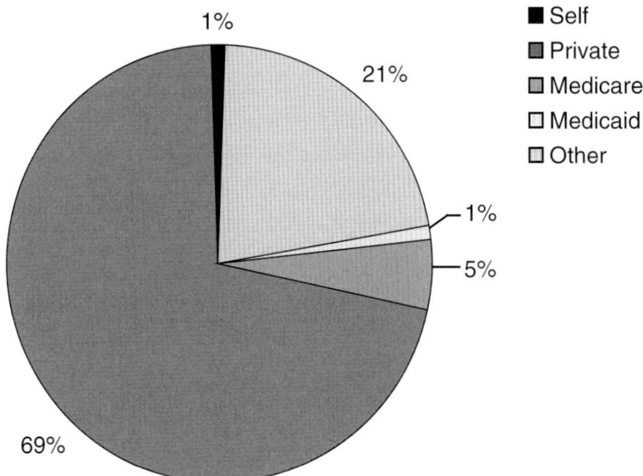

Figure 140.3 Nursing home payment source: long-term stay >90 days: United States, 2004. Source: Jones AL, Dwyer LL, Bercovitz AR and Strahan GW. The National Nursing Home Survey: 2004 overview. National Center for Health Statistics. *Vital Health Stat* 2009;**13**(167):1–155.

stay in an inpatient hospital department and 96% were discharged to their own home situation. Only 7% lived permanently in special institutions for chronic care, including residential care or nursing home care. Persons with physical disability or with progressive dementia, who have impaired activities of daily living (ADLs) and who need more complex continuing care beyond the range of home care services in a residential homes, are admitted to a nursing home. The number of nursing home beds is 3.6 per 1000 persons (in 2003), with a total of 330 nursing homes with ~26 000 beds designed primarily for persons with physical problems and 32 000 beds in psychogeriatric wards for persons with dementia. Nursing home care is covered by a mandatory national insurance system, the Exceptional Medical Expenses Act. In addition to the funds from this national insurance, income- and household-dependent out-of-pocket payments are obligatory for persons admitted to nursing homes.[11]

In the UK, the number of patients in private or voluntary homes rose from 18 200 in 1983 to 148 500 in 1994.[12] The number of institutional care beds for older persons doubled to 563 000 between 1980 and 1995. National Health Service beds accounted for less than 10% of the total in 1995 compared with 23% in 1980, while private and voluntary (not-for-profit) residential and nursing home beds increased to 76%.[13]

Persons in the UK receiving long-term care provided in care homes are required to meet financial means testing. Those who have assets, including the value of their homes (with some exceptions), above a limit (£23 250 in 2011) are required to pay the care home's fees in full. Those with assets below the limit make a co-payment that is usually less than the full fee. For those with the lowest income and assets, this payment may be met from Income Support, the UK's means-tested welfare benefit. Almost all older people who own their home would be required to meet care home fees in full. The same approach exists in France. The children are also constrained by a law obligating them to pay if the payment cannot be met by the resident.

Means testing dates back to 1948 in the UK and has changed little in the many years since then. However, the growing numbers of older persons and increasing home ownership have stressed the means test. Local public authorities are responsible for payment for long-term care for older persons who meet means test requirements, whether in a care home or in the person's own home. For care services delivered at home, the value of an older person's home is disregarded in determining how much he or she contributes. An older home owner is, therefore, likely to incur considerably more – and the public budget correspondingly less – of the cost of care in a residential setting than of the equivalent cost of care at home. The result is a financial incentive for public authorities to arrange for a home owner's care to be provided in an institution rather than in their own home. The financial incentive works in the opposite direction for older home owners themselves. Whether the likelihood of entry to a care home is increased or decreased by the level of an individual's economic resources would seem to depend on whether individual choice or the policy of the local public authority dominates.[14]

Resident demographics

In the USA, 43% of persons who were 65 years of age in 1990 will enter a nursing home in their lifetime. Of these, 55% will stay for at least one year and 21% will stay for five years or longer.[15] The percentage of retired patients who will pass through a nursing home during their lifetime is nearly double in some European countries.

Nursing home use is strongly associated with age, even after adjusting for disability. This suggests that the future need for nursing home care will increase as the population increases in life expectancy. By 2030, the need for nursing home beds in the USA is projected to increase to 5 million.[16,17]

Most nursing home admissions are for short-stay residents. About 2.5 million residents are discharged after an average length stay of 272 days. Long-stay residents remain in the nursing home for an average of 873 days.

In France, 70% of nursing home admissions come from hospital. Most of the time, the mean length of stay does not reflect the rapid turnover of a small proportion of the nursing home residents who died after a short stay while others stay for a longer period.[1] The changes in acuity and

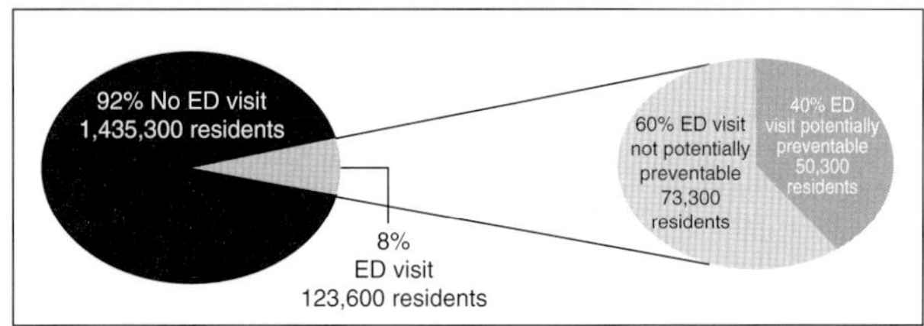

Figure 140.4 Percentage of nursing home residents with a potentially preventable emergency department (ED) visit in the past 90 days: United States, 2004. Source: CDC/NCHS, National Nursing Home Survey, 2004, http://www.cdc.gov/nchs/data/databriefs/db33.pdf (last accessed 7 November 2011).

dependence in most countries[18] result in increased needs such as care in the emergency department (Figure 140.4).[1,3]

Residents in nursing homes do not reflect the demographics of the general population. In the USA, most nursing home residents (71%) are female. Some 88% were aged 65 years and older and 45% were aged 85 years and older. The average length of time from admission for all nursing home residents was 835 days in 2004. The median length of time from admission was 463 days. Among nursing home residents aged 65 years and older, time from admission was less than 3 months for 19% of residents, 3 months to less than 1 year for 24% of residents and 1 year or more for 56% of residents. More than half of all nursing home residents were either totally dependent or required extensive assistance in bathing, dressing, toileting and transferring. In France, the mean age is about 84 years in a nursing home.

Nursing homes provide extensive services to residents. Almost all nursing homes reported providing nursing services (100%), medical services (97%) and personal care services that included ADLs (97%). Non-medical services most frequently offered by nursing homes include nutrition (99%), social services including assistance to residents and their families in handling social, environmental and emotional problems (98%) and physical therapy (97%). The least frequently offered services include hospice services (72%) and home health services (23%).

Nursing home regulation

In the USA, nursing homes are licensed by each state and require a certificate of need to operate. Each State regularly surveys nursing homes for compliance with State regulations. In addition, the Federal government contracts with each State to survey nursing homes for compliance with Federal regulations if the home receives payments from Medicare or Medicaid sources. Nearly all nursing homes (96%) have some form of certification. More than three-quarters of all facilities were certified by both Medicare and Medicaid. Only 4% of the 16 000 nursing homes were not certified.

Federal regulations are contained in two Congressional Acts, the Omnibus Budget Reconciliation Act of 1987 (OBRA '87) and the Balanced Budget Act of 1997 (BBA '97). OBRA '87 had a major impact on general nursing care, including the introduction of the Minimum Data Set (MDS), requirements for a Medical Director and the reduction in physical and chemical restraints. Regulations based on BBA '97 initiated the Prospective Payment System and consolidated billing. These Federal regulations have created standards of care in nursing facilities. The regulations resulting from OBRA '87 are divided into two parts. First, the law is stated. These statements are labelled by 'F-tags' and a number. An 'F-tag' is jargon for the actual law published in the Federal Register. Second, an interpretive guideline follows the regulation. The guidelines comprise the instructions used by surveyors to determine compliance with the law. Failure to comply with State or Federal regulations can result in fines or in decertifying the facility from participation in Federal programmes. A comparison of Federal quality-of-care indicators is published on the Internet and updated at intervals.

In the autumn of 2009, a new Minimum Data Set (MDS version 3.0) was implemented in the USA. Residents, families, providers, researchers and policymakers had expressed concerns about the reliability, validity and relevance of MDS 2.0. Some argued that because MDS 2.0 fails to include items that rely on direct resident interview, it fails to obtain critical information and effectively disenfranchises many residents from the assessment process. The new version MDS 3.0 was designed to improve the reliability, accuracy and usefulness of the MDS, to include the resident in the assessment process and to use standard protocols to evaluate nursing home residents.

A national testing of the MDS 3.0 was conducted in 71 community nursing homes in eight US States and in 19 Veterans' Administration nursing homes. The evaluation tested data reliability, the validity of new cognitive, depression and behaviour items, response rates for interview items, user satisfaction and feedback on changes and time to complete the assessment.

Improvements incorporated in MDS 3.0 produced a more efficient assessment with greater reliability and shorter completion time. A key component of MDS 3.0 was a focus on direct interviewing of the resident. For areas such as cognition, mood, preferences and pain, studies have repeatedly shown that staff or family impressions often fail to capture the resident's (or any adult's) real condition or preferences. Published measures of clinical conditions were incorporated into MDS 3.0 to increase validity. A direct-interview pain assessment, the Geriatric Pain Assessment,[19] uses resident self-report to obtain pain information. The pain severity items include the 0–10 scale, a recognized scale that is used in other settings, and the verbal descriptor scale, which may be easier to answer for some residents with cognitive impairment. Depression is assessed using the PHQ-9 instrument.[20] The Brief Interview for Mental Status[21] assesses cognitive function. The Confusion Assessment Method[22] evaluates delirium, an exceptionally common problem in nursing home residents.

In the UK, nursing homes are required to report on their quality-of-care activities each year and are also regularly visited by Health Care Inspectorate personnel.

Medical care

Care of residents in a nursing home is overseen by a physician. Each nursing home is required to have a physician Medical Director, who oversees the quality-of-care in the facility. Each resident is seen by their physician, who either visits them in the facility or arranges for clinic visits. The frequency of visits is dictated by medical necessity, but cannot be less frequent than once every 30 days for the initial 3 months following admission or less than once every 60 days thereafter. Physician extenders or nurse practitioners may also see residents in a facility, but may not be used to meet this minimum standard. In France, each nursing home is supposed to be coordinated by a geriatrician on duty two days per week. He or she is mainly responsible for the comprehensive geriatric assessment and the community health policy of the nursing home. However, their role is limited as the referring general practitioner of each resident is in charge of prescribing their treatment.

The number of physicians who see residents in a facility is small. Only one in 10 of US primary care physicians provides care in a nursing home; 77% of all physicians report spending no time in a nursing home. Only 15% of specialists spend any time in a nursing home. Among physicians who report seeing patients in a nursing home, a majority have spent less than 2 h per week with residents.[23] Contributing to this minimal involvement, over one-third of surveyed physicians report inadequate training in geriatric syndromes such as falls, incontinence, dementia, nutrition and chronic pain.[24]

Medical care in nursing homes focuses on chronic disease and geriatric syndromes, owing to resident comorbid conditions. Functional impairment is the final common pathway of most chronic disease, especially in older persons with multiple advanced disorders.[25] Nursing home residents in the USA are becoming older, increasingly female and more functionally impaired. In these conditions, the challenge is to put the 'home' back in nursing home and not to transform the nursing home into a small hospital.[26]

An estimated 59% of adults with five or more ADL impairments will be admitted to nursing homes.[27] In general, functional status declines with time. Older adults in nursing homes with substantial functional impairment show poorer function at the end of the 6 months than those with higher function[28] and a shorter life expectancy in the nursing home than institutionalized adults of the same age who are less impaired.[29] Functional status is the most sensitive clinical indicator with which to follow disease progression or response to therapy in the elderly. Improvement in function rather than cure of disease is the major therapeutic goal of nursing home care.

Other chronic conditions affect the care of residents in long-term care facilities. Between 45 and 70% of the estimated 1.6 million nursing home residents fall annually.[30] Of these, 30–40% will fall two or more times and 11% will sustain a serious injury as a result of the fall.[31] Urinary incontinence affects approximately half of nursing home residents.[32] Dementia of various types is present in over 60% of typical nursing home residents,[33,34] many of whom exhibit behavioural disturbances.[35] The prevalence of pressure ulcers is higher in long-term care settings.[36] In Medicare-certified nursing home beds, one-quarter of residents receive enteral feeding.[18,37] Weight loss and undernutrition frequently complicate the care of older adults.[38] The prevalence of chronic conditions and interacting comorbid conditions increase the medical complexity of caring for nursing home residents. Several guidelines for the evaluation and management of common clinical problems in the nursing home have been published.[39,40]

Comparison of nursing homes in different countries

In 1997, *Age and Ageing* published a supplement comparing nursing homes in multiple different countries utilizing the data collected by the Resident Assessment Instrument.[41–45] Most of the data were collected in the early 1990s. These findings are summarized in Table 140.1. Some recent data collected using the Resident Assessment Instrument in the USA from 2005 are also included in the table. As can be seen, there is a large variability between countries.

Iceland and Denmark have over 50% of their nursing home population over 85 years of age, whereas in Italy and Japan it is under 40%. Sweden and the USA have over 20% of the nursing home population staying for less than 30 days, whereas none of the Japanese population stay for such a short period. Except in Japan, fewer than one-third of residents are cognitively intact. In the USA, this has changed remarkably in the 10 years since the survey, with now over half of patients being cognitively intact. This almost certainly represents the shift from shorter length of stay in hospitals and more rapid discharge to nursing homes for rehabilitation. Of interest is that in the 1990s, more residents in Japan and Iceland were receiving therapy than were residents in the USA, despite the fact that these two countries had the smallest number of residents staying for less than 30 days.

Table 140.1 Comparisons between nursing homes across countries.

Data collected	Denmark 1992–1993	Italy 1992–1994	Japan 1993	Sweden 1990–1993	Iceland 1994	France 1993	USA 1993	USA 2005
Age								
<65	4.2	4.5	4.6	3.8	1.8	10.2	6.5	–
65–84	45.7	56.1	60.3	52.6	46.6	45.5	53.9	–
85+	50.1	39.3	35.2	43.5	51.5	44.3	47.2	–
Length of stay								
≤ 30 days	2.6	–	0	22.8	0.7	3.8	20.9	–
>2 years	49.4	–	48.5	30.8	60.6	43.8	45.7	–
Cognitively intact	21.8	15.3	32.7	19.7	28.5	11.0	18.5	53.4
Low ADLs	49.0	55.0	42.0	–	38.0	–	48.0	–
Residents receiving rehabilitation	23.0	14.0	30.0	–	31.0	–	11.0	17.2
Restraints	2.2	16.6	4.5	15.2	8.5	17.1	16.5	7.6
Incontinence								
Urine	52.2	54.4	42.9	61.6	56.5	65.2	46.4	55.8
Bowel	22.4	45.3	30.6	39.5	23.0	55.5	29.5	45.8
Participate in activities	52.0	20.0	43.0	–	44.0	–	50.0	–
Nursing time per patient	–	–	84.4	133.7	–	–	118.3	–

There was a low rate of use of physical restraints in Denmark and Japan. The use of physical restraints has halved in the USA in the last decade. In Spain, 39.6% of residents were restrained. As all the evidence shows that restraints do more harm than good, it is extremely puzzling why nursing homes continue to use this form of maltreatment. Of the five countries where social engagement was measured, only Italy had a very low level (20%); in the other countries it varied between 43 and 52%.

In the USA, it is now regulated that all residents have at least some form of social engagement every week.

Nursing time spent with each resident (patient) is highest in England and Wales at 155.5 min and lowest in Japan (84.4 min). In the USA, only 7.5% of the care was given by registered nurses compared with 53.2% in England and Wales. Registered nurses in Japan, Sweden and Spain provided between 14 and 18.2% of the care.

Overall, these studies stress the differences between patient mix and care in different countries. Asian nursing homes in Taiwan showed a moderate level of satisfaction with care, with a monotonous pace of life, inadequate privacy and lost items being the major problems. The average Functional Index Measure (FIM) score was 49.2, which is similar to those seen in the USA in residential care facilities; 74.7% of patients had severe cognitive impairment, physical restraint use was as high as 54%, pressure ulcers varied from 5.3 to 12.1% and the prevalence of stool impaction was 29.4%.[46] As the MDS is more widely used throughout the world, it will become possible to compare nursing homes throughout the world and to develop a gold standard for high-quality nursing homes.

Special nursing home programmes

About half of nursing home residents are diagnosed with dementia.[1] The number of nursing home residents with cognitive dysfunction increased from 39% of long-stay residents in 2004 compared with 25% in 1999.

Dementia is often accompanied by problem behaviours, which can be verbal or physical in nature and can be aggressive or non-aggressive.[47] Good practice in the management of patients with dementia with behavioural symptoms provides an effective alternative to neuroleptics.[48] Special Care (or Needs) Units have been developed in the USA to take care of persons with behavioural problems associated with dementia. These are usually locked units and have a higher staff-to-resident ratio. Many also offer a higher level of recreational therapy. Some of these offer special programmes such as pet or music therapy. Overall, studies have failed to show a major advantage of these units over general nursing home care.

In France, about 44% of the nursing homes have a Special Care Unit. These wards take care of Alzheimer's disease residents with behavioural disturbances, are locked and receive additional funding for organizing non-pharmacological treatment. Innovative strategies such as telemedicine may also be a relevant approach in the nursing home.[49]

Snoezelen is a multisensory therapy that provides easy to-do activities in an enabling environment. It provides a high level of interaction and is both stimulating and relaxing. Although in some nursing homes staff have found it useful, high-quality-controlled studies of its efficacy do not exist. At this time, the small number of available research projects and the small number of participants in each research

Table 140.2 Example of facility quality measure/indicator report.

Facility name______________						**Run date**______________		
City/State______________						**Report period**______________		
Provider number____________						**Comparison group**____________		
Login/Internal ID____________						**Report version number**_________		
		Facility				**Comparison group**		
Measure ID	Domain/ **measure description**	**Num**	**Denom**	**Observed percent (%)**	**Adjusted percent (%)**	**State average (%)**	**National average(%)**	**State percentile**
Chronic care measures								
	Accidents							
1.1	Incidence of new fractures	6	198	3.0	–	2.2	2.0	74
1.2	Prevalence of falls	33	215	15.3	–	15.2	13.0	55
	Behaviour/emotional patterns							
2.1	Residents who have become more depressed or anxious	27	215	12.6	–	12.9	16.0	55
2.2	Prevalence of behaviour symptoms affecting others: Overall	34	215	15.8	–	19.5	18.7	42
2.2-HI	Prevalence of behaviour symptoms affecting others: High risk	26	115	22.6	–	23.5	21.8	51
2.2-LO	Prevalence of behaviour symptoms affecting others: Low risk	8	93	8.6	–	8.2	8.0	63
2.3	Prevalence of symptoms of depression without antidepressant therapy	14	215	6.5	–	4.4	5.4	78
	Clinical management							
3.1	Use of 9 or more different medications	105	215	48.8	–	63.1	61.3	14
	Cognitive patterns							
4.1	Incidence of cognitive impairment	1	107	0.9	–	10.9	12.9	23
	Elimination/incontinence							
5.1	Low-risk residents who lost control of their bowels or bladder	49	123	39.8	–	35.7	47.1	64
5.2	Residents who have/had a catheter inserted and left in their bladder	13	215	6.0	5.1	7.6	8.0	39
5.3	Prevalence of occasional or frequent bladder or bowel incontinence without a toileting plan	51	51	100.0	–	27.5	44.5	100[a]
5.4	Prevalence of faecal impaction	0	215	0.0		0.2	0.1	0
	Infection control							
6.1	Residents with a urinary tract infection	13	215	6.0	–	9.6	9.5	33
	Nutrition/eating							
7.1	Residents who lose too much weight	36	208	17.3	–	10.0	10.9	89
7.2	Prevalence of tube feeding	26	215	12.1	–	4.7	7.2	92[a]
7.3	Prevalence of dehydration	1	215	0.5	–	0.6	0.5	74
	Pain management							
8.1	Residents who have moderate to severe pain	15	215	7.0	5.5	8.6	7.8	45
	Physical functioning							
9.1	Residents whose need for help with daily activities has increased	26	193	13.5	–	16.1	18.3	47
9.2	Residents who spend most of their time in bed or in a chair	16	215	7.4	–	3.2	5.5	92[a]
9.3	Residents whose ability to move in and around their room got worse	9	158	5.7	6.2	15.1	17.1	18
9.4	Incidence of decline in ROM	4	214	1.9	–	7.1	8.6	18
	Psychotropic drug use							
10.1	Prevalence of antipsychotic use, in the absence of psychotic or related conditions: Overall	28	188	14.9	–	22.8	21.9	21

ROM, range of motion
Dashes represent a value that could not be computed.
[a]Above or below national average.

Table 140.3 Comparison between quality assurance and continuous quality improvement.

Quality assurance	Continuous quality improvement
Retrospective	Prospective/continuous
Lays blame	No blame
Administrator lead	Team lead
Opinion driven	Data driven
Problem focused	Customer focused
Snapshot	Continuous
Resistant to change	Seeks change

Table 140.7 The most frequent legal allegations of malpractice against nursing homes.

1 Fall
2 Negligent care
3 Pressure ulcers
4 Lack of care
5 Abuse/assault
6 Dehydration/malnutrition
7 Elopement/wandering

Table 140.4 Problems in the nursing home most amenable to quality improvement.

Depression
Polypharmacy
Pressure ulcers
Undernutrition
Falls
Incontinence
Osteoporosis
Behaviour problems
Lost items
Food quality
Customer satisfaction
Skin tears

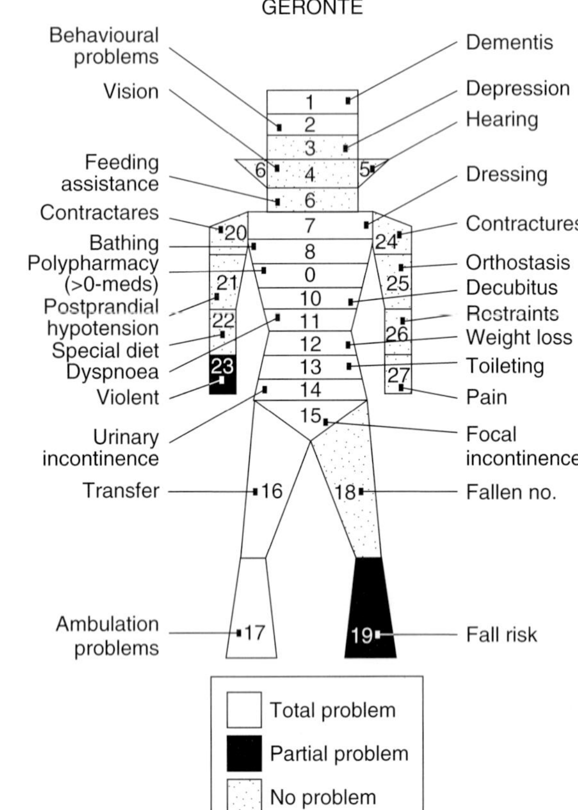

Figure 140.5 A visual communication device: the Geronte, as used by LifeCare Centers of St Louis and the Division of Geriatrics, Saint Louis University.

Table 140.5 Pharmacy quality assurance report for an academic skilled nursing facility.

	Jan	Feb	Mar	Apr	May	Comparison group[a]
Routine meds(n)	9.2	9.4	9.4	9.3	9.7	9.8
PRN meds(n)	1.9	1.8	1.6	1.5	1.5	6.5
Antipsychotics(%)	11	7	5	6	4	12.2
Anxiolytics(%)	9	8	11	15	9	22.0
Sedative/ hypnotics(%)	14	7	8	11	9	24.4

[a]Comparison group is to skilled nursing beds in the same city.

Table 140.6 Measurement of quality in a skilled nursing facility utilizing the Functional Index Measure (FIM).

Level of function	Home	Discharge to hospital	Residential care facility
At home prior to event	106	82	106
On admission	77	55	53
At discharge	96	64	69

project prevent a confirmation of this method as a valid therapeutic intervention.[50]

Adapted exercise programmes seem to slow the functional decline[51] and the decline in health-related QOL among institutionalized elderly persons with dementia.

The Eden Alternative involves the introduction of a variety of animals to the nursing home and also the provision of an environment where the residents can be involved in gardening. These environments can improve the home-like

Table 140.8 The IAGG Task Force recommendations.

No.	Recommendation
Recommendation 1	Effective leadership structures are established, that where possible include an expert physician (Medical Director) and an expert registered nurse (Nursing Director) and skilled administrator
Recommendation 2	An international alliance is formed to develop nursing home leadership capacity and capabilities
Recommendation 3	To showcase international exemplars of excellence in nursing home practice to raise awareness of the demonstrable benefits for older people and high standards achieved through expert practice
Recommendation 4	To create positive working conditions for nursing home practitioners with attractive career development opportunities, recognition and similar rewards enjoyed by healthcare workers in comparable roles within the acute care services
Recommendation 5	That nursing home quality indicators are developed that are sensitive to clinical and care needs and the right of older people to care that is dignified and respectful
Recommendation 6	The use of physical and chemical restraints should be reduced to those that are absolutely indispensable
Recommendation 7	That 'meaningful activities' be offered to residents to provide physical and mental exercise and opportunities to participate within the nursing home and in community life, enhancing personal autonomy, social relationships (including intergenerational relationships) and social support
Recommendation 8	That evidence informed pain assessment and management programmes are introduced into all nursing homes
Recommendation 9	That evidence-informed end-of-life and palliative care programmes are introduced into all nursing homes
Recommendation 10	National drug approval agencies consider requiring drug trials that are age appropriate and inclusive of nursing home residents before they are approved
Recommendation 11	IAGG develop international certification courses for nursing (care) home health professionals
Recommendation 12	Pilot the use of 'Community of Practice Models' as a practice improvement method for nursing homes; utilizing both face-to-face interdisciplinary training and virtual team support
Recommendation 13	A universal ethical approach to obtaining informed consent and monitoring the appropriateness of research is developed
Recommendation 14	Develop nursing home research capacity in developing nations
Recommendation 15	An investment is made in research priorities that address major public health problems and inequalities that affect older people receiving long-term care. Research priorities for which a high need is recognized include: a A worldwide survey of different models of care, nursing home structure and issues in improving quality of care is undertaken b A worldwide survey of older persons and their families is undertaken to determine their preferences for long-term care c A cross-national, prospective epidemiological study measuring function and quality of life in nursing homes d Development of culturally appropriate standardized assessment instruments including those involving social participatory methods e A function-focused approach of the prevalence of geriatric syndromes, their impact on function and development of strategies to improve care for these syndromes needs to be developed f Research that evaluates the impact of different models of care against trajectories of physical and cognitive function

quality of the nursing home and encourage visits by young children. Again, however, quality studies demonstration efficacy do not exist.

The measurement of quality of care is fraught with difficulties. Fahey *et al.* compared the quality of medical care for elderly residents in nursing homes with that of elderly people living at home in the Bristol area in the UK.[52] They found that in the nursing home only 74% of those persons with heart disease and 62% of those with diabetes mellitus had had their blood pressure measured within the previous year. In France, 76% of the nursing home women and 60% of men had known hypertension and over 91% of the patients were receiving antihypertensive treatment; 51% of the treated hypertensive patients were well controlled.[53]

In contrast, in the USA, it is the expectation that blood pressure is measured monthly and in persons in Bristol, UK, living at home the rate of measurement was 96%. Only 38% of residents in nursing homes had been prescribed a β-blocker following a myocardial infarction. Nursing home residents were less likely than people living at home to have received a pneumonococcal vaccination, although the rate of nursing home vaccination was similar.

In the USA, studies using the MDS have demonstrated that residents who are incontinent are unlikely to be on a documented scheduled toileting regimen.[54] Troyer found that Medicaid residents had a slightly higher death rate than privately funded residents.[55] Much of this difference was associated with the resident and also the market they were in. Stevenson found that consumer complaints concerning nursing homes, when made to State Survey agencies, were associated with low nurse aide staffing levels and the number of deficiencies found on the State Survey.[56] Persons who receive potentially inappropriate medications in the nursing home have a much higher chance of subsequent hospitalization or death.[57] Finally, it should be recognized that general practitioners who work in nursing homes will have a higher death rate in their patients than those who work only in the community, making it essential to establish a different standard for these practitioners.[58]

The big picture as given by the recounting above can be reduced to statistics for a single facility so that it can assess its quality and improve its care. Facilities in the USA can use their data as reported in the On-Line Survey Certification and Reporting (OSCAR) and the MDS Quality Indicator data to compare their facility with others in their region, State and the nation (Table 140.2).

The best method to improve care is to put in place a Continuous Quality Improvement plan where data are collected and presented to the interdisciplinary team leaders and staff representatives monthly. When an unacceptable variation in the data is seen, a plan is put in place to determine the reason and to fix the problem. The same data are evaluated each month to allow the team to determine their success at fixing the problem. The differences between continuous quality improvement and old-fashioned quality assurance programmes are delineated in Table 140.3. Areas in the nursing home that are highly amenable to continuous quality improvement programmes are set out in Table 140.4. Examples of monitoring of data in the nursing home for prescribing and efficacy of therapies are given in Tables 140.5 and 140.6. The keys to continuous quality improvement resulting in improved nursing home care are administrative buy-in, team empowerment to fix the problem and continuous collection and feedback of data.

Legal issues in the nursing home

There has been a marked increase in lawsuits against nursing homes in the USA over the last 5 years. In many cases they are frivolous and rely on the fact that the fear of large awards by a jury and the cost of litigation make the nursing home chains settle without going to court. The largest awards are made for elopement (average $860 000) and pressure ulcers (average $293 000). Table 140.7 lists the most frequent allegations against nursing homes.

Visualizing the resident

Communication between all the members of the interdisciplinary team and the physician is often limited. The Geronte is a visual communication device originally developed in France. This single sheet provides a snapshot of the problems that the resident has. Problem areas can be coloured in by any staff member (Figure 140.5).

Improving nursing home care

The International Association of Gerontology and Geriatrics (IAGG) Task Force, in concert with the World Health Organization, has developed a blueprint for improving nursing home care worldwide (Table 140.8).

Key points

- Nursing home facilities are more unique than similar.
- The Minimum Data Set provides a method to compare nursing homes worldwide.
- Nursing homes have short-stay residents who are predominantly there for rehabilitation and long-term residents who require custodial care.
- The introduction of special programmes, for example, the Eden Alternative, increased involvement of physicians and continuous quality improvement methods have improved quality of care in nursing homes.

References

1. Rolland Y, Abellan van Kan G, Hermabessière S *et al.* Descriptive study of nursing home residents from the REHPA network. *J Nutr Health Aging* 2009;**13**:679–83.
2. Jones A. The National Nursing Home Survey: 1999 summary. National Center for Health Statistics. *Vital Health Stat* 2002;**13**(152):1–116.
3. Jones AL, Dwyer LL, Bercovitz AR and Strahan GW. The National Nursing Home Survey: 2004 overview. National Center for Health Statistics. *Vital Health Stat* 2009; **13**(167):1–155.
4. Gabrel CS. An overview of nursing home facilities: data from the 1997 national nursing home survey. *Adv Data* 2000;(311):1–12.
5. American Nursing Association. Staff shortages hurting nursing homes the most. *Am J Nurs* 1991;**91**:85–90.
6. Caudill ME and Patrick M. Costing nurse turnover in nursing homes. *Nurs Manage* 1991;**22**:61–4.
7. Castle NG, Engberg J and Men A. Nursing home staff turnover: impact on nursing home compare quality measures. *Gerontologist* 2007;**47**:650–61.
8. Levit KR, Lazenby HD, Cowan CA and Letsch SW. National health care expenditures. *Health Care Financ Rev* 1991; **13**:29–54.
9. Sonnenfeld ST, Waldo DR, Lemieux JA and McKusick DR. Projections of national health expenditures through the year 2000. *Health Care Financ Rev* 1991;**13**:1–27.

10. Komisar HL, Feder J and Kasper JD. Unmet long-term care needs: an analysis of Medicare-Medicaid dual eligibles. *Inquiry* 2005;**42**:171–82.
11. Schols JMGA, Crebolder HFJM and van Weel C. Nursing home and nursing home physician: the Dutch experience. *J Am Med Dir Assoc* 2004;**5**:207–12.
12. Black D and Bowman C. Community institutional care for frail elderly people. Time to structure professional responsibility. *BMJ* 1997;**315**:441–2.
13. Kavanagh S and Knapp M. The impact on general practitioners of the changing balance of care for older people living in institutions. *BMJ* 1998;**317**:322–7.
14. Hancock R, Antony A, Jagger C and Matthems R. The effect of older people's economic resources on care home entry under the United Kingdom's long-term care financing system. *J Gerontol B Psychol Sci Soc Sci* 2002;**57**: S285–93.
15. Kemper P and Murtaugh CM. Lifetime use of nursing home care. *N Engl J Med* 1991;**324**:595–600.
16. Zedlewski SR, Barnes RO, Burt MK *et al. The Needs of the Elderly in the 21st Century*, Urban Institute Press, Washington, DC, 1990.
17. Doty PJ. The oldest old and the use of institutional long-term care from an international perspective. In: R Suzman, DP Willis and KG Manton (eds), *The Oldest Old*, Oxford University Press, New York, 1992, pp.251–67.
18. Shaughnessy PW and Kramer AM. The increased needs of patients in nursing homes and patients receiving home health care. *N Engl J Med* 1990;**322**:21–7.
19. Ferrell BA, Stein WM and Beck JC. The Geriatric Pain Measure: validity, reliability and factor analysis. *J Am Geriatr Soc* 2000;**48**:1669–73.
20. Kroenke K and Spitzer RL. The PHQ-9: a new depression diagnostic and severity measure. *Psychiatr Ann* 2002; **32**:509–15.
21. Callahan CM, Unverzagt FW, Hui SL *et al*. Six-item screener to identify cognitive impairment among potential subjects for clinical research. *Med Care* 2002;**40**:771–81.
22. Wei LA, Fearing MA, Sternberg EJ and Inouye SK. The Confusion Assessment Method: a systematic review of current usage. *J Am Geriatr Soc* 2008;**56**:823–30.
23. Katz PR, Karuza J, Kolassa J and Hutson A. Medical practice with nursing home residents: results from the national physician professional activities census. *J Am Geriatr Soc* 1997;**45**:911–7.
24. Darer JD, Hwang W, Pham HH *et al*. More training needed in chronic care: a survey of US physicians. *Acad Med* 2004;**79**:541–8.
25. Thomas DR. Focus on functional decline in hospitalized older adults. *J Gerontol A Biol Sci Med Sci* 2002;**57**: M567–8.
26. Morley JE and Flaherty JH. Putting the 'home' back in nursing home. *J Gerontol A Biol Sci Med Sci* 2002;**57**: M419–21.
27. Guralnik JM, Simonsick EM, Ferrucci L *et al*. A short physical performance battery assessing lower extremity function: association with self-reported disability and prediction of mortality and nursing home admission. *J Gerontol A Biol Sci Med Sci* 1994;**49**: M85–94.
28. Buttar A, Blaum C and Fries B. Clinical characteristics and six-month outcomes of nursing home residents with low activities of daily living dependency. *J Gerontol A Biol Sci Med Sci* 2001;**56**: M292–7.
29. Donaldson LJ, Clayton DG and Clarke M. The elderly in residential care: mortality in relation to functional capacity. *J Epidemiol Commun Health* 1980;**34**:96–101.
30. Thappa PB, Brockman KG, Gideon P *et al*. Injurious falls in nonambulatory nursing home residents: a comparative study of circumstances, incidence and risk factors. *J Am Geriatr Soc* 1996;**44**:273–8.
31. Rubenstein LZ, Josephson KR and Robbins AS. Falls in the nursing home. *Ann Intern Med* 1994;**121**:442–51.
32. Ouslander JG and Schnelle JF. Incontinence in the nursing facility. *Ann Intern Med* 1995;**122**:438–49.
33. Jakob A, Busse A, Riedel-Heller SG *et al*. Prevalence and incidence of dementia among nursing home residents and residents in homes for the aged in comparison to private homes. *Z Gerontol Geriatr* 2002;**35**:474–81.
34. Rovner BW, German PS, Broadhead J *et al*. The prevalence and management of dementia and other psychiatric disorders in nursing homes. *Int Psychogeriatr* 1990;**2**:13–24.
35. Thomas DR. Who's going to cause me trouble? Predicting behavioral disturbances in demented patients. *J Am Med Dir Assoc* 2002;**3**:204–5.
36. Thomas DR. Age-related changes in wound healing. *Drugs Aging* 2001;**18**:607–20.
37. Haddad RY and Thomas DR. Enteral nutrition and tube feeding: a review of the evidence. *Gastroenterol Clin North Am* 2002;**18**:867–82.
38. Thomas DR, Zdrowski CD, Wilson MM *et al*. Malnutrition in subacute care. *Am J Clin Nutr* 2002;**75**:308–13.
39. Ouslander JG and Osterweil D. Physician evaluation and management of nursing home residents. *Ann Intern Med* 1994;**120**:584–92.
40. Evans JM, Chutka DS, Fleming KC *et al*. Medical care of nursing home residents. *Mayo Clin Proc* 1995;**70**:694–702.
41. Fries BE, Schroll M, Hawes C *et al*. Approaching cross-national comparisons of nursing home residents. *Age Ageing* 1997;**26**(Suppl 2):13–8.
42. Berg K, Sherwood S, Murphy K *et al*. Rehabilitation in nursing homes: a cross-national comparison of recipients. *Age Ageing* 1997;**26**(Suppl 2):37–42.
43. Ljunggren G, Phillips CD and Sgadari A. Comparisons of restraint use in nursing homes in eight countries. *Age Ageing* 1997;**26**(Suppl 2):43–7.
44. Sgadari A, Topinkova E, Bjornson J and Bernabei R. Urinary incontinence in nursing home residents: a cross-national comparison. *Age Ageing* 1997;**26**(Suppl 2):49–54.
45. Schroll M, Jonsson PV, Mor V *et al*. An international study of social engagement among nursing home residents. *Age Ageing* 1997;**26**(Suppl 2):55–9.
46. Yeh S-H, Lin L-W and Lo SK. A longitudinal evaluation of nursing home care quality in Taiwan. *J Nurs Care Qual* 2003;**18**:209–16.
47. Cohen-Mansfield J and Mintzer JE. Time for change: the role of nonpharmacological interventions in treating behavior problems in nursing home residents with dementia. *Alzheimer Dis Assoc Disord* 2005;**19**:37–40.
48. Fossey J, Ballard C, Juszczak E *et al*. Effect of enhanced psychosocial care on antipsychotic use in nursing home

residents with severe dementia: cluster randomised trial. *BMJ* 2006;**332**:756–61.

49. Mitka M. Telemedicine eyed for mental health services: approach could widen access for older patients. *JAMA* 2003;**290**:1842–3.

50. Lotan M and Gold C. Meta-analysis of the effectiveness of individual intervention in the controlled multisensory environment (Snoezelen) for individuals with intellectual disability. *J Intellect Dev Disabil* 2009;**34**:207–15.

51. Rolland Y, Pillard F, Klapouszczak A *et al*. Exercise program for nursing home residents with Alzheimer's disease: a 1-year randomized, controlled trial. *J Am Geriatr Soc* 2007; **55**:158–65.

52. Fahey T, Montgomery AA, Barnes J and Protheroe J. Quality of care for elderly residents in nursing homes and elderly people living at home: controlled observational study. *BMJ* 2003;**326**:580–3.

53. Benetos A, Buatois S, Salvi P *et al*. Blood pressure and pulse wave velocity values in the institutionalized elderly aged 80 and over: baseline of the PARTAGE study. *J Hypertens* 2010;**28**:41–50.

54. Schnelle JF, Cadogan MP, Yoshii J *et al*. The minimum data set urinary incontinence quality indicators: do they reflect differences in care processes related to incontinence ? *Med Care* 2003;**41**:909–22.

55. Troyer JL. Examining differences in death rates for Medicaid and non-Medicaid nursing home residents. *Med Care* 2004;**42**:985–91.

56. Stevenson DG. Nursing home consumer complaints and their potential role in assessing quality of care. *Med Care* 2005;**43**:99–101.

57. Lau DT, Kasper JD, Potter DE *et al*. Hospitalization and death associated with potentially inappropriate medication prescriptions among elderly nursing home residents. *Ann Intern Med* 2005;**165**:68–74.

58. Mohammed MA, Rathbone A, Myers P *et al*. An investigation into general practitioners associated with high patient mortality flagged up through the Shipman inquiry: retrospective analysis of routine data. *BMJ* 2004;**328**:1474–7.

CHAPTER 141

Geriatric occupational therapy: achieving quality in daily living

Karen F. Barney
Saint Louis University, St Louis, MO, USA

Overview

Humans are occupational beings

The science underlying the occupational therapy (OT) profession views humans as *occupational beings*.[1,2] Globally, humans are typically identified by their *occupations*. In other words, *who we are* is often determined by *what we do*. What we do are the *activities (occupations)* that comprise our lives. Thus, the focus of OT interventions with and on behalf of older adults is to address their unique needs and preferences for *what they need and want to do in addition to what they are expected to do*, typically concurrently with age-related changes and acute and/or chronic conditions. These p*otential or actual changes in the ability to perform necessary and desired activities (occupations)* impact how elders conduct their everyday lives and present a threat to their overall health and identity.[2–4] Typically, the identity and sense of wellbeing of the elders is expressed through their participation in the activities/occupations that comprise the roles, habits and routines that encompass their lives. These patterns of participation represent who they have been throughout their lives, who they are today and who they may yet become. Participation in society to the extent needed and desired by elders is fundamental to their perception of the quality of personal life and also a basic component of the World Health Organization (WHO) current disability model, the International Classification of Functioning, Disability and Health (ICF).[5]

Conceptual foundations of geriatric occupational therapy

With a simultaneous focus upon intrinsic and extrinsic factors that impact elders' participation in expected, desired and meaningful activities, OT personnel work in partnership with the individual or organizational client to promote the enablement of ageing adults to pursue a meaningful quality of life (QOL) at all levels of care. The WHO conceptual model and OT services interface intimately, as noted in Figure 141.1.

OT interventions centre on enabling elders to pursue the activities, tasks, habits and routines that are personally important and meaningful to them. All of these activities and occupational components contribute to the elders' perception of their QOL. The WHO ICF is the currently accepted model for systematically grouping consequences associated with health conditions. Level of ability, function and/or disablement are seen as a dynamic interaction between the individual's health condition and their personal environmental contextual factors. These intrinsic and extrinsic factors affect the individual's ability to pursue the needed and desired activities that comprise their lives and to participate in individual and group societal functions. If impairments and contextual factors are incompatible, this set of circumstances in turn affects the individual's overall sense of wellbeing and personal perceptions of their QOL.[5]

Person–Environment–Occupation–Performance/Participation model

Figure 141.2 presents the OT Person–Environment–Occupation–Performance/Participation (PEOP) model that is complementary to the WHO ICF model.[6] The PEOP model depicts wellbeing and QOL as a function of the relationship of the personal/intrinsic factors, the environmental/extrinsic factors, occupation/activity and occupational performance/participation in activity and society.[6] These components are shown as being totally interdependent. Figure 141.2 and the following model

Principles and Practice of Geriatric Medicine, Fifth Edition. Edited by Alan J. Sinclair, John E. Morley and Bruno Vellas.

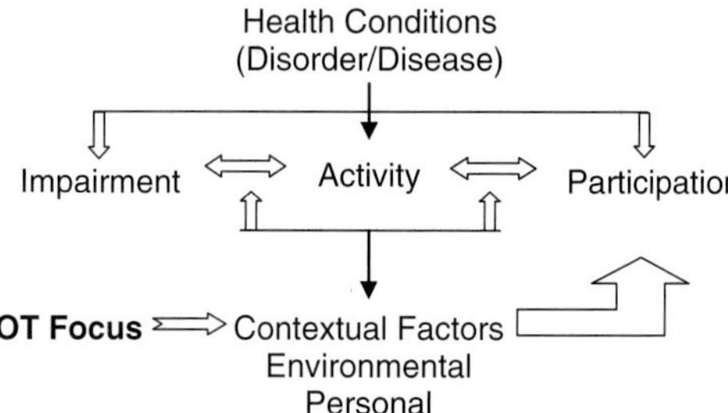

Figure 141.1 WHO ICF model. Adapted from *International Classification of Functioning, Disability and Health (ICF)*, World Health Organization, Geneva, 2001, Figure 1.

express the *P–E–O–P* relationship:

$$\text{Elder Quality of Life} = f\begin{pmatrix}\text{Personal Attributes} + \text{Environmental} \\ \text{Factors} + \text{Occupational Performance} \\ + \text{Participation}\end{pmatrix}$$

where 'elder quality of life' is dependent upon and a function of the *person's* unique health status and functional abilities, plus the degree to which their *environment* supports the *occupations/activities* that they need and want to pursue and allows them to *perform/participate* in society, to meet their requisite needs and desires.

Person (intrinsic factors)

Occupational therapists assess and intervene to enable elders to cope with normal and inherent age-related changes known as *intrinsic factors*. These factors include physiological, motor, cognitive, spiritual, neurobehavioural and psychological components of human function. The older adult's level of motivation, and also roles, habits and routines that comprise their lifestyle, are an integral part of occupational performance and QOL. Hence the capacity for life-long homemakers to continue cooking and taking pride in their culinary creations may be compromised by diminishing olfactory and gustatory ability. In addition, the elders' individual beliefs about themselves and their life experiences – past, current and potential – impact their execution of self-maintenance, work, service, leisure and other activities.

Environment (extrinsic factors)

Extrinsic or environmental/contextual determinants of occupational performance include social support, social and economic systems, culture and values, technology, the built environment and also the natural environment.[6,7] Typically, intrinsic age-related changes in vision, hearing, olfaction, vestibular functions, musculoskeletal and other systems may alter the individual's ability to cope with any or all of these extrinsic environmental factors. The elder's physical surroundings may not adequately support their performance of necessary and desired activities because of age-related changes that they experience. Therefore, in order for elders to continue to live independently (if culturally appropriate) and participate as fully as possible, the inherent changes in sensory and other systems, and also in cognition, may require changes in their physical environment and other external support systems.

Occupation (activity)

What humans do consists of occupation(s). Occupations, better known as *activities*, include all abstract and observable types, and comprise the everyday lives of people of all ages around the world.[8] They also assist individuals in understanding who they are, as humans often define themselves by what they do. When younger adults are asked, 'What do you do?', they may respond by stating their role as student, the type of worker/vocation they pursue or their role as homemaker or parent. When elders are asked the same question, they may respond differently, depending upon what is important to their sense of identity at this later point in life. Nevertheless, occupation/activity in all conceivable forms is the fabric of human existence.

Participation

Active involvement in daily life and various life situations comprises *participation*. This concept includes the ability to perform roles at home, work and in the community. Various factors may hinder an individual's ability to function in one or more of these environments, due to lack of support, attitudes, and physical, social and/or societal barriers.[7,9,10] Throughout their lifespan, individuals encounter different forms of access or barriers to participate in activities that are necessary and meaningful to them.[5,11–14] In the latter years of life, elders may encounter limits to their participation due to decline in age-related or functional abilities, ageism or policies that limit continuation of involvement in activities such as employment or driving.

Scope of occupational therapy services

OT services are provided at three different levels: (1) directly with individuals and/or family/caregiver(s), (2) consultation and administration with community organizations and (3) consultation and/or administration with governmental and/or international agencies. Historically, the majority of services have been provided for individual patients and clients; however, a growing number of community-level OT services have been established during the past several decades. Overall, geriatric OT services are designed to sustain or improve

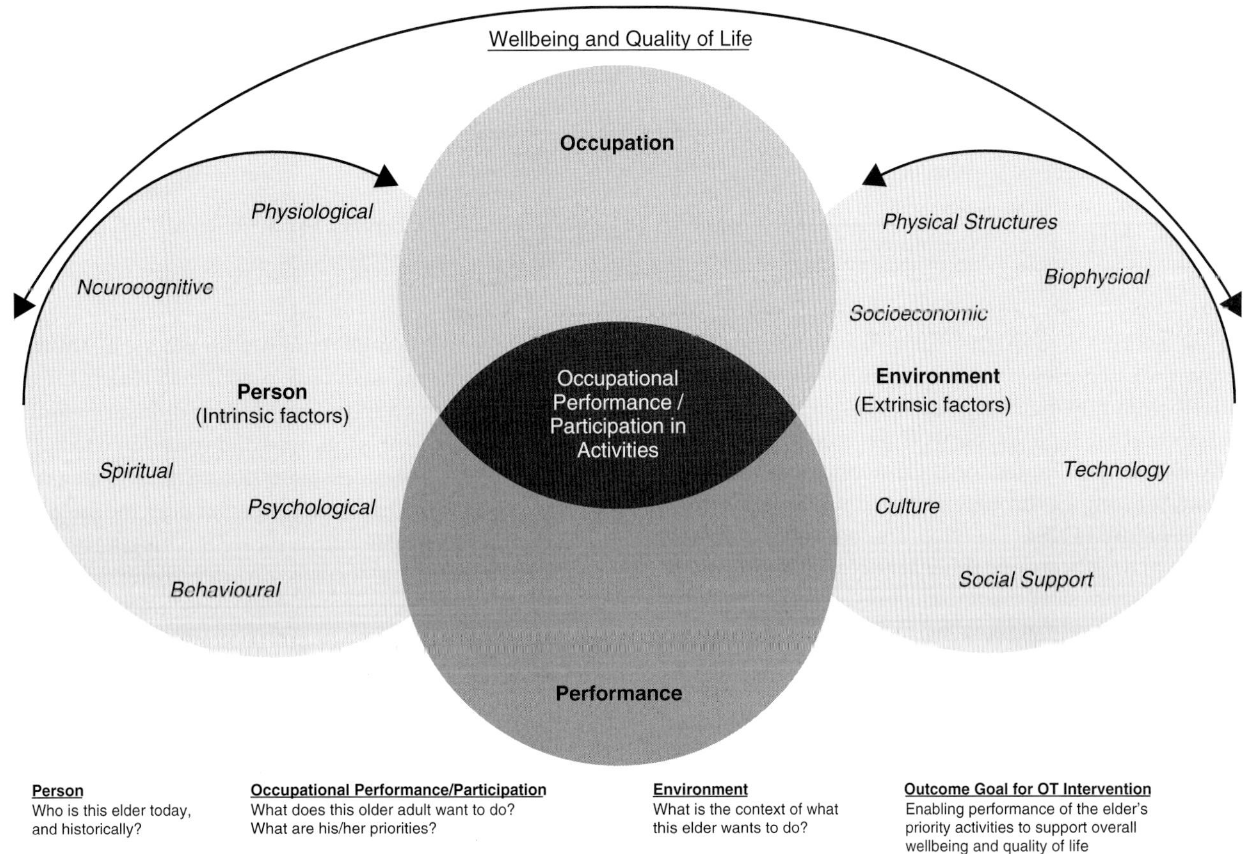

Figure 141.2 Person–Environment–Occupation–Performance/Participation (PEOP) model applied to geriatric OT practice. Adapted from Christiansen *et al.*[6]

the everyday activity-related wellbeing and QOL of older adults. In addition, services aim to enable families, non-governmental organizations and government agencies to mobilize efforts that promote the health of elders, prevent deterioration of function associated with age-related changes, restore functions that are impaired by organic disease, impairment or disability, and/or provide compensatory techniques necessitated by age or disability-related changes. In providing services, OT personnel collaborate with older adults, medical providers and organizations, in order to sustain or improve the ability of elders to perform necessary and meaningful activities, taking into consideration their overall health status, personality, lifestyle, family and/or other support systems. Thus, whether administered with an individual, group or population, OT interventions aim to ensure a QOL commensurate with the elders' priorities, and also those of their family members, carers and their communities.

OT assessment and intervention services are provided collaboratively with or on behalf of older adults who are at risk for or experience limitations due to disease, acute or chronic illness, injury, developmental disability, ageing with an existing disability (e.g. cerebral palsy, spinal cord injury, post-polio) and/or the ongoing ageing process. For example, a person who has sustained a stroke may receive OT services in order to relearn how to dress or to feed themselves. Furthermore, an older adult with dementia may benefit from interventions that simplify tasks and routines, maintain safety within the environment and also support the daily routines and wellbeing of the carer. These services are provided throughout the continuum of care, to address the full range of daily activity (occupation) and participation needs of older clients or patients, as shown in Figure 141.3. The levels and forms of OT services range from the needs of older adults living in the community to the needs of those experiencing end-of-life circumstances.

Hence primary, secondary and/or tertiary settings are included in this continuum of OT services. Primary care OT interventions include provision of health promotion and health protection services within communities, and also for individuals. Examples of these types of services include programmes on home safety to prevent falls and other injuries and driver screening, assessment and retraining, as elders experience age-related changes in function. Secondary care OT interventions include individual, group and/or community approaches for management of health conditions

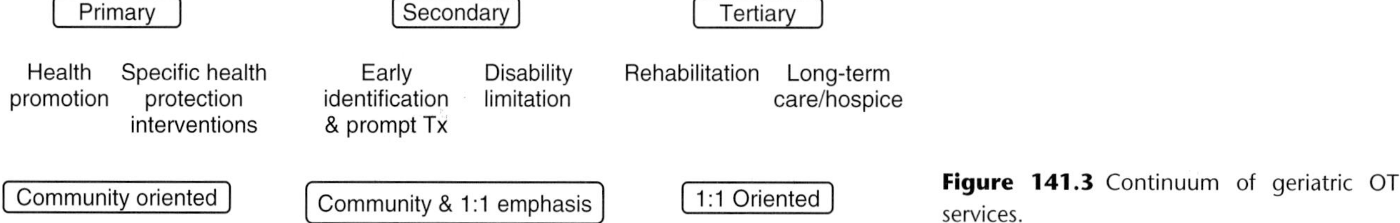

Figure 141.3 Continuum of geriatric OT services.

such as arthritis and Alzheimer's disease. Figure 141.4 displays the categories of services that OTs provide to older adults, their family members, and/or carers.

This topical list depicts typical OT services and is not completely exhaustive. Professional OT services are provided in a range of settings throughout the continuum of care, as shown in Figure 141.5. OT services are coordinated with the providers of healthcare and other services, including physicians, nurses, physical therapists, speech therapists, social workers, community and public health agencies and others, whenever indicated and available. When services are provided on an individual basis, family members and/or other available support systems often become an integral component of the OT service team, to ensure successful intervention outcomes. Furthermore, in addition to working with the older adult, OT personnel provide services to their carers, in order to maximize efficiency, diminish stress and support the health and wellbeing of the carers.

Occupational therapy process

Assessment and intervention

Wherever possible, an evidence-based process is applied to the determination of what should be included in the OT assessment and intervention with elders, as shown in Figure 141.6. In the standard practice in which OT personnel work with an individual older adult, a three-phase process of assessment is followed and considered to be 'best practice'.[15] The first assessment objective is to determine who this individual has been and what does the individual need and want to do, in both a short- and long-term period. The second objective focuses on identifying where and how the relevant current activities, tasks, routines or other occupations can and/or should be done. The third area of concentration in assessment is to determine the biological, psychological and/or social barriers to the elder's achievement of their desired activities. Other individuals or groups may also contribute to the compilation of information on occupational performance issues for the elderly. The Occupational Therapy Practice Framework (OTPF) is the guiding protocol for the OT assessment and intervention process.[6,8]

Occupational profile

The initial step in the OT assessment process determines the client's occupational history and experiences (e.g. summary of activities that have comprised their life to date), and also current patterns of daily living, interests, values

• Transition Planning • Meaningful Engagement • Employment / re-employment • Retirement • Loss of spouse/partner • End of life • Development of leisure activities • Establishing/ re-establishing occupational (activity participation) balance • Relationships • Physical activity/ fitness/exercise • Sexuality • Spirituality • Community service • Use of technology	• Lifelong learning • Assistive product development • Home design & accessibility • Home management • Home safety • Shopping • Use of alternative/public transportation • Driving skills • Energy conservation • Joint protection • ADL • IADL • Care management • End-of-life activities	Compensatory activity approaches for: • Age-related sensory changes including: Presbyopia Presbycusis • Tremors • Incoordination & balance • Weakness • Low endurance • Arthritis • Joint replacements • Amputations • CVA, TIA • Spinal cord injuries • Traumatic brain injuries • Dementias, including Alzheimer's disease • Pain • Terminal illness • Family/carer/staff skills and coping

Figure 141.4 Geriatric OT services.

Community Based

- Individual homes/apartments
- Senior centres
- Senior housing
- Retirement centres
- Naturally occurring retirement communities (NORCs)
- Elder continuum of care centres
- Learning centres
- Shopping centres
- Parishes, temples, churches and other religious congregations
- Private practices
    - Home modification services
    - Assistive technology/devices interventions
    - Care management
    - Lifestyle redesign programmes
    - Re-employment services
    - Worksite evaluation and remediation
    - Driving skills
- Local, regional, and/or national private or public agencies

Institution Based

- Acute care
- Subacute care
- General medicine services
- Rehabilitation
- Adult day services
- Group homes
- Assisted living
- Intermediate care
- Skilled care
- Palliative care
- Hospice care

Figure 141.3 Geriatric OT service settings.

and needs. The client's problems and concerns about performing daily and other relevant life activities are identified, the client's priorities are determined and plans of care and/or management focus on these collaboratively determined priorities.[7] The approach is top-down and client-centred, where enabling participation in personally and culturally relevant and meaningful activities is the focus of planning.[8,16]

Occupational performance assessment

This step in the evaluation process specifically determines the client's biopsychosocial assets, needs, problems or potential problems, based upon results of reliable and valid standardized evaluation instruments. Preferably, the therapist observes the performance of selected activities in order to identify what supports or hinders performance. This skilled observation includes all aspects of the individual's abilities, including affect, cognitive/executive and motor functions. Ideally, the assessment process takes place in the elder's usual environment, typically at home, since performance in an unfamiliar environment may be different. Performance skills, performance patterns, contexts, activity demands and client factors are all considered, but only aspects that are specifically relevant to the desired activities may be assessed. Targeted outcomes are identified, based upon the elder's expressed interests and needs.

The OT assessment of the client's occupational performance takes into consideration all pertinent individual and environmental factors. These factors may include the individual's age, gender, socioeconomic background and current status, racial/ethnic/cultural and/or religious background, developmental status, health history and current status, as well as educational and vocational histories. Interviewing the patient/client and/or the family, whenever feasible, is combined with standardized and other evidence-based performance assessments to determine the individual's profile from which to construct the individualized intervention plan.[17–19] Inquiry covers the following areas:

1 What roles, routines, habits and/or new activities does the patient/client *want to perform (elder priorities)*?

2 What may be done to facilitate the patient/client in the range of activities that they *do perform (current activities)*?

3 What is the patient/client currently *able to perform (intrinsic ability)*?

4 If the individual depends upon a support system, *what activity supports are provided and to what extent*?

5 *Does/do the carer(s) also need OT intervention in order to carry out their support effectively*?

The environment, scope of activities/occupations and roles in which elders typically engage are shown in Figure 141.7. The knowledge of the context, activities and those that comprise the roles that the elder assumes assists OT personnel in collaborative assessment and intervention with elderly clients, their carers, families and other support systems.

Where multiple environmental factors serve as barriers to participation in necessary and desired activities and thereby impact the wellbeing of older adults, OT practitioners collaborate with other disciplines in evaluating the individual's circumstances and planning appropriate interprofessional interventions. On an independent basis, OT personnel frequently evaluate facilities or the elder's home, in order to facilitate PEOP compatibility. The evaluations compare the elder's activity needs and priorities with their functional abilities and the physical environment in which they function, in order to determine and predict the likelihood of their success in being able to perform these activities. The identified deficiencies are then targeted in the intervention plan.

OT is concerned with how elders perform in their daily lives and how performance affects their engagement in occupations (activities). These occupations typically are components of performance that support their participation in the habits, routines and roles that provide meaning to their lives. Thus, the evaluation process determines what the patient/client needs and wants to do, what are their functional capabilities, and what are the barriers or supports needed to perform those priority occupations.[8]

When interventions are indicated, due to a poor PEOP fit, OT personnel work with the elder and family or other support systems to improve these factors. Recommendations may include specific changes to the physical environment, compensatory changes in their routines and activities and/or assistive equipment to permit successful

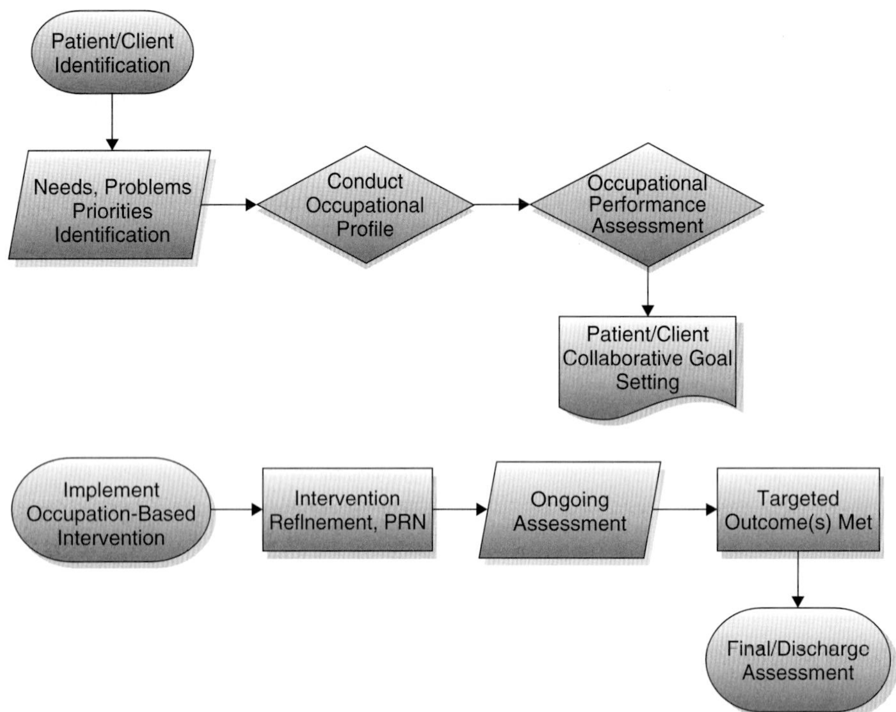

Figure 141.6 OT process.

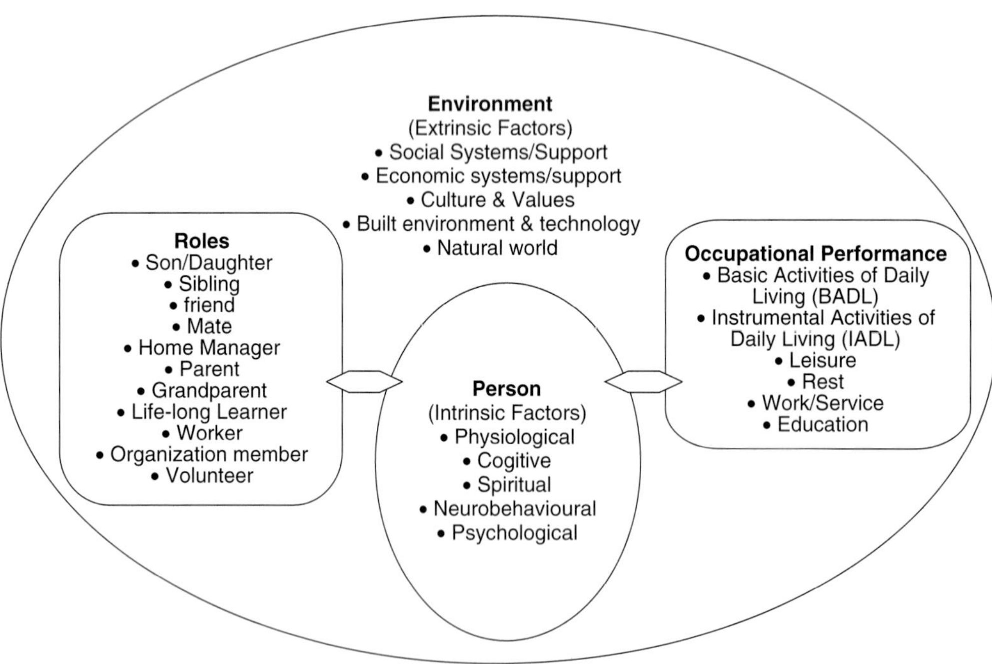

Figure 141.7 OT assessment and intervention components.

occupational performance. These needs are often overlooked completely or underestimated when the individual is being discharged from one level of medical care to another or to their home. When this insight is lacking, the gaps in environmental support may put the older adult at increased risk for dependency, in addition to falls and other injuries.

Intervention

Development of the intervention plan

OT personnel individually tailor the interventions to the patient/client's needs in order to promote optimal outcomes. The intervention plan is thus developed collaboratively with the client and their family, if indicated, so that appropriate strategies, specific interventions and targeted outcomes are included and mutually agreed upon. Therefore, the approach utilized to increase functional level in ADLs, IADLs and also self-esteem, socialization and a sense of personal competence in whatever is pursued is unique to each patient/client.

Intervention implementation via client-centred care

Utilizing goal-directed activities that are meaningful to the patient/client, depending upon the nature of their health status, the OT assists the individual to adapt temporarily or permanently to the physical and social environment that circumscribes their life. This approach promotes mastery of essential living skills, and also those skills that represent the patient/client's other priority interests. As a group, elders exemplify highly diverse lifestyles and interests. Therefore, OT personnel identify modalities and activities that are motivating to the patient because they are relevant to their particular lifestyle. Collaboration with the patient/client, known as *client-centred care*, facilitates and enables the mobilization of the individual's internal psychological resources. This process then promotes greater participation in the intervention, which in turn optimally assists in restoring or enhancing function where functional change or decline has occurred or is threatened. If indicated, family members or other carers are included in planning and implementation, depending upon the needs of all relevant members. All interventions are continually documented, monitored, re-evaluated and adapted or discontinued, based upon the client's overall status.

OT interventions may include any or all of the following categories.

Use of occupation to enhance quality of life

Health promotion

Most individuals' lives are comprised of a variety of self-maintenance, productive, leisure and/or service activities. Thus OT personnel utilize occupations (activities), tasks, roles, routines and/or habits as therapeutic agents in achieving long-term and short-term goals toward adaptation and habilitation, restoration of function and/or enhancing the individual's QOL. Many health promotion programmes are provided in the community; however, OT personnel integrate health promotion perspectives in services throughout the continuum of care[4,8,20,21] (see Figures 141.3–141.5).

End of life

The latter applies also to OT's promotion of QOL and independence in daily occupations with terminally ill patients, to the extent possible for as long as possible. OT also facilitates maintenance of ADLs, pain management, joy, life review and other meaningful closure activities at the end of life by assisting the elder and their family members to participate in meaningful activities with terminally ill individuals.

Community-level instruction and patient/client education

In community settings, OT personnel provide health promotion and other training programmes for the elders, family members, carers and agency employees.[20,21] The content is tailored to the needs of the target group, just as when interventions are implemented for individuals. Subjects covered include those identified or related to those given in Figure 141.4.

In acute or subacute care, rehabilitation and home healthcare, collaborating with the older patient/client in basic skills training or retraining in functional occupations (e.g. ADLs and/or IADLs) are standard components of OT practice. Interventions may also focus on making positive transitions in overall lifestyle based on physical, emotional, and/or retirement, continuing employment and service needs of elders.[1,2] Furthermore, the OT personnel collaborate, wherever indicated, with other healthcare providers in the rehabilitation team as well as community agencies to promote optimal patient/client outcomes.[8,22,23]

Since older adults and their support systems may not be aware of age-related physiological and psychological changes, OT may also employ education or training in these areas to facilitate adaptation to deterioration of function and adjustments in relationships. Topics may include the use of compensatory strategies, recommendations for equipment and other methods to compensate for loss of function and ensure the ability to participate in meaningful occupations. Health promotion teaching strategies may include the following: [20]

- Prevention of physical deterioration through the use of age-appropriate approaches for participation in activities:
  - body mechanics
  - joint protection
  - energy conservation
  - activity and exercise guidelines

- Prevention of psychosocial deterioration through the use of occupation:
  - adjustment of lifestyles to accommodate age-related, role and other changes in life
  - the role of purposeful, balanced activities in maintaining health and overall wellbeing
  - overall time management
  - self-esteem, empowerment, mastery strategies
  - interpersonal skills and socialization activities
  - an emphasis on positive aspects of living in promoting a healthy lifestyle

Remediation strategies for functional decline

OT interventions to compensate for sensorimotor occupational performance deficits focus on enabling the elder to participate in the activities identified for maintenance of function and/or improvement of function. These activities include sitting and standing balance, strengthening, endurance, range of motion and coordination. Therapeutic approaches employed in all of these occupational performance skills areas are related in the intervention process to ADL and IADL participation, including related tasks and roles performed by and meaningful to the individual.

Furthermore, comorbidities that the older adult experiences are simultaneously factored into the intervention approaches. Interventions are individualized to accommodate cognitive, behavioural and affective changes that occur following a stroke and/or other neurological conditions, as in dementias or Parkinson's disease. When oral–motor dysfunction, muscular rigidity, joint pain, bradykinesia or other symptoms impede direct intervention, OT practitioners utilize facilitatory techniques and positioning approaches. These interventions focus on enabling the elder to participate in functional, meaningful activities that accomplish the desired mobilization and overall rehabilitation goals. OT personnel also develop therapeutic programs in a wide variety of settings, which are shown in Figure 141.5.

Physical environment adaptations

Because of normal age-related changes, OT consultation and implementation of specific environmental adaptations and modifications may be indicated for most elders, in order to facilitate their continued participation in the activities that are important to them. Where individual or comorbid conditions limit participation, personally relevant physical environmental modifications may be recommended. Additional lighting, railings, ramps, grab bars and assistive devices may be indicated, in order to promote accessibility and independence in mobility and the ability to pursue the elder's necessary and desired occupations. OT interventions also include methods to compensate for cognitive, memory and psychological changes. These compensatory accommodations that can be implemented in existing or new facilities may make the difference between the elders' dependence and their meaningful participation. OT personnel also provide suggestions for environmental adaptations relative to therapeutic programming and activities for persons with dementia, including cognitive integration, orientation, memory, safety and pursuit of meaningful activities.

Technological aids and devices

Both low and high technological assistive devices may be recommended to enhance the elder's occupational performance and participation in solitary, group or community activities. Low vision aids and assistive devices for hearing loss are examples of equipment that may be recommended for use if sensory deficits result in occupational performance deficits. OT personnel often recommend assistive devices for individuals who demonstrate limitations in sensorimotor function, range of motion, strength, coordination and endurance. Different types of assistive devices may be suggested for persons who demonstrate occupational performance deficits in their cognitive abilities. Overall, devices are recommended only if they support improved participation in the activities that are important to the elder and/or their family or other support system.

Intervention review

As noted earlier and depicted in Figure 141.6, OT interventions are continually reviewed and refined, as indicated. Periodic reassessment of the client's status, including ongoing inputs from the elder and/or their carers, family members and other support systems are integrated into any alterations in the intervention plan. When the targeted outcomes are met, or it is determined that the elder may not be able to achieve the outcomes despite refinement of the intervention plan, the elder undergoes a final assessment process and is discharged or discontinued from OT services.

Outcomes (engagement in activity to support participation)

Outcome assessment information determines the extent to which the targeted goals and objectives of the intervention were met. This information is used to plan future collaborative therapy with the client, discontinue services, and evaluate the service programme.

Case examples

Case 1

An 86-year-old Caucasian woman, Irene, was admitted to a local acute-care hospital following a right hip fracture sustained when she fell from a chair while trying to change a light bulb. She was scheduled for a hip replacement.

OT intervention

During her hospitalization, OT personnel met Irene and completed an occupational profile that informed the therapist about this elderly woman – in particular, her lifestyle and the activities that she needed and wanted to do. She was provided with a long-handled reaching device to enable her to more easily reach items in her hospital room and at home, once she was discharged. The OT learned that Irene enjoyed knitting and recommended that her daughter bring her mother's current knitting project to the hospital during her stay. Knowing that her right hip mobility would likely be limited for the weeks during her recovery from the hip replacement surgery, the OT worked with Irene on donning her socks, using a sock-aid, and continually reinforcing postsurgical hip precautions. During her hospital stay and immediately prior to discharge, the OT reviewed all ADL and IADL implications, and also other high-priority activities that Irene identified during her initial occupational profile. Irene agreed to have the OT arrange for her to have an elevated toilet seat with attached rails, a tall shower stool, a handheld shower and grab bars for her home shower for her use following discharge from the hospital. Additional recommendations were made regarding the height of the furniture that Irene would use at home for sitting, eating and knitting. Irene's daughter agreed to obtain extensions for the legs of Irene's favourite easy chair, so that she would be able to sit and rise from the chair easily. At the time of discharge, Irene's daughter stated that she felt that her mother was well prepared to manage at home during the remainder of her recovery and, most important, Irene agreed.

Case 2

A 65-year-old African man, Kwesi, who completed initial acute care and rehabilitation treatment for a cerebral vascular accident (CVA) with left-side hemiparesis and mild expressive aphasia, was referred for continued OT upon discharge to his home.

OT intervention

His wife and the OT collaborated with Kwesi in determining the priorities of his current activities and target goals. At this point, he was dependent upon his wife for assistance with toileting, bathing and dressing and was not performing IADL tasks that he had assumed prior to his CVA. These activities, plus rejoining his men's group, were very important to him. Therefore, over the next several weeks, his OT worked with him to upgrade his independence. Since organizing and sequencing the steps within those activities were still difficult, the OT provided him and his wife with strategies to enable him to relearn the steps that were problematic. These included transfer assistance to the toilet and into the bathtub with the use of a bath bench, organizing clothes within easy reach and by colour groups to identify appropriate combinations easily, and relearning his use of the telephone. The OT also worked with his wife to help her realize more success and improved coping with her husband's condition, in addition to having more time for the activities that were important to her. Throughout this process, the OT coordinated the intervention plan with Kwesi's physician and other healthcare providers.

Case 3

A 75-year-old immigrant from Bosnia, Soofi, was found wandering several miles from her neighbourhood. Her family, with whom she lived, was referred to neurological/psychiatry services for her to receive a complete work up for probable dementia.

OT intervention

Following her evaluation by a neurologist, Soofi was referred to OT for assessment and intervention. The occupational therapist therefore scheduled a time to meet with Soofi and her family at their home, in order to obtain the most accurate information regarding her occupational performance within her usual environment. In addition, the OT would observe and discuss the nature of the support that Soofi needed and that the family provided for her. This would also provide an opportunity for the OT to adapt approaches to address cultural needs, if indicated. Results of the assessment process indicated that Soofi had difficulty with sequencing her hygiene maintenance and dressing and she also typically awakened in the early hours of the morning, rummaging through her room and the kitchen trying to find items and creating enough noise to awaken the household. The OT worked with the family over several sessions in the home to assist them in simplifying the organization of Soofi's room and the kitchen. Part of the approach involved mounting pictures of the types of clothing in her dresser on the drawers and also on the outside of the kitchen cabinets, so she could better associate the items she was seeking in the relevant location. Furthermore, the OT worked with the family to adjust Soofi's routine to facilitate a more predictable schedule. The family was also informed of the supportive resources provided by the local Alzheimer's Association.

Conclusion

OT focuses on the elder's ability to participate in the activities that comprise their lives and that are important to them. The aims of interventions are to (1) collaborate with the older adult to plan client-centred care, (2) tailor the approaches to meet the elderly patient's/client's activity needs and (3) address the elder's continued participation in society in a manner that is appropriate and meaningful to that individual, thus affecting their overall wellbeing and quality of life. Fundamental concerns of OT practitioners include supporting the elder's autonomy in setting priorities and making decisions regarding their participation and maintaining a level of mastery and control over their environment and lifestyle. OT personnel foster an enabling therapeutic relationship with older adults of all ability levels throughout the continuum of care, together with their families and/or other support systems. The emphasis of OT on the elder's ability to participate in meaningful occupations promotes cost-effective care, individual competence and optimal quality of life.[1,2]

Key points

- Humans throughout their lives are *occupational beings*. Thus, *who we are* is typically framed by *what we do*. OT is patient/client centred, collaborative and focuses on what the individual *needs* and *wants to do*.
- OT services aim to sustain or improve the elders' ability to perform necessary and meaningful activities (*occupations*), whether they are long term and historically a part of the elder's life, newly acquired interests and roles or future desired activity goals.
- OT identifies the strengths and priorities of the patient/client and partners with the individual and their family members or other support systems to ensure their participation in the occupations that sustain their overall health and quality of life.
- OT interventions focus on supporting age-related changes and/or comorbidities that affect the elder's ability to participate in desired activities/occupations. Interventions thus target the individual's biopsychosocial occupational performance abilities and often include adaptive approaches and assistive devices that compensate for any existing occupational performance deficits.
- OT services are provided throughout the continuum of care, from primary care health promotion and wellness approaches to interventions in tertiary, long-term care, palliative and hospice settings.

References

1. Clark F, Azen SP, Zemke R *et al*. Occupational therapy for independent living older adults: a randomized controlled trial. *JAMA* 1997;**278**:1321–6.
2. Clark F, Azen SP, Carlson M *et al*. Embedding health-promoting changes into the daily lives of independent-living older adults: longterm follow-up of occupational therapy intervention. *J Gerontol B Psychol Sci Soc Sci* 2001;**56**:P60–3.
3. Csikszentmihalyi M. *Finding Flow: the Psychology of Engagement with Everyday Life*, Harper Collins, New York, 1997.
4. Wilcock, A. *Occupation and Health*, 2nd edn, Slack, Thorofare, NJ, 2006.
5. World Health Organization. *International Classification of Functioning, Disability and Health (ICF)*, World Health Organization, Geneva, 2001.
6. Christiansen CH, Baum CM and Bass-Haugen J (eds). *Occupational Therapy: Performance, Participation and Well-Being*, Slack, Thorofare, NJ, 2005.
7. Law M, Polatajko H, Baptiste W and Townsend E. Core concepts of occupational therapy. In: E Townsend (ed.), *Enabling Occupation: an Occupational Therapy Perspective*, Canadian Association of Occupational Therapists, Ottawa, 1997, pp. 29–56.
8. American Occupational Therapy Association. *The Occupational Therapy Practice Framework*, 2nd edn, American Occupational Therapy Association, Bethesda, MD, 2008.
9. Whiteneck G and Holicky R. Expanding the disablement model. In: M Brabois S, Garrison, K Hart and L Lehmkuhl (eds), *Physical Medicine and Rehabilitation: the Complete Approach*, Blackwell Science, Malden, MA, 2000, pp. 19–25.
10. Fougeyrollas P. Documenting environmental factors for preventing the handicap creation process: Quebec contributions relating to the ICIDH and social participation of people with functional differences. *Disabil Rehabil* 1995;**17**:145–53.
11. Antonovsky A. *Health, Stress and Coping*, Jossey-Bass, San Francisco, 1979.
12. Antonovsky A. *Unraveling the Mystery of Health: How People Manage Stress and Stay Well*, Jossey-Bass, San Francisco, 1987.
13. Frankl VE. *Man's Search for Meaning*, Simon & Schuster, New York, 1963.
14. Frankl VE. *Man's Search for Ultimate Meaning*, Plenum Publishing, New York, 1997.
15. Dunn W. *Best Practice Occupational Therapy in Community Service with Children and Families*, Slack, Thorofare, NJ, 2000.
16. Kielhofner G. *A Model of Human Occupation: Theory and Application*, 2nd edn, Williams & Wilkins, Baltimore, 1995.
17. Birren JE, Lubben JE, Rowe JC and Deutchman DE (eds). *The Concept and Measurement of Quality of Life in the Frail Elderly*, Academic Press, San Diego, 1991.
18. Steiner A, Raube K, Stuck A and Aronow H. Measuring psychosocial aspects of well-being in older community residents: performance of four short scales. *Gerontologist* 1996;**36**:54–62.
19. Stewart AL and Ware JE. *Measuring Functioning and Well-Being: the Medical Outcomes Study Approach*, Duke University Press, Durham, NC, 1992.
20. Hay J, LaBree L, Luo R *et al*. Cost-effectiveness of preventive occupational therapy for independent-living older adults. *J Am Geriatr Soc* 2002;**50**:1381–8.
21. Rothman J and Levine R. *Prevention Practice: Strategies for Physical Therapy and Occupational Therapy*, Saunders, Philadelphia, 1992.
22. Mullins LL, Balderson BHK, Sanders N *et al*. Therapists' perceptions of team functioning in rehabilitation contexts. *Int J Rehabil Health* 1997;**3**:281–8.
23. Reilly C. Transdisciplinary approach: an atypical strategy for improving outcomes in rehabilitative and long-term acute care settings. *Rehabil Nurs* 2001;**26**:216–20.

CHAPTER 142

Geriatric medicine education in Europe and the United States

Antonio Cherubini[1], Philippe Huber[2], Jean-Pierre Michel[2] and Miguel A. Paniagua[3]

[1]Perugia University Medical School, Perugia, Italy
[2]University Hospital of Geneva, Geneva, Switzerland
[3]Saint Louis University School of Medicine, St Louis, MO, USA

Introduction

During the twentieth century there was a remarkable increase of >30 years in life expectancy in developed countries.[1] It has been recently estimated that the majority of babies born since 2000 in these countries will reach 100 years of age if the current gain in life expectancy continues during the twenty-first century.[1] As a consequence of this fast process of ageing of the population, a new category of patients has appeared, characterized not only by advanced age but also by the simultaneous occurrence of multimorbidity, disability and frailty.[2] A cross-sectional analysis conducted on a random sample of more than one million Medicare beneficiaries aged 65 and older living in the United States in 1999 revealed that 65% had multiple chronic conditions.[3] Older patients with multimorbidity tend to have more rapid declines in health status and a greater likelihood of disability.[4,5] A recent Italian study of older patients cared in acute care wards, home care and nursing homes in Italy confirmed that the majority of these patients are aged >80 years, suffer from multiple diseases and have severe disability in ADL.[6]

Unfortunately, there is still a huge gap between the healthcare needs of these patients and the ability of the healthcare system to satisfy them. Part of the responsibility of the current healthcare crisis lies in the medical education, which has traditionally focused on single diseases, and particularly on acute conditions requiring hospital care, and therefore is more and more inadequate in preparing physicians for their future practice, which will often consist of providing effective healthcare for patients suffering from multiple chronic diseases, i.e. mainly the older patients.[7]

The failure of medical education to adequately prepare physicians for the care of older patients has been acknowledged for the last 20 years,[8] but the situation has not significantly improved, except for the slow and heterogeneous diffusion of geriatric medicine in undergraduate and postgraduate medical curricula.

In this chapter an overview of current geriatric education in Europe and United States will be provided.

Geriatric education in Europe

The Council of Europe includes 45 state members, while the European Community, limited until May 2004 to 15 countries, includes nowadays 27 different countries, with varying degrees of industrialization, economic benefits and employment. These initial remarks highlight that it is not possible to consider Europe as a homogeneous group of countries. The wide variation of demographic data is probably the best way of showing the 2008 disparity among the European countries.[9]

– Birth rate: the highest is in Iceland (2.2/woman) and the lowest in Slovakia (1.3/woman);
– Mortality rate during the first year of life: the highest is in Turkey (16.0/1000) and the lowest in Luxembourg (1.8/1000);
– Life expectancy at birth for men: the highest is in Liechtenstein (79.9 years) and the lowest in Lithuania (66.3 years);
– Life expectancy at birth for women: the highest is in Switzerland (84.6 years) and the lowest in the former Yugoslav Republic (76.5 years).

However, in more developed European countries, life expectancy at birth continues to increase: there is actually a 3-month 'bonus' of life for each year of life.[10] In 2008, the European Union (EU) (27 countries) had a total population of 501 million inhabitants, of which 17% were over 65 years. Between 2010 and 2050, the EU (27 countries) dependency rate (ratio between people over the age of 65 and people

Principles and Practice of Geriatric Medicine, Fifth Edition. Edited by Alan J. Sinclair, John E. Morley and Bruno Vellas.

between the ages of 15 to 64.9) is expected to increase from 25.9 to 59.4.

The number of nonagenarians, centenarians and supercentenarians (over 110 years) will continue to increase.[11] While the healthy life expectancy is longer than ever in developed countries, still many older subjects spend the last years of their life suffering from chronic diseases and increasing disability, which explains why a large percentage of patients requiring healthcare belong to this age-group.

In this context, the promotion of training in geriatric medicine should be a priority in every European medical schools with the following aims: (1) to improve the understanding and integration of the ageing process within the life cycle, (2) to increase the basic and more specialized knowledge of chronic and disabling diseases, (3) to perform comprehensive assessment of the ageing and aged old persons in order to guarantee a better follow-up of the patient, and (4) to guarantee more suitable care, including the appropriate use of drugs in older subjects, neglecting neither ethical nor costs of care issues.[12,13]

In the 1990s, a first European geriatric education survey was performed by a small group of professors of medical gerontology whose three goals were: (1) to establish the basis of a consensual undergraduate core curriculum, (2) to be politically active in order to obtain the creation of a chair of geriatric medicine in each European medical school, and (3) to set up a long-life training course to teach and train the future academics in geriatric medicine.[14] Fifteen years later, an update was realized to evaluate the degree of achievement of these goals, the real situation at the beginning of a new millennium and the needs of professional academic specialists to better cope with the increasing care demand of the future older subjects.[15] In this chapter a further update of the data of these two surveys will be provided.

Among the 31 European countries included in the 2008 survey, Geriatrics is:
– a medical speciality in 16 countries (Belgium, Bulgaria, Czech Republic, Denmark, Finland, France, Germany, Hungary, Italy, Lithuania, Macedonia, Malta, the Netherlands, Spain, Sweden and United Kingdom);
– a medical subspeciality in 9 other countries (Iceland, Ireland, Norway, Poland, Serbia and Montenegro, Slovakia, Switzerland, Turkey and Ukraine);
– not recognized as a specialty in 6 countries (Austria, Estonia, Greece, Luxembourg, Moldavia and Slovenia).
It is interesting to point out that the existence of geriatric nurses is recognized only in 13 European countries (mainly those in which geriatrics is considered as a medical speciality). However, recognition of the existence of a specialty does not imply that gerontology and geriatrics are included in the medical education curricula.

In seven European countries a chair of Geriatrics exists in all medical schools; the chair is most often filled but in a few cases the chairperson has not been nominated yet or is in the process of being appointed (Belgium, Finland, France, Iceland, Norway and Sweden). In several European countries, a chair of Geriatrics exists in some medical schools (80% Switzerland, 70% in Italy, 50% in the Netherlands and Serbia, 33% in Denmark and Austria, 36% in Spain and only 16% in Germany and Portugal). Moreover, no chair of Geriatric Medicine exists in Estonia, Greece, Luxembourg, Malta, Macedonia, Moldavia and Slovenia. It is interesting to notice that two countries (Macedonia and Malta) do not have a geriatric chair even if Geriatrics is recognized as a medical speciality.

Undergraduate geriatric medicine education in Europe

Although the European Union of Medical Specialists – Geriatric Medicine Section (GMS-UEMS) has produced an undergraduate curriculum in geriatric medicine in 2003, which has been approved by a number of national geriatric societies, there is no evidence that this curriculum has been implemented in the majority of EU countries.[16]

Undergraduate teaching of geriatric medicine is organized in 25 countries, but it is mandatory in only 9, and nonexistent in 6 of the 31 surveyed European countries. The existing teaching activities are based on European/National core curriculum in only 2 countries, while in general, the content is independently determined by each medical school. Thus, variability is high both in teaching hours and curriculum. The mean number of teaching hours devoted to geriatrics varies considerably from one to another country, with a maximum of 100 hours in Norway, 60 hours in Serbia and Spain, 50 hours in Italy, Slovenia and Slovakia, 40 hours in Finland and Iceland, 30 hours in France, Hungary and Poland, 20 hours in Denmark and Germany, between 10 to 15 hours in Belgium, Czech Republic, Lithuania, Malta and Turkey and less than 10 hours in Ireland and Luxembourg. Within each country variability is also high. In 10 of these countries, geriatric teaching takes place at different times of the medical studies. Again, the differences are wide from one country to the other, but in most cases, geriatric teaching takes place in the second half of the medical studies, i.e. between the 4th and the 6th year. Moreover it is important to notice that the teaching methodology is 'problem-based learning' in nearly 50% of cases. Undergraduate teaching activities are organized in all medical schools of only 14 countries of the 31 surveyed, while clerkships are available in 16 of these countries (11 mandatory and 5 elective).

Geriatric medicine teaching at the postgraduate level

Postgraduate teaching activities are specifically organized by geriatricians in 16 European countries (Belgium, Czech Republic, Finland, France, Hungary, Ireland, Italy, Lithuania, Malta, the Netherlands, Norway, Poland,

Slovak Republic, Spain, Sweden and United Kingdom) and in collaboration with internal medicine in 6 other countries (Germany, Iceland, Serbia, Switzerland, Turkey and Ukraine). Geriatric postgraduate teaching does not exist in 9 countries. In countries organizing postgraduate teaching activities, students are selected on a pre-requisite basis (N = 9) and the course is based on a pre-established core curriculum (N = 16). A final mandatory examination takes place at the end of the course in 13 countries and a mandatory re-validation is needed in only 8 countries.

Continuing medical education

Continuing medical education (CME) in geriatrics is organized in 18 different European countries, but is mandatory in only 11 of them (Austria, Belgium, Czech Republic, Finland, Hungary, Italy, the Netherlands, Poland, Slovakia, Switzerland and Ukraine).

Undergraduate geriatric education in the United States

Even as the post-World War II 'baby boom' generation ages and requires more medical care, the United States (USA) is facing a critical shortage of geriatricians. In the USA, there have been ongoing efforts to increase medical students' early exposure to geriatrics in the hope of increasing the number of students selecting a career in geriatric medicine. However, to ensure that ageing Americans have access to adequate medical care, for over 20 years the American Association of Medical Colleges (AAMC) has recommended that all physicians should be educated and trained to treat geriatric patients, even if not as a specific specialty focus.[17,18]

Even though only 10% of all US medical schools had a required geriatric medicine clinical rotation in 2001, 92% of medical schools included geriatrics education within some required course. By 2005, this proportion grew to 98%.[19] Additionally, a growing number of US medical schools are reporting having identifiable geriatrics curricula. Most schools have sections or divisions of geriatrics or gerontology in departments of internal medicine or family practice. However, few medical schools in the USA have a dedicated department of geriatrics.[19] Ongoing foundational and government-supported programmes such as the John A. Hartford Foundation or the Donald W. Reynolds Foundation also aim to increase exposure to geriatrics in medical school in the USA.

Postgraduate geriatric education in USA

Residency

Primary care Graduate Medical Education (GME) in the USA has traditionally had a paucity of specific training in the comprehensive management of geriatric patients. Nearly two-thirds of America's internists report being undertrained in chronic care management as a result. In 1993, the Institute of Medicine (IOM) recommended that primary care residency programmes should include at least nine months of geriatric training.[17] As a result, internal medicine residency programmes have increased their geriatric training, with over 90% of programmes requiring dedicated geriatric training of at least two weeks' duration. Despite this, only a minority of internal medicine residencies require six or more weeks of geriatrics training, which mostly exist in the form of block rotations. More than 95% of family medicine residency programmes now have a required curriculum, not just a curricular component, in geriatrics. However, only one quarter of family medicine residencies require four or more weeks of geriatric medicine training during their residency.[20]

Fellowship

According to the IOM report, there are approximately 7100 geriatricians, and the numbers are declining – even as the US population rapidly ages. Because the number of geriatricians has grown slowly over time and nowhere near the rate of the ageing population, in 1998 the American Boards of Internal Medicine and Family Practice reduced from two years to one the duration of the fellowship required for eligibility to sit for the qualifying examination for the Certificate of Added Qualification (CAQ) in Geriatric Medicine. This reduction resulted in the elimination of educational methods, research and leadership from the training of most geriatrics.[21] Despite this, the rate of unmatched geriatric fellowship positions has been rising, in part due to the relatively poor reimbursement rates for geriatricians in practice compared to procedure-based specialties and the increased burden of student loans for graduating students in the USA. Discussions at the national level to promote entry into primary care specialties, and subsequently the field of geriatric medicine, are underway and include loan repayment programmes as well as enhanced reimbursement systems for geriatric care.[20] The recruitment of high-quality US medical school graduates into geriatric medicine continues to be a challenge.

Initiatives for improving undergraduate and postgraduate geriatric education: United States

The Donald W. Reynolds Foundation has undertaken a major effort to strengthen the training in geriatrics of medical students, residents, practicing physicians and affiliated healthcare professionals. During the past decade, the Foundation has provided support to 2 departments of geriatrics, 30 medical schools to improve medical education

Table 142.1 Minimum geriatric competencies for medical students (USA).[18]

Medication Management

1. Explain impact of age-related changes on drug selection and dose based on knowledge of age-related changes in renal and hepatic function, body composition and central nervous system sensitivity.
2. Identify medications, including anticholinergic, psychoactive, anticoagulant, analgesic, hypoglycaemic, and cardiovascular drugs, that should be avoided or used with caution in older adults, and explain the potential problems associated with each.
3. Document a patient's complete medication list, including prescribed, herbal, and over-the-counter medications, and, for each medication, provide the dose, frequency, indication, benefit, side effects, and an assessment of adherence.

Cognitive and Behavioural Disorders

4. Define and distinguish among the clinical presentations of delirium, dementia and depression.
5. Formulate a differential diagnosis and implement initial evaluation in a patient who exhibits dementia, delirium, or depression.
6. In an older patient with delirium, urgently initiate a diagnostic workup to determine the root cause (aetiology).
7. Perform and interpret a cognitive assessment in older patients for whom there are concerns regarding memory or function.
8. Develop an evaluation and non-pharmacological management plan for agitated demented or delirious patients.

Self-care Capacity

9. Assess and describe baseline and current functional abilities (instrumental activities of daily living, activities of daily living, and special senses) in an older patient by collecting historical data from multiple sources and performing a confirmatory physical examination.
10. Develop a preliminary management plan for patients presenting with functional deficits, including adaptive interventions and involvement of interdisciplinary team members from appropriate disciplines, such as social work, nursing, rehabilitation, nutrition and pharmacy.
11. Identify and assess safety risks in the home environment, and make recommendations to mitigate these.

Falls, Balance, Gait Disorders

12. Ask all patients over 65 years old, or their caregivers, about falls in the last year, watch the patient rise from a chair and walk (or transfer), and then record and interpret the findings.
13. In a patient who has fallen, construct a differential diagnosis and evaluation plan that addresses the multiple aetiologies identified by history, physical examination and functional assessment.

Health Care Planning and Promotion

14. Define and differentiate among types of code status, healthcare proxies, and advance directives in the state where one is training.
15. Accurately identify clinical situations where life expectancy, functional status, patient preference, or goals of care should override standard recommendations for screening tests in older adults.
16. Accurately identify clinical situations where life expectancy, functional status, patient preference, or goals of care should override standard recommendations for treatment in older adults.

Atypical Presentation of Disease

17. Identify at least three physiological changes of ageing for each organ system and their impact on the patient, including their contribution to homeostenosis (the age-related narrowing of homeostatic reserve mechanisms).
18. Generate a differential diagnosis based on recognition of the unique presentations of common conditions in older adults, including acute coronary syndrome, dehydration, urinary tract infection, acute abdomen and pneumonia.

Palliative Care

19. Assess and provide initial management of pain and key non-pain symptoms based on patient's goals of care.
20. Identify the psychological, social and spiritual needs of patients with advanced illness and their family members, and link these identified needs with the appropriate interdisciplinary team members.
21. Present palliative care (including hospice) as a positive, active treatment option for a patient with advanced disease.

Hospital Care for Elders

22. Identify potential hazards of hospitalization for all older adult patients (including immobility, delirium, medication side effects, malnutrition, pressure ulcers, procedures, peri- and postoperative periods, and hospital acquired infections) and identify potential prevention strategies.
23. Explain the risks, indications, alternatives, and contraindications for indwelling (Foley) catheter use in the older adult patient.
24. Explain the risks, indications, alternatives, and contraindications for physical and pharmacological restraint use.
25. Communicate the key components of a safe discharge plan (e.g., accurate medication list, plan for follow-up), including comparing/contrasting potential sites for discharge.
26. Conduct a surveillance examination of areas of the skin at high risk for pressure ulcers, and describe existing ulcers.

at their institutions, and 4 consortium schools aimed at developing faculty to teach geriatrics. Overall, it appears this funding strategy was has been successful in achieving its goals of enhancing geriatrics education. The investment of the Reynolds Foundation in the development of geriatrics curricula, programmatic development and training at US medical schools continues to influence undergraduate, graduate and practising physician education.[22]

The John A. Hartford Foundation has had a longstanding commitment to geriatrics education at all levels of learners including the surgical and related specialties. With the AAMC, the Hartford Foundation has advanced geriatric and gerontology studies through integrative and innovative curricula. Forty of the 126 eligible medical schools received a total of $100 000 each for two years to create and implement a four-year undergraduate curriculum incorporating geriatrics education.

The Health Resources and Services Administration (HRSA), an agency of the US Department of Health and Human Services, is the primary federal agency for improving access to healthcare services for people who are uninsured, isolated or medically vulnerable, including elders. Through Geriatric Education Centers (GEC), as well as the establishment of Geriatric Academic Career Awards (GACA), HRSA has helped educate, train and retain health professional faculty, students and practitioners in the diagnosis, treatment and prevention of disease, disability and other health problems of the aged.

At the 2007 Geriatrics Consensus Conference, hosted by the AAMC, more than 450 experts in geriatric medicine including medical professionals, educators, experts and leaders devised a set of 26 competencies in 8 domain areas for evaluating the quality of the geriatric curriculum and its benefits, entitled 'Geriatric Competencies for Graduating Medical Students' (see Table 142.1). This effort has been a major first step in setting the standard of care of elders for US healthcare providers.[18]

Conclusion

In Europe as well as in the USA undergraduate and postgraduate training programmes in geriatrics are varied in content and format and in general are inadequate to provide physicians with the knowledge and skills that are necessary to provide effective healthcare to older patients. Restructuring the educational process taking into account the healthcare needs of the ageing societies can no longer be deferred. Otherwise, there is a risk of a progressive collapse of European and American healthcare systems under the burden of the multimorbidity and disability of the rapidly increasing older population.

Key points

- Ageing of the population has been very fast in Europe and the United States during the last century and it will continue in the next decades. Whereas the majority of older people live healthy and independent lives, the risk of morbidity, ill health and disability increases with age.
- The frail elderly population with its specific medical and psychosocial needs requires high-quality geriatric care: this can be provided only if appropriate geriatric training is guaranteed to all categories of healthcare professionals and, particularly, doctors.
- In many European countries and in the USA, undergraduate training in gerontology and geriatrics is not adequately developed and is not integrated into the medical curricula, particularly with basic and preclinical disciplines.
- Postgraduate training in geriatric medicine is available in the USA and in some European countries, but not in others. In general, the number of geriatricians is still inadequate to match the increasing number of older patients with multimorbidity and disability requiring healthcare.

References

1. Christensen K, Doblhammer G, Rau R, Vaupel JW. Ageing populations: the challenges ahead. *Lancet* 2009;**374** (9696):1196–208.
2. American Medical Association White Paper on Elderly Health. Report of the Council on Scientific Affairs. *Arch Intern Med* 1990;**150**:2459–72.
3. Wolff JL, Starfield B, Anderson G. Prevalence, expenditures, and complications of multiple chronic conditions in the elderly. *Arch Intern Med* 2002;**162**:2269–76.
4. Verbrugge LM, Lepkowski JM, Imanaka Y. Comorbidity and its impact on disability. *Milbank Q* 1989;**67**:450–84.
5. Fried LP, Bandeen-Roche K, Kasper JD, Guralnik JM. Association of comorbidity with disability in older women: the Women's Health and Aging Study. *J Clin Epidemiol* 1999;**52**; 27–37.
6. Lattanzio F, Mussi C, Scafato E *et al*. Health care for older people in Italy: The U.L.I.S.S.E. Project (Un Link Informatico sui Servizi Sanitari Esistenti per l'anziano – A Computerized Network on Health Care Services for Older People). *J Nutr Health Aging* 2010;**14**:238–42.
7. Holman H. Chronic disease – the need for a clinical education. *JAMA* 2004;**292**:1057–9.
8. Schroeder SA, Zones JS, Showstack JA. Academic medicine as a public trust. *JAMA* 1989;**262**:803–12.

9. European demographic data. Eurostat. http://epp.eurostat.ec.europa.eu/portal/page/portal/population/data/main_tables (last accessed December 2011).
10. Oeppen J, Vaupel JW. Demography. Broken limits to life expectancy. *Science* 2002;**296**:1029–31.
11. Robine JM, Paccaud F. Nonagenarians and centenarians in Switzerland, 1860–2001: a demographic analysis. *J Epidemiol Community Health* 2005;**59**:31–7.
12. Michel JP, Gold G. Coping with population aging in the old continent – the need for European academic geriatrics. *J Gerontol A Biol Sci Med Sci* 2001;**56**: M341–39.
13. Duursma S, Castleden M, Cherubini A *et al.* European Union Geriatric medicine Society Position paper on geriatric medicine and the provision of health care for older people. *J Nutr Health Aging* 2004;**8**:190–5.
14. Stähelin HB, Beregi E, Duursma SA *et al.* Teaching medical gerontology in Europe. Group of European Professors in Medical Gerontology (GEPMG). *Age Ageing* 1994;**23**:179–81.
15. Michel JP, Huber P, Cruz-Jentoft AJ. Europe-wide survey of teaching in geriatric medicine. *J Am Geriatr Soc* 2008;**56**: 1536–42.
16. Geriatric Medicine Section of the European Union Medical Specialists. Undergraduate training www.uemsgeriatricmedicine.org (accessed May 2010).
17. Institute of Medicine. *Retooling for an Aging America: Building the Health Care Workforce*, National Academy Press, Washington DC, 2008.
18. Leipzig RM, Granville L, Simpson D *et al.* Keeping Granny safe on July 1: A consensus on minimum geriatrics competencies for graduating medical students. *Acad Med* 2009;**84**: 604–10.
19. Boult C, Christmas C, Durso SC *et al.* Perspective: Transforming chronic care for older persons. *Acad Med* 2008;**83**:627–31.
20. Warshaw GA, Bragg EJ. The training of geriatricians in the United States: Three decades of progress. *J Am Geriatr Soc* 2003;**51**: S338–S345.
21. Warshaw GA, Bragg EJ, Shaull RW *et al.* Geriatric Medicine Fellowship Programs: A National Study from the Association of Directors of Geriatric Academic Programs' Longitudinal Study of Training and Practice in Geriatric Medicine. *J Am Geriatr Soc* 2003;**51**:1023–30.
22. Reuben DB, Bachrach PS, McCreath H *et al.* Changing the course of geriatrics education: An evaluation of the first cohort of Reynolds Geriatrics Education Programs. *Acad Med* 2009;**4**:619–26.

CHAPTER 143

Systems of healthcare: the United States

Julie K. Gammack
Saint Louis University School of Medicine, and St Louis VA Medical Center, Geriatric Research Education and Clinical Center, St Louis, MO, USA

Introduction

The extraordinary growth in life expectancy at birth in nearly all countries of the world reflects an ongoing revolution in longevity. This revolution has resulted in both survival of individuals to older ages and a changing age distribution of the entire population. The impact of the longevity revolution has been pervasive and profound. The impact is felt financially, socially and politically throughout the United States (USA). This trend has resulted in significant healthcare changes, both on an individual and societal level.

Developed nations across the world have approached the ageing population and need for expanded health services in a variety of ways. Home health, hospital-based and nursing home care have experienced a profound increase in complexity over the last quarter century. This complexity of care is reflected in the expansion of funding arrangements, number of service providers, and geographic service areas. Governmental expenditures for healthcare services have continued to rise but are not sustainable at the current rate. The development and passage of the Health Care Reform Bill has attempted to slow the rise in spending while promoting increased quality and universal access to care healthcare services.

Institutes of higher learning have evolved to support the growing fields of gerontology and geriatric medicine. Educating the medical providers, workforce and community on the needs of older adults has become an area of profound interest within and outside of the academic environment. It is important to draw older people into the processes of developing the services and new technologies that they themselves and others of their generation will use. By developing these new healthcare opportunities, the greatest gains may be made in health, independence and quality of life (QOL) in old age.

Overview of healthcare demographics

The USA spends over 15% of the GDP, 2.5 trillion dollars, on healthcare expenditures. This is more than any other industrialized nation.[1–3] Healthcare expenditures have doubled in the past 10 years; however, 16% of population does not have health insurance. The provision of healthcare is equally split between private insurance, Medicare/Medicaid and other sources including out-of-pocket payers.

The annual number of hospitalizations has remained relatively stable at 11 per 100 population, and the average length of hospital admission has dropped consistently over the last 10 years to an average length of stay of 4.6 days.[3,4] Despite this trend, hospital expenditures have risen 50% in the last 10 years.[3] Outpatient encounters have increased by 40% over that same time.[4] About one-third of healthcare resources are spent on hospitalization and one-quarter on physician services. Individuals age 65 or older utilize one quarter of outpatient encounters, one third of hospitalization, and one third of the total healthcare expenditures.

Currently 13% of the US population is aged 65 or older. This population is projected to reach 21% by 2050.[5] These trends have caused great concern both economically and socially. The healthcare budget cannot sustain the current growth rate of medical expenditures. Methods to provide cost-effective, quality healthcare for an ageing population are being addressed on a system-wide level. Research funding, educational efforts and clinical care models are being developed to better serve the healthcare needs of the geriatric population.

Development of geriatric medicine

In the USA, geriatrics came into the medical consciousness through the writings of Dr Ignatz Nascher. Although born

Principles and Practice of Geriatric Medicine, Fifth Edition. Edited by Alan J. Sinclair, John E. Morley and Bruno Vellas.

in Austria, he was raised in the USA and received his medical degree from New York University. In 1909 at the age of 46, Dr Nascher published his first geriatrics article titled 'Longevity and Rejuvenescence'. In this work he proposes that 'geriatrics' be added to the medical vocabulary and that it be considered a distinct aspect in medicine. Over the next five years he authored more than 30 articles on ageing and the first American geriatrics textbook titled *Geriatrics: The Diseases of Old Age and Their Treatment*. This text focused dually on the physiology and pathophysiology of ageing. Nascher touched on a multitude of topics including organ system physiology, pharmacology, diseases of ageing, and psychosocial aspects of medicine. With an optimistic view, he wrote in 1926 that, 'Geriatrics is now firmly established as a special branch of medicine ... '.

Unfortunately, geriatrics was not yet widely accepted and the growth of this specialty was quite slow through the 1930s and 1940s. The mid-1900s were notable for the establishment of two medical societies. Malford W. Thewlis founded the American Geriatrics Society in 1942, and the Gerontological Society (now called The Gerontological Society of America) was established in 1945.

Research in ageing was championed by Dr E. Vincent Cowdry who received his PhD in anatomy from the University of Chicago in 1913. During his 65-year career spent predominantly at Washington University School of Medicine, Dr Cowdry focused his research efforts on cancer and the cytological changes of ageing. During the latter half of his career he authored several books including *The Problems of Ageing: Biological and Medical Aspects* (1939), *The Care of the Geriatric Patient* (1958), and *Aging Better* (1972).

Geriatrics in the United States developed as much through the establishment of governmental socioeconomic programmes as it did from the work of prominent physicians. In 1861, a military pension plan was established to support the Civil War era veterans. After the Civil War, many states established veterans' homes to provide disability and medical care services. These services were consolidated through the development of the Veterans Administration in 1930. By 1935, a rapidly increasing population of impoverished older adults led to the formation the Social Security Board which reorganized in 1946 to become the Social Security Administration. This programme provides a retirement benefit to individuals upon leaving the workforce. Although state and federal subsidies for healthcare services were sporadically available in the 1920s, the first private hospital insurance plan (Blue Cross) was not provided until 1933. Further discussion and development of government-sponsored health insurance for the elderly spanned five presidential administrations and more than three decades.

In 1950, through efforts by President Truman, the Federal Security Administration held a national conference on ageing to assess the challenges posed by the changing population. No immediate programmes were initiated, but this conference spurred the development of an advisory committee on ageing that eventually lead to the first White House Conference on Aging in 1961. The conference resulted in the expansion of Social Security benefits and support for the later development of Medicare and Medicaid. In 1965, insurance was finally guaranteed to older adults, the disabled and the impoverished through the passage of Medicare and Medicaid programmes.

During the mid 1900s, the US Government was the primary financial sponsor of healthcare research and scientific programmes. The National Institute of Health (NIH) was formed in 1930 and later became a consortium of institutes and centres dedicated to healthcare research. The National Institute on Aging (NIA) was formally established out of the National Institutes of Health (NIH) in 1974, but the roots of the NIA can be traced back to the 1940s and 1950s with the Unit on Aging, Gerontology Branch, and Section on Aging subsections of NIH programmes.

The NIA receives substantial funding for the advancement of ageing research. Through NIA support, the 30 Alzheimer's Disease Centers, 15 Claude D. Pepper Older American Independence Centers, and numerous Edward R. Roybal Centers for Research on Applied Gerontology sponsor investigations into the biological, behavioural and clinical aspects of ageing.[6,7] During the last quarter century, there has been a growth in the private support of geriatric medicine research and education. Hundreds of millions of dollars have been provided by The John A. Hartford, Donald W. Reynolds and other agencies dedicated to the care of the ageing population.

Home healthcare

For most of history, medical care has been provided in the home by a physician. In the mid 1900s 40% of all patient–physician encounters took place at home. With the growth of hospital and office-based care, fewer than 1% of healthcare visits took place at home by 1980.[8] Home healthcare (HHC) began growing again in the 1980s as new models of home assessment developed and the delivery of home care evolved into an organized, multidisciplinary business. The current HHC model primarily utilizes nursing, therapy and personal care providers to deliver healthcare services; however, physician house calls still remain under-utilized as a means of caring for frail older adults.

Home visits are an effective method for delivering medical assistance for the aged and chronically ill homebound individuals. House calls have most often demonstrated benefit in chronic and relapsing diseases such as congestive heart failure and emphysema. Regular visits by a medical professional can improve disease control and reduce hospitalizations.[9,10] This translates to a societal cost savings, which has prompted Medicare, Medicaid and private insurance agencies to continue the funding of home care services.

Medicare and Medicaid provided nearly 80% of HHC coverage in the US between 1990 and 1997, HHC expenditures grew almost sixfold to $18 billion. The growth of HHC utilization prompted a change in reimbursement from a fee for service to a prospective payment system reimbursement model. Despite the change in funding, the expenditure on HHC has continued to increase and has more than doubled since 1997.[11] For each 60-day certification period, agencies are reimbursed around $2300 per enrollee, adjusted for geographic region and intensity of care provided.[12] This initially resulted in a reduction in the enrolment length and frequency of HHC visits, but over the past several years, the number of home healthcare recipients has increased. In 2007 nearly three million individuals received over 114 million home care visits from 9000 certified agencies.[13–15]

To qualify for HHC, an agency must receive a physician order, document that a recipient is homebound (a definition that has remained vague) and provide a skilled intervention by a nurse or therapist. Common uses of HHC include medication management, disease assessment, wound care, home safety evaluation, physical and occupational therapy, and patient/family education. The average number of visits per enrollee is 37.[14]

When personal care is needed at home, aides can be hired for in-home assistance with laundry, housekeeping, meal preparation and personal care needs. Medicare does not pay for personal care aides, nor do most private insurance plans. Individual case management and social services are available to seniors based on resources and needs. Services such as meals-on-wheels, transportation, and legal aid are often provided on a sliding fee-scale basis. The availability of these services varies by community.

Hospice care is another service traditionally provided in the home, although there is a growing use of hospice in the nursing home setting. In 2009, over 5000 hospice agencies provided care to 1.5 million individuals through Medicare, an increase of 20% over four years. Forty percent of these patients were served at home and 19% resided in nursing homes. Eighty percent of hospice recipients are age 65 or older and just over half are female. The average length of service is 69 days but 34% of hospice recipients die within 7 days of enrolment. This suggests that hospice services are largely under-utilized for those deemed to have 'less than 6 months to live'.[15] In addition to nursing, hospice provides therapy, social service and family support in the home. Hospice agencies are not capable of providing continuous 24-hour personal care.[15,16]

British physician Dame Cicely Saunders first coined the term hospice in 1967. Yale School of Nursing Dean Florence Wald subsequently adopted this care model in the United States. It was not until 1979 that the Health Care Financing Administration (HCFA) funded 26 hospices as a demonstration programme. In 1982 hospice care was added as a benefit under the Medicare and Medicaid programmes and has since become a standard benefit provided by all health insurance plans. To qualify for hospice a physician must certify an estimated life expectancy of six months or less. Half of the hospice enrollees have a terminal diagnosis of cancer. Cancer diagnoses have dropped 10% in the last three years due to a rise in use of hospice care for non-malignant terminal illnesses such as dementia and emphysema.

Nursing home care

The number of nursing homes in the United States has dropped slowly since the early 1980s, although the total number of residents in nursing homes has increased almost 10% during that time. In 2004 the number of licensed nursing home beds dropped to 1.7 million from 1.9 million in 1999. The average bed capacity increased slightly to an average of 108 residents per facility.[17] Seventy percent of nursing home residents are female and 85% are Caucasian. The average length of stay is 2–3 years. Despite common misconceptions of the elderly population, less than 5% of citizens over the age of 65 reside in nursing homes. Less than 20% of adults over age 85 live in nursing homes.

Most nursing homes certify a portion of their beds (25–35%) for post-acute care, skilled nursing services. These residents receive intensive nursing, therapy and medical services after an acute medical illness with the hope of regaining lost function. Medicare funds most of the skilled nursing care in the United States but private insurance also covers post-acute rehabilitation services. Medicare beneficiaries receive up to 100 days of skilled nursing care before other insurance or private pay must shoulder costs. The average length of skilled nursing care is 27 days.

Medicare and most private insurers do not pay for non-skilled (custodial) care in nursing homes. The bulk of custodial care is paid for by Medicaid once individuals have 'spent down' their personal resources to the point of qualifying for this jointly state-federal sponsored healthcare coverage. The Medicaid qualification level varies by state. An individual generally must have a monthly income less than or equal to the federally designated poverty level ($902/ month in 2010) and net personal resources of only a few thousand dollars.[18] The average yearly cost of nursing home care is roughly $70 000.[19] Nursing home insurance is becoming available but in general is costly and is not widely purchased by the general population.

Nursing home care has improved dramatically in the past 20 years. The Omnibus Budget Reconciliation Act (ORBA), passed in 1987, was instrumental in changing the management and oversight of nursing home care in the United States. Unfortunately, past abuses have resulted in a highly regulated and punitive system of ensuring the current quality of institutional patient care. Nursing homes are surveyed annually by the State regulatory agency. Deficiencies and fines are applied liberally and are a matter of public record. The State has the authority to immediately close down any facility that is found to have practices that place residents in 'immediate jeopardy' of harm. Areas that are frequently cited include unnecessary use of physical restraints and psychotropic medication, weight loss, development of pressure ulcers and fall-related injuries.

As hospital length of stay shortens and the severity of illness of newly admitted residents increases, nursing homes have become more comprehensive in providing medical and therapy services. Most facilities offer intravenous antibiotics and fluids. Gastric tube feeding, suctioning and oxygen treatment are routine. Facilities contract with mobile laboratory and radiology agencies. Physical, occupational and speech therapists, nutritionists and consulting pharmacists are on-staff or consult on a regular basis. Nurses are being challenged to perform more sophisticated care and more rigorous assessments while faced with limited staffing ratios and a high rate of nursing turnover.

Assisted living facilities are assuming some of the rôle that nursing homes played 20 years ago. 'Well' elderly who require only some assistance with daily activities live semi-independently in studio-type apartments with or without a kitchenette. Facilities vary in size from several dozen to over one hundred residents in a single building. A licensed nurse is usually available during most of the day and may pass meds, perform assessments, inject insulin, check glucoses and perform other skilled tasks based on resident needs. The provision of meals, light housekeeping and social activities is usually included in the cost of room and board.

The cost of care is partly based on the level of services designated by the patient/family. Assisted living costs are highly variable but range from $30 000–40 000 or more per year.[19] Almost universally, the cost of assisted living is incurred out-of-pocket by the resident and/or family. Despite being less costly, most long-term care insurance providers will not reimburse assisted living as an alternate to nursing home care. Assistance with ADLs, IADLs, safety checks and other personal care are provided by 24-hour per day nursing assistants at the facility. At this time 900 000 residents reside in approximately 40 000 assisted living facilities. Most assisted living residents receive medical care in the office of medical providers as opposed to on-site as in nursing homes. There are currently very few governmental regulations or requirements in assisted living facilities.

Hospital care

Hospitals in the United States are evolving to provide specialty services for the ageing patient with the hope of improving patient outcomes and reducing adverse health events. Programmes such as adult day care, palliative care and home healthcare, offered through the hospital system, address a wide variety of needs for elderly patients both during and after hospitalization. The American Hospital Association (AHA) publishes the prevalence of these services annually. Over time, utilization of hospital-based skilled nursing units has dropped and use of free standing post-acute skilled nursing facilities has increased.[20] This is likely a result of decreased reimbursement of in-hospital skilled nursing care. In the subsequent years, the frequency of hospital-based services for care of older adults has declined steadily as seen in Table 143.1. The only geriatric programmes which have increased significantly, are palliative care and case management with 28.8% and 80.6% of hospitals having these services respectively in 2007.[21,22] It is interesting that neither an Acute Care for the Elderly (ACE) unit nor a stroke unit are used as markers in this consumer-evaluation model, but both are accepted by the field of geriatric medicine as beneficial interventions.

ACE units

The ACE unit is a growing model for comprehensive and multidisciplinary care of the older hospitalized adult. An ACE unit is a hospital-based ward which emphasizes a comprehensive, multidisciplinary approach to acute care of older adults. These units are usually associated with a university hospital, 15–20 beds in size, and admit patients with a variety of medical conditions.[23] The 'ACE' concept and term were developed in the early 1990s with key elements of the model being (1) environment alterations, (2) patient-centred care, (3) interdisciplinary planning for discharge, and (4) medical care review. Important components of an ACE unit structure are detailed in Table 143.2.[24] The goal of this model is to reduce the functional impairments which so often develop in acutely ill, hospitalized elders.

Table 143.1 Hospital facilities and services trends.[21,22]

Special services offered	% of hospitals 2007	% of hospitals 2003
Skilled nursing care unit	28.5	33.4
Intermediate care unit	9.8	10.2
Adult day care services	6.2	8.1
Assisted living	4.5	5.3
Case management	80.6	75.5
Geriatric services	38.4	40.4
Home health services	32.7	37.4
Hospice	23.5	23.3
Meals on wheels	10.4	12.8
Psychiatric-geriatric services	29.4	30.4
Palliative care programme	28.8	22.2

Table 143.2 Components of an Acute Care for the Elderly (ACE) unit.

Interdisciplinary Team
Medical Director
Physician
Nursing staff
Social work/Case management
Pharmacist
Pastoral care
Palliative care
Therapy services
Physical
Occupational
Speech
Dietician
Regular team meetings
Daily updates
Interdisciplinary participation
Daily assessment
Physical
Cognitive
Functional
Specialty geriatrics training/education
Staff
Patients/families
Physicians
Comprehensive discharge planning
Home discharge emphasis
Coordination with home care services
Communication with caregivers
Assessment for geriatric syndromes
Delirium
Dementia
Depression
Polypharmacy
Falls
Incontinence
Functional decline
Frailty
Environmental modifications
Communication aids
Reorientation strategies
Restraint reduction protocols
Assistive devices
Sleep hygiene
Higher nurse:aide ratio

Two philosophical differences are employed in the ACE model of care. First, care management is shifted toward a biopsychosocial rather than a biomedical model. The hospitalization and discharge planning process focuses on the relationship between the patient and the social structures that are needed for effective treatment. Barriers to successful recovery and risks for ongoing functional decline are identified early in the hospitalization. Appropriate interventions such as reduction in polypharmacy, nutritional assessment, social support evaluation, and physical and occupational therapy assessment are initiated for each patient. Discharge plans ensure that the patient transitions to an appropriate environment and with appropriate social services in place.

Second, a functional-based rather than disease-based approach is used in medical decision-making. Many elders suffer from multiple, chronic medical conditions that will not be cured. Goals of care focus on maximizing function in the context of disease management rather than solely marking improvement by measures of disease severity. With this method, functional status and QOL measures become the markers for successful recovery from illness.

The implementation of an ACE unit has consistently resulted in improved functional status and increased discharge to home compared with usual care wards.[24–26] Despite the additional interventions applied by the multidisciplinary team, the total cost of hospital care is not higher on the ACE unit. The benefits of teamwork in caring for the complexity of frail older adults translates to a more efficient and thorough treatment plan for both the hospital and the patient, without resulting in excess cost. Despite these potential benefits, the growth of ACE units and research in this area has not increased substantially in the past 5–10 years.

Stroke units

Death from cerebrovascular disease is the third leading cause of death and more than two thirds of strokes occur in patients over the age of 65. Despite longstanding use of stroke units outside of the USA, and strong evidence demonstrating the morbidity and mortality benefit of this strategy, comprehensive stroke management models are just beginning in the US healthcare system.[27,28] Previous literature on the benefit of an organized inpatient stroke care team comes almost universally out of the United Kingdom and Northern Europe. For over 20 years, patients with acute stroke in these countries have been managed on a dedicated stroke unit: either on a discrete stroke ward or by a stroke team working exclusively with stroke patients. The focus of a stroke unit can include acute stroke care, subacute rehabilitation or a combination of strategies.

To improve the consistency and quality of stroke care across the United States, the 'Brain Attack Coalition' (BAC) was convened in 2000 to establish recommendation for hospital care of stroke patients. The BAC recommended a two-tier organization for hospital-based stroke care: Primary Stroke Centres (PSCs) and Comprehensive Stroke Centres (CSCs). The major criteria for a PSC or CSC are listed in Table 143.3.[29] PSCs provide the basic emergency

Table 143.3 Requirements for Stroke Centre Certification.[29]

Primary Stroke Centre	Comprehensive Stroke Centre

Acute Stroke Team
  24-hour coverage
  15-minute response time
Written Protocols
  Diagnostic steps
  Therapeutic steps
Emergency Medical Services (EMS)
  Coordination with hospital
  Communication during transport
Emergency Department
  Trained staff
  Coordination with Stroke Team
  Coordination with EMS
Stroke Unit
  Specialized monitoring
  Specialized services
Neurosurgical Services
  Available within 2 hours
Commitment
  Hospital administration
  Medical staff
Neuroimaging
  CT scanning with 25 minutes
  Radiology review within 20 minutes
24-hour Diagnostic Services
  Laboratory
  ECG
  X-ray
Quality Improvement
  Stroke registry
  Outcome database
Annual Educational Programmes
  8 hours staff continuing education
  2 community programmes
	Expert Personnel
	  Vascular specialists
	  Neurology
	  Neurosurgery
	  Surgery
	Interventional Specialists
	  Radiology
	  Neuroradiology
	Advance Practice Nurses
	Stroke nurses
	Critical Care Physicians
	Physiatrists
	Rehabilitation Therapists
	  Physical
	  Occupational
	  Speech
	  Respiratory
	Invasive Therapies
	  Carotid endarterectomy
	  Aneurysm treatments
	  Reperfusion therapies
	Infrastructure
	  Stroke unit
	  Intensive care unit
	  24-hour coverage
	  24-hour operating room
	  Interventional services
	  Stroke registry
	Diagnostic techniques
	  MRI with angiography
	  CT with angiography
	  Cerebral angiography
	  Transcranial Doppler
	  Carotid ultrasound
	  Transoesophageal echo
	Educational Programmes
	  Community
	  Professionals
	  Patients

evaluation and stabilization, while complex cases requiring specialty imaging and intervention should be referred to a CSC. Although over 600 hospitals have accreditation as a PSC, this represents less than 15% of US hospitals.[30]

Academic geriatrics

The development of academic geriatric programmes and medical training has lagged behind the demand for a larger and more skilled geriatric medicine healthcare workforce. This is in part due to the lack of universal acceptance of Geriatrics as a unique discipline within the medical profession. With the increasing age, functional impairment and psychosocial complexity of older adults, the mantra that 'I'm a geriatrician because most of my patients are elderly', is fading, but slowly.

In 1982, Mount Sinai School of Medicine established the first Department of Geriatrics. At this time most of medical schools have some form of a geriatrics programme. The vast majority of the 132 academic geriatrics programmes are organized as Divisions or Sections within a Department of Internal or Family Medicine.[31] Few institutions have the financial capability of supporting independent departments of geriatric medicine. Two thirds of geriatrics programmes have been in existence for less than 20 years. The average programme has 10 faculty members. Fifty percent of programme leaders have been in that position for less than eight years.[32] The first professorship in geriatric medicine was granted at Cornell University in 1977.

Dr Les Libow at Mount Sinai School of Medicine offered the first geriatric medicine fellowship programme in 1966. Since that time the number of trainees and training sites remained fairly limited until the early 1980s. In the 1970s, the Veterans Administration was charged with the task of increasing the understanding of ageing and passing this knowledge to healthcare providers. Funding was provided in 1975 for the first VA Geriatric Research Education and Clinical Center (GRECC). Twenty GRECCs are currently active through the VA.[33] GRECCs began offering geriatric medicine fellowship training opportunities in 1978.

In 1988 the Accreditation Council for Graduate Medical Education began accrediting geriatric medicine fellowship training programmes. 1988 was also that year that an examination became mandatory to attain the Certification of Added Qualification (CAQ) in Geriatrics after at least two years of fellowship training. Until the mid 1990s, most fellows in geriatric medicine engaged in two or more years of training. Extended training was vital for the development of an academic and research career in geriatrics. In 1995, the training requirement for CAQ in geriatrics was reduced to one year and geriatric medicine became an independent subspecialty with board certification status.

Currently there are 105 Internal Medicine and 45 Family Medicine accredited geriatric medicine fellowship training programmes.[34] Despite an increasing number of medical student graduates in the United States, almost one third of fellowship slots go unfilled each year. Although the number of fellowship training programmes has increased, the total number of board certified geriatricians and number of graduates from fellowship training have not increased substantially in the past 10 years. There is significant concern that the increased need for geriatric specialists will not meet the population needs in the next two decades. Significant changes in the healthcare structure and workforce will be needed to ensure that adequate care for older adults can be provided in the US healthcare system.

Conclusion

In the next 50 years, the population demographic in developed countries will change substantially. Up to a quarter of the citizens will be over age 65 with the highest growth rate in age seen in the oldest age groups. Older adults are the highest consumers of healthcare resources and are usually supported, at least in part, by local and national governmental medical programmes. With healthcare costs rising, the United States continues to explore alternate means of caring for the ageing population.

Home healthcare includes a wide variety of programmes and services, most of which are not physician-directed. Traditional physician house calls remain a small portion of the home care encounters performed today. The provision of medical and non-medical services allows individuals to remain independent and in their homes for a longer period of time. Many services are community based and thus help individuals maintain a connection with society.

Nursing home care has increased substantially in cost and complexity over the past 20 years. In an effort to control escalating long-term care costs, intermediate care settings have evolved to allow individuals more autonomy in a less costly setting. Resources and supervision are provided to individuals on an as-needed basis in most of these facilities. For individuals in need of comprehensive supervised care, nursing homes still provide the maximal degree of therapy, social work and nursing support.

Hospital care has evolved to focus more on the delivery of quality healthcare to the elderly individual. Stroke units are well established as an effective model for managing hospitalized older adults. ACE units are now growing in the same manner. It is apparent that quality care for complex elderly patients requires a team of medical providers working together toward common goals.

Academic geriatrics has grown substantially over the past 50 years with most medical schools and academic centres establishing a department or section of geriatric medicine. The role of geriatricians, relative to general practitioners, is still evolving in the care of the older adult. As the older population expands there is an ongoing need to training physicians, both generalists and specialists, in the principles of geriatric medicine.

Key points

- The elderly will account for over 20% of the US population in the next half century.
- Services for the elderly have grown most extensively in the realm of home healthcare.
- Geriatric wards, stroke units, and Acute Care for the Elderly (ACE) units are well-developed and effective models of hospital care for the elderly.
- The growth of nursing home care has slowed and is shifting to 'intermediate-care' service models.
- Geriatrics as a unique field of medicine has developed over the past half century.

References

1. Charting the Economy. Health Care Expenditures as a % of Gross Domestic Product, 8 April 2009. http://chartingtheeconomy.com/?p=526 (last accessed December 2011).
2. American Hospital Association. Chapter 1. Trends in the Overall Health Care Market. Chartbook. Trends Affecting Hospitals and Health Systems. Last update 8 June 2010. http://www.aha.org/aha/research-and-trends/chartbook/ch1.html (last accessed December 2011).
3. Facts and Figures 2007 – Section 4. Table of Contents. Healthcare Cost and Utilization Project (HCUP), September 2009. Agency for Healthcare Research and Quality, Rockville, MD. www.hcup-us.ahrq.gov/reports/factsandfigures/2007/section4_TOC.jsp (last accessed December 2011).
4. National Center for Health Statistics. Health, United States, 2009, With Special Feature on Medical Technology. http://www.cdc.gov/nchs/data/hus/hus09.pdf#listtables (last accessed December 2011).
5. US Census Bureau. US Population Projections. National Population Projections, 2009. http://www.census.gov/population/www/projections/2009cnmsSumTabs.html (last accessed December 2011).
6. National Pepper Center Website. Claude D. Pepper Older Americans Independence Centers (OAIC) Programs. https://www.peppercenter.org/public/home.cfm (last accessed December 2011).
7. National Institute of Aging. Alzheimer's Disease Research Centers. http://www.nia.nih.gov/Alzheimers/ResearchInformation/ResearchCenters/ (last accessed December 2011).
8. Leff B, Burton JR. The future history of home care and physician house calls in the United States. *J Gerontol Med Sci* 2001;**56A**:M606–608.
9. Rich MW, Beckham V, Wittenberg C *et al.* A multidisciplinary intervention to prevent the readmission of elderly patients with congestive heart failure. *N Engl J Med* 1995;**333**: 1184–9.
10. Stewart S, Marley JE, Horowitz JD. Effects of a multidisciplinary, home-based intervention on unplanned readmissions and survival among patients with chronic congestive heart failure: a randomized controlled study. *Lancet* 1999; **28**:613–20.
11. US Department of Health and Human Services. Centers for Medicare and Medicaid Services. National Health Expenditure Data. Table 2: National Health Expenditures Aggregate Amounts and Average Annual Percent Change, by Type of Expenditure: Selected Calendar Years 1960–2009. Last Modified: 11/04/2011. http://www.cms.gov/NationalHealthExpendData/downloads/tables.pdf (accessed 8 December 2011).
12. Federal Register. Vol. 75, No. 141. Friday, July 23, 2010. Centers for Medicare and Medicaid Services. Part II. 42 CFR Parts 409, 418, 424, *et al.* Home Health Prospective Payment System Regulations and Notices. http://edocket.access.gpo.gov/2010/pdf/2010-17753.pdf (last accessed December 2011).
13. CDC/National Center for Health Statistics National Home and Hospice Care Survey, Current Home Health Care Patient and Annual Hospice Care Discharge Trends. Page last updated 4 March 2010. http://www.cdc.gov/nchs/nhhcs/nhhcs_patient_trends.htm (last accessed December 2011).
14. Medicare Home Health Agency Utilization by State Calendar Year 2007. Centers for Medicare and Medicaid Services. Page last modified 23 January 2009. http://www.cms.gov/MedicareFeeforSvcPartsAB/Downloads/HHAst07.pdf (last accessed December 2011).
15. National Hospice and Palliative Care Organization. NHPCO Facts & Figures: Hospice Care in America. Last modified 1 October 2010. http://www.nhpco.org/files/public/Statistics_Research/Hospice_Facts_Figures_Oct-2010.pdf (last accessed December 2011).
16. Centers for Medicare and Medicaid Services. Medicare Utilization for Part A. Medicare Hospice Utilization By State Calendar Year 2008. Page last modified: 2 December 2009. http://www.cms.gov/MedicareFeeforSvcPartsAB/02_MedicareUtilizationforPartA.asp#TopOfPage (last accessed December 2011).
17. Centers for Disease Control. Vital Health and Statistics. Series 13, Number 167. June 2009. The National Nursing Home Survey: 2004 Overview. http://www.cdc.gov/nchs/data/series/sr_13/sr13_167.pdf (last accessed December 2011).
18. Centers for Medicare and Medicaid Services. 2010 Poverty Guidelines. http://www.cms.gov/MedicaidEligibility/Downloads/POV10Combo.pdf (last accessed December 2011).
19. MetLife Mature Market Institute. The 2009 MetLife Market Survey of Nursing Home, Assisted Living, Adult Day Services, and Home Care Costs, October 2009. http://www.metlife.com/assets/cao/mmi/publications/studies/mmi-market-survey-nursing-home-assisted-living.pdf (last accessed December 2011).
20. White C, Seagrave S. What happens when hospital-based skilled nursing facilities close? A propensity score analysis. *Health Serv Res* 2005;**40**:1883–97.
21. Health Forum LLC/American Hospital Association. *Hospital Statistics*, Healthcare InfoSource, Chicago, 2005, Table 7, pp. 151–64.
22. Health Forum LLC/American Hospital Association. *Hospital Statistics*, Healthcare InfoSource, Chicago, 2009, Table 7, pp. 153–69.
23. Siegler EL, Glick D, Lee J. Geriatric nursing. Optimal staffing for Acute Care of the Elderly (ACE) Units 2002;23:152–5.
24. Landefeld CS, Palmer RM, Kresevic DM *et al.* A randomized trial of care in a hospital medical unit especially designed to improve the functional outcomes of acutely ill older patients. *N Engl J Med* 1995;**332**:1338–44.
25. Asplund K, Gustafson Y, Jacobsson C *et al.* Geriatric-based versus general wards for older acute medical patients: a randomized comparison of outcomes and use of resources. *J Am Geriatr Soc* 2000;**48**:1381–8.
26. Counsell SR, Holder CM, Liebenauer LL *et al.* Effects of multicomponent intervention on functional outcomes and

process of care in hospitalized older patients: a randomized controlled trial of Acute Care for Elders (ACE) in a community hospital. *J Am Geriatr Soc* 2000;**48**:1572–81.

27. Stroke Unit Trialists' Collaboration. Collaborative systematic review of the randomised trials of organised inpatient (stroke unit) care after stroke. *BMJ* 1997;**314**:1151–9.
28. Stroke Unit Trialists' Collaboration. Organised inpatient (stroke unit) care for stroke. *Cochrane Database Syst Rev* 2002;**1**:CD000197.
29. Alberts, MJ, Hademenos G, Latchaw RE *et al*. Recommendation for the Establishment of Primary Stroke Centers. *JAMA* 2000,**283**:3102–9.
30. The Internet Stroke Center. Stroke Center Directory. Internet Stroke Center at Washington University, St Louis, MO. http://www.strokecenter.org/strokecenters.html (last accessed December 2011).
31. American Geriatrics Society. Geriatrics Workforce Policy Studies Center. Academic Geriatric Programs in Allopathic Medical Schools 2008–2009, Table 2.1. Copyright © 2010, University of Cincinnati. http://129.137.5.214/GWPS/files/Table%202_1.pdf (last accessed December 2011).
32. American Geriatrics Society. Geriatrics Workforce Policy Studies Center. Academic Staff in Geriatric Programs (Full-Time Equivalents) in 2001, 2005, 2007 and 2008 (Data presented as mean), Table 2.3. Copyright © 2010, University of Cincinnati. http://129.137.5.214/GWPS/files/Table%202_3.pdf (accessed 2 January 2012).
33. Geriatric Research Education and Clinical Centers. US Department of Veterans Affairs Washington, DC. Reviewed/Updated Date: 21 September 2011. http://www1.va.gov/grecc/(last accessed December 2011).
34. Accreditation Council for Graduate Medical Education. Number of Accredited Programs for the Current Academic Year (2010–2011). http://www.acgme.org/adspublic/(last accessed December 2011).

CHAPTER 144

Systems of healthcare: Australia

Gideon A. Caplan

Prince of Wales Hospital, Sydney, Australia

Overview of healthcare demographics

Australia has an ageing population comparable to most developed countries. In 2005, 13.1% of the 20 million residents were age 65 and over. With a life expectancy of 79.2 for males and 83.7 for females, it is estimated that one quarter of the Australian population will be over age 65 by the year 2051. At that time, the projected life expectancy will be 83.3 for males and 86.5 for females. In this population, dementia is the leading cause of disease burden by a factor of two. Dementia accounts for 16.7% of years of life lost to disability. Currently, over 160 000 Australians have dementia and this rate is predicted to increase over 250% by 2041. While vascular disease and cancer remain the two leading causes of death, mortality rates from these diseases in older people have decreased markedly over the last decade.[1]

While the health of the Australian population has generally been improving, the health of indigenous people, the Aborigines and Torres Strait Islanders (ATSI) has not improved at the same rate. These groups suffer death rates of two to three times that of the general population. The leading causes of death in these individuals remain vascular disease, respiratory illness, injury and cancer. While aged care services for most Australians are targeted toward the population over age 70, for ATSI people these same services are provided for those over age 50.

Australia spent 9.8% of the GDP on healthcare in 2004–2005 (AUD $87.3 billion). Although health spending has grown as the population has aged, this is mainly attributed to spending on new technology and pharmaceuticals, rather than on the increasing number of older individuals. The percentage of GDP spent on healthcare is lower than the United States, comparable to Canada and European countries, but higher than the United Kingdom. The Australian health system is tortuous in its complexity, particularly for the consumer. The services and care for older adults have been particularly complicated.

Development of geriatric medicine

The speciality of Geriatric Medicine in Australia is generally considered to have started in 1950 when the Hospital Commission of New South Wales (NSW) requested the Royal Newcastle Hospital to survey the known people with multiple sclerosis in the Hunter Valley, with a view to setting up a hospital clinic for those patients. Dr Richard Gibson and Miss Grace Parbery, a social worker, were appointed to conduct the survey and identified the need for medical, nursing and domestic care at home for the chronic sick in general. It took another five years to institute these outreach services and subsequently hospital rehabilitation services as well. Rudimentary services started soon after in other states but the independent origins led to different patterns of development.

Australia was founded in 1901 as a federation of six states each of which had a slightly different history and health system. Each state government retained control of existing health services, mainly hospitals. Over the years, the growth of national government taxation revenue has resulted in the initiation of new healthcare programmes, mainly non-hospital services. Many of these services were developed in response to genuine healthcare deficiencies but as a result, Australia has a dually administered health system through a partnership of the national and state governments. The Australian National Government generally retains primary control over the newly established healthcare services or programmes. The national government pays for community health, nursing home and visits to doctors' offices, but the level of control over these programmes varies. The Australian Government pays for visits to doctors under the Medicare scheme of universal health insurance. Medicare is partially funded by a 1.5% levy on income tax and a 1% surcharge from those earning at least AUD $50 000. Additional revenue for the physician may be generated from the patients, who are responsible for paying

Principles and Practice of Geriatric Medicine, Fifth Edition. Edited by Alan J. Sinclair, John E. Morley and Bruno Vellas.

when the physician decides to charge an extra fee. Medicare reimburses physicians 85% of the established *Schedule Fee*, an amount derived from a survey of fees in the early 1970s. The schedule fee has been under-adjusted for inflation over time, with a resulting 30% drop in reimbursement rates. This has prompted some physicians to pass on increasing co-payment fees to their patients. At this time, the percentage of GP consultations entirely paid for by Medicare has declined to about 70%.

Most medical care for older people is administered by GPs. Medicare disproportionately rewards GPs for shorter office-based consultations, which favours younger, single problem patients. General practice has also seen a shift toward corporatization, where companies employ GPs in multidoctor practices and generally discourage non-office work. These trends have resulted in a decrease in the number of GPs who perform home or nursing home visits. In 1999 a range of longer, better-remunerated consultations were introduced to encourage adequate consultations with frail, older people, including annual health assessments, multidisciplinary care planning and case conferencing. These have recently been augmented to also cover residential aged care; however, these measures have not been adequately assessed to determine whether they provide any benefit.

The Australian Government under the Pharmaceutical Benefits Scheme (PBS) pays for medications with some co-payments charged to patients. Rapid increases in the cost of the PBS of around 15% per year have led to a variety of measures to decrease costs. One method is to limit the number of new drugs coming onto the PBS. Patients have also been required to pay the full cost of many new drugs. In other situations, drug companies will negotiate to cap payments for a new pharmaceutical agent on the basis of the projected medication expenditures for that agent.

Geriatric Medicine is a relatively new, but growing speciality. A survey of all specialist consultant physicians found that there were 185 practising geriatricians in 2003. One third also practises general medicine. This provides Australia with approximately one geriatrician per 5900 people aged 75 and over.[2,3] Because geriatric medicine attracts a higher proportion of female specialists in Australia, and over a lifetime, females work approximately 75% of the hours of male graduates, access to geriatricians is more limited than what is actually calculated. The demand for geriatricians is increasing, but not currently met by the supply of trainees. In 2007 specific long and comprehensive consultations exclusively for geriatricians were introduced which meant that a geriatrician could be reimbursed by Medicare at a higher rate than any other physician, to appropriately reflect the complexity of consultations with frail older patients.

The profession, healthcare industry and the government continue to grapple with this problem.

Home healthcare

Home care services have become increasingly complex in the types of care provided, the funding arrangements, and number of service providers. The healthcare needs of patients are also more complex due to greater functional and physical dependency. Medical care at home has traditionally been provided by GPs for patients who were too acutely or chronically unwell to attend office visits. However, the relatively poor reimbursement by Medicare and the increasing demand for home visits has led many GPs to abandon them altogether. Because many aged care assessment teams (ACATs) now include a geriatrician or other medical officer, they may provide medical home visits as part of an initial assessment, but not as part of routine care.

Government-sponsored community services existed as early as the 1940s, including emergency housekeeper service and meals-on-wheels, delivered by women volunteers on bicycles. The Australian Government began funding home nursing services in 1956. Although the management and structure varies considerably between states, there is general availability of visiting registered nurses to provide nursing services in the home. Most commonly these services are time limited and based on the individual needs of the client and family. There are separate but generally parallel services for war veterans and individuals in the private sector. Home and Community Care (HACC) services expanded in 1969 to support housekeeping or other domestic assistance, senior citizens centres and welfare officers. Home care was further enhanced with the passage of the Home and Community Care Act in 1985 to include personal care such as bathing and dressing. Demand almost perpetually outstrips supply, because of under-funding, lack of gate keeping at entry, and inadequate exit strategies for maintenance services. A common assumption by service providers is that clients will not significantly improve and thus need prolonged enrolment in the programme. Home care recipients assume that services are difficult to access and thus attempt to retain services long term rather than re-request assistance at a later date.

HACC also funds meals-on-wheels, transportation, home maintenance and modification, counselling, social support, centre-based day care, allied health services, provision of aids, respite care and laundry. HACC services are not exclusively for older people, with 23% of their clients being under age 65, but usage rates do increase with age. The most commonly used service is domestic assistance (usually housekeeping). In 2007–2008, 8 million hours of domestic assistance were provided under the HACC programme. The programme was jointly funded by the state (40%) and national government at $1.65 billion in 2007–2008.

ACATs are a network of 128 regionally based multidisciplinary teams that provide comprehensive geriatric assessment at home or in hospital, facilitate access to the best possible combination of services at home, and determine eligibility for residential and complex community care. ACATs often provide health advice and support for the common conditions, which afflict older people, such as dementia and incontinence. ACATs may assume the additional therapeutic role of rehabilitative therapy. ACATs assess approximately 1 in every 10 people over age 70 every year. ACATs have a key role in assessing older people at home in complex situations, such as when elder abuse is suspected or if guardianship is being considered. If residential placement is recommended, the ACAT works with the client and their caregiver to negotiate entry. Staffing varies but generally includes nursing and allied health, social workers, physiotherapists, occupational therapists and psychologists. Increasingly ACATs have access to a geriatrician, particularly when they are co-located with a hospital aged care service, and sometimes even a psychogeriatrician. In non-metropolitan areas, the medical officer is usually a GP (family medicine practitioner) with an interest in aged care.[4]

Referral to ACAT is from any source, including self-referral. ACATs perform a standardized initial assessment using a minimum data set, with subsequent assessments according to identified problems. Occasionally, ACATs must assess younger people with disabilities for eligibility to enter residential aged care if no suitable alternatives exist. The shift away from institutional care has led to ever more complex packages of care being introduced into the community. The Community Options Programme was established in the late 1980s to provide case management and brokerage funds in the community to a small group of clients that is up to 10 times the average level of funding for other HACC clients, and also as recognition of the wide [illegible] in the community.

Community aged care packages (CACPs) were introduced in 1992 and support people at home with up to 14 hours of care per week as a substitute for admission to a hostel. Assistance with personal care such as bathing, domestic assistance with laundry, shopping, meal preparation, gardening and transportation outside the home are provided. The median length of time on the programme is just under a year. Two-thirds of people who leave the programme are admitted to residential care or die. More than half (56%) of all recipients live alone and only 8% live with their children. Recipients pay up to $7.69 per day, with the Australian Government providing $35.41 per day per recipient.

Extended Aged Care at Home (EACH) packages were introduced in 1998 to support people at home who are eligible for nursing home placement. Clients receive an average of 16.1 hours of care per week. These recipients tend to be younger (32% under age 75) and more cognitively intact (31% diagnosed with dementia, compared to 80% in nursing homes) than most nursing home residents. The government subsidy for EACH Dementia packages is $130.54 per day. The more complex packages of care require ACAT assessment of need.[5] By June 2006, about 48 000 people were receiving CACP or EACH packages with the governments plan to make available 18 CACP per 1000 persons over the age of 70. By comparison, over 236 000 were staying in residential aged care, although 37 000 were there temporarily in respite care.[6]

Transition Care Programmes (TCP) commenced in 2005 to provide up to 12 weeks of care for frail older people who had not recovered sufficiently, after an acute hospital stay and usually some rehabilitation, to manage independently at home and thereby were at risk of permanent institutionalization. The National Evaluation suggested that TCP reduced the risk of entering an institution (hospital and residential aged care) during six months of follow-up.

Although the spectrum of home care appears broad and comprehensive, it can also be cumbersome and complex. In practice, 17 separate programmes are funded by the Australian Government and delivered by a myriad of 1000 different service providers. Most state governments fund additional services, particularly for post acute care at home after hospitalization. The result is a complicated health delivery system with patchy coordination and insufficient communication, particularly for consumers and their caregivers. In theory, one assessment by ACAT should be sufficient for any other service but, in practice, each service provider makes its own assessment. That this plethora of providers does not meet the needs of older disabled people and their caregivers was demonstrated by a study of dementia sufferers in Victoria. Data revealed that over 40% of demented individuals do not make use of any community or respite services. When asked why they did not make use of various community services, 77-88% of individuals stated that the services were not needed, although many caregivers were not managing well as evidenced by poor self-reported health and high levels of strain.[7] Since 1972, caregivers have been subsidized by a domiciliary nursing care benefit to care for a disabled person at home who would otherwise require institutional care. The patient must be over the age of 16 and certified by a medical practitioner to require continuing care.

Nursing home care

The development of residential aged care dates back to the poor houses of the nineteenth century. In NSW, the first state, government asylums for the aged and destitute were built to house the aged poor. By 1890, these homes had become 'practically hospitals for chronic and incurable diseases as well as homes for the infirm and indigent'. However the introduction of a pension plan in 1909 allowed more aged poor to continue living in the community and institutional care was used only for marked disability or poverty.[8] Essentially all residential care was provided by the charitable and public sectors until the mid-1950s, but not-for-profit organizations still provide 63% of all residential care places.

In 1954, there was a swing back to residential aged care when the Australian government passed the Aged Persons Homes Act that provided subsidies to charities (and later to private operators) that built or purchased homes for needy older people. This prompted a surge in construction of nursing homes that continued for three decades. In the early 1970s, a quota of 50 nursing home beds per 1000 population of age 65 and over was introduced. An intermediate level of care, called *hostel*, was announced in an attempt to reduce the number of nursing homes being built, particularly by the private sector. Hostels were aimed at people who needed assistance with IADLs while nursing homes were designed for people who needed assistance with basic ADLs. A 1978 survey found that 30% of nursing home residents could easily be treated at home with minimal services.[9] In 1986, a government review pointed out that the cost of institutional care had risen tenfold in 10 years, from $100 million to $1 billion per annum, and the percentage of the Department of Health's budget paid to nursing homes had increased from 9 to 25% over 20 years. By the mid 1980s nearly 90% of all aged care funding was going to residential care. The rate has now been reduced to about 75% with a commensurate increase in community care. In 2004, there were 175 000 allocated residential care sites and 30 000 community care sites. On the basis of the truism that most people prefer to remain in their own homes, the government changed the quota for nursing home beds to 72.6 per 1000 people over age 70. In 1985, the multidisciplinary ACATs were charged with developing more stringent entry criteria, which resulted in a 35% decrease in admissions to nursing homes. HACC services were also strengthened in order to maintain people at home.[10] Over the years, the government has changed the ratio of nursing homes and hostel places to increase the availability of home support, but this has been complicated by the growth of the population over age 70. Individuals over age 85 are most likely to require nursing home placement and are the fastest growing segment of the population. A decrease in funding for residential care has caused many facilities to close down. Ninety licensed residential care beds are now allocated per 1000 population over age 70. These transformations have meant significant increases in disability in hostel care, as well as increased average disability in nursing homes.

A further series of reforms took place in 1997 with the introduction of the Aged Care Act. The two levels of care were unified under one legislative framework with an integrated Resident Classification Scale (RCS) and quality assurance framework. The levels were renamed high (nursing home) and low (hostel) care. The 1997 reforms also introduced a small amount of deregulation and emphasized greater contributions to the cost of health and welfare services by those with the capacity to pay. In general, the provision of residential aged care remains a controversial issue in Australia. Approximately one in three people who reach 65 years of age will spend some time in residential aged care, but whether the cost should be met more by the community or by the individual and their family is a matter of equity, ethics and finances.

Hospital care

In 1993, a government survey of 942 Australian hospitals found that 32% operated a geriatric service. These were almost exclusively based in the public sector, and usually consisted of visiting care services.[11] Only 13% of programmes included a geriatrician. Replication of the survey in 2001 found that 31% of 778 hospitals had a geriatrician providing inpatient care.[12]

The distribution of geriatric services varies between states. Those states with more acute geriatric medical beds typically provide care to patients admitted through the emergency department. New South Wales, Western Australia and South Australia have the highest ratio of acute geriatric beds (0.67–0.85 beds per 1000 people over age 70 in 2002). In Victoria and Western Australia there are more designated aged care rehabilitation beds (0.62–0.63 per 1000 people) than in the other states. The extent of geriatric services vary by hospital, with 11% reporting a day hospital, 7% having bed-based psychogeriatric services, and only 4% having orthogeriatric services. Orthogeriatric services provide coordinated orthopaedic and geriatric management for older traumatic and elective orthopaedic patients. The type of geriatric services available to patients tends to mirror the hospital environment. Where the hospital focuses on acute-care and managing emergency admissions, more attention is devoted to improving assessment and management of older people in the emergency department and on acute hospital wards. Where the hospital has developed a stand-alone rehabilitation centre, more emphasis is placed on managing chronic conditions, such as dementia, Parkinson's disease and incontinence. However, with time the scope of available services is increasing and differences between states are receding.

Stroke units are becoming increasingly popular, although geriatrician involvement is not universal. A recent study found that only 40% of all strokes were treated in stroke units.[13] Hospital in the home for older patients is increasing in popularity, but is essentially in its infancy as a model of healthcare. This service provides patient-centred care in the patient's home or a residential care facility, while decreasing the risk of hospital associated adverse events.

Major geriatric complications were less likely to occur in the hospital in the home model compared with the traditional hospital model.[14]

Public hospitals, which are the majority, are under the control of state governments.

Only about 30% of hospitals are private and these concentrate on elective procedures. Almost all large and teaching hospitals are public, so that the vast majority of acute and more complicated medical or surgical work is done in public hospitals. Admission to a public hospital as a public patient is free to Australian residents. However, if a patient wants a choice of doctor, they must enter as a private patient. Owing to tax incentives, about 43% of the population has private insurance for hospital care. Public hospitals receive about half their budget from the national government and half through the state governments.

This dichotomy of control of the health system has led to lack of coordination, and incentive to cost shift between the hospital and non-hospital sectors. There are also limited health services run by local government (the third tier), religious and charitable organizations, individuals and private commercial interests.

Academic geriatrics

In NSW, geriatric medicine originated in the Royal Newcastle Hospital, an acute public hospital and later became an acute speciality hospital. Lidcombe Hospital in NSW was another early centre of geriatric medicine that evolved away from the mainstream, having originally been an asylum which developed into an acute hospital, but retained a large group of long-stay chronic patients. Many of the doctors involved there went on to be national leaders in geriatric medicine. In Victoria, South Australia, and Queensland the speciality started in chronic hospitals, which developed out of the poor houses, and continues as a rehabilitation hospital model, though it now also interacts with acute hospitals. In Victoria, the Mount Royal Hospital was a custodial institution for elderly people where the state hospital and charities commission decided to open a geriatric centre, aimed at rehabilitation. Though the initial director was only part-time, the centre flourished and also became a centre for ageing research. The Australian Association of Gerontology was formed in the early 1960s as a multidisciplinary organization interested in later life, and the doctors involved went on to form The Australian and New Zealand Society for Geriatric Medicine (ANZSGM) to meet the special needs of medical practitioners. Many geriatricians take a leading role as advocates for older people together with consumers and other service providers.

The Royal Australasian College of Physicians (RACP) recognizes geriatric medicine as a speciality. Trainees must complete 3 years of advanced training in geriatric medicine, though 1 year of this may include working in another speciality or in full-time research. Advanced training can only be undertaken after successfully completing the demanding written and oral basic physicians' examination, which is generally attempted 4–5 years post-graduation from medical school. Only about two-thirds of candidates are successful in this exam. Almost all basic physician trainees, who later go on to various internal medicine subspecialities, have some exposure to working in geriatric medicine. This is most beneficial for attracting trainees for advanced training. However, workforce issues are as much a problem in terms of shortages in the supply of doctors for older people, as well as nurses and allied health professionals.

The first full professor of geriatric medicine was appointed at the University of Melbourne in 1975, though early professorships were often in 'community medicine and geriatrics'. Now each medical school boasts of at least one professor and there are research institutes dedicated to age-related research in the larger states.

Many other research institutes also have some interest in age-related research. Clinical research is also conducted in many teaching hospitals. Most research funding derives from the National Health and Medical Research Council that does not yet have a section devoted to ageing. However, in 2002 the Australian Government released a national strategy for ageing research and identified national research priorities which included 'promoting and maintaining good health' whose goals include 'ageing well, ageing productively'. This led to the establishment of two research networks designed to encourage and seed fund collaborative interdisciplinary research into ageing.

Key points

- The speciality of geriatric medicine in Australia is generally considered to have started in 1950.
- Extended Aged Care at Home (EACH) packages were introduced in 1998 to support people at home who are eligible for nursing home placement.
- Geriatric medicine is a relatively new, but growing speciality. A survey of all specialist consultant physicians found that there were 185 practicing geriatricians in 2003. One third also practises general medicine. This provides Australia with approximately one geriatrician per 5900 people aged 75 and over.
- ACATs are a network of 128 regionally based multidisciplinary teams that provide comprehensive geriatric assessment at home or in hospital, facilitate access to the best possible combination of services at home, and determine eligibility for residential and complex community care.

References

1. Australian Health & Ageing System: The Concise Factbook, October 2007. http://www.health.gov.au/internet/main/publishing.nsf/Content/concisefactbook-june2011-introduction (accessed December 2011).
2. Dent O. *Clinical Workforce in Internal Medicine and Paediatrics in Australasia*, The Royal Australian College of Physicians, 2004.
3. Australian Medical Workforce Advisory Committee. *The Geriatric Medicine Workforce in Australia: Supply and Requirements 1996–2007*, AMWAC Report 1997.5, AMWAC, Sydney, 1997.
4. Lincoln Gerontology Centre. *Aged Care Assessment Program National Minimum Data Set Report July 2000–June 2001*, September 2002. http://www.health.gov.au/internet/main/publishing.nsf/Content/ageing-reports-acapmds.htm/$FILE/acapmds01.pdf (accessed December 2011).
5. Extended Aged Care at Home (EACH) Update Newsletter. Aging and Aged Care Division. Issue 1, 2002. http://www.health.gov.au/internet/wcms/Publishing.nsf/Content/ageing-commcare-each-eachnews.htm/$file/each1.pdf (accessed April 2005).
6. National Evaluation of the Transition Care Program. http://www.health.gov.au/internet/main/publishing.nsf/Content/BDA22E555921E4A1CA2574BB001634B8/$File/ExecutiveSummary.pdf (accessed February 2010).
7. Thomson C, Fine M, Brodaty H. Carers' Support Needs Project: Promoting the Appropriate Use of Services by Carers of People with Dementia, 1997; Research consultancy for the New South Wales Ageing and Disability Department as part of the New South Wales Action Plan on Dementia.
8. Dickey B. Care for the aged poor in Australia, 1788–1914. *Community Health Studies* 1983;**8**:247–55.
9. Bennett C, Wallace R. At the margin or on average: some issues and evidence in planning the balance of care for the aged in Australia. *Community Health Studies* 1983;**7**:35–41.
10. Warne RW. Issues in the development of geriatric medicine in Britain and Australia. *The Medical Journal of Australia* 1987; **146**:139–41.
11. Dorevitch M, Gray L. *National Survey of Hospital Geriatric Services: A Study of Hospital-based Geriatric Services in Australia*, Australian Government Publishing Service, Canberra, 1993.
12. Gray L, Dorevitch M, Smith R et al. *Service Provision for Older Australians in the Acute - Aged Care Sector: Final Report 2002*. http://www.health.gov.au/internet/main/publishing.nsf/Content/health-minconf.htm/$FILE/1bfinalreport.pdf (accessed December 2011).
13. Lee AH, Somerford PJ, Yau KKW. Factors influencing survival after stroke in Western Australia. *The Medical Journal of Australia* 2003;**179**:289–93.
14. Caplan GA, Ward JA, Brennan N et al. Hospital in the home: a randomised controlled trial. *The Medical Journal of Australia* 1999;**170**:156–60.

CHAPTER 145

Systems of healthcare: the United Kingdom

Simon Conroy
University of Leicester, UK

Introduction

The growth in life expectancy at birth in much of the Western world reflects an ongoing revolution in longevity. This revolution encompasses both survival of individuals to older ages and changing age profiles of the entire population. In particular, the growth of the oldest old has resulted in significant healthcare changes, both on an individual and at societal level. Developed nations across the world have approached the ageing population and need for expanded health services in a variety of ways. Home health, hospital-based and nursing home care have experienced a profound increase in complexity of care needs over the last quarter century. This complexity of care is reflected in the expansion of funding arrangements, number of service providers and geographic service areas. Governments have expanded healthcare spending and broadened the scope of medical care. The development of health insurance programmes in some countries has allowed a greater number of individuals to access medical services. Institutes of higher learning have evolved to support the growing fields of gerontology and geriatric medicine. Educating the medical providers, workforce and community on the needs of older adults has become a major area of interest within and outside of the academic environment. It is important to draw older people into the processes of developing the services and new technologies that they themselves and others of their generation will use. By developing these new healthcare opportunities, the greatest gains may be made in health, independence and quality of life (QOL) in old age.

Overview of healthcare demographics

The proportion of UK citizens aged >80 years is set to increase from 2.7 million in 2008 to 6.7 million in 2050; at the same time the proportion of younger citizens will fall, with the result that the dependency ratio[1] will rise from 25% today to 38% in 2050.[1] By 2060, healthcare spending will take up 8.3% of gross domestic product (GDP), and long-term care 0.7% of GDP.[1] The rapid growth in the oldest old, with the associated frailty and the apparent failure to compress morbidity into the final year or two of life, means that the health and social care of frail older people will continue to be a major challenge for the UK Government.

Healthcare spending in the United Kingdom has grown more quickly than other economic expenditures, reaching 8.1% of the gross domestic product (GDP) in 2007. Even in the harsh climate of post-recession Britain, healthcare spending remains an important part of the overall UK budget, which continues to support publicly funded health and social care. Public healthcare expenditure increased by £5.1 billion (8%) in 2002 compared with £700 million (5%) in private health expenditures. All individuals residing in United Kingdom are entitled to receive treatment from the National Health Service (NHS), which is free at the point of delivery. The NHS, established in 1948, is the third largest employer in the world after the Chinese Army and Indian Railways respectively.

Development of geriatric medicine

For various historical reasons, specialist geriatric services developed as an integral part of the NHS in the United Kingdom earlier than in any other area of Europe. Marjorie Warren established geriatric medicine in Britain in the late 1930s. Her message was the need for assessment and rehabilitation of older disabled people, education of medical students, and research into the problems of ageing and old age.[2,3] This derived from her work in the workhouse infirmary associated with the West Middlesex

[1]The dependency ratio is the ratio of people aged 65+ in relation to people aged 15–64, expressed as a percentage.

Principles and Practice of Geriatric Medicine, Fifth Edition. Edited by Alan J. Sinclair, John E. Morley and Bruno Vellas.

Hospital in London. Her methods (careful medical and social assessment, medical treatment and rehabilitation) were described in a series of publications.[2–4] The general conclusion was that older patients should be treated in a dedicated area of general hospitals because:

- geriatrics is an important subject to teach medical students;
- geriatrics should be an essential part of the training of student nurses;
- general hospital facilities are necessary for correct diagnosis and treatment;
- research on diseases of ageing can only be undertaken with the full facilities of a general hospital.

These were visionary proposals in 1943 but continue to resonate in current discussions about managing older people. The emerging recognition of the needs of older people in an ageing society led to a number of major surveys and resulted in the collection of planning data for the introduction of new healthcare services. Curran and colleagues (1946) published data on about 1000 males over age 65 and females over age 60 and who lived in poorer areas of Glasgow, all of whom received home visits. A social and medical survey of people in England over age 65 was also performed by the Nuffield Foundation in 1943. The results were published in two reports: *Old People* (1947) and the *Social Medicine of Old Age* (1948).[5,6] The British Medical Association (BMA) set up a working group in 1947 to review care of the elderly and infirm and to make general healthcare recommendations.[7] Of the 21 BMA members, four were active in the new speciality of Geriatrics (Amulree, Brooke, Cousin, Warren). Dr Trevor Howell, originally a general practitioner (GP), became interested in geriatric medicine after becoming responsible for Chelsea pensioners. He was appointed consultant physician at Battersea and subsequently opened one of the first geriatric units.[8–10] In 1947, he called a meeting to bring together physicians who had a special interest in older people and skills in rehabilitation, incontinence management and domiciliary assessment. This meeting launched the Medical Society for the Care of the Elderly, the society was renamed the British Geriatrics Society in 1959. These pioneering physicians persuaded the Minister of Health to appoint more geriatricians as part of the hospital consultant expansion of the new NHS. Dr Tom Wilson was appointed the first consultant geriatrician in 1948 at Cornwall, which marked the introduction of this new medical speciality. By 2008, there were 1111 consultant geriatricians in the United Kingdom, but increasing subspecialization (for example into stroke medicine) and the feminization of the workforce means that the long-term aim of having one whole time equivalent geriatrician per 40 000 of population is still some way off.

The NHS has recognized the value of Geriatrics, now the largest medical speciality in the UK, and has invested significant time and resources to improve services and standards of care for older people. During the 1980s and much of 1990s, the trend in United Kingdom was for geriatric practice to become more closely identified with acute general internal medicine and to be less involved with rehabilitation and long-term care. The improved access to acute diagnostic facilities for older people was welcomed. The rise in consumerism and desire for choice have resulted in the public having a higher expectation of all services. Inadequacies and inequalities in the healthcare of older people have had a major influence on current heath policy, now in part being addressed by the National Institute for Heath and Clinical Excellence (NICE – http://www.nice.org.uk/). A campaign started by a national newspaper and an older people's charity (Help the Aged) led the government to commission an independent inquiry into the care of older people. As a result of the finding, a National Service Framework (NSF) containing standards of care for older people was published in 2001 in order to apply to the NHS for implementation. The NSF was a 10-year healthcare improvement programme implemented through local health and social care partners, and national underpinning programmes. It was the first framework to establish standards for social as well as healthcare. The NSF established new national standards, service models and social services for all older people, whether they lived at home, in residential care or in hospital. This was achieved through the single assessment process, integrated commissioning arrangements and integrated provision of services. Ten years later, whilst there is still much to be done, the NSF has facilitated major improvements in the care of frail older people. In response to older peoples' demands for care close to home,[11,12] there is a growing move to shrink the acute hospital sector whilst increasing community services for older people. In the UK at least, it seems as though we have come full circle and are now rediscovering the art of geriatric medicine in community settings as pioneered by Marjorie Warren in the 1940s.

Home healthcare

The practice of seeing patients in their own homes has been an essential component of geriatric practice since its early stages when consultants inherited large panels of patients with long waiting lists. However, there has been something of a demise in domiciliary visits in the last decade, relating in part to the growing purchaser-provider split in the NHS. But as acute care episodes are shrinking, there is a growing need for geriatric expertise to support acute care in the community setting. This is especially true for intermediate care settings – either patients being 'stepped-up' from their own home to a more supportive environment in the context of a crisis (usually medical) or patients being 'stepped-down' from acute care (early supported discharge). Community services have developed massively in the last few years, and include residential or home-based intermediate care, community matron services and other therapy and social services. Geriatricians are increasingly integrating with such teams to deliver comprehensive geriatric assessment.

In addition to services aimed at supporting medical and social crises, there are a growing number of falls prevention services and other out-patient type activities being provided in the community, which traditionally would have been delivered in hospital outpatients or geriatric day hospitals. Despite their popularity with staff and patients, day hospitals have come under increasing pressure to close as they are perceived as being too expensive.

Psychogeriatric services have developed along the lines described above, with reciprocal roles in the acute and community sector, and the recent focus on expanding memory clinics. However, acute hospital care for people with mental health issues in non-psychiatric settings is significantly underdeveloped. More recently there is a growing interest in developing dedicate units for patients with mental health issues, analogous to the development of stroke and orthogeriatric services.

Preventive care in the community rests very much in the hands of general practitioners, with focused efforts to increase the uptake of vaccinations and screening for common treatable conditions such as diabetes and hypertension. Access to falls services remains somewhat *ad hoc*, though NICE guidance does request that older people are asked about falls with a view to accessing falls prevention services. Older people are currently excluded from the common cancer screening programmes (colorectal cancer and breast cancer), but this is being hotly debated and may change.

There is a growing awareness of the benefits of exercise in older people, not just in terms of preventing falls and functional decline, but also for the psychological and metabolic benefits. A great deal of work remains to be done to identify the optimal methods of engaging older people (as well as younger people!) in healthy living activities.

Nursing home care

The care home sector in the UK has largely taken over the role of the long-term care wards from the 1940s. There are around 5700 nursing homes in England providing 186 800 beds. Individuals admitted to nursing homes tend to be heavily dependant and require regular nursing care (for example for care of pressure sores). Individuals in residential homes will require some help with activities of daily living, but should not require daily access to nursing care. In practice there is considerable overlap within homes, as many are registered to provide both nursing and residential care. There are dedicated nursing homes for those with psychiatric disorders, including dementia, which may also be registered to provide residential care. All state-funded individuals should now undergo a continuing care assessment prior to entry into long-term care to determine their need for nursing care.

The majority of care homes are in the hands of the private sector, with most being run as a relatively small business with no more than 20–30 residents. Healthcare input is variable, and it is not unusual for residents in one care home to be managed by their original general practitioner, rather than a single GP service taking over the care of all residents. This results in rather fragmented care and relatively little support for social care staff who are left managing the most complex, frail older people. This may in part explain the substantial number of care home residents admitted to acute care with a crisis that might have been reasonably managed in the care home had the support mechanisms been in place. It is interesting to contrast a UK care home with models such as those used in Holland, with larger units and greater medical and therapy input.[13]

The ideal approach to the comprehensive management of care home residents would see a collaborative effort between the geriatricians and the GP providing day-to-day care in the nursing home setting in conjunction with other health and social care professionals. However, geriatricians have been criticized for a relative lack of attention to the long-term care and community-based care needs of frail older people. Greater attention is now being focused on care home medicine.[14] Newer models (or the re-birth of old models) such as interface geriatrics[15] – combining acute hospital geriatrics with community geriatrics are starting to emerge.

Hospital care

Various models of acute hospital care exist throughout the UK, ranging from age-based services (though these are becoming less and less prevalent following the focus on ageism in the NSF), needs-related (based on geriatric syndromes) or a more integrated approach. A common goal is to discharge patients (sometimes too quickly) from such wards either to their own homes or to other appropriate settings. Patients requiring ongoing nursing care for irremediable conditions are referred for nursing home admission.

A major factor in the delivery of acute hospital care is the European Working Time Directive, which mandates the number of hours that a doctor can work in a single day and over a week. Most hospitals now operate a shift system, with a loss in continuity of care. Despite efforts to improve medical handover of patients, there is still significant disruption. Older people, especially those with cognitive impairments, may suffer more at the hands of this new system than their more autonomous younger counterparts. Given that older people occupy around two-thirds of all hospital beds, this raises major concerns about the quality and by inference the efficiency of acute hospital care. On a more positive note, multidisciplinary working is now widespread, not just within geriatric medicine units. Overt age discrimination is rare and will soon be the subject of legislation, but subvert age discrimination in the form of inadequate assessments and the attribution of functional decline to age rather than a medical diagnosis remains a major challenge to be tackled.

One of the areas of geriatric medicine that has perhaps had the greatest success (some might argue to the detriment of other areas) is stroke medicine. Stroke medicine has gone from being a cinderella speciality to becoming a priority, both in hospital care (through the provision of thrombolysis services and acute stroke units, etc.) and in primary care (early supported discharge and daily access to clinics for patients with possible transient ischaemic attacks).

Academic geriatrics

The first academic chair of Geriatric Medicine was established in 1965 in Glasgow, Scotland. The first professor of geriatric medicine was William Ferguson Anderson (1914–2001). There is concern amongst some geriatricians that conventional academic geriatric posts are withering on the vine[16] and that opportunities for funding geriatric research, as opposed to ageing research, are inadequate. This view is fuelled by concerns that many chairs in Geriatric Medicine have been 'lost' or remain unfilled. Combined with concerns about undergraduate geriatric education,[17–19] might lead one to become despondent about the future of any would-be academic geriatricians. But there are now around 50 geriatricians holding professorial chairs throughout England and Wales, and many geriatricians hold important roles in undergraduate education throughout the country, albeit not necessarily university-based posts. Now, more than ever before, Geriatrics is the mainstream speciality. Geriatricians are no longer seen as second-class physicians, but are becoming increasingly valued for their generalist approach and ability to manage complex patients, whether in acute care settings, rehabilitation settings, in end-of-life care and other scenarios both in primary and secondary care. Few other specialities can bring such breadth of knowledge and skills to their patients. Teaching of the geriatric giants is now commonplace on most medical school curricula. Several geriatricians have leading roles in the Royal College of Physicians and the Department of Health as well as other august bodies. In terms of research, ageing is now one of the top three priority areas for the Medical Research Council, and the rationalization of NHS funding should lead to a greater focus of research on priority areas for the NHS – of which ageing and frailty is surely one.

Higher medical training in geriatric medicine is well established, and there are currently around 400 trainees nationally. Applicants for higher medical training (HMT) should have completed a minimum of two years general professional training and have to pass a competitive interview to enter further medical training before choosing a speciality (Figure 145.1)

Clinical training in geriatric medicine is usually undertaken in parallel to training in general internal medicine and lasts five years. There are dedicated training structures for clinical academics which can take longer. Whilst such clear pathways are to be welcomed, they do rather impose an early choice on relatively junior doctors (Figure 145.2), which may be a concern for geriatric medicine – typically a mature or late choice for career physicians.

Conclusion

In the next 50 years, the population demographic in developed countries will change substantially. Up to a quarter of the citizens will be over age 65 with the highest growth rate in age seen in the oldest age groups. Older adults are the highest consumers of healthcare resources and are usually supported, at least in part, by local and national government medical programmes. With healthcare costs rising, countries like the United Kingdom, United States and Australia are exploring alternate means of caring for the ageing population. Home care encompasses a wide variety of programmes and services, most of which are not physician-directed. Traditional community geriatrics dropped substantially in the early 1990s and despite a recurrence in interest, is still nascent. The provision of medical and non-medical services should allow individuals to remain independent and in their homes for a longer period of time. Many services are community based and thus help individuals maintain a connection with society. As the ageing population expanded, health expenditures increased tremendously. In an effort to control escalating long-term care costs, intermediate care settings have evolved to allow individuals more autonomy in a less costly setting. Resources and supervision are provided to individuals on an as-needed basis in most of these facilities. For individuals in need of comprehensive supervised care, nursing homes still provide the maximal degree of therapy, social work and nursing support. Hospital care has evolved to focus more on the delivery of quality healthcare to the elderly individual. Stroke units are well established as an effective model for managing hospitalized older adults. ACE units are now growing in the same manner. It is apparent that quality care for complex older patients requires a team of medical providers working together toward common goals. Academic geriatrics has grown substantially over the past 50 years with most medical schools and academic centres establishing a department or section of geriatric medicine. The role of geriatricians, relative to GPs, is still evolving in the care of the older adult. As the

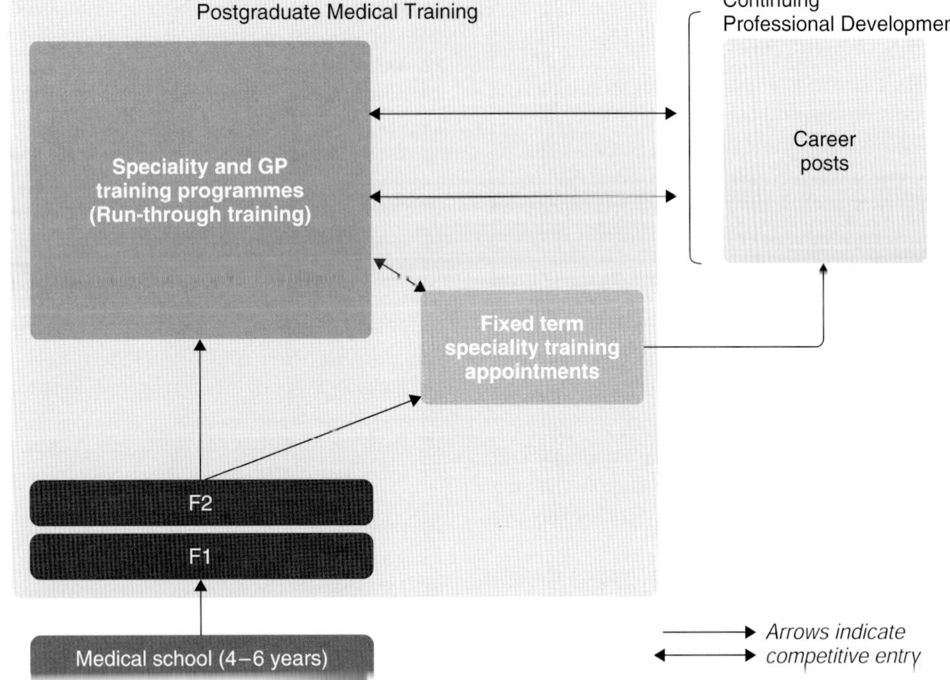

Figure 145.1 Training structure for medicine in the United Kingdom.

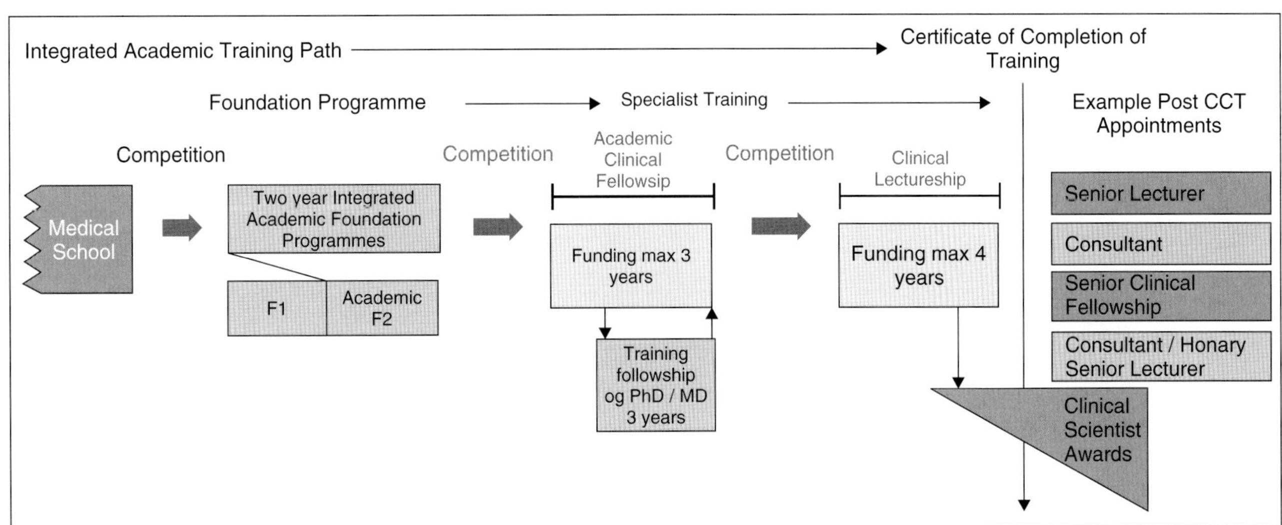

Figure 145.2 Academic training in the United Kingdom.

older population expands there is an ongoing need to train physicians, both generalists and specialists, in the principles of geriatric medicine.

Key points

- Older people will account for over 20% of the United Kingdom, United States and Australian population in the next half century.
- Services for older people have grown most extensively in the realm of home healthcare.
- Geriatric wards, stroke units and Acute Care for the Elderly (ACE) units are well developed and are effective models of hospital care for older people.
- The growth of nursing home care has slowed and is shifting to 'intermediate care' service models.
- Geriatrics as a unique field of medicine has developed over the past half century.

References

1. Anon. Communication from the Commission to the European Parliament, the Council, the European Economic and Social Committee and the Committee of the Regions. *Dealing with the impact of an ageing population in the EU (2009 Ageing Report)*, 2009.
2. Warren MW. Care of chronic sick: a case for treating chronic sick in blocks in a general hospital. *BMJ* 1943;**ii**:822–3.
3. Warren MW. Care of the chronic aged sick. *Lancet* 1946;**i**: 841–3.
4. Warren MW. The role of a geriatric unit in a general hospital. *The Ulster Medical Journal* 1949;**18**:3–12.
5. Nuffield Foundation. *Old People*, Oxford University Press, Oxford, 1947.
6. Sheldon JH. *The Social Medicine of Old Age*, Oxford University Press, Oxford, 1948.
7. British Medical Association. *The Care and Treatment of the Elderly and Infirm*, Report of a Special Committee of the British Medical Association, 1947.
8. Adams GF. Eld health. Origins and destiny of British geriatrics. *Age and Ageing* 1975;**4**:65–8.
9. Irvine RE. *Forty Years On*, BGS Annual Report, 1986–1987.
10. Howell TH. Origins of the BGS. *Age and Ageing* 1974;**3**:69–72.
11. Philp I. A new ambition for old age: Next steps in implementing the National Service Framework for Older People, Department of Health, 2006.
12. Department of Health. *Our health, our care, our say: a new direction for community services: A brief guide*, 2006.
13. Conroy S, Van Der Cammen T, Schols J *et al.* Medical services for older people in nursing homes – comparing services in England and the Netherlands. *Journal of Nutrition, Health & Aging* 2009;**13**:559–63.
14. Donald IP, Gladman J, Conroy S *et al.* Care home medicine in the UK – in from the cold. *Age Ageing* 2008: 37:618–20.
15. Conroy S, Ferguson C, Banerjee J. Interface geriatrics: an evidence based solution for frail older people with medical crises. *Br J Hosp Med* 2010;**71**:98–101.
16. Jackson S. BGS Academic and Research Strategy, British Geriatrics Society, 2004.
17. Bartram L, Crome P, McGrath A *et al.* Survey of training in geriatric medicine in UK undergraduate medical schools. *Age & Ageing* 2006;**35**:533–5.
18. Fletcher P. Will undergraduate geriatric medicine survive? *Age & Ageing* 2007;**36**:358–60.
19. Lally FC P. Undergraduate training in geriatric medicine: getting it right. *Age & Ageing* 2007;**36**:366–8.

CHAPTER 146

Geriatric medicine in China

Leung-Wing Chu
Sau Po Centre on Ageing, University of Hong Kong, and Queen Mary Hospital, Hong Kong

Introduction

The elderly population in China

China is a developing country. It has undergone a rapid economic growth recently, and is now the world's third-largest economy. In the past 60 years, China has made great achievements in controlling infectious diseases and improving public health. A direct indicator is the demographic transition from a young population into an ageing population. In 1999, the proportion of elderly people aged 60 years and over was already more than 10%. In the 5th National Population Census of 31 provinces, autonomous regions and municipalities of mainland China in November 2000, the population was 1 265 830 0010. There were 88 110 000 persons aged >65 years. This represented 7% of the population.[1] In the 2005 One-percent Population Survey, the total population of China was 1 306 280 0010. The number of persons >65 years had increased to 100 450 000, which constituted 7.7% of the whole population. In 2005, average life expectancy at birth was 71.0 years for males and 74.0 years for females. (Tables 146.1, 146.2 and 146.3).[2]

There are several special features regarding population ageing in China. The number of elderly is huge and represents 20% of the world's elderly population and 50% of the Asian elderly population, and the growth is rapid. From 1982 to 1999, the proportion of elderly persons aged >60 years increased from 7.64% to 10.1%. Such a demographic transition occurred within 18 years in China but the same change took several decades in developed Western countries. China has now moved into an accelerated phase of population ageing and is becoming an ageing society in an underdeveloped economy. While Western countries have become both 'old' and 'rich', China has become 'old' before getting 'rich'. This constitutes a burden on economic growth. Another characteristic is the regional difference in the demographic transition. Population ageing occurs more rapidly in the developed coastal cities than in the underdeveloped inner rural areas within China. Urban cities show a higher proportion of elderly people than rural areas. For example, in 2005 Shanghai had the highest percentage of elderly people (11.94%) while Qinghai province had the lowest (6.04%).[2] Amongst elderly population subgroups, the growth of those aged >80 years is fast and increasing at a rate of 5.4% per year. This subgroup increased from 8 million in 1990 to 11 million in 2000 and is projected to reach 27.8 million by 2020.[1,3] With an ageing population, the prevalence of chronic diseases, which include diabetes mellitus, hypertension, stroke, coronary heart disease and chronic obstructive pulmonary disease, has also increased. For example, 1.5 million patients are newly diagnosed with stroke every year in China. Heavy medical expenses are required and these diseases constitute an important burden. Although the life expectancy of women is higher than men, women survive longer but are less healthy than men.[1–6] The birth control and one-child policy has had a great impact on family size in China.[7] The Chinese family has decreased from 4–5 to 3–4 person households in recent years. Family size is largest in rural areas and small in city areas. This trend has been affecting the foundation of traditional family support of the elderly population.

The elderly population in Hong Kong SAR, Macau SAR and Taiwan

In 2009, 0.89 million persons in Hong Kong were aged 65 years and over, which represented 12.8% of the total Hong Kong population. The proportion of Hong Kong elderly will increase to 26.4% by 2036.[8] This increase will place an enormous demand on long-term care and healthcare services. The ageing demographic change is related to a decrease in births in Hong Kong.[9–12] The elderly dependency ratio, which is defined as the number of persons aged 65 years and over per 1000 persons aged 15–64 years, will increase from 382 in 2001 to 562 in 2031. In 2009, average life expectancy at birth was 79.5 years for men and 85.2 years for women (Tables 146.1, 146.2 and 146.4). Life expectancy is closely related to the healthcare needs of the elderly. In 2009, at age 60, the average life expectancy was 22.3 years

Principles and Practice of Geriatric Medicine, Fifth Edition. Edited by Alan J. Sinclair, John E. Morley and Bruno Vellas.

Table 146.1 China's population (including Hong Kong SAR, Macau SAR, Taiwan).

	Mainland China (1 Nov. 2005; One-percent Population Survey)	Hong Kong SAR (2009)	Macau SAR (2008)	Taiwan (2009)
Total population	1 306 280 0010	7 003 700	549 200	23 069 000
No. of elderly (>65 years)	100 450 000	893 500	39 500	2 406 097
% of elderly (>65 years)	7.69% (Increase of 0.73% compared with 2000 Census)	12.8%	7.19%	10.43%
Average life expectancy at birth, years	All = 73.0		All = 82.0	
	Male = 71.0	Male = 79.5	Male = 79.0	Male = 75.6
	Female = 74.0	Female = 85.2	Female = 84.8	Female = 81.9

Table 146.2 China major cities' population in 2005, Hong Hong in 2009.

	Beijing (2005)	Shanghai (2005)	Hong Kong SAR (30 June 2009)
Total population	15 360 000	17 780 000	7 003 700
No. of elderly (>65 years)	1 660 000	2 120 000	893 500
% of elderly (>65 years)	10.79% (increase of 2.37% compared with 2000 Census)	11.94% (increase of 0.48% compared with 2000 Census)	12.8% (increase of 1.8% compared with 2000 Census)

Table 146.3 Declining birth and death rates in mainland China.

Year	Mainland China (Overall)		Beijing		Shanghai	
	Natural birth rate (per 1000 pop.)	Natural death rate[a] (per 1000 pop.)	Natural birth rate (per 1000 pop.)	Natural death rate[a] (per 1000 pop.)	Natural birth rate (per 1000 pop.)	Natural death rate[a] (per 1000 pop.)
1949	36	20	–	–	–	–
1970	33.43	7.6	–	–	–	–
1980	18.21	6.34	–	–	–	–
1990	21.06	6.67	13.35	5.43	11.32	6.36
2001	13.38	6.43	6.1	5.3	5.02	5.97
2002	12.86	6.41	6.6	5.7	5.41	5.95
2003	12.41	6.40	–	–	–	–
2006	12.09	6.81	6.26	4.97	7.47	5.89

[a]Natural death rate=crude death rate

for men and 26.9 years for women, and at age 80, this was 8.3 years and 10.6 years for men and women, respectively. The increased life expectancy is related to improvements in public health and nutrition, and also to improved medical care for very elderly patients.[8–12] However, improved survival may not mean normal health without disability or functional impairment. Elderly persons have multiple chronic diseases, functional impairments and need for regular medical services.[13–15]

Macau SAR is a small city in China. In 2008, it had a population of 0.55 million. The natural birth and death rates have fallen over recent decades and the population is also ageing. In 2008, the elderly aged >65 years constituted 7.19% of its population. Average life expectancy at birth for males and females was 79.0 years and 84.8 years, respectively (Tables 146.1 and 146.4).[16]

Taiwan has also experienced a rapid demographic transition. The fertility rate has decreased from 5.9 children per woman in 1949 to 1.77 in 1997. Thus, the ratio of adult children to older parents will fall greatly in the coming years. A decline in the death rate has resulted in an increase in average life expectancy at birth. Between 1951

Table 146.4 Declining birth and death rates in Hong Kong SAR, Macau SAR and Taiwan.

Year	Hong Kong SAR		Macau SAR		Taiwan	
	Natural Birth Rate (per 1000 pop.)	Natural Death Rate (per 1000 pop.)	Natural Birth Rate (per 1000 pop.)	Natural Death Rate (per 1000 pop.)	Natural Birth Rate (per 1000 pop.)	Natural Death Rate (per 1000 pop.)
1946	20.1	20.1	–	–	–	–
1956	37.0	37.0	–	–	–	–
1966	25.5	25.5	–	–	–	–
1976	16.9	16.9	–	–	–	–
1986	13.1	13.1	–	–	–	–
1990	12.0	5.2	20.5	4.4	15.5	5.6
1995	11.2	5.1	14.1	3.2	13.8	5.7
2000	8.1	5.1	8.8	3.1	11.7	5.7
2002	7.1	5.0	7.2	3.2	11.0	5.7
2003	6.9	5.4	–	–	–	–
2006	9.5	5.5	–	–	–	–
2008	11.3	6.0	5.4	3.2	8.6	6.2

and 2008, average life expectancy at birth has increased from 53.4 years to 75.6 years for males, and from 56.3 years to 81.9 years for females. These changes have led to an increase in the elderly population (>65 years) from 2.5% in 1950 to 10.4% in 2008. This percentage is projected to increase to 24% by 2030. The increase of those aged 80 and over is very fast. In 1960, 9.2% of the elderly population belonged to the >80 group. By 2036, almost one-quarter (24%) of the elderly population will be in this group.[17–19] (Tables 146.1 and 146.4).

Policies toward ageing in mainland China

Officially, the basic principle of China's ageing policy is to maintain sustainable development by setting up a support system partnership involving the state, community, family and the individual. The priorities in meeting the challenge of population ageing in China are to develop China's economy, to set up an old age security system, to speed up the establishment of a community-based care system, to set up a legislative system to protect the rights of the elderly (the Law of the People's Republic of China on Protection of the Rights and Interests of the Elderly was enacted in 1996), to establish safety networks for the elderly, to raise their living standards, and to create an environment for healthy ageing. In the past decade, China has set up five guiding principles for the work on ageing. These are 'Elderly people should be supported, have medical care, be contributive to society, be engaged in life-long learning and live a happy life'. In 1994, the China Development Outline on the Work of Ageing was formulated with a view to gradually upgrading living standards of the elderly and to enrich their cultural life.[20]

As formal care services are limited, many older persons rely on the support of family members, particularly in rural areas. Family support functions include financial support (income security), care-giving tasks (physical care) and comforting tasks (psychological care). Most of the younger population still maintain that taking care of elderly family members is their responsibility. However, more and more young people are unable to provide all of these functions, and require some assistance from the government, policy-makers and community services providers.[4,6]

It is projected that the rapid ageing in China will lead to only 2 working age people for every senior citizen by 2050, compared with 13 to 1 now. Pension support is of great concern. As of March 2008, the Chinese pension system covered 205 million people, which represents 15% of the population. In rural areas, the pension system started in 1990 and covers only about 10% of the rural labour force. A further one-third drop in the number of pension participants occurred between 1999 and 2004. This was a setback attributed to the government's shortsightedness, as it was assumed that families would take care of rural elderly. Family support is declining, as younger family members migrate to work as labourers in factories, construction sites or other employment in cities. There is a plan to expand urban and rural pension coverage which aims at changing the present system to help migrant workers who change jobs frequently to maintain their retirement benefits.[21] There are other initiatives, including four 'demonstration bases' in the cities of Beijing, Tianjin and Chongqing, and in Jiangsu Province. The total investment would amount to 500 million yuan (Chinese dollars) each year. These centres would provide a model for the industry on care for the elderly. With regard to public commitment to long-term care, there will be an increase in the number of nursing homes. For example, Beijing plans to add 15 100 nursing home beds in 2010, that is, an increase of 43%.[21]

Health of the elderly in mainland China and Hong Kong SAR

In mainland China in 2008, the top killer diseases included cancer, cerebrovascular diseases, respiratory diseases, heart diseases, injuries and poisoning. Chronic diseases included hypertension, cerebrovascular diseases and coronary heart disease (CHD). Diabetes mellitus and CHD are more common in urban city areas than in rural areas.[22–25] (Table 146.5). All these fatal and chronic diseases occur predominantly in elderly persons.

In the Hong Kong SAR, the top killer diseases in the elderly include cancer, heart diseases and pneumonia,[12] while common chronic diseases include arthritis, hypertension and diabetes mellitus[13,15,27–30] (Table 146.6).

Healthcare services in mainland China

China's healthcare delivery system is organized in a three-tier fashion. In urban areas, it consists of street health stations, community health centres and district hospitals. In the economically less-developed rural areas, village stations, township health centres and county hospitals are responsible for healthcare delivery. Doctors in the village stations receive only six months training (i.e. no formal medical school) after junior high school and receive an average of 2–3 weeks ongoing education every year. Township health centres usually have 10–20 beds and are looked after by a physician with 3 years of medical school education after high school. They are supported by assistant

Table 146.5 Causes of death and common chronic diseases in China (all ages), 2008.

City	County
Top killer diseases in 2008:	**Top killer diseases in 2008:**
Male	*Male*
1 Cancer	1 Cancer
2 Cerebrovascular diseases (stroke)	2 Cerebrovascular diseases (stroke)
3 Heart diseases	3 Respiratory diseases
4 Respiratory diseases	4 Heart diseases (incl. HT heart disease)
5 Injury and poisoning	5 Injury and poisoning
6 Diseases of the digestive system	6 Diseases of the digestive system
7 Endocrine, nutrition and metabolic diseases (e.g. diabetes mellitus (DM))	7 Endocrine, nutrition and metabolic diseases (e.g. diabetes mellitus (DM))
8 Kidney diseases (nephritis, nephrotic syndrome, etc.)	8 Kidney diseases (nephritis, nephrotic syndrome, etc.)
Female	*Female*
1 Cancer	1 Cerebrovascular diseases (stroke)
2 Heart diseases (incl. HT heart disease)	2 Cancer
3 Cerebrovascular diseases (stroke)	3 Respiratory diseases
4 Respiratory diseases	4 Heart diseases (incl. HT heart disease)
5 Injury and poisoning	5 Injury and poisoning
6 Endocrine, nutrition and metabolic diseases (e.g. diabetes mellitus (DM))	6 Endocrine, nutrition and metabolic diseases (e.g. diabetes mellitus (DM))
7 Diseases of the digestive system	7 Diseases of the digestive system
8 Kidney diseases (nephritis, nephrotic syndrome, etc.)	8 Kidney diseases (nephritis, nephrotic syndrome, etc.)
Common chronic diseases:	**Common chronic diseases:**
1 Hypertension	1 Hypertension
2 Diabetes mellitus	2 Gastroenteritis
3 Cerebrovasclar diseases	3 Rheumatoid arthritis
4 Coronary heart disease	4 Intervertebral disc disease
5 Intervertebral disc disease	5 Cerebrovasclar diseases
6 Gastroenteritis	6 Chronic obstructive airway disease
7 Rheumatoid arthritis	7 Choleltih and cholecystitis
8 Chronic obstructive airway disease	8 Diabetes mellitus
9 Choleltih and cholecystitis	9 Coronary heart disease
10 Peptic ulcers	10 Peptic ulcers

Source: Ministry of Health of China. *China Health Statistics* [Abstract], 2008.[25]

Table 146.6 Mortality and morbidity of the elderly in Hong Kong.

Leading causes of death in the elderly in 2001:

1. Cancer
2. Heart diseases (incl. HT heart disease)
3. Pneumonia
4. Cerebrovascular diseases (stroke)
5. Chronic lower respiratory disease
6. Kidney diseases (nephritis, nephrotic syndrome, etc.)
7. Diabetes mellitus (DM)
8. Injury and poisoning

Common chronic diseases:

1. Arthritis
2. Hypertension
3. Bone fracture
4. Peptic ulcers
5. Diabetes mellitus
6. Coronary heart disease
7. Hyperlipidaemia
8. Dementia
9. Hyperthyroidism
10. Chronic obstructive airway disease
11. Stroke
12. Asthma

Source: Chu, 1998[13]; Woo, 1997[15]; Chiu, 1998[27]; Chu, 2005[28]; Lau, 1997[29]; Leung, 1997[30]

physicians and village doctors. County hospitals usually have 250–300 beds and are staffed by physicians with 4–5 years of medical training after high school. They are assisted by nurses and technicians.[5,22,31]

Healthcare costs in old age are an important problem for the poor and those living in rural areas. If they cannot afford the costs, they will be denied access to healthcare. In the olden days, the rural Cooperative Medical System (CMS) schemes primarily provided funding and organized prevention, primary care and secondary healthcare for the rural population. After 1950, a mutual assistance mechanism was established to provide access to basic drugs and primary healthcare. During the Cultural Revolution (1966–1976), the CMS was given a political priority. The rural CMS then organized health stations, paid village doctors to deliver primary healthcare, provided drugs and partially reimbursed patients for services received at township centres and county hospitals. China's relative success in extending healthcare to the rural population has played a key role in improving the health status of the population. However, the CMS suffered from problems of poor management and a small risk-pooling base, contributing to the downfall of these early cooperative financing schemes after the initiation of agricultural reforms in 1980. The CMS has gradually disintegrated in most rural areas. In 2004, fewer than 10% of China's villages had a CMS scheme. In addition, many village doctors have left to go into farming or to become private practitioners. Township health centres and county hospitals are largely financed by fee-for-service and out-of-pocket payment. Access to healthcare in many areas is principally governed by the ability to pay rather than the need for healthcare. Many elderly persons in villages face bankruptcy if they have a major illness and have to be hospitalized. For example, the cost of one average hospitalization would exceed the average annual income of 50% of the rural population. The insurance coverage level of the primarily village-based community financing schemes in rural areas is severely limited. Poverty after an illness and the related treatment expenses continues to be a serious problem for the rural elderly, and they are often deprived of the needed medical care because of their inability to pay. Reform of the rural CMS is needed. In May 1997, the State Council issued a special document emphasizing that CMS reform was a major direction for China's rural health reform.[31]

The healthcare costs of elderly retired government officials or workers from large corporations are paid from either the Government Insurance Scheme (GIS) or Labour Insurance Scheme (LIS), which have been effective in ensuring equity of access to healthcare. In urban areas, GIS and LIS will pay the healthcare costs for most elderly persons. Exceptions are those who do not belong to these two groups, who have to be financed by fee-for-service and out-of-pocket payment. Again, access to healthcare amongst these persons is determined by the ability to pay. In recent years, the government and other enterprises are facing increasing difficulty in supporting GIS and LIS medical expenditures. With the rapid introduction of high-technology medical services, increasing incomes drive up the demand for healthcare. Without an effective controlling mechanism on the medical service consumers or providers, China now faces a serious problem of inflation in medical costs. The primary weaknesses of GIS and LIS programmes are the relative inefficiency in health resource allocation and healthcare provisions as well as the lack of risk-pooling across enterprises or local governments. Each organization under GIS and LIS systems is self-insured. If an enterprise is running a deficit, it will not be able to reimburse the medical expenses of the employee or the retired employee, rendering the individual uninsured.[6,31]

Healthcare for the elderly requires government provision and support. However, the distribution of healthcare resources including healthcare professionals in China is very uneven. Geographical variations exist between cities and rural areas as well as coastal and inland areas. Eighty percent of healthcare resources are allocated to the cities, of which two-thirds are allocated to big hospitals. Primary health organizations in rural areas are severely insufficient. The healthcare utilization rate is very low, largely related to inadequate supply and access. The level of healthcare resources in mega-cities like Beijing and Shanghai may match those in developed countries. However, primary healthcare has not adequately developed. The charging system for healthcare is through insurance from government for government officials and for employees of large companies. These are also applicable to retired older persons who have previously worked in government institutes or major companies. Ordinary elderly people without these insurance supports have to pay the medical costs out of their own pocket. A government financial subsidy policy is usually not available, which is not reasonable.[31]

Healthcare financing reforms have recently started in some pilot cities. In 1994, Jiujiang in Jiangxi Province and Zhenjiang in Jiangsu Province were selected as pilot reform cities. A combination of individual saving accounts and social risk-pooling formed the basis for financing medical expenditures. This model emphasized individual responsibility with social protection through citywide risk-pooling for GIS and LIS. These reforms had some success in controlling the escalation of medical costs and in expanding coverage to those who were previously uninsured or underinsured. In 1996, it was decided that the pilot scheme should be extended to over 50 cities in 27 provinces and administrative regions.[31]

The coverage and financing of healthcare has been an ongoing difficult problem in China. Realizing the weaknesses of the public Government Insurance Schemes (GIS) and the Labour Insurance Scheme (LIS) the Chinese Government combined the two schemes into one. Currently, 180 million urban employees are covered under this new scheme.[32]

Since 2003, a new rural cooperative medical scheme (NRCMS) has also been launched in rural areas. This is essentially a basic health insurance scheme. In the ensuing five years, this scheme became increasingly adopted by citizens in rural areas, and by September 2007, 730 million rural citizens were included. A similar version of basic health insurance was also implemented in city and town areas. By 2007, over 30 000 000 persons were covered by this scheme.[24,32]

Community health services

According to the Chinese National Committee on Ageing, China has limited resources to set up comprehensive facilities to meet the increasing needs of the elderly. However, community service is considered to be an attractive way to complement the role of the family in caring for elderly persons. Over the past decade, there has been a great development in community service. By 1997, there were 930 000 community service facilities, 5055 community centres and 1.01 million community service stations throughout the whole country. Eighty-five percent of these facilities primarily serve the elderly persons in the local community, and 5.4 million volunteers have provided services. The community service embraces several groups of service providers including care services for daily living (e.g. home help, lunch, household work, shopping, escort, etc.), cultural activities (e.g. activity centres, lifelong learning, universities of the third age), legal assistance (i.e. when the legal right of an elderly member is violated) and day care services. Day care services are provided by either homes for the elderly or day care centres. The latter also provide simple medical services like clinical check-ups, intravenous saline treatment (as 'health maintenance') and family hospital beds. The medical service components are derived from the earlier street health stations and community health centres in urban areas. 'Doctors' in these centres usually receive basic training only and do not have formal geriatric medicine training.[33]

The Chinese Government's most pressing concern is how to provide equal access to basic healthcare for all Chinese people. Implementing basic medical and healthcare services for all would include public health, rural healthcare services, urban community healthcare services, and traditional Chinese medicine. Increasing the commitment of the central, provincial and local governments must be achieved. Development of basic healthcare facilities with basic medical technology, training for basic healthcare manpower, and making the basic drugs available to all urban and rural residents should be implemented. These reforms should also include changes in healthcare financing. Government spending needs to be increased, but resources from corporations and individuals should also be mobilized. Since China's economic reform in 1979, national healthcare spending has increased from 11 billion yuan in 1978 to 984.3 in 2006.[32]

Putting reform into practice, the roles of preventive healthcare and community health services are increasingly recognized by China's health authority. From 2003 to 2008, community health services were further developed to cover 93–98% of city areas and 50% of town areas. By 2008, approximately 24 000 community health service units had been set up in city and town areas. Meanwhile, there was an emphasis on improving healthcare services in rural areas, which included programmes to improve the training of local health professionals as well as attracting doctors from city areas to serve in rural areas.[24]

Regarding long-term care for the elderly population, nursing home care is an inevitable care model for frail older persons in China. Currently, approximately 1.5% of the elderly population live in nursing homes and apartments for older people.[34] As mentioned above, the one-child policy has resulted in a rapid decrease in family size in China, and a decline in the family support tradition for older family members is expected in the coming years. Hence, the demand for nursing home care will continue to increase, particularly in big cities. For example, Beijing city added 15 000 nursing home beds in 2010 – an increase of 43%![32]

Geriatric medicine in China and Hong Kong SAR

Geriatric medicine has been defined as a branch of general medicine which deals with the clinical, rehabilitative, psychosocial and preventive aspects of illness in elderly people. Despite an emphasis on the impact of the ageing population, geriatric medicine has not yet been developed in China. Traditionally, there is a group of doctors who practice 'geriatrics'. They are responsible for the delivery of medical care to 'elderly' and senior government officials in China. With the increasing number of retired senior government officials, the demand for their clinical services has also increased. Most of these doctors are well trained and specialized in one particular organ-based discipline (e.g. cardiology, respiratory medicine, neurology). Their training and clinical practice in 'geriatrics' are different from geriatricians in other parts of the world. Their research works are primarily targeted at an organ-based approach which includes cardiac diseases in the elderly, dementia, osteoporosis, biological mechanisms of ageing and anti-ageing drugs. However, there is a lack of research in geriatric syndromes such as falls or clinical models of geriatric care.

Medical education and training programmes in geriatric medicine and gerontology

As the elderly population increases, professional care in geriatric medicine and gerontology has an important role to play. There is a great need to provide education and training programmes in this area for doctors, nurses, social workers and allied health professionals. The current provision is grossly inadequate in China. There is only one undergraduate educational programme on social gerontology at the tertiary education level at the People's University of China, which was started in 1994.[4]

Basic undergraduate medical training in Chinese medical schools includes both a general and a shorter special diploma curriculum. The duration of the general comprehensive curriculum is usually 5 years, but may be 6–7 years in some schools. In terms of scope, this is comparable to primary medical training in other countries. In 1999, there were 21 university-based medical schools and 69 independent medical schools.[35]

High-school graduates may also study the special diploma programmes, which usually take four years. These medical training programmes are not comprehensive and each focuses on one special area only (e.g. oral health, hygiene, child health, physiology, pharmacology, chemistry, clinical medicine, physics, basic medical sciences, Chinese medicine, preventive medicine, medical imaging, acupuncture, etc.). In 1999, there were 20 medical diploma schools and 15 colleges with medical diploma courses.[35]

Geriatric medicine educational programmes in mainland China

Geriatric medicine education is lacking in most medical schools. In the undergraduate medical training in China, teaching of geriatric medicine is included in the curriculum of only 2.9% of medical schools. Most doctors in China are not equipped with knowledge in this area when they graduate from medical schools. This policy is not in keeping with the needs of an ageing population in mainland China and is different from many parts of the world. In Hong Kong SAR, United Kingdom, Europe and other developed countries, geriatric medicine is included in the core teaching of the undergraduate medical curriculum. In the United States, 60% of medical schools have included geriatric medicine as either a core or compulsory module, while 40% include this as an optional module.[35]

In mainland China, there are as yet no formal clinical post-graduate educational programmes for doctors or allied health professionals in geriatric medicine. This indicates that although China has paid great attention to family planning and population control, the university education system has not adapted to the needs of an ageing society. Compared to the widespread availability of post-graduate medical training in geriatric medicine in countries such as the United Kingdom, United States, Canada, Europe, Hong Kong, Australia and New Zealand, it is clear that this lack should be rectified.[6,10,11,35–37]

Specialty status for doctors in China primarily follows their research degrees (e.g. Master's and PhD degrees) as well as their publications in those specialty areas (e.g. geriatric cardiology, osteoporosis, basic science in ageing mechanism, dementia). There is no formal clinical specialist training for physicians in a subspecialty (e.g. cardiology, neurology, or geriatric medicine). Thus, most professors in current geriatric departments usually have a research interest in diseases that are prevalent in old age.[38,39]

The Chinese Geriatrics Society has been publishing the *Chinese Journal of Geriatrics* since 1982. The papers published can be categorized into disease-based research findings, biological mechanisms of ageing and anti-ageing interventions. There is a lack of publications on clinical geriatrics services, geriatric assessment, models of geriatric care and inter-disciplinary interventions. The summary report of the Fourth Committee meeting of the Chinese Geriatrics Society of the Chinese Medical Association emphasizes mainly research works on ageing, anti-ageing, anti-ageing drugs, longevity, geriatric cardiology, geriatric respiratory diseases, dementia and molecular biology, etc. The report also describes future problems which include epidemiology research in diseases in the elderly, basic scientific research, clinical research on common geriatric diseases and health promotion.[40] Unfortunately, the problems of the lack of clinical services in geriatric medicine and the need to train specialists have not yet been fully appreciated. The current trend of continued development of pure organ-based specialists to look after frail geriatric patients who have multiple problems is detrimental to the quality of care and the healthcare cost for most geriatric patients. This will perpetuate fragmentation of care, neglect of atypical presentations of diseases in the elderly, unnecessary investigations, iatrogenesis related to the duplication of drugs and potential interactions related to multiple medical care providers.

Clinical service in geriatric medicine

Geriatrics departments have existed in China for a long time. The traditional role of doctors in these departments is to provide hospital care for senior government officials (working or retired). The range of specialty skills in this group of doctors may range from neurologist, cardiologist, intensive care physicians, urologist, and so on. The focus is still on organ-based hospital specialists. This is very different from the practice of geriatric medicine in other parts of the world.[36,41–45] See also Chapters 143–145 on systems of healthcare in the United States, Australia and the United Kingdom. The principles of geriatric assessment and interdisciplinary intervention are not practiced. Geriatric rehabilitation is also not available in the clinical service programmes of these departments.

The health and long-term care system for the elderly in Hong Kong SAR

All Hong Kong citizens are entitled to inexpensive health and social care services. Moreover, for those who are on the Comprehensive Social Security Allowance (CSSA) Scheme, service fees are waived. The latter scenario is common among frail elderly patients in public hospitals. Together with escalating healthcare costs and an ageing demography, the annual budget of the Hong Kong Hospital Authority has increased by 19% from HK$27 801 million in 2004/2005 to HK$33 041 million in 2009/2010. With this magnitude of funding increase, the Hong Kong Hospital Authority has no deficit currently.[46,47]

The Social Welfare Department has been responsible for policy and funding of social services up to now. At present, social services for the elderly are categorized into community support (non-residential) and residential care services.[48] In the past, long-term care services for the elderly referred primarily to residential care services, which are largely provided by non-government organizations (NGOs). Over the past decade, the private old people's home industry has been developing rapidly and private homes now form the main service group for residential care of the elderly in Hong Kong. Meals delivery and personal care services are the key non-residential home care services available to those living in their own homes. The great demand for long-term residential care services has been a problem for many years and the magnitude of this problem is on the increase. At present, institutional care is quite commonly utilized and approximately 8% of the elderly in Hong Kong now reside in residential care homes for the elderly (RCHEs) and the hospital infirmary.[14,48–50] The majority of the RCHEs in Hong Kong are low-quality private homes, and a minority are government-funded and self-financing.

History of the development of geriatric medicine in Hong Kong SAR

On the basis of the British model, Hong Kong established its first geriatric unit in 1975. In the initial 10 years, development of geriatric medicine was slow. However, in recent years, the importance of geriatric service to the elderly community has been gradually recognized. At present, there is at least one geriatric service per hospital cluster (Tables 146.7 and 146.8).[14]

Lack of a systematic approach in acute geriatrics care in Hong Kong SAR

A fundamental and serious problem in the present organization of hospital care for the elderly is the lack of a systematic approach to acute geriatrics care. While a multidisciplinary, multidimensional geriatric assessment is frequently practiced in extended care hospitals, there is a general lack of an acute geriatrics service in most acute care hospitals. At present, only 3 out of 15 acute hospitals have designated acute geriatric wards (Table 146.7).[14]

The number of elderly in acute care hospitals is a huge case load. To be cost-effective, acute care for the elderly has to be focused. To attain a cost-effective healthcare model, targeting of the frail elderly patients in the acute geriatrics care programmes is necessary. These targeted patients would be physically, cognitively, and/or psychosocially frail. The settings of screening geriatric assessment would be at the sites where the frail elderly are present (i.e. medical, surgical, orthopaedic and emergency room settings). Concurrent with acute treatment of the presenting medical disease, geriatric assessment and intervention should be started simultaneously to prevent and reverse functional decline.

The unit for development of acute care for the elderly should include several core elements in its programme: targeting of frail elders (i.e. in the emergency department, general medical, orthopaedic, neurosurgical and surgical wards with particular attention to those elderly who

Table 146.7 Geriatric service in the Hong Kong Hospital Authority by hospital clusters.

Year	Cluster	Hospital	Unit/Ward/Team
1994	Hong Kong (HK) West	Queen Mary Hospital (QMH)	Geriatric Team
1994		Fung Yiu King Hospital (FYKH)	Geriatric Department
2002		Tung Wah Hospital (TWH)	Geriatric Team
2004		Grantham Hospital (GH)	Geriatric Department
1990	Hong Kong (HK) East	Rutonjee and Tang Siu Kin Hospitals (RTSKH)	Geriatric Department
1995		Pamela Youde Nethersole Hospital (PYNEH)	Geriatric Team
1996		Tung Wah East Hospital (TWEH)	Geriatric Team
1995		Wong Chuk Hang Hospital (WCHH)	Geriatric Department
1995		Saint John Hospital (SJH)	Geriatric Department
1996		Cheshire Home Chung Hom Kok (CCH)	Geriatric Team
1974	Kowloon East	United Christian Hospital (UCH)	Geriatric Ward
2000		Tseung Kwan O Hospital (TKOH)	Geriatric Team
1991		Haven of Hope Hospital (HOHH)	Geriatric and Rehabilitation Unit
1975	Kowloon West	Princess Margaret Hospital (PMH)	First formal Geriatric Department
1978		Caritas Medical Centre (CMC)	Geriatric Department
1982		Kwong Wah Hospital (KWH)	Geriatric Unit
1994		Yan Chai Hospital (YCH)	Geriatric Team
1995		Our Lady of Maryknoll Hospital (OLMH)	Geriatric Team
1995		Wong Tai Sin Hospital (WTSH)	Geriatric Team
1993	Kowloon Central	Queen Elizabeth Hospital (QEH)	Geriatric Team
1995		Kowloon Hospital (KH)	Geriatric and Rehabilitation Unit
2003		Buddhist Hospital (BH)	Geriatric Team
1985	New territories (NT) East	Prince of Wales Hospital (PWH)	Geriatric Team
2001		Shatin Hospital (SH)	Geriatric Unit
1997		Alice Ho Miu Ling Nethersole Hospital (AHMLNH)	Geriatric Team
1998		Tai Po Hospital (TPH)	Geriatric Team
1990	New Territories (NT) West	Tuen Mun Hospital (TMH)	Geriatric Department

are residents from old people's homes), comprehensive geriatric assessment, case-based conference by interdisciplinary team, and intervention. The interdisciplinary management should include a 'Prehab' programme to prevent functional decline with an appropriately designed acute care ward environment and then a 'Rehab' programme to reverse functional decline and improve activity of daily living. Discharge planning (i.e. predischarge planning and postdischarge support with appropriate placement) with a case management approach should be implemented. Clinical outcomes must be optimized while unnecessary hospital admissions prevented.[36,51]

Inadequate rehabilitation after acute illness is also a problem and the waiting time for Geriatric Day Hospital (GDH) is long. Inadequate GDH transportation is another obstacle to providing adequate day rehabilitation for the frail elderly. Because of moderate disability, they usually require transportation support (e.g. Non-emergency Ambulance Transport) from home to the GDH.[14]

Issues in primary healthcare for the elderly in Hong Kong SAR

For the general population, primary healthcare is largely provided by the private healthcare sector, and the government is responsible for approximately 10% of this service. The latter is provided by the general outpatient clinic. In the elderly, the proportion of private doctor consultation is less than in the young and approximately 70% of them consult general outpatient clinics for primary healthcare problems.[52] Most of the patients attending these clinics are either old or financially poor. Primary care providers are mostly private doctors who can manage episodic health problems well, but are inexperienced in detecting and managing chronic geriatric problems and syndromes. For

Table 146.8 Geriatric services in the Hong Kong West Hospital Cluster.

Acute hospital care	QMH (Integrated model) GH (Direct transfer from Emergency Room)
Convalescent care	FYKH TWH GH
Geriatric rehabilitation beds	FYKH TWH GH
Long-stay infirmary beds for geriatric patients	FYKH TWH
Pre-discharge programme and post-discharge support	QMH, TWH, FYKH,GH
Geriatric Day Hospital as day rehabilitation centre	FYKH TWH
Geriatric Specialist Clinics	QMH Geriatric Specialist Out-Patient Department QMH Memory Clinic QMH Falls Clinic QMH Nutrition Clinic FYKH Continence Clinic
Hong Kong West (HKW) Community Geriatric Assessment Team (CGAT)	Outreach Geriatric Doctor Clinics in >60 years old people's homes (Subsidized Care & Attention homes, private old people's homes, day care centres) Visiting Medical Officer (VMO) under CGAT-VMO programme Central Infirmary Waiting List (CIWL) clients pre-admission assessment Domiciliary visits: medical, nursing, physiotherapy and occupational therapy Educational and training programme for carers and community elders Health education programmes with community partners

Note: For hospital name abbreviations, please refer to Table 146.7.

example, dementia is sometimes referred to as a 'normal ageing phenomenon' without appropriate investigation and treatment.

Health promotion to improve lifestyles (e.g. quit smoking, healthy diet, exercise, etc.), disease prevention (e.g. falls prevention and influenza vaccination for the elderly), and early chronic disease identification and control are important. These measures would improve the health of the whole population and decrease geriatric health problems and the need for long-term care in the years to come. Seasonal influenza vaccinations for the elderly with chronic diseases can decrease the chance of influenza-related complications as well as reducing the rate of hospitalizations.[53]

The Department of Health's Elderly Health Service (EHS) provides a health promotion programme for elderly members at their centres.[54] However, data regarding improvement of the health status of elderly participants in these programmes have not yet been reported. Moreover, elderly citizens who are not members of these centres do not have access to the programmes.

Geriatric healthcare at residential care homes for the elderly (RCHES) in Hong Kong SAR

Those elderly living at home and alone constitute 12.4% of the over 65 year olds (11.2 and 13.6% for elderly men and women respectively).[55] While community and primary healthcare is largely provided by private family doctors and general outpatient clinic (GOPC) doctors, specialist geriatric services at old people's homes are provided mainly by a Community Geriatric Assessment Team (CGAT) and partly by Community Health Nurses (CNS).[56,57] A new programme of Visiting Medical Officers (VMOs) was started in October 2003 to improve areas of infection control and provide ad hoc primary or geriatric medical care for frail elders in old people's homes. Approximately 100 VMOs have been appointed as part-time HA staff to upgrade the previously inadequate primary and geriatric care in over 100 old people's homes in Hong Kong.[46,58] The success of this VMO programme has led to its implementation throughout Hong Kong. Recent evaluations also showed that the VMO programme has reduced the number of emergency hospital admissions from old people's homes and hospitalization-related healthcare costs.[59,60]

Service gap and duplication issues for health and long-term care of the elderly

Multiple and continuous gaps in our traditional care models may lead to the 'falling through the cracks' phenomenon.[61] The fragmentation of care can lead to frustration of the elders and caregivers and cause potential harm to patients, for example, being subjected to either 'multiple repeated or similar drugs' (multiple doctors) or 'no drugs' (waiting for new case appointment). The latter is a common transitional care problem for the elderly in Hong Kong.

In the community, the single frail elder commonly receives multiple healthcare services (e.g. the private family doctor, VMO, orthopaedic doctor, ophthalmologist, cardiologist, endocrinologist, etc.) as well as multiple social services (e.g. members of several multiservice or social centres for the elderly, home help services, etc.). The current problems include fragmentation of care, service gaps, overlapping of services, poor communication and coordination. It is believed that an integrated geriatric health and long-term care team across both health and social sectors would be able to overcome these undesirable issues substantially.

Unfortunately, the current financing and public policy do not facilitate this development. Moreover, the present public health and social policy still lead to unhealthy competition for clients as well as creating some important gaps in services for the elderly. At present, separate service providers are under different budget holders in the Department of Health's Elderly Health Service (EHS of DH), Hospital Authority (HA), Social Welfare Department (SWD) and NGOs. Most elders use the public health and social long-term care services. Only a small proportion of the elderly population seeks services from private hospitals, clinics and social services. In general, the objectives and policies of different service organizations differ. The policy on service directions may also be different. In terms of collaboration between different elderly service providers, a service purchase model among different organizations is in operation, but this has great limitations on breaking the gaps or eliminating service overlaps. For example, frontline staff have difficulty in working together as an integrated team despite overlapping of services (e.g. EHS of DH and Geriatric Service of HA). Loose collaboration is the practice at present, which is not ideal.

For the interface issue between public and private health sectors, there is a slow development. Communications have improved and private doctors can obtain a discharge summary of their patients from HA if they have preregistered. The recent public–private collaboration with VMOs in the Caritas Evergreen Home is one of the successful pilot projects implemented by the author in the Hong Kong West (HKW) Hospital Cluster.[58]

The present organization of healthcare for the elderly indirectly gives rise to an overuse of hospital care services as against community care services. The trend for cost containment would shift hospital care from acute to subacute hospital care, and shorten the length of hospital stay in the acute care hospital per episode of admission. This is a consequence of concentrating only on the activity figures. There is no cost incentive to decrease unnecessary hospital readmissions. Moreover, there has been an overemphasis on specialty-led and organ-based disciplines, which are all very costly.

Thus, alternative health and long-term-care service models for the elderly with an appropriate healthcare financing policy are needed urgently. Effective solutions should be explored and implemented in the near future to avoid catastrophic incidents in both health and social care services for the elderly.

Financing of the public healthcare system for the elderly in Hong Kong is inadequate. Most elderly persons in Hong Kong are poor and obviously would choose to use public healthcare services (under Hospital Authority and Department of Health) rather than the private sectors. The financial status of current and next-generation older persons is definitely not good or optimistic. Recently, the Hong Kong SAR Government has implemented a pilot health voucher scheme with a view to reducing the imbalance of public–private healthcare services utilization. Under this scheme, all elderly citizens aged 70 or over are entitled to consult private doctors, who would be reimbursed the consultation fees with a ceiling of HK$500 per year. The scheme was launched on 1 January 2009. By the beginning of December 2009, 40% (0.26 million) of elderly people had enrolled in the scheme, and over 321 000 doctor consultation reimbursements had been processed.[62]

Recommendation for an integrated health and social care delivery system in Hong Kong SAR

A comprehensive long-term and geriatric healthcare programme is needed for the elderly in Hong Kong SAR. This programme can be subdivided into regional teams. The geriatric health and social long-term services must be fully integrated. We need to improve on the present interface and collaboration models further. Financial incentives are crucial for the success of this model. Merging different organizational structures to form an integrated long-term and geriatric care team is a cost-effective and sustainable way of providing targeted care to the frail elderly among the elderly population of Hong Kong.

Conclusions

The population of China is rapidly ageing. Declining birth and mortality rates and 25 years of the one-child policy are the main reasons for this phenomenon, particularly in urban cities like Shanghai, Beijing and Hong Kong SAR. Recently, the Chinese Government has implemented healthcare reforms to improve healthcare coverage and the insurance system, particularly for rural areas. However, the practice of geriatric medicine with an interdisciplinary intervention is the most suitable clinical management approach for frail older persons in China. Unfortunately, this has not yet started in most parts of China except the Hong Kong SAR. To cope with the demands of an ageing population, there is a definite and pressing need to develop clinical geriatric services together with geriatric medicine educational programmes. Research in local clinical geriatrics care models is also essential for a proper evaluation of their effectiveness. In Hong Kong SAR, further improvement in the practice of geriatric care is needed. The fragmentation of health and long-term care services needs to be rectified in the near future. Integration of geriatric services with social long-term care services for the elderly is recommended.

Key points

- The population of China is ageing and the proportion of elderly >60 years is over 10%; in the 2005 population survey, the elderly population aged >65 years was already >100 million.
- Geriatric medicine has not been developed in most parts of China except the Hong Kong SAR.
- Educational programmes in geriatric medicine at undergraduate and graduate levels and clinical training programmes for doctors are greatly needed in most parts of China.
- Clinical geriatric service with an interdisciplinary team approach should be developed in China. Research in these clinical geriatric care models has to be performed simultaneously.
- The issue of inadequate healthcare insurance for older persons in China, particularly those in rural areas, has improved but needs further development. Financial contributions from the government, the older persons and families are needed.
- The basic principle in China's ageing policy is to maintain sustainable development by setting up an elderly support system partnership involving the state, the community, the family and the individual.

References

1. National Bureau of Statistics of China. 5th National Population Census of China (No. 1), 2004. http://www.stats.gov.cn/tjgb/rkpcgb/qgrkpcgb/t20020331_15434.htm (accessed April 2010).
2. National Bureau of Statistics of China. Population survey of China (One-percent sample), 2006. http://www.stats.gov.cn/tjgb/rkpcgb/qgrkpcgb/t20060316_402310923.htm (accessed April 2010).
3. Lee L. The current state of public health in China. *Annu Rev Public Health* 2004;**25**:327–39.
4. Du P, Guo ZG. Population ageing in China. In: DR Phillips (ed.), *Ageing in Asia-Pacific Region. Issues, Policies and Future Trends*, Taylor & Francis, London, 2000, pp. 194–209.
5. Ministry of Health of China, 2004. China Health Statistics [Abstract]. http://www.moh.gov.cn/statistics/digest04/tt.htm (accessed September 2004).
6. Woo J, Kwok T, Sze FKH, Yuan HJ. Ageing in China: health and social consequences and responses. *Int J Epidemiology* 2002;**31**:772–5.
7. Festini F, de Martino M. Twenty-five years of one-child family policy in China. *J Epidemiol Commun H* 2004;**58**:358–60.
8. Census and Statistics Department, HKSAR. *Hong Kong Population Projections 2007–2036, Census and Statistics Department*, HKSAR, Hong Kong, 2009.
9. Census and Statistics Department, HKSAR. *Vital Statistics of Hong Kong*, Census and Statistics Department, HKSAR, Hong Kong, 2009.
10. Chow N, Chi I. Ageing in Hong Kong. In: SK Lam (ed.), *The Health of the Elderly in Hong Kong*, Hong Kong University Press, Hong Kong, 1997, pp. 173–92.
11. Chow N. Ageing in Hong Kong. In: DR Phillips (ed.), *Ageing in Asia-Pacific Region. Issues, Policies and Future Trends*, Taylor & Francis, London, 2000, pp. 158–73.
12. Hospital Authority, HKSAR. *Hospital Authority Statistical Report 2007–2008*, Hospital Authority, HKSAR, Hong Kong, 2009.
13. Chu LW, Kwok KK, Chan S *et al*. A Survey on the Health and Health Care Needs of Elderly People Living in the Central and Western District of the Hong Kong Island [Report], Central and Western District Board of Hong Kong, Hong Kong, 1998.
14. Chu LW, Chi I. Long-term care and hospital care for the elderly. In: GM Leung, J Bacon-Shone (eds.), *Hong Kong Health Care System: Reflections, perspectives and visions*, Hong Kong University Press, Hong Kong, 2006, pp. 223–52.
15. Woo J, Ho SC, Chan SG *et al*. An estimate of chronic disease burden and some economic consequences among the elderly Hong Kong population. *J Epidemiol Commun H* 1997;**51**: 486–9.
16. Macau SAR Government, 2010. http://www.gcs.gov.mo/files/factsheet/geography.php?PageLang=E (accessed April 2010).
17. Barlett HP, Wu SC. Ageing and aged care in Taiwan. In: DR Phillips (ed.), *Ageing in Asia-Pacific Region. Issues, Policies and Future Trends*, Taylor & Francis, London, 2000, pp. 210–22.
18. Council for Economic Planning and Development, Taiwan, 2010. http://www.cepd.gov.tw/encontent/m1.aspx?sNo=0001457 (accessed in April 2010).
19. Statistics Department, Ministry of the Interior, Taiwan. *Statistical Yearbook 2008*. http://www.moi.gov.tw/stat/english/year.asp (accessed April 2010).
20. Liang HC. The health management of the aged in China. Presented at The 5th Asia Oceania Regional Congress of Gerontology, Hong Kong, 19–23 November 1995.
21. China National Committee on Ageing. China begins to address a coming wave of elderly; http://www.cnca.org.cn/en/index.html (accessed May 2010).
22. Editorial Committee of China Health Annual. *China Health Annual 2003* [in Chinese] (Zhongguo Weisheng Nianjian), People's Health Publishing, Beijing, China, 2004.
23. Editorial Committee of China Health Annual. *China Health Annual 2008* [in Chinese] (Zhongguo Weisheng Nianjian), People's Health Publishing, Beijing, China, 2009.
24. Editorial Committee of China Health Annual. *China Health Annual 2009* [in Chinese] (Zhongguo Weisheng Nianjian), People's Health Publishing, Beijing, China, 2010.
25. Ministry of Health of China. *China Health Statistics* [Abstract], 2008. http://www.moh.gov.cn/publicfiles//business/htmlfiles/wsb/index.htm (accessed April 2010).

26. Hospital Authority, HKSAR. *Hospital Authority Statistical Report 2007–2008*, Hospital Authority, HKSAR, Hong Kong, 2009.

27. Chiu HF, Lam LC, Chi I *et al*. Prevalence of dementia in Chinese elderly in Hong Kong. *Neurology* 1998;**50**:1002–9.

28. Chu LW, Chi I, Chiu A. Incidence and predictors of falls in the Chinese elderly. *Ann Acad Med Singapore* 2005;**34**:60–72.

29. Lau CP, Lok N. Prevalence of coronary heart disease and associated risk factors in ambulant elderly. In: SK Lam (ed.), *The Health of the Elderly in Hong Kong*, Hong Kong University Press, Hong Kong, 1997, pp. 99–110.

30. Leung EMF, Lo MB. Social and health status of elderly people in Hong Kong. In: SK Lam (ed.), *The Health of the Elderly in Hong Kong*, Hong Kong University Press, Hong Kong, 1997, pp. 43–61.

31. China Medical Association. http://www.chinamed.org.cn/healthcare2.htm (accessed September 2004).

32. Cheng TM. China's latest health reforms: A conversation with Chinese Health Minister Chen Zhu [Interview]. *Health Affairs* 2008;**27**:1103–10.

33. Zhang WE. The Ageing of Population and the Policies of China [Monograph]; Chinese National Committee on Ageing, Beijing, 2003.

34. Chu LW, Chi I. Nursing homes in China. *J Am Med Dir Assoc* 2008;**9**:237–43.

35. Higher Education Office of China Ministry of Education Reform and Development of Higher Medical Education in China [in Chinese], People's Health Publishing, Beijing, 2004.

36. Chu LW, Lam SK. Geriatric medicine in Hong Kong. In: SK Lam (ed.), *The Health of the Elderly in Hong Kong*, Hong Kong University Press, Hong Kong, 1997, pp. 1–20.

37. Hong Kong College of Physicians. Guidelines for higher training in geriatric medicine. In: Hong Kong College of Physicians (ed.), *Guidelines for Higher Training in Internal Medicine*, Hong Kong College of Physicians, Hong Kong, [illegible]

38. Luk WW. Geriatric health care of Shanghai in the 21st century. Presented at The 2000 Hong Kong-Shanghai Geriatrics Scientific Forum, Hong Kong Geriatrics Society and Renji Hospital of Shanghai, Renji Hospital, Shanghai, 11–14 May 2000.

39. Zhu HM. Epidemiology of bone fracture and its influence on life quality in the elderly. *Chinese Journal of Geriatrics* 1993; **12**:168–72.

40. Wong ST. A summary report of the 4th committee meeting of the Chinese geriatrics society of the Chinese medical association. *Chinese Journal of Geriatrics* 1999;**8**: 197.

41. Fox RA, Puxty J. Geriatrics and the problem-solving approach. In: RA Fox, J Puxty (eds), *Medicine in the Frail Elderly. A Problem-oriented Approach*, Edward Arnold, London, 1993, pp. 1–13.

42. Hall MRP, Rowe MJ. The United Kingdom. In: MSJ Pathy (ed.), *Principles and Practice of Geriatric Medicine*, 3rd edn, John Wiley & Sons, Ltd, Chichester, 1998, pp. 1523–34.

43. Isaacs B. The giants of geriatrics. In: B Isaacs (ed.), *The Challenge of Geriatric Medicine*, Oxford University Press, Oxford, 1992, pp. 1–5.

44. Lindsay RW, Barker WH. The United States of America. In: MSJ Pathy (ed.) *Principles and Practice of Geriatric Medicine*, 3rd edn, John Wiley & Sons, Ltd, Chichester, 1998, pp. 1535–48.

45. Swift CG. The problem-oriented approach to geriatric medicine. In: MSJ Pathy (ed.) *Principles and Practice of Geriatric Medicine*, 3rd edn, John Wiley & Sons, Ltd, Chichester, 1998, pp. 251–68.

46. Hospital Authority, HKSAR. Hospital Authority Annual Plan 2004–2005, Hospital Authority, HKSAR, Hong Kong, 2004.

47. Hospital Authority, HKSAR. Hospital Authority Annual Plan 2009–2010, Hospital Authority, HKSAR, Hong Kong, 2010.

48. Social Welfare Department, HKSAR, 2004. http://www.info.gov.hk/swd/texeng/ser sec/serelder/ (accessed July 2004).

49. Social Welfare Department, HKSAR, 2010. http://www.info.gov.hk/swd/text_eng/ser_sec/ser_elder/ (accessed April 2010).

50. Hospital Authority, HKSAR. HA Monthly Statistical Report on Central Infirmary Waiting List on 30 June 2004, Hospital Authority, HKSAR, Hong Kong, 2004.

51. Palmer RM, Landefeld CS, Kresevic D, Kowal J. A medical unit for the acute care of the elderly. *J Am Geriatr Soc* 1994; **42**:545–52.

52. Census and Statistics Department, HKSAR. *Special Topics Report No. 27: Social data collected via the General Household Survey*, Census and Statistics Department, HKSAR, Hong Kong, 2001.

53. Hui SL, Chu LW, Peiris JSM *et al*. Immune response to influenza vaccination in community-dwelling Chinese elderly persons. *Vaccine* 2006;**24**:5371–80.

54. Department of Health, HKSAR. *Annual Report of the Department of Health 2001–2002*, HKSAR, Hong Kong, 2004.

55. Census and Statistics Department, HKSAR. *Thematic Report – Older Persons 2002*, Census and Statistics Department, HKSAR, Hong Kong, 2002.

56. Leung JYY, Yu TKK, Cheung YL *et al*. Private nursing home residents in Hong Kong – how frail are they and their need for hospital services. *Journal of the Hong Kong Geriatrics Society* 2000;**10**:65–9.

57. Luk JKH, Chan FHW, Pau MML, Yu C. Outreach geriatrics service to private old age homes in Hong Kong West Cluster. *Journal of the Hong Kong Geriatrics Society* 2002;**11**:5–11.

58. Chu LW, Ho C, Chan F *et al*. A new model of primary medical and specialist care for the elderly in residential care homes for the elderly. A public-private interface collaboration project. Presented at The Hong Kong SARS Forum and Hospital Authority Convention, Hong Kong, 8–11 May 2004.

59. Chau KM, Luk JKH, Choi A *et al*. Phase III CGAS/CVMO Collaboration Scheme in HKWC – a novel care model to reduce A&E attendance and hospitalization in institutionalized elderly. Presented at the Hospital Authority Annual Convention, 8–9 May 2006 [Abstract].

60. Luk JKH, Chau KM, Choi A *et al*. Reduction of hospitalization cost after implementation of CVMO programme in Hong Kong West Cluster – The first year result. Presented at the Hospital Authority Annual Convention, Hong Kong Convention and Exhibition Centre, 7–8 May 2007 [Abstract].

61. Coleman EA. Falling through the cracks: challenges and opportunities for improving transitional care for persons with continuous complex care needs. *J Am Geriatr Soc* 2003; **51**:549–55.
62. Department of Health, HKSAR. Health voucher scheme, 2010. http://www.news.gov.hk/en/category/healthandcommunity/091216/html/091216en05012.htm (accessed May 2010).

Further Reading

Hong Kong SAR Government, 2010. http://www.info.gov.hk/censtatd/eng/hkstat/index.html (accessed May 2010).

CHAPTER 147

Ageing in developing countries

Renato Maia Guimarães
Hospital Universitário de Brasília, Universidade de Brasília, Brazil

Introduction

The number of older people in many developing countries is growing more rapidly than those in industrialized nations. However, population ageing also reveals social inequality. In South Africa it is interesting to note that only 7% of the blacks, people of colour and Indians (who constitute 89% of the total population) are old people, whereas 14.2% of the minority white population are 60 years and over.[1] Other determinants rather than the Gross National Product (GNP) have a strong influence on life expectancy. Cuba, Costa Rica, Barbados and Sri Lanka are low-income countries with life expectancy similar to North America and many industrial countries of Europe.

The usual view of the developing world held by people living in the West, namely that of families with many children and high infant mortality rates, nowadays applies only to the least developed countries, mainly in Africa. Major fertility reductions in the developing world took place over the last three decades of the twentieth century. From 1950–1955 to 2005–2010, the total fertility rate in the developing world dropped by almost 60%, from 6.2 to 2.7 children per woman.[2] In 2009 the fertility rate in Brazil was similar to the rate in France (1.9 children per woman). Children begging in the streets of some Latin America countries for instance, reveal a lack of adequate social policies despite the reduction in fertility.

There are several possible explanations for the recent demographic scene in the developing world; these include urbanization, improvement in basic sanitary conditions and education, better health assistance and economic growth. Dissemination of information and access to the health system, including distribution of oral contraceptive pills, have strongly contributed to the decline in family size. Greater female participation in the labour market has also played a key role. The size of families parents wish to have has declined, as the cost of raising a child has risen and child survival has increased.[3] In China, government intervention consisted of the coercive and unpopular one-child policy.

Demographic development poses widespread social and economic challenges for societies. The total dependency ratio is a measure of potential social support needs. It represents the ratio of children (persons under age 15) and older persons aged 65 and over to the number of potential working people aged 15 to 64, expressed per 100 population. In developing countries there will be a fast shift from young to old age dependency, since the number of children is declining and the proportion of older persons is increasing rapidly. In African countries with a high prevalence of HIV/AIDS the supposed support given by potential working adult people does not always apply. Many older Africans find themselves in a double-bind. They constitute the majority of the community in the rural areas, responsible for the care of their ill and dying relatives. After sick relatives pass way, older people are often left with grandchildren to support with no middle-age generation present. In Africa alone, 12 million orphaned children grow up without their parents and very often live with their grandparents.[1]

One of the key challenges confronting developing countries with an increasingly ageing population is to guarantee to the whole elderly population an adequate level of income, without placing excessive demands on younger generations and national economies. This dilemma has direct implications for social security systems. Many countries do not have a full pension scheme covering all the working population, mainly those in informal activities or living in rural areas. The increasing life expectancy has not been fully considered by social security schemes in many countries, and a move from early retirement would require a major change in sociocultural model attitudes. In developed and developing countries, early withdrawal from the labour market is currently seen as both desirable and acceptable, even for people in full possession of their faculties and in sound health.[4] At the same time in nations with low and middle economies, elderly people who did not make any contribution to social security are left without any income. However, it is estimated that at least 50 developing

Principles and Practice of Geriatric Medicine, Fifth Edition. Edited by Alan J. Sinclair, John E. Morley and Bruno Vellas.

countries provide social pensions for their elderly citizens, defined as non-contributory cash income.

Social security systems will also be stretched in response to the new demands made by the health needs of older persons.

Ageing and health

The epidemiological transition is the correlate of demographic transition in health. Deaths due to communicable disease are declining and there is a worldwide increase in deaths due to chronic disease, mainly cardiovascular disorders, cancer and diabetes. Despite this trend, it is appropriate to consider that developing countries are facing an epidemiological polarization. Communicable disease remains an important cause of morbidity and mortality, notwithstanding the predominance of deaths due to chronic disorders. Increased vulnerability, a hallmark of the poor and the elderly, and inequity make the risk of infectious disease unfairly high, depriving this section of the population of benefits of human progress achieved as long as a century ago.

In 2002, chronic diseases were responsible for 46% of all deaths in developing countries, a figure that is projected to grow to 59% by 2030.[5] However, the increased risk of chronic diseases is not simply a result of a reduction in infectious disease mortality, nor due to an ageing population alone. Life-course epidemiology reminds us of a new approach to chronic disease. Subnutrition and an unhealthy environment in early life may increase the incidence of chronic disease in later life. So, today's epidemiological scene in developing countries may also reflect past conditions of people who survived despite sub- or malnutrition and poor health conditions in early life.[6] There is a significant association between economic status and good, basic and advanced functional ability. Geriatric functional ability is closely associated with income not only in developing countries, but also in developed countries.[7]

Behavioural risks are estimated to account for 30–60% of chronic disease. In developing countries experiencing economical growth without a corresponding increase in the education level, new behaviours can be imposed by poorly controlled publicity inducing the consumption of tobacco, alcoholic beverages and junk foods.

At the same time as the world is shocked by images of starvation in African countries at conflict, the current trend in developing countries toward higher fat, more refined diets that augment the risk of chronic disease is increasing. Obesity is particularly high in Latin America and the Caribbean. On the other hand, a lack of policies to meet the nutrition needs of the elderly is placing the senior population at even greater risk of food insecurity and malnutrition.[8]

Mortality statistics reveal a limited scope of the health pattern of a population. Chronic disease is by definition a long duration disorder that, before causing death, can impact the patient's life in several ways. The Disability Adjusted Life Year or DALY is a health gap measure that extends the concept of potential years of life lost due to premature death (PYLL) to include equivalent years of 'healthy' life lost by virtue of being in states of poor health or disability. DALYs for a disease or health condition are calculated as the sum of the years of life lost due to premature mortality (YLL) in the population and the years lost due to disability (YLD) for incident cases of the health condition. According to the Global Burden of Diseases estimates for 2004, 68% of the 751 million years lived with disability (YLD) worldwide are attributable to chronic non-communicable diseases, and 84% of the burden of chronic disease arises in countries with low and middle incomes.[9] Although the prevalence and incidence of most chronic diseases are strongly age dependent, only 20% of the disability burden caused by chronic disease in countries with low and middle incomes occurs in people aged 60 years and older, compared with 36% for high-income countries, where demographic ageing in much more advanced.[10] Thus health conditions of old people living in developing countries tend to be worse than those who live in high-income countries, reflecting also adversities in early life, nutrition problems, unhealthy lifestyle and lifelong insufficient healthcare. Differentials in education contribute to prevalence of disability at ages >65 years independently of disease.[11] Thus education remains the most important correlate to health with tough consequences in old age. Whereas the current generation of older adults in much of the developing world is characterized by low and gender-segregated levels of education, offspring have higher levels of education and the gender gap has closed considerably. It may therefore be expected that older adults are exposed by their children to a new set of beliefs and an expanding knowledge base that may alter and expand available resources.[12]

In the next 30 years developing countries will pay for their tormented past even if socioeconomic growth continues. There will be a dramatic shift in the distribution of death from younger to older age and from communicable to non-communicable causes. Most developing countries are not sufficiently equipped to meet the needs of the older population, mainly the leading causes of YLD: eye disease, hearing loss, dementia, musculoskeletal disease and heart disease. Although it is not so difficult to implement healthcare for cataracts and hearing loss, for example, the demands of the three latter disorders are complex and more difficult to attend.

Health care and geriatric medicine

To be elderly in middle- and low-income countries is to have a high chance of being in adverse health conditions. This reveals the challenge that countries with a recent history of demographic 'shock' will face. Lives are not saved, rather death is postponed. Thus developing countries will have to deal with the expensive and complex demands related to the care of the 'survivors' of the socioeconomic traps imposed by poverty and ignorance, contrasting with the simple and less expensive (per capita) investment made in sanitation, vaccines and the use of antibiotics that allowed children and young adults to survive into old age.

Health systems in less developed countries are not uniform. There are very well-equipped institutions in most countries; however, primary care attention is somewhat deficient. In countries like Cuba where there is comprehensive healthcare, life expectancy is high. In the developing, and also in the developed world, geriatric medicine has a long way to go. In Africa only some northern countries have a few geriatric centres. China, as the country with the greatest elderly population, is reorganizing its public health system. Their Medicare system coverage is not available to two fifths of employees in cities and towns, and even less to workers living in rural areas.[13] It is difficult to assume that a high standard of medical care for those above the age of retirement will soon be available. Many Indian geriatricians have made important contributions to the quality of geriatric care in the United Kingdom, whereas in India, work in geriatric medicine has mostly been an application of the principles of general medicine to disorders and conditions related to old age. Departments of geriatric medicine are just beginning to come into being.[14]

In Latin America the geriatric societies are very active but the incorporation of the principles of geriatric medicine by the public health system is far from satisfactory. Although the health services are under pressure due to the new demands of the older population, there is very little or nothing specifically to meet their needs. The rather poor teaching of geriatric medicine in medical schools has, as a consequence, the under-diagnosis of problems of elderly patients, making the 'iceberg phenomenon' a common condition at the same or at a higher level than it was 50 years ago in the United Kingdom.[15]

It took a long time for health systems to set up assistance to acute problems. Although in many countries this assistance is criticized, a new challenge is on the table: to increase the capacity of health systems in transforming systems from acute to chronic care. In many countries the unsatisfactory response of the public sector has led to the increasing privatization of healthcare. In this context, it must be underlined that elderly individuals when sick, have higher expenses in the face of lower incomes and that the transition from public to private responsibilities carries some risks – the 'cream skimming' of private sectors selecting those younger and wealthier, and thus selective exclusion of women, the less well-off, and the elderly who tend to remain under the public sector's responsibility.[16]

As formal care for geriatric patients has to be improved or even built from scratch, more is expected from informal care, especially that provided by families. However, families in the developing world are far from the romantic model of supposed grandparents being respected for their contribution to society and for their wisdom, who live surrounded by happy grandchildren begging for another story.[17] India is a country with a hoary past, with traditions of family care of the elderly, but this traditional care is in jeopardy of disruptive influences from modernization, migration and dual careers, thus posing a direct challenge to the policy-makers.[1] Most family care in developing countries involves women; so the inclusion of female in the labour sector is another reason for the reduction of traditional care in developing countries.

Population ageing does not always mean reaching 65 years of age. In developing countries a significant proportion of the elderly population is represented by people of 75 years and over. There are more than 10 million people aged 75 years or over in Africa, and almost twice this number in Latin America and the Caribbean. In this age group it is imperative to plan long-term care. The percentage of elderly people living in institutions is as low as 0.1% in Iran, 0.6% in Botswana, nearly 1% in Brazil and Mexico compared to 7.5% in Switzerland. Ironically this lack of infrastructure opens the way to create alternative, community-based long-term care systems.[16] Data indicate there will be a rising need of long-term care even in developing countries in the future. Higher relative percentages of oldest olds with more *activities of daily living* (ADL) impairments, rising costs and fewer sources of informal care will stretch countries' resources to the limits. Economic privatization efforts will only push more of the costs back onto the families, where the greatest burden of care already lies, especially among those caring for the elderly with diseases such as Alzheimer's.[18]

Specific increases in costs and health needs for the population, and the subsequent pressure that will be placed on formal and informal healthcare systems will depend on factors such as incidence and prevalence, rates of health disorders and how these change concurrently with an ageing population.[12] In developing countries the project pressure will be high since the compression of mortality into old age does not necessarily mean that compression of morbidity will also be achieved.

Key points

- There are more than 10 million people aged 75 years or over in Africa, and almost twice this number in Latin America and the Caribbean.
- One of the key challenges confronting developing countries with an increasingly ageing population

is to guarantee to the whole older population an adequate level of income, without placing excessive demands on younger generations and national economies.

- Most developing countries are not sufficiently equipped to meet the needs of the older population, mainly the leading causes of years lost due to disability (YLD): eye disease, hearing loss, dementia, musculoskeletal disease and heart disease.

References

1. Ramamurti PV. Ageing in developing countries. *Ageing International* 2000;**25**:13–15.
2. United Nations (UN). World Population Ageing. UN Department of Economic and Social Affairs, Population Division, New York, 2007.
3. Bongaarts J. Human population growth and the demographic transition. *Phil Trans R Soc* 2009;**364**:2985–90.
4. Sigg R. A Global Overview on Social Security in the Age of Longevity. UN Expert Group Meeting on Social and Economic Implications of Changing Population Age Structures, United Nations, New York, 2005.
5. Stuckler D. Population causes and consequences of leading chronic diseases: A comparative analysis of prevailing explanations. *The Milbank Quarterly* 2008;**86**:273–326.
6. Barker JP. *Mothers, Babies and Health in Later Life*, 2nd edn, Churchill Livingstone, Edinburgh, 1998.
7. Okumyia K, Wada T, Ishine M. Close association between geriatric functional ability and economic status in developing and developed countries. *J Am Geriatr Soc* 2005;**53**:1448–9.
8. Tucker K, Buranapin S. Nutrition and aging in developing countries. *J Nutr* 2001;**131**:2417S–2423S.
9. Murray CJL, Lopez AD (eds). *The Global Burden of Disease. A comprehensive assessment of mortality and disability from diseases, injuries and risk factors in 1990 and projected to 2020*, Harvard University Press, Cambridge, MA, 1996.
10. Souza RM, Ferri CP, Acosta D *et al*. Contribution of chronic diseases to disability in elderly people in countries with low and middle incomes: a 10/66 Dementia Research Group population-based survey. *Lancet* 2009;**28**:1821–30.
11. Jagger C, Matthews R, Melzer D *et al*. Educational differences in the dynamics of disability incidence, recovery and mortality: Findings from the MRC Cognitive Function and Ageing Study (MRC CFAS). *Int J Epidemiol* 2007;**36**:365–7.
12. Zimmer Z, Martin LG. Key topics in the study of older adults' health in developing countries that are experiencing population ageing. *J Cross Cult Gerontol* 2007;**22**:235–41.
13. Pen D, Hui Y. China. In: EB Palmore, F Whittington, S Kunkel (eds), *The International Handbook on Aging*, ABC-CLIO, Santa Barbara, 2009.
14. Ramamurti PV, Jamuna D. India. In: EB Palmore, F Whittington, S Kunkel (eds), *The International Handbook on Aging*, ABC-CLIO, Santa Barbara, 2009.
15. Williamson J, Stokoe IH, Gray S *et al*. Old people at home, their unreported needs. *Lancet* 1964;**1**:1117–23.
16. Gutiérrez- Robledo LM. Looking at the future of geriatric care in developing countries. *Journal of Gerontology: Medical Sciences* 2002;**57A**: M162–M167.
17. Van Dullemen C. Older people in Africa: New engines to society. *NWSA Journal* 2006;**18**:99–105.
18. Arnsberger P, Fox P, Zhang X, Gui S. Population aging and the need for long-term care: A comparison of the United States and the People's Republic of China. *J Cross Cult Gerontol* 2002;**15**:2007–227.

CHAPTER 148

Geriatric medicine in the European Union: towards unification of diversity

Alfonso J. Cruz-Jentoft
Hospital Universitario Ramón y Cajal, Madrid, Spain

Introduction

Europe has a landmass of 9 938 000 km^2, 6.7% of the total land area on earth. Unlike the United States of America, Europe is not a federation of states with a unifying governmental structure, but a continent that groups 49 very diverse countries, with long and diverse history, languages, climates, customs, traditions, cultures, populations and governments. However, in the last century the European Union (EU) has provided a certain amount of integration between the member states in terms of laws, trade and governmental policies. At present, the EU has expanded to 27 member states, and a number of other countries have applied to become members. In 2010, the EU had 499 million inhabitants – the world's third largest population after China and India – and includes many of the countries with the world's highest proportions of older people.

The EU developed after World War II, with the aim of ending the frequent and bloody wars between neighbours, and has been growing in number of countries and depth of understanding ever since. EU citizens have freedom of movement of goods, services, people and money within their countries. Passports are not needed to move within most countries, and many share now a common currency, the Euro. The EU brings many unifying initiatives, but countries have the right not to join many multilateral EU initiatives, which helps to explain the present heterogeneity of the Union. Active debate is ongoing on the need for a European constitution.

The EU is not a traditional federation of countries, neither is it a common organization for cooperation between governments, like the United Nations. Member states of the EU remain independent nations but they delegate some of their decision-making powers to shared institutions, so that decisions on specific matters of joint interest can be made democratically at European level. The EU has a complex structure, where three main institutions participate in decision-making. The *Council of the European Union*, which represents the individual member states, is the main decision-making body, where ministers from each member state can commit their government to various EU policies. The *European Parliament* represents the EU's citizens, its members being elected directly by voters in each state. The *European Commission*, based in Brussels, Belgium, is the civil service of Europe, and is independent of national governments. Its job is to represent and uphold the interests of the EU as a whole. It is split into various directorates which each have an appointed political head combined with an overall Commission President. The Commission has responsibility for proposing European legislation (the Parliament and Council decide on adoption of new laws), implementing agreed policy (together with national governments), enforcing EU law and representing the EU at international level.

Healthcare is not included in the list of common policy areas, only public health is, and this has a critical impact on the provision of healthcare and the organization of healthcare systems around Europe. Each EU country is free to decide on the health policies best suited to national circumstances and traditions, although they all share common values. These include the right of every citizen to the same high standards of health and equity in access to quality healthcare. The EU is also committed to taking into account the implications of health in all its policies and decisions.

Demography

The EU compiles statistics from member states through its agency Eurostat (epp.eurostat.ec.europa.eu), including a great wealth of population- and health-related parameters. However, Eurostat does not collect data directly, but rather collates and tries to harmonize data obtained from national agencies, so problems may arise with the uniformity of their

Principles and Practice of Geriatric Medicine, Fifth Edition. Edited by Alan J. Sinclair, John E. Morley and Bruno Vellas.

collection, not only in terms of completeness but also their comparability and quality. Most relevant statistical data are open access and regularly updated.

Bearing in mind the above, it appears that Europe's population has been ageing steadily for a long time. The total EU population is projected to rise by 5% between 2008 and 2030, and the median age is likely to increase in all but seven out of the 281 European regions, due to the combined effect of three factors: the existing population structure, fertility lower than replacement levels, and steadily rising numbers of people living longer.[1] The proportion of the total population aged 65 or over is projected to increase considerably in the near future, from 17.1% in 2008 (87 million) to 23.5% (123 million) in 2030. The number of very old, aged >80 years, is already 22 million (4.4% of the population), and in 11 of the former EU-15 member states, at least 10% of their population will be aged 80 or over by 2050. Gender differences in ageing are considerable, as life expectancy for women is currently more than six years longer than for men.

These global figures may disguise major variations across the EU countries, both in population growth and in ageing rates. Life expectancy at birth varied in males in 2007 from 64.9 years in Lithuania to 78.9 years in Sweden, and in females from 76.1 years in Romania to 84.4 years in France. The share of the population aged 65 years or over in the 27 EU countries ranged in 2008 between 10.9% in Ireland and 20.1% in Germany (Figure 148.1). Regional variation is even higher, ranging between 9.1% (in Inner London, UK) and 26.8% (in Liguria, Italy). Contrary to expectations, these differences are not diminishing, but are expected to increase in the near future, ranging in 2030 between 10.4% (again in Inner London, UK) and 37.3% (in Chemniz, Germany). The proportion of citizens >80 years in 2008 ranged between 2.7% in Ireland and 5.5% in Italy.

In parallel with these changes, the working population over the same time frame is projected to decrease significantly. The old age dependency ratio, defined as the projected number of persons aged 65 and over expressed as a percentage of the projected number of persons aged between 15 and 64, is projected to increase from 25.9 in 2010 to 38.0 in 2030. This has been called a 'demographic time bomb' and has considerable implications for health and social care planning across the EU.

Major differences between EU member states also exist in active life expectancy (life expectancy with no disability). As

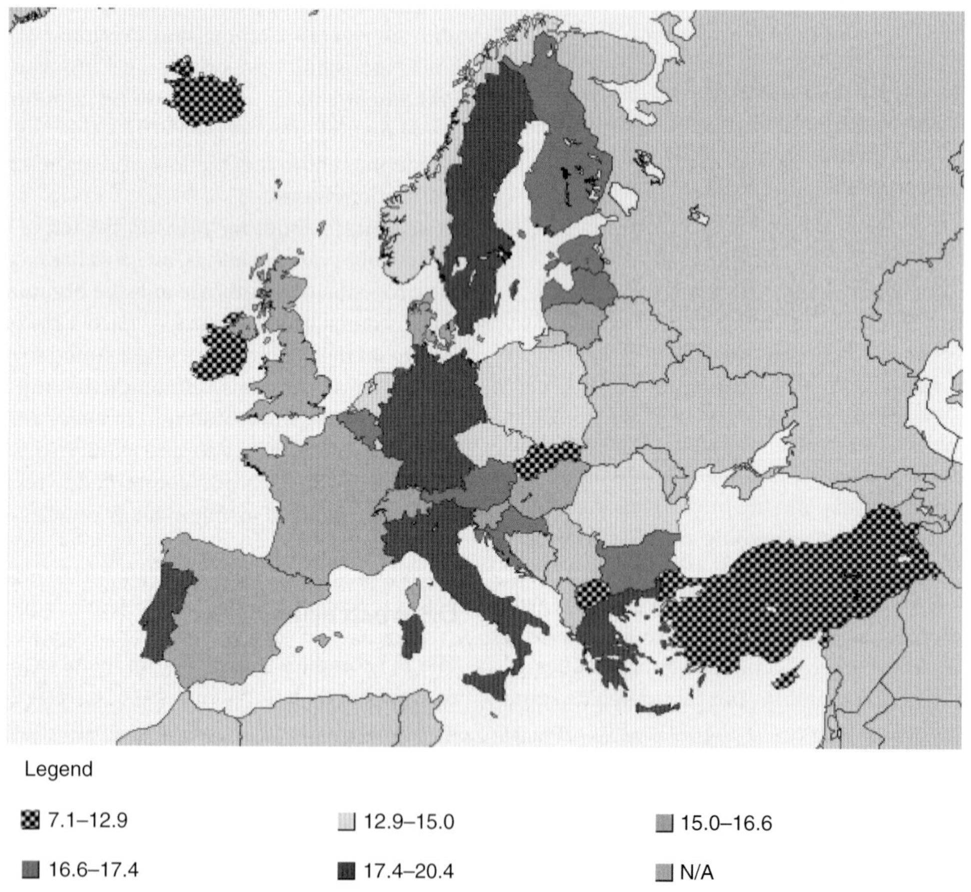

Figure 148.1 Proportion of population aged 65 and over (% of total population). See plate section for a colour version of this image.

a whole, in 2007 men in the EU were expected to live 80.9% of their life without disability, but this ranges from 89.3% in Norway to 71.9% in Germany. Women in the EU could expect to live 75.8% of their lives free of disability, ranging from 87.3% in Malta to 66.2% in Slovakia. Since 2003, the measurement of *Healthy Life Years* is considered a structural indicator on health in the EU, which is a very relevant step forward for geriatric prevention and care planning.

Healthcare and health systems

Medicine has developed in Europe for more than 25 centuries: Hippocrates of Kos (Greece) is considered to be the father of modern medicine, and over the centuries many milestone advances have been made in European countries. There is a centuries-old tradition of medical care, and all the EU member states have systems in place that offer complete, or near complete, rights to healthcare for people residing within their borders. High-quality health services are considered a priority issue for European citizens, and rights to healthcare are recognized in the Charter of Fundamental Rights of the EU. Most countries jealously guard management of their own healthcare systems, so it is no surprise that, with the exception of public health, states retain competence for health policies and health systems, and do not delegate these under EU instances. However, and very recently, health systems policies across the EU countries seem to be more interconnected, due to public expectations, movement of patients and health professionals across countries, and information and medical technology. The EU holds responsibility to complement the work of member states (i.e. in patient mobility or international health threats) and to reduce health inequalities, fostering cooperation between countries.

Healthcare systems in the EU are financed in two broad ways, either through general taxation, or using systems based on social health insurance, although in highly variable proportions. Taxation predominates in some countries (e.g. Denmark, Italy, Spain, Sweden and the United Kingdom), while social health insurance contributions are the predominant source in others (e.g. the Czech Republic, France, Germany and the Netherlands).[2] Both systems usually limit their liability to pay the full cost of treatments, such that expenditure borne by households amounts to 20–30% in the majority of member states. The difference is made up either through direct contributions or via supplementary private insurance. It is, however, clear that public-sector funding makes up a significant proportion of health expenditure in all the EU member states: this proportion being lowest in Greece (56%) and rising to a high 95% in the Netherlands.

Although in most states universal access to healthcare is granted, including for older, impoverished or immigrant populations, the reliance on a degree of financial participation may adversely affect some groups' access to healthcare as they are unable to afford the costs. This is particularly true of older people who may have both lowered incomes and considerable comorbidity. Thus some member states have enacted methods to target older people either by reducing their financial liability or ensuring that they are regularly screened by relevant health professionals. However, the universal access approach is putting a great deal of financial pressure on the sustainability of the whole care system.

The impact of ageing on health and long-term care systems is considered to be one of the most significant challenges for the economies and welfare systems of European countries. According to OECD Health Data 2010, total health expenditure in EU countries in 2008 ranged from 6.1% of gross domestic product in Estonia to 11.2% in France. This contrasts with 16% in the same period in the United States. As most experts predict that increases in healthcare expenditures will continue over the next 50 years, finance is a major issue for most countries. Thus, the economic and financial affairs directorate is carefully examining this currently, estimating and modelling the size and timing of projected changes in expenditure and their underlying driving factors, in order to assess sustainability. Many publications have appeared recently feeding a public policy debate which may force changes in the near future.[3]

Health and ageing trends

Life expectancy has been steadily growing in the EU over the last century, and this trend has not stopped in recent years (Table 148.1). A European citizen aged 65 years may expect to live more than 19 years into 'old age'. This could theoretically mean that diseases and disabilities of old age are steadily increasing, although this is actually challenged.[4] Changes in lifestyles, risk factor management, public health and healthcare have pushed for a slow but steady reduction in some of the main causes of mortality in old people, such as diseases of the circulatory system (a 27.4% reduction in the last 10 years), stroke (32.2% reduction) or cancer (7.8% reduction). However, mental health disorders (particularly dementing diseases and depression) seem to be increasing rapidly during the same time period (an increase of 26.7%), not only in mortality but especially in morbidity.

An enormous variability is also found in the health needs of individual countries within the EU, and differences have increased with the new countries that have recently joined. For instance, the standardized death rate by 100 000 inhabitants for ischaemic heart disease in 2008 ranges from only 33.8 in France to 321.3 in Lithuania, and crude death rates by 100 000 inhabitants from suicide in those aged 85 and over range from 1.9 in Ireland to 64.8 in Hungary in the same year. Thus, health planning in each country

Table 148.1 Health trends in European Union member states in the last 10 years.

	1998	2008	Percent change
Basic demographic indicators			
Population, millions	479.8	496.4	3.5
% of population aged 65+ years	15.33	16.93	10.4
Mortality indicators			
Life expectancy at birth, years	76.84	79.43	3.4
Life expectancy at age 65, in years	17.32	19.06	10.0
Disability-adjusted life expectancy, in years	70.35[a]	71.7[b]	1.9
SDR, diseases of circulatory system, 65+ per 100 000	2437.99	1771.04	−27.4
SDR, ischaemic heart disease, 65+ per 100 000	896.26	638.22	−28.8
SDR, cerebrovascular diseases, 65+ per 100 000	646.54	438.06	−32.2
SDR, suicide and self-inflicted injury, 65+ per 100 000	21.1	17.45	−17.3
SDR, malignant neoplasms, age 65+ per 100 000	1055.71	973.55	−7.8
SDR, mental disorders and diseases of the nervous system and senses	153.31	194.53	26.9
Healthcare resources			
Hospitals per 100 000	2.87	2.62	−8.7
Hospital beds per 100 000	647.61	530.53	−18.1
Acute care hospital beds per 100 000	462.21	378.18	−18.2
Physicians per 100 000	284.91	323.71	13.6
General practitioners per 100 000	82.50	85.59	3.7
Nurses per 100 000	687.96	775.24	12.7
Healthcare utilization and costs			
Average length of stay, all hospitals	10.14	8.72	−14.0
Average length of stay, acute care hospitals only	7.51	6.74[b]	−10.3
Outpatient contacts per person per year	6.69	6.86[b]	2.5
Total health expenditure, % of gross domestic product	7.94	9.01	13.5
Total health expenditure, $ per capita	1661.12	2877.54	73.2

[a]1999
[b]2007
SDR: standardized death rate
Source: European Health for All Database, WHO Regional Office for Europe, Copenhagen, Denmark.

needs to take account of these differences, providing health promotion and care systems that are more prone to have an impact on relevant health outcomes in each country.

One of the main problems researchers in geriatric care are faced with when studying illness in older people in the EU is the lack of good morbidity data of geriatric interest. Health statistics are available for communicable diseases, for some chronic diseases, for health habits and lifestyles, and for disease related mortality. However, there are no reliable data regarding geriatric diseases and syndromes (delirium, hip fracture, urinary incontinence), nor in disease related physical and mental disability. Data are fragmented, come from different years and sources, are gathered with different criteria and are not systematically collected. Good age-specific data for older subjects are especially sparse. Research and progress in this area is urgently needed, and several research initiatives funded by the EU are trying to fill this gap.

For instance, research in health and social implications of ageing has been fostered through the *Survey of Health, Ageing and Retirement in Europe* (SHARE, www.share-project.org), a multidisciplinary cross-national database on health, socioeconomic status and social and family networks of individuals over the age of 50. Data collected include health variables (including physical functioning, cognitive functioning, health behaviour and use of healthcare facilities), psychological, economic and social support variables.

Changes in the characteristics of disease in older people are transforming the paradigm of healthcare. Healthcare was developed a long time ago for the care of single, acute diseases, usually unexpected, with cure and self-sufficiency as the usual outcomes. However, older patients usually have multiple, chronic morbidities (sometimes with acute exacerbations), where disease course can be expected, with dependency as a very frequent outcome. Unfortunately, healthcare systems in Europe, very efficient for acute care, have evolved only slowly and in a very irregular and heterogeneous mode, even within different regions of the same country, to be able to manage chronic diseases in dependent people. This lack of efficiency may explain why per capita health expenditure increases sharply after the age of 65 and even more sharply after the age of 80. Responses to tackle this change of paradigm are still naïve in the EU. Recent moves to promote a comprehensive approach in tackling chronic diseases, including cardiovascular disease, cancer, mental health problems, diabetes mellitus, chronic respiratory disease and musculoskeletal conditions, are still organ-based rather than individual-centred.

Over the last three decades, the number of hospitals and hospital beds has been diminishing, including those used for acute care, while the number of general practitioners, nurses and primary care units has not grown at the same rate. Intermediate and long-term hospital beds have suffered a slower reduction, and rehabilitation and palliative care services for older people are scarce and irregularly distributed, not only between countries, but within different areas of the same country.

In common with other developed countries the member states see the need to recruit staff appropriately trained in the needs of older people and also to create post-acute rehabilitation facilities and other healthcare settings to assist a multidisciplinary approach to treatment with the goal of re-ablement and settlement in the community.[5] Unfortunately, too often these rehabilitation units are adrift from main acute centres in the mistaken belief that rehabilitation can wait till the conclusion of an acute episode of care.

Long-term care has been seen for a long time as mainly a social risk. Recently, it has been acknowledged that long-term care is inadequate in many EU countries and suffers from labour shortages and low quality. Long-term care depends on national governments, so the EU has started a new programme that promotes the coordination of national long-term care policies with a particular focus on universal and equal access to different long-term care services, quality and sustainability, as spending on long-term care is expected to grow fast in view of population ageing.[6] Long-term care services are now judged to be crucial to the welfare of older people, and the importance of these services in terms of numbers of clients and expenditures is expected to grow. Steps to ensure the long-term sustainability of public financing are now being discussed.

Public health, depending on the EU institutions, seems to be focusing more on other ages and groups, not on older citizens. Only a couple of initiatives, including a growing emphasis on nutrition and age, and the promotion of healthy ageing by the development of an integrated holistic approach to health in later life, seem to be gaining momentum in recent years. The debate on the redefinition of the age of retirement, forced by the economic crisis, has provoked an unprecedented public debate on some age-related issues.

Geriatric medicine

Geriatric medical care, as may be expected is also extremely diverse within the EU.[7,8] Geriatric Medicine is recognized in many European countries, either as a lone standing speciality or as a subspecialty of Internal Medicine.[9] It is an official specialty accepted by the EU, but it is not yet available in every country: only 18 of the 27 countries had, in 2006, established the mechanism for mutual recognition of the speciality (Table 148.2), which requires a minimum length of training of four years. However, this list may not present a fair picture of Geriatric Medicine in Europe. In some countries (Belgium, Germany) this discipline has a wide distribution, with academic hospital departments and specific geriatric training programmes, even when mutual recognition has not been achieved. In other countries, even when formally present, Geriatric Medicine is very poorly developed. European geriatricians are working hard to promote recognition of the specialty and development of geriatric medicine departments in every EU country. This comes not without its problems.[9]

It might be expected that a medical speciality department would be somehow similar around Europe, so similar up-to-date procedures will be applied to any patient admitted to a medical department of a hospital, i.e. Cardiology or Gastroenterology. However, this is not completely true for Geriatric Medicine,[10] although very little systematic data exist. Excellent geriatric departments exist in most EU countries, but citizens living in different places will have different access rights to these departments, and a significant proportion of older people in the EU will not have access to geriatric medicine. This is not due to lack of evidence, as very solid evidence exists about the benefits of most levels of geriatric care, but to discrimination against old people by political decision-makers.[5] Primary care is almost universally available for the older population in the EU, but many general practitioners are not prepared to manage this special population due to a lack of academic leaders and continuing professional development in geriatric medicine.

Education in geriatric medicine in Europe is also extremely variable, both at undergraduate and postgraduate level, although it seems to be improving. In a recent survey, only six European countries had an established Chair of Geriatric Medicine in each of their medical schools.[11] Undergraduate teaching activities were not present in many countries and had a highly variable number of hours, and all levels of geriatric teaching were

Table 148.2 Mutual recognition of Geriatric Medicine in the European Union.

Country	Name of discipline
Belgique/België/ Belgien	
България	Гериатрична медицина
česká republika	Geriatrie
Danmark	Geriatri eller alderdommens sygdomme
Deutschland	
Eesti	
Ελλάς	
España	Geriatría
France	
Ireland	Geriatric medicine
Italia	Geriatria
Κύπρος	Πηριατρική
Latvija	
Lietuva	Geriatrija
Luxembourg	Gériatrie
Magyarország	Geriátria
Malta	Gerjatrija
Nederland	Klinische geriatrie
Österreich	
Polska	Geriatria
Portugal	
România	Geriatrie şi gerontologie
Slovenija	
Slovensko	Geriatria
Suomi/Finland	Geriatria/geriatri
Sverige	Geriatrik
United Kingdom	Geriatrics

Source: Council Directive 2006/100/EC of 20 November 2006 adapting certain Directives in the field of freedom of movement of persons, by reason of the accession of Bulgaria and Romania. *Official Journal of the European Union*, 20.12.2006.

heterogeneously organized from country to country and within each country.

Traditionally, family members have accepted a high degree of responsibility in the care of older people in most of Europe, especially the Mediterranean countries. This is changing, with the growing numbers of older people and a reduced ability of weaker family networks to care for them, when they depend on others. This is helping to increase the need for long-term care in different settings (home care, long-stay units or nursing homes). Such care has not been regularly covered by health systems, and it is not a universal right within the EU, in contradistinction to acute healthcare. In many cases it depends on private systems, although some countries are now trying to regulate by law the care of dependent citizens. Nursing home use and availability is also diverse across the EU: rates are close to 10% of people 65 or older in some northern countries (Sweden, Holland) and lower than 3% in some Mediterranean countries (Spain, Portugal), with a gradient from north to south that is not only explained by economic reasons, but depends more on people preferences and family networks.

A last area of concern in geriatric care is the lack of solid research in medicines used by older people. The European Medicines Agency recently acknowledged this was a problem, especially in the very old and frail, and is now actively discussing, under the lead of several scientific organizations, changes that need to be made in the approval process of medicines for older persons.[12]

Geriatric organizations

Europe has a very long tradition of national geriatric societies: for instance, the British Geriatrics Society (BGS) was founded in 1947, the Spanish Geriatric and Gerontology Society (SEGG) in 1948, and the Italian Geriatric and Gerontology Society (SIGG) in 1950. The first World Congress of Gerontology took place in Liège (Belgium) in July 1950, and the *International Association of Gerontology and Geriatrics* (IAGG) was founded at that congress, under the lead of Professor Lucien Brull. The European Region section of the IAGG (www.iagg-er.org) is an umbrella organization of national societies, with a multidisciplinary approach and an aim to foster research, education and cooperation in all branches of Gerontology.[13]

The need to improve specific aspects of geriatric medicine led in 2001 to the creation of the European Union Geriatric Medicine Society (EUGMS, www.eugms.org), a blossoming medical society that is now very active in fostering the development of geriatric medicine in all the member states of the EU, trying to achieve availability of these services to all citizens of the EU, promoting education with very successful annual scientific meetings, and developing documents and guidelines.[14]

The official instance for representations of geriatricians before the European authorities is the Geriatric Section of the European Union of Medical Specialists (UEMS, www.uemsgeriatricmedicine.org). This organization has been able to provide a consensus definition of Geriatric Medicine, documents on accreditation for specialist training and undergraduate training, and is part of the European Accreditation Council for Continuing Medical Education.

The need to raise the level of academic geriatric medicine and to promote leadership both in teaching and research led in 1995 to the creation of the European Academy for Medicine of Ageing (EAMA, www.eama.eu), an organization that is being extremely successful in fostering leading geriatricians.[15] The model of this institution has been exported to Asia and South America.

Recent developments in EU policy

Public health policy and the promotion of a high level of human health is a relevant part of the EU Treaty. Recent developments in the care of older people have been fostered by the European social policy agenda. In March 2000, the European Council in Lisbon set out a ten-year strategy (the Lisbon Strategy), a commitment to bring about economic, social and environmental renewal in the EU to make the EU the world's most dynamic and competitive economy. Under this strategy, social policies that ensure sustainable development and social inclusion were to be fostered, together with improved coordination of teaching and research looking for a knowledge-based society. These policies were based, in many cases, on an improved cooperation between member states, respecting the principle of subsidiarity. However, a mid-term look at the Lisbon strategy found that the outcomes were disappointing.[16]

Healthcare of older people was not seriously considered at the European level until 2001, when the Goteborg Council asked for an initial report on orientations in the field of healthcare and care for the elderly, in conformity with the open method of coordination (a method used to improve coordination in some policy areas, allowing member states to challenge common problems, defining their own national strategies and benefiting from experiences of other member states). This request resulted in a report that carefully analysed the impact of demographic ageing on healthcare systems; expenditure; the growth of new technologies and treatments; an improved wellbeing and a better standard of living; the diversity of national systems and the contribution of the EU. Access to healthcare is considered a fundamental right and an essential element of human dignity that must therefore be guaranteed for all EU citizens, regardless of income or wealth. The need for special protection is recognized for dependency and old age, and the need to improve quality to reduce diversity and variation is also underlined. Financial viability is needed to sustain health and social systems of care in the future. This request finished with a resolution of the European Parliament on the future of health and social care of older people, calling for improvements in accessibility, quality and financial viability.

Later, in 2004, the European Commission issued a new report that sought to outline a common framework to support member states in the reform and development of healthcare and long-term care using the open method of coordination. This report proposed common objectives for healthcare provision that would add to similar ongoing coordinating processes in three social policy areas: pensions, social inclusion and employment. The most relevant aspects of this document related to Geriatric Medicine are outlined in Table 148.3.

These steps by the European Commission are a promising move for geriatric care. Nevertheless, it must be remembered that the Commission can only suggest action lines, which have to be agreed and implemented by member states, and this seems not to be happening at the expected

Table 148.3 Recent European Union action lines related to geriatric medicine.*

- Health systems have a role in combating the risk of poverty and disease, contributing to social cohesion and fighting the consequences of demographic ageing.
- The principles of accessibility of care for all (taking into account the needs and difficulties of the most disadvantaged groups and individuals), high-quality care for the population (which keeps up with the emerging needs associated with ageing) long-term financial sustainability of this care have to be met.
- The provision and funding of health and long-term care are key elements of the economic and social modernization strategy of the EU.
- To meet the challenges posed by demographic trends and technological progress, it is vital to have a sufficient number of trained professionals and to give them quality jobs.
- Demographic ageing will mean more age-related illnesses and more people in long-term care; and a growing number of old people living alone. The response to the needs of this population group will include developing a wide range of services, including care at home, and specialized institutions, as well as closer coordination between care providers.
- The social protection systems need to be reformed in an integrated and coordinated way to meet these challenges. Health and elderly care is one of the areas where coordination in the field of social protection should be streamlined.
- Access to high-quality care based on the principles of universal access, fairness and solidarity must be ensured, providing a safety net against poverty or social exclusion associated with ill health, accident, disability or old age, for both the beneficiaries of care and their families. Particular attention will have to be paid to persons requiring long-term or expensive care, to those with particular difficulties accessing care and those on low incomes. Financial and physical accessibility of care systems for disabled persons has to be ensured, and specific care for elderly people offered, based in particular on closer coordination between the social services, primary carers, hospital services and specialized institutions.
- The system should be properly funded, in order to meet the new challenges posed by ageing, changes in society and technological progress. Responsibility for the organization and funding of the healthcare and elderly care sector rests primarily with the member states.

*Extracted from *Modernising social protection for the development of high-quality, accessible and sustainable health care and long-term care: support for the national strategies using the 'open method of coordination'*. EU COM 304 final, April 2004.

rates. European and national organizations of geriatric medicine specialists have a long way to go to ensure that their older patients have the best multidisciplinary care in the most optimal setting.[5]

European countries are facing a rising demand for health and social services as a result of an ageing population and higher income levels, although the funding available remains limited. At the same time, citizens have higher expectations and the mobility of patients and of health professionals has increased. One of the ways the EU is using to tackle this situation is the development of e-Health systems and services, trying to reduce costs, improve productivity, reducing medical error, cutting down on unnecessary care, and improving the quality of healthcare. These measures may have an impact on geriatric care.[17] Today at least four out of five European doctors have an Internet connection, and a quarter of Europeans use the Internet to get information about diseases and health matters. These encouraging figures indicate that e-Health systems and services will develop rapidly. Estimates suggest that by 2010 up to 5% of health budgets are being invested in e-Health systems and services.

Finally, an important issue that is now actively being pursued is the reform of universities. Despite reasonably good teaching quality, European universities are not using their full potential, and investment in higher education is insufficient. Europe must strengthen education, research and innovation, and universities are essential in these three aspects, so there is a need to invest more, modernize and improve the quality of universities as a direct investment in the future of Europeans.[18] Here, Geriatric Medicine can find its way into teaching geriatric principles to all health professionals, not only to physicians.

Key points

- European countries are facing a rising demand for health and social services as a result of an ageing population and higher income levels, although the funding available remains limited.
- The European Commission is trying, through the open method of coordination, and with the support of many European institutions, to improve access to healthcare, quality of care, and financial sustainability of health and social care systems.
- One of the main problems facing researchers in geriatric care when studying illness in older people in the EU is the lack of good morbidity data of geriatric interest.
- Education in geriatric medicine in Europe is extremely variable, both at the undergraduate and postgraduate level, although it seems to be improving.

Acknowledgements

Professor Paul Knight (Glasgow, UK) contributed in a similar chapter written for the previous edition of this book.

References

1. Giannakouris K. (2010) *Regional population projections EUROPOP2008: Most EU regions face older population profile in 2030*. Catalogue number: KS-SF-10-001-EN-N. European Union.
2. Elias Mossialos E, Dixon A. Funding health care: an introduction. In: E Mossialos, A Dixon, J Figueras, J Kutzin (eds), *Funding Health Care: Options for Europe*, Open University Press, Buckingham, 2002, pp. 1–30.
3. Ageing Report: Economic and budgetary projections for the EU-27 Member States (2008–2060). European Economy 2/2009. Office for Official Publications of the European Communities, Luxembourg, 2009.
4. Christensen K, Doblhammer G, Rau R, Vaupel JW. Ageing populations: the challenges ahead. *Lancet* 2009;**374**:1196–208.
5. Cruz-Jentoft AJ, Franco A, Sommer P *et al*. Silver paper: the future of health promotion and preventive actions, basic research, and clinical aspects of age-related disease – a report of the European Summit on Age-Related Disease. *Aging Clin Exp Res* 2009;**21**:376–85.
6. European Commission. *Long-term Care in the European Union*. Office for Official Publications of the European Communities, Luxembourg, 2008.
7. Hastie IR, Duursma SA; Geriatric Medicine Section of the European Union of Medical Specialists. Geriatric medicine in the European Union: unification of diversity. *Aging Clin Exp Res* 2003;**15**:347–51.
8. Duursma S, Castleden M, Cherubini A *et al*. European Union Geriatric Medicine Society. Position statement on geriatric medicine and the provision of health care services to older people. *J Nutr Health Aging* 2004;**8**:190–5.
9. Meinck M, Lübke N, Plate A. Auf- oder Abbau geriatrischer Versorgungsstrukturen in Deutschland? Kritische Analyse zur Aussagekraft der amtlichen Statistik und anderweitiger Erhebungen [Expansion or reduction of geriatric care structures in Germany? A critical analysis on the significance of the official statistics and other surveys]. *Z Gerontol Geriatr* 2006;**39**:443–50.
10. Michel JP, Rubenstein LZ, Vellas BJ, Albarede JL. *Geriatric Programs and Departments around the World*, Serdi, Paris, 1998.
11. Michel JP, Huber P, Cruz-Jentoft AJ. Europe-wide survey of teaching in geriatric medicine. *J Am Geriatr Soc* 2008;**56**: 1536–42.
12. Cherubini A, Del Signore S, Ouslander J *et al*. Fighting against age discrimination in clinical trials. *J Am Geriatr Soc* 2010;**58**:1791–6.
13. Baeyens JP. Development and organization of gerontology and geriatrics in Europe. *Eur Geriatr Med* 2010;**1**: 141.
14. Baeyens JP, Cruz Jentoft AJ, Cherubini A. The success story of the European Union Geriatric Medicine Society (EUGMS). *Eur Geriatr Med* 2010;**1**:137–40.
15. Swine C, Michel JP, Duursma S *et al*. Evaluation of the European Academy for Medicine of Ageing 'Teaching the

Teachers' programme (EAMA course II 1997–1998). *J Nutr Health Aging* 2004;**8**:181–6.

16. Barroso J. Communication to the Spring European Council. Working together for growth and jobs: A new start for the Lisbon Strategy. COM (2005) 24 final. Available in most European languages at http://eur-lex.europa.eu (last accessed December 2011).

17. e-Health – making healthcare better for European citizens: an action plan for a European e-Health Area. COM (2004) 0356 final. Available as above.

18. Mobilising the brainpower of Europe: enabling universities to make their full contribution to the Lisbon Strategy. COM (2005) 152 final. Available as above.

APPENDIX

Function assessment scales

John E. Morley
Saint Louis University School of Medicine and St Louis Veterans' Affairs Medical Center, St Louis, MO, USA

Components of the geriatric assessment

Dimension	Screening test	Assessment tests
Advanced directives	Do you have an advanced directive or living will?	Detailed discussion Document desires in chart Discuss ventilation separately from cardiac resuscitation Discuss feeding tube Discuss long-term beliefs if the person becomes cognitively impaired Assess the person's ability to make appropriate decisions
Affective	Are you sad?	Geriatric Depression Scale
Alcohol abuse	Do you drink alcohol?	CAGE Michigan Alcohol Screening Test – 9
Blood pressure	In older persons all blood pressures need to be measured at a minimum of sitting and standing	Check for postural hypotension at one and 3 minutes after standing If the person falls, is dizzy, syncopal or has a stroke or myocardial infarction within 2 hours of a meal, check for postprandial hypotension Both orthostatis and postprandial hypotension are more common in the morning Because of arteriosclerotic occlusion of vessels older persons often have a higher blood pressure in one arm than the other. Always treat the higher blood pressure Arteriosclerosis can lead to pseudohypotension. This can be screened for by the Osler Manoeuvre but as it has poor sensitivity and specifically intra-arterial blood pressure may need to be obtained 'White-coat' hypertension is common so always obtain home blood pressures A wide pulse pressure has a poor prognosis in older persons
Caregiver burden	Is the caregiver having problems coping?	Geriatric Depression Scale Caregiver Burden Inventory, looks at time, developmental needs, social burden and emotional burden
Dehydration	How much fluid do you drink each day?	Check serum osmolality Remember elevated BUN to creatinine ratio occurs with renal failure, liver disease, heart failure and gastrointestinal bleeding

(*continued overleaf*)

Principles and Practice of Geriatric Medicine, Fifth Edition. Edited by Alan J. Sinclair, John E. Morley and Bruno Vellas.

Dimension	Screening test	Assessment tests
Delirium	Is the person confused? Does the level of confusion fluctuate?	Confusion Assessment methodology (acute onset, fluctuates, lack of attention, disorganized thinking including illusions, delusions and hallucinations; hyperalert or lethargic)
Dental	Do you have false teeth? Do you have sores in your mouth or gum disease? Do you often have bad breath?	DENTAL screening tool
Dizziness	Do you get dizzy or does your head spin around?	Check for postural hypotension Hallpike Manoeuvre for Benign Paroxysmal Positional Vertigo (BPPV) Haemoglobin Geriatric Depression Scale
Driving assessment	Do you drive? How do you meet your transportation needs?	If poor vision, cognition or motor function refer to a Driving Rehabilitation Specialist to test in either a driving simulator or on-road driving test. This may include monitoring driving when alone utilizing a GPS device. If this is refused. the physician needs to report the patient to the Department of Motor Vehicles as unsafe to drive
Economic	Do you have enough money to pay your bills and purchase medicines and food?	Health Insurance Medicare Part D Can a cheaper drug replace a more expensive one?
Fatigue	Are you easily exhausted (tired)?	Bioavailable testosterone (in males) C-reactive protein, haemoglobin, TSH and vitamin B_{12} Epworth Sleep Inventory for sleep apnoea Fried Frailty Test (see Chapter 113, Frailty)
Function	Do you need help at home?	Barthel Index Katz Activities of Daily Living (ADL) Lawton Instrumental Activities of Daily Living (IADL) More sophisticated testing includes giving a person a medicine bottle and asking them how they would take the medicines, opening and shutting a variety of small doors, putting beans in a tin can, putting on a jacket or buttoning a shirt Social Activities Inventory
Hearing	Do you have trouble hearing especially in a noisy environment?	Hearing Handicap Inventory for the Elderly Audioscope Remove wax Consider hearing frequency testing
Incontinence	Do you wet yourself?	Urine for cells and culture Does it occur when coughing, sneezing (stress) Do you get the urge to go and have to go immediately (urge) Urodynamics
Insomnia	Do you have trouble sleeping? Are you tired during the day? Does your partner say that you stop breathing when sleeping?	Full sleep history including daytime napping, pain at night, nocturia, time going to sleep and environment Consider overnight sleep test for sleep apnoea

Dimension	Screening test	Assessment tests
Masked renal failure	Loss of muscle mass leads to normal serum creatinine levels in the face of severe renal failure	Use Cockcroft–Gault formula or measure serum cystatin-C
Memory	Do you have problems remembering anything or do any of your family or friends think you are having problems?	Saint Louis University/VA Mental Status Examination (SLUMS) If positive, TSH, vitamin B_{12} and homocysteine Consider MRI in some cases
Mobility/balance	Do you have trouble walking or lose your balance? Have you had a fall? Do you have a fear of falling?	Get up and go from a chair (may ask to do so holding a glass of water) Gait speed over 10 metres Stand on one foot with eyes open and shut Observe walking with a turn or dance with the patient. This should also be done while distracting the patient Measure stride length and variability
Nutrition	Have you lost weight? Height? Weight? Simplified Nutrition Assessment Questionnaire (SNAQ)	Body mass index Mini nutritional assessment Use 'meals on wheels' mnemonic to look for treatable causes
Osteoporosis	What was your height when 25 years old? Compared it with measured height now	Bone mineral density All women should have first at 50 years and men by 65 years of age. If results are borderline it should be repeated in 2 years during the same season 25-OH-vitamin D levels should be greater than $30\,\mathrm{mg\,dl^{-1}}$ All persons with a hip fracture should have calcium, vitamin D and bisphosphonates, unless a contraindication, e.g. renal failure
Pain	Do you hurt? Does your medicine relieve your pain?	Pain scale (faces better than Likert Scale) Full pain history If muscle pain, check ESR for polymyalgia rheumatica If temporal headache, check neck muscles for cramping
Polypharmacy	Are you on 7 or more medications? Is the person on any inappropriate medicines using the Beers Criteria?	Add history of herbal and over-the-counter medications Ask why they are taking all medications, are they compliant, who prescribed them and are there any side effects Check for orthostasis
Prostate	Do you have difficulty initiating your urine stream or dribble afterwards?	International Prostate Symptom Score Rectal examination Prostate-specific antigen
Sexuality	Are you having sexual relations? Do you want to have sex? How is your sexual desire? Then only; are you impotent?	*For women:* Ask about dyspareuria (pain on intercourse) Poor vaginal lubrication, itching or burning Are intimacy needs being met? *For men:* ADAM Questionnaire for low testosterone; if positive, bioavailable testosterone

(*continued overleaf*)

Dimension	Screening test	Assessment tests
		Discuss erectile dysfunction, including soft erections *For both:* Does their partner's or their health cause sexual difficulty? Are they using appropriate protection from sexually transmitted diseases?
Skin assessment	Do you have any new sores, rashes or growths on your body? Are you itching? Are any of your moles growing?	Full body examination Braden Scale to determine risk of pressure ulcers
Social support	Who lives with you? Who helps you?	Older American Resources and Services OARS Social Resources Scale explores fully the available helpers and strength of relationships
Spells	Do you have spells? Have you fainted (lost consciousness)? Have you fallen recently?	Orthostasis (if present, BUN, glucose, creatinine, sodium, haemoglobin) Carotid sinus massage Echocardiography Event monitor EKG Consider partial complex seizures (often missed in the elderly) and if likely need EEG
Vaccinations	Have you been vaccinated for flu, pneumonia and tetanus?	Influenza – yearly Pneumonia – every 5 years Tetanus – every 10 years Herpes zoster – once
Vision	Do you have trouble seeing?	Snellen eye chart Useful field of vision Dark adaptation Fundus examination

Activities of daily living (ADLs) and instrumental activities of daily living (IADLs)

Basic ADLs	IADLs
Bathing	Using the telephone
Dressing	Shopping
Toileting	Food preparation
Transfers	Housekeeping
Continence	Laundry
Feeding	Transportation
	Taking medicine
	Managing money
ADL Score:____/6	IADL Score:____/8

Dental

Screening assessment for dental conditions that may interfere with proper nutritional intake and possibly dispose a person to involuntary weight loss.

D̲ry mouth (2 points)
E̲ating difficulty (1 point)
N̲o recent dental care (1 point) (within 2 years)
T̲ooth or mouth pain (2 points)
A̲lterations or change in food selection (1 point)
L̲esions, sores or lumps in mouth (2 points)

A score of $\geq$3 points could indicate dental problems. Patient may need evaluation by a dentist.

Hallpike Manoeuvre

With the patient sitting, turn their head to 45° on one side. Hold the head at this angle while rapidly lowering the patient so that their head is 30° below the level of the examining table. Watch for nystagmus that comes on a few seconds after lowering them; lasts less than 30 seconds and decreases with repeated testing. Also ask if their symptoms are reproducible.

Osler Manoeuvre for pseudohypertension

Pump the blood pressure cuff up until you can no longer feel the pulse. Run your finger along the artery. At this stage it should have collapsed. If you can still feel the artery this is suggestive of arteriosclerosis and pseudohypertension.

Simplified Nutrition Assessment Questionnaire (SNAQ)

1 My appetite is
- A very poor
- B poor
- C average
- D good
- E very good

2 When I eat
- A I feel full after eating only a few mouthfuls
- B I feel full after eating about one-third of a meal
- C I feel full after eating over half of a meal
- D I feel full after eating most of the meal
- E I hardly ever feel full

3 Food tastes
- A very bad
- B bad
- C average
- D good
- E very good

4 Normally I eat
- A less than one meal a day
- B one meal a day
- C two meals a day
- D three meals a day
- E more than 3 meals a day

Instructions: Complete the questionnaire by circling the correct answers and then tally the results based upon the following numerical scale: A = 1, B = 2, C = 3, D = 4, E = 5.
Scoring: If the score is less than 14, there is a significant risk of weight loss.

The Mini-Nutritional Assessment (MNA) Scale

Last name: ____________ First name: ____________ Sex: ________ Date: ________

Age: ________ Weight, kg: ________ Height, cm: ________ I.D. Number: ________

Complete the screen by filling in the boxes with the appropriate numbers.
Add the numbers for the screen. If score is 11 or less, continue with the assessment to gain a Malnutrition Indicator Score.

Screening

A Has food intake declined over the past 3 months due to loss of appetite, digestive problems, chewing or swallowing difficulties?
- 0 = severe loss of appetite
- 1 = moderate loss of appetite
- 2 = no loss of appetite ☐

B Weight loss during the last 3 months
- 0 = weight loss greater than 3 kg (6.6 lbs)
- 1 = [illegible]
- 2 = weight loss between 1 and 3 kg (2.2 and 6.6 lbs)
- 3 = no weight loss ☐

C Mobility
- 0 = bed or chair bound
- 1 = able to get out of bed/chair but does not go out
- 2 = goes out ☐

D Has suffered psychological stress or acute disease in the past 3 months
- 0 = yes 2 = no ☐

E Neuropsychological problems
- 0 = severe dementia or depression
- 1 = mild dementia
- 2 = no psychological problems ☐

F Body Mass Index (BMI) (weight in kg) / (height in m)²
- 0 = BMI less than 19
- 1 = BMI 19 to less than 21
- 2 = BMI 21 to less than 23
- 3 = BMI 23 or greater ☐

Screening score (subtotal max. 14 points) ☐ ☐

12 points or greater Normal – not at risk – no need to complete assessment
11 points or below Possible malnutrition – continue assessment

Assessment

G Lives independently (not in a nursing home or hospital)
- 0 = no 1 = yes ☐

H Takes more than 3 prescription drugs per day
- 0 = yes 1 = no ☐

I Pressure sores or skin ulcers
- 0 = yes 1 = no ☐

J How many full meals does the patient eat daily?
- 0 = 1 meal
- 1 = 2 meals
- 2 = 3 meals ☐

K Selected consumption markers for protein intake
- At least one serving of dairy products (milk, cheese, yogurt) per day? yes ☐ no ☐
- Two or more servings of legumes or eggs per week? yes ☐ no ☐
- Meat, fish or poultry every day yes ☐ no ☐

[illegible]
0.5 = if 2 yes
1.0 = if 3 yes ☐.☐

L Consumes two or more servings of fruits or vegetables per day?
- 0 = no 1 = yes ☐

M How much fluid (water, juice, coffee, tea, milk...) is consumed per day?
- 0.0 = less than 3 cups
- 0.5 = 3 to 5 cups
- 1.0 = more than 5 cups ☐.☐

N Mode of feeding
- 0 = unable to eat without assistance
- 1 = self-fed with some difficulty
- 2 = self-fed without any problem ☐

O Self view of nutritional status
- 0 = views self as being malnourished
- 1 = is uncertain of nutritional state
- 2 = views self as having no nutritional problem ☐

P In comparison with other people of the same age, how do they consider their health status?
- 0.0 = not as good
- 0.5 = does not know
- 1.0 = as good
- 2.0 = better ☐.☐

Q Mid-arm circumference (MAC) in cm
- 0.0 = MAC less than 21
- 0.5 = MAC 21 to 22
- 1.0 = MAC 22 or greater ☐.☐

R Calf circumference (CC) in cm
- 0 = CC less than 31 1 = CC 31 or greater ☐

Assessment (max. 16 points) ☐ ☐.☐

Screening score ☐ ☐

Total Assessment (max. 30 points) ☐ ☐.☐

Malnutrition Indicator Score

17 to 23.5 points	at risk of malnutrition	☐
Less than 17 points	malnourished	☐

Saint Louis University social activities assessment

1 How often do you go out socially?
  - **a** daily
  - **b** twice a week or more
  - **c** weekly
  - **d** monthly
  - **e** rarely

2 How often do you garden?
  - **a** at least an hour daily
  - **b** less than an hour daily
  - **c** twice a week or more
  - **d** weekly
  - **e** rarely

3 How often do you go to church/synagogue/mosque?
  - **a** more than once a week
  - **b** weekly
  - **c** at least once a month
  - **d** only on religious holidays
  - **e** never

4 How often do you talk to friends or family on the telephone?
  - **a** more than once a day
  - **b** daily
  - **c** 2 to 4 times a week
  - **d** weekly
  - **e** rarely

5 How often do you go to a restaurant to eat?
  - **a** daily
  - **b** twice a week or more
  - **c** weekly
  - **d** monthly
  - **e** rarely

6 How often do you go for a walk?
  - **a** daily
  - **b** twice a week or more
  - **c** weekly
  - **d** monthly
  - **e** rarely

7 How often do you go dancing?
  - **a** daily
  - **b** twice a week or more
  - **c** weekly
  - **d** monthly
  - **e** rarely

8 How often do you go to a concert/theatre/movie?
  - **a** daily
  - **b** twice a week or more
  - **c** weekly
  - **d** monthly
  - **e** rarely

9 How often do you play with your grandchildren?
  - **a** daily
  - **b** twice a week or more
  - **c** weekly
  - **d** monthly
  - **e** rarely

10 How satisfied are you with the time spent and quality of your social activities?
  - **a** extremely satisfied
  - **b** very satisfied
  - **c** satisfied
  - **d** somewhat satisfied
  - **e** not at all satisfied

The Confusion Assessment Method (CAM) diagnostic algorithm

The diagnosis of delirium by the Confusion Assessment Method (CAM) requires the presence of features 1 and 2 plus either 3 or 4.

Feature 1: *Acute onset and fluctuating course*. This feature is usually obtained from a family member or nurse and is shown by positive responses to the following questions: Is there evidence of an acute change in mental status from the patient's baseline? Did the (abnormal) behaviour fluctuate during the day, that is, tend to come and go or increase and decrease in severity?
Check appropriate box: Present ☐ Absent ☐

Feature 2: *Inattention*. This feature is shown by a positive response to the following question: Did the patient have difficulty focusing attention, for example, being easily distractible or having difficulty keeping track of what was being said?
Check appropriate box: Present ☐ Absent ☐

Feature 3: *Disorganized thinking*. This feature is shown by a positive response to the following question: Was the patient's thinking disorganized or incoherent, such as rambling or irrelevant conversation, unclear or illogical flow of ideas or unpredictable switching from subject to subject?
Check appropriate box Present ☐ Absent ☐

Feature 4: *Altered level of consciousness*. This feature is shown by an answer other than 'alert' to the following question: Overall, how would you rate this patient's level of consciousness? Alert (normal); Vigilant (hyperalert overly sensitive to environmental stimuli, startled very easily); Lethargic (drowsy, easily aroused); Stupor (difficult to arouse); Coma (unarousable); Uncertain
Check appropriate box Present ☐ Absent ☐

Type of delirium
Hyperalert ☐ Hypoalert ☐ Mixed ☐

Reference: Inouye S, van Dyck C, Alessi C *et al*. Clarifying confusion: the confusion assessment method. *Ann Intern Med* 1990;**113**:941–8.

Saint Louis University

Mental Status (SLUMS) Examination

Name ______________________ Age ______________________

Is patient alert? ______________________ Level of education ______________________

__/1 ❶ **1. What day of the week is it?**

__/1 ❶ **2. What is the year?**

__/1 ❶ **3. What state are we in?**

4. Please remember these five objects. I will ask you what they are later.

Apple Pen Tie House Car

5. You have $100 and you go to the store and buy a dozen apples for $3 and a tricycle for $20.

❶ **How much did you spend?**

__/3 ❷ **How much do you have left?**

6. Please name as many animals as you can in one minute.

__/3 ⓪ 0-4 animals ❶ 5-9 animals ❷ 10-14 animals ❸ 15+ animals

__/5 **7. What were the five objects I asked you to remember?** 1 point for each one correct.

8. I am going to give you a series of numbers and I would like you to give them to me backwards. For example, if I say 42, you would say 24.

__/2 ⓪ 87 ❶ 649 ❶ 8537

9. This is a clock face. Please put in the hour markers and the time at ten minutes to eleven o'clock.

❷ Hour markers okay

__/4 ❷ Time correct

__/2 ❶ **10. Please place an X in the triangle.**

❶ **Which of the above figures is largest?**

11. I am going to tell you a story. Please listen carefully because afterwards, I'm going to ask you some questions about it.

Jill was a very successful stockbroker. She made a lot of money on the stock market. She then met Jack, a devastatingly handsome man. She married him and had three children. They lived in Chicago. She then stopped work and stayed at home to bring up her children. When they were teenagers, she went back to work. She and Jack lived happily ever after.

❷ **What was the female's name?** ❷ **What work did she do?**

__/8 ❷ **When did she go back to work?** ❷ **What state did she live in?**

_______ **TOTAL SCORE**

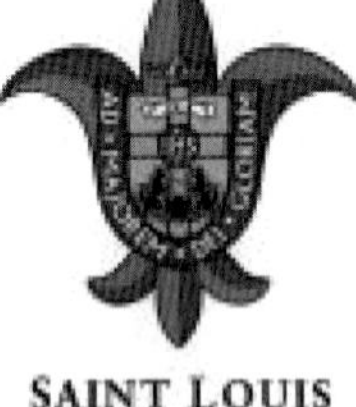

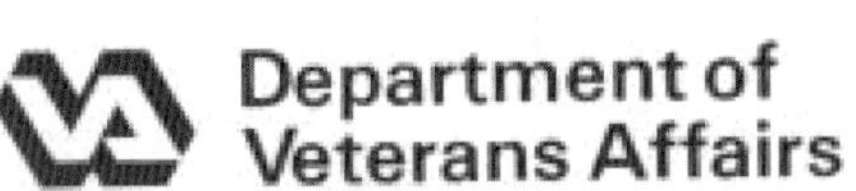

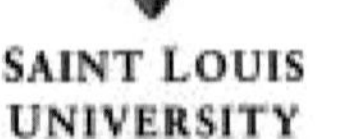

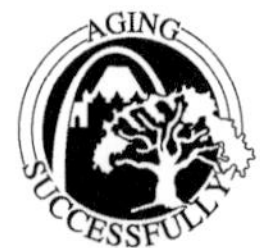

SCORING

High School Education		Less than High School Education
27-30	Normal	20-30
20-26	MCI	15-19
1-19	Dementia	1-14

WA Banks and JE Morley. Memories are made of this: Recent advances in understanding, cognitive impairment, and dementia. *J Gerontol Med Sci* 2003;58A:314-21.

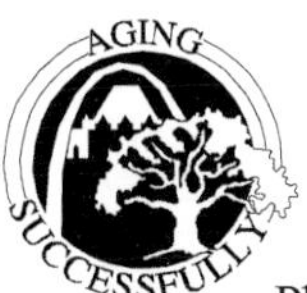

Saint Louis University Division of Geriatrics

Passport to Aging Successfully*

SAINT LOUIS UNIVERSITY

Please complete this questionnaire before seeing your physician and take it with you when you go.

NAME ______________________ **AGE** ________

BLOOD PRESSURE laying down: ________ standing: ________

WEIGHT now: ________ 6 months ago:________ change: ________

HEIGHT at age 20: ________ now: ________

CHOLESTEROL LDL:________ HDL: ________

VACCINATIONS ☐Influenza (yearly) ☐Pneumococcal ☐Tetanus (every 10 years)

TSH Date: ________ **FASTING GLUCOSE** Date: ________

Do you SMOKE? ________

How much ALCOHOL do you drink? ______ per day

Do you use your SEATBELT? ________

Do you chew TOBACCO? ________

EXERCISE: How often do you

do endurance exercises (walk briskly 20 to 30 minutes/day or climb 10 flights of stairs) _____ /week

do resistance exercises?_____ /week do balance exercises? _____ /week

do posture exercises? _____ /week do flexibility exercises? ____ /week

Can you SEE ADEQUATELY in poor light? ________

Can you HEAR in a noisy environment? ________

Are you INCONTINENT? ________

Have you a LIVING WILL or durable POWER OF ATTORNEY FOR HEALTH? ________

Do you take ASPIRIN daily (only if you have had a heart attack or have diabetes)?________

Do you have any concerns about your PERSONAL SAFETY? ________

When did you last have your STOOL TESTED for blood? ________

When were you last screened for OSTEOPOROSIS? ________

Are you having trouble REMEMBERING THINGS? ________

Do you have enough FOOD? ________

Are you SAD? ________

Do you have PAIN? ________

If so, which face best describes your pain?

0 1 2 3 4 5

MALES

Do you have trouble passing urine?______

Have you discussed PSA testing with your doctor? ______

What is your ADAM score?________

FEMALES

When was your last pap smear? ________

When was your last mammogram?________

Do you check your breasts monthly?________

Are you satisfied with your sex life?________

Now, please answer the four questionnaires on the next page.

* This questionnaire is based on the health promotion and prevention guidelines developed by Gerimed® and Saint Louis University Division of Geriatric Medicine.

Passport to Aging Successfully

Please fill out these forms before seeing your physician and take them with you when you go.

Geriatric Depression Scale	(circle one)
Are you basically satisfied with your life?	YES NO
Have you dropped many of your activities and interests?	YES NO
Do you feel that your life is empty?	YES NO
Do you often get bored?	YES NO
Are you in good spirits most of the time?	YES NO
Are you afraid that something bad is going to happen to you?	YES NO
Do you feel happy most of the time?	YES NO
Do you often feel helpless?	YES NO
Do you prefer to stay at home, rather than going out and doing new things?	YES NO
Do you feel you have more problems with memory than most?	YES NO
Do you think it is wonderful to be alive?	YES NO
Do you feel pretty worthless the way you are now?	YES NO
Do you feel full of energy?	YES NO
Do you feel that your situation is hopeless?	YES NO
Do you think that most people are better off than you are?	YES NO

Sheikh JI, Yesavage JA. Geriatric Depression Scale (GDS): Recent evidence and development of a shorter version. *Clinical Gerontologist* 1986;5:165.

CAGE

Have you ever considered **C**utting down on your alcohol intake? ________________

Do people **A**nnoy you by criticizing your drinking? ________________

Have you ever felt bad or **G**uilty about your drinking? ________________

Have you ever had an alcoholic drink first thing in the morning (**E**yeopener) to steady your nerves or get rid of a hangover? ________

ADAM (Men only)

1. Do you have a decrease in libido? ________
2. Do you have a lack of energy? ________
3. Do you have a decrease in strength and/or endurance? ________
4. Do you have a decreased enjoyment of life? ________
5. Are you sad? ________
6. Are you grumpy? ________
7. Are your erections less strong? ________
8. Have you noticed a recent deterioration in your ability to play sports? ________
9. Are you falling asleep earlier after dinner? ________
10. Has there been a recent deterioration in your work performance? ________

Epworth Sleepiness Questionnaire

How likely are you to doze off or to fall asleep in the following situations, in contrast to just feeling tired? This refers to your usual way of life in recent times. Use the following scale to choose the most appropriate number for each situation.

0–would never doze	1–slight chance of dozing
2–moderate chance of dozing	3–high chance of dozing

Situation	Chance of dozing
Sitting and reading	
Watching TV	
Sitting inactive in a public place	
As a passenger in a car for an hour	
Lying down to rest in the afternoon	
Sitting and talking to someone	
Sitting quietly after a lunch without alcohol	
In a car while stopped for a few minutes	
Total	____ / 24

Index

Page numbers in *italics* denote figures, those in **bold** denote tables.

Principles and Practice of Geriatric Medicine, Fifth Edition. Edited by Alan J. Sinclair, John E. Morley and Bruno Vellas.